Anesthesia Bridges

Sharif Mohamed • Raymond Graber
Amr Abouleish • Edwin Avery IV
Jeffrey Kirsch • Catherine Marcucci
Editors

Anesthesia Bridges

Wisdom for Your Personal and Professional Journey

Volume I

Springer

Editors
Sharif Mohamed
Department of Anesthesiology
The University of Texas Medical Branch
Galveston, TX, USA

Amr Abouleish
Department of Anesthesiology
The University of Texas Medical Branch
Galveston, TX, USA

Jeffrey Kirsch
Department of Anesthesiology and Pain Medicine
University of Washington School of Medicine,
Seattle, WA, USA

Raymond Graber
Department of Anesthesiology and Perioperative
Medicine
University Hospitals Cleveland Medical Center
Cleveland, OH, USA

Edwin Avery IV
Department of Anesthesiology and Perioperative
Medicine
University Hospitals Cleveland Medical Center
Cleveland, OH, USA

Catherine Marcucci
Department of Transfusion Medicine,
Clinical Center
National Institutes of Health
Bethesda, MD, USA

ISBN 978-3-032-08293-0 ISBN 978-3-032-08294-7 (eBook)
https://doi.org/10.1007/978-3-032-08294-7

This Springer imprint is published by the registered company Springer Nature Switzerland AG
The registered company address is: Gewerbestrasse 11, 6330 Cham, Switzerland

Editors

Sharif Mohamed: To my parents Samy and Safy and to my wife Lobna. And also to my kids Lina, Amr, Ali, and Hamza—your support is my lifeline.

Ray Graber: To my wife, Mary, who lovingly keeps our household running. To our sons, Luke and Colin, who are both launched and finding success in their careers. To Bridget and Lauren—so great to have you with us in the family. And to Aubrie, who is growing into a lovely young woman and college student.

Amr Abouleish: To my most important mentors—my parents, Ezzat and Atiya Abouleish. I am who I am because of them.

Ed Avery: To my wife Lauren who is our family's always vigilant safety officer. To my daughter, Nicole, whom I am so proud of for her hard work at Northwestern University, and to my son, Edwin, who is a top student in his class.

Jeff Kirsch: To my granddaughters Noa, Romi, and Mika and to my grandson Dylan, who give me hope for a better tomorrow. And to my grandson, Daniel, whose tragic death indelibly revealed that medicine can and must do better. I love you all.

Cathy Marcucci: To Charlie and Lisa, as always! Being your Mom is the best thing that ever happened to me. And to Neil—many thanks for helping with yet another book.

Contributing Editors (Alphabetical)

Mike Axley: To my twin brother Chris, who is my personal hero. He is just a really thoughtful, caring person. I always try to live by his immortal words, "Could you, please, just attempt to be cool?"

Ron Bank: To my parents, Barron and Lois, whose support and encouragement carried me through to becoming a physician. To my family who support me and tolerate my long hours. To my patients, who entrust me with their lives—an honor greater than any other.

Andrew Barker: To my wife—I am forever grateful for your support and love. Your patience and belief in me are sustaining. To my wonderful children, whose curiosity and energy inspire me every day.

John Briggs: To KB, the real hero, love of my life, and forever partner. Thank you, JB and MB, for always leading by example and I am forever grateful. JB and WB—may the future be bright. I love you all.

Carol Bodenheimer: First, to my family who keep things busy and interesting, always! And to Temple University School of Medicine and Temple University Hospital staff, who taught me the importance of lifelong learning and professionalism.

Kirk Lalwani: To my wife Seema, who always puts family first and has cheerfully supported me through the years. To my kids Nikita and Rohan, as they forge their paths to adulthood and inspire me to be the best Dad I can.

Dan McCoy: To my mother, Peggy, who taught me, word by word, how to listen, how to think, and how to write. Your example of kindness and work ethic guides and inspires me to this day.

Raj Nathwani: To my wife Laura for keeping life together so that I can pursue medicine; to my children Ary, Zubin, and Kamy for keeping the sunshine flowing in; and to my parents for all their sacrifices.

Steve Orebaugh: To anesthesia trainees everywhere. We hope that this book can enhance your ability to care for perioperative patients and keep them safe!

Amy Robbins: To my parents, Gary and Marilyn Robbins, who instilled the pursuit of education and a long-lasting love of learning into me as a young child.

Neil Sandson: To my wife, Cathy Marcucci (you may have heard of her), and my children, Charlie and Lisa. Thank you for bringing purpose and richness to my otherwise bland life.

Jake Seagull: To Judy and my son Daniel, and our canine family member, Sasha, for their unfailing support, love, and tail wagging—although only one of them wags.

Brandon Togioka: To my father, a model of servant leadership and to my mother, who taught me how to write. To my wife Jennifer—my source of inspiration and support.

Jennifer Tripi: To my husband, for his unwavering love, patience, and support. To my sisters for their devoted friendship. And to my parents for their constant encouragement and guidance through life.

Brant Wagener: To my wife and kids whose love and support make my life possible.

David Zvara: To Bharathi—an amazing wife, mother, and companion; my driving inspiration.

We also thank Contributing Editors **Albert Liao** *and* **Kristin King Liao** *for their advice and assistance with the manuscript.*

In Memoriam

Saundra E. Curry, MD *1952–2024*

Richard A. Jaffe, MD PhD *1947–2023*

John S. Rogoski, DO *1961–2024*

Highland Park Bridge—Pittsburgh, PA

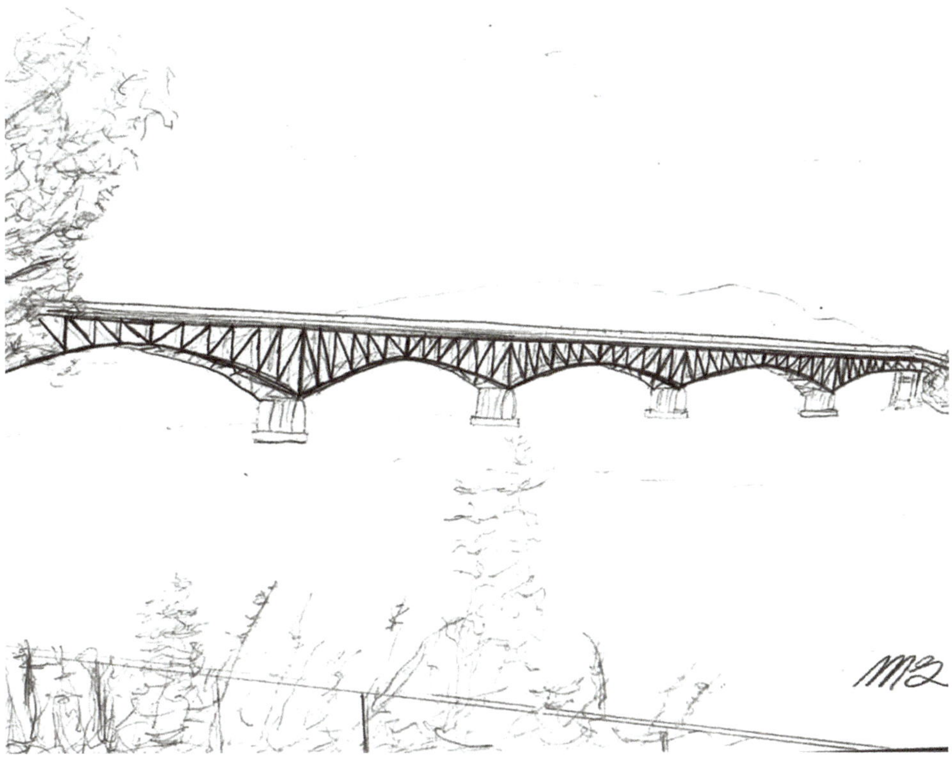

Author **Neil Sandson** chose the Highland Park Bridge in Pittsburgh as his favorite. He tells us that growing up in the Squirrel Hill section of the city but going to school in Fox Chapel meant that he crossed the bridge at least twice a day—thousands of times in total. The bridge was constructed between 1937 and 1939. It carries vehicular traffic across the Allegheny River between the Pittsburgh neighborhood of Highland Park and the suburb of Aspinwall northeast of the city.

Neil and the *Anesthesia Bridges* editors thank **Mitchell Godett** of The Architectural Team in Boston, MA, for his charming pencil drawing that perfectly captures the bridge in its riparian setting. We were delighted when Mitchell also sent us a detailed drawing of the bridge's trusses, below.

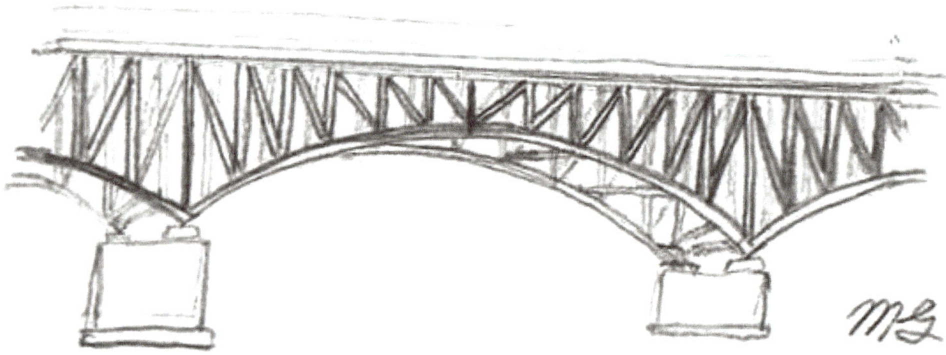

The steel truss design was created by the same engineer who was responsible for Pittsburgh's South Tenth Street and Homestead High Level Bridges. It replaced a much smaller streetcar bridge and was designed to handle "heavy commuter traffic." Construction costs were about $2.5 million (1930s dollars).

Foreword

I've always had a deep interest in thinking about how we can better support the professional development of anesthesiology trainees and those in practice with an eye toward understanding how we can more effectively guide individuals throughout their careers—no matter what trajectories, twists, or turns they might take. So when the editors of *Anesthesia Bridges* told me about their concept for a new book, I was immediately excited to learn more.

While I have been in continuous practice since finishing residency in 2008, I have also integrated a number of nontraditional activities into my professional portfolio. Since finishing training, I've served in combat deploying overseas as US Navy Commander, led the American Medical Association as its chair and president, developed novel artificial intelligence algorithms that have been deployed at scale across the globe, served on both for-profit and not-for-profit boards, overseen the launch of six tech-enabled healthcare companies, and currently direct a $560 million health philanthropy. Throughout my career, I've always yearned for a reference that could give me perspective on how to seek, prioritize, and best position myself for to look for and receive new opportunities. This book is that reference I have longed for.

On the surface, this book is a collection of 200+ essays spread out in ten sections: Communication, Professionalism, Leadership, Academic Promotion and Career Planning, Education and Training, Doctor-Patient Relations, Clinical Wisdom, More Wisdom on Clinical Anesthesia Practice, Personal Stories, and Life Stories. But the sum is very much greater and more powerful than the parts. Taken together, these stories, anecdotes, and pearls of wisdom provide the reader with an opportunity to reflect on how to bring their best self to the bedside, the profession, apply it, and look for the unexpected opportunities to impact the world around us.

While many of the authors are either known to me, or personal friends, I cannot remember a time when I so enjoyed reading the words of my colleagues because of the deeply personal nature of this work. I invite you to enjoy it, reflect on it, and let it guide you to the next chapter of your professional success.

Jesse Ehrenfeld, MD MPH
Professor of Anesthesiology
Senior Associate Dean
Medical College of Wisconsin
Milwaukee, WI, USA

Artists

Edwin Avery

Claiborne Pell Bridge

Ed is a professor of anesthesiology with a subspecialty in cardiothoracic anesthesiology. He immensely enjoys both detailing his sports car and traveling in his off time; a favorite getaway spot of his is the island of Providenciales in Turks and Caicos. He regularly gives lectures to his Turks and Caicos medical colleagues as well as sponsors free blood pressure clinics for the islanders when he visits.

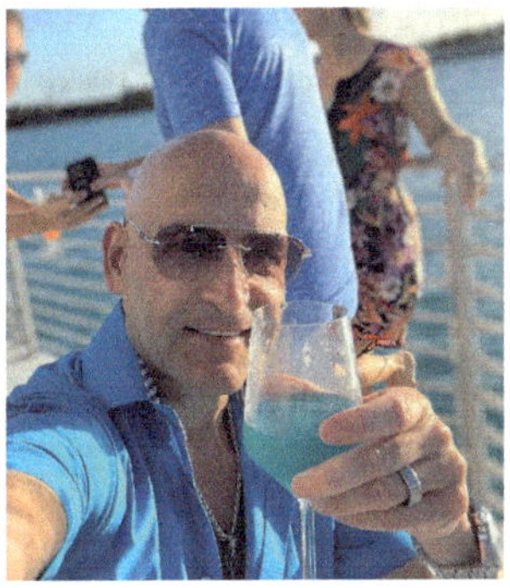

Nina Babbitt

Newport Bridge

Nina Babbitt holds a BS and a Master of Architecture degree from Wentworth Institute of Technology. She currently works at The Architectural Team in Boston. She enjoys working on a range of projects from historic rehabilitations to new builds. She especially likes to be involved in the schematic phase of the design process, studying how architecture can be woven into the fabric of a place. When she is not at work, she loves to travel, practice yoga, and spend time in the ocean.

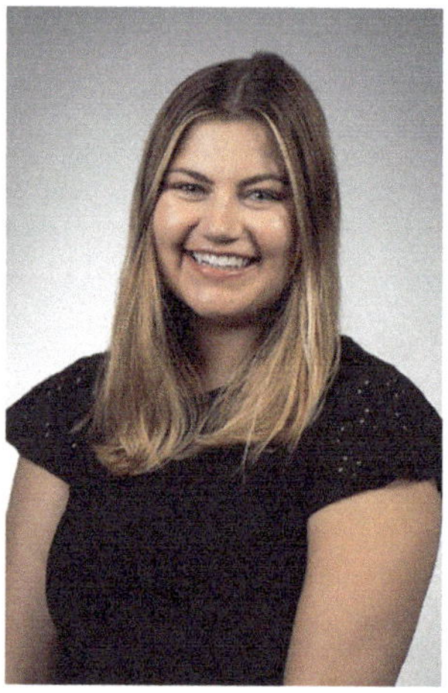

Niamh Curry

A Stone Bridge, Pennsylvania

Niamh Curry was born in Ireland and raised in Massachusetts. She has always been passionate about art and architecture, and is proud to work at The Architecture Team based out of Chelsea, MA. She graduated from the University of Massachusetts Amherst, in 2022 with a Bachelor of Science in Architecture. Her favorite projects to work on usually involve rehabilitations of old buildings.

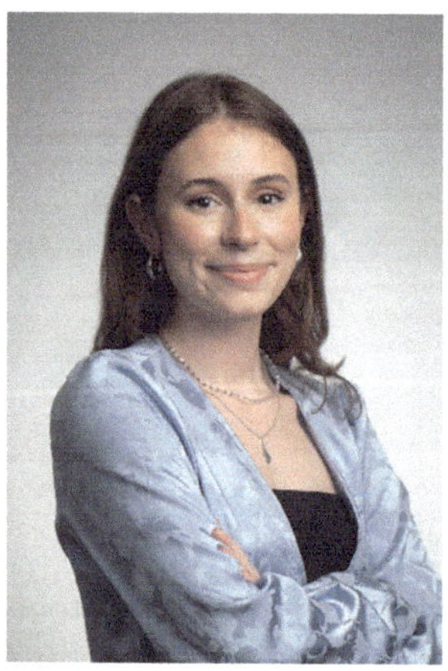

John Giacalone

Harrisburg Railroad Bridge

John Giacalone is an employee at The Architectural Team and former student of Roger Williams University. He is an enthusiast of modern architecture, and some of his favorite architects include Le Corbusier and Frank Lloyd Wright. Outside of architecture, his interests include staying active with things such as snowboarding and martial arts, as well as watching and performing stand-up comedy.

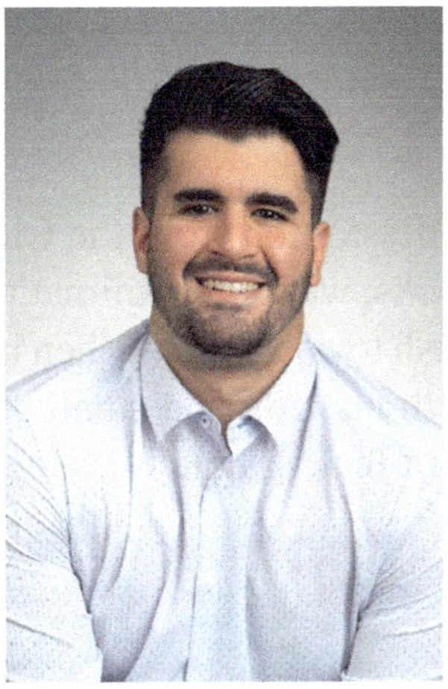

Mitchell Godett

Highland Park Bridge

Mitchell Godett was born and raised in New England. Since a young age, he has enjoyed spending time outdoors whether it be skiing in the mountains of New Hampshire or fishing Massachusetts's coastline. He has particular interest in the historic preservation of local architecture, and currently works as a project designer in Chelsea, Massachusetts, after receiving his master's degree from Northeastern University. He also brings the aspect of reusing something old to make something new into his passion for woodworking.

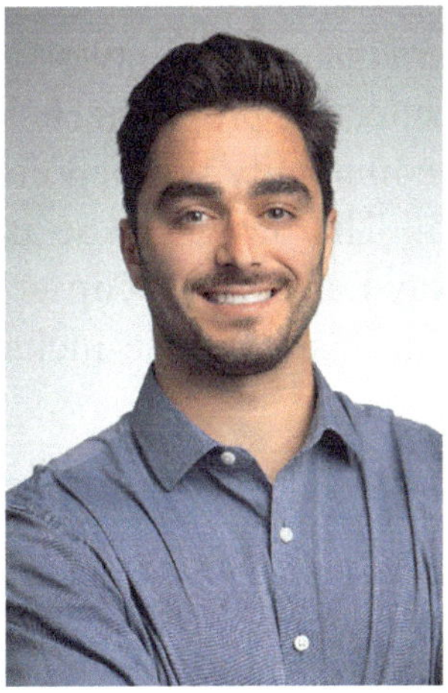

Luke Graber

Anatomic Drawings

Luke Graber has a BFA in illustration from the Cleveland Institute of Art. He has illustrated children's books, worked in animation, developed board games, and currently works as a plush toy designer. When he isn't doing creative work, he enjoys spending time with his wife and small dog at home and looking for new ways to create fun out of their simple lives together.

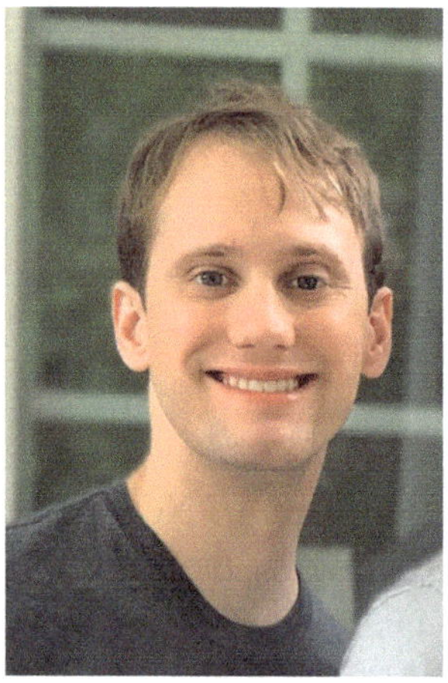

David Howe

Cooper River Bridge

David Howe is a recent graduate of Wentworth Institute of Technologies Bachelor and Master of Architecture program. He has a strong passion for creating designs that enhance community ties and create a more equitable environment through built form. The designers he is most inspired by include Renzo Piano, Charles and Ray Eames, Olaf Gipser to name a few. Some of the hobbies he partakes in during his free time include yoga, reading, furniture making, and antiquing.

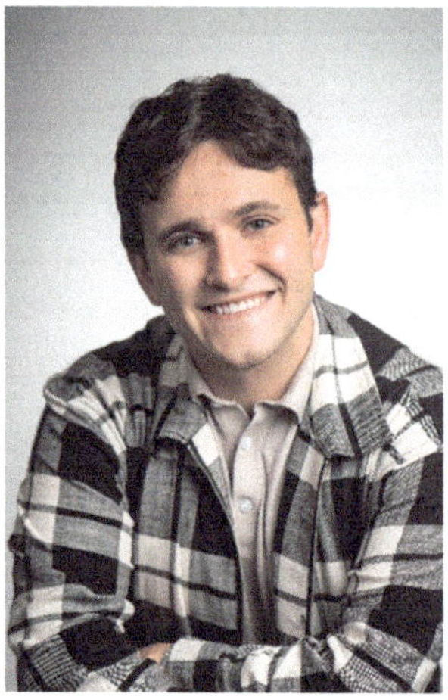

Mark Liu

Ambassador Bridge, Ankle Block

Mark is pursuing a fashion design program at Savannah College of Art and Design. His interests include photography and film. He is particularly interested in street fashion, a sensibility which is reflected not only in his admiration for avant garde designers such as Yohji Yamamoto but also in his extensive knowledge of underground hip hop and personal relationships he has developed with musical artists such as MF Grimm.

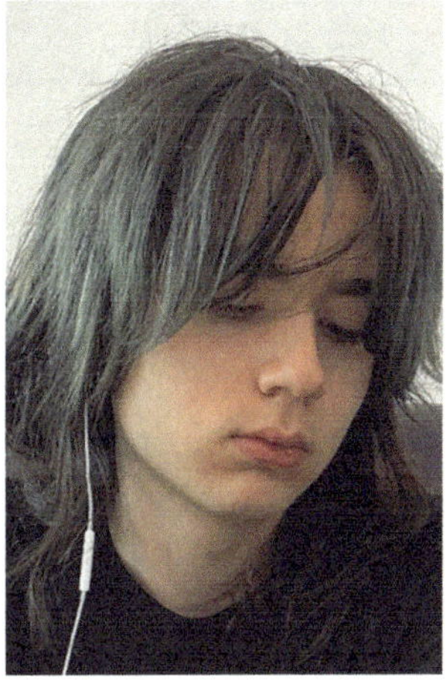

Michael Liu

Stari Most (Old Bridge)

Michael Liu is (emeritus) Senior Partner and Design Principal at The Architectural Team, Inc. where he has directed the design of numerous significant building and master plan commissions. He has been active in the recruitment and cultivation of staff and has been a regular guest design critic at the University of Notre Dame, Roger Williams and Northeastern schools of architecture. His design tastes are eclectic and include both contemporary and traditional architectural expressions. He particularly enjoys sketching buildings and urban venues in his overseas travels.

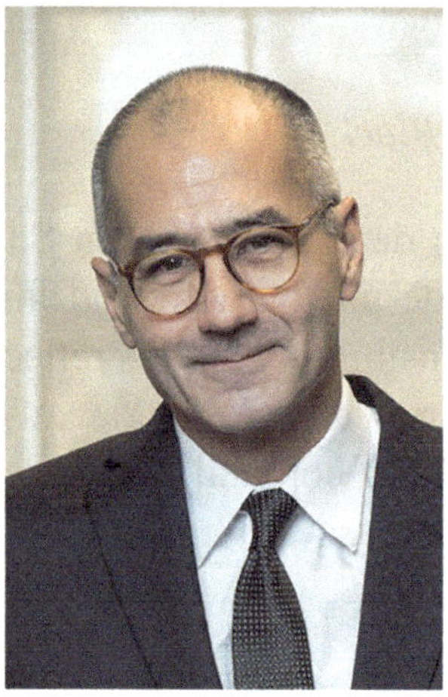

Daniel Nemec

Chesapeake Bay Bridge

Daniel Nemec is a designer and artist located in Boston, Massachusetts. Holding a master's degree in architecture from Northeastern University and a bachelor's degree from Roger Williams University, his work is focused around social-ecological design. Utilizing 2D and 3D mediums, the artwork explores their intersectionality through combining orthogonal and natural forms.

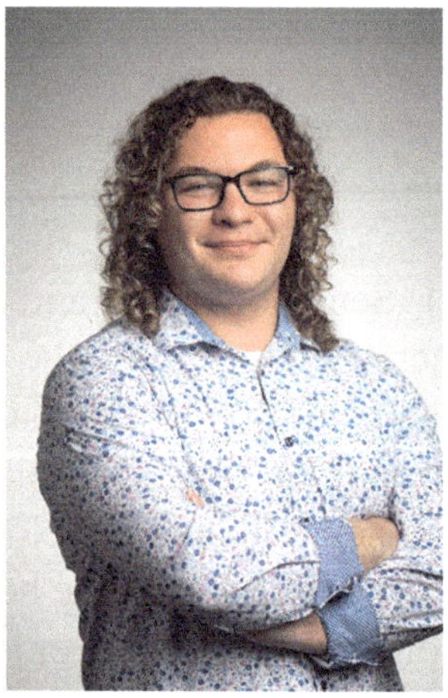

Kelsey O'Connor

Zakim Bunker Hill Memorial Bridge

Kelsey O'Connor, NCIDQ, is a designer located in Boston, Massachusetts. She earned a BFA in interior design from Suffolk University. She draws much of her inspiration from the built environment and the way that we experience space.

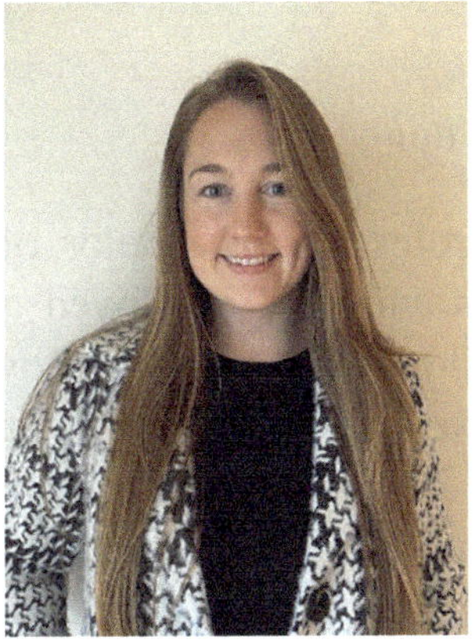

Craig Riley

Thurston Avenue Bridge

Craig Riley was drawn into the field of architecture at a young age due to his fascination of playing with Legos and Lincoln Logs. In order to pursue an education within architecture, he elected to attend the University of Massachusetts Amherst. There, he was able to harness his skills of elaborate designing and constant puzzle-solving.

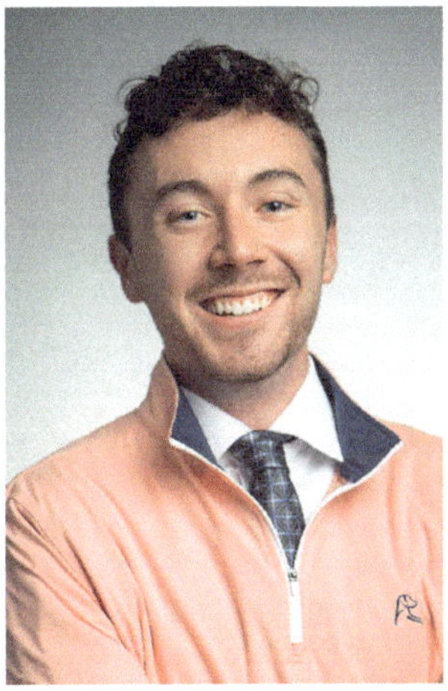

Lisa Sandson

Tiny Bridge on Yellow Mountain

Lisa Sandson holds the professional bachelor of architecture degree from Syracuse University and is currently employed at Cummings Properties in Boston, a unique design/build firm. She grew up loving the arts and has a background in realistic drawing and oil painting. She has always been interested in bridges, as they are the perfect example of a spatialized threshold. She has a black belt in martial arts and loves cooking, travel, and dogs.

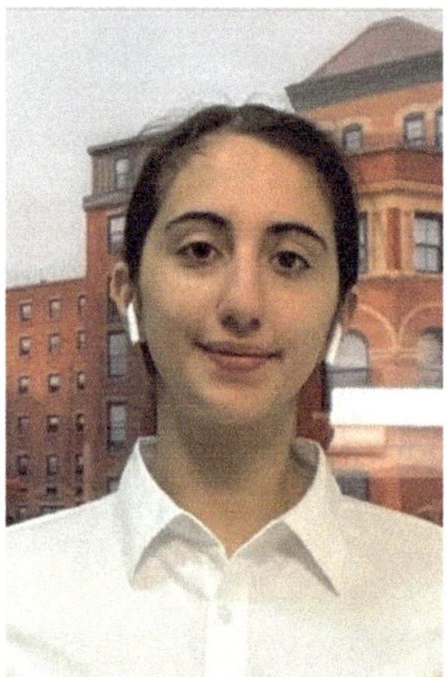

Photographers

Daniel Asher

Operating Room Panorama

Daniel is a cardiac anesthesiologist who actively seeks opportunities for creativity in his daily life. When he's not gardening or cooking, you will probably find him right next to his kids drawing sailboats in crayon or designing a new technological process for his hospital's actively evolving EMR.

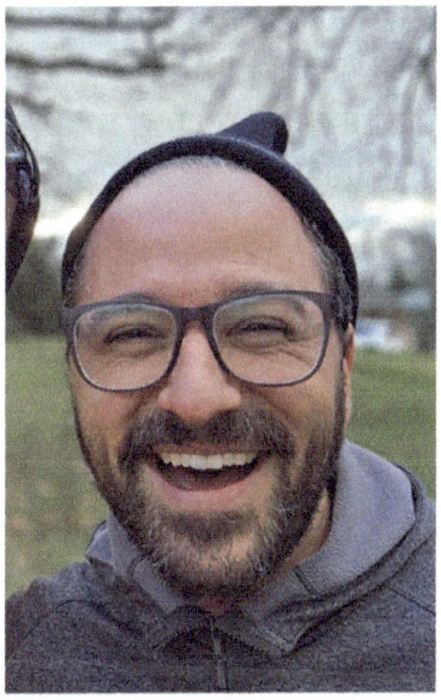

Michael Axley

Microscope, Gladstone Bag, Sellwood Bridge

Michael is an anesthesiologist in private practice with Oregon Anesthesiology Group. He lives in Portland, OR, with his wife, Kimberly Malek, and his three children. He has lived in Portland since he came out to go to school at Reed College and considers himself fortunate to make that wonderful city his home. His hobbies include general aviation, fishing, and the beach.

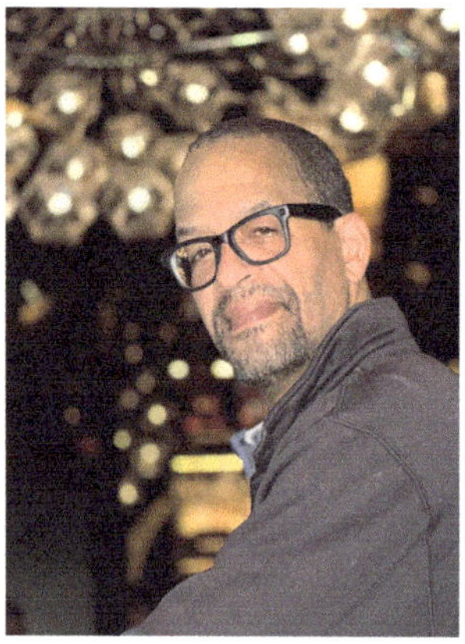

Jordan Bank

Memorial Bridge

Jordan is a student in the metropolitan Washington DC area with special interests in American, world, and aviation history. He is a very serious baseball player and participates in an intense showcase league. He is also a certified SCUBA diver, with multiple dive specialties in many different skill sets. In his remaining spare time, he is deeply interested in animal advocacy and writes for his local animal rescue newsletter.

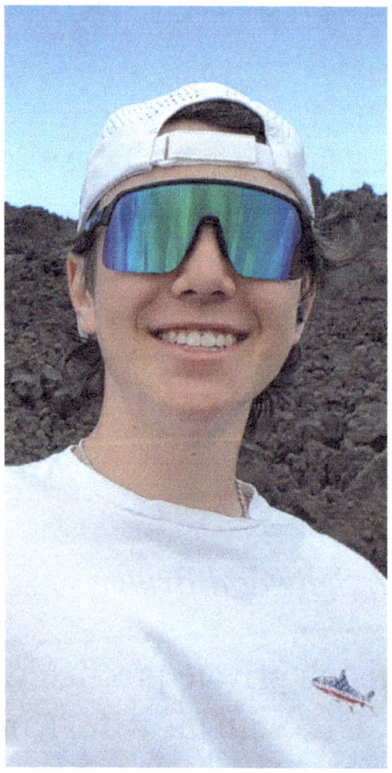

Emma Bailey

Benson Bridge

Emma Bailey is the creator of "Pines & Vines"—a Pacific Northwest travel blog with a focus on outdoor recreation. She is passionate about helping people connect with nature regardless of physical ability or previous experience. She enjoys hiking, photography, and nerding out about the local geology. She lives in Portland, OR.

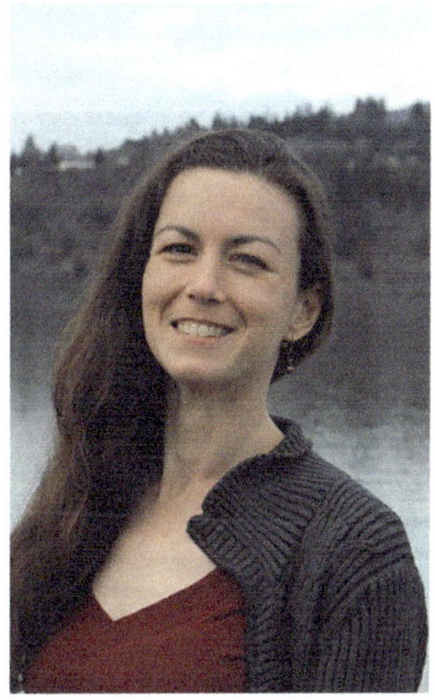

Marlee Chamberlain

The Tilikum Crossing

Marlee is a medical student at Oregon Health and Science University (OHSU). She obtained a BS in biology at Oregon State University, then went on to achieve an AS in paramedicine at OHSU and an MS in biomedical sciences at the University of Northern Colorado. She worked as a paramedic in Portland, and with a love of hiking and traveling, takes pictures where she travels or when she was stationed in an ambulance waiting for a call.

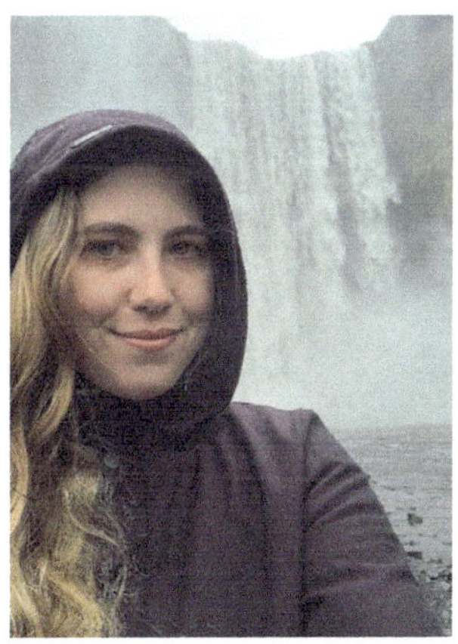

Harriet Chen

Jekyll Island Bridge, Porto Bridge, Boston Bridge

Formerly a NICU nurse and always a devoted mother of two, Harriet has been creating portraits for over 28 years. She absolutely loves connecting with people and allowing special and fun moments to happen naturally. Passionate about capturing light and reflecting the beauty in everyone, her images are original, organic, and have a bit of a documentary flair. She works both in the studio and on location. She currently lives in Alabama with her husband, five cats, and their dog.

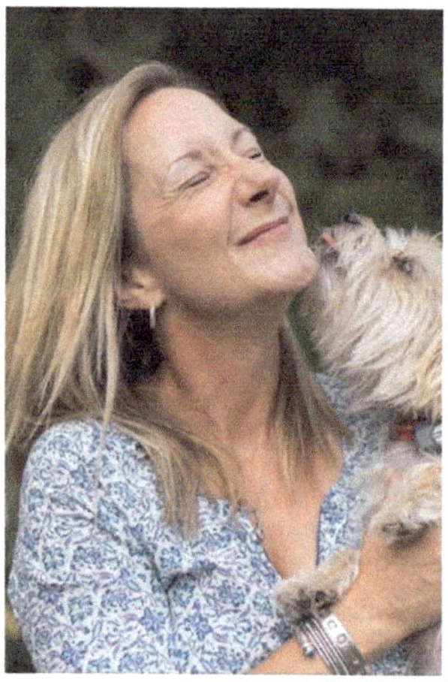

Laura Chess

St John's Bridge, Oregon

Laura is a double-boarded emergency and critical care physician in Portland, OR. She trained in Detroit but is grateful to now live so close to the ocean and mountains. When she is not spending time with her husband and three kids, she enjoys hiking, surfing, cooking, wine tasting, playing polo, and skiing.

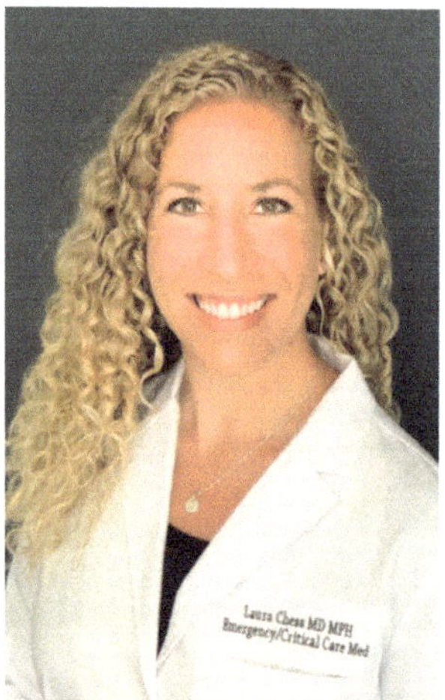

Benjamin Conner

Glen Canyon Navajo Bridge, Grand Canyon Silver Bridge

Ben is currently a physical medicine and rehabilitation resident at Spaulding Rehab Hospital in Boston, where he is already mentoring medical school students and applicants. When he is not spending time with his beloved wife and their animals, he enjoys a healthy balance of outdoor adventures and reclining seats at the movie theater.

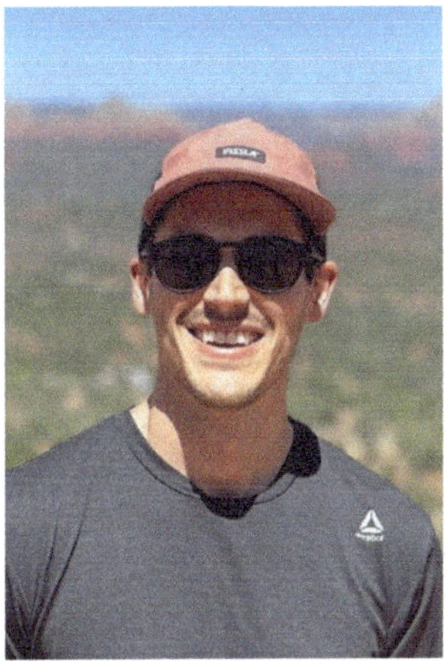

Lois Connolly

Earpiece

Lois is a professor of anesthesiology and medical director of the Master of Science in Anesthesia program at the Medical College of Wisconsin, Milwaukee. Additionally, in the ASA she serves as vice president for professional affairs. She deeply believes that the culture of our environment where we spend a great part of our day influences our health. Healthy clinician = healthy patients; meaning better patient outcomes. Lois and Patrick enjoy traveling the world experiencing cultures and history.

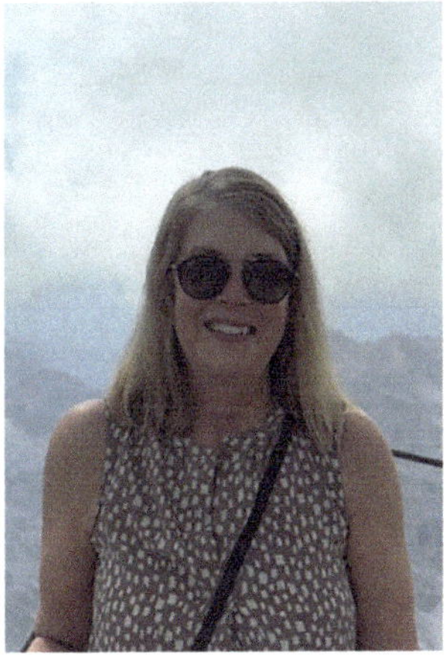

Abigail Crawford

Alaskan Bridge

Abigail is a graduate of the University of Alaska where she obtained a BS degree in natural sciences and a minor in psychology. She attends the University of Washington School of Medicine. Her hobbies include most things outdoors in the beautiful state of Alaska—she loves to hike, bike, kayak, camp, fish, play tennis, ski, and snow machine. She has also volunteered at Project Hope, which makes free naloxone kits for the state of Alaska.

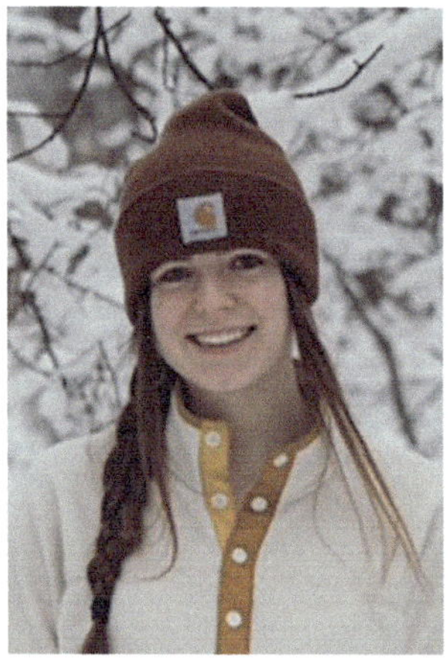

Isabella Giglio

Philadelphia Walkway Bridge

Isabella Giglio is a busy medical student at Sydney Kimmel Medical College pursuing her interest in surgery. She attended University of California Santa Barbara for her undergraduate degrees where she has dual degrees in Aquatic Biology and Sociology. She enjoys combining her passions of medicine and art through photography.

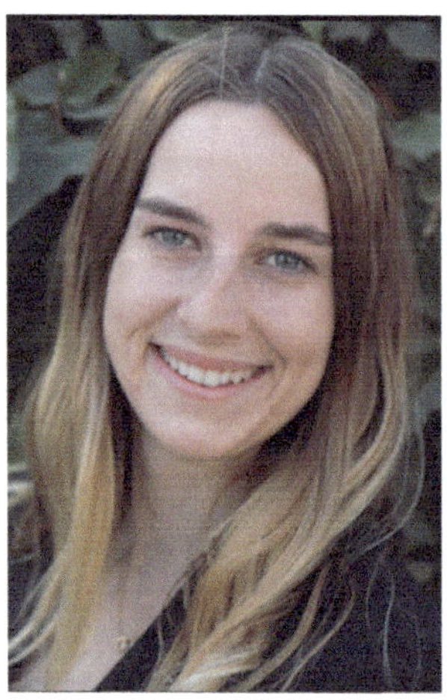

Aubrie Graber

Medical Text Books

Aubrie is a Cleveland native and cat aficionado who loves to chronicle life around her through photos and video. She is a former long time competitive cheer flyer and also varsity cheerleader. She developed a passion for doing sports photography at her high school, including for basketball, lacrosse, and wrestling. She is studying communications and media production at the University of Dayton.

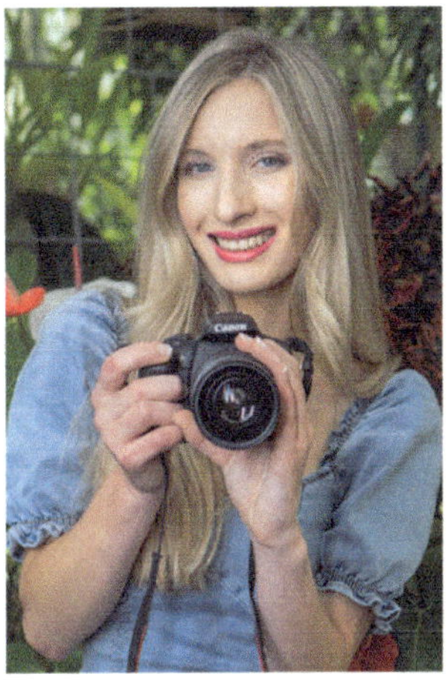

Mary Graber

London Tower Bridge

Mary graduated with a BA in interior design from Ashland University and formerly worked as a wallpaper designer. She is also the proud mother of three amazing children. In her spare time, she enjoys traveling, photography, decorating, gardening, biking, yoga, baking, and many other creative projects, but she especially treasures spending time with her family and three cats: Theodore, Tulip, and Angel.

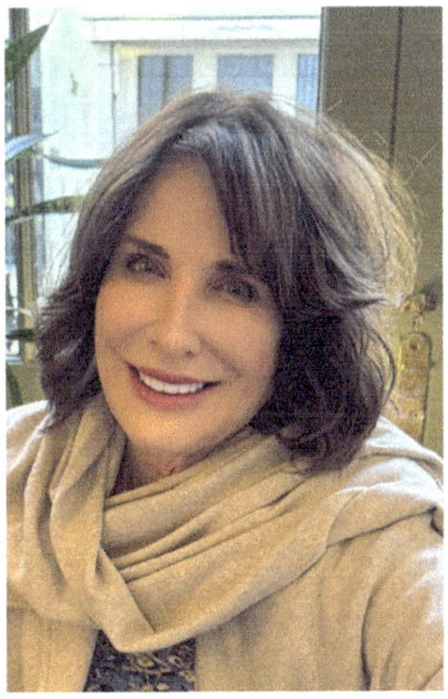

Gavin Hess

Bamboo Slide Rule

Gavin is a busy college student at Auburn University where he is majoring in business and finance and enjoying getting to know that part of the country. He enjoys traveling with his family, especially Hawaii and the beautiful South Carolina beaches. He is a sports and outdoors enthusiast and was a competitive wrestler throughout his school years.

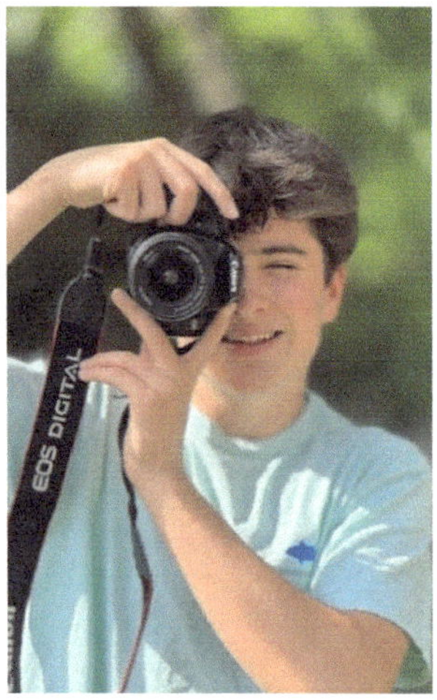

Harriet Hopf

Heaphy Track Pedestrian Bridge

Harriet is a professor of anesthesiology and biomedical engineering and president of the Academic Senate at the University of Utah. Her local and national leadership roles have positioned her for her current focus on nurturing career and leadership success in the next generation. Her husband Leo is an expert in strategy and decision-making and a peerless peer mentor. McKinley, their off spring, recently received a MA in history from the U of Utah and is busy reinventing the way history is told.

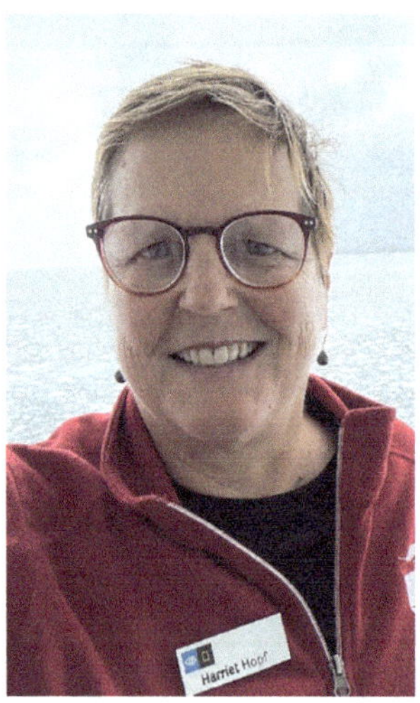

Scott Hull

Wheelhouse of the tugboat George L. Ostrander, Mackinac Bridge

Scott has been a chief engineer in the US Merchant Marine for the past 40 years, formerly on the Bering Sea and the Gulf of Alaska, but now sailing on commercial vessels in the Great Lakes. Home is a small lake in central Indiana, where he boats and rides his Indian motorcycle with wife and *Anesthesia Bridges* author Conni Walkup Hull. He also enjoys painting and photography in his shop while rocking out to Joan Jett and Blondie.

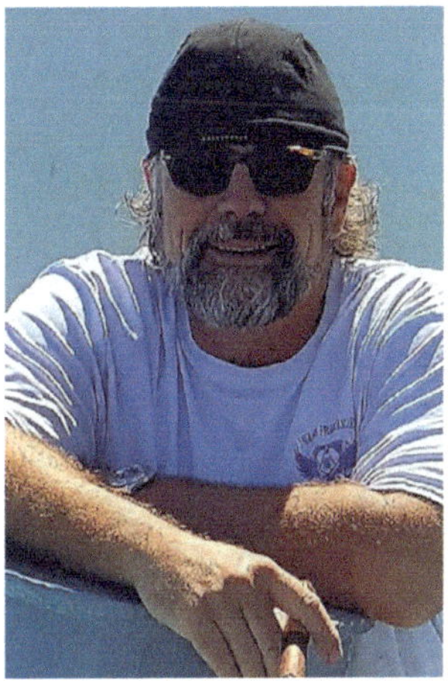

Hailey James

Sedona, Flying Dog Lennon

Hailey James is originally from Arizona. She still loves the Southwest but loves dogs more and relocated to East Texas several years ago to begin her career in dog rescue. She considers it the hardest but most worthwhile thing she has ever done. The 24/7 nature of dog rescue precludes a lot of free time, but she continues to enjoy doing photography when she can. Her photo of Lennon (below) won several contests and landed him a loving home in Canada.

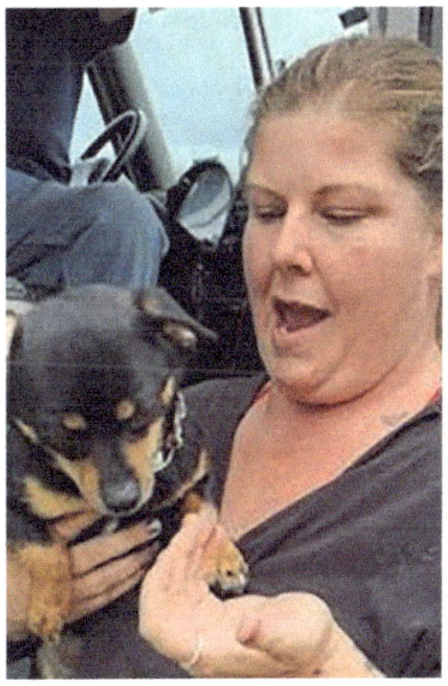

Randy Jensen

RJ Acres Farm Pictures

Randy Jensen lives and farms in Blair, NE, on a beautiful and historic 900-acre property. A devoted family man, he spends as much time as possible with his grown children and their spouses and his four beautiful grandchildren. He also enjoys volunteering at his church, traveling both in the US and internationally, and rooting for the Nebraska Cornhuskers.

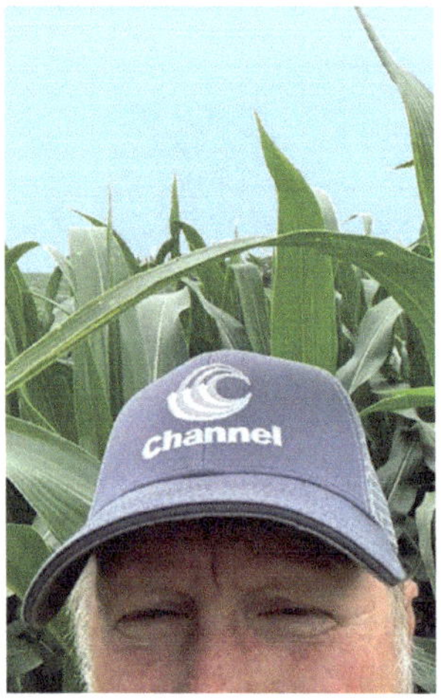

Ruth Jensen

RJ Acres Farm Pictures

Ruth's professional accomplishments include working for over four decades as a senior chemical engineer and engineering executive and holding an office in her family's farm corporations, all while never losing sight of her pre-eminent role as a mother and now grandmother. She is a dedicated churchwoman, expert cook, and world traveler. She also collects and has been asked to exhibit her beautiful antique jewelry.

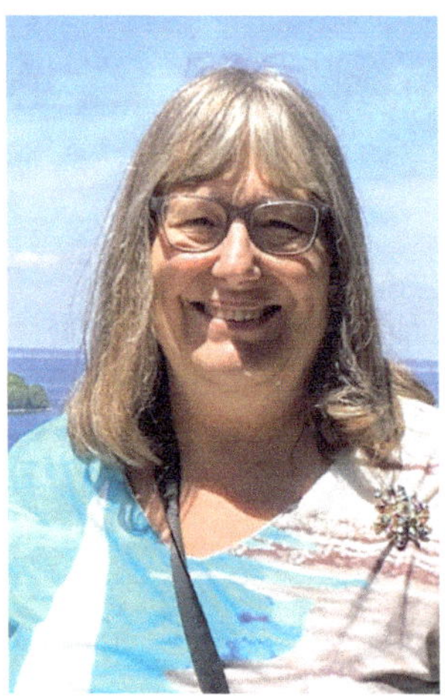

Bo Johns-Hennessy

C&O Canal Bridge, Arlington Memorial Bridge

Bo is a native Washingtonian and resides there with his husband and their Shih Tzu, Wally. He finds joy in exploring and photographing the wider DC area. He is a devoted volunteer, serving in leadership positions with GO BO GO Fund, the Foundation for Community Betterment, and Lehigh University. He was a consultant at McKinsey & Company before founding his own firm to collaborate with real estate and technology clients to shape the built environment.

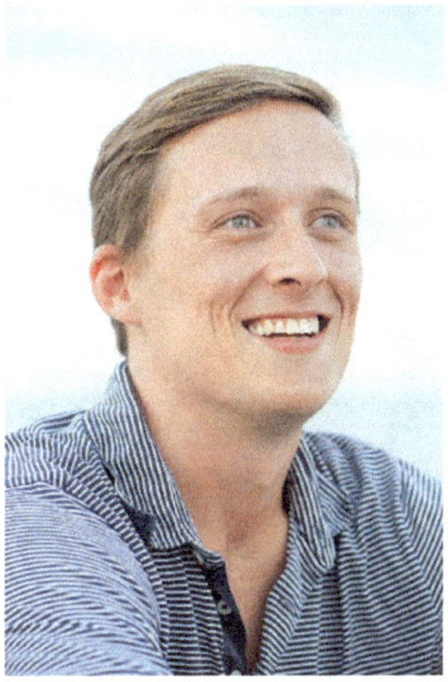

Caroline Koloski

Pullen Park Bridge

Caroline is from Charlotte, NC. She has a BA in psychology and is now a premed student. When she isn't hanging out with her cat Blackie, she can be found on the golf course or going to concerts with her friends. She also loves spending time with her large family. After finishing a study abroad semester in Florence, Italy, she is now an EMT and preparing for medical school.

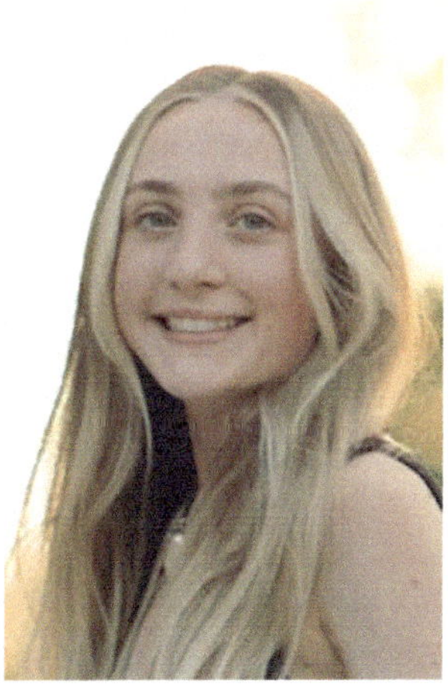

LouAnn Kopenhaver

Hanover Walkway

LouAnn is a retired reading specialist and literacy coach, having earned a BS in Education from Millersville University and an MEd in psychology of reading from Temple University. Since retiring, her favorite pastime is spending time with her grandkids, family, and friends, but she also enjoys golf, reading (of course), and traveling with her husband.

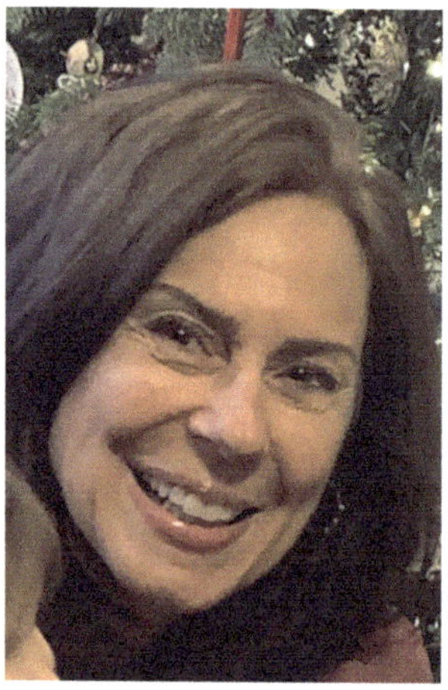

John Liao

Liao Gladstone Bag

John is an honors student, talented artist, musician, and aspiring pilot. He has studied violin for eleven years and has formally studied visual art for three years. He enjoys oil painting, sculpture, and drawing and is currently studying color theory. His many other interests include running cross country, engineering, space, film, science fiction, history, and anything to do with airplanes. He is the grandson of Dr. Schue-Yuan Liao.

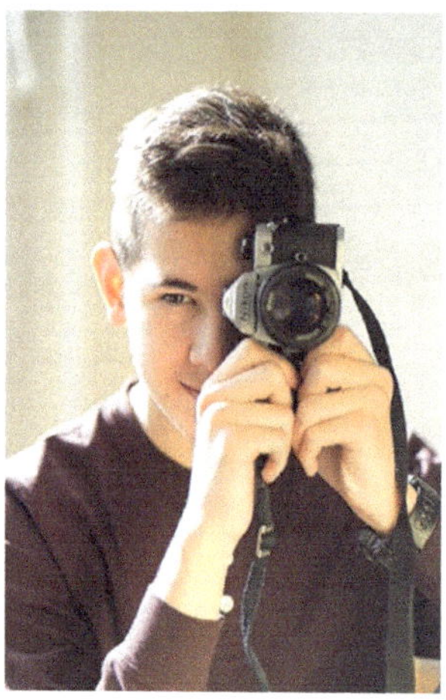

Catherine Marcucci

Rain Bridge in the Mt. Washington Arboretum, Brandywine River Bridge, Olentangy River Bridge

Cathy thinks of herself more as an editor than photographer, but she snaps a photo here and there. Her professional careers have been in engineering, anesthesiology, and transfusion medicine. Her abiding personal interest is her family and when she can find the time, she also enjoys traveling, swimming, minor league baseball, duplicate bridge, and helping out dog rescues.

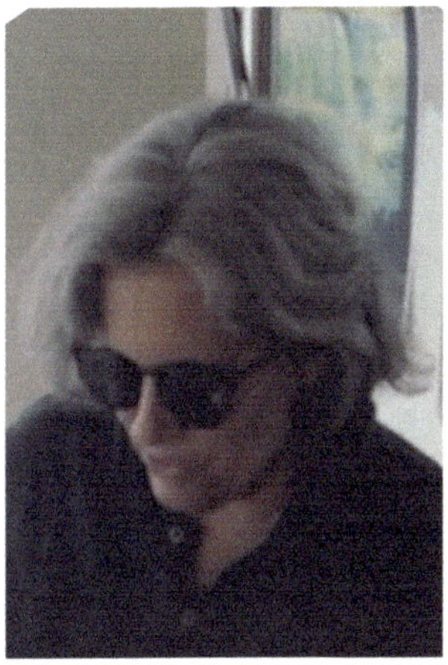

Elaine Matte Mut

St. Louis Arch

Elaine is a Houston-based amateur photographer who began her photography journey in earnest as a volunteer publicity photographer for three Houston public schools, as well as local community events. She has been fortunate to have her photography published in local papers and magazines and exhibited at several local galleries. Her main passion in retirement is traveling with family to areas with abundant wildlife and natural surroundings.

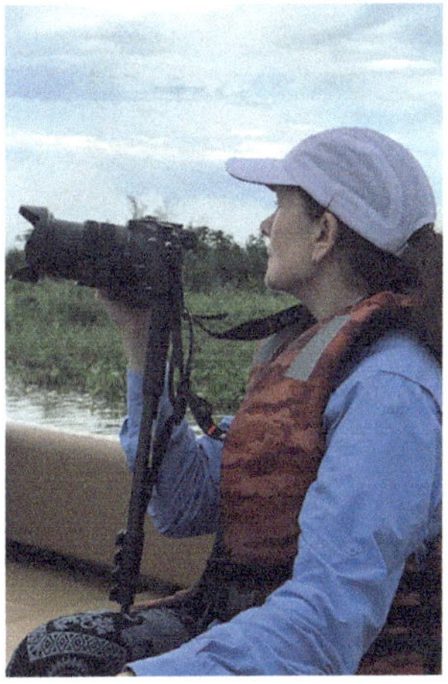

Kathleen Naughter

Washington Park Bridge

Kathleen received her BS in studio art from the College of St. Rose in Albany, New York, where she worked as an assistant in the photography lab back in the days of 35 millimeter film. She considers her greatest accomplishment to be raising her three wonderful sons, John, Patrick, and James. Her newest role is grandmother, and she is looking forward to spending time with Lucille, the most beautiful baby in the world.

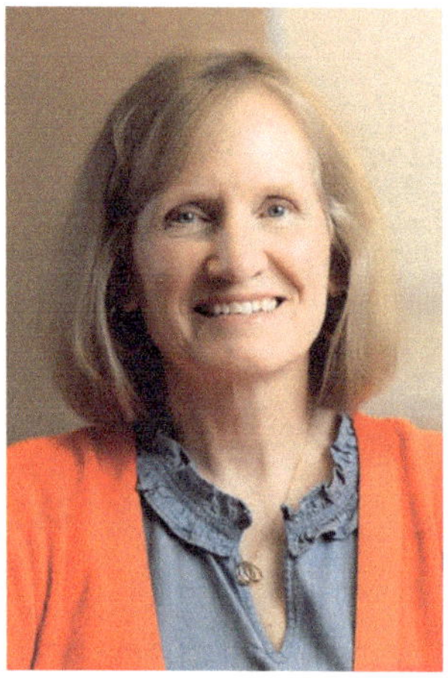

James Nguyen

Philadelphia Walkway Bridge

James is from Newport Beach, California, and is now a busy fourth year medical student at Thomas Jefferson University in Philadelphia who is in the residency interviewing process. In his free time, he enjoys exploring Chinatown and other Philadelphia neighborhoods as well as raising his kitten, Boh.

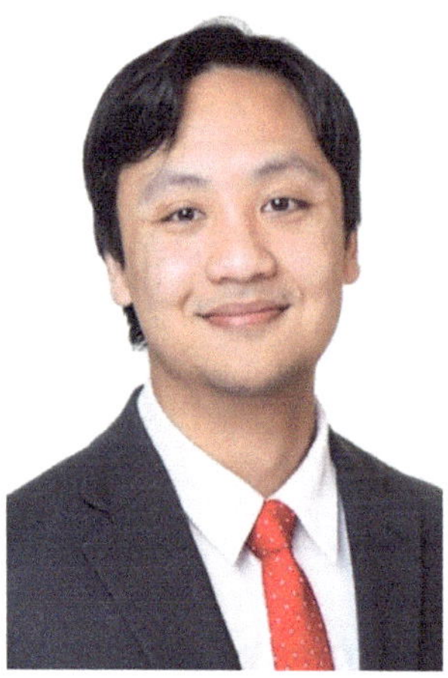

Anthony Passannante

UNC Skyway Bridge

Tony is a professor and executive vice-chair of anesthesiology at UNC Chapel Hill, and assistant dean for admissions for UNC SOM. His focus in anesthesiology practice has been vascular anesthesia and operating room management. His hobbies include hiking and traveling. His family continues to grow with two recent weddings and two grandchildren growing up at an astonishing pace.

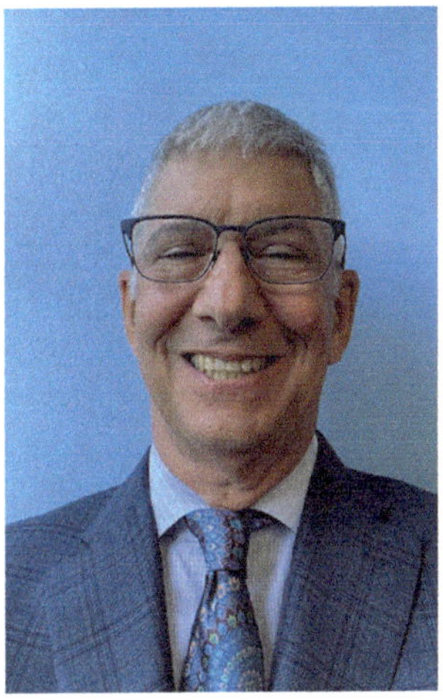

Alex Pelayo

Montgomery County Bridge

Alejandra is a San Francisco native who completed a research fellowship at the National Institutes of Health. She graduated from the University of Redlands with degrees in sociology and biology. She is passionate about diversifying medicine and science and has served on several boards. She is now an MBA student and is seriously considering medical school to follow.

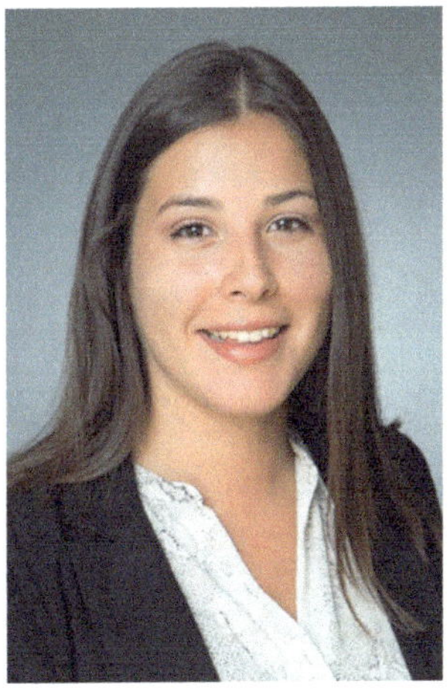

Amy Robbins

Aqueduct of Segovia

Amy is an anesthesiologist and medical executive who specializes in palliative medicine and cancer pain management. She remains deeply committed to both clinical work and the development of healthcare safety, quality, and clinical decision supports for best practices. She lives in NC with her husband, two dogs, and two cats. Her passions include her family, travel, animal rescue, and collecting art.

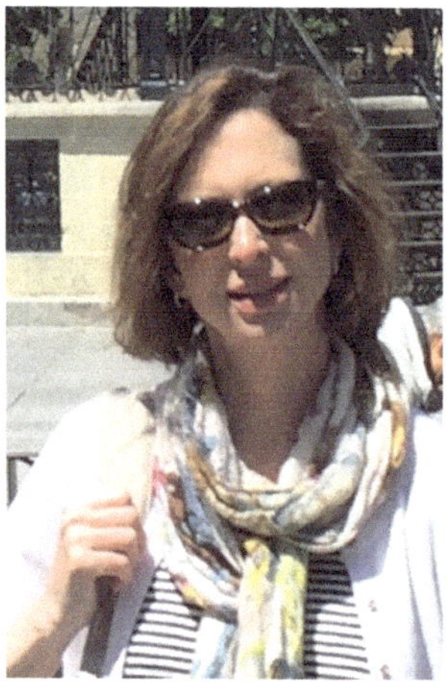

Neil Sandson

Stick Bridge

Neil Sandson is a psychiatrist, proud husband and father, and lifelong squash and duplicate bridge player, gamer, and science fiction buff. Fortunately, none of that distracted him from his newfound passion for the art and science of bridge building, edible or otherwise. He was especially honored to be asked to make a cheese bridge.

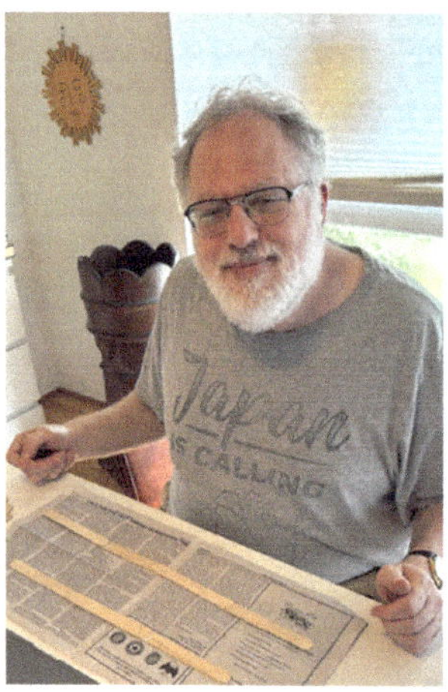

Daniel Sessler

Harbor Bridge, Sydney

Dan is a senior anesthesiologist who has authored more than 980 research papers. He has been a principal or co-investigator on grants totaling $100 million. He founded and directs the Outcomes Research Consortium—the world's largest anesthesia research group; it publishes a full paper every other day, for a total of more than 2000 papers. In his previous life, he was a photographer and still enjoys great images.

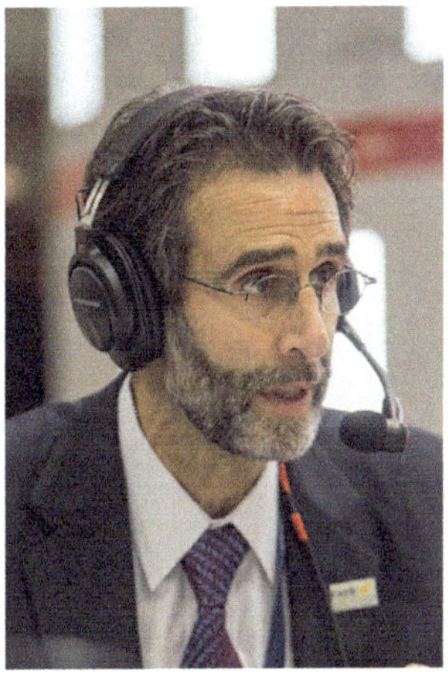

Richard Sheffield

Abril Bridge in Lisbon, Portugal

Richard is a retired technologist and is now fully occupied as a writer and author. After graduating from Georgia Tech, he learned that understanding the latest wave of high-tech gadgets and being able to write about them is a rare and valuable skill. He splits time between the heat of Atlanta and the more heat of Miami, where he loves spending time with his plastic surgeon girlfriend.

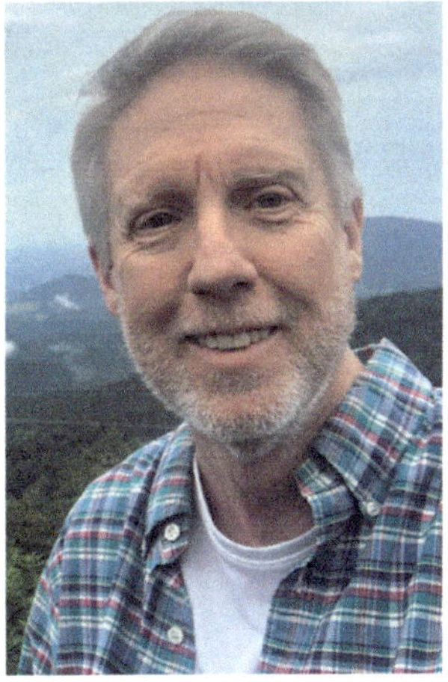

Dillon Shook

Gottschalk Bag

Dillon Shook is a software engineer working primarily on the web for the last decade. His other hobbies include photography and getting inspiration from other photographers like Albert Dros, Irene Rudnyk, and Markus Reugels, playing guitar and listening to lots of music, game development, cooking, gardening, and not having enough time in the day.

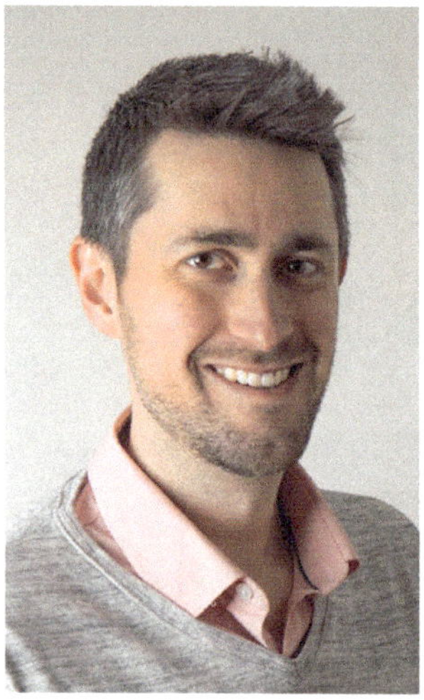

Joshua Stich

The High Line, New York City

Born in Atlanta, Georgia, Joshua grew up both there and on the Gold Coast, Australia. He attended New York University, where he majored in neural science and chemistry. He is now a medical student at Albert Einstein where he is naturally already interested in anesthesiology. In his spare time, he plays all the ice hockey he can, volunteers with a number of organizations, and travels.

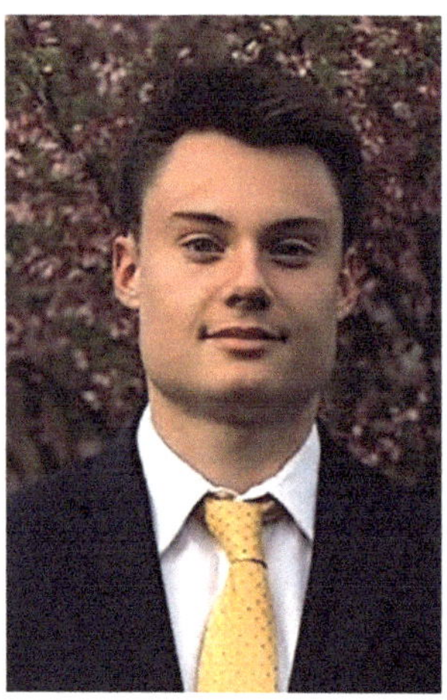

Jennifer Tripi

UNC Skyway Bridge

Jennifer (Jen) completed her obstetric anesthesia fellowship at UNC Hospitals at Chapel Hill this year and joined the Ohio State team as a general and obstetric anesthesiologist. When she isn't busy at the hospital, she enjoys spending time with her husband, family, and friends. She also loves exploring and hiking our country's beautiful national parks, traveling the world, playing board games, and interior designing.

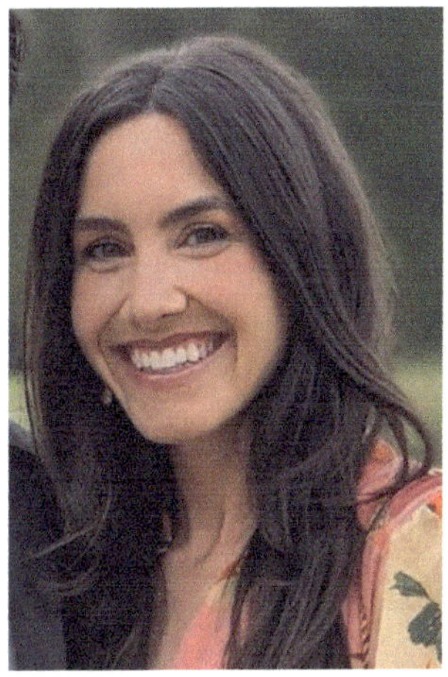

Chloe Wagener

The Natural Bridge

Chloe Landon Wagener loves to travel, reads voraciously, and writes short stories. When she has time away from her studies, she is working on the basics of a novel. She is endeared to all animals, especially dogs, and loves chocolate. She is a percussionist and pianist and wants to pursue a career in medicine or law.

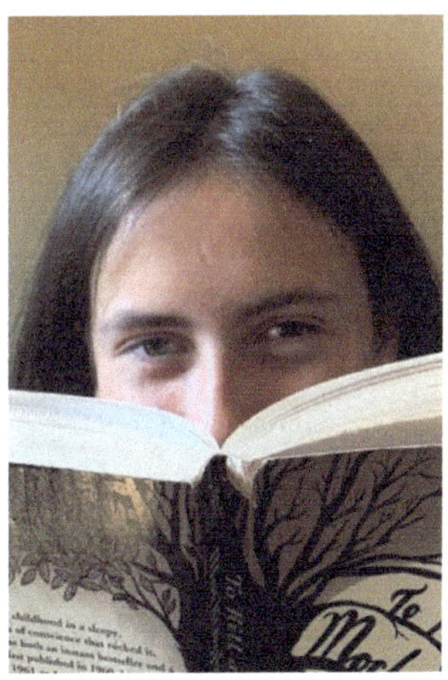

James Wyatt Wagener

Footbridge

James Wyatt is an energetic soul like his mother. He loves to try everything at least once like his dad. He loves to travel, wants to learn to cook, and dances like a fiend. He plays the violin and is learning the clarinet. He wants to learn the saxophone so he can play in the jazz band and is a member of the mountain biking team.

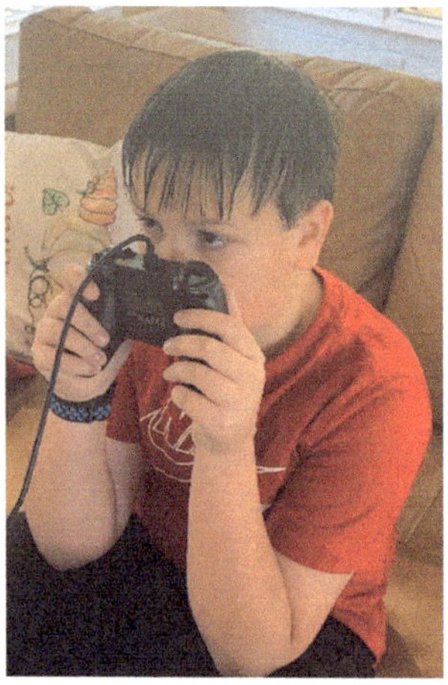

Nathaniel R. Wagener

National Bridge Park

Nathaniel Ryan is a boy's boy. His current love is soccer, and he idolizes Lionel Messi. He also loves to play games on his Nintendo Switch with his brother and is learning to play Pokémon with the help of his dad. He plays the piano when he has to and is a math wizard.

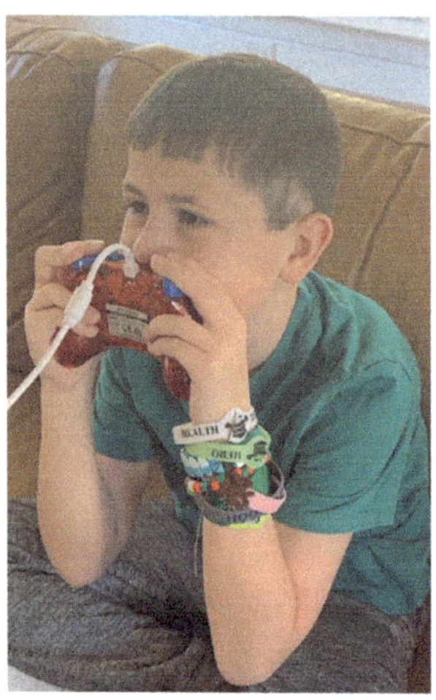

Daniel Walker

Alaskan Wooden Footbridge

Danny is a student in suburban Philadelphia, PA. He enjoys taking photos while working summers on his grandfather's commercial fishing boat in Southeast Alaska and already has a large collection of striking nature photos. Danny also enjoys sports, running cross country, traveling, soccer, and playing his cello.

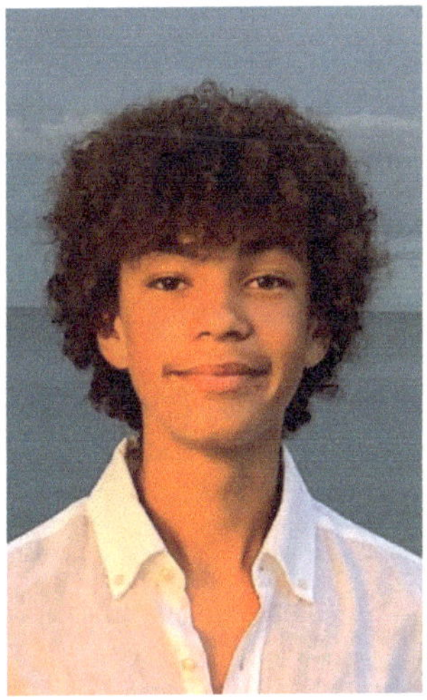

John Walker IV

Fairmont Park Bridge

John is a busy student at Drexel University. He is a premed major and is also taking extra coursework in psychology. He enjoys sports of all kinds, spending time with his family, exploring the most interesting places in Philadelphia, traveling, playing rugby for his school club team, distance running, and playing cello.

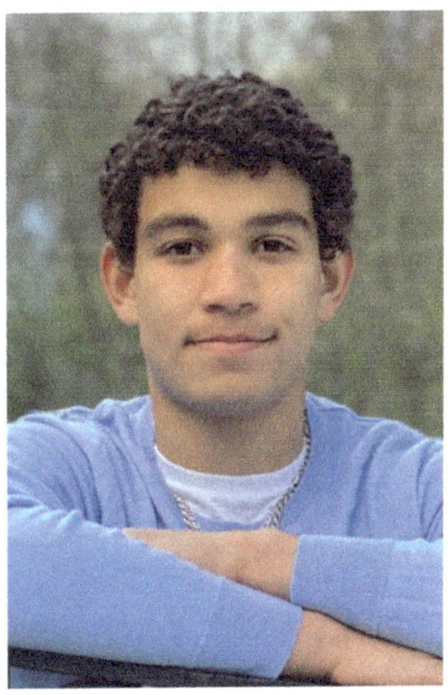

Marilyn Walker

Little Island at Pier 55

Marilyn was born and raised in Atlanta, Georgia. As someone with a strong passion for the sciences, she carried this interest into her undergraduate studies, where she pursued degrees in psychology and chemistry at New York University. As an intern at the Sigurdsson Neuroscience lab at NYU Langone, she hopes to continue to advance the field of medicine.

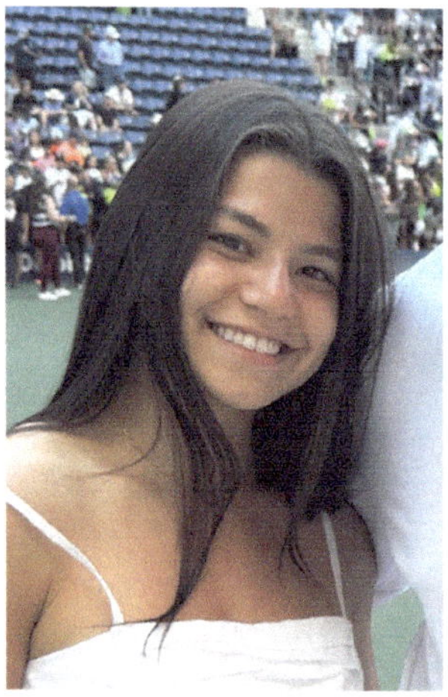

Christie Waters

Sandstone Natural Bridge, Jordan

Christie is a mostly retired chemical engineer and STEM educator who enjoys spending as much time outdoors as the upstate New York weather permits. In addition to taking too many photos of her grandkids, she tries to capture both the simple and the stunning beauties she encounters while traveling.

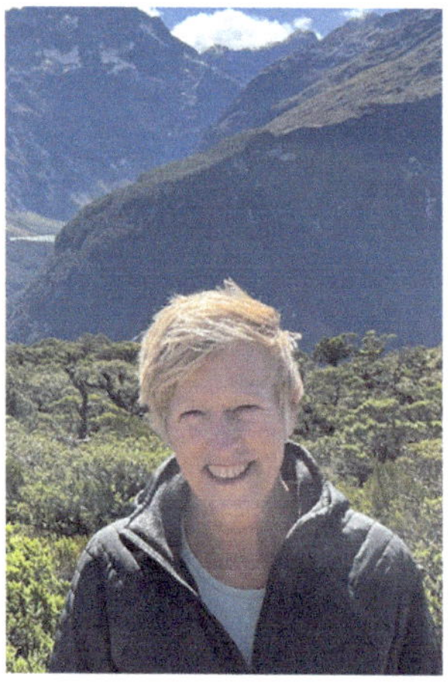

Toby Weingarten

Cold Creek Bridge

Toby Weingarten is a professor of anesthesiology at the Mayo Clinic and has been a member of their faculty since 2005. He has been very active in researching anesthetic outcomes with over 250 peer-reviewed publications, numerous abstracts, and book chapters. When he is not in the hospital, he is almost always outside, bird watching, fishing, gardening, tapping maple trees, or playing with his bees.

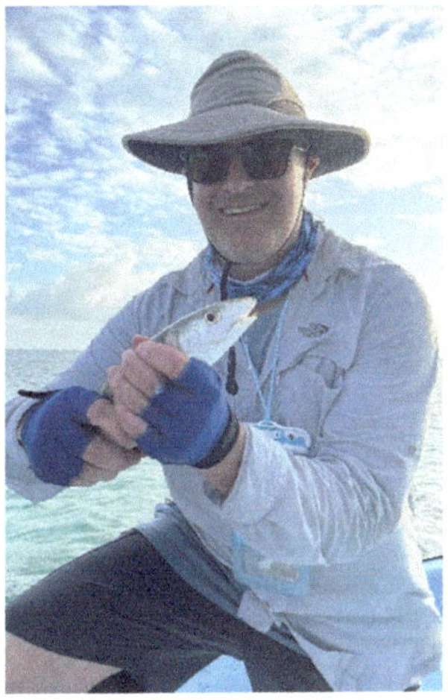

Brad Winters

BNSF Freight Train

Brad is a senior anesthesiologist and intensivist at Johns Hopkins. He is a devoted family person whose outside interests include hiking and mountain climbing, kayaking, ice climbing, mountain and road biking, movies, travel, collecting vintage slide rulers and antique microscopes, and of course trains.

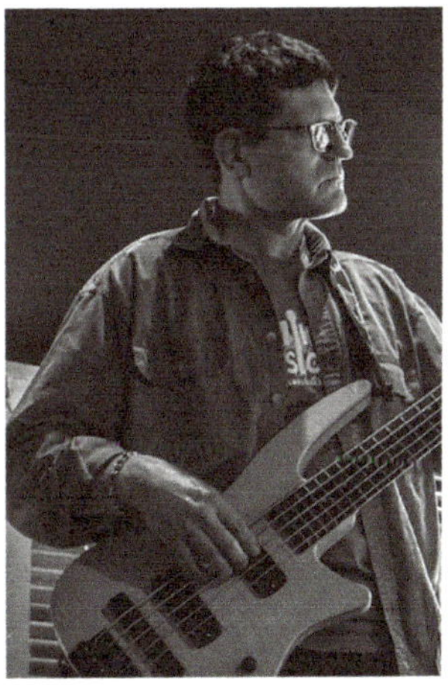

Eli Wright

Student Walkway at Towson U

Eli lives in the Baltimore area and is a busy executive and entrepreneur in the automotive industry, with expertise in the European luxury models. He followed the creation of this book from the start and finally agreed to join the project after several requests. In his very rare spare time, he enjoys music, sports, and photography.

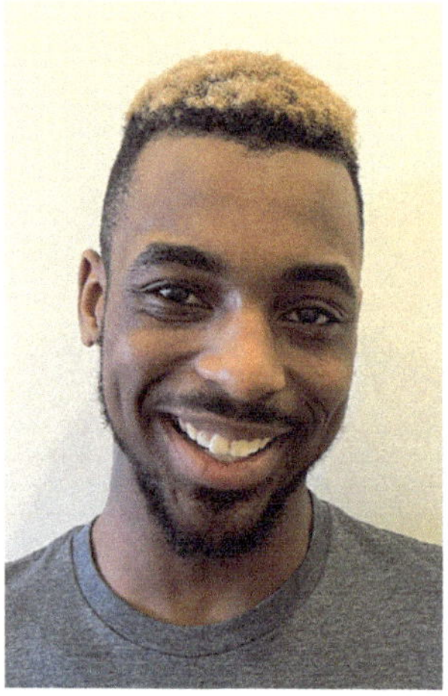

Charles Yeo

Philadelphia Main Line Bridges

Charlie Yeo is an internationally known pancreas surgeon and the eighth Samuel D. Gross Professor and chairman of the Department of Surgery at the Sidney Kimmel Medical College of Thomas Jefferson University. He is a sports fan, loves rock and roll music, and is an avid reader. He and his wife have a new puppy, Paxton—and many of their recent photos have been of him, of course.

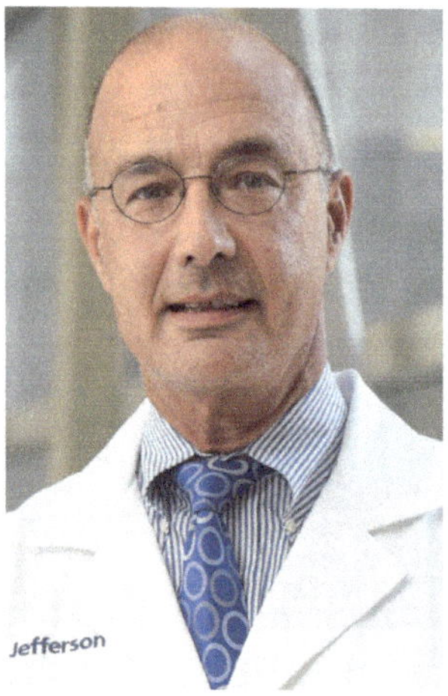

David Zvara

North Carolina Bridge

David is an avid iPhone photographer, capturing over 8664 images to include the grandkids' birthdays, grandkids' soccer, grandkids' first day of school, more grandkids with pets. In short, endless sources of creative inspiration! To date, the commercial translation of this work has fallen short of expectations, but opportunity abounds as the grandkids star in school plays nearly every weekend of the year.

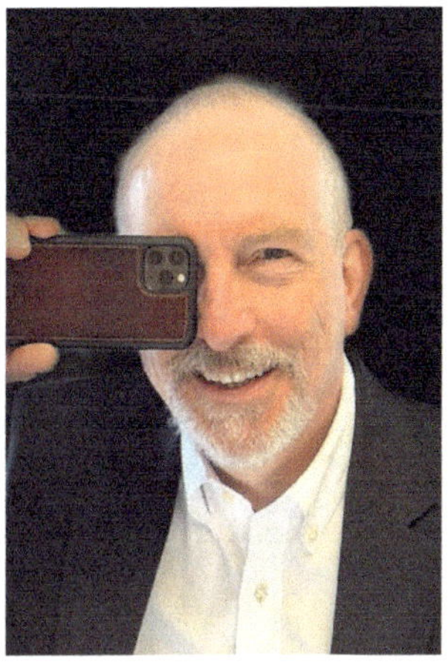

Jessica Zvara

Natural Log Bridge over Creek with Exuberant Dog

Jessica is a faculty anesthesiologist at the University of Virginia, where she specializes in cardiothoracic anesthesiology. Outside of the operating room, she loves romping around the woods with her two kids, her husband, and her dog Hobbes. A little late to the game, she is beginning to dabble in the art of baking and is currently loving homemade English muffins.

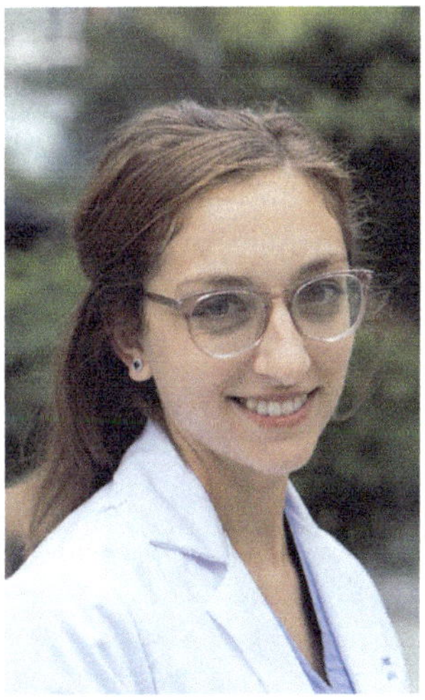

The editors also thank (in alphabetical order) the Abouleish family, the Altose family, the Auers-Jensen families, the Bank family, Barking Mad Animal Refuge, Inc, Amberly Hall Brown, Austin Brown, Hon. Christopher C. Conner, the Dalal-Taylor family, the DeCaria-Lupa family, Steven M. Frank MD, the Gottschalk family, the Graber family, the Harrison-Jordan-Marcucci family, Vincent L. Hoellerich MD, the Leffert family, the Lessinger-Wiener family, the Lien-Brinzac family, Sharon L. Milgram PhD, the Peterson family, the Prischak family, the family of Gary and Marilyn Robbins, the Robbins-McGahey family, Matthew Rorie, the Sandson family, F. Jacob Seagull PhD, the Togioka family, the Tung family, and the Zvara family for sending us photos and images from their personal files and collections.

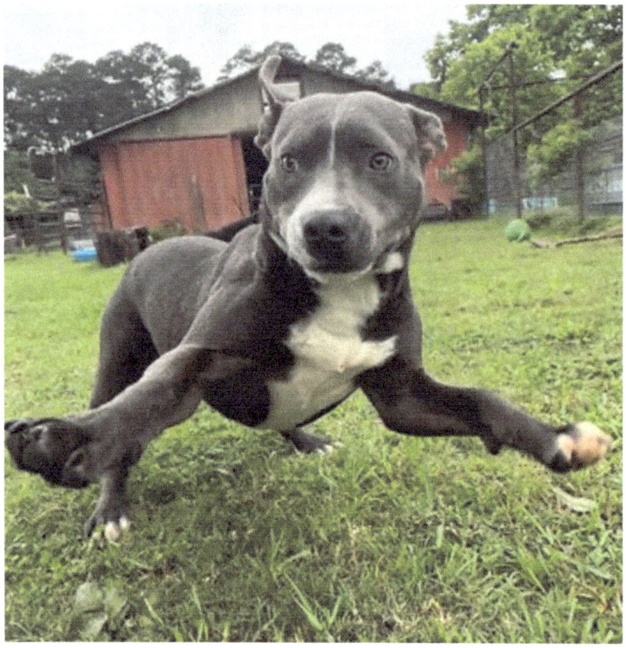

This is Lennon at **Barking Mad Animal Refuge** in Hemphill, Texas. He's such a handsome dog and a bit of a celebrity, having won several contests for best dog photo. Plus, he can fly! If you have room in your hearts and lives, please consider the millions of abandoned animals in rescues and sanctuaries who desperately need help. Fortunately for Lennon, a wonderful family saw this photo and offered him a loving home. **Photo: Hailey James**

BMAR *is online at barkingmadanimalrescue.com*

The Newport Town Bridge—Newport, Wales

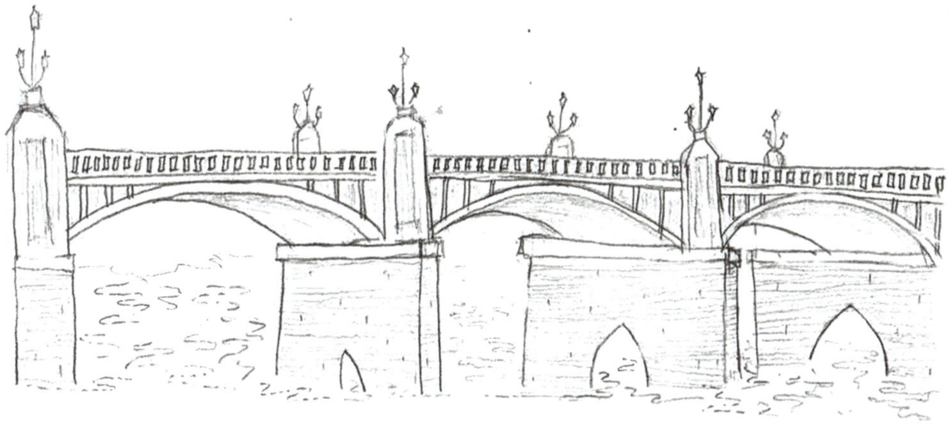

This charming little bridge in Wales is known to the locals as Town Bridge. It was selected as a favorite bridge by consensus of the editors. It opened in 1927 and spans the River Usk, connecting the High Street with Newport Castle. The five-span bridge replaces earlier wood and stone bridges.

The famous escape artist Harry Houdini jumped off the stone version in 1913 with his hands manacled and his feet shackled. He was arrested the next week for holding a public entertainment on the bridge and obstructing traffic. Four of the pillars of the current bridge are decorated with a painted stone cherub and shield design that has found its way onto British merchandise and even album covers.

The *Anesthesia Bridges* editors thank **Nina Babbitt** from The Architectural Team in Boston, MA, for her lovely original drawing that captures the romantic quality of the 1920s architecture.

Statement of Disclaimer

The views expressed herein are solely the authors' and contributors' own personal and professional opinions and experiences and should be used only to foster thought, reflection, and (we hope) lively discussion and further inquiry.

They do not represent superseding clinical mandates and should not be construed as the official statements, instructions, guidelines, recommendations, or positions of any employer, educational and/or academic institution, business, or professional clinical group including but not limited to the American Board of Anesthesiology, the American Society of Anesthesiologists, the Society for Pediatric Anesthesia, the American Society of Regional Anesthesia and Pain Medicine, the Society for Pediatric Anesthesia, the Anesthesia Quality Institute, the Closed Claims Program, the Anesthesia Patient Safety Foundation, and the Foundation for Anesthesia Education and Research.

The authors' opinions and advice also do not represent any official administrative, clinical, or academic position of any other company, institution, group, or practice, whether mentioned by name or not.

No aspect of this book represents the official positions of the National Institutes of Health, the US Food and Drug Administration, the Department of Health and Human Services, the Department of Veterans Affairs, the Department of Defense, or any other civilian or military entity or agency of the United States government.

Finally, the content and the proffered opinions in this book should not substitute for the appropriate legal, financial, or medical advice.

There is no disclaimer needed concerning the kindness, interest, and enthusiasm that the staff of Towson Hot Bagels in Timonium, Maryland, had for this project as they saw senior editor Cathy Marcucci every weekend for breakfast for **at least** three years (Fig. 1). As soon as she trudged up to the counter with her laptop the counter staff would automatically start her usual order—plain bagel toasted with a fried egg and sausage, no cheese. The staff even followed along closely enough to ask how specific chapters were coming along! Many thanks to the breakfast crew with the bagels!

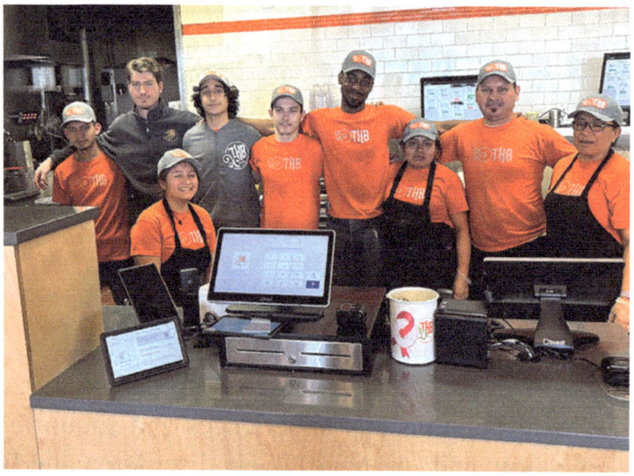

Fig. 1 The Saturday morning crew at Towson Hot Bagels in Timonium, MD

We once gave the THB crew a page of quotations planned for the book and asked them which were their favorites. They selected the important life wisdom below.

From Conni Walkup Hull: If you bleed in the water, sharks will come. It's the way of things. But it's a waste of time to blame the sharks - it's what they are. It's up to us not to look like a tasty snack.

From Neil Sandson and Coach Ed Serues: Never change a winning game, always change a losing game.

Acknowledgments

The practice of anesthesiology is more than a science, it is also an art. Several years ago, we realized that there was a generation of supremely wise and superbly competent anesthesiologists who were at or near retirement age. As these wonderful clinicians and mentors moved on to the next phases of their lives, we saw that an entire encyclopedia of knowledge, experience, wit, and wisdom would go with them. The science would still be found in the pages of the journals and the textbooks, but the art would be lost.

Our lead editor Sharif Mohamed had the great idea to develop a book project to build a wisdom bridge from that generation of practitioners to the junior people coming up behind us. But this bridge would not be made of concrete and steel, rather it would be constructed piece by piece with thoughts, advice, stories, and perhaps a gentle admonishment and warning or two. And so, the *Anesthesia Bridges: Wisdom for Your Personal and Professional Journey* project was created. Additional editors and a huge number of contributors were recruited and what followed were several years of emails, texts, and interviews as hundreds of the best physicians and clinicians (and nicest people!) in our specialty took the time the help us. As we began talking to and corresponding with the most senior and retiring anesthesiologists, we also spoke with many anesthesiologists who are still at the full pinnacle and prime of their careers and began to gather up and collate their wisdom and knowledge to pass on as well.

And so, this book became a heartfelt gift from the community of senior anesthesiologists to our junior physician colleagues.

The manuscript is organized into the topics that pertain to the life and careers of an anesthesiologist. Each section has essays ranging from short, pithy pieces of advice to longer contemplative pieces in a conversational style, as if you were chatting with the experts themselves. Each section ends with a collection of additional words of wisdom and short sayings. This book is not intended to be a clinical anesthesia handbook but of course some clinical topics found their way into the manuscript. They do not comprise comprehensive clinical coverage of any one topic but perhaps a clinical pearl or two will resonate and stay with the reader.

In every book project, there are always those individuals who go above and beyond. Co-editor Ray Graber has done a heroic amount of work on this book, especially in the middle third of the project, when he really kept the snowball rolling down (up?) the hill and the juggling pins in the air. Left to his own devices, he would eschew special mention, nonetheless the editorial group feels strongly that his absolutely critical contributions must be mentioned—there would be no book without him. We also thank senior editor Cathy Marcucci for devoting her time and focused effort to the project over many months and lending us her advice, expertise, and the benefit of her network. We appreciate having her wisdom in developing what we hope is a fun, easy-to-read book that is still packed with valuable content.

We would also like to give special mention to our colleagues who took on extra subjects and topics on short notice. These friends were hugely helpful in consulting on editorial decisions and even developing entire sections of the book by writing, editing, reviewing, and finding authors for us. Each of them fully deserves their positions as consulting and contributing associate editors. And so, we thank (in alphabetical order) Michael S. Axley MD, Ronald S. Bank MD, Andrew Barker MD, Carol F. Bodenheimer MD, John C. Briggs MD, Kirk Lalwani MD, Albert Liao LAc, Kristin King Liao LAc, Daniel J. McCoy MD '26, Rajen V. Nathwani MBBS BSc, Steven L. Orebaugh MD, Amy J. Robbins MD MBA, Neil B. Sandson MD, F. Jacob Seagull PhD, Jennifer N. Tripi MD, Brandon M. Togioka MD, Brant Wagener MD PhD, and David Zvara MD.

Neil Sandson, Carol Bodenheimer, and Jake Seagull are three of the best friends the anesthesiology community ever had. They all reviewed numerous chapters and provided expert addenda and comments. We couldn't imagine doing a book without them. The same is true of Kirk Lalwani, who has to be one of the best people in the entire country to do a large writing project with. David Zvara lent us his wisdom and advice at crucial points in the manuscript development and sent us his brilliant essay for beginning physicians.

Amy Robbins is a superb clinician who has boarded in anesthesiology and two anesthesiology subspecialties and who always replied within two minutes with suggestions, advice, and content. Brandon Togioka also was always immediately available and always correct and helped us immeasurably with his special expertise in obstetrical anesthesia. Steve Orebaugh was unfailingly generous with his expertise in two of major areas of the practice of anesthesiology—airway management and regional anesthesia. The University of Alabama at Birmingham associate editors—Andrew Barker, Brant Wagener, and John Briggs, were a rock-solid resource and sent us important content, great ideas and suggestions, and encouragement. Similarly, Al and Kristin Liao provided important editorial support on our acupuncture content.

Raj Nathwani popped onto our radar early in the project and provided us with such valuable content and advice that he was invited to join the editorial group on the spot. Mike Axley, who was a writer and journalist before going into medicine, was our go-to person for all questions and problems of that nature. A special acknowledgment and thanks goes out to Ron Bank, who wasn't involved in the earliest stages of the project but who instantly understood what we were trying to do and sent us pages and pages of ideas, suggestions, edits, clinical pearls, and words of wisdom, all while meeting the demands of a busy clinical practice. Finally, Jen Tripi had the firepower to undertake full editorial duties by recruiting contributors and developing content even while being a busy anesthesiology trainee.

Throughout this project, we were fortunate to draw on the knowledge and expertise of a number of guest authors, who are not part of the anesthesia community. We thank them for taking time from their studies and professional communities to contribute to ours. First, we thank Harvey Alter MD, who is the 2020 Nobel Laureate in Medicine or Physiology for the discovery of the Hepatitis C virus. There are many demands for Dr. Alter's attention, nonetheless he took the time to help develop a chapter on blood donation (and insisted that he appear only as a middle author) and write us a short essay on his life's priorities. We also thank James K. Gilman MD (Maj. Gen. ret.) who was the Director of the Clinical Center of the National Institutes of Health for sending us both clinical and life wisdom advice.

Other guest authors and contributors who assisted with content and from whom we learned much are (in alphabetical order):

Brian Adolph, Robert Adolph, Abdullah Alswied MD, Miya R. Asato MD, CJ Barilleaux-Badger, A.M. Coleman (Cole) Bank, Amberly Hall Brown, Austin Brown, Marina Bueno MLS (ASCP) SBB, Melissa Butynski MEM, Karen M. Byrne MDE MT (ASCP) SBB, Kathleen (Cathy) Conroy-Cantilena MD, Marlee Chamberlain MD '26, Richard W. Childs MD, Herbert Chen MD, Leonard N. Chen MD PhD, Xiaopo Cheng MS PhD, Anthony A. Chico III DO, Robert Christian MD, Ariana S. Cogan MT (ASCP)^{CM}, Benjamin C. Conner MD PhD, Hon. Christopher C. Conner, Emma R. Cooley BA, Abigail J. Crawford MD '28, Edward J. Damrose MD FACS, David Daniel MD, Willy A. Flegel MD, Deborah Gerson MS CCC-SLP, Chelsea L. Gottschalk MD, Laura M. Gottschalk MSW MPH, Michael D. Graham PhD, John Matthew Hess BS ME, Theodore C. Houk MD, Conni Walkup Hull JD, Jane B. Jacobs Esq, Randy G. Jensen BAnimSc, Ruth A. Jensen PE, Deb Waterman Johns BS, Shelley Sahu Kalsi MD, Oliver Karam MD PhD, Caroline C. Koloski BA, LouAnn Kopenhaver BS MEd, Stephen D. Lasday DPM FACFAS, Patricia Lee DO JD, Olivia Liao BA '28, Yafet T. Mamo MD, Daniel J. Marcucci PhD MLA AICP, Daniel J. McCoy MD '26, Carolyn B. Metzler PhD, Sharon L. Milgram PhD, Robert E. Minahan MD, Scott D. Mist PhD LAc, Logan Olson PharmD BCCCP,

Alejandra Pelayo, Marc P. Pelletier MD, Linda M. Peterson MD FAPM, Kailey L. Peterson, Kelsey Peterson Ostergren MPH CIC, Herleen Rai MD, Emily Rhinehart BS, Captain W. Mitchell Robbins BSAE MS, Matthew Rorie BS AgEcon, Charles H. Sandson BS IME, Joseph M. Schwartz MD, Richard Sheffield BS MA, Linda Song MD MPH, Valentina Baez Sosa MD, Joshua L. Stich MD '28, Grant Taylor MD, Nicholas B. Taylor MD, Zachary R. Taylor BS, Megan E. Terek MD, Patricia Togioka MA, Robert Togioka MA, Tsung-Lin Tsai MD PhD, Joanna L. Walker MD, John R. Walker IV, Marilyn X. Walker BS, Jenny Wang MD MBA, Kamille West-Mitchell MD, Hon. Jennifer P. Wilson, and Charles J. Yeo MD FACS.

We must also give a big shout-out to the artists and photographers who donated their original work to our project. There is a separate acknowledgment for each of these talented people in the pages that follow. Special thanks go to Michael E. Liu AIA NCARB, for arranging to have the talented young architectural designers at The Architectural Team do such beautiful drawings for us.

We also send our deep thanks to Jesse Ehrenfeld MD MPH for writing our Foreword.

Finally, we are extremely grateful for the superb skills and superb patience of everybody at Springer especially Sinchu Mohan, Nithiya Vadivazhagan, and Greg Sutorius. Thanks for hanging in there with us – the whole team was great to work with at all times!

As we developed the manuscript, each of the editors chose to acknowledge the special person or persons who built the bridges that we ourselves crossed in our personal and professional development. Sharif, of course, gets the lead-off acknowledgment. He is honoring his father, Dr. Samy Mohamed Rezk, a prominent OB-GYN in Saudi Arabia and Egypt (Fig. 2). Sharif credits his dad with being his first mentor and teacher and the most important life role model he has ever had.

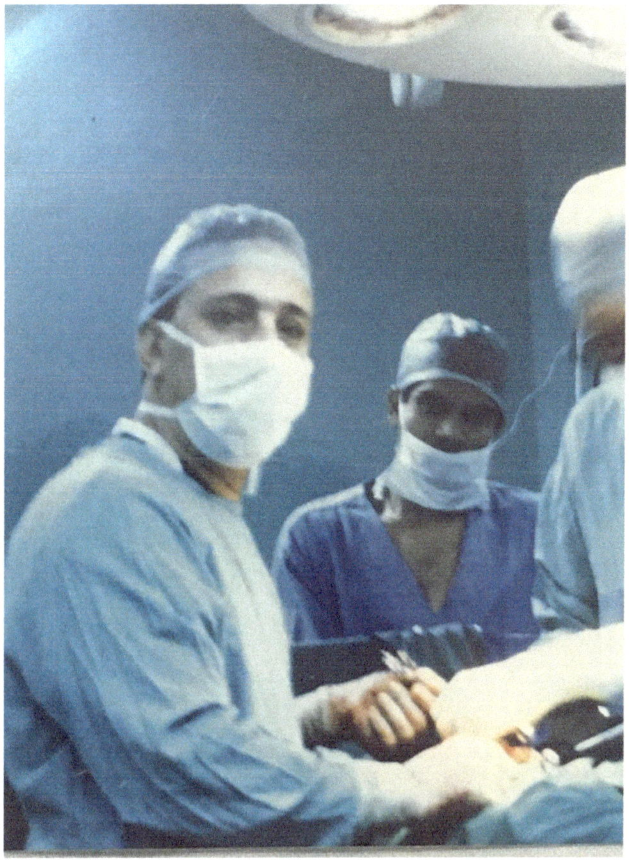

Fig. 2 Dr. Samy Mohamed Rezk operating on a large fibroid tumor in 1986 at Al Noor Specialist Hospital in Saudi Arabia. Dr. Rezk now lives in Dokki, Giza, Egypt, with his spouse (and Sharif's mom) Safy Ezzat. As we went to press, he was still in clinical practice! When not busy running his fertility clinic, he enjoys spending time with his 4 children, 12 grandchildren, fishing in the Nile, and leading the congregation at his local mosque

Finally, we thank our contributors and editors for their outstanding generosity to the Foundation for Anesthesia Education and Research—every person who contributed to this book instantly agreed that all royalties from this project be pledged in perpetuity to FAER. We are humbled and honored to be associated with and learn from this generous and caring group of professionals and providers.

Galveston, TX, USA — Sharif Mohamed, MD
Cleveland, OH, USA — Raymond G. Graber, MD
Galveston, TX, USA — Amr E. Abouleish, MD
Cleveland, OH, USA — Edwin G. Avery, MD
Seattle, WA, USA — Jeffrey R. Kirsch, MD
Bethesda, MD, USA — Catherine Marcucci, MD

Contents of Voume I

Contents of Voume II

Contributors

James H. Abernathy, MD MPH Department of Anesthesiology and Critical Care Medicine, Johns Hopkins School of Medicine, Baltimore, MD, USA

Amr E. Abouleish, MD MBA Department of Anesthesiology, John Sealy School of Medicine, The University of Texas Medical Branch, Galveston, TX, USA

Brian Adolph Adolph Citgo, Timonium, MD, USA

Robert Adolph Adolph Citgo, Timonium, MD, USA

Konstantinos Alfaras-Melainas, MD MSc Department of Anesthesiology and Perioperative Medicine, University of Pittsburgh School of Medicine, Pittsburgh, PA, USA

Abdullah Alswied, MD Center for Cellular Engineering, Department of Transfusion Medicine, Clinical Center, National Institutes of Health, Bethesda, MD, USA

Harvey J. Alter, MD Department of Transfusion Medicine, Clinical Center, National Institutes of Health, Bethesda, MD, USA

Michael D. Altose, MD PhD Department of Anesthesiology and Perioperative Medicine, University Hospitals Cleveland Medical Center, Case Western Reserve University School of Medicine, Cleveland, OH, USA

Gregory K. Applegate, DO Department of Anesthesiology and Perioperative Medicine, University Hospitals Cleveland Medical Center, Case Western Reserve University School of Medicine, Cleveland, OH, USA

Miya R. Asato, MD Departments of Neurology and Pediatrics, Johns Hopkins School of Medicine, Baltimore, MD, USA

Daniel I. Asher, MD Department of Anesthesiology and Perioperative Medicine, University Hospitals Cleveland Medical Center, Case Western Reserve University School of Medicine, Cleveland, OH, USA

Edwin G. Avery IV, MD Department of Anesthesiology and Perioperative Medicine, University Hospitals Cleveland Medical Center, Case Western Reserve University School of Medicine, Cleveland, OH, USA

Michael S. Axley, MD Oregon Anesthesiology Group, Portland, OR, USA

A. M. Coleman Bank, BS Medical Assistant, Pre-Medical Candidate, Fairfax, VA, USA

Ronald S. Bank, MD FASA Department of Anesthesiology, INOVA Fairfax Hospital, Falls Church, VA, USA
UVA School of Medicine INOVA Campus, Falls Church, VA, USA

David W. Barbar, MD BayCare Clinic, Green Bay, WI, USA

C. J. Barilleaux-Badger Barking Mad Animal Refuge, Hemphill, TX, USA

Andrew B. Barker, MD Department of Anesthesiology and Perioperative Medicine, Heersink School of Medicine, University of Alabama at Birmingham, Birmingham, AL, USA

Rodger E. Barnette, MD FCCM (Retired) AIC Kijabe Hospital, Kijabe, Kenya
Department of Anesthesiology, Lewis Katz School of Medicine, Temple University, Philadelphia, PA, USA

Brian P. Barrick, MD DDS Department of Anesthesiology, University of North Carolina at Chapel Hill School of Medicine, Chapel Hill, NC, USA

Mark J. Baskerville, MD JD MBA MA Department of Anesthesiology and Perioperative Medicine, School of Medicine, Oregon Health & Science University, Portland, OR, USA

James Berry, MD Department of Anesthesiology and Pain Management, UT Southwestern Medical Center, Dallas, TX, USA

Meena Bhatia, MD Department of Anesthesiology, University of North Carolina at Chapel Hill School of Medicine, Chapel Hill, NC, USA

Ali Bilal, MD Department of Internal Medicine, University of Texas Medical Branch, Galveston, TX, USA
John Sealy School of Medicine, University of Texas Medical Branch, Galveston, TX, USA

Nicholas V. Bishop, MD US Anesthesia Partners, Seattle, WA, USA
Department of Anesthesiology and Perioperative Medicine, School of Medicine, Health & Science University, Portland, OR, USA

Carol F. Bodenheimer, MD H. Ben Taub Department of Physical Medicine and Rehabilitation, Baylor College of Medicine, Houston, TX, USA
Spinal Cord Injury Care Line, Michael E. DeBakey VA Medical Center, Houston, TX, USA

Mark V. Boswell, MD PhD MBA Department of Anesthesiology, University of Toledo College of Medicine, Toledo, OH, USA

Denis L. Bourke, MD (Retired) Baltimore VA Medical Center, Baltimore, MD, USA
(Retired) Department of Anesthesiology, University of Maryland, Baltimore, MD, USA

John C. Briggs, MD MHSA Department of Anesthesiology and Perioperative Medicine, Heersink School of Medicine, University of Alabama at Birmingham, Birmingham, AL, USA

Amberly Hall Brown Austin Brown Music, Nashville, TN, USA

Austin Brown Austin Brown Music, Nashville, TN, USA

Marina Bueno, MLS (ASCP) SBB Department of Transfusion Medicine, Clinical Center, National Institutes of Health, Bethesda, MD, USA

Melissa Butynski, MEM PhD'28 Department of Biology, University of British Columbia, Kelowna, BC, Canada

Karen M. Byrne, MDE MT(ASCP)SBB (retired) Department of Transfusion Medicine, Clinical Center, National Institutes of Health, Bethesda, MD, USA

Michelle J. Capdeville, MD Department of Cardiothoracic Anesthesiology, Anesthesiology Institute, Cleveland Clinic, Cleveland Clinic Lerner College of Medicine, Case Western Reserve University, Cleveland, OH, USA

Christine Garcia Cattaneo, MD MBA Anne Arundel Medical Center, Annapolis, MD, USA
TeamHealth, Inc., Knoxville, TN, USA

Marlee Chamberlain, MD '26 School of Medicine, Oregon Health & Science University, Portland, OR, USA

Herbert Chen, MD Department of Surgery, O'Neal Comprehensive Cancer Center at UAB, Birmingham, AL, USA
Heersink School of Medicine, University of Alabama at Birmingham, Birmingham, AL, USA

Leonard N. Chen, MD PhD Department of Transfusion Medicine, Clinical Center, National Institutes of Health, Bethesda, MD, USA

Xiaopo Cheng, MS PhD Department of Chemical & Biologic Engineering, University of Wisconsin, Madison, WI, USA
Artificial Intelligence Technology, NVIDIA, Santa Clara, CA, USA

Anthony A. Chico III, DO FAPA Veterans Affairs Maryland Health Care System, Private Practice, Baltimore, VA, USA

Richard W. Childs, MD Commissioned Corps of the U.S. Public Health Service, Bethesda, MD, USA
Laboratory of Transplantation Immunotherapy, National Heart Lung and Blood Institute, National Institutes of Health, Bethesda, MD, USA

Katya H. Chiong, MD Department of Anesthesiology and Perioperative Medicine, University Hospitals Cleveland Medical Center, Case Western Reserve University School of Medicine, Cleveland, OH, USA

Robert J. Christian, MD Transfusion Medicine, Department of Pathology and Laboratory Medicine, School of Medicine, Oregon Health & Science University, Portland, OR, USA
Blood Baking/Transfusion Medicine, University of Washington/Bloodworks NW/ Seattle Children's Hospital, Seattle, WA, USA

Rose Christopherson, MD PhD Department of Anesthesiology, Portland VA Medical Center, Portland, OR, USA

Ariana S. Cogan, MT (ASCP)CM Department of Transfusion Medicine, Clinical Center, National Institutes of Health, Bethesda, MD, USA

Neal Cohen, MD MPH MS Anesthesia and Perioperative Medicine and Medicine, University of California, San Francisco School of Medicine, San Francisco, CA, USA

Norman A. Cohen, MD (Retired) Department of Anesthesiology and Perioperative Medicine, School of Medicine, Oregon Health & Science University, Portland, OR, USA
Committee on Late Career and Retired Members, American Society of Anesthesiologists, Portland, OR, USA

Daniel J. Cole, MD David Geffen School of Medicine at UCLA, Los Angeles, CA, USA
American Society of Anesthesiologists, Los Angeles, CA, USA

Christopher M. Conley, MD Boston University School of Medicine, Department of Anesthesiology, Boston Medical Center, Boston, MA, USA

Benjamin C. Conner, MD PhD Department of Physical Medicine and Rehabilitation, Spaulding Rehabilitation Hospital, Harvard Medical School, Boston, MA, USA

Hon. Christopher C. Conner Middle District of Pennsylvania, Harrisburg, PA, USA

Lois A. Connolly, MD Department of Anesthesiology, Medical College of Wisconsin/Froedtert Hospital, Milwaukee, WI, USA

Kathleen (Cathy) Conroy-Cantilena, MD Department of Transfusion Medicine, Clinical Center, National Institutes of Health, Bethesda, MD, USA
MedStar Washington Hospital Center, Washington, DC, USA
MTF Biologics, Edison, NJ, USA

Emma R. Cooley, BA Brand Experience Design Group, Charlotte, NC, USA

Catherine Cooper, MD Stony Point Endoscopy Center, Department of Anesthesiology, Virginia Commonwealth University School of Medicine, Richmond, VA, USA

Dane Coyne, MD Department of Anesthesiology and Perioperative Medicine, University Hospitals Cleveland Medical Center, Case Western Reserve University School of Medicine, Cleveland, OH, USA

Abigail J. Crawford, MD '28 School of Medicine, University of Washington, Seattle, WA, USA

Saundra E. Curry, MD Department of Anesthesiology, Columbia University Roy and Diana Vagelos College of Physicians and Surgeons, New York, NY, USA

Niloofer F. Dalal, MD Emory Clinic, School of Medicine Faculty, Emory Health Care, Atlanta, GA, USA

Edward J. Damrose, MD FACS Department of Otolaryngology - Head and Neck Surgery, Department of Anesthesiology, Perioperative and Pain Medicine, Stanford University School of Medicine, Stanford, CA, USA

David Daniel, MD Division of Transfusion Medicine, Department of Pathology, Johns Hopkins School of Medicine, Baltimore, MD, USA
Department of Transfusion Medicine, Clinical Center, National Institutes of Health, Bethesda, MD, USA

Beth Darnall, PhD Department of Anesthesiology, Perioperative and Pain Medicine, Stanford University School of Medicine School of Medicine, Stanford, CA, USA

Dawn Dillman, MD Department of Anesthesia, Carver College of Medicine, University of Iowa, Iowa City, IA, USA

David R. Dininny, MD Department of Anesthesiology and Perioperative Medicine, University Hospitals Cleveland Medical Center, Case Western Reserve University School of Medicine, Cleveland, OH, USA

Anis Dizdarevic, MD Department of Anesthesiology, Columbia University Roy and Diana Vagelos College of Physicians and Surgeons, New York, NY, USA

Sarah E. Dodd, MD Department of Anesthesiology and Perioperative Medicine, Mayo Clinic, Rochester, MN, USA

Karen B. Domino, MD MPH Department of Anesthesiology & Pain Medicine, University of Washington School of Medicine, Seattle, WA, USA

Susan D. Dumas, MD Obstetric Anesthesia Division, Department of Anesthesiology, Vanderbilt University Medical Center, Vanderbilt University, Nashville, TN, USA

Zeyd Ebrahim, MD Anesthesiology Institute, Cleveland Clinic, Cleveland Clinic Lerner College of Medicine, Case Western Reserve University, Cleveland, OH, USA

Charles W. Emala, Sr. MS MD Department of Anesthesiology, Columbia University Roy and Diana Vagelos College of Physicians and Surgeons, New York, NY, USA

Brenda G. Fahy, MD FCCP MCCM University of Florida College of Medicine, Gainesville, FL, USA

Joel M. Feinstein, MD University Hospitals, Heersink School of Medicine, University of Alabama at Birmingham, Birmingham, AL, USA

Brian C. Fitzsimons, MD Department of Anesthesiology and Perioperative Medicine, University Hospitals Cleveland Medical Center, Case Western Reserve University School of Medicine, Cleveland, OH, USA

Willy A. Flegel, MD Department of Transfusion Medicine Clinical Center, National Institutes of Health, Bethesda, MD, USA
Georgetown University Medical Center, Washington, DC, USA
Huazhong University of Science and Technology, Wuhan, Hubei, China

Lee A. Fleisher, MD Leonard Davis Institute for Health Economics, Department of Anesthesiology and Critical Care, Philadelphia, PA, USA
Department of Medicine, Perelman School of Medicine of the University of Pennsylvania, Philadelphia, PA, USA
Center for Clinical Standards and Quality, Center for Medicare and Medicaid Services, Baltimore, MD, USA

Patrick J. Forte, MD Department of Anesthesiology & Perioperative Medicine, University of Pittsburgh, Pittsburgh, PA, USA

Steven M. Frank, MD Johns Health System Blood Management Program, Center for Bloodless Medicine and Surgery, Department of Anesthesiology and Critical Care Medicine, Johns Hopkins School of Medicine, Baltimore, MD, USA

Sarah N. Fribance, MD Department of Anesthesiology and Perioperative Medicine, University of Pittsburgh School of Medicine, Pittsburgh, PA, USA

Daniel M. Frohwein, MD Interventional Pain Management, Orlando Orthopedic Center, Orlando, FL, USA

William R. Furman, MD MMHC (Retired) Department of Anesthesiology, Vanderbilt University Medical Center, Nashville, TN, USA
Physician Hospital Surveyor, The Joint Commission, Boston, MA, USA

Harley S. Geller, MD Senior Anesthesiologist, Charlotte, NC, USA

Deborah Gerson, MS CCC-SLP (Retired) Speech and Language Pathologist, Timonium, MD, USA

Brian T. Gierl, MD Neuroanesthesiology and Neuroanesthesiology QI, UPMC Presbyterian, Department of Anesthesiology & Perioperative Medicine, University of Pittsburgh School of Medicine, Pittsburgh, PA, USA

James K. Gilman, MD Office of the Director, Clinical Center, National Institutes of Health (Retired), Adjunct Professor of Medicine, Uniformed Services University of the Health Sciences, Bethesda, MD, USA

Allan Gottschalk, MD PhD Department of Anesthesiology and Critical Care Medicine, Department of Neurosurgery, Johns Hopkins School of Medicine, Baltimore, MD, USA

Chelsea L. Gottschalk, MD Lexington Eye Associates, Lexington, MA, USA

Laura M. Gottschalk, MSW MPH Health Promotions, American Lung Association, Chicago, IL, USA

Lindsey N. Gouker, MD Anesthesia Services Chatham Hospital, Department of Anesthesiology, The University of North Carolina at Chapel Hill School of Medicine, Chapel Hill, NC, USA

Raymond G. Graber, MD Department of Anesthesiology and Perioperative Medicine, University Hospitals Cleveland Medical Center, Case Western Reserve University School of Medicine, Cleveland, OH, USA

Michael D. Graham, PhD Department of Chemical and Biological Engineering, University of Wisconsin-Madison, Madison, WI, USA

Jeffrey A. Grass, MD MMM (retired) Department of Anesthesiology and Perioperative Medicine, University Hospitals Cleveland Medical Center, Case Western Reserve University School of Medicine, Cleveland, OH, USA

Ronald L. Harter, MD Department of Anesthesiology, Wexner Medical Center at The Ohio State University, American Society of Anesthesiologists, Columbus, OH, USA

Maya Jalbout Hastie, MD EdD Department of Anesthesiology, Columbia University Roy and Diana Vagelos College of Physicians and Surgeons, New York, NY, USA

Judith Hellman, MD Department of Anesthesia and Perioperative Care, University of California, San Francisco School of Medicine, San Francisco, CA, USA

Mada F. Helou, MD Department of Anesthesiology and Perioperative Medicine, University Hospitals Cleveland Medical Centerz, Cleveland, OH, USA

John Matthew Hess, BS Tessco Technologies, Inc., Hunt Valley, MD, USA

Jeremy C. Hoban, MD Department of Anesthesiology and Perioperative Medicine, University Hospitals Cleveland Medical Center, Case Western Reserve University School of Medicine, Cleveland, OH, USA

Vincent L. Hoellerich, MD Central Carolina Hospital, Sanford, NC, USA
Duke Health Community Division of Anesthesia, Raleigh, NC, USA

Jeffrey T. Hopcian, MD Department of Anesthesiology and Perioperative Medicine, University Hospitals Cleveland Medical Center, Case Western Reserve University School of Medicine, Cleveland, OH, USA

Harriet W. Hopf, MD Department of Anesthesiology, University of Utah, Salt Lake City, UT, USA
Member of the Board of Directors, Women in Anesthesiology, Salt Lake City, UT, USA

Theodore C. Houk, MD (Retired) St. Joseph's Hospital, University of Maryland Medical System, Towson, MD, USA

Mark E. Hudson, MD MBA Department of Anesthesiology and Perioperative Medicine, University of Pittsburgh School of Medicine, Pittsburgh, PA, USA

Conni Walkup Hull, JD Law Office of Conni L. Walkup, Columbia City, IN, USA

Michael P. Hutchens, MD MA Surgical Intensive Care Unit, Portland Veterans Administration Medical Center, Portland, OR, USA

Jane B. Jacobs, Esq Tarter Krinsky and Drogin LLP, New York, NY, USA

Jeremy Jaffe, MD SEPA Pain & Spine, Horsham, PA, USA

Richard A. Jaffe, MD PhD Department of Anesthesiology, Perioperative and Pain Medicine, Stanford University School of Medicine, Stanford, CA, USA

Randy G. Jensen, BS RJ Acres, Inc., Blair, NE, USA

Ruth A. Jensen, BS RJ Acres, Inc., Blair, NE, USA

Vesna Jevtovic-Todorovic, MD PhD MBA Department of Anesthesiology, School of Medicine, University of Colorado Anschutz Medical Campus, Aurora, CO, USA

Shawn Y. Jia, MD Department of Anesthesiology, The University of North Carolina at Chapel Hill School of Medicine, Chapel Hill, NC, USA

Deb Waterman Johns, BS Scout, Get Dressed, FIFI, Washington, DC, USA

Daniel M. Joseph, MD Emory Clinic, School of Medicine Faculty, Emory Health Care, Atlanta, GA, USA

Vilma A. Joseph, MD MPH FASA Department of Anesthesiology, The University Hospital of Albert Einstein College of Medicine, Montefiore Medical Center, New York, NY, USA

Tymoteusz J. Kajstura, MD PhD Cardiac Anesthesia Division, Department of Anesthesiology and Critical Care Medicine, Johns Hopkins School of Medicine, Baltimore, MD, USA

Shelley Sahu Kalsi, MD Hematology Graduate Medical Education and Consult Service Section, Division of Intramural Research, National Heart, Lung, and Blood Institute, National Institutes of Health, Bethesda, MD, USA

Inas Kamel, MD PhD Department of Anaesthesia and Intensive Care, Cairo University, Cairo, Egypt

Sharon T. Kapulek, MD Department of Anesthesiology, University of North Carolina at Chapel Hill School of Medicine, Chapel Hill, NC, USA

Patricia A. Kapur, MD Anesthesiology and Perioperative Medicine, David Geffen School of Medicine at UCLA, Los Angeles, CA, USA
Anesthesiology and Critical Care, Perelman School of Medicine, University of Pennsylvania, Philadelphia, PA, USA

Oliver Karam, MD PhD Department of Pediatrics, Yale School of Medicine – Yale University, New Haven, CT, USA
Pediatric Critical Care, Yale New Haven Children's Hospital, New Haven, CT, USA

Evan D. Kharasch, MD PhD Department of Anesthesiology, Duke University School of Medicine, Durham, NC, USA

Jeffrey R. Kirsch, MD FASA Department of Anesthesiology and Pain Medicine, University of Washington School of Medicine, Seattle, WA, USA
(Emeritus) Anesthesiology and Perioperative Medicine, School of Medicine, Oregon Health & Science University, Portland, OR, USA

Rachel Kirsch, MD Department of Anesthesia and Perioperative Care, University of California-San Francisco School of Medicine, San Francisco, CA, USA

Ziyad O. Knio, MD Division of Critical Care Medicine, Department of Anesthesiology, Columbia University Roy and Diana Vagelos College of Physicians and Surgeons, New York, NY, USA
Department of Anesthesiology, University of Virginia School of Medicine, Charlottesville, VA, USA

Lynn Knox, MD Department of Anesthesiology, John Sealy School of Medicine, The University of Texas Medical Branch, Galveston, TX, USA

Caroline C. Koloski, BA Velocity Clinical Research, Raleigh, NC, USA

LouAnn DePalma Kopenhaver, BS MEd (Retired) Capital Area Intermediate Unit, South Western School District, Hanover, PA, USA

Alexander S. Kuo, MD Department of Anesthesiology, Harvard Medical School, Massachusetts General Hospital, Boston, MA, USA

Julia K. Labovski, MD Department of Perioperative Medicine, Clinical Center, National Institutes of Health, Bethesda, MD, USA

Kirk Lalwani, MD FRCA MCR FASA Department of Anesthesiology and Perioperative Medicine, School of Medicine, Oregon Health & Science University, Portland, OR, USA

Meghan B. Lane-Fall, MD MSHP FCCM Department of Anesthesiology and Critical Care, Vagelos College of Physicians and Surgeons, Columbia University, New York, NY, USA

Stephen D. Lasday, DPM FACFAS Sarasota Memorial Hospital, Sarasota, FL, USA
West Coast Podiatry Center, Sarasota, FL, USA

Kathryn K. Lauer, MD Department of Anesthesiology, Medical College of Wisconsin/Froedtert Hospital, Milwaukee, WI, USA

Patricia Lee, DO JD Department of Transfusion Medicine, Clinical Center, National Institutes of Health, Bethesda, MD, USA

Sarah K. Lee, MD Department of Anesthesiology, Lewis Katz School of Medicine, Temple University, Philadelphia, PA, USA

Lisa Leffert, MD Department of Anesthesiology, Yale School of Medicine – Yale University, New Haven, CT, USA

Marc Leib, MD JD Healthcare Consultant, Phoenix, AZ, USA

Mark J. Lema, MD PhD Department of Anesthesiology, Roswell Park Comprehensive Cancer Center, SUNY Distinguished Service Professor and Chair, Jacobs School of Medicine & Biomedical Sciences, American Society of Regional Anesthesia, American Society of Anesthesiologists, Buffalo, NY, USA

Michael C. Lewis, MD FASA Department of Anesthesiology, Pain Management, & Perioperative Medicine, Henry Ford Hospital, Henry Ford Health System, Detroit, MI, USA

Albert Liao, LAc Liao Acupuncture, Towson, MD, USA

Kristin King Liao, LAc Liao Acupuncture, Towson, MD, USA

Olivia Liao, '28 Carnegie Mellon University, Pittsburgh, PA, USA

Cynthia A. Lien, MD Department of Anesthesiology, Medical College of Wisconsin/Froedtert Hospital, Milwaukee, WI, USA

Michael Lin, MD John Sealy School of Medicine, The University of Texas Medical Branch, Galveston, TX, USA

M. Concetta Lupa, MD Departments of Anesthesiology and Pediatrics, Department of Anesthesiology, The University of North Carolina at Chapel Hill School of Medicine, Chapel Hill, NC, USA

Yafet T. Mamo, MD Department of Transfusion Medicine, Clinical Center, National Institutes of Health, Bethesda, MD, USA

Andrew Mannes, MD ME MBA Department of Perioperative Medicine, Clinical Center, National Institutes of Health, Bethesda, MD, USA

Asad Mansoor, MD Department of Anesthesiology, University of Michigan Medical School, Ann Arbor, MI, USA

Catherine Marcucci, MD Department of Transfusion Medicine, Clinical Center, National Institutes of Health, Bethesda, MD, USA

Daniel J. Marcucci, PhD MLA AICP Center for Leadership in Global Sustainability, Virginia Polytechnic Institute and State University, Blacksburg, VA, USA

David P. Martin, MD PhD Department of Anesthesiology and Perioperative Medicine, Mayo Clinic, Rochester, MN, USA

David C. Mayer, MD Department of Anesthesiology, Department of Obstetrics and Gynecology, University of North Carolina at Chapel Hill School of Medicine, North Carolina Society of Anesthesiologists, Chapel Hill, NC, USA

Daniel J. McCoy, MD'26 The University of Arizona College of Medicine – Phoenix, Phoenix, AZ, USA

K. A. Kelly McQueen, MD MPH FASA Department of Anesthesiology, University of Wisconsin School of Medicine and Public Health, Madison, WI, USA

Rita B. Merman, MD Department of Anesthesiology and Perioperative Medicine, University Hospitals Cleveland Medical Center, Case Western Reserve University School of Medicine, Cleveland, OH, USA

Jay Mesrobian, MD MBA FASA TeamHealth Anesthesia, Milwaukee, WI, USA

Berend Mets, MB ChB PhD FRCA FFA(SA) Department of Anesthesiology and Perioperative Medicine, Penn State College of Medicine, Penn State Milton S. Hershey Medical Center, Hershey, PA, USA

Carolyn B. Metzler, PhD Senior Mathematician and Analyst, Gaithersburg, MD, USA

Lucas Meuchel, MD PhD Department of Anesthesiology and Perioperative Medicine, School of Medicine, Oregon Health & Science University, Portland, OR, USA

Frederick G. Mihm, MD Division of Critical Care Medicine, Department of Anesthesiology, Perioperative and Pain Medicine (Critical Care), Stanford University School of Medicine, Stanford, CA, USA

Sharon L. Milgram, PhD National Institutes of Health, Bethesda, MD, USA

Robert E. Minahan, MD Real Time Neuromonitoring Associates, Glen Burnie, MD, USA

Scott D. Mist, PhD LAc Department of Anesthesiology and Perioperative Medicine, School of Medicine, College of Nursing, Oregon Health & Science University, Portland, OR, USA

Sharif Mohamed, MD Department of Anesthesiology, John Sealy School of Medicine, The University of Texas Medical Branch, Galveston, TX, USA

Hanan Mohamed Mostafa, MD Anesthesia, Surgical Intensive Care, Pain Medicine, Kasr AlAiny School of Medicine, Cairo University, Cairo, Egypt

Ahmed Mukhtar, MD PhD Department of Anaesthesia and Intensive Care, Cairo University, Cairo, Egypt

Bryant A. Murphy, MD, MBAFASA Department of Anesthesiology, The University of North Carolina at Chapel Hill School of Medicine, Chapel Hill, NC, USA

Rajen V. Nathwani, MBBS BSc Department of Anesthesiology and Pain Medicine, University of Washington School of Medicine, Harborview Medical Center, Seattle, WA, USA

Mark Nelson, MD MEd Department of Anesthesiology, Virginia Commonwealth University School of Medicine, Richmond, VA, USA

David J. Ninan, DO FAOCA CPE Kansas College of Osteopathic Medicine, Wichita, KS, USA
Department of Anesthesiology, Riverside University Health System, Western University of Health Sciences, Pomona, CA, USA

Matthew P. Norcia, MD Department of Anesthesiology and Perioperative Medicine, University Hospitals Cleveland Medical Center, Case Western Reserve University School of Medicine, Cleveland, OH, USA

Mark C. Norris, MD Boston University School of Medicine, Boston Medical Center, Boston, MA, USA

Logan M. Olson, PharmD BCCCP PGY2 Critical Care, Nebraska Medical Center, Nebraska Medicine, Omaha, NE, USA

Steven L. Orebaugh, MD Department of Anesthesiology & Perioperative Medicine, University of Pittsburgh School of Medicine, Pittsburgh, PA, USA

Maria K. Orlic, MD Department of Anesthesiology and Perioperative Medicine, School of Medicine and Dentistry, University of Rochester Medicine, Rochester, NY, USA

Kelsey Peterson Ostergren, MPH CIC Health Policy Initiatives, Michigan Health & Hospital Association, Okemos, MI, USA

Anthony N. Passannante, MD Department of Anesthesiology, UNC School of Medicine, University of North Carolina at Chapel Hill School of Medicine, Chapel Hill, NC, USA

Alejandra Pelayo, BS National Institutes of Health, Bethesda, MD, USA

Marc P. Pelletier, MD Division Chief of Cardiac Surgery, Yale School of Medicine, New Haven, CT, USA

Nicholas L. Pesa, MD Department of Anesthesiology and Perioperative Medicine, University Hospitals Cleveland Medical Center, Case Western Reserve University School of Medicine, Cleveland, OH, USA

Linda M. Peterson, MD FAPM McLaren Greater Lansing Hospital, Lansing, MI, USA

Kailey L. Peterson Kohler Company, Kohler, WI, USA

William P. Peterson, MD Cardiac, Thoracic, and Vascular Anesthesia, University of Michigan Health, Sparrow Health System, Lansing, MI, USA

Emily T. Poynton, MD Department of Anesthesiology and Perioperative Medicine, University Hospitals Cleveland Medical Center, Case Western Reserve University School of Medicine, Cleveland, OH, USA

Donald S. Prough, MD Department of Anesthesiology, John Sealy School of Medicine, The University of Texas Medical Branch, Galveston, TX, USA

Marcelo J. Quezado, MD MedStar Medical Group Anesthesiology, Medstar Union Memorial Hospital, Baltimore, MD, USA

Herleen Rai, MD Division of Transfusion Medicine, Department of Pathology, Clinical Pathology Residency, The Johns Hopkins School of Medicine, Baltimore, MD, USA

Michael A. Ramsay, MD FRCA Department of Anesthesiology and Pain Management, Baylor University Medical Center, Dallas, TX, USA

Mojica Remskar, MD PhD MACM Department of Anesthesiology, University of Minnesota Medical School, Minneapolis, MN, USA

Emily C. Rhinehart, BS Pre-Medical Candidate, Fallston, MD, USA

LeeAnn Rhodes, MD Pain Medicine Interventionalist (Anesthesiology), Maryland Brain, Spine and Pain, Annapolis, MD, USA

Amy J. Robbins, MD MBA Stanson Health, a Premier Inc. Company, Atrium Health, Carolinas Palliative Care and Hospice Group, Charlotte, NC, USA
Atrium Health, Carolinas Palliative Care and Hospice Group, Charlotte, NC, USA

Wendye Robbins, MD Incendia Therapeutics, Boston, MA, USA
Blade Therapeutics, Inc., South San Francisco, CA, USA

W. Mitchell Robbins, BS MS Pilot and Airline Captain, Ponte Verda, FL, USA

John S. Rogoski, DO Department of Anesthesiology, College of Medicine, Wexner Medical Center, The Ohio State University, Columbus, OH, USA

Matthew L. Rorie, BS RJ Acres, Inc., Blair, NE, USA

Richard W. Rosenquist, MD Department of Pain Management, Anesthesiology Institute, Cleveland Clinic, Cleveland Clinic Lerner College of Medicine, Case Western Reserve University, Cleveland, OH, USA

Frank Rosinia, MD MHCM Department of Anesthesiology, Joe R. & Teresa Lozano Long School of Medicine, UT Health San Antonio, San Antonio, TX, USA

Charles H. Sandson, BS ZS Associates, Washington, DC, USA

Lisa L. Sandson, BArch Cummings Properties, LLC, Woburn, MA, USA

Neil B. Sandson, MD Department of Psychiatry, University of Maryland School of Medicine, Baltimore, MD, USA
VA Maryland Health Care System, Baltimore, MD, USA

H. David Sanusi, MD Physician Specialists in Anesthesia, PC, Atlanta, GA, USA

Joseph M. Schwartz, MD Senior Psychiatrist, Baltimore, MD, USA

F. Jacob Seagull, PhD Center for Bioethics and Social Science in Medicine, Michigan Medicine (University of Michigan Medical School), Ann Arbor, MI, USA

Troy G. Seelhammer, MD Department of Anesthesiology and Perioperative Medicine, Mayo Clinic, Rochester, MN, USA

Daniel I. Sessler, MD Department of Anesthesiology, Center of Outcomes Research, UTHealth, Houston, TX, USA

Ahmed Shash, MD Department of Anaesthesia and Intensive Care, Cairo University, Cairo, Egypt

Richard G. Sheffield, BS IM MA (Retired) Blog – Spend Your Retirement Money!, UPS.com, Atlanta, GA, USA

Kenneth T. Shelton, MD Division of Critical Care, Department of Anesthesia, Critical Care and Pain Medicine, Heart Center, ICU, Harvard Medical School, Massachusetts General Hosptial, Boston, MD, USA

Cobin Soelberg, MD JD Master of Bioethics Bend Anesthesiology Group, Bend, OR, USA

Linda H. Song, MD MPH MD Anderson Cancer Center, Houston, TX, USA
Department of Transfusion Medicine, Clinical Center, National Institutes of Health, Bethesda, MD, USA

Ziyan Song, MD Division of Cardiothoracic Anesthesiology, Division of Perioperative Medicine, Department of Anesthesiology, Adult Cardiothoracic Anesthesia, Heersink School of Medicine, University of Alabama – Birmingham, Birmingham, AL, USA

Valentina Baez Sosa, MD National Heart Lung Blood Institute, Bethesda, MD, USA
Department of Transfusion Medicine, Clinical Center, National Institutes of Health, Bethesda, MD, USA

Juraj Sprung, MD PhD Department of Anesthesiology and Perioperative Medicine, Mayo Clinic, Rochester, MN, USA

Joshua L. Stich, MD '28 Albert Einstein College of Medicine, New York, NY, USA

M. Christine Stock, MD FCCM FCCP Department of Anesthesiology, Northwestern University Feinberg School of Medicine, Chicago, IL, USA

Louise Y. Sun, MD Cardiac Anesthesiology, University Medical Line, Anesthesiology, Perioperative, and Pain Medicine, Stanford University School of Medicine, Stanford, CA, USA
Institute for Clinical Evaluative Sciences, Toronto, ON, Canada

Christopher E. Swide, MD Department of Anesthesiology and Perioperative Medicine, School of Medicine, Health & Science University, Portland, OR, USA

Edwin Tavarez, MD Department of Anesthesiology, Montefiore Medical Center, The University Hospital of Albert Einstein College of Medicine, New York, NY, USA

Grant Taylor, MD Wellstar Douglas Surgical Associates, Douglasville, GA, USA

Nicholas B. Taylor, MD General Surgery Residency Program, Jefferson Abingdon Hospital, Abingdon, PA, USA

Zachary R. Taylor, BS Chemist, Philadelphia, PA, USA

Megan E. Terek, MD Cardiac Intensive Care Unit, INOVA Fairfax Hospital, Falls Church, VA, USA

Michael M. Todd, MD Department of Anesthesiology, University of Minnesota School of Medicine, Minneapolis, MN, USA

Brandon M. Togioka, MD Department of Anesthesiology and Perioperative Medicine, School of Medicine, Oregon Health & Science University, Portland, OR, USA

Patricia M. Togioka, MA (Retired) Oregon School for the Deaf, Certified Interpreter for the Deaf and Hard of Hearing, Salem, OR, USA

Robert D. Togioka, MA (Retired) Oregon School for the Deaf, Certified Interpreter for the Deaf and Hard of Hearing, Salem, OR, USA
American Sign Language, Salem-Keizer School District, Keizer, OR, USA

Jennifer N. Tripi, MD Obstetric Anesthesiology, The University of North Carolina at Chapel Hill School of Medicine, Chapel Hill, NC, USA

Paul A. Tripi, MD Department of Anesthesiology and Perioperative Medicine, Division of Pediatric Anesthesiology, Rainbow Babies & Children's Hospital, Case Western Reserve University School of Medicine, University Hospitals Cleveland Medical Center, Case Western Reserve University, Cleveland, OH, USA

Christopher A. Troianos, MD FASE FASA Anesthesiology Institute, Cleveland Clinic, Cleveland Clinic Lerner College of Medicine, Case Western Reserve University, Cleveland, OH, USA

Tsung-Lin Tsai, MD PhD Bloodworks NW, Seattle, WA, USA
Department of Transfusion Medicine, Clinical Center, National Institutes of Health, Bethesda, MD, USA

Elizabeth A. Ungerman, MD MS Anesthesiology Residency Program, Department of Anesthesiology & Perioperative Medicine, University of Pittsburgh School of Medicine, Pittsburgh, PA, USA

Kamila Vagnerova, MD Department of Anesthesiology and Perioperative Medicine, School of Medicine, Oregon Health & Science University, Portland, OR, USA

Brant M. Wagener, MD PhD Division of Critical Care Medicine, Division of Molecular and Translational Biomedicine, Birmingham, AL, USA
Department of Anesthesiology and Perioperative Medicine, Heersink School of Medicine, The University of at Birmingham, Birmingham, AL, USA

Joanna L. Walker, MD Clinical Dermatology, Rare and Advanced Skin Cancer Clinic, Perelman School of Medicine, University of Pennsylvania, Philadelphia, PA, USA

John R. Walker IV Drexel University, Philadelphia, PA, USA

Marilyn X. Walker, BS Sigurdsson Laboratory, NYU Langone, New York, NY, USA

David A. Wallace, MD Department of Anesthesiology and Perioperative Medicine, University Hospitals Cleveland Medical Center, Case Western Reserve University School of Medicine, Cleveland, OH, USA

Jenny Wang, MD MBA VA Maryland Health Care System, Baltimore, MD, USA

Jonathan H. Waters, MD Department of Anesthesiology & Perioperative Medicine, University of Pittsburgh School of Medicine, Pittsburgh, PA, USA
Blood Management Program, University of Pittsburgh Medical Center (UPMC), Pittsburgh, PA, USA

Anesthesia Services, Magee Women's Hospital of UPMC, Pittsburgh, PA, USA
Department of Bioengineering, Swanson School of Engineering, University of Pittsburgh, Pittsburgh, PA, USA

Toby N. Weingarten, MD Department of Anesthesiology and Perioperative Medicine, Mayo Clinic, Rochester, MN, USA

Ronald H. Wender, MD Department of Anesthesiology, Cedars-Sinai Medical Center, Los Angeles, CA, USA

Kamille A. West-Mitchell, MD Blood Services Section, Department of Transfusion Medicine, Clinical Center,National Institutes of Health, Bethesda, MD, USA

Charles Whitten, MD Department of Anesthesiology and Pain Management, University of Texas Southwestern Medical Center, Dallas, TX, USA

Jeanine Wiener-Kronish, MD Harvard Medical School, Massachusetts General Hospital, Boston, MA, USA

Hon. Jennifer P. Wilson Middle District of Pennsylvania, Harrisburg, PA, USA

Bradford D. Winters, MD PhD FCCM Adult Critical Care Medicine, Department of Anesthesiology and Critical Care Medicine, Johns Hopkins Hospital Surgical ICUs, Bayview Medical Center Surgical and Burn ICUs, Baltimore, MD, USA
The Armstrong Institute for Patient Safety and Quality, Baltimore, MD, USA
RESQ Committee for Johns Hopkins Hospital, Baltimore, MD, USA
Johns Hopkins School of Medicine, Baltimore, MD, USA

Susan Wong, BS Office of Scientific Resources, Office of Research Services, National Institutes of Health, Bethesda, MD, USA
Friends of Rabbits, Columbia, MD, USA

Lee C. Woodson, MD PhD Department of Anesthesiology, John Sealy School of Medicine, University of Texas Medical Branch, Galveston, TX, USA

Charles J. Yeo, MD FACS Department of Surgery, Sidney Kimmel Medical College, Enterprise Surgery, Jefferson Health, Philadelphia, PA, USA
Pancreas, Biliary, and Related Cancer Center, Thomas Jefferson University, Philadelphia, PA, USA

David A. Young, MD MEd MBA FASA Department of Anesthesiology, Baylor College of Medicine, Texas Children's Hospital, Houston, TX, USA

Jordan S. Zunder, BSC MSC BMBS FRCPC University of Ottawa, Ottawa, ON, Canada
Department of Anesthesiology and Pain Medicine, The Ottawa Hospital, Ottawa, ON, Canada

Department of Anesthesiology and Pain Medicine, University of Washington School of Medicine, Harborview Medical Center, Seattle, WA, USA

David A. Zvara, MD FASA FAHA (Emeritus) Department of Anesthesiology, The University of North Carolina at Chapel Hill School of Medicine, Chapel Hill, NC, USA

Jessica Zvara, MD Vascular Anesthesia Division, Department of Anesthesiology, University of Virginia School of Medicine, Charlottesville, VA, USA

Part I

Communication

The Cooper River Bridge—Charleston, SC

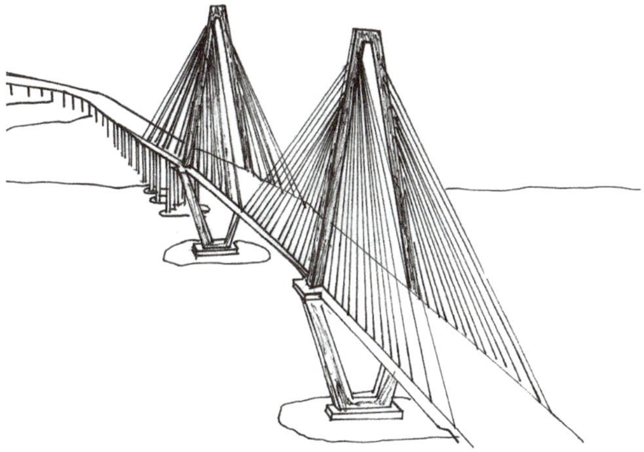

The Arthur Ravenel Jr. Bridge, also known as the Cooper River Bridge, is a cable-stayed bridge over the Cooper River in South Carolina, connecting Charleston to Mount Pleasant. It is one of editor **Amy Robbins'** favorite bridges.

The bridge has a total length of 13,200 ft, a main span of 1546 ft, and height of 575 ft. It was completed in 2005. The bridge structure is designed to withstand shipping accidents and the natural disasters that have historically plagued the Charleston area. The span is designed to endure wind gusts in excess of 300 mph, and to withstand an earthquake of approximately 7.4 on the Richter scale without total failure. The towers are flanked by one-acre rock islands to protect from errant ship collisions. The roadway consists of eight 12-ft lanes, four in each direction plus a 12-ft bicycle and pedestrian path, which overlooks the Charleston Harbor and the Atlantic Ocean.

Amy and the editors of *Anesthesia Bridges* thank **David Howe** from The Architectural Team in Boston, MA, for his wonderful drawing showing the strong yet elegant design of the bridge.

1 Introduction

Catherine Marcucci

We don't live in bubbles. We live and work in communities of families, neighbors, and co-workers. One of the things that will determine how successful we will be in our personal lives and careers is how well we can communicate. Communication is such a broad concept—it's not just what you say, but how you say it, when you say it, and why you say it. Communication is spoken and written, and nowadays often "observed" because includes all kinds of social media avenues that we couldn't imagine when our careers started out. If you can't get your points across successfully, your ability to lead and advance your career will be compromised.

In this section, we present a mix of chapters on both verbal and written communication. We are reminded of the importance of listening, of knowing names, of paying attention to your body language, of tailoring your message appropriately to the audience you are trying to reach, and of not responding in anger in times of conflict. You will also read about writing styles, writing letters, and being open to writing about things that occur in the day-to-day practice of anesthesiology. We hope that our authors have provided our readers with some food for thought in these areas. There truly is magic everywhere.

Author

Cathy Marcucci is a senior academic anesthesiologist and inveterate anesthesiology educator. She is also fellowship-trained in transfusion medicine. When not taking care of patients and/or putting the latest book together, she dedicates her time to mentoring junior colleagues, writing copy for animal rescues, and travel.

C. Marcucci (✉)
Department of Transfusion Medicine, Clinical Center, National Institutes of Health, Bethesda, MD, USA

S. Mohamed et al. (eds.), *Anesthesia Bridges*, https://doi.org/10.1007/978-3-032-08294-7_1

Bridges as Inspiration and Metaphor

2

Rachel Kirsch and Michael S. Axley

Mistakes are the usual bridge between inexperience and wisdom.
—Phyllis Grissim-Theroux

Introduction

In a very literal sense, bridges are the groundwork of prior generations that allow for future generations to progress. At times, we may not even notice these bridges, especially when they become familiar, yet we would instantly notice if a well-used bridge were gone. When that happens, we must start over, rebuilding the infrastructure that had already been painstakingly built by our predecessors and rebuilding our forward momentum. We are fortunate to have these bridges at our disposal, yet we must take the time ourselves to learn how to craft these pathways, if we are to prevent mistakes that lead to collapse.

Arkadiko Bridge and Roman Arched Bridges

Consider one of the oldest arched bridges: Arkadiko Bridge, located in Southern Greece (Figs. 2.1 and 2.2). This bridge was built an estimated 3300 years ago and is still in use today. For thousands of years, this bridge has supported progress and connections, a process that continues to this day. Imagine the millions of people who must have crossed over this bridge, all thanks to the ingenuity and knowledge of this long-past group of builders. The architects of this span likely experienced many collapsed attempts before the sturdy stone structure supported the chariots for which it was built.

Through many generations, the craft of arched bridges was eventually perfected by the Roman Empire, who unlocked the secrets of the keystone—a single central stone in an arch that allows for the distribution of weight through every stone, making the sum far stronger than the individual. A bridge made of the strongest granite would crumble without its central keystone, yet a single stone can produce a struc-

R. Kirsch
Department of Anesthesia and Perioperative Care, University of California-San Francisco School of Medicine, San Francisco, CA, USA

M. S. Axley (✉)
Oregon Anesthesiology Group, Portland, OR, USA

S. Mohamed et al. (eds.), *Anesthesia Bridges*, https://doi.org/10.1007/978-3-032-08294-7_2

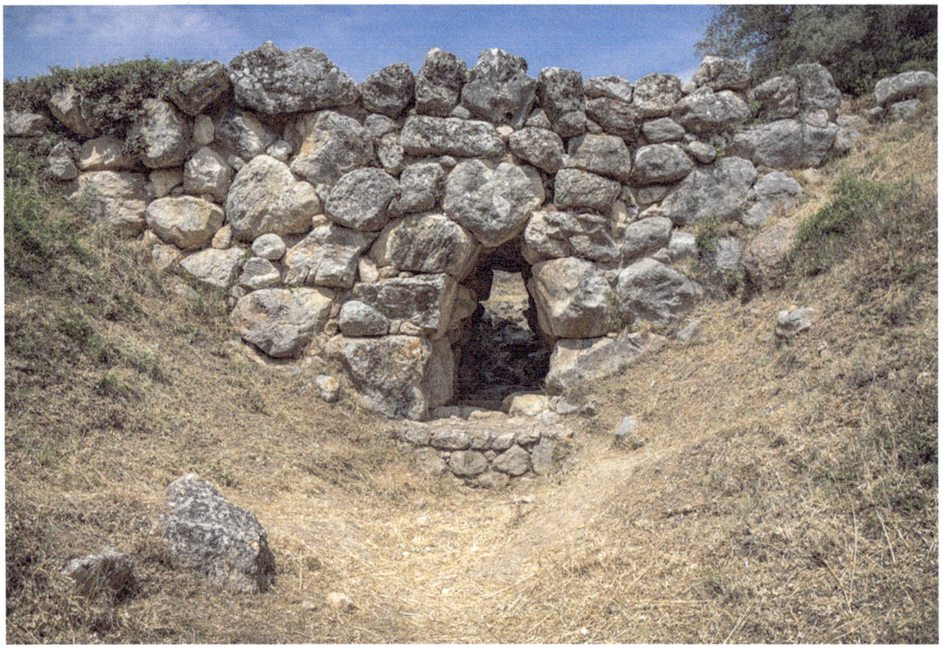

Fig. 2.1 The Arkadiko Bridge—a Mycenaean corbel arch bridge in Greece. Not the most beautiful or graceful bridge, but one of the oldest bridges in the world, still in use and the oldest stone arch bridge in Europe. It was originally one of four bridges in a road network between two Bronze Age towns. Photo: Image used under standard license from stock.adobe.com

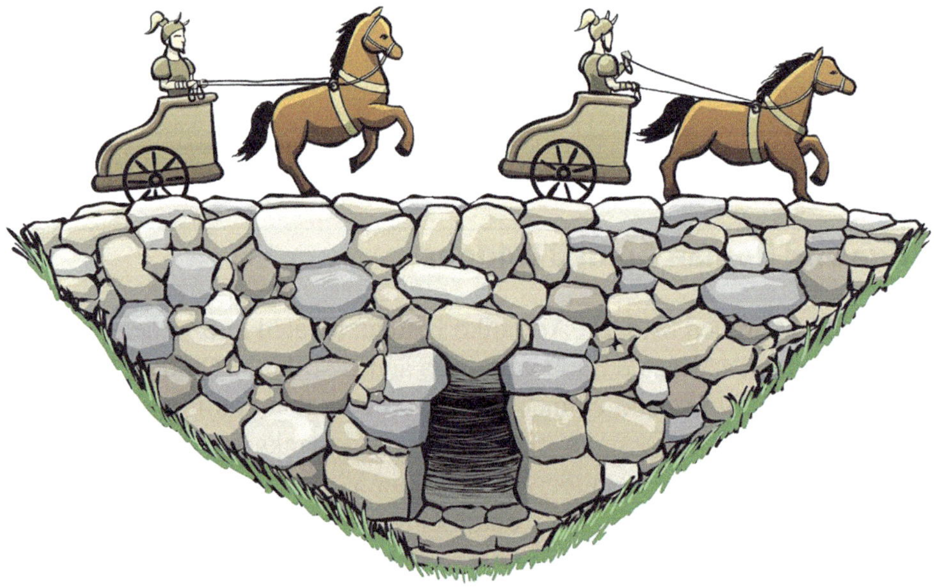

Fig. 2.2 The Arkadiko Bridge was used for carts, commerce, chariots, and other military equipment 3300 years ago. It is still intact and strong enough for car traffic. Wild to think about, isn't it? Illustration: Luke Graber

ture that stands for millennia. With the keystone-anchored bridge at their disposal, the Romans launched a civilization that would remain a dominant force for many generations.

We Depend on the Knowledge Base Built by Others

There are numerous bridges in our profession that have been constructed, stone by stone, through experience, and at the center of each bridge sits the anesthesiologist as the keystone. While they remain in the field, younger generations of anesthesiologists utilize their experience to make decisions and care for patients. Yet as many older anesthesiologists leave, they take their keystones with them, and their bridges will collapse in the wake of their departure if the younger generation has not learned from their experiences. It is vital that we preserve these passages and tap into this wealth of knowledge that will soon be lost. Without this preservation, each generation is compelled to rebuild, repeating past errors and struggling to forge pathways that had previously been established.

Though technology and medicine are evolving rapidly, these advances are always built on a foundation of knowledge laid by the physicians and innovators of generations past. How could anyone build a ventilator if they first had to rediscover electricity? It is equally important to build new experiences upon the foundation of the errors and triumphs of those who came before us. Preserving these stories—reinforcing these keystones—will allow each generation to propel confidently forward and reach destinations yet unknown.

Lessons Learned

- Civilizations could not and would not have progressed without bridges. It is astonishing that there are any bridges left from antiquity, but there are.
- Bridges can serve as a metaphor for just about everything in life, professional and otherwise.

Authors

Rachel Kirsch began her career as an anesthesia technician in her hometown of Chicago at Northwestern Memorial Hospital. She moved to Chapel Hill, NC, with her husband, Alan, and eventually started medical school at the University of North Carolina. She has seen the field of anesthesiology as a technician, as a patient, as a medical student, and now as a resident in anesthesiology. She is excited to begin this new chapter as an anesthesia provider and experience yet another side of a field that has captivated her so thoroughly. She resides in the San Francisco area with her family.

Mike Axley worked as an investigative journalist for a variety of news outlets in Oregon for the first part of his career, and then went east for medical school at Cornell. After medical school, he spent a year earning his master's degree at the graduate journalism school of Columbia University, then headed back to Oregon. As an anesthesiologist, he enjoyed the academic life at Oregon Health & Science University for ten years before joining the staff of the Providence St. Vincent anesthesiology group, where he is now chair of the department. He lives in southwest Portland with his partner Kim and their three children and enjoys some of Oregon's great recreational opportunities—fishing, golfing, and skiing.

3 Communication Basics!

Emma R. Cooley and Michael S. Axley

Introduction

It's often said to young professionals that it's not what you know but who you know. But really, the value lies in *how* you communicate *what* you know to *who* you know. Communication is not just about sending out information. It's the way in which that information is conveyed and understood. Being able to communicate effectively is an essential skill for every area of your life, both personal and professional. It is key to building successful relationships and core to how you present yourself to the world. Commit to being a strong communicator, and you will not only enable your interpersonal relationships to thrive but equip yourself with the power to shape how others perceive you.

Your Personal Reputation Starts with Communication

How you portray yourself to others, or your "personal brand," is more important now than ever before. Technology has taken away many of the face-to-face conversations that teach people to interact with one another in real life. Meaning is lost in a constant overload of information, making it imperative for you to take thoughtful and purposeful steps to close that gap when communicating in person.

Though just a single one-on-one conversation may seem insignificant, people will naturally develop impressions based on these small moments, and so these individual interactions form a larger experience that directly impacts how they remember you when you walk away. You may offer the same service as your peers, but if you can carefully manage how you communicate and how you make others feel, you will stand out and draw people in. Evolving your communication style and defining your personal brand take effort and intention. It's constant work in progress but lay the foundation early and you will only grow and improve over time.

E. R. Cooley
Brand Experience Design Group, New York, NY, USA

M. S. Axley (✉)
Oregon Anesthesiology Group, Portland, OR, USA

S. Mohamed et al. (eds.), *Anesthesia Bridges*, https://doi.org/10.1007/978-3-032-08294-7_3

1. **Be authentic.** Differences make us human. Staying true to yourself and embracing your quirks will make you more relatable and genuine. People can sense if you are putting on a show or faking it. When first meeting someone, ask their name and then use it immediately and repeatedly, but naturally. This quickly establishes sincerity and mutual understanding, which earns others' trust.

2. **Be confident.** If you are confident in what you are saying, people are more likely to listen to you and believe you. Look people straight in the eye and speak with a strong, steady voice.

3. **Be direct.** Clarity and concision are central to avoiding misunderstanding. Be straightforward and transparent. Don't beat around the bush. Filling your message with unnecessary information will only make room for confusion.

4. **Be consistent.** Convey the same uniform message through your words, your tone, and your body language. If your facial expression does not match what you are saying, you may come off as dishonest. If you act like a completely different person in various situations, people will be wary of who you really are.

5. **Be flexible.** Adapt to your environment. Know your audience and put yourself in their shoes. Read the room and tailor your language accordingly to ensure your message is understood. If you are shaking someone's hand, stand up. If you are initiating a serious conversation, sit down with the other person.

6. **Be respectful.** From the moment you enter a room to the time you exit, be polite and considerate. Especially as a young adult, displaying respect toward others will help you gain theirs in return. Knock before opening a closed door. Never check your phone during a conversation. Even if you are the expert in the situation, be receptive to the ideas and input of others.

7. **Be attentive.** Listen more than you speak. Take notes if you need. Do not interrupt. Wait for people to finish what they're saying but insert "hmmm" and "okay" when appropriate to signal you are listening. Active listening makes the other person feel heard and gives you a deeper understanding of them.

8. **Be engaged.** Focus completely on the other person. Multitasking will cause you to miss essential verbal and nonverbal cues. Ask questions. Being inquisitive is the easiest way to get people to open up and shows you are interested and paying attention. Summarize your takeaways before leaving the conversation and confirm it is correct, so all parties are on the same page.

9. **Be patient.** Think before you speak and speak slowly (slower than what feels natural). You may need to repeat things. Even if you are in a rush, take the time to check that your message has been received.

10. **Be positive.** Smile. Regardless of what else is going on, set those emotions aside when you enter a new conversation. Maintain a pleasant demeanor, even if you disagree or do not like what you're hearing. Your attitude can heavily influence the other party. If you speak calmly and gently to someone who is stressed or anxious, it will instill in them a sense of peace.

Life Lessons

- Small moments count when people communicate, they truly do. Especially when those communications are face-to-face.
- Your communication style should reflect who you really are but is also worth working at.
- The editors agree with all ten of the authors' points above! To us, prime among these equal factors are to be authentic, be respectful, and be positive.

Authors

Emma Cooley grew up in Charlotte, NC, and studied communication and studio art at Wake Forest University. She is actively involved in animal rescue organizations, fostering kittens, and rehoming cats with special needs. She works as a strategist for a national branding agency, and when not busy planning a new design project, Emma enjoys spending time with her own rescue cat, exploring new places, and keeping active with yoga and running.

Mike Axley worked as an investigative journalist for a variety of news outlets in Oregon for the first part of his career and then went east for medical school at Cornell. After medical school, he spent a year earning his master's degree at the Graduate Journalism School of Columbia University, then headed back to Oregon. As an anesthesiologist, he enjoyed the academic life at Oregon Health & Science University for ten years before joining the staff of the Providence St. Vincent anesthesiology group, where he is now chair of the department. He lives in southwest Portland with his partner Kim and their three children and enjoys some of Oregon's great recreational opportunities—fishing, golfing, and skiing.

Names Matter

4

Amr E. Abouleish

Introduction

My name is not the usual American name. It's not easy to pronounce by simply looking at the spelling. So, I try to introduce myself to my co-workers. In return, I want to also address my co-workers by their name. In order to do this on a regular basis, first, I am willing to say, "I'm sorry, I know we have met, but please tell me again your name." I'm not embarrassed since I want to know their name. If I call someone by the wrong name, my response is, "I don't even call my own children by the right name the first time!"

"Anesthesia" Is Not a Name!

This issue with names has also come up when a surgeon refers to me or my team as "anesthesia." We have a name! Similarly, I will never call a radiology technician "Xray" or a respiratory therapist "respiratory." I ask them for their name first. This modus operandi of always wanting to know someone's name before asking for something became famous among the ICU nurses when I was a resident. My rule was that I would not give a verbal order if I did not know the nurse's name. So, the nurses figured out that if I was moving too fast in managing a patient in the ICU, they just stopped telling me their name, especially a new nurse that I had not worked with before! I had to wait till they were ready for the next order and willing to tell me their name.

Names are important. And acknowledging everyone is also important. My first jobs in healthcare were summer jobs during college. I was first a phlebotomist, and then the next summer I was a physical therapy aide (basically a transportation person). I saw firsthand how some physicians did not see those around them. This was in stark difference to when I visited my father at the hospital. My late father was an academic obstetrical anesthesiologist. I remember going to work with him, and as he walked into the hospital and labor and delivery, and I distinctly remember that he said hello to everyone—from the man mopping the floor, to the unit secretary, to the nurses. Even when we went to the cafeteria, the workers there knew him because he always greeted them.

A. E. Abouleish (✉)
Department of Anesthesiology, The University of Texas Medical Branch, Galveston, TX, USA
e-mail: aaboulei@UTMB.EDU

S. Mohamed et al. (eds.), *Anesthesia Bridges*, https://doi.org/10.1007/978-3-032-08294-7_4

The final reason why I try to learn everyone's name is to acknowledge that my success as a physician is a team effort. I cannot do what I do and provide the best care to my patients without the contribution of everyone.

Lessons Learned

- Co-workers appreciate being known by name.
- When you know people by name, it enhances team building and comradery.

Author

Amr Abouleish joined UTMB Galveston in 1993 as the first chief of pediatric anesthesiology. He has simplified the pronunciation of his name for Americans to "Ahm" since the "A" when pronounced in his first language is a vowel not found in English. His mentor professionally and in life is his late father, Ezzat Abouleish MD, who was a well-known academic obstetric anesthesiologist. Please see Chap. 5 for more about the senior Dr. Abouleish.

The Esteemed Dr. Ezzat Abouleish

5

Raymond G. Graber and Catherine Marcucci

Contributor:

Amr. E. Abouleish, MD MBA

Introduction

In the previous chapter, **Amr Abouleish** mentions his late father, Ezzat Abouleish MD (1931–2014), and his dad's amazing ability to connect with people. The senior Dr. Abouleish also possessed an innate sense of humility and humanity. He worked with many of the leading figures in anesthesiology, such as Sir Robert Macintosh, but never stopped learning. He is one of the people who inspired this project, and we thought our readers would like to know a bit more about him—the examples he set and the bridges he built for his family and the specialty of anesthesiology, especially the field of obstetric anesthesiology.

Early Years

Ezzat was born in Egypt and received his medical degree from Ain Shams University in Cairo in 1954, and also completed his residency training in anesthesiology there. He stayed on and joined the anesthesiology department faculty and eventually was promoted to associate professor. He immigrated to the United States in 1968 and initially worked as a senior instructor in anesthesiology at Case Western Reserve University Hospital for two years. He next joined the staff of what is now UPMC Magee-Womens Hospital in Pittsburgh—as the director of obstetric anesthesia (Fig. 5.1). He served 12 years in Pittsburgh, eventually reaching full professor status. In 1982, Dr. Abouleish left Pittsburgh to join the faculty of the University of Texas-Houston, where he served again as a full professor of anesthesiology till 2001, and then as professor emeritus during his retirement (Fig. 5.2).

R. G. Graber
Department of Anesthesiology and Perioperative Medicine, University Hospitals Cleveland Medical Center, Cleveland, OH, USA

C. Marcucci (✉)
Department of Transfusion Medicine, Clinical Center, National Institutes of Health, Bethesda, MD, USA

S. Mohamed et al. (eds.), *Anesthesia Bridges*, https://doi.org/10.1007/978-3-032-08294-7_5

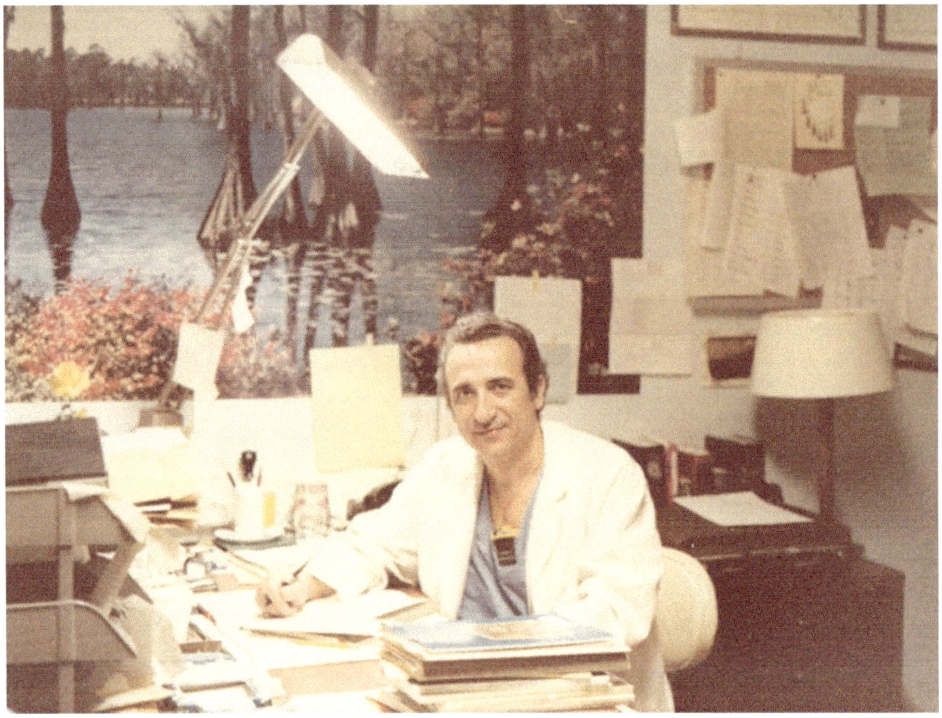

Fig. 5.1 Dr. Ezzat Abouleish at Magee-Womens Hospital where he revolutionized the care of women in labor. Photo: Amr Abouleish

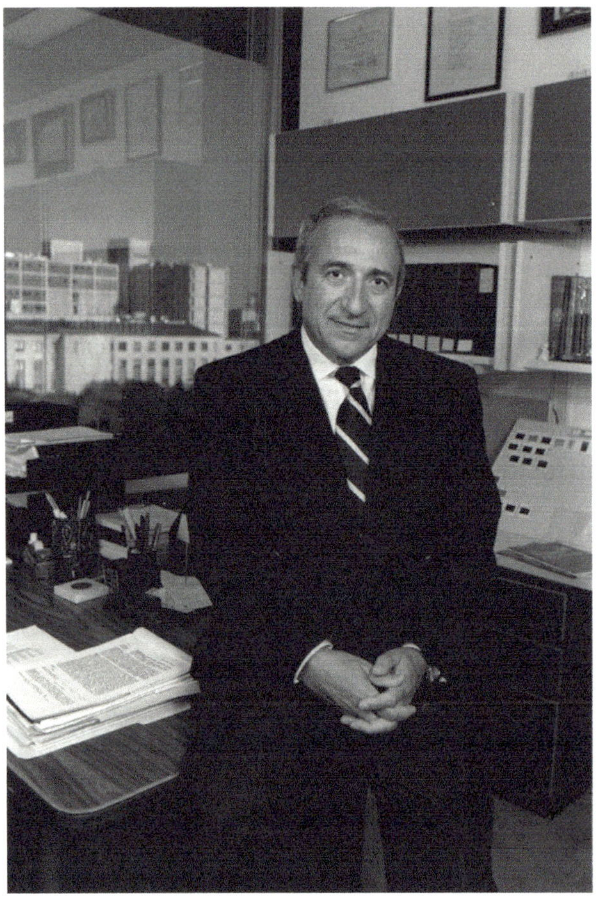

Fig. 5.2 One of Atiya Abouleish's favorite photographs of her husband—Ezzat Abouleish, MD, at the University of Texas-Houston. Here, he continued his pioneering clinical work and teaching in obstetrical anesthesia, including the introduction of the combined spinal-epidural technique. Photo: Amr Abouleish

Medical Pioneer and Academic Anesthesiologist

Dr. Abouleish was a pioneer in the field of obstetric anesthesiology. In fact, he was the first anesthesiologist to place an epidural for labor analgesia at Magee-Womens Hospital in 1972. Of note, that first patient was his wife. This successful first labor epidural was instrumental in reducing resistance to this new technique at Magee-Womens and paved the way for generations (and millions!) of women to receive labor epidural analgesia. He went on to teach this technique to a multitude of residents and his peers.

Dr. Abouleish was also known to perform the "double catheter technique"—where dual caudal and epidural catheters were placed at the same time. The catheters were then utilized according to the stage of labor, with the caudal catheter primarily used during the latter stage and delivery. At UT Houston, he pioneered the combined spinal epidural (CSE) technique for labor analgesia and received a patent for a spinal catheter that could be used in labor. In 1985, he founded the annual meeting Texas Anesthesia Conference for Obstetrics (TACO). He then worked with Dr. Tom Joyce at Baylor to make TACO an annual meeting that was co-sponsored by UT Houston and Baylor. In 1999, Dr. Abouleish was honored to be selected by the Society for Obstetric Anesthesiology and Perinatology (SOAP) to give the Gertie Marx Lecture and receive the Nils Löfgren Award (Fig. 5.3).

Dr. Abouleish was a prolific author. He was the author or co-author of over 70 peer-reviewed original journal articles, almost 20 book chapters, and five books. Some notable publications include *Childbirth…A Joy Not A Suffering* (1975)—a book written specifically for the lay public that discussed all the analgesic methods available for labor and delivery—and *Pain Control in Obstetrics* (1977)—a classic anesthesiology textbook.

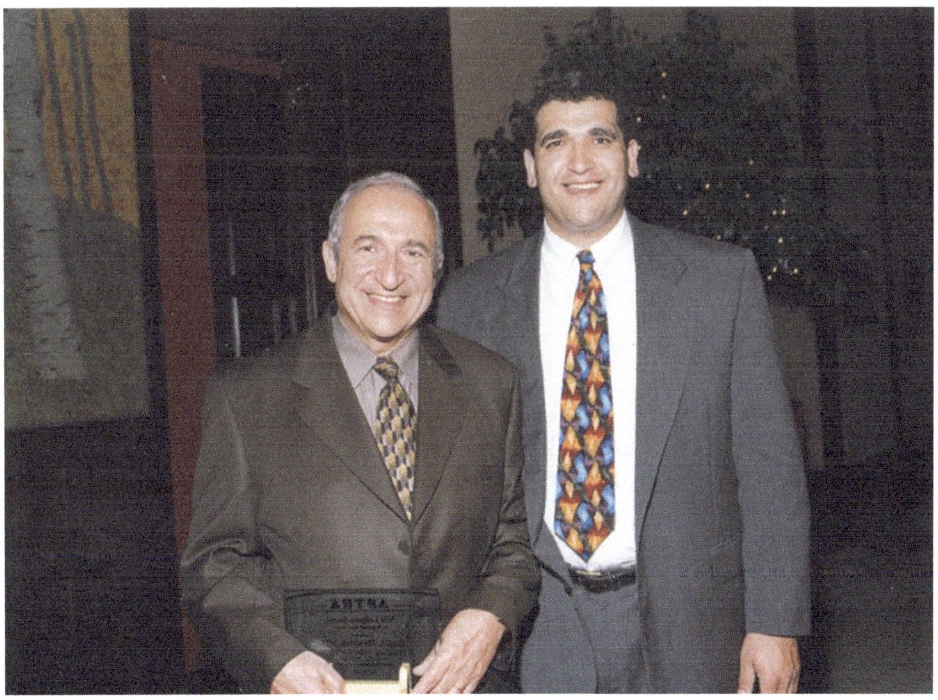

Fig. 5.3 Dr. Ezzat Abouleish with son and *Anesthesia Bridges* editor Dr. Amr Abouleish receiving the prestigious SOAP award. Photo: Amr Abouleish

Artist and Family Man

In addition to his medical accomplishments, Ezzat Abouleish was a respected artist and calligrapher. Although it was a lifelong hobby, this passion became a full-time endeavor during his retirement. He was a regular contributor to the ASA annual meeting art exhibit, where his work won several awards. His artwork has been exhibited throughout the United States and won many awards both in classical fine and Islamic art. In 2006, he was one of the main artists contributing to the project "Painting for Peace" that was displayed at Rice University in Houston and the University of Houston Main Campus.

Dr. Abouleish was also a devoted family man and a mentor and friend to many residents and faculty during his long career. He and his wife, Atiya, raised three children and were the proud grandparents of eight grandchildren (Figure 5.4). He is truly a role model for us all to emulate. In the SOAP Summer 2014 Newsletter, colleagues memorialized him as follows:

> Ezzat Ibrahim Abouleish was a true renaissance man—artist, author, philosopher, scientist, physician—as well as a wonderful husband, father, grandfather—but more importantly a great friend to all. Dr. Abouleish truly made this world more beautiful, fun, and happy. In all his life, Ezzat's compassion for his fellow man and woman was evident. From being integral in making obstetric anesthesia safe for the laboring woman, to advocating for peace and understanding among all people, to sharing his art and calligraphy with the world, and his love of God, Ezzat touched many lives with love and humor. He will be missed by his many friends, colleagues, and family. [1]

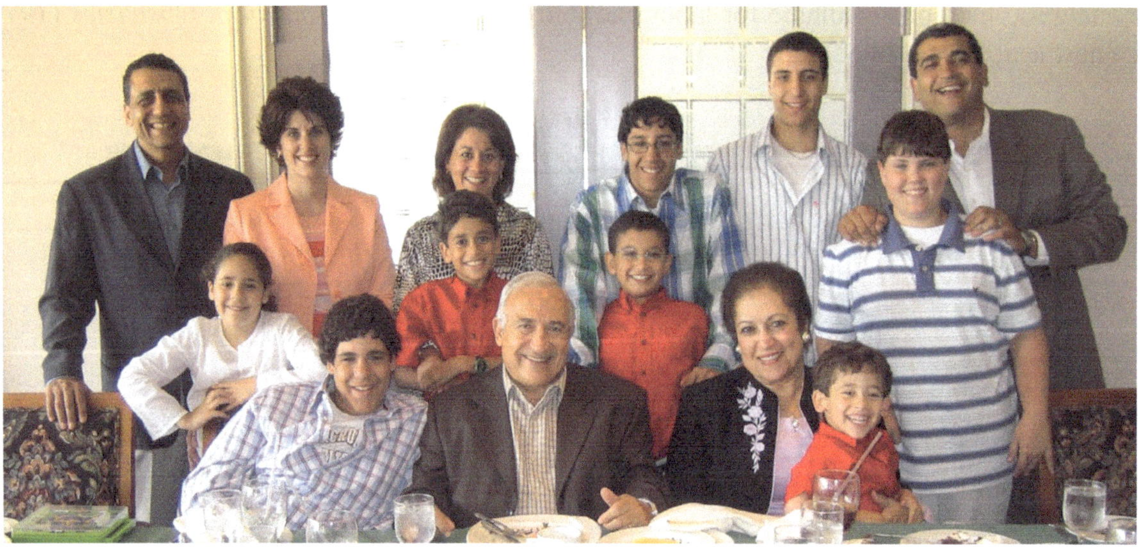

Fig. 5.4 Dr. and Mrs. Abouleish in 2004, surrounded by their children and eight beautiful grandchildren. *Anesthesia Bridges* coeditor Amr Abouleish is standing upper right. Photo: Amr Abouleish

Lessons Learned

- Dr. Abouleish's professional and personal lives can serve as an example to us all. What comes through in the tributes to him by the people who knew him best is the zest and generosity he brought to whatever endeavor he undertook. While being a giant in the field of OB anesthesia—imagine being the original proponent of epidural labor analgesia—he took care not to neglect his personal life or outside interests and was the head of a large and close family.

- Dr. Abouleish was first and last a communicator. Whether he was interacting with patients, colleagues, students, trainees, or staff, his goal was to establish the human connection, whether through his medical practice, research, writings, or paintings.

- Ezzat had a fascinating post-retirement life, filled with writing and art. He took his lifelong interests and developed them into a fulfilling second career. His paintings are spectacular in their use of line and color. We asked Amr if he happened to know who owns one of the most captivating paintings—blue flowers on a black ground (Fig. 5.5). That one is especially cherished by the family and hangs today in Mrs. Abouleish's home.

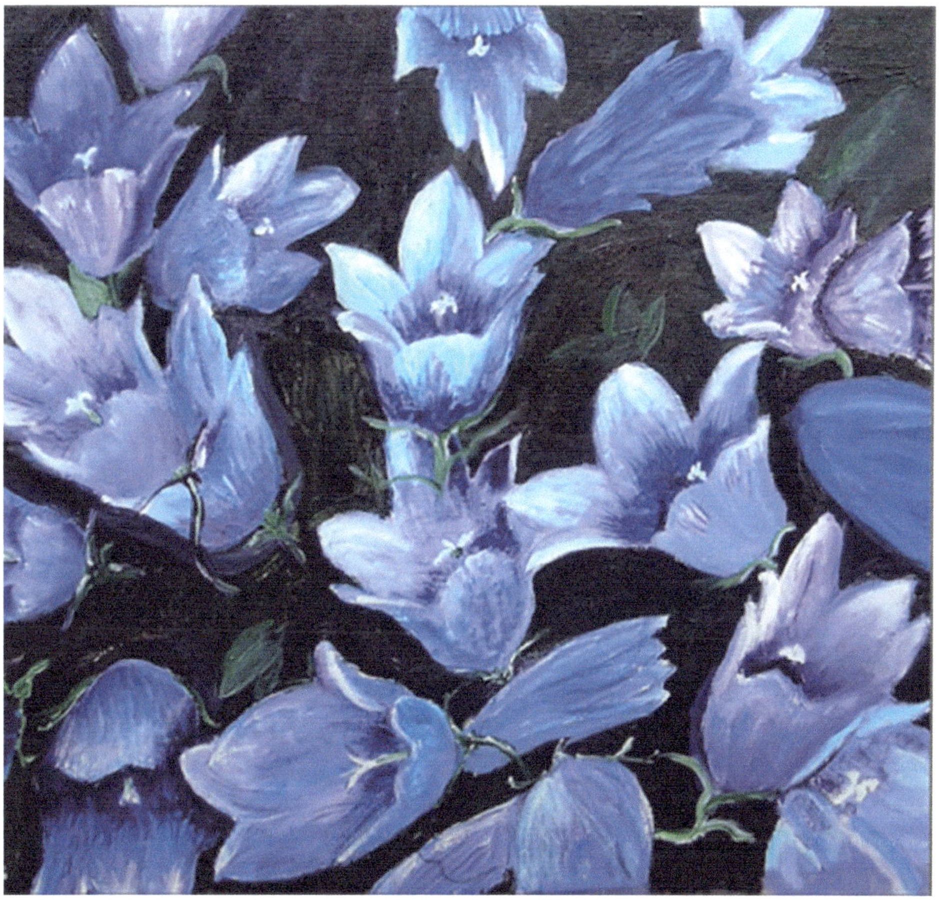

Fig. 5.5 A beautiful painting by Dr. Ezzat Abouleish. Photo: Amr Abouleish

Reference

1. Vallejo MC, Silip AT, Camann WR. In Memory of Ezzat I. Abouleish. SOAP Newsletter, Summer; 2014.

Authors

Ray Graber and **Cathy Marcucci** were honored to peek into the Abouleish family photo album and to compile this brief tribute to the senior Dr. Abouleish. It was a pleasure to learn more about his life and work. They regret that they never had the opportunity to meet him.

6 Listening

Lois A. Connolly

Murmur

Irregular

Wheezy or Clear Breath Sounds

Vigilantly Monitoring

Listen

Many anesthesiologists new to practice may not recognize this device (Fig. 6.1). The earpiece was connected to either a precordial stethoscope or esophageal probe to constantly monitor the patient's heart rate, rhythm, murmurs and breath sounds. The earpiece was made professionally during the first weeks of anesthesia residency training. The device was used to vigilantly monitor the patient throughout a procedure.

The earpiece was a symbol of an anesthesiologist. Why did we lose this listening device? Listening enables us to gather information and gain understanding. Listening enables early action or intervention in patient care. Listening is an essential element in leadership and emotional health. Listening develops empathy. Stephen R. Covey, author of *The 7 Habits of Highly Effective People,* states: "Most people do not listen with the intent to understand; they listen with the intent to reply." Listen without bias. Listen with curiosity. Listen.

L. A. Connolly (✉)
Department of Anesthesiology, Medical College of Wisconsin/Froedtert Hospital, Milwaukee, WI, USA
e-mail: connolly@mcw.edu

S. Mohamed et al. (eds.), *Anesthesia Bridges*, https://doi.org/10.1007/978-3-032-08294-7_6

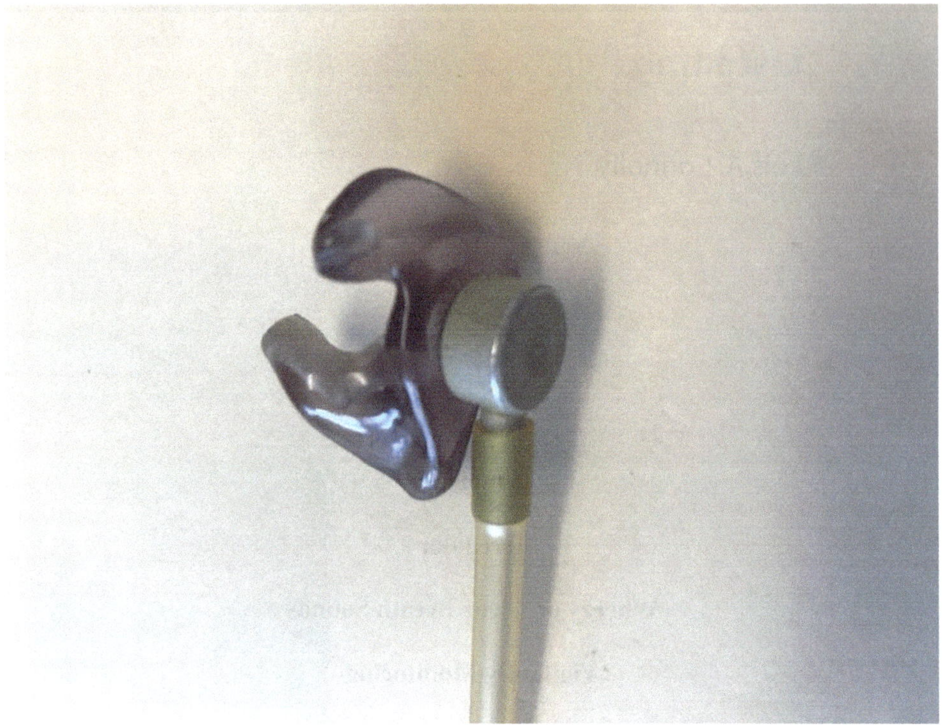

Fig. 6.1 A custom-molded anesthesia earpiece. Photo: Lois Connolly

Lessons Learned

- If you can take the time to really listen to and understand what people are trying to tell you, you will be a better partner and leader.

Author

Lois Connolly pursued a long career in academic medicine and is a tenured professor at the Medical College of Wisconsin (MCW), Department of Anesthesiology. She provides clinical care and resident education as a neuro and liver transplant anesthesiologist. Lois serves as the medical director of MCW's Master in Anesthesia Program. In addition to her academic career, she contributes her time to many ASA committees and boards. After raising two successful children, she and her husband, Patrick, enjoy road biking and have traveled to over 40 different countries, exploring the local culture by biking or hiking.

Write What You Mean

7

Daniel I. Sessler

Introduction

Dan Sessler is the founder and director of the *O*utcomes *R*esearch Consortium. The group just celebrated its 30th anniversary and is the world's largest clinical anesthesia research group. The Consortium has published more than 1700 full papers and publishes a new one every 2.5 days. We asked him to tell us who his earliest mentors were and the best writing and publishing advice he ever received, given his prodigious career. We also asked him to let us know what his favorite bridge is, and he might just get the prize for sending us the best bridge picture. Here are Dan's submissions in a nutshell.

Dr. Andrew M. Sessler

My primary mentor was my father, Andrew Sessler, a famous theoretical physicist and noted humanitarian and environmentalist. He directed the Lawrence Berkeley National Laboratory and was a member of the National Academy of Sciences. My mother was also a physicist, and both taught me much about writing. I will never forget my father's all-to-apparent frustration, telling me over and over, "write what you mean, write what you mean." It was great advice and, of course, requires first figuring out exactly what you do mean. And once you know, write just that; don't write "around the topic," requiring readers to guess what you're trying to say, because too often, they will guess wrong and lose the thread of the logic.

And from my mother, I learned to write concisely. Two rules—first, always use the most precise word to convey as much information as possible and, second, if a word can be removed from a sentence without changing its meaning, that word shouldn't be there.

One evening, my father and I worked through about five pages of complex differential equations describing heat flow through tissues under various circumstances. My father did the work; I just struggled to vaguely understand what he was doing. The result was a relatively simple equation based on measurable inputs that could be used experimentally. The next morning, my father called me in abject apology for losing a factor-of-two somewhere in the pages of calculations. Personally, I thought being within a

D. I. Sessler (✉)
Department of Anesthesiology, Outcomes Research Consortium, Houston, TX, USA
e-mail: ds@OR.org

S. Mohamed et al. (eds.), *Anesthesia Bridges*, https://doi.org/10.1007/978-3-032-08294-7_7

factor-of-two after so much math was great. But I realized afterwards, that for my father to be off by a factor-of-two, was like me forgetting to give oxygen. We fixed the error and then co-authored a series of anesthesiology papers based on that and related derivations.

***Note from the Editors:** We asked Dan Sessler to tell us about his favorite bridge. He just happened to have this beautiful picture in his personal photo files! (Fig. 7.1)

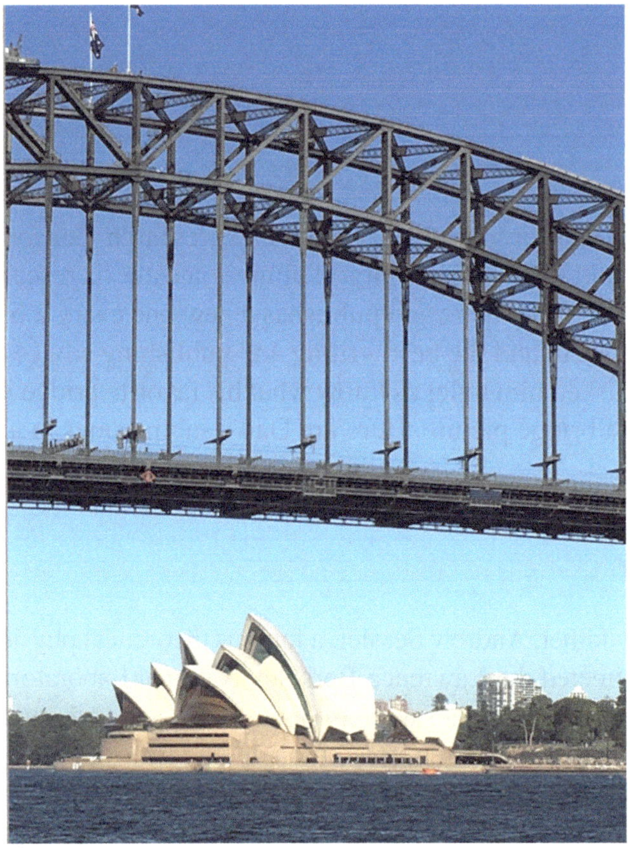

Fig. 7.1 The Harbor Bridge, from McMahons Point, Sydney, Australia. This beautiful bridge opened in 1932 and is a steel arch bridge that is nicknamed "The Coat Hanger" because of its rounded shape. It carries rail, vehicular, and pedestrian/bicycle traffic. The view is considered one of the most iconic man-made visual snapshots on the planet. Photo: Dan Sessler

Lessons Learned

- The key to writing is to first know exactly what you want to say. Be humble and diligent—keep working until you have solved this problem, and don't be afraid to go back over your conclusions and calculations.
- When you start writing, direct your efforts precisely to this subject; don't write around your topic.
- Write as concisely as possible. Consider whether each word has earned its place in your work.

Author

Dan Sessler is the vice-president for clinical outcomes and research and professor of anesthesiology at UT Health. He was an editor for *Anesthesiology* for nine years and serves as a reviewer for more than 65 journals. His grants total more than $85 million. Dr. Sessler has published more than 900 full research papers, which have been cited more than 60,000 times—making him the world's most published and cited anesthesiologist, and among the top 0.02% cited authors in all scientific fields. His awards include a Fulbright Fellowship and the ASA Excellence in Research prize.

8 How to Handle Requests for Recommendations and References, and How to Make Sure Your Own Requests Are Well Received

Raymond G. Graber, David A. Zvara, Jeffrey R. Kirsch, Cynthia A. Lien, and Rodger E. Barnette

Introduction

As you become more senior and advance in your career, residents and colleagues will start coming to you and requesting letters of recommendation. This can be an easy (and even fun) endeavor when you are writing to support someone you really like and have a high opinion of. However, this won't always be the case. Sooner or later, you will get asked to write a letter for someone who just doesn't measure up to your standards.

Alternatively, you might get asked to write a letter for someone that you have no real knowledge of. Is it your duty to support everyone who asks you for a reference, or should you be selective about who you write for? How do you write letters for people who were once in your department but have since moved on? In other words, you know them from the past, not the present. We asked several wise current or former department chairpersons to give us their takes on these questions.

R. G. Graber (✉)
Department of Anesthesiology and Perioperative Medicine, University Hospitals Cleveland Medical Center, Cleveland, OH, USA
e-mail: raymond.graber@uhhospitals.org

D. A. Zvara
(Emeritus) Department of Anesthesiology, The University of North Carolina at Chapel Hill School of Medicine, Chapel Hill, NC, USA

J. R. Kirsch
Department of Anesthesiology and Pain Medicine, University of Washington School of Medicine, Seattle, WA, USA

(Emeritus) Anesthesiology and Perioperative Medicine, School of Medicine, Oregon Health & Science University, Portland, OR, USA

C. A. Lien
Department of Anesthesiology, Medical College of Wisconsin/Froedtert Hospital, Milwaukee, WI, USA

R. E. Barnette (Retired)
AIC Kijabe Hospital, Kijabe, Kenya

S. Mohamed et al. (eds.), *Anesthesia Bridges*, https://doi.org/10.1007/978-3-032-08294-7_8

Be Honest

David Zvara discusses his personal solutions to the issue of references for those that are less than stellar:

- Be honest with the applicant and tell them at the time of their asking that you cannot give a favorable or glowing recommendation. Truth hurts, but this immediately avoids future problems.
- Do not agree to give a recommendation and then sabotage the applicant. That's worse than telling them you're not going to write one.
- When blindly asked for a recommendation—the applicant did not ask your permission—and it is unfavorable, ask yourself, "Is he/she so bad that I can't say anything positive?" Usually, there are positives. Think hard before denying someone an opportunity.
- Still, be honest. If there are truly damning comments and opinions, it is best handled by phone. My response is to write back, "Please call me about this applicant." Anything in writing, unfortunately, is discoverable. Be careful what you write.
- Remember, personality issues must be separated from performance issues. You may not "like" someone, but can they do the job? In any recommendation, set aside all personal feelings. Stick to the facts. If they can do the job, say so.
- If there are true issues of performance, professionalism, attendance, or reliability, then say so. Your reputation is on the line with this colleague.
- Grace is always a good default. Someone who underperformed at your institution may be a better fit at another. Give them a chance.
- Remember that life is about balance and finding out what works.

***Note from the Editors:** Just as we were putting this chapter together, we received this photo from a dear friend who was on vacation in Jordan. We think this bridge perfectly illustrates balance and grace (Fig. 8.1).

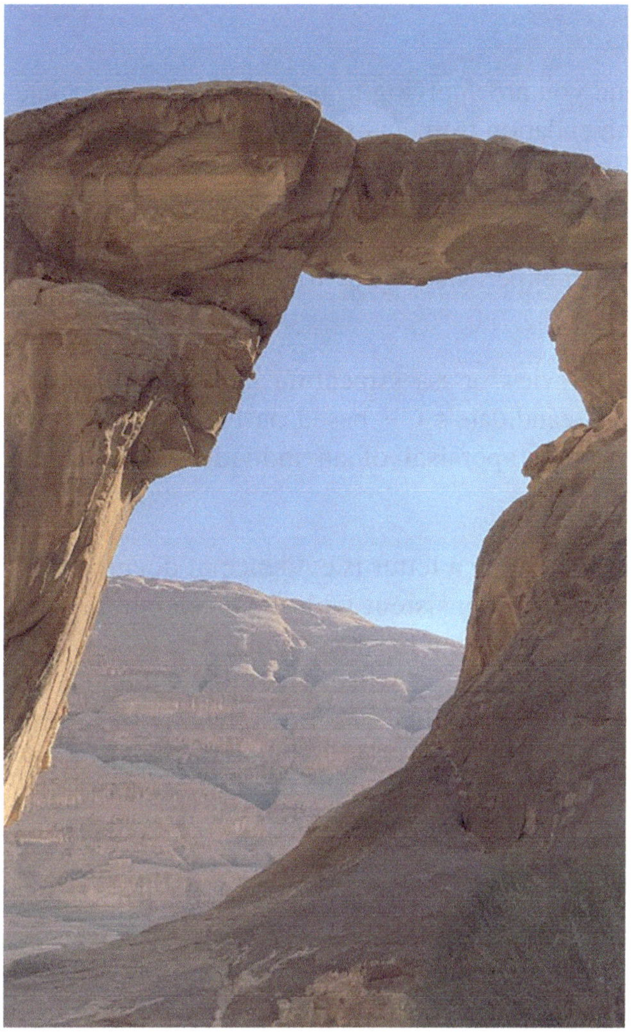

Fig. 8.1 A beautiful natural sandstone bridge in Wadi Rum Jordan, where much of the movie *Lawrence in Arabia* was filmed. Photo: Christie Gilmartin Waters

Simply Decline

Jeff Kirsch advises short but honest responses that still courteously spare feelings when asked to provide a reference that he is not comfortable with:

- If I'm asked by a third party, I simply decline. Depending on the situation, I either indicate that I cannot support the person if they are someone seeking promotion that I do not support, or just indicate that I don't have the time.

- If I'm asked by the individual, I just apologize and tell them that I am too busy to be able to write a good letter for them.

A number of our senior anesthesia colleagues also mentioned a slightly different technique to us—they write a brief but inclusive outline or list of the pros and cons that would appear in the (lukewarm or worse) recommendation, and then show it to the requester to ask if they should proceed. This might seem a bit harsh, but it is nothing if not honest, and both parties know where the other stands. This can also be done with a friendly but frank conversation.

External References

As your career advances and you are applying to be promoted to associate or full professor, you may need to get letters of recommendation from an external referee. An external referee is typically defined as an individual who is independent of the candidate, who is an expert in the candidate's field, and who is able to provide an objective appraisal of the candidate's work.

Cynthia Lien tells us about her experience in that role and what she looks for:

- I frequently write letters of review or assessment for individuals I do not know. The letters typically are a reorganization of the candidate's CV based on the institution's requirements for promotion. While they provide an honest appraisal of an individual's work, these letters tend to be very impersonal.
- What I look for in agreeing to write a letter is evidence of documented productivity since the person was last promoted, which is consistent with the academic mission. Rather than considering promotion to be a reward for work that has been done, I view it as an opportunity to look at what has been done and determine whether it is likely that the individual will make more contributions to our specialty—this will depend on their success in having seen projects through, their publication in high impact journals as first or last author, and their reputation—national and international.

Write Contemporaneous References for the Record

Rodger Barnette discusses an interesting approach to the problem of being asked to write letters for former department members who have moved on:

- When I was chair at Temple, I started the practice of writing letters of recommendation as residents, fellows, and even faculty members left the institution.
- When asked later (sometimes years later) for letters of recommendation, I would send a copy of the letter written when they left—and include a cover letter. The cover letter would state that since the individual had left, I was no longer familiar with his/her current practice, academic activities, etc. I would make clear that this was not intended to be pejorative, but was simply a statement of fact, and was the standard practice in our department.
- I might add that this practice over the long haul reduces the work and time involved in writing such letters. And I used this practice for all third-party requests for credentialing, etc.
- Finally, all of us can write letters that do not have much content, though they read smoothly. I did not write many such letters, but whenever I received one, I would pick up the phone.

***Note from the Editors:** Rodger Barnette has lived part-time in Kenya for many years, so in his honor, we selected this wonderful railway bridge through the Nairobi National Park (Fig. 8.2).

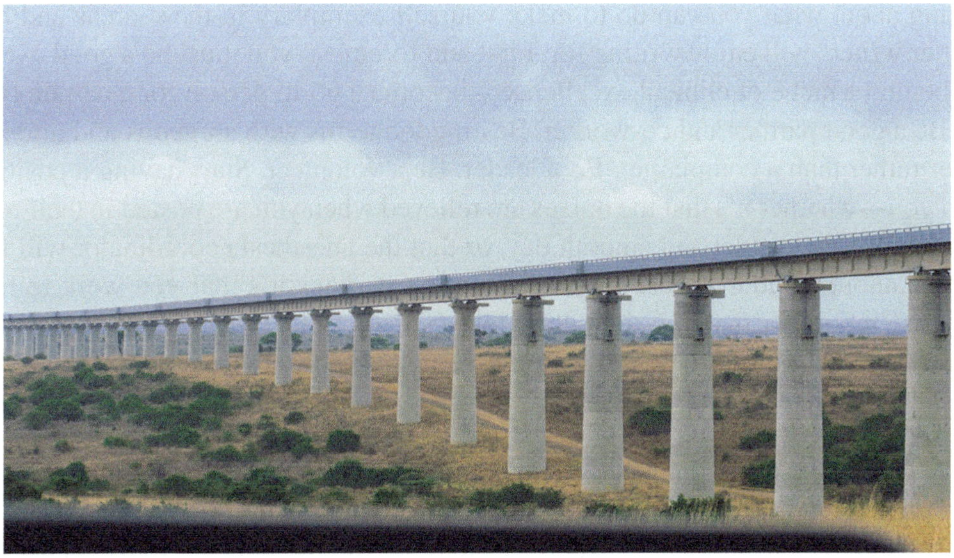

Fig. 8.2 This beautiful railway bridge spans the terrain in Nairobi National Park. The bridge was specifically built at a height of 6.5 meters so that large animals such as giraffes and elephants could easily pass through. Sometimes, who crosses under a bridge is just as important as who crosses on the topside of the bridge. Please see Chap. 206, "Animals Need Bridges, Too", for more information on this important subject. Photo: Image used under standard license from stock.adobe.com

Don't Compromise Your Own Reputation

All the suggestions above notwithstanding, it is usually true that most of us would rather say nice things and support those who come to us, because we want to be "nice," and it is hard to say "no." However, our wise consultants remind us that we don't want to compromise our own reputations by padding someone else's. There is a tendency to write references that are better than they ought to be when you are younger, but everybody we discussed this topic with became less and less willing to do that as they became more senior.

And remember, no matter what is written, a significant amount of "referencing" is done by phone. You don't want to be in the position of saying one thing in writing, and another thing when speaking—that isn't fair to either the subject or the end-recipient of the reference. And that sort of two-faced way of dealing with references will eventually catch up to you.

Make it Easy for Your Future Reference Writers

Now, here are some thoughts for the more junior folks. How do you make sure that you are never in a position where a request for a reference is not welcome? First, consider what the ultimate reader of the reference really wants to know. It comes down to four basic things: your clinical competence, whether you can work well with others, whether you will bring your new location to grief in any way, and whether you can pass any required exams.

So start thinking about what you can do to make yourself exemplary in these areas and be the type of person that letter writers will enjoy writing for. First and foremost, you must be a good overall clinician, and then maybe find a niche of clinical excellence—become a go-to person for a certain type of case or subspecialty. Be a good partner and co-worker. Be on good terms with surgeons and nursing staff. Be a problem solver rather than a complainer. Be a leader. Be a volunteer. Start having a positive impact on people around you—whether it's that the nurses are relieved when you are posted in their rooms because they know they will have a quiet and smooth day, or that the anesthesia coordinator will not encounter undue resistance about an add-on case in your room. Or perhaps it's that you work to include others when writing case reports or that you do a good job on a committee that no one wanted to be on. You don't always have to work hard to advertise these activities to reference writers—word has a way of getting around.

There's no way to stop the telephone back channels mentioned above, so you might as well accept this and make sure that the conversations about you are going to be favorable. In our experience, the telephone is how surgeons often communicate about a candidate among themselves, but also with the anesthesia departments at their respective institutions. We're aware of cases where the surgeons put cold water on an anesthesiologist applicant, and the same is true in reverse. So think about that the next time your OR is a bit thick with tension.

Remediate on an Immediate Basis

If you *have* done something that might impact a future reference, start remediating that immediately. It happens—everybody makes mistakes in their professional demeanor and conduct to some degree at some point. Unless it is a serious clinical issue, these can usually be repaired. First, go to the person or persons directly involved and try to make amends. A sincere apology is a good start. If you have been a gigantic grouch, find the person as soon as you can and say, "Please accept my apology for being testy and inappropriate."

Then, go to one of your department leaders (who later might be turning the incident over in their minds when considering a reference for you) and acknowledge that you have created a problem for yourself and them. You can just simply state, "I would like to be known as a person who is courteous and calm in all situations, and unfortunately. on Friday, I was neither of those things."

Then state any mitigation efforts, "I could have and should have done this differently. We had a really difficult case, and instead of discussing it with the ICU in that light, an argument resulted. But I went and talked to the team, apologized, and asked them to join me on a case report." This simple, straightforward approach to interpersonal mistakes allows the reference writer to get past having to deal with a blow-up they heard about and instead credit you with maturity, integrity, and resilience. This is important as future employers will be interested in how you react and perform under stress as well as when everything goes smoothly.

Lessons Learned

- Assume that suspiciously bland letters of reference are going to generate phone calls.
- Be honest! This is just so important. Don't go out on a limb for someone you do not feel strongly positive about. Your own reputation for truthful integrity is ultimately up for consideration with every reference you write.
- Be kind wherever and whenever possible. Not always, of course, but occasionally a person's less-than-excellent performance might actually have been a matter of fit.
- Consider writing reference letters in a contemporaneous time frame. It's when your impressions are freshest and will ultimately save time.
- Junior people should start thinking long and hard about becoming the person they themselves would like to give a reference for. There are many common-sense ways to do this. And remember that later in your career, you may need objective references that are not going to be about how much the reference-writer likes you on a personal basis.
- You will never be able to beat the telephone. The anesthesia community is just not that big. Somebody wanting a reference about you will most probably be able to get the whole story on you and everything you've done, good and bad, in less than three phone calls.
- Don't assume that one mistake will tank a reference from someone. We believe that what you did can be balanced by how you recovered.
- Blind requests for references put the writer in a bind. Don't do it.
- The authors would like to thank Catherine Marcucci, MD, for her ideas and assistance with this chapter.

Authors

Ray Graber is a vice chair and associate professor of anesthesiology at University Hospitals Cleveland Medical Center.

David Zvara is a professor of anesthesiology and a former chairperson at the University of North Carolina at Chapel Hill. He has served as the COO for UNC faculty physicians. At present, he is also the CMO for UNC Hospitals.

Jeff Kirsch is the chair emeritus of the OHSU Department of Anesthesiology and Perioperative Medicine and formerly associate dean of Faculty Affairs and professor of anesthesiology at the Medical College of Wisconsin. He is currently a professor and the department head of Anesthesiology and Pain at the University of Washington's Harborview Medical Center.

Cynthia Lien is the chairperson and professor of anesthesiology at the Medical College of Wisconsin.

Rodger Barnette is the former chairperson and emeritus professor of anesthesiology at the Lewis Katz School of Medicine at Temple University. He is a consultant at AIC Kijabe Hospital in Kijabe, Kenya.

9 Communication—The Little Things Really Matter!

David A. Young

Introduction

Your ability to communicate impacts practically every aspect of your professional and personal life. I wish that I had fully appreciated the significance of this topic at a younger stage in my career. I am hoping to convince you that emphasizing effective communication skills in all aspects of your practice can result in better outcomes, additional opportunities, and reduced conflicts.

Details!

As the title suggests, small details really matter when it concerns communication. Many small details can add up to make a significant impact. Although we typically think about communication as being what we write or speak, it also occurs through more subtle methods, such as our body and facial expressions. In fact, most people that we interact with are actively and also subconsciously observing our body language while we communicate. This includes patients, staff members, and your colleagues. I'm sure that you can easily think of an example of a facial expression that you interpreted to suggest a positive response (for example, a smile). However, do you really know the actual reason for this nonverbal reaction?

The same argument holds true for a perceived negative response, like shrugged shoulders. It may be possible that this person was upset by a comment you previously made or perhaps is upset from a recent email (unrelated to you). We display these types of responses many times throughout our day, and you can see the potential for a confusing mixed message when our body language does not match our intended message.

In addition, people can misunderstand or misinterpret the actual content of what we say or write, and there are times when we completely forget to communicate. How many times have you interpreted a text message incorrectly due to the limited information given? Have you ever received an incorrect message that was passed on from another person? As you can see, ineffective communication can occur in a variety of circumstances and be interpreted inaccurately.

D. A. Young (✉)
Department of Anesthesiology, Texas Children's Hospital, Houston, TX, USA
e-mail: davidy@bcm.edu

S. Mohamed et al. (eds.), *Anesthesia Bridges*, https://doi.org/10.1007/978-3-032-08294-7_9

Challenges and Barriers

Now that we have discussed the importance of effective communication, we should also consider some of the challenges and barriers to providing accurate communication. Some of these common challenges include time pressure, appropriate framing of the actual message, and perhaps having the forethought to do so. Time pressure is a significant factor in many of our daily professional activities. Our profession uses different staffing models, including the supervision of residents, fellows, and perhaps anesthetists; this means that we frequently are overseeing several individuals simultaneously. This can result in feeling under pressure to provide effective communication to multiple team members while also performing at a high productivity rate.

Any message should also be formatted in a manner that is accurate and comprehensible to the receiving individual. This requires that our terminology be understood by the receiving individual. For example, an anesthesiologist may need to explain to an anesthesia technician that there is an urgent need for a fiberoptic scope to be brought to the operating room for a procedure uncommonly performed at that institution. In addition, this communication may occur by phone or via another person, such as having the secretary page the anesthesia technician to perform a particular task, such as setting up a fiberoptic scope.

*__Note from the Editors:__ Speaking of challenges and barriers, remember that bridges don't always have to cross over landscape obstacles. Sometimes they can provide a wonderful way to travel through nature (Fig. 9.1).

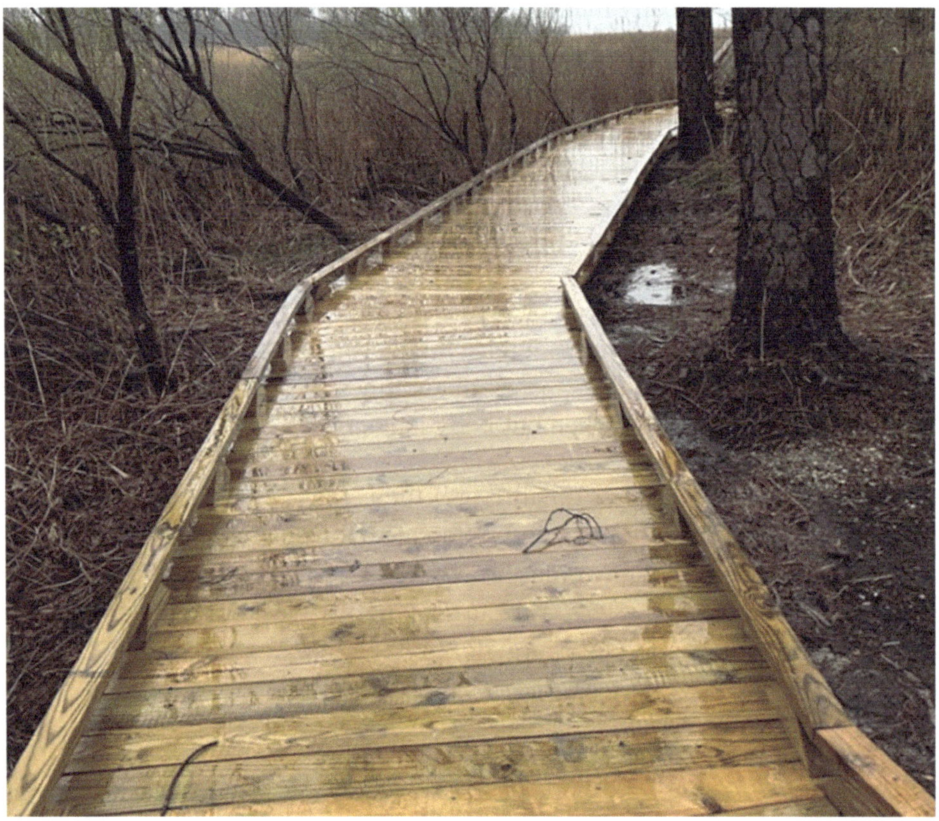

Fig. 9.1 This little elevated bridge walkway traverses a tiny, flat section of the Eastern Neck National Wildlife Refuge. Photo: Cathy Marcucci

Thinking Ahead

Perhaps the most difficult communication issue to deal with is having the forethought to generate a specific communication. This can result from a variety of factors, such as production pressure, cognitive overload, assuming others have the same assumptions as you do, or other intraoperative distractions. The key point from all of these examples is to recognize that providing effective communication takes a significant and continuous amount of effort. It's always good practice to repeat and/or verify an important request, such as giving heparin during a cardiac case. If you are not sure someone has heard your own statement, repeat it and verify that the message has been heard.

Day-to-Day Communications Strategies

I hope that you now recognize and accept that on a daily basis, you can work to improve your communication skills, and that this can result in better outcomes for yourself and your patients. I believe that everyone wants to do a good job and provide the best possible patient care. I've learned over the years that despite what you may think someone is thinking, you really never know for sure until you ask them.

Throughout our average day, we make many assumptions about why people are acting and talking the way they do without really actually knowing the true and complete story. For example, you asked a staff member to obtain a certain item for you and then found out that the item was not acquired. The reasons for the item not being brought to you could be many. This can range from the staff member not knowing where it is located, or they were already tasked with other important things to do, or the item was out of stock. Initially, your internal reaction may be the same—frustration, anger, etc.—but actually knowing the reason could substantially modify your sentiment.

One of the best strategies to adopt to improve your interactions in the workplace is to stay calm while communicating. In the previous example, you could follow up regarding the status of the item in a non-judgmental manner. As we all know, there are many ways to ask a question in terms of the actual words used, but don't minimize the effect of the tone of your voice and facial expressions. In my daily practice, I have taken the position that most of my colleagues and ancillary employees are sometimes overwhelmed in terms of production pressure and system complexity. I know it's not uncommon for someone to say that they were unaware of a new policy or are unfamiliar with a current guideline or workflow process.

Checklists

Another way to improve communication and patient care in certain situations is to use checklists. Regular training using well-accepted checklists and algorithms are two very effective strategies to improve performance, particularly in complex and/or unfamiliar situations. In addition, improved personal performance can likely lead to enhanced team functioning. Most anesthesiologists are familiar with the American Heart Association's Advanced Cardiac Life Support algorithms as well as the American Society of Anesthesiologists' Difficult Airway Algorithm.

There are also other anesthesiology-specific checklists, such as The Society for Pediatric Anesthesia Critical Events Checklist and the Stanford Emergency Manual: Cognitive Aids for Perioperative Critical Events. All of these cognitive aids are best utilized if the learner has had previous exposure and training in how to use them. The aids can both be utilized to verify the steps of well-known guidelines (such as the order for chest compressions and defibrillation) and also be used as guides for the treatment of conditions the provider may be less familiar with, such as dantrolene dosing for malignant hyperthermia. These cognitive aids also have the secondary benefit of improving team performance and team communication during a medical crisis. Regardless of the tool selected, the best way to have effective communication is to use direct and specific statements as much as possible.

Simulation

Medical simulation can also be a very useful tool to improve communication among providers during a wide range of encounters. These encounters can be designed to improve competency during commonly performed psychomotor tasks, used to promote critical thinking during rare but possible situations, and can be used to system test new processes. All of these activities involve various forms of communication. System testing actually uses the provider to test the practical usefulness of a new process and/or area; it is not designed to examine the knowledge or performance of the actual provider. The results of the system test can also be used to modify many aspects of the system, including building design, personnel workflow, administrative processes, and so forth. Algorithms and checklists can also be incorporated into the medical simulation activities.

Summary

In summary, effective communication is the key to successful performance in the anesthesiology environment. Providing effective communication requires a sustained and positive effort. Remember that communication occurs in many forms and can easily be misinterpreted. Algorithms and checklists can both be used to enhance the communication of the individual and of the entire team. Educational tools such as medical simulation can be used to provide training in communication for the individual, team, and entire system. Regardless of the type of communication, the best way to have an effective message is to use the most direct and specific statement that considers the background and knowledge of the intended individual.

Lessons Learned

- Communication impacts practically every aspect of your profession and daily life.
- Providing effective communication takes a significant and continuous amount of effort.
- Acquiring effective communication skills can result in better outcomes, additional opportunities, and reduced conflicts.

Author

David Young received all his education and training at the University of Miami/Jackson Memorial Hospital. This was followed by serving in the US Army as an anesthesiologist prior to relocating to Houston, Texas. Dr. Young's main interests include medical simulation, medical education, pediatric trauma, and pediatric resuscitation.

10 Communication—Up, Down, Lateral

Charles Whitten

Introduction

In my leadership journey, I have realized the importance of different styles of communication related to subject matter and audience. My guiding principle has been to always tell the truth; therefore, you don't have to remember what you said!

Different Styles for Different Situations

In communications with senior physician leaders, it is of vital importance to be succinct and remain at a high level. You need to focus on selling them concepts. Succinct tables, graphs, and charts can be of great assistance. In follow-up, it is always necessary to educate senior leaders' subordinates within the organization regarding the path forward. They will be the individuals who assist you in developing the deliverables. *Educate! Educate! Educate!*

In communications with senior nonphysician administrative leaders, I have learned it is of importance to be succinct, provide medical justification, and have high-level detail to support your requests. This generally involves multiple follow-up conversations to outline the details.

In communications with subordinates, it is of vital importance to be open and honest. Make sure that you use "lingo" specific to their frame of reference. Go to great lengths to outline the details. Subordinates need to understand how they will directly be impacted. Take the time and be willing to engage in a back-and-forth discussion until all issues are addressed.

In communications with colleagues within your specialty, it is of vital importance to state "why" and provide answers to "why" certain things are being changed or the justification for a new path forward. Alterations of policy or procedure should always be determined via input from all stakeholders. Every voice needs the opportunity to land on a set of "soft ears." This will lead to buy-in from all parties. The collective wisdom is the best wisdom!

C. Whitten (✉)
Department of Anesthesiology and Pain Management, University of Texas Southwestern Medical Center, Dallas, TX, USA
e-mail: charles.whitten@utsouthwestern.edu

S. Mohamed et al. (eds.), *Anesthesia Bridges*, https://doi.org/10.1007/978-3-032-08294-7_10

In communications with colleagues outside your specialty, verbalize distinctly from a consultant's frame of reference and make sure that you specifically address the questions or issues directed to your attention.

> **Always tell the truth. If you tell the truth, you never have to remember what you said.**—Chuck Whitten

Lessons Learned

- It is important to tailor your message to the type of audience you are speaking with.
- If you are able to communicate effectively with your target audience, you are more likely to get buy-in and achieve your goals.

Author

Chuck Whitten is a native of Missouri but considers himself a Texan. Following receipt of his BSEE at SMU, he has spent the last 41+ years at UT Southwestern in a multiplicity of capacities. His wife, Cheri, is the greatest positive force in his life. His current professional passions include physician leadership development and collaborative projects related to the economics of academic anesthesiology practice. If you play golf, you are his friend!

11 Be Mindful in Your Communication

Jay Mesrobian

Early in my career, our practice's attorney and I had the following exchange:

David Summer, Esq.: "Hey, Jay, do you know what the 'e' in 'email' stands for?"

Jay: "Electronic?"

David: "Evidence and Eternal!"

We all have hit the 'Send' button too quickly and, more broadly, had communications—verbal, email, text—that we wish we could take back. Communication that is not well thought out and mindful can have serious negative consequences upon both our personal and professional relationships, consequences that can impact your group's reputation and performance.

Lessons Learned

What would I tell my 35-year-old self?

- Always pause before hitting 'Send' and ask yourself, should this communication best occur via email or text?
- If a text is longer than two sentences, pick up the phone.
- If an email is longer than a paragraph, pick up the phone.
- *Two ears, one mouth.* Take time to listen before offering advice that may or may not be wanted.

J. Mesrobian (✉)
TeamHealth Anesthesia, Milwaukee, WI, USA
e-mail: jay_mesrobian@teamhealth.com

S. Mohamed et al. (eds.), *Anesthesia Bridges*, https://doi.org/10.1007/978-3-032-08294-7_11

- Be a giver, not a taker. Support others without expectation of anything in return.
- Assume best intentions from all parties unless there is clear evidence to the contrary.
- Take a deep breath before responding to a hostile or negative communication. There simply is too much to lose by responding in kind.

Author

Jay Mesrobian is a native of Chicago but has spent the past 20+ years living behind the "cheddar curtain" in Milwaukee, Wisconsin, and the prior nine years in Columbia, South Carolina. He is passionate about patient experience, the development of young physician leaders, and defining ways anesthesiologists can drive improvements in patient care. He has advocated in both state and national organizations, including serving as ASA Assistant Treasurer, and is eternally thankful to the mentors and partners who encouraged him along that path. He and his wife Beth have two adult daughters and a Newfoundland named Dilly.

Principles of Academic Writing

12

Olivia Liao, Raymond G. Graber, and Catherine Marcucci

Introduction

A good academic medical writer is first and foremost a writer who understands the universal principles that underpin good writing of any stripe. Historically, writing has been the most powerful form of communication available to mankind. Its best practitioners have always understood that we write first in the hopes that other people might find our writing and read it. And then perhaps, if we are lucky, what we have written prompts the reader into further thinking. The ultimate victory happens when something is set in motion in the future—one of your themes sticks with the readers for the rest of their lives, or they will use your writing as a reference in their own work.

Why Write?

The three main purposes of writing are to *inform, persuade, and entertain* the intended audience, and these goals are not mutually exclusive. Before beginning to write, an author should sit down and conceptualize his or her writing mission—what will be the proportions of each of these in the finished piece? Deep and clear thought is called for, and a formal outline is even better.

Most often, of course, the medical reader reads to learn new information. This is obvious. But what isn't always so apparent is whether readers are likely to be reading about a topic that's entirely new to them or reading to gather information that either reinforces or contradicts an existing belief of theirs. And hence it behooves the medical writer to have the firmest grasp on how to communicate the methods through which the content was obtained. The discussion section of a medical paper takes the most finesse and nuance, perhaps, but the methods section is really the sine qua non when writing to inform the medical reader.

O. Liao
Carnegie Mellon University, Pittsburgh, PA, USA

R. G. Graber
Department of Anesthesiology and Perioperative Medicine, University Hospitals Cleveland Medical Center, Cleveland, OH, USA

C. Marcucci (✉)
Department of Transfusion Medicine, Clinical Center, National Institutes of Health, Bethesda, MD, USA

S. Mohamed et al. (eds.), *Anesthesia Bridges*, https://doi.org/10.1007/978-3-032-08294-7_12

Develop Your Skill Sets

Writing to persuade and writing to entertain—each requires its own skill sets for academic medical writers. The best persuasive writing of any type is usually backed up by personal experience because sharing parts of your world or worldview with your readers gives them the chance to relate and empathize with you. Really skilled persuasive writers have nearly always done extensive reading of their own about their subject matter, and their stories and examples must be believable. A reader who can understand why you think the way you do is easier to persuade than one who can't. Remember that writing is all about sharing and that people learn through experiences and examples.

Writing to entertain is the least common objective in academic medical writing, but still has its place, of course. Elements of humor and storytelling not infrequently appear in academic medical writing, including in all our previous books. When writing to entertain, we feel that it is of utmost importance to be respectful of your readers' time and to tell stories and use examples that are concise, relatable, and not too far-fetched. Even a quick read for fun and laughs uses valuable time, something that seems to be in short supply for all physicians these days.

Permanence

Another important concept for the writer to acknowledge and master is the drive for "permanence." Once you write an idea down, it has the potential to last forever. The past can influence the future, but only if we can remember the past. Ideas taken from the Magna Charta and England's Bill of Rights were woven into the United States Constitution, and the only reason that was possible is because physical written evidence of those documents existed. So, remember that writing is first and foremost physical evidence. Make your piece as excellent as time and expediency allow. You never know who will read it decades down the road.

Procrastination...

Finally, there is the problem of procrastination. Early in our careers, we would perform elegant, thoughtful experiments and assemble complicated data sets and statistical analyses. And then we would sit stumped and stymied by the stark, shall we say, even bleak, challenge of an empty discussion section. Cathy Marcucci was once so flummoxed by what she had yet to write on a grant application that she resorted to distracting and comforting herself with online searches about writer's block, hoping to find answers and motivation. By far, her favorite has remained this gem from E.B. White (Fig. 12.1), the masterful writer of some of the best children's books ever written:

> Delay is natural to a writer. He is like a surfer – he bides his time, waits for the perfect wave on which to ride in. Delay is instinctive with him. He waits for the surge (of emotion? of strength? of courage?) that will carry him along.

These are reassuring words for any writer. If procrastination plagued a giant like E.B. White, why would lesser mortals think they could escape unscathed? No, it's best to just accept and plan for it as a natural occurrence and hazard and not fight against the tide more than necessary.

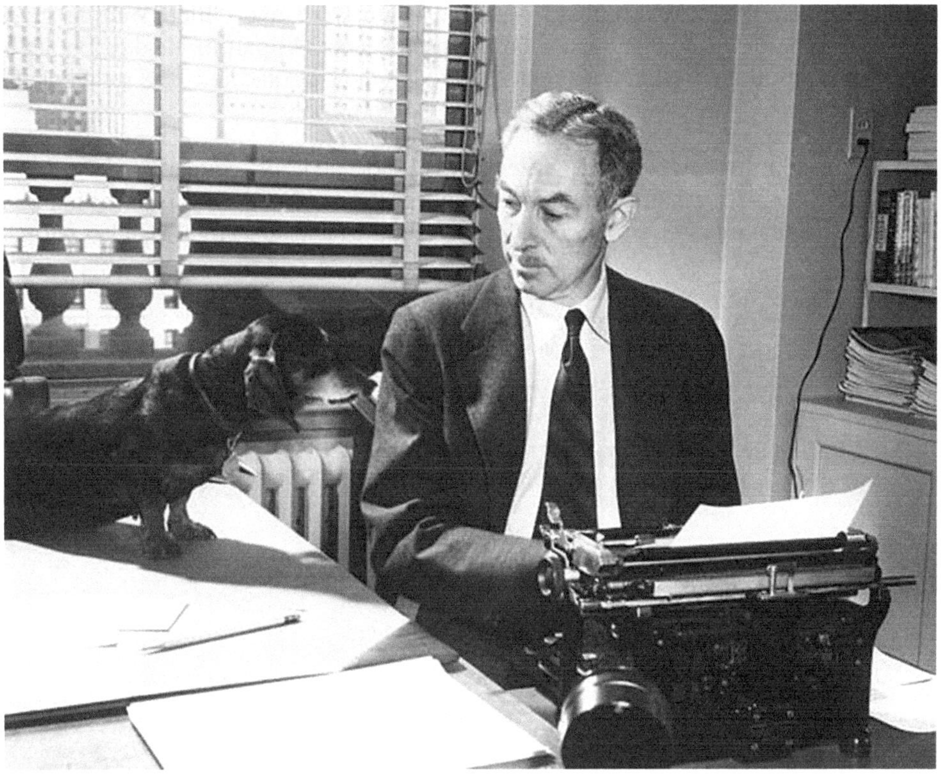

Fig. 12.1 E.B. White at the typewriter. "Andy" wrote essays, the news, magazine articles, literary criticism, poems, and the immortal classics *Stuart Little* and *Charlotte's Web*. Photo: Image purchased by Catherine Marcucci

Lessons Learned

Courtesy of Elwyn Brooks White, who would be turning 127 this year:

> Writers do not merely reflect and interpret life; they inform and shape life.
>
> Although there is no substitute for merit in writing, clarity comes closest.
>
> Use the smallest word that does the job.
>
> A writer has the duty to be good, not lousy; true, not false; lively, not dull; accurate, not full of error. He should tend to lift people up, not lower them down.
>
> The best writing is rewriting.

Authors

Olivia Liao is a college and liberal arts student at CMU. She is a multiple published author who has enjoyed story telling for as long as she can remember. She likes to read in between college courses, other literary work, and sleep, and it's rare that she's seen without a book in hand. Currently, her favorite genre is mystery, and she's partial to any story involving ghosts or written by Jonathan Stroud. Her first novel is titled *The Enemy of My Enemy Is My Step-Sibling* and is for sale on Amazon.

Ray Graber enjoys the writing process and finds it to be a great creative outlet. Writing gives him a chance to really nail down what he knows, and that makes him a better teacher. As part of his day job, he has spent a lot of time writing educational material for his residents rotating through their cardiac and TEE rotations. Ray has benefited from collaboration with multiple authors during the production of this book.

Cathy Marcucci has been a lifelong reader, writer, and editor and, of course, a fan of fellow Cornellian E.B. White. Rumor has it that she lived in the same dorm suite that Andy White had roomed in 58 years earlier. The *Wind in the Willows* by Kenneth Grahame and *Bleak House* by Charles Dickens are also in her permanent library.

13 There Is Magic Everywhere, So Write What You Can

Olivia Liao and Catherine Marcucci

Introduction

Cathy Marcucci's academic anesthesiology career tilted a bit when she had her children. In her early married days, she did the typical Johns Hopkins junior faculty program—fellowship, then instructor, then assistant professor. She had the good fortune to work in Brett Simon's lab, and he wrote an incredible RO1 grant proposal that was accepted on their first application. A major paper in the *Journal of Applied Physiology* followed and then several smaller papers, which were also well received.

From Cathy: Life and Luck Happen

But then it was four years and two kids later. I transferred to the Baltimore VA, which provided rewarding clinical work and my desired work-life balance, but what to do for academic satisfaction? I didn't want to go from Hopkins to no academic output whatsoever. Plus, I firmly believe that if you care about your patients and colleagues, you have to leave your medical specialty better than you found it. But full-time clinical physicians in the VA system generally don't have protected research time and, by official policy, can't hold the extramural funding that requires it.

Fortunately, I was lucky again, on two counts. First, my husband's boss had once mentioned to him that every single major advancement in his own distinguished career was directly traceable to something that he had written, and Neil passed that mentoring advice onto me. So, I doubled down on my determination to let go of a career that involved traveling and speaking but to keep writing, if at all possible.

O. Liao
Carnegie Mellon University, Pittsburgh, PA, USA

C. Marcucci (✉)
Department of Transfusion Medicine, Clinical Center, National Institutes of Health, Bethesda, MD, USA

S. Mohamed et al. (eds.), *Anesthesia Bridges*, https://doi.org/10.1007/978-3-032-08294-7_13

Eyes Open!

Second, **Denny Bourke** was the chief of anesthesia services at the VA at that time. Denny was endlessly knowledgeable and supportive in teaching me how to keep my eyes open and take something interesting and unusual that happened in the OR and translate it into a concise short article or case report—first and foremost by assuming that if it was a subject that we hadn't previously seen and needed to read up on, everybody else would as well. We accepted that we weren't doing major manuscripts for the top basic science journals, but we were going to write what was accessible and available to us and publish clinically relevant pieces in the top anesthesiology journals. I was to find that this would be an equally valuable and satisfying way to do an "academic" career.

Denny's next maxim was to always remember that you have to answer the reader's most basic question—why should I take this particular minute of my valuable time to read this? He especially pushed me to develop manuscripts when I had a really great illustration or picture as the lead-in to the case report or letter. It was also in those early years at the Baltimore VA that I learned how to do multi-disciplinary publishing projects. If our clinical event had a cardiology slant to it, we just called up the cardiologists and asked if someone would be interested in reviewing and helping for a decent spot in the author list. They always were.

And if you finish your manuscripts and give people a fair stake in the credit, pretty soon you won't have to look that hard for interesting material—and so we were all too happy to write up the interesting patients that both of our preoperative nurse practitioners made us aware of. I repeated this process over and over, and it eventually expanded into my being the developer and the lead editor of the *Avoiding Common Errors in Anesthesia* and *A Case Approach to Perioperative Drug-Drug Interactions* books.

And Then....

But even more interesting is what happened in late 2019 when I was interviewing at the National Institutes of Health. Background—in 2006, I was taking over a case at the Baltimore VA when the anesthesiologist signing out said, "Don't use that unit of plasma, I refused it. It's going back to the blood bank to be trashed. Looks like pea soup—bacterial contamination." I thought, hey, wait, do we know that for sure? Denny walked over with his camera to take a picture, of course.

I carried that picture around for months, then decided to write it up, because it turns out that those units of green plasma are almost always okay to use. By this time, I was at the Philadelphia VA, and since it was a blood bank paper, I decided that we needed a blood bank author. My coauthor said to me, "You can't just call up the Penn-Jersey Red Cross, they're not going to help us with a manuscript." And I said, "Oh yes, we can call them and, yes, they will help us." And they did. A little Letter to the Editor titled "Green Plasma—Revisited" was duly published in *Anesthesiology* [1]. And we also had fun publishing a second transfusion medicine paper in a different journal.

So, 11 years later, I was down interviewing at the National Institutes of Health and one of the people I spoke to said, "Your CV came across my desk last week and I said to my colleagues, I know who this is. Because we've taught the fellows the material in your green plasma letter for years – see, here it is on my desktop in a 2012 folder."

You could have knocked me over with a feather. Talk about "magic everywhere!" I was simply dumbfounded that the NIH had found it and archived it for teaching. The interviewer laughed a bit and went on with the interview, and the manuscript wasn't mentioned for the rest of the interview day. I got that job offer, and I will always have the unshakeable belief that those 800 words, on something that had crossed my path for a minute in a routine sign-out more than a decade prior, were part of the reason why.

Lessons Learned

- Write whatever and whenever you can!
- Don't dismiss your own ideas because the people around you aren't as interested or motivated as you are. There is always going to be someone out there in the wider community who can benefit from reading your findings.
- On the flip side, it's also important to keep the intended audience's interests and available time in mind so they stay engaged. A great picture helps.
- Remember that what you are writing now can create great opportunities for future collaborations.

Reference

1. Elkassabany NM, Meny GM, Doria RR, et al. Green plasma – revisited. Anesthesiology. 2008;108(4):764–5.

Authors

Olivia Liao is a college student at CMU. Her first novel is titled *The Enemy of My Enemy Is My Step-Sibling* and is for sale on Amazon. She is also an accomplished violinist and is a competitive fencer. In her rare free time, she is an inveterate film buff and has set herself the goal of seeing every important movie ever made.

Cathy Marcucci is an academic anesthesiologist and anesthesia textbook author and editor. She loves nothing more than collaborating and networking on anesthesia writing projects and has been on the lookout for publishable material for 35+ years.

How It Began, Where It Went

14

Denis L. Bourke, Olivia Liao, and Catherine Marcucci

How It Began

When I first started my anesthesiology residency at the University of Pennsylvania in 1970, I had no ambition of staying in academic medicine. I very soon discovered that practically every fourth patient at Penn was enrolled in one study or another. Some of the studies were extensive and complicated, while others were simple and were directed at answering questions that came up in daily practice. It wasn't long before I began to develop ideas for clinical studies of my own.

In the early 1970s, the concept of hemodilution in clinical practice was just starting to garner interest. The practicality of hemodilution at that time was somewhat difficult inasmuch as real-time access to hemoglobin and hematocrit values was not always available. I decided to run around the operating rooms collecting blood samples and data on estimated blood volumes, estimated blood loss, and crystalloid and colloid fluids administered in hopes of developing a table or graph that might guide others during hemodilution.

Ultimately, I collected about 100 data sets from approximately 30 patients and put the information into tabular and graphic form to distribute to the other residents and staff. When I showed my work to my mentor, Ted Smith, he suggested I develop a formula based on the data. I was surprised that I hadn't thought of the idea, but that is what mentors are for. With my math background and master's degree, it wasn't very difficult to set up a differential equation that theoretically described hemodilution and very closely fit my data. This resulted in my first published paper [1].

Where It Went

I think this first simple clinical study spurred me to spend the rest of my career in academic medicine. I've always encouraged residents and other staff to pursue interesting incidents in and around the operating room. I think I've been fortunate to be able to encourage others to think more about some of the

D. L. Bourke
Anesthesia Services, Baltimore VA Medical Center, Baltimore, MD, USA

Department of Anesthesiology, University of Maryland, Baltimore, MD, USA

O. Liao
Carnegie Mellon University, Pittsburgh, PA, USA

C. Marcucci (✉)
Department of Transfusion Medicine, Clinical Center, National Institutes of Health, Bethesda, MD, USA

S. Mohamed et al. (eds.), *Anesthesia Bridges*, https://doi.org/10.1007/978-3-032-08294-7_14

interesting occurrences in our daily practice. Of course, this has benefited me by becoming a coauthor of publications that I was able to encourage others to pursue. More importantly, I hope I have been able to successfully encourage many of my residents to pursue academic careers.

An interesting coincidence, similar to Cathy Marcucci's, occurred while I was on the staff at Johns Hopkins: The blood bank director asked me to participate in a study of immediate preoperative hemodilution blood salvage for re-transfusion during or after surgery. The blood bank director's fellow, who planned to participate in this study, spoke up and said, "It won't be hard, you can predict what the results will be. Here's an article with a differential equation." She then handed me a copy of my article from 25 years before—without realizing that I was the author.

Lessons Learned

- Your goals and ambitions can change. The expectations you have going into a situation can be vastly different by the time you come out of it, and that's okay. That first "mathematics" anesthesiology paper that I published was built on skills that I already had, but led to an entire career.
- Keep your eyes open! Taking notice of the patterns and information that you see around you now can lead to big things in the future.
- Discussing your ideas with your colleagues and mentors is always beneficial because they can bring things and ideas to light that you hadn't thought about at first. Helping you develop publishing content is the sign of a great mentor.

Reference

1. Bourke DL, Smith TC. Estimating allowable hemodilution. Anesthesiology. 1974;41:609–12.

Authors

Denny Bourke lives in the Baltimore area with his wife Connie, an accomplished writer and editor in her own right. He received his MA in mathematics from the University of Michigan before segueing into a medical career. He did his anesthesiology training at the University of Pennsylvania and was on faculty at the University of Pennsylvania, Tufts University, University of Texas, Boston University, Johns Hopkins University, and University of Maryland/Baltimore VAMC, where he published over 170 manuscripts. He considers his mentoring relationships with dozens of junior physicians in multiple specialties to be among his greatest accomplishments.

Olivia Liao is currently studying literary arts, linguistics, and liberal arts at Carnegie Mellon University. She recently published her first novel, a superhero fantasy adventure story that has been very well received by readers of that genre. She's grateful for the opportunity to collaborate with knowledgeable academic writers from the medical field.

Cathy Marcucci worked for Denny Bourke as a resident at Hopkins and then again as a staff anesthesiologist and faculty at the Baltimore VA and the University of Maryland Department of Anesthesiology. Dr. Bourke remains one of her most esteemed anesthesia colleagues and personal friends. Their collaborative articles and case reports are her favorite publications.

A Minute Is Measured by Which Side of the Bathroom Door You Are On

15

Amr E. Abouleish

Introduction

Knowing how to distract someone is not only essential for a magician but it is also a great skill for everyone. Parents use distraction therapy when on trips or in line with their kids. Physicians use distraction therapy when doing procedures. And anesthesiologists use distraction therapy clinically during inhalational induction in children … and when the resident does not turn off the anesthetic gas early enough. We use distraction therapy on the surgeons and the OR staff, so they don't appreciate how long it is taking to wake the patient up. I've always said that is why a good anesthesiologist has to be able to tell jokes!

In fact, here is one of my favorite jokes:

> Back in the early 1700s, a treasure ship was on its way back to port. The crew on deck yelled, "Captain, Captain, come up here." The captain, who was in his cabin, runs up to the deck. He pulls out his spyglass and looks out where the crew is pointing. He sees one pirate ship approaching.
>
> "Captain, Captain, what do we do?" asked the first mate. "First mate," said the captain, "go to my cabin, open my sea chest, and bring me my red shirt." The first mate did so.
>
> Wearing his bright red shirt, the captain exhorted his crew to fight. So inspiring was he, in fact, that the pirate ship was repelled without casualties.
>
> A few days later, the ship was again approached, and the same thing happens.
>
> "Captain, Captain, come up here." The captain, who was in his cabin, runs up to the deck. Pulls out his spyglass and looks out where the crew is pointing. He sees **three** pirate ships approaching.
>
> "Captain, captain, what should we do?" "First mate," said the captain, "go to my cabin, open my sea chest, and bring me my red shirt."
>
> Wearing his bright red shirt, the captain exhorted his crew to fight. So inspiring was he, in fact, that the pirate ships were repelled without casualties.

A. E. Abouleish (✉)
Department of Anesthesiology, The University of Texas Medical Branch, Galveston, TX, USA
e-mail: aabouleí@UTMB.EDU

S. Mohamed et al. (eds.), *Anesthesia Bridges*, https://doi.org/10.1007/978-3-032-08294-7_15

The next day, the first mate asked the captain the secret of his bright red shirt.

"It's simple, first mate. If I am wounded, the blood does not show, and the crew continues to fight without fear."

A week passed, and they were nearing their home port, when the same thing happens again.

"Captain, Captain, come up here." The captain, who was in his cabin, runs up to the deck. Pulls out his spyglass and looks out where the crew is pointing. He sees TEN pirate ships approaching.

"Captain, captain, what should we do?" "First mate," said the captain, "go to my cabin, open my sea chest, and bring me my brown pants."

Lessons Learned

- Humor can be a useful tool. It can help build relationships and can be used clinically in the right situation.
- And we wouldn't be surprised if, after the publication of this book, "bring me my brown pants" becomes a clinical anesthesia meme when the situation in the OR starts to get really dicey……

***Note from the Editors:** Amr Abouleish and Sharif Mohammed gave us a short list of their favorite bridges. The beautiful Stanley Bridge in Egypt was on it (Fig. 15.1).

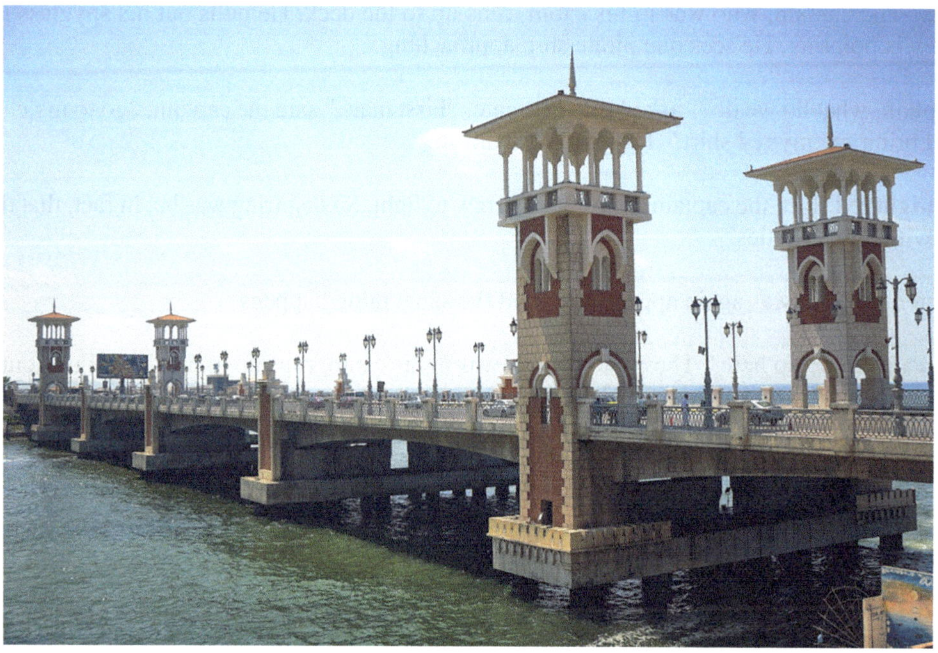

Fig. 15.1 The Stanley Bridge in Alexandria, Egypt. This stunning structure is the first Egyptian bridge to be built over the sea. It was constructed in the late 1990s over Stanley Bay in Alexandria as part of the reconstruction and decoration of the beach area of this beautiful and historic Mediterranean Sea city. It is anchored by four exquisite towers in the Islamic style and carries vehicular and pedestrian traffic. Photo: Image used under standard license from Shutterstock.com

Author

Amr Abouleish joined UTMB Galveston in 1993 as the first chief of pediatric anesthesiology. His motto for teaching pediatric anesthesia to residents is "every month is July!" He is also a national speaker on economics in healthcare, especially for anesthesiology departments.

How to Give Feedback and Have Difficult Conversations

16

Catherine Marcucci, Neil B. Sandson, and Sharon L. Milgram

Introduction

Anesthesiologists receive continual feedback at every level of training and experience. Whether the feedback is from a supervisor, physician peer, junior trainee, patient, or patient's family, you will receive a constant stream of information concerning what you did or did not do and with what level of competence, skill, and dexterity. The information below is presented largely from the viewpoint of supervisory feedback—giving and receiving—but the principles are applicable to a variety of situations.

Types of Feedback

But first, what is "feedback?" Of course, it's simply the process of giving specific information about a person's current behavior. That's universally understood. What isn't as well understood is how to do it well.

There are generally four types of feedback. The easiest, and most fun, is feedback given in appreciation of a personal trait or performance. This type of feedback is given to reinforce positive attributes or events and to elicit more of the same. The second type is coaching feedback. Because people generally have difficulty modifying their personal characteristics, what is sought with coaching is modification of behavior. It does not necessarily imply a negative to the person receiving the feedback, just that a change is desired. The third type is evaluation feedback and generally involves an assessment of current circumstances—"here's where you stand." The fourth type of feedback is the performance review. This is larger in scope than a simple evaluation and seeks to provide an overall assessment of standing and progress. This type of comprehensive feedback often has a balance of positive and negative features.

C. Marcucci (✉)
Department of Transfusion Medicine, Clinical Center, National Institutes of Health, Bethesda, MD, USA

N. B. Sandson
Department of Psychiatry, VA Maryland Health Care System, Baltimore, MD, USA

University of Maryland, Baltimore, MD, USA

S. L. Milgram
Office of Intramural Training and Education, National Institutes of Health, Bethesda, MD, USA

S. Mohamed et al. (eds.), *Anesthesia Bridges*, https://doi.org/10.1007/978-3-032-08294-7_16

- *Feedback is difficult to give.* Except for feedback given in appreciation, most people who have to provide feedback experience some difficulty doing it, at least at first. We want to be liked, even by the people we are supervising and evaluating. We often don't have a lot of practice at giving feedback and haven't had good role models for this skill. Also, it's hard to walk the line between commentary on personal vs. professional attributes.

- *Feedback is also difficult to receive.* There is a *lot* of psychic tension between wanting growth/development and acceptance in the person receiving feedback. It can stimulate distortions and projections in the person receiving feedback, and in extreme cases, it can be triggering/retraumatizing.

If and When to Give Feedback

A key question is how to decide when feedback is necessary. In general terms, the answer is when the *harm of not addressing the issue exceeds the harm of addressing it.* This applies to positive or reinforcing feedback as well as corrective feedback. Do you have a person in your system who has been going above and beyond expectations and is just about ready to toss it in due to a lack of recognition? Feedback is urgently needed. Is there a risk of imminent harm to the patients? Feedback is urgently needed and probably action as well. In less dire situations, an array of factors should be considered, though circumstances may require a more rapid calculation than would be ideal. Whenever possible, the decision to provide feedback should be made deliberately and calmly.

Before you start a feedback conversation, make sure that you, as the evaluator, are clear about your own biases, blind spots, and vulnerabilities. Have the circumstances impacted your own issues in a personal way? Are you seeking to redress a type of harm that was done to you at some previous point? These are situations in which somebody else should perhaps be giving the feedback. Otherwise, you may be entering conversations in which you may provide ineffective or even punitive feedback that has the potential to do greater harm than good.

Next, you must consider the "extenuating circumstances." The times being what they are, is the person receiving the feedback dealing with diagnosed or undiagnosed mental illness and/or substance use/abuse issues? Although these do not necessarily excuse behaviors and events, they may shed light on the explanations and reactions to the feedback. Has the person already taken self-corrective action? Although it is important to be aware that people generally have a limited ability to self-recognize a problem and self-correct. Is there regret and remorse?

Remember, feedback is ultimately about interface, building bridges, closing loops, and lighting the way (Fig. 16.1).

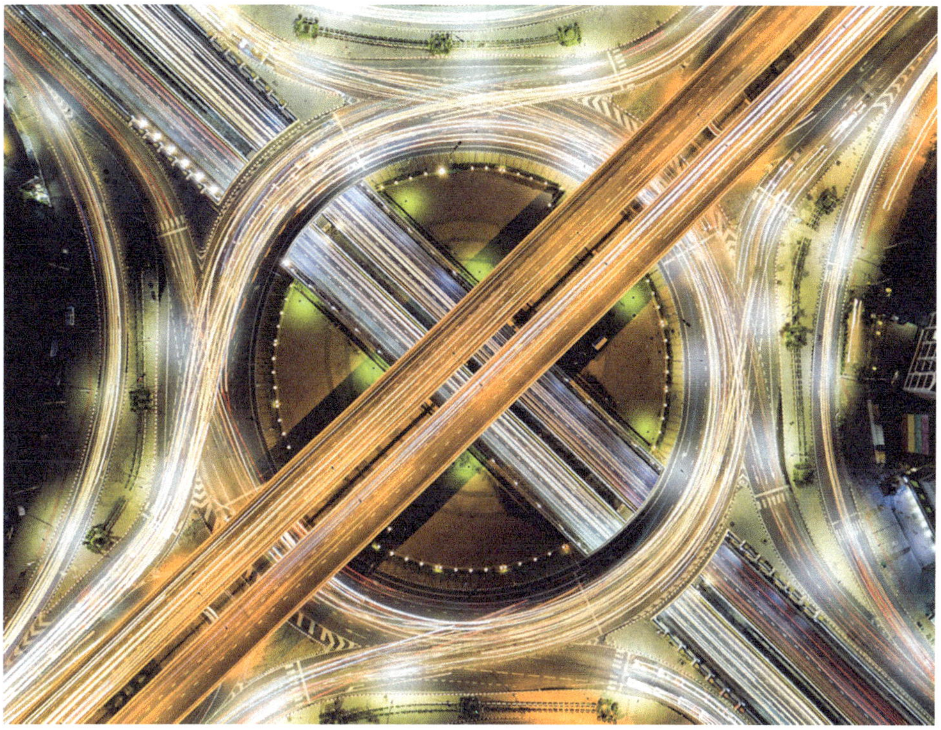

Fig. 16.1 A great illustration of the components of superlative feedback. Photo: Image used under standard license from stock.adobe.com

How to Give Feedback

To give effective, successful feedback, it is very important to strive for collaboration, even while acknowledging individual positions. Always use an approach that is based on an "us working together on a problem" as opposed to a "you did this bad thing" paradigm, unless/perhaps, you are firing the person. And it is *critical* that people giving feedback be able to monitor and moderate their own behavior in tense/emotional positions. If you think that you are going to get angry in a feedback conversation, don't have it then and there.

Remember that we are all storytellers! It is human nature to make assumptions about observed behaviors. Thoughts, emotions, and behaviors all occur in real-time, and we fill in the blanks (unknowns) in order to construct narratives regarding the connections between these things that make sense to ourselves. However, we are not always accurate when we come to such conclusions without consulting other involved parties. This is why mental health professionals are taught to simply say, "Can you help me understand why you did that?" Especially when opening a conversation about an incident of difficult or problematic behavior.

When you start the feedback, be aware that you will be discussing three points (past, present, and future) on the "event timeline" (Fig. 16.2). Strive to acquire the data and complete the conversation for each point of the timeline before moving on to the next. It is sometimes difficult to stay organized in your feedback discussion, as a stressed or upset person may purposely or involuntarily jump around the timeline during the discussion, but you must have a firm grip on the agenda of the feedback presentation to keep things on track. You are driving this bus.

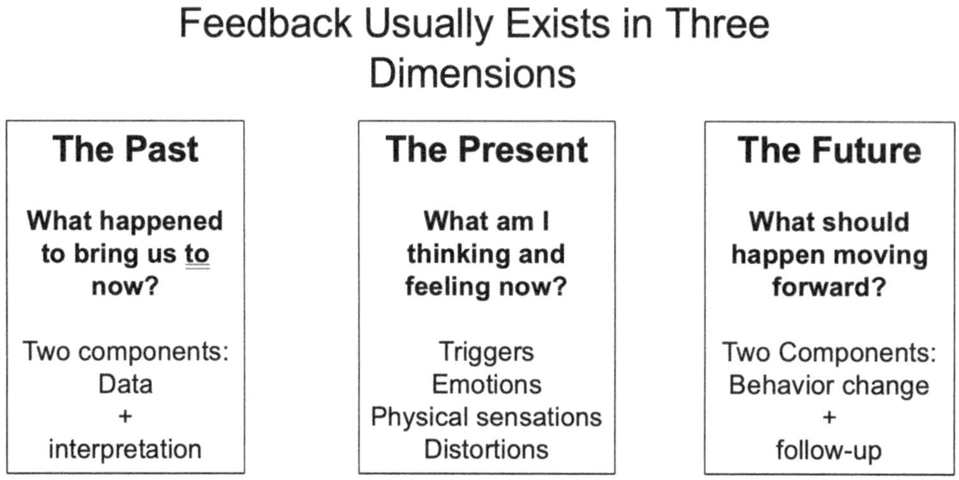

Fig. 16.2 Feedback concerns multiple points on an event timeline. Figure courtesy of Sharon Milgram

- When discussing the past in a feedback conversation—*ask, don't interpret*. Be specific in introducing past events to the conversation and be open to new information. Remember that you have likely already told yourself a story about what happened, and your internal story may be distorted due to your own assumptions and biases.

- When moving from a review of what happened to the present time, consider pausing and regrouping. If necessary, the rest of the feedback conversation can take place later. It's fine to give the other party notice of your current feelings as long as you are drawing on your highest level of emotional intelligence. They should also be given the chance to state their feelings as well.

- When discussing what should happen in the future, set specific dates/times/goals. Also acknowledge that feedback is stressful. During the feedback conversation, take several small steps to repair the relationship.

- At every step in a feedback conversation, focus on the behavior, not the person! Be specific and descriptive. Avoid over-statements like "always" and "never."

Examples

- *Poor feedback:* "You are always over-confident. It gets you and the patient in trouble all the time."

- *Better feedback:* "I've noticed that you often delay too long in calling me about a problem with the patient. Or you call me and tell me that you've got the situation under control, and then you miss the chance to get my help in time to make changes or interventions in the patient's anesthesia plan."

- *Poor feedback:* "Please be more professional next time you are working in the preop clinic."

- *Better feedback:* "I expect that you will wear khakis or dress pants and a button-down shirt or clean scrubs with a white coat on your preop center rotation. Also, please do not chew gum or stop to answer social media when seeing patients in the preop center."

- *Suboptimal feedback:* "Nice job on your talk!"

- *Better feedback:* "Your slides were clear and concise, you appeared poised and confident, you really handled the questions well, especially…."

And remember, metacommunication matters! There are many nonverbal and para-language cues that carry meaning and can either enhance or negate what we say in words. These include our tone of voice, body language, gestures, and facial expressions, whether we are on our phone, looking at our screen, reading while "listening," whether we sit down with someone or "talk down" to them, and whether we sit across a desk or next to them.

Of course, giving effective and successful feedback is part of successful management skills. Anesthesiologists who are superb clinicians often don't see themselves in a supervisory or management role. But consider that every time you staff a case with a trainee, you are essentially the CEO of that little anesthesia team. You may also need to give feedback to other members of the anesthesia care team, or to trainees/supervisees, if you are the program or fellowship director or running a department. As you become more senior and more experienced at giving feedback, hopefully you will develop a feedback culture in which feedback represents a valued opportunity rather than something to fear. What are some ways to do this?

- Talk about feedback as part of the "selection and orientation" process. Let your new people know how many times and when they will get feedback. Or, in the day-to-day setting, when you are discussing your cases the night before with your residents, you can say, "let's meet in the back corner of the PACU at the end of the day, and we'll debrief the cases for five minutes." Then keep it to five minutes!

- Give feedback often, especially at the outset.

- Make sure there's a healthy dose of appreciation and coaching feedback. Really look for reasons to give positive feedback, and this should be specific rather than general.

- Ask others for feedback on yourself—making it clear that feedback is being used as a tool for growth.

- *Never give feedback when you are angry or emotional.* Whatever you say can so easily be outweighed by the damage that will be done.

- Give feedback in private, with exceptions.

- Always give the chance for verbal feedback to accompany written evaluations or feedback.

- Most importantly, when others respond well to your feedback and successfully modify their behavior(s), provide explicit recognition and appreciation for their efforts in accomplishing this, thus creating an effective and positive feedback loop. This is the very opposite of a toxic work culture.

Bonus Content! Coauthor Sharon Milgram has graciously loaned the anesthesia community her template for statements that you can actually use (Fig. 16.3). Everybody should practice these from time to time!

General Scaffold For Difficult Conversations

State the purpose	To help us work together better, I wanted to talk about ..... I wanted to give you some feedback in the hopes that.... I feel we need to talk about....
Describe what you observed	"When you were.... , you ..... ; Yesterday I observed you..... When XXXX asked you to ..., you said ....
Describe the impact	"I was ..... ; I felt ...... ; As a result..... ; The samples.....
Give the individual time to ask questions and respond	Would you like to share your perspective on this? Is there anything you are not sure you agree with? Is there anything you want to add? Is there something I should know?
Ask for and offer specific suggestions	My strategy for dealing with XXX, is YYY. Perhaps.... Have you considered... Would you like help finding... Do you have any thoughts about... I want to encourage you to reach out to...
Summarize and express support	I think we agree.... I appreciate your effort in .... and know you will continue to improve.

Fig. 16.3 Suggestions for difficult conversations. Figure courtesy of Sharon Milgram

Lessons Learned

- Feedback is difficult to both give and receive.
- Understand clearly, when going into a feedback conversation, the type of feedback you are giving. Consider giving the smallest aliquot of feedback that gets your goal accomplished.
- The person receiving the feedback has rights! They deserve to be treated with dignity and respect, and a lack of excess emotion.
- Feedback should involve three points on the event timeline—what happened, what is the status/view/assessment of that event in the present, and what future plans or actions are necessary.
- Everything in the metacommunication space counts—tone of voice, choice of language and descriptors, body posture, even seating arrangement.
- Work hard to develop a constructive feedback culture. That includes yourself.
- We don't generally advocate for the technique of criticism sandwiches.
- We've included some specific phrases and statements to help you with your difficult conversations. Practicing them, even in front of a mirror, will help build your skills.

The *Anesthesia Bridges* editors thank Dr. Milgram for her generosity in loaning her lecture materials and slides for this chapter.

Authors

Cathy Marcucci is a senior anesthesiologist who has been known to be on the receiving end of a feedback conversation or two in her medical career, not to mention feedback from her kids about her parenting style. ☺ Her personal style when giving feedback tends to be warm and effusive. She *particularly* loves to write thank you notes to her authors and editors after finishing an anesthesia textbook project.

Neil Sandson is a psychiatrist at the University of Maryland and the VA Maryland Health Care System. He has been a clinical supervisor of physicians and other medical professionals, a training supervisor, and a physician educator for many years. He is a frequent consultant for the national anesthesia community. He lives in suburban Baltimore with his wife Cathy Marcucci, and has two young adult children.

Sharon Milgram is a cell biologist by training and the director of the Office of Intramural Training and Education at the National Institutes of Health. She is passionate about the development and delivery of career/professional development programs for students interested in biomedical, behavioral, and social science careers. Dr. Milgram is a sought-after speaker and educator on career management and mentoring for biomedical professionals. She lives with her wife in Silver Spring, MD.

More Wisdom on Communications

17

James K. Gilman, Amy J. Robbins, Ronald S. Bank, Neil B. Sandson, and Catherine Marcucci

Contributors:

Edwin G. Avery IV, MD (EGA)

Herbert Chen, MD

Mark J. Lema, MD PhD (MJL)

Sharon L. Milgram, PhD (SLM)

Neil B. Sandson, MD (NBS)

Joseph M. Schwartz, MD (JMS)

F. Jacob Seagull, PhD (FJS)

Grant Taylor, MD

Patricia M. Togioka, MA (PMT)

Disclaimer: Several of the contributors to this chapter are or were federal employees. The views expressed herein are solely the authors' own and do not represent the positions, official or otherwise, of the United States of America, the Department of the Army, the Department of Veterans Affairs, the Department of Health and Human Service, or the National Institutes of Health.

J. K. Gilman
Office of the Director, Clinical Center, National Institutes of Health (Retired), Adjunct Professor of Medicine, Uniformed Services University of the Health Sciences, Bethesda, MD, USA

A. J. Robbins
Stanson Health, a Premier Inc. Company, Charlotte, NC, USA

Atrium Health, Carolinas Palliative Care and Hospice Group, Charlotte, NC, USA

R. S. Bank
Department of Anesthesiology, INOVA Fairfax Hospital, UVA School of Medicine, INOVA Campus, Falls Church, VA, USA

N. B. Sandson
Department of Psychiatry, VA Maryland Health Care System, Baltimore, MD, USA

University of Maryland, Baltimore, MD, USA

C. Marcucci (✉)
Department of Transfusion Medicine, Clinical Center, National Institutes of Health, Bethesda, MD, USA

S. Mohamed et al. (eds.), *Anesthesia Bridges*, https://doi.org/10.1007/978-3-032-08294-7_17

Robert D. Togioka, MA

David A. Wallace, MD (DAW)

Charles J. Yeo, MD

Introduction

There is a constant need to communicate effectively and well with all of the constituents of the anesthesia service—patients, families, nurses, surgeons, and among ourselves. Rarely, however, do anesthesiologists receive much formal training in communication skills. Much of the wisdom below was learned, not so much the hard way, but perhaps we could say by trial and error. We hope that by passing on our wisdom, we speed your acquisition and deployment of top-notch communication skills.

General Wisdom

- I have never been in an organization where those at the grass roots level would say that there was really good communication. When leaders hear that they assume that there is a need for a better webpage or a better newsletter. They think they need more video productions and webcasts. They look for established methods of *broadcasting* information. My unproven hypothesis is that those who think the communication is poor want (more often than not) to know that someone *listens* to them. That IS a big problem for leaders because listening is often very inefficient, and staff members want to know that their individual voices are heard. Listening requires enormous amounts of energy but when leaders no longer have the energy to listen enough, they cease to lead.—**JKG**

- I avoided more medical errors by listening to nurses than by anything I learned in medical school, residency, or fellowship.—**JKG**

- There is a recognized skill set for active listening. First, encourage open communication. Then avoid judgment—show that you are open to hearing explanations and perspectives by stopping to listen and asking curious/clarifying questions. Validate others by showing appreciation for the other person's efforts to address an issue and affirm their feelings and give space for their emotional expressions.—**SLM**

- The best advice comes from Covey's original text on *The 7 Habits of Highly Effective People*—Seek to first understand and then be understood. We often try to drive our point home before realizing what is at the core of the issue.—**MJL**

- Jeff Kirsch told me once to always find a way to tell the truth.—**CM**

- Always do your best to provide a good letter of recommendation for a colleague who asks you for one but be honest with them about the strength of recommendation that you can provide.—**EA**

- Try to meet one new person in the hospital each day. Or if you can't manage that, try for one new person a week. Just introduce yourself to anybody—even if they don't introduce themselves back.

You can just say, "Hey, hi, I'm Jim Hernandez from anesthesia, nice to meet you," to the cashier in the cafeteria. All great physicians know the support staff—that's one thing that makes them great. Dr. Ezzat Abouleish, who is featured in Chap. 5 was known for being able to say hello by name to everybody in the hospital.—**Editors**

- Once, when I was still at Hopkins and walking over to Wilmer to do a quick case on call, I saw the late legendary physician and geneticist Victor McKusik leaning on the counter of the parking attendant, his briefcase on the floor, in deep conversation with the person manning the parking desk. When I finished the case and walked back, Dr. McKusik was still talking with the garage attendant. They were so engrossed in their conversation that neither person even glanced at me.—**CM**

- Another time I was standing in line in the coffee shop, and I saw Dr. Gilman, the CEO of the Clinical Center at the NIH, pause in the main hallway to speak to a federal police officer and then greet by name the next four people that walked by. But you can also seek people out. For instance, just walk over to the office of a surgeon that you work with and spend 30 seconds saying hello to their office staff. That's all you have to do. Over the years, this will pay big dividends.—**CM**

***Note from the Editors**: Two of the most fascinating bridges in all of military history (and world history) were the WW II floating roadway bridges and harbors at Omaha Beach and Arromanches on the Normandy coast. They were temporary pontoon bridges, but traces of the bridges still remain (Fig. 17.1). The bridge at Omaha Beach was destroyed in a storm only days after it was erected but the bridge at Arromanches remained intact and within days was the ingress to one of the busiest shipping ports in the world.

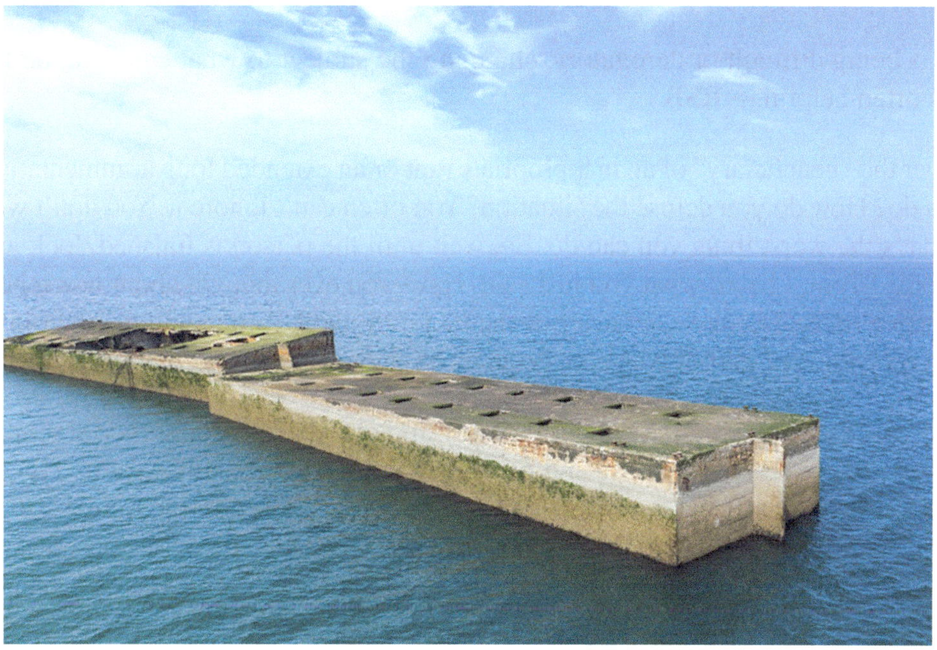

Fig. 17.1 Remnants of the floating roadway bridge in the English Channel at Arromanches on the Normandy Coast. Two bridges were designed by British engineers and constructed in 1943-44 in secrecy in separate locations in the United Kingdom. Up to 50,000 workers participated in the fabrication of the bridge and roadway sections, which were then towed to Normandy and were ten miles long when assembled. In the ten months after D-day, 2.5 million men, half a million vehicles, and 4 million tons of supplies drove across the roadway shown above and into France to supply Allied troops. Photo: Florent Martin, image used under standard license from iStock.com

- Two things that are not easy to do and can be liberating are to say, "*I don't know*" and "*I was wrong*." Then you can correct the deficit.—**DAW**

- Dave Wallace is correct! One day, when I was a resident, an attending tore into me for something I hadn't done. About thirty minutes later he came over to me and said simply, "Please accept my apologies for being testy and inappropriate." And I did and that was the end of that. That simple, sincere apology without an attempt to rationalize or justify insured that I never even held one molecule of a grudge against that person.—**CM**

- Practice finding ways and things to say to defuse tension, such as "I am looking to shed light here, not heat." "This feels a bit tricky to discuss because usually we are on the same side of most questions."—**Editors**

- Here is a way to approach the situation where you are getting pushback for being too fussy about an incremental lab value—"Yes, I understand that this seems like there isn't that much difference between a potassium of 2.9 and 3.2. And perhaps there isn't. But what I'm trying to do here is establish a safe clinical practice with a reasonable margin of safety."—**Editors**

- Here is something I've been thinking about. About five years ago, I noticed that a colleague never used the term "Down syndrome." He always said, "Trisomy 21." Finally, I asked him why. He reported that this was out of respect for and solidarity with his Asian colleagues who did not prefer to memorialize John Langdon Down as he was the first to introduce the term "mongoloid" to describe this disability. It should be noted that the World Health Organization still uses the term Down syndrome in its publications, as do national and international foundations that serve this community. But the use of medical eponyms is steadily going out of favor. Could it be time to retire this one and use the more medically descriptive term Trisomy 21? Just sayin'.—**CM**

- If someone is being difficult or derogatory, changing the subject to what can be done for this patient right now is often helpful.—**RSB**

- If you are ever the "beneficiary" of an inappropriate rant or an extended long argumentative monologue, what do you do? How do you defuse the situation? You often can't ignore it. You don't want to argue or rant back, that's the worst thing you can do. So, wait until the person is finished, look at them calmly, and say quietly, "Tom, I heard what you just said. Have you ever thought about law school?" Or say it to a third party who is also the beneficiary of the rant—"I think Tom would be great in a courtroom." Then just go on with your part of whatever needs to be said or done. This works, try it.—**Editors**

- Early in my career, I developed the habit of quickly and quietly reminding the surgeons of important information before the start of the case and have been thanked many times for it. This is even before the huddle. Or after the huddle. Or even after the drapes go up. It's a simple thing to quietly say, "Just to remind you, the patient's not under general anesthesia." Or while the surgeons are scrubbing, "Just wanted to remind you that the patient has hepatitis C and HIV." It's appreciated because it shows the surgeons that you care that they do not find themselves in an avoidable untoward situation.—**CM**

- Please be oh-so-careful about your email hygiene. There is a ubiquitous mantra that email never disappears and it's tempting to think, oh that's not going to happen to me, nobody is going to fish up my old emails. Everybody knows this and has heard this a million times. Nobody really believes it. *But we've seen it!* We are aware of a situation in which an email from eight years previously that stated (we are paraphrasing), "I come to work furious, and I leave work furious" was fished up and used to support a disciplinary action of "disruptive physician." It's best to practice defensive emailing—like defensive driving. Be safe and assume that others won't. Treat emails you create like a telegram—just the facts, as brief as possible. And no identifying patient information! No anger or negative emotions, *ever.* Just remember that this type of "telegram" can never just be crumpled up and tossed in the wastebasket.—**FJS and Editors**

- People in business are taught to make **NO** editorial comments about any aspect of an online meeting until *the meeting is over*, meaning the screen-is-dark-over, or they are in another room. And untoward comments get made as frequently before the meeting starts as during and after the meeting. Everybody thinks they are in full control of their mute button, and everybody has slipped up at least once.—**Editors**

- It's sometimes said that it's not possible to overcommunicate. This is not true. When the volume of communication displaces the ability to act in the service of what is being communicated, then it has become excessive. Over-redundancy can be disruptive to individuals and derail efficient system operations.—**NBS**

- Consider clearing your email inbox every 24 hours. Even if you email back and say that the email was received, and a longer response is coming in the next day. Because don't you yourself dislike it when you send an email and then don't get a response?—**Editors**

- Consider also using the same form of address and signature for all email correspondence. We've noticed the surgeons do this. They tend to sign their emails with their initials above their formal signature block. This way the "tone" of an email is kept neutral and even, regardless of who he recipient is. Everybody gets the same courteous greeting and sign off, which is a good thing and causes less trouble over time.—**Editors**

- Always use closed loop communication for important events such as giving heparin, protamine, etc.—**RSB**

- There are six basic human emotions—*happy, sad, angry, fearful, disgusted, and surprised.* Humans can recognize these emotions in others based on a variety of static and dynamic facial expressions. It seems that observers focus on specific facial domains for each emotion. For example, in one study, the eye region was looked at earlier and longer for angry and sad faces; the mouth region, for happy faces; and the nose/cheek region, for disgusted faces; the eye and the mouth regions attracted attention in a more balanced manner for surprise and fear [1]. Humans can also register and recognize tiny changes in facial expressions and positions—on the order of millimeters. When listening to and speaking with others, it is critical that you be aware of the amount of information that is telegraphed by your body language and face. Your non-verbal communication is as important as what you are saying.—**Editors**

- Several of the editors have practiced in the VA Health Care System where there are lots of veterans on staff. Those staff people use "spelling alphabets" constantly. They are sometimes also called phonetic alphabets—for our purposes these terms are interchangeable because we are not radio or military communications experts. By whatever name, these alphabets are good policy for all OR and ICU staff as these are noisy places (see below).—**Editors**

- The history of spelling alphabets is fascinating. The first spelling alphabets were developed in English. British signal operators used a partial rudimentary spelling alphabet in the very late 1890s. The first true complete spelling alphabets were used when the first wired (early telephone) networks were built, just over 100 years ago. They were further developed for two-way radio use by the military and have been in ubiquitous military use since then. Various national militaries had their own alphabets and sometimes different branches of the same military had unique alphabets. After World War II, there was a concerted research and institutional effort to study and standardize a "universal" spelling alphabet.—**Editors**

- The alphabet below is the one used at present by NATO, the US Federal Aviation Administration, and the International Amateur Radio Union. As global distances decrease and linguistic diversity in every country increases there have been articles and editorials calling for the next major update. Consider that the word "Lima" also is the word for "five" in Tagalog (Philippines), which is similar to the word "rima," which means five in both Seediq (Taiwan) and Maori. These are all similar to the word "dimy" which means five in Malagasy (Madagascar). Research and revisions are surely coming, but for now, the most common standardized spelling alphabet is below.—**Editors**

A: Alfa	N: November
B: Bravo	O: Oscar
C: Charlie	P: Papa
D: Delta	Q: Quebec
E: Echo	R: Romeo
F: Foxtrot	S: Sierra
G: Golf	T: Tango
H: Hotel	U: Uniform
I: India	V: Victor
J: Juliett	W: Whiskey
K: Kilo	X: X-ray
L: Lima	Y: Yankee
M: Mike	Z: Zulu

- In some ways, good communication is really an act of empathy. Of course, you must be clear, but that's where your communication efforts start, not end. Because you should also always keep in mind what your listener or recipient might need to receive the communication to the fullest benefit. Do you as the messenger need to either include or dispense with jargon? Do you need to adjust for educational level or provide examples? Does your listener need a certain tone in your voice? Do they need to receive the communication in person? Do they need a smile? Do they need a certain measured pace to the communication or some preliminary explanation? Does the communication need to be repeated and if so, how many times? Do they need to reply and, if so, how much time do they need to make that reply? And remember, what your listeners need to best receive and understand the communication is their determination to make, not yours.—**NBS**

- What about “criticism sandwiches”—a feedback style that involves giving praise, then criticism, then praise? It was all the rage and taught in business schools and management courses a while back. Honestly? We are not completely sold on this technique as a blanket or universal approach. Criticism sandwiches can feel gimmicky—too forced—and muddy the message. Most individuals hear only the good or only the bad. This is because all or none thinking is basic human nature in times of stress. Criticism sandwiches can come off as inauthentic and a bit of a mind game when the feedback giver is frustrated, upset, or angry and the “praise” is mild or vague. It is human nature to be resistant and resentful to “being played.” Criticism sandwiches are difficult to reframe as a connection to the future. You’ve told the person a lot about what you think of them, but not much about the way forward.—**SLM and Editors**

- That said, there may be some utility to the criticism technique—good/bad/good—as part of a strengths-based approach for more complex situations, like a debrief after a big event or sitting down with your mentor for a major review of your long-term career plan when things are going reasonably well.—**Editors**

- As a practicing psychiatrist, I am always amazed at how professionals and other educated and high-functioning people think so carefully and strategically about their workplace communication style yet so utterly let go of all communication principles and finesse when interacting with the people at home and in their close personal circles. Those people deserve the exact same, or better, communication courtesies as those you give to your colleagues, patients, and patients’ families.—**NBS**

- The most important communication is with yourself. Practice extreme self-awareness. Force yourself to look straight at situations, including your problems, and tell yourself the truth about what is going on and, even more important, how you feel about what is going on.—**Editors**

- Don’t use sarcasm, ever. It is a terrible reflection on the person who uses it. First, it’s so rude. Second, it’s not very clever, being nothing more than a clumsy attempt at an interpersonal verbal power play. You will accomplish nothing more than marking yourself as a narcissistic jerk.—**Editors**

- Don’t swear! At least until you are in your car on your way home.—**Editors**

*__Note from the Editors:__ Another of the world’s most fascinating bridges is the Pont Neuf or “New Bridge” in Paris (Fig. 17.2). Despite the name, which arose because it replaced older wooden structures, it is the oldest standing stone bridge in Paris. Work on the bridge commenced in 1578, although the bridge was not opened until 1607, the difficult times being what they were. It has undergone several extensive refurbishments in the ensuing centuries.

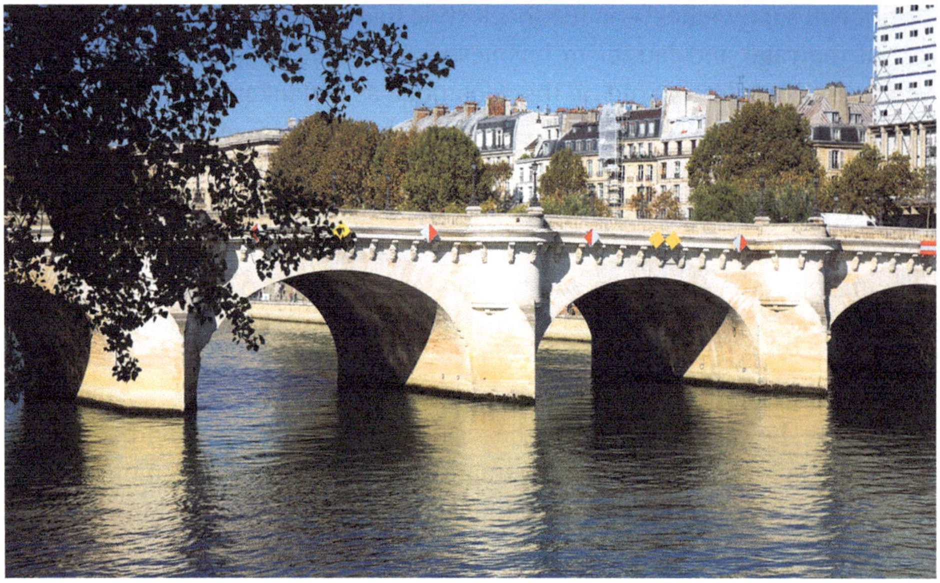

Fig. 17.2 The Pont Neuf in Paris. It is a two-span bridge with 12 stone arches and is a Paris landmark. The bridge was cutting-edge for its time, as it was one of the first European bridges built with the spans at a slight angle to each other to better withstand the dynamics of the river flow. Also, it was one of the first bridges to be built without houses on the spans and had pedestrian lanes designed into the roadway as part of the original design. The bridge is famous for the hundreds of *mascarons*, or stone masks that decorate the sides of the bridge. The originals of these masks were removed when the bridge was rehabbed in the 1850s, today's *mascarons* are exact copies. Photo: Image used under standard license from shutterstock.com

- I am not a huge fan of the "elevator pitch." Junior folks are taught, even exhorted to write, and practice a 30–60 second sales pitch involving an introduction, ask, and close. When I am asked about them or for help in developing one, I tell trainees if they don't feel they want to do this or wouldn't be good at it, then not to bother or feel guilty about it. Artfully delivered, elevator pitches can be okay, but often they are *not* artfully delivered. Think about it—there are dozens of dimensions along which you need to titrate your abilities and approaches, such as vocal tone, emotional tone, level of conciseness or expansiveness, listening vs talking. To me, the elevator pitch represents a particularly trendy and gimmicky formulation of directness and conciseness and faux interpersonal connection. Remember, if you are talking during that elevator ride, you are not listening. If you have 30 s to meet with someone new, a nice thing to do is introduce yourself simply and politely and then pause and find out a little bit about the person you are speaking with. Basically, just the manners you were taught early in life.—**NBS**

- Business consultant and coach Dorothea Hendricks writes the following cautionary words in an online article entitled *Ditch the Elevator Pitch: "Name one person who likes to be talked at, dumped on, bombarded with information, and sold to*."—**Editors**

- I met *Anesthesia Bridges* author Logan Olson when I got into an Uber at the zoo—not joking. I said, "Do you like being a ride share driver and how did you get into this line of work?" He replied that *actually* he was the PharmD for one of the ICUs at the university hospital and was doing some ride-share driving to pay off student loans before the birth of his first baby. We struck a deal during that 15 minutes ride to collaborate on some projects! This all happened because I asked about him instead of talking about myself.—**CM**

- One of the most effective communicators I have seen was somebody I just met this past weekend in a social setting. This person was actually quite quiet—he only said maybe 30 words every hour, but I was struck that every comment he made was either to offer a pithy observation that got right to the heart of the subject under discussion or was hysterically funny. There was such value to every single word he said. It's a great standard for *everybody* to strive for.—**NBS**

- It's been said that email and texting are over-used, but we actually think they are under-used. Use them both to always report and document your tasks and targets in writing. Don't believe or trust or stake your safety on a verbal communication. Ask people to send you emails with follow-up details and deadlines.—**Editors**

- Create an incontrovertible record of the communications you receive and make when on call from home. Several years ago, a not-very-professional physician colleague tried to slam one of us and transfer blame about a patient who had not done well. This physician tried to create a narrative that it had taken over an hour to make the necessary phone calls, talk to the team, and give the order. Nope. Not allowing that accusation to stand. It took 8 minutes. There was a preserved log of the time-stamped phone calls—happy to type it up and circulate to her boss, the medical staff office, and the QA and Trigger Tool groups if everybody would find that helpful.—**Editors**

- Give as many talks as you can. But try to make them as practiced and professional as possible. Videos always work well in a talk if they are not too long. Be careful about using audience queries, though, as some people find them annoying. Always, always, always do a full-dress rehearsal and time yourself. It is better to have a talk that is five minutes too short than five minutes too long.—**Editors**

- Think carefully about who you are representing when you give a talk. Is it just yourself? Or are you officially or unofficially representing your department—such as presenting at a symposium your department is hosting or a QA proceeding of any type? Invest a bit of extra time if it is the later. You don't want to fluff it if you are acting as the voice of your group.—**Editors**

- Similarly, if you are a trainee who is giving a talk to the senior physicians, work hard on that. It's your first chance to present yourself to the faculty as one of them and you also want to make your mentor for the talk look good. You might not hurt your young career if it doesn't go well, but you can certainly help it if it does. The faculty tends to remember who the good presenters are and this gets mentioned in formal and informal references.—**Editors**

- In this day and age, gentle humor, a cartoon, or one or two personal pictures is acceptable and even welcomed in a talk.—**Editors**

- If you don't have your own data to present, look for opportunities to give seminar-style talks on a subject that interests you. Try to write seminar-style talks such that they can be given or easily adapted to be given at least three times.—**Editors**

Special Topic 1—Conferring and Communicating With the Surgeons

- We want to tread a bit lightly here. But to start this topic, it bears stating—it's sometimes said that we are at the mercy of the surgeons. However, it's also true that they are at our mercy as well. It must cause anxiety to know that you can do the most successful and technically elegant surgery, but if the patient is cold and vomiting and under-resuscitated and in pain, on some level the family is always going to feel that the surgery didn't go that well—when actually it was the anesthetic plan that didn't go well.—**Editors**

- The operating room can be a place of conflict. You might as well just acknowledge this and so start to get to work on the problem. This is because, at least in the US, there are two independent services sharing the primary care of the patient. It's been said that there are a minimum of four conflicts or points of disagreement occurring during each surgery—not that every conflict becomes a tense stand-off or a full argument.—**Editors**

- We use the airplane analogy. Co-sharing the care of the patient is like having two large airplanes tethered together and trying to fly in parallel. Each airplane has the power to crash the other. To make it more challenging, the anesthesia airplane takes off several minutes before and lands several minutes later than the surgical airplane.—**Editors**

- Do not make the mistake of placing all the responsibility for conflict on the surgeons! There are other services directly or indirectly present in an operating room—nursing staff, other technical staff, the room turnover staff, and the blood bank and pathology staff. Conflict often happens within the members of a team, as well.—**Editors**

- Get to know your surgeons, get to know their family relationships and their interests. Common and familiar chit chat in the OR operating room can help to build trust when you know your surgeon and you know the situation and you know the personality better. Always try, if they are willing, to develop a rapport —that can only strengthen your relationship when it comes to dealing with patient care when you are picking your battles.—**AJR**

- We are in total agreement with Amy Robbins above. As stated above, the OR environment is a set-up for conflict. The trick is to not let differences in opinion about clinical care develop into longitudinal relationship conflict.—**Editors**

- Over the years, a number of surgeons have confided in us that they are more aware of what is going on with the anesthesia team than we might think. We are not just the nameless, faceless "anesthesia" people. They often know who the really, really good anesthesiologists are and who the merely-okay-good people are. They feel far better walking into an OR when the know the attending anesthesiologist and at least recognize the anesthesia resident. They understand, of course, that this doesn't always happen in a large teaching hospital, but it's what they prefer. And they really don't like at all to see or even get the sense that there is tension and disagreement on the anesthesia team.—**Editors**

- We know a senior surgeon who cheerfully refers to the surgical drapes as the "other blood-brain barrier." You have to respect the surgeons for a willingness to poke a little fun at themselves.—**Editors**

- It's also "incredibly important" to the surgeons that the anesthesiologist has some notion of the operation, the anticipated blood loss, and the particularly difficult elements of the surgery. They don't mind us looking over the drapes at all. They are somewhat concerned about it when we don't.—**Editors**

- Ever wondered what the surgeons exactly and precisely want? Ask them! We did a little survey and asked several people that we know well. The pretty simple and easy answers came back right away:

  - From **Herb Chen**—chair of surgery at UAB. Things I want from my anesthesiologist:

    - *ON* time start
    - Deep extubation to minimize cough (to reduce the chance of hematoma)
    - Parathyroid hormone draws at 5, 10, and 15 minutes
    - Fun OR day

  - From **Charlie Yeo**—chair of surgery at Jefferson. I welcome communication with our anesthesiologists. What is important to us:

    - A timely start.
    - As much advance notice as possible if there is a problem with a patient (this includes before and during the case) and a proposed plan to deal with the problem. What's helpful to us is to know what you are thinking and why.
    - If it's a big case, I appreciate hearing from the anesthesiologist, even if there are no problems that will hold the surgery up. It's nice to get just a quick check-in about what the outlines of their plan are, such as what lines are planned, what the blood bank has to say, etc.
    - Recognition and assistance with the patient's longitudinal issues throughout the perioperative period—such as postoperative pain.
    - Also, my group has published on excessive fluid administration impacting outcomes, and we sometimes will bring papers to the OR for the anesthesia team—we greatly appreciate it if the anesthesiologist will read and discuss.
    - Courteous interactions in the OR.

  - From **Grant Taylor**—private practice general surgeon. My needs and wishes with respect to my anesthesiologists are really pretty basic. What is important/ideal to me:

    - Just working with somebody I know and who knows how our medical system works. My smaller hospital does hire agency and locum tenens anesthesiologists, but I prefer working with somebody that I have had a chance to develop a rapport with.

- My job is to help my private practice patients get their surgical problems fixed and get them back to their lives as quickly as possible. I prefer to have an anesthesiologist who sees this as a team effort and who is available and interested in solving perioperative problems with me.

- This may seem ridiculous to say, but I need a basic level of competence and the ability to respond calmly and effectively in emergencies. Unfortunately, in my long career in private practice at several locations, I have seen several instances where the anesthetic care did not seem up to snuff to me (and I have my own anesthesia consultant at home, so I am pretty sure I am correct).

So, these all seem pretty reasonable, don't they? There's nothing the slightest bit demanding about any of the above points that are important to these three surgeons, and their basic message is that they just want to be able to *talk* to their anesthesiologists. Above and beyond those basics, each surgeon will know and be able to tell you instantly what else is important to them and working with them on these issues, this will go a long way towards creating a happy room. So ask! It's much better to do a difficult case in a happy room than an easy case in an unhappy room.—**Editors**

- Similarly, once I was the call attending at Hopkins, and I got a call on a Saturday night in the early evening from one of our favorite junior surgeons—now a chairperson at a major academic department. He had a severe calendar pressure of some sort—might have been a plane to catch—and was hoping to do an elective case at 5 AM the next morning, a Sunday, when we typically didn't do elective cases. He didn't try to bully us into doing the case. He didn't post it as an urgent case and demand it be done. He just called us and was completely honest and straightforward about the scheduling pressures and asked if we would consider doing the case. We said yes and did it the next morning.—**CM**

- The above points remind me of a case I did when I was first in private practice. I had anesthetized a 7-year-old girl for tonsillectomy and adenoidectomy. The ambulatory center was closing down, and the patient, her mother, a nurse, and I were the only people in the facility. She started bleeding from the mouth and nose, and I called the surgeon at his office. I reported profuse bright red blood. He recommended that we give Afrin, which did not help. Then he said, "Have the mother drive her to my office and I will take a look." I was not comfortable with this. I knew there was no way I would allow her to leave the surgery center. I was in consideration of transfer to the ED for further evaluation. So, I said to this surgeon, "Respectfully, Sir, I am not comfortable with your plan. If you cannot come back to the surgery center, I will call for transport to the ED." Guess what? He heard me, speaking with *respect and firmness*, and he arrived 5 minutes later to evaluate the girl. Moral of this story—speak with respect, for your own position as well as the surgeon's, and you are more likely to be taken seriously.—**AJR**

*__Note from the Editors:__ Herb Chen is a Stanford graduate and loves the San Francisco area. Several of our contributors chose the Golden Gate Bridge as their favorite, but Herb has been a good friend of the anesthesia community since at least the early 1990s at Hopkins, so we told him he could have it (Fig. 17.3).

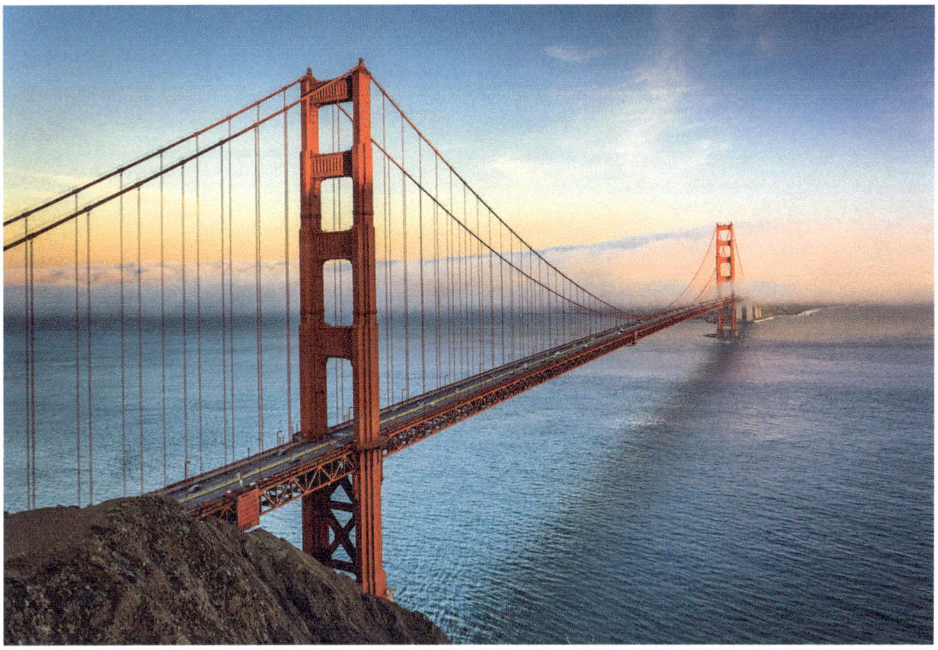

Fig. 17.3 It has been said that the Golden Gate Bridge is one of the most dramatic and beautiful structures ever built. We agree! Photo: Image used under standard license from shutterstock.com

Special Topic 2—*Ad Hominem* Verbal Attacks: What to Do

- *Ad hominem* attacks are sort of the verbal version of a chart war, which we describe how to handle in a previous book. This sort of ultra-personal attack—upon one's character, intelligence, medical competency, work ethic, or what have you—still happens, in spite of nearly ubiquitous workplace training modules. We have been attacked in front of patients, families, our anesthesia colleagues, nursing staff, medical students, and residents. It's happened to all of us at some point.—**Editors**

- We must first advise two incredibly important things about *ad hominem* attacks. *First, you need to be aware of your professional environment.* Will you be supported in advocating for oneself in such a situation, or are you expected to just absorb attacks in the moment and address the matter later (or not even that)? Will you receive censure for standing up for yourself? These are critical questions to know the answers to *before* deciding on a specific course of action in such a situation.—**NBS and Editors**

- Second, *do not ever* engage the attacker and "return fire" in front of the patient (Fig. 17.4) because all you will do is create tension and torch your communication bridges! As we teach with dealing with a chart war, you are going to take action but not in front of the patient.—**Editors**

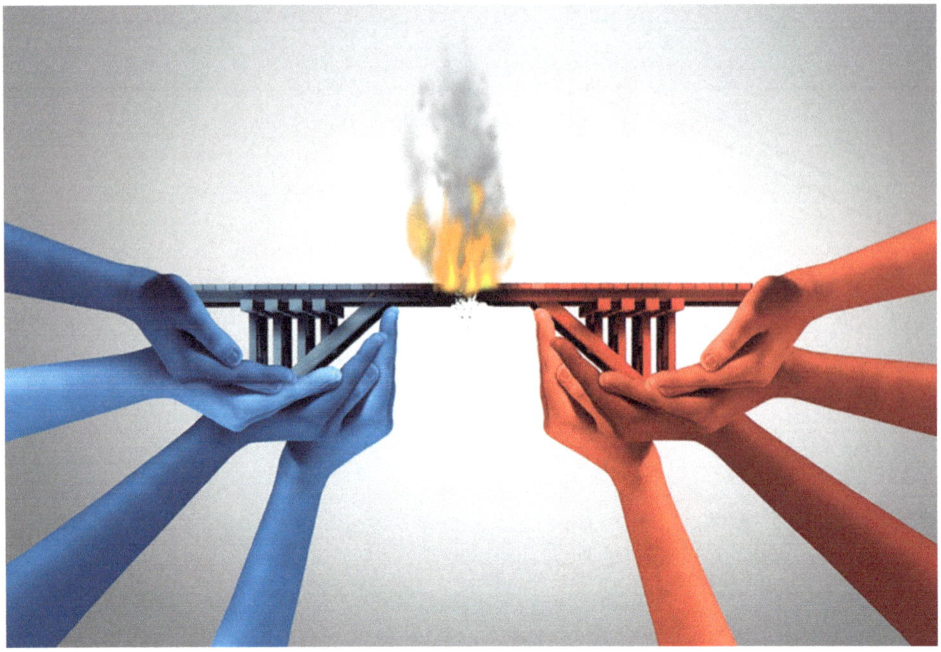

Fig. 17.4 Do not *ever* return the verbal assault or respond angrily—it's the biggest mistake you can make. You are going to respond but not in the moment. Photo: Image used under standard license from shutterstock.com

- *Sometimes a hostile verbal attack just comes out of nowhere*. We've have been involved in incidents when we have been talking to patients in the preop center for only 60 seconds, having just been told a case was being put in our rooms, and had someone approach and start belittling and insulting about delaying the case. We've been walking down the hall and been shouted at to stop the passive-aggressive act and get in the room and the case started when we weren't even posted in the OR that day, we were on a research day. Once somebody called one of our houses and yelled at our spouse and then hung up. But often there has been a bit of a build up to the attack or insult. If it has gotten to this point, de-escalation has probably failed, or is arguably too late. The most important thing to realize at this point is that this person doesn't like you. We tend not to yell or even become hostile with people we like. It seems a cliché to say that, but it's a basic law of human nature. You are not going to be able to rely on friendliness to get you through this tense interpersonal exchange because the attacker isn't your friend. You will have to deploy scrupulous business courtesy instead.—**NBS and Editors**

- Unless the patient is actively trying to die, gross breaches of professionalism do need to be addressed, but quietly. Plan to do this in two steps. First, take defensive actions to end the attack. Then, decide what your next action will be. But always, always, always take the high road, which is the professional approach. It's the only way to come out "the winner" in such a situation.—**Editors**

- *If the patient is present*, try to politely ignore the speaker. If you can't ignore somebody standing on the other side of the stretcher, try a 2-4 word answer such as, "Yes, okay, thank you." Or, "Thank you, Dr. Jones." This can be repeated several times. Or state an obvious fact in a mild voice, "I'm just putting the IV in." If you get really pushed, you might say, "Dr. Jones, this is Mrs. Smith."—**Editors**

- If the patient isn't present, here's what you want to *ultimately* communicate:

  I do not believe that calling me not qualified to take care of complicated patients because I told you that the patient has a harsh machinery murmur that wasn't appreciated on the preop exam is either professional or appropriate. I would like to collaborate with you on the care of this patient, but I cannot do so if you continue to direct inappropriate and insulting language at me. If necessary, I will make the best decision I can for the patient with what I know now.

- You may feel that you would have institutional support to say this at the time of the attack. You may end up writing this in a memo and/or saying it in a meeting. This will depend on institutional culture.—**Editors**

- We do not advise you delay the care of a patient to settle this dispute. If you are an attending, then you may make whatever clinical care call that you need to make. It's better if you do it in a collaborative way with other staff, but if they won't collaborate, then you may make your decisions unilaterally. Whoever is angry or insulting you may not like it, and you may be later called to justify them, but they can't overrule your clinical decisions. You are not fundamentally the consultant for the surgical or ICU services, you have legal autonomy over and responsibility for your medical decisions. You can't be ordered to start an anesthetic or take any medical action against your medical judgment.—**Editors**

- One exception is if the belligerent party is obviously impaired or under the influence of a substance. In that instance, you do stop the progress of the case. Sadly, it has happened. Quite a few of us know of cases where the verbal attack was actually a drunken verbal attack.—**Editors**

- If you are a trainee, call your attending at the soonest possible second, regardless of the level of the person who is yelling at you and whether or not the patient is present. In this case, your response is, "I'll call my attending." And then, as much as possible, try to bring things back to the care of the patient: "I've called Dr. Senior Person. I'm going to get back to taking care of the patient."—**JMS and Editors**

- Don't excuse or discuss or explain the background of the incident to the patient if the perpetrator retreats. You don't have to apologize for what somebody else did and you are not responsible for what comes out of somebody else's mouth. It's not up to you to adjudicate the matter in front of, or with, the patient. If the patient asks about what was going on it is probably due to their own anxiety. Reassure them that you will do everything in your power to insure they will receive good care. It's fine to make a low-key transition statement such as, "With your permission, I'm going to continue to finish the preoperative discussion and put your IV in."—**Editors**

- Whatever you do, stay calm and collected and composed. It can be difficult to do that, but remember, it is our job to be calm and effective in emergencies. Consider this an interpersonal emergency.—**Editors**

- Do not expect that the entire staff present will file immediate memoranda supporting you. If they do, that's great—but rather rare.—**Editors**

- Also, expect that if a hostile and insulting person has retreated, they may be making phone calls and trying to tell their story elsewhere. You can't stop this. Keep your attention focused on your patient.—**Editors**

- You "prevail" in these situations based on how successfully you've managed previous confrontations, as much as you managed the current one. The person who has the *a priori* reputation for being a hothead or unprofessional is not in a good starting position should the incident be adjudicated one way or the other. It is so helpful to have an impeccable reputation and record of interpersonal skills and interactions.—**Editors**

- You also advantage yourself by meticulous record keeping. We can't give any advice as to how to pursue final adjudication of the incident—does it get dropped, developed into a formal complaint, etc. These are big, big questions and specific to the situation. But what we can advise is that the subject of the attack should write a careful memo—to their personal files at the very least—with names, dates, and details while the incident is still fresh.—**Editors**

- Although abusive/insulting language is never acceptable in the workplace, one does need to consider the possibility that a colleague is sharing an uncomfortable kernel of truth with you, albeit in a highly inappropriate way. Is there a way to extract something of value, in terms of improved insight, from this highly negative interaction?—**JMS**

- Be willing to forgive, although perhaps not forget. Once one of our authors was just torn apart in a difficult trauma case in the middle of the night. There was actual screaming, although not by her. All she managed to say over the drapes was, "I don't think this is fair." Later, she was in her other room when she was called overhead to go back to the trauma case. It was with trepidation and palpitations that she went, but she was the anesthesiologist of record. When informed that the surgeon of record wanted to speak to her, what could she do? When she arrived, the surgeon stated that he wanted to make a public apology to her in front of everybody who had witnessed the event. The apology was accepted, and she never had so much as a difficult word with that surgeon again.—**Editors**

- I agree with the above statement. Some of the firmest and fondest professional relationships that I've forged have arisen in the context of someone appropriately confronting another's inappropriate behavior, and the confronted party (original offender) promptly acknowledging that their behavior was inappropriate and apologizing on the spot. Both parties subsequently developed a strong respect for each other going forward. Strange but true!—**NBS**

- A few more suggestions for neutral statements to consider when you need something to defuse and deflect a personal attack are below.—**NBS**

  Why are you speaking to me in this fashion and with this volume and tone?

  Are you okay?

  Yelling isn't okay.

  Dr. Johnson, you are kind of yelling.

  Dr. Johnson, are you being sarcastic on purpose?

  The patient isn't in any danger (or is stable) so let's talk later and we can review these issues.

  I need to take a metaphorical and literal step away from this interpersonal situation.

  The old saying applies here and that is connect before you correct, so let's try to find some common ground before we attempt to set each other straight. Note: This one is best said with a smile.

Special Topic 3—Noise in the OR

- Noise in the OR is a fascinating topic. It is a great area for projects, research, and training. One reason is because quite a bit of human factors and occupational health work has already been done, so you can get into this area without inventing the wheel.—**Editors**

- Another reason that noise research in the perioperative period would be a fun area to work in is that there are so many constituents for noise interventions—anesthesiologists and anesthesia team members, surgeons, nurses, and patients of all ages and types—pediatric patients through the elderly. Then you could study the different types of noise and effects of when the noise occurs. And the effects of noise on the learning environment of trainees at different levels. You could repeat your basic study design for the different types of anesthetics. And different types of patients, such as patients with sensory processing disorders. And *then* you have all of the different stages of the perioperative period, from the preop assessment through the OR through the PACU and ICU through discharge. For example, do patients understand and remember their preop instructions better if there is classical music playing? We don't think it's ever really been determined. More than one of us has said, man, I'd think about getting into this area of research if I was younger. We hope that at least one person who reads this might be inspired to do so. ☺—**Editors**

- And all of the above study ideas would be great to do a cross-disciplinary projects with the nurses and/or surgeons!—**Editors**

- Yet another thing to study might be when noise is *helpful*. For instance, schizophrenic patients often welcome headphones or even ambient noise as it serves to drown out the voices.—**NBS**

- Remember, it's been said that the most requested song by WW II soldiers was the Brahms lullaby. Do patients getting general anesthesia do better on induction if a lullaby is playing? It wouldn't be that hard to design a study. Same with "extubation music."—**Editors**

- There is a tendency to assume that most of the excess noise in an OR is from the music that the surgeons want. Some of it definitely is. However, we probably will not be able to get the surgeons to stop listening to music during cases. We saw a mention online that, in the Spotify and streaming era, today over 90% of surgeons and surgical trainees listen to music, up from about 70% in 2008. There is some literature that listening to music increases focus and that listening to specific music, especially classical music, can improve spatial task performance. This last benefit of music listening is known as the Mozart effect. Of course, no type of music will be beneficial if played at a volume that is known to represent noise pollution.—**Editors**

- We really don't know any anesthesiologists who insist on music once the anesthesia case has started. We do know anesthesia providers who use music very effectively in the pre-induction period to relax and distract (in a beneficial way).—**AJR**

- The "average" OR has a noise level of 65–70 decibels, about the same as a washing machine or driving inside a car going 60 mph.—**AJR**

- A "busy" OR has a mean noise level of about 70–80 decibels or the noise level of a mid-size Airbus jet during flight.—**AJR**

- What is the source of this noise? All kinds of noise-generation contribute to the total decibels. For one, the air flow in an OR is noisier than any other place in the hospital. There is considerable noise from the handling of metal instruments. The number of people talking in an operating room will also increase noise. And then there are the saws and surgical instruments, which can push the noise level over 130 decibels.—**AJR**

- In general, OSHA mandates noise management programs in work locations that have a time-averaged noise level of 80 decibels over 8 hours.—**Editors**

- Spend a bit of time reading the literature about what happens when noise reduction programs are implemented. The noise papers are fascinating.—**Editors**

- The best times to target noise reduction is during intubation, extubation, surgical count, and critical moments during the operative procedure such as placing an aneurysm clip.—**Editors**

- There are wall monitors and handheld noise dosimeters that will give a visual readout of the ambient noise level (Fig. 17.5). Is it fair to ask the surgeons to accept having the music off during these critical times if the decibel level is above a certain threshold number? It might be. Another approach that is used is to create a "sterile" cockpit with respect to noise during these intervals in the perioperative period.—**Editors and AJR**

- A very cool study in 2014 by Engelmann et al looked prospectively at the effects of a noise reduction on the surgeons [2]. The study measured noise levels before and after a reduction program and recorded operative complications and the surgeons' biometric data including salivary cortisol and electrodermal activity. Stress perception was captured via questionnaires. The intervention reduced noise by about 50%, significantly improved the complication rate, and decreased stress responses in the surgeons, especially surgeons who were noted to be "responders" or sensitive to noise.—**Editors**

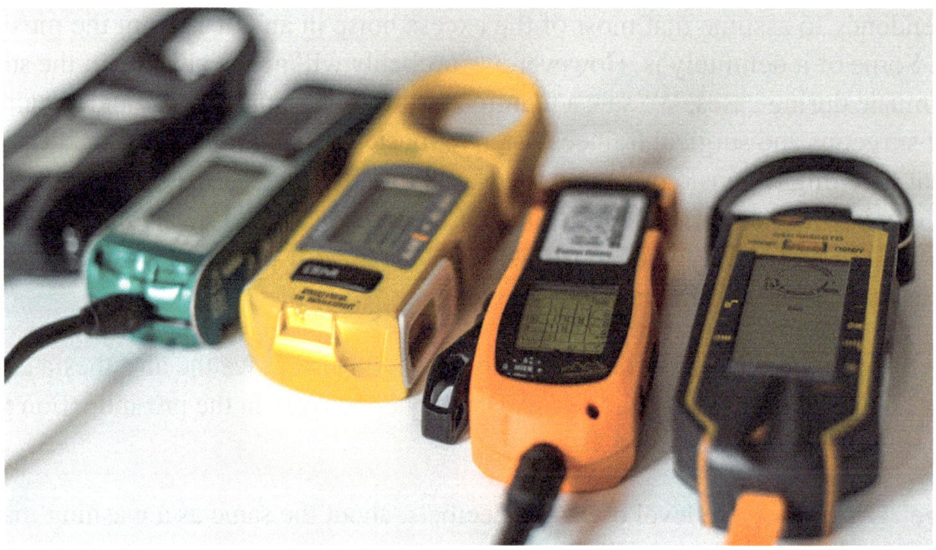

Fig. 17.5 An array of noise dosimeters to measure occupational or recreational ambient noise. Photo: Image used under standard license from adobestock.com

Special Topic 4—Language Barriers Including Names

- The first principle when facing a language barrier is courtesy, courtesy, courtesy. There are multiple ways to express this, the barriers in verbal communication notwithstanding.—**Editors**

- The language professionals who are helping you with your patients who are not proficient in English are *interpreters*, not translators. I was recently corrected—in front of the patient, who did speak some English—when I absentmindedly used the wrong term.—**CM**

- The requirements and certification for medical interpreters varies. The National Board of Certified Medical Interpreters offers certification in six languages—Cantonese, Mandarin, Korean, Russian, Spanish, and Vietnamese. There is both a written exam and an oral exam and the pass rates are as low as 65% for the oral exam. The certification must be renewed every five years.—**Editors**

- If you are at a new hospital, try to get experience in using that hospital's interpretation service as soon as you can. Some hospitals use a device that's basically a tablet on a stand—you pick a language, and a videoconference is immediately set up with an interpreter. But other (government?) hospitals sometimes have an older, slightly clunkier telephone interpreter system, especially on the floors. You don't want to be in the situation of needing to have an important conversation and you haven't used the service yet.—**Editors**

- This should be well-known by now, but always speak directly to the other person, not to the interpreter.—**Editors**

- Unfortunately, mistakes in interpretation do happen. We are aware of a case (we weren't personally involved) when the word "prognosis" was substituted for "diagnosis" in a medical interpretation involving American Sign Language. If you, as the medical provider, become aware of a gap in comprehension, do not be afraid to ask for a redo.—**PMT and CM**

- Due to dialects and regional accents and *face masks*, language barriers can still arise even when all speakers are fluently speaking the same language. Don't get flustered. Just try the following approach, "You may not be understanding me because of my North Carolina/Boston/Philadelphia/wherever accent. Would you mind if I jotted down a bit of what I am saying?" This gives you the opening to ask them if they can write down what they are saying.—**Editors**

- If the person who you are speaking with is discussing the recent hospital town hall meeting or what to order for lunch and you aren't understanding everything, you can do the occasional nod-and-smile. However, if a patient or other medically important topic is under discussion, you *must understand* every word of what the other person is saying.—**Editors**

- People who are deaf or have hearing impairment will often not indicate that they have not comprehended what is being communicated to them. In order to make sure that this is not happening, it is okay to ask them to communicate back their understanding of the information.—**PMT**

- We think it's okay to learn a simple greeting and just a very few simple words in the languages that are common to your patients. Again, courtesy.—**Editors**

- I *always* ask people to tell me the exact pronunciation of their name. My Italian last name has been mispronounced a million times in my life and I don't really mind. But I do appreciate it when people take the time to get it right.—**CM**

- You can also use this if you have forgotten somebody's name. It's sometimes awkward to say, "I've forgotten your name." You can say, "Can you tell me again the exact pronunciation of your name? I thought I heard somebody mispronounce and I want to get it right."—**Editors**

- Do not, however, assign people nicknames, especially those derived from their formal names or body habitus or attributes. This can be a personal and sensitive issue. If I meet somebody new who is being called by a nickname, I usually ask them if they prefer to go by that before I start using it. More than once, I've been told that the individual actually doesn't care for that name.—**NBS**

- As we mentioned above, we advise that you learn a couple of words in the languages that are prevalent in your patient population. Even if these words are just "hello" and "thank you." Or even words such as "reading," which is what you may have the patient do with the consent form. Below, Brandon Togioka's fun and cool parents demonstrate a few words in American Sign Language (ASL) (Figs. 17.6, 17.7, and 17.8). The photos below are from the collection of the Togioka family.—**Editors**

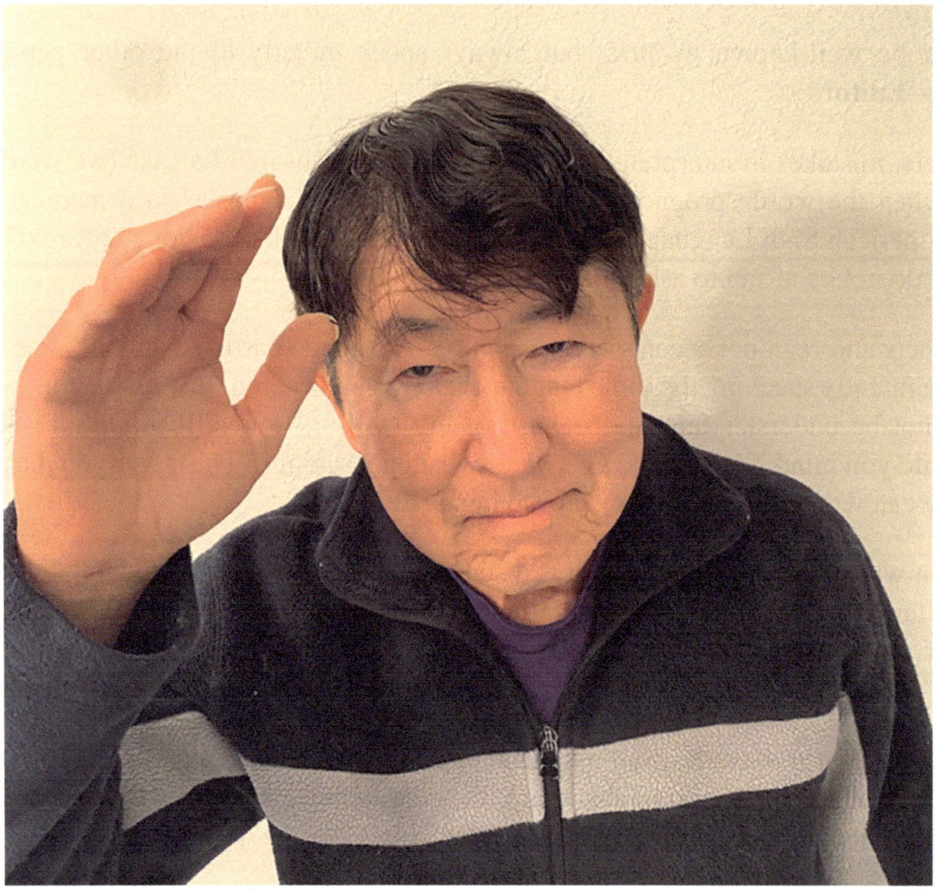

Fig. 17.6 Bob Togioka says "hello" in American Sign Language. Learn to say hello in 50 languages, if you have to

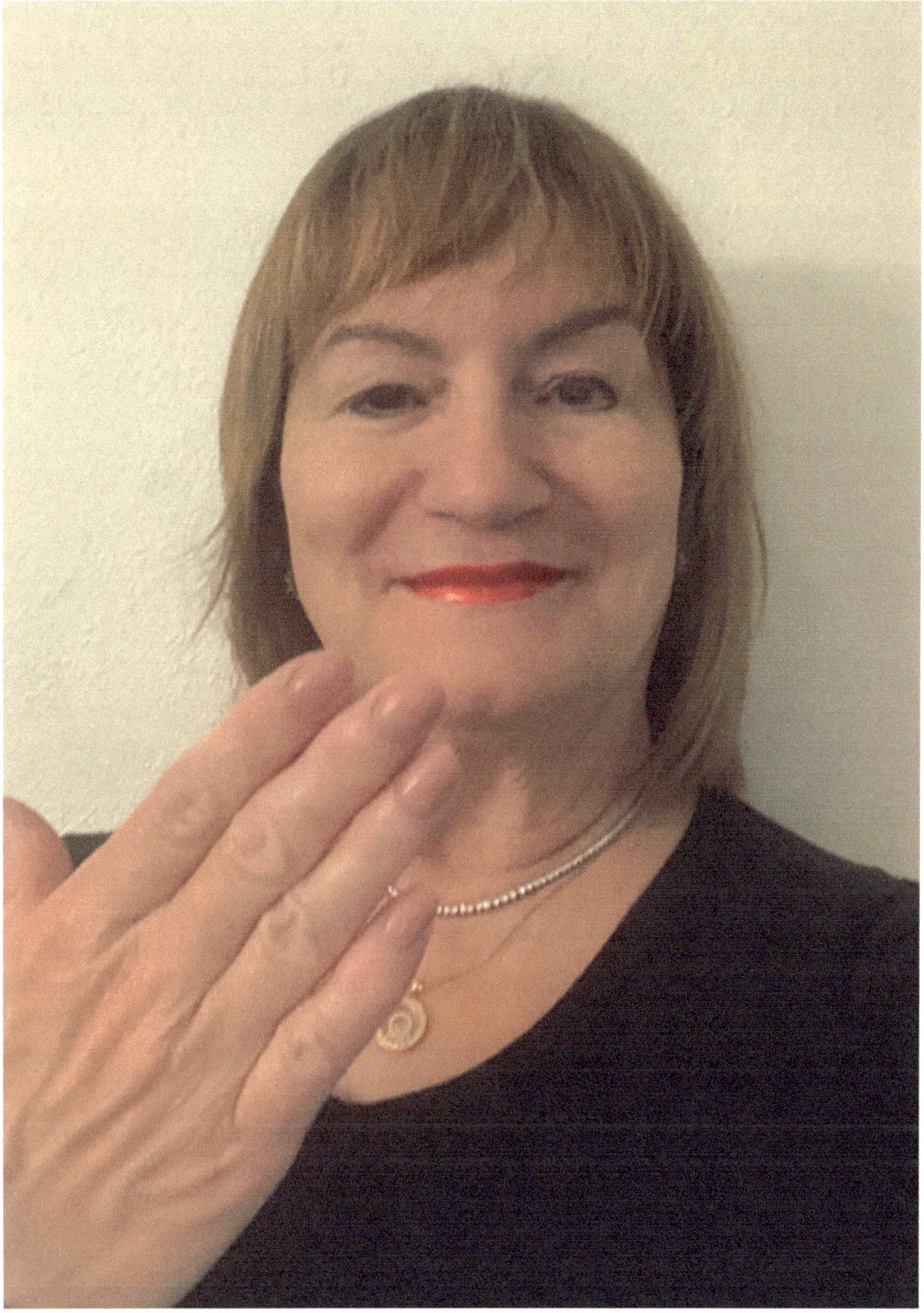

Fig. 17.7 Patti Togioka shows us the words "thank you" in American Sign Language. Good to use at any point in communicating with the patient or family

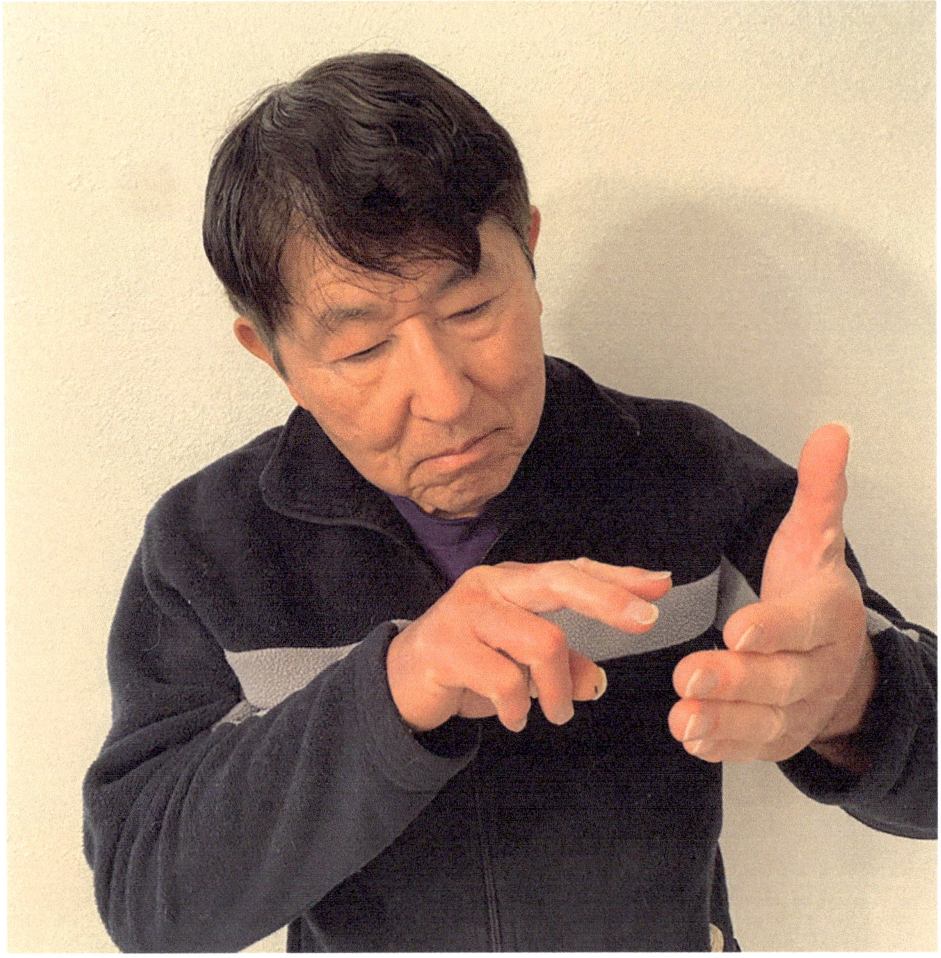

Fig. 17.8 Bob shows us the ASL sign for "reading." You might use this sign to introduce the anesthesia consent to the patient

Note: The editors thank Drs. Gilman, Chen, Yeo, and Taylor, Ms. Togioka, and Mr. Togioka for contributing to this chapter. And as we said above in ASL, many thanks for reading this section and chapter on the basics and nuances of communication.

References

1. Calvo MG, Fernandez-Martin A, et al. Selective eye fixations on diagnostic face regions of dynamic emotional expressions: KDEF-dyn database. Sci Rep. 2018;8:17039. Published online 2018 Nov 19.
2. Englemann CR, Neis JP, et al. A noise-reduction program in a pediatric operation theatre is associated with surgeon's benefits and a reduced rate of complications: a prospective controlled clinical trial. Ann Surg. 2014;259(5):1025–33.

Authors

James Gilman is a cardiologist by training, the former chief executive officer of the Clinical Center at the National Institutes of Health, and a retired U.S. Army Major General. Among his U.S. Army commands were Walter Reed Health Care System and Brooke Army Medical Center. James Gilman was known at the NIH Clinical Center for his accessibility, including personally replying to emails and his common-sense and down-to-earth "weekly updates from the CEO's Office."

Amy Robbins is a health care executive in Charlotte, NC and also maintains an active clinical practice in palliative and hospice medicine. She is an accomplished (and constant) presenter, writer, and editor.

Ron Bank is a cardiac and trauma anesthesiologist at INOVA Fairfax. He has been known since residency for his friendly interpersonal style and as a great presenter. He recently participated in the "Residents in a Room" podcast series for the American Society of Anesthesiologists.

Neil Sandson is a senior psychiatrist and physician educator in Baltimore, Maryland. He is a frequent consultant for and collaborator with the national anesthesia community. He has lectured and published widely. In addition to his clinical work, Neil has held a variety of administrative, supervisory, and executive positions and has adjudicated many workplace disputes in both a formal and informal capacity.

Cathy Marcucci received a "Chatty Cathy" doll for Christmas in 1961, and the rest is history. It has been said that she missed her true calling in life, which would have been talk show host.

Part II

Professionalism

Claiborne Pell Bridge—Newport, RI

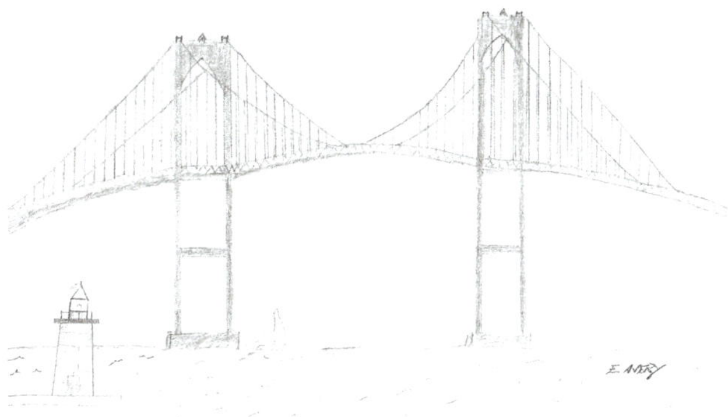

Editor **Ed Avery** selected the Claiborne Pell Bridge as his favorite and then sent us a sketch he had done himself! Pretty dang impressive for a cardiac anesthesiologist, if you ask us, because this is exactly what the Claiborne Pell looks like. It's an awesome bridge, and we totally understand why it is Ed's favorite.

The bridge, commonly known by its previous name as the Newport Bridge, is a suspension span that crosses the East Passage of the Narragansett Bay in Rhode Island. The bridge connects the city of Newport on Aquidneck Island and the Town of Jamestown on Conanicut Island. The main span of the Newport Bridge is 1601 ft, ranking it number 87 among the longest suspension bridges in the world and making it the longest suspension bridge in New England. The overall length of the bridge is 11,247 ft. Its main towers reach 400 ft above the water surface, and the roadway height reaches as high as 215 ft. It is four lanes wide, two in each direction. The bridge opened in 1969 to great fanfare and is featured on the Rhode Island State quarter. It significantly impacted the lifestyle, demographics, and economy of Conanicut Island. It was renamed for Senator Pell in 1992.

The editors of *Anesthesia Bridges* thank Ed Avery for his charming drawing and for demonstrating that the "A" in Anesthesiologist can also stand for Artist if the need arises.

18 Introduction

Edwin G. Avery IV

Professionalism in the practice of medicine is a key concept, whether we are considering our interactions with other anesthesiologists, surgeons, nonphysician anesthesia care providers, nurses, or any of the other clinical care teams we may interact with in the hospital. This section brings forward many important and recurring themes in the practice of medicine that we hope our readers can benefit from reviewing.

Importantly, much of this section relates to how we as medical professionals respectfully communicate and interact with our peers as well as how we present ourselves. There are also robust essays on how we as physicians may successfully transition into new leadership roles when moving to an unfamiliar institution, an exercise that can be a "make it or break it" time for a prospective leader. We have included insights into the importance of promoting efficiency in the hospital and an excellent primer on medical malpractice. Finally, we offer what is likely the strongest value in this section—copious examples of various dimensions of professionalism from individual leaders in anesthesiology who carry with them several collective lifetimes of clinical and leadership experience.

Author

Ed Avery IV is a New Englander who trained and worked at the MGH for over a decade before being recruited to Cleveland. He is a cardiac anesthesiologist with multiple areas of interest—including blood pressure control, the coagulation system, and improving patient outcomes. He has served as chief of cardiac anesthesia, vice chair for research, and chair of the transfusion committee during his time at University Hospitals Cleveland Medical Center.

E. G. Avery IV (✉)
Department of Anesthesiology and Perioperative Medicine, University Hospitals Cleveland Medical Center, Cleveland, OH, USA

S. Mohamed et al. (eds.), *Anesthesia Bridges*, https://doi.org/10.1007/978-3-032-08294-7_18

19 "I'll Be Right There": A Life-Long Lesson

Michael M. Todd

Introduction

I was a third-year medical student at the University of Chicago on my first clinical rotation. About a week after starting, our team was called to the ER to admit a 16-year-old lifeguard who had drowned during a training swim in Lake Michigan. He was in full arrest when pulled from the water, but was resuscitated by a physician who happened to be on the scene. I don't remember doing much in the ER for this cold, intubated young man—although I do remember seeing an arterial blood gas with a pH of <7.00.

The Patient

The patient was transferred to our tiny 4-bed medical ICU. He was in severe respiratory failure, ventilated with an old Bennett MA1—and doing very poorly. Another medical student and I were tasked as "runners"—hand-delivering blood samples to the various laboratories every hour. We were being directed by our second-year medical resident, while our attending physician basically sat at a desk building and filling out hand-written flow sheets. I do not remember hearing anything from him.

Several hours after the patient's arrival, a small "respiratory consult team" from the Department of Anesthesiology arrived, led by Dr. Christian Rattenborg.* I knew too little about respiratory medicine at that point to understand what he did—but within a very short while, the patient's respiratory status dramatically improved. I just remember thinking "this is very interesting."

The patient remained relatively stable for much of the next day and actually woke up, but still required full mechanical ventilation. Now I was tasked as the "chest physical therapist"—turning him, doing chest percussion, suction, and so forth. I basically never left the ICU.

M. M. Todd (✉)
Department of Anesthesiology, University of Minnesota School of Medicine, Minneapolis, MN, USA
e-mail: mmtodd@umn.edu

S. Mohamed et al. (eds.), *Anesthesia Bridges*, https://doi.org/10.1007/978-3-032-08294-7_19

The Phone Call

Late that night, he began to rapidly deteriorate. Nobody seemed to have any idea of how to respond—so my resident turned to ME and said, "call Dr. Rattenborg." This was around 2:00 AM—so being an obedient student, I contacted the hospital operator and asked her to call Dr. Rattenborg at home. Please note—Dr. Rattenborg *was not on call* for anything.

The call went through, a very sleepy Dr. Rattenborg answered the phone, and I explained what was going on. And his response has been burned into my brain ever since—as the mark of the most professional man I ever met. He simply said, "I'll be right there...." No discussion, no questions, no arguments—just "I'll be right there....."

Since he lived in the neighborhood, he arrived in about 20 minutes. Again, I didn't really understand what he did—but like magic, everything improved. And I knew from that night forward that I wanted to be an anesthesiologist.

I was lucky enough to work with Dr. Rattenborg many more times over my remaining time at the University of Chicago.

And I have never forgotten that part of what it means to be a physician is to "be right there" when asked.

Lessons Learned

- An important part of being a physician is to be readily available when your expertise is needed.
- Keep in mind that students and residents are watching and listening to us. We need to continuously strive to be excellent role models for them.

***Note from the Editors:** We didn't know much about Dr. Rattenborg when we received Dr. Todd's essay and went straight to the literature and the internet to find out more. It is fascinating to see what he and his colleagues in an earlier generation of anesthesiologists were thinking about and working on when today's senior anesthesiologists were in elementary school (Fig. 19.1).

But Dr. Rattenborg wasn't just working on ventilation and pulmonary mechanics and publishing in *Anesthesiology*. He was also working on acid–base issues, the effects of hemorrhage, and laryngeal anatomy—and publishing in the European anesthesiology journals, the surgical journals, and the *New England Journal of Medicine*. And he was apparently a go-to person for none other than Dr. Joseph Artusio, one of the legendary pioneers of modern anesthesiology. No wonder that he became an exemplar for Mike Todd. How the rest of us wish we could have met him.

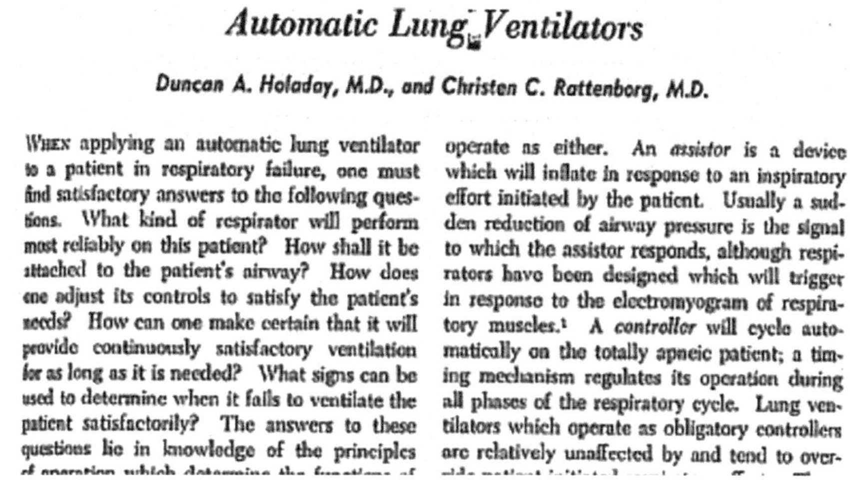

Automatic Lung Ventilators

Duncan A. Holaday, M.D., and Christen C. Rattenborg, M.D.

WHEN applying an automatic lung ventilator to a patient in respiratory failure, one must find satisfactory answers to the following questions. What kind of respirator will perform most reliably on this patient? How shall it be attached to the patient's airway? How does one adjust its controls to satisfy the patient's needs? How can one make certain that it will provide continuously satisfactory ventilation for as long as it is needed? What signs can be used to determine when it fails to ventilate the patient satisfactorily? The answers to these questions lie in knowledge of the principles

operate as either. An *assistor* is a device which will inflate in response to an inspiratory effort initiated by the patient. Usually a sudden reduction of airway pressure is the signal to which the assistor responds, although respirators have been designed which will trigger in response to the electromyogram of respiratory muscles.[1] A *controller* will cycle automatically on the totally apneic patient; a timing mechanism regulates its operation during all phases of the respiratory cycle. Lung ventilators which operate as obligatory controllers are relatively unaffected by and tend to over-

Fig. 19.1 An influential paper with Dr. Rattenborg as senior author in *Anesthesiology* in July 1962, Vol. 23, pp. 493–506. Photo: Image used with permission under license from Wolters-Kluwer Health, Inc.

Author

Mike Todd is a professor and vice chair at the University of Minnesota—after over 30 years at the University of Iowa. He's spent a lifetime in academic anesthesia, with a few intermixed years as a department chair, as editor in chief of *Anesthesiology*, a clinical trialist, and a devoted "neuro guy" in the OR.

You Are the Rank of Who You Argue With

20

Amr E. Abouleish

Introduction

The transition from resident to faculty is a major milestone. When I joined my department, the most profound advice I received was from my chair. During morbidity and mortality conference one week, a case was being presented, and the major issue was a lack of surgical faculty and to anesthesiology faculty communication. My chair said to the whole conference, "You are the rank of who you argue with."

Advice for New Faculty

It was directed to the new faculty on the case. He was a new faculty member. He did not feel the patient was optimized for surgery, but the surgical resident argued and pressured the anesthesiology faculty to proceed with the surgery. Instead, the anesthesiologist should have insisted that the surgical resident have his faculty call him directly. This sage advice is especially valuable for new faculty who were residents in the same department. Surgeons, residents, nurses, and others may still view the faculty as a resident. My advice to these new faculty, "You are the rank of who you argue with!"

Lessons Learned

- Attending-to-attending communication is the best way to deal with any conflicts with our surgical colleagues.

Author

Amr Abouleish joined UTMB Galveston in 1993 as the first chief of pediatric anesthesiology. His motto for teaching pediatric anesthesia to residents is "every month is July!" He is also a national speaker on economics in healthcare, especially for anesthesiology departments.

A. E. Abouleish (✉)
Department of Anesthesiology, The University of Texas Medical Branch, Galveston, TX, USA
e-mail: aaboulei@UTMB.EDU

S. Mohamed et al. (eds.), *Anesthesia Bridges*, https://doi.org/10.1007/978-3-032-08294-7_20

More Thoughts About Authority and Responsibility

21

F. Jacob Seagull and Catherine Marcucci

Introduction

In the previous chapter, Amr Abouleish relates some extremely valuable advice that applied to a young anesthesiology attending in conflict with a surgical resident.

General Principles

This advice can be generalized to the larger work environment. People in work contexts, including the clinical arena, often find themselves in uncomfortable, stressful situations when their responsibility exceeds their authority. They are responsible for completing a major task, but do not have the proper authority to do the requisite steps in the task.

For example, when residents make decisions, they are operating under the medical authority of an attending. They do not have the ultimate authority in the care of the patient. They may feel the weight of responsibility for taking care of a patient and providing safe care, but the attending is officially the one responsible. Add to this lack of authority that they **SHOULD NOT** be making difficult decisions. Judgement calls should be the domain of experts. Trainees are, by definition, not experts. Residents don't have the perspective, experience, or expertise to properly make a judgement call. We can say that perhaps the residents' lack of authority is a good thing.

It makes sense to avoid two unqualified people arguing over something neither one is sure of. Two residents should not engage in a power struggle. Neither of them hold actual power, nor should they. An argument among residents wastes time and is not in the patient's best interests—the time is better spent in quickly taking the dispute to the appropriate level for resolution of the clinical care issues and questions at hand.

F. J. Seagull
Center for Bioethics and Social Science in Medicine, University of Michigan Medical School, Ann Arbor, MI, USA

C. Marcucci (✉)
Department of Transfusion Medicine, Clinical Center, National Institutes of Health, Bethesda, MD, USA

S. Mohamed et al. (eds.), *Anesthesia Bridges*, https://doi.org/10.1007/978-3-032-08294-7_21

Take It to the Attendings

Two attendings can more productively engage in a discussion of what is best for the patient for a number of reasons:

1. They are the same rank, and there is no inherent power differential. We cannot state too clearly—power differentials can lead to bad decisions and bad outcomes.

2. They are both experts and will likely have a broader perspective on the situation and understand the context/complexities better.

If you feel yourself getting into an argument with somebody at your (junior) level, a good way to approach it is to say, "I'll tell you what. I think it's best if we take this to the attendings. It will be faster that way and the resolution will be more expert and reliable for the patient." Stay pleasant and then disengage from the other junior person. Then just place a quick call to your attending and let them know the basic factors without a long-winded recitation.

Be very careful about being given the task to take a message or a final decision back to the other junior person or their attending. The discussion should happen with the attendings together, not a series of messages and a decision/discussion by proxy. You might catch a bit of flak if you refuse to act as the messenger, but it's better than being the proverbial messenger who gets shot. And remember, no matter who you are talking to—**stay brief and stay polite!** A smile and a calm and courteous attitude are always good ways to conduct any interaction.

Lessons Learned

- Two residents in a dispute: rookie arguing with a rookie—no authority, no experience (bad).
- Resident arguing with attending: power differential (bad).
- Attending to attending: makes sense to have two experts discuss a complex issue on equal footing (better!).
- A friendly demeanor and courteous attitude *are essential.*
- If you are a resident, passing the discussion along to your attending *is* taking part in the problem-solving and dispute reconciliation. You have not shirked your responsibility, so don't let anyone portray it as otherwise.
- Be careful about getting into situations at any point in your career where you don't have the authority to accomplish your responsibilities.

Authors

Jake Seagull holds a PhD in psychology and is a recognized expert in how and why people do what they do in stressful and challenging situations. Over his career, he has published and lectured widely on topics pertaining to how physicians and other medical practitioners react to each other and their environments.

Cathy Marcucci is an anesthesiologist and transfusion medicine physician. She wishes that she could state that she had never been drawn into a debate outside her authority and responsibility. However, she does happily report that she has collaborated with Jake Seagull over many years with nary a tense moment or word.

22 A New Surgeon Comes to Town (Part 1)

Marc P. Pelletier

Introduction

In this chapter, we hear from a cardiac surgical colleague about what it's like to move to a new practice setting and work with a new anesthesia and surgical team, and how this transition can be successfully navigated.

The Cardiac Surgery OR

The operating room is a beehive of activity in most hospitals, and nothing epitomizes this more than a cardiac surgery operating room. When one walks into this room, the excitement of a multidisciplinary team is on full display. There may be ten or more healthcare workers working together at any given time, all with their own particular roles that are crucial to the success of the operation. It is a place where lives are saved, and miracles happen. It's also a place where people die and where we sometimes leave feeling sad and heartbroken.

As with any team, the cardiac team has members with different roles and responsibilities. While each role is vitally important, there is ultimately a hierarchy and different levels of leadership. In nearly all cases, both cardiac surgeon and anesthesiologist will need to exert strong and positive leadership, and for much of the procedure, will serve as "Captains of the Ship."

Therefore, when a new cardiac surgeon arrives in a hospital, especially to a well-established team, it can be both an exciting time but also a very disruptive one for all involved. While there is excitement and anticipation, there is also concern and anxiety. How do we support this transition? How do we make sure the team and the onboarding surgeon are in harmony? The answer lies in structure and communication. Individuals cannot control all aspects of their environment, but they can control how they behave and how they prepare.

M. P. Pelletier (✉)
Division of Cardiac Surgery, Department of Surgery, Yale School of Medicine, New Haven, CT, USA
e-mail: marc.pelletier@Yale.edu

S. Mohamed et al. (eds.), *Anesthesia Bridges*, https://doi.org/10.1007/978-3-032-08294-7_22

The New Surgeon

Before discussing structure, consider what happens when a new cardiac surgeon is recruited. Even before that first day, questions abound: What is he like? Is she nice? Does he have a temper? Is she good technically? It's not that the surgeon is the only important person, but in reality, much of the tenor and tone of an operation will be dictated by that individual's skill and personality. There are typically weeks of preparation required to onboard a new surgeon, verifying preferences, procedures, and instruments.

While this new arrival may cause anxiety among the team, the surgeon will also typically experience similar feelings. It's important for the surgeon to realize that his/her arrival may be very disruptive to a team that has already achieved a level of stability. At the core of this disruption is the relationship with anesthesia, which must be a successful collaboration if good outcomes are to be achieved.

One can easily see that it is incumbent upon the surgeon to have a plan of action and to act accordingly for the onboarding process to be successful. How can this be accomplished? In my experience, there are a few strategies that work that are applicable to most aspects of our lives. They have certainly served me well when onboarding into a new cardiac surgery team.

Strategies for success

- Behave respectfully
- Develop structure
- Set goals and write them down
- Don't look back
- Show up

The chances are quite good that when any surgeon joins a new team, both sides are hoping for a smooth transition. It is always hoped that the new surgeon will have a high EQ and be able to interact positively, in the respectful and professional manner of any excellent physician. Imagine a situation where a new surgeon starts with a new team, is angry with the scrub nurse, yells at the perfusionist, and is rude to the anesthesia team. How will that be perceived? Chances are that it will set a negative tone that will be difficult to overcome. The new surgeon will benefit by being positive and engaging, by being likeable and respectful. First impressions are important, and most will be watching carefully, scrutinizing early moves and actions.

***Note from the Editors:** Marc Pelletier partially trained at McGill University. We went looking to see if McGill was in any way in the bridge business, and they are! Below is the logo and online excerpt of a most interesting university group (Fig. 22.1). We bet this is a bunch of smart people. They compete with students from other universities and the event is hosted by Concordia University.

> The McGill Bridge Building Team (MBBT) is a fully student-run engineering design team. We design and build wooden bridges for the annual Troitsky Bridge Building Competition. Our aim is to bridge (haha) theory and practice by engaging our members in all aspects of solving an engineering problem.

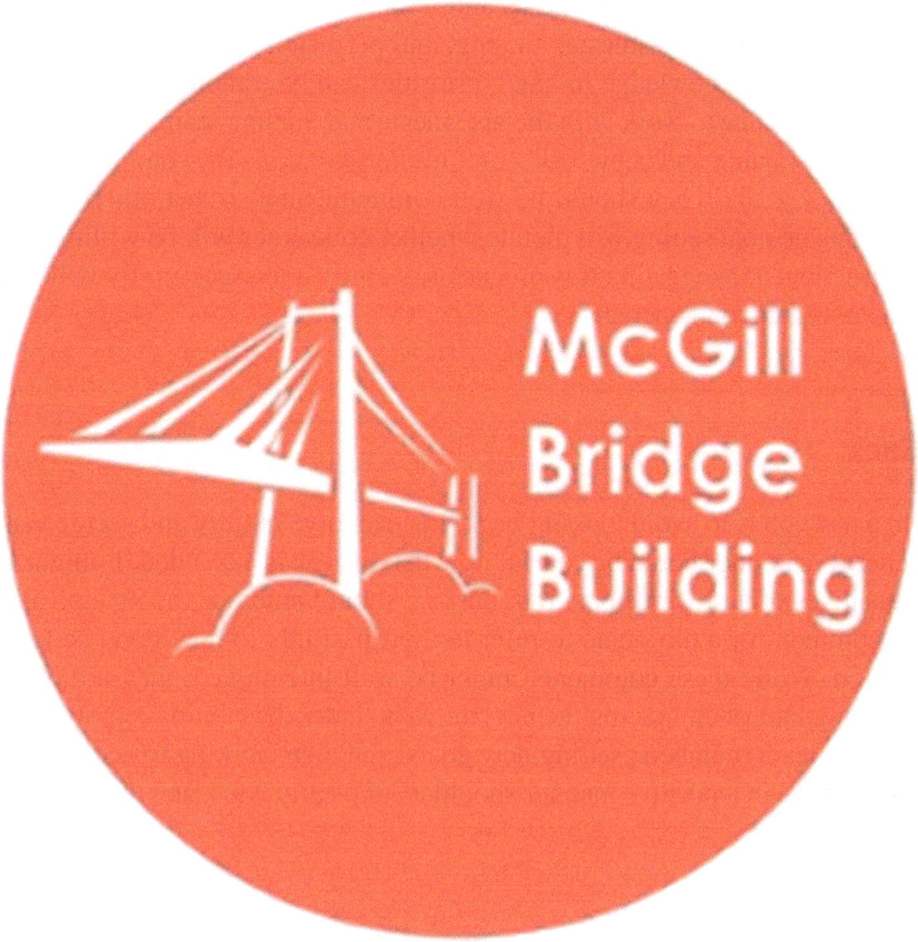

Fig. 22.1 Logo of the McGill Bridge Building Team, a student-led engineering design group that reflects teamwork, structure, and innovation. These qualities are also essential in surgical practice. Illustration: Reproduced with permission from the McGill Bridge Building Team, Department of Civil Engineering, McGill University

Strategies for Stress Reduction

This can be a stressful time. Much of this stress can be alleviated by reviewing and developing structure. A new surgeon should attempt to do as much prearrival preparation as possible and ideally start working on this at least 90 days before the actual start date. This will help to ensure that the surgical team is well prepared when the first surgical day finally arrives and will hopefully reduce stressful surprises. One should take time to meet with the cardiac anesthesiology, perfusion, and nursing teams well ahead of the first surgical day. It is important to connect with nursing staff to review instruments and preference lists. If possible, do a mock case with the assistants and the nurses. It's incredible what one can learn from this exercise. Another good idea is to scrub into cases (as an assistant) with new surgical colleagues, to observe, and possibly learn new tricks. One should take time to review how nurses set up their tables, and to review the sutures and needles and any implants that might be needed. This level of engagement will be seen favorably and should ensure a positive start.

The next important strategy is to set some goals and write them down. Consultation with new surgical colleagues and leadership of the anesthesia, nursing, and perfusion teams will be key to understanding current challenges. With this knowledge in hand, priorities can be established, and goals can be developed. It is of prime importance to work with the anesthesia and nursing teams during this process. Make sure these goals are reasonable and achievable, and limited in number—you don't want to overwhelm the team with too many goals. They should be well communicated so that others will understand and support them. Reasonable goal setting will dictate whether colleagues will be willing to help or whether they might be obstructionist. Navigating this process gracefully and successfully will have an important impact on how the new surgeon is perceived.

Don't Look Back

A key mindset in a new job is to avoid looking back. Instead, dive in fully and secure early wins. Moves require a lot of energy, and one should be careful how that energy is expended. It might be normal to try to replicate the positives of a previous position, but one should embrace the new position and its challenges. It's quite common for a physician to refer to their past job, to how good certain things were at their prior institution. While these comments might be well intentioned, they are often viewed negatively by the new team. Part of embracing the new move includes developing relationships, reaching out to new colleagues and team members, setting new goals, and then working to accomplish them. Setting realistic goals and starting in a positive manner should lead to early wins, and these should be celebrated with the team.

Just Be There!

The last strategy is perhaps the most basic one in all aspects of life: **Just show up**. This might sound overly simplistic, but it's not. Showing up, both physically and emotionally, is such an important trait. Like all qualities, this ability is not necessarily innate and can be improved upon. There are many days when we might be tired or overwhelmed, but those can be the most rewarding when something positive is accomplished at the end of the day. A major aspect of being present, whether in the OR or in committee meetings, is having good communication skills.

When interacting with my anesthesia colleagues, this may start with planning discussions in the preoperative phase, especially for more complicated cases. In the OR, we want to have clear dialogue during huddles and during procedures, with ongoing discussion of patient status, echo findings, bleeding issues, etc. And lastly, toward the end of procedures, any remaining problems are communicated to ensure a smooth transition out of the operating room. Throughout all interactions between cardiac surgery and anesthesia, there should be mutual respect and a give and take of ideas. Both parties want the case to be efficient and successful, and to be of the highest quality. If this relationship is not functioning in a positive and symbiotic nature, achieving success will be difficult (Fig. 22.2).

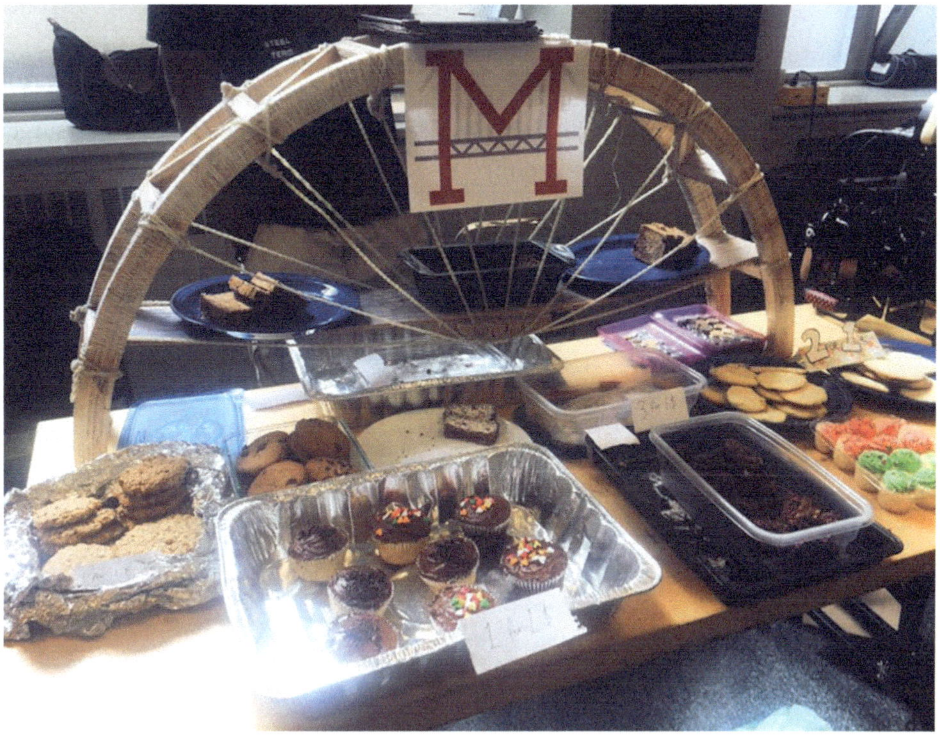

Fig. 22.2 The McGill Bridge Building Team is a true student-led organization, complete with bake sales to raise money for competition expenses. Here is one of their wonderful McGill-built bridges. Photo: Image used with permission from the McGill Bridge Building Team, Department of Civil Engineering, McGill University

Summary

When a new surgeon comes to town, there is both excitement and trepidation. There is excitement about adding to the team, and there is the potential for new and better things. However, this comes with trepidation, concern, and anxiety for all involved. The surgeon should focus on what he or she can control. By being likeable, developing structure, setting clear and achievable goals, simply showing up both physically and emotionally, and by developing a strong relationship with his anesthesia colleagues, the new surgeon will have a strong foundation upon which to join and build a new team, and the transition should be successful.

Lessons Learned

- The arrival of a new surgeon can potentially be disruptive and anxiety producing for all members of the surgical team. This can be reduced by everyone working together to develop new relationships, good structure, and achievable goals.
- Being cordial and respectful and having excellent communication skills will go a long way toward achieving team success.

Author

Marc Pelletier is a cardiac surgeon trained at McGill and Stanford. He has practised in both the United States and Canada, in vastly different climates and healthcare systems. He served as the head of cardiac surgery at University Hospitals Cleveland Medical Center and has been appointed to be chief of cardiac surgery at Yale as of March 1, 2025, so he will continue to put these principles to good use in his own career. He and his wife are proud parents of four boys, which means that other than the operating room, he can often be found on an ice rink, ski hill, tennis court, or golf course.

A New Surgeon Comes to Town (Part 2)

23

Raymond G. Graber

Introduction

You are a cardiac anesthesiologist. You've been working for a while at your institution. Things are going reasonably well. You have developed good working relationships with your surgeons, perfusionists, and nursing staff. Everything is comfortable. Sure, there will always be stressful times and cases, but you know and trust the people you are working with, and you can predict how people will respond in difficult situations.

Always the Possibility of Someone New

Then one day, you hear that the cardiac surgical chief has taken another job. Maybe some of the people he has recruited leave, too. Before you know it, a new cardiac surgical chair has been recruited, and he's starting any day now. Let's talk about some of the issues that can come up, and how we can ease the transition.

In all types of surgery, the anesthesia and surgical teams need to work together. However, this is even more the case in cardiac surgery. There is constant communication about hemodynamic issues, TEE findings, TEE guidance of cannula insertions, and coagulation issues. In a highly functioning cardiac OR, all team members have developed a level of trust that everyone is doing their job and doing it correctly.

Expect Changes

The first step toward developing a trusting relationship is to initiate introductions. It is very helpful to have some sort of meet and greet prior to the first day of surgery. This can be supplemented with written information about who the various team members are, and maybe some background information about

R. G. Graber (✉)
Department of Anesthesiology and Perioperative Medicine, University Hospitals Cleveland Medical Center, Cleveland, OH, USA
e-mail: raymond.graber@uhhospitals.org

S. Mohamed et al. (eds.), *Anesthesia Bridges*, https://doi.org/10.1007/978-3-032-08294-7_23

them. However, face-to-face time is very important in the initial phases of developing a relationship. It is an excellent idea to exchange contact information. You will then be able to text or call your surgeon when the need arises, and vice versa.

Your new surgeon may have different ways of doing things. Maybe the new surgeon is doing more minimally invasive approaches that utilize different incisions, different cannulation strategies, and require lung isolation. Maybe they will do more radial artery harvesting. These things affect us—what type of endotracheal tube will be required, where we place are arterial lines, etc. There can be monitoring preferences—some surgeons like PA catheters in all their patients and some like to utilize cerebral oximetry. There are preferences for minimal hemoglobin levels. There may be preferences for inotropic or vasoconstrictor therapy. These things will all have to be worked out with input from both sides.

Sharing Is Caring (and Courteous and Collegial)

For complex cases such as heart and lung transplants, it is helpful to share current protocols. When we share this type of information, it helps demonstrate to the surgeon that he is working with thoughtful, competent people who have a plan and aren't just winging it. This also can be the start of a dialog—a chance for the surgeon to give his input regarding any potential changes or improvements. As you learn about the techniques and preferences of your new surgeon, share this information with your colleagues so that each individual is not just starting from scratch. Write up these details and email to all members of your cardiac anesthesia team, including attendings and anesthetists. We show ourselves to be a competent team when we can adapt to change.

***Note from the Editors:** On the subject of sharing and caring, the Graber family frequently relaxes and enjoys family time by travelling together. Ray tells us that a recent family trip to London was "pretty close to a 10" due to Mary's detailed and thoughtful planning (Fig. 23.1).

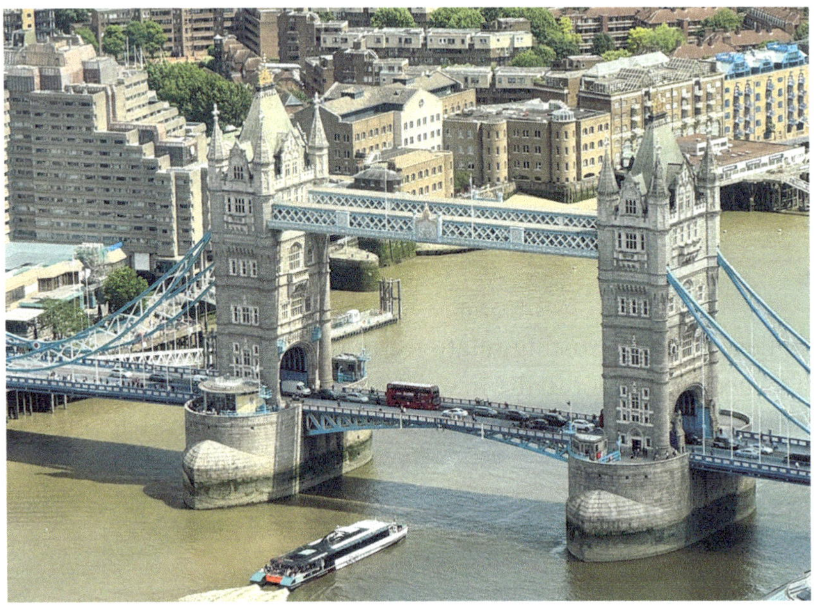

Fig. 23.1 The London Tower Bridge is as stunning in real life as in the picture books. This view is from the 52nd floor of the Shard building, near the south bank of the Thames River in London. Photo: Mary Graber

Communications

Excellent communication is a key part of developing and maintaining a relationship with your new surgeon. As you develop a relationship, you will develop a feel for what information the surgeon wants to hear. At our institution, as at most places, we "huddle" prior to induction, and discuss all aspects of the surgical and anesthetic plan. Often the surgeon will leave while we place lines and induce the patient. I text my surgeons to keep them up to date—when lines are done, chest is prepped, and any other concerns. During the case, we review TEE findings pre- and post-pump. We teach our residents to repeat back all surgeon requests—"call and response." When there is a second case for the day, I will set a room turnover goal with the team and inform the surgeon of the plan—so he or she can plan their time accordingly. I also think that everyone deserves positive feedback after a job well done—including surgeons. This is all routine basic stuff but nevertheless is important.

Another important thing to remember is that good communication reduces the risk of errors. Leaders who seek input, are respectful, and willing to listen are more likely to receive valuable input from other members of the operating room team. By speaking up and speaking freely, team members can contribute important information to the team as a whole and enable the team to learn from and prevent future mistakes. We need to continually develop these communication skills in ourselves and also encourage our surgeons to do the same.

Borrowing from Business

In the business literature, there has been much written about the development of and the qualities found in highly performing teams. There is an evolutionary process that teams must go through, which has been summarized below [1].

- **Forming:** getting to know each other and forming a commitment to the team
- **Storming:** challenging the leader and each other, and working through issues and conflicts
- **Norming:** starting to work together
- **Performing:** moving toward shared goals

We, as leaders in the operating room, can facilitate this process by using open and clear communication, by getting input from all team members, by creating an atmosphere of mutual trust and respect, by managing conflict (dealing with conflict openly and respectfully and not allowing grudges to build up and hinder team morale), and by contributing to a positive atmosphere.

It can take some time to develop a good working relationship with a new surgeon. By being efficient, competent, communicative, sharing, caring, and appreciative, we can shorten this process and do great work together. Although we have focused on cardiac surgery here, these same traits will serve you well when working with any surgical service.

Lessons Learned

- Good communication is the key to success.
- Share case management protocols with your new surgeon, so new processes can be co-developed.
- Share what you have learned about your new surgeon's technique and style with your co-workers, so they can learn from your experience.
- The stages in the successful formation of a team are forming, storming, norming, and performing. Don't spend any **extra** time in "storming" but always don't be excessively worried if you encounter a bit of stormy weather. It's a stage your team is moving through.

Reference

1. Tuckman BW. Development sequence in small groups. Psychol Bull. 1965;63(6):384–99.

Author

Ray Graber's fellowship training was in regional anesthesia, but he always enjoyed cardiac physiology and thus has also worked as a cardiac anesthesiologist since 1988. On the job training! He is now working with his fifth, soon to be sixth, cardiac surgical chief.

The Art of Changing Medical Practices: Collaboration, Adaptation, and Resilience

24

Susan D. Dumas

Introduction

Twenty years in an anesthesia practice, preceded by four years of residency, and two years of medical school—all at the same institution—is a long time. In many minds, it is considered an "era." While these extended professional intervals were common during the beginning of my career, they are no longer considered the norm as families become more transient and changing medical practices become more commonplace. Never having considered the possibility that I would change locations 20 years into my career, my husband was presented with an opportunity to move with his company to a new city. What would this mean for me as an anesthesiologist after such a long tenure? I would soon answer this question as we packed up our home of over 20 years and moved to Nashville.

Cleveland

Shortly after my husband completed law school, we got married and made the joint decision to stay in my hometown of Cleveland, Ohio. Cleveland was home to my family and provided great opportunities for both of us to find employment. It was affordable, which was important as we worked to start careers and a family and soon became a home location we cherished. As I finished medical school, we had our first child and followed with two more over the next several years. My husband and I were very busy with work, raising a family, and enjoying long-lasting friendships both inside and outside of work.

As I moved up in the department from junior to senior faculty and subsequently became part of the leadership team, I became settled. I knew everyone from the ambulance staff and paramedics that brought our patients through the emergency room doors to hospital administrators who helped support our policy and management needs. It was not just a job with coworkers, but a professional home with a family working to support each other every day. One can only imagine the difficulty I faced when I said my good-byes and moved to a new city with a new job, new colleagues, and a different way of achieving my own professional goals.

S. D. Dumas (✉)
Department of Anesthesiology, Vanderbilt University Medical Center, Nashville, TN, USA
e-mail: Susan.d.dumas@vumc.org

S. Mohamed et al. (eds.), *Anesthesia Bridges*, https://doi.org/10.1007/978-3-032-08294-7_24

Nashville

During my first weeks in Nashville, I spent time working to assimilate into the new culture. Orientation came and went, the pace of the job picked up quickly, and I was off to a rapid start in a new and unfamiliar place. As medical director of obstetric anesthesiology, I was also tasked with many administrative responsibilities that added to my daily responsibilities. Despite my experience in the field, it proved to be a bit of a learning curve for me as I got to know the processes and hierarchy of a large institution that served as a major referral center for three contiguous states.

Unlike a resident, who has the opportunity to listen and learn the norms of a new hospital and rely on their attending, as a seasoned anesthesiologist I had to learn a lot while on the job. In the thick of the moment, I was expected to be completely knowledgeable. I also came to realize that some of the phrases I used—which I had considered to be common terminology—seemed foreign to my new co-workers. For example, I received peculiar looks when I asked, "Who is my frontliner?" or "Was the Kefzol given?" In my new setting these terms were replaced with "in-room provider" and "Ancef." Thus, I soon learned that even my language could be a barrier to effective communication and leadership.

***Note from the Editors:** The John Seigenthaler Pedestrian Bridge in Nashville is a sentimental favorite of Susan's and is best viewed from Riverfront Park (Fig. 24.1).

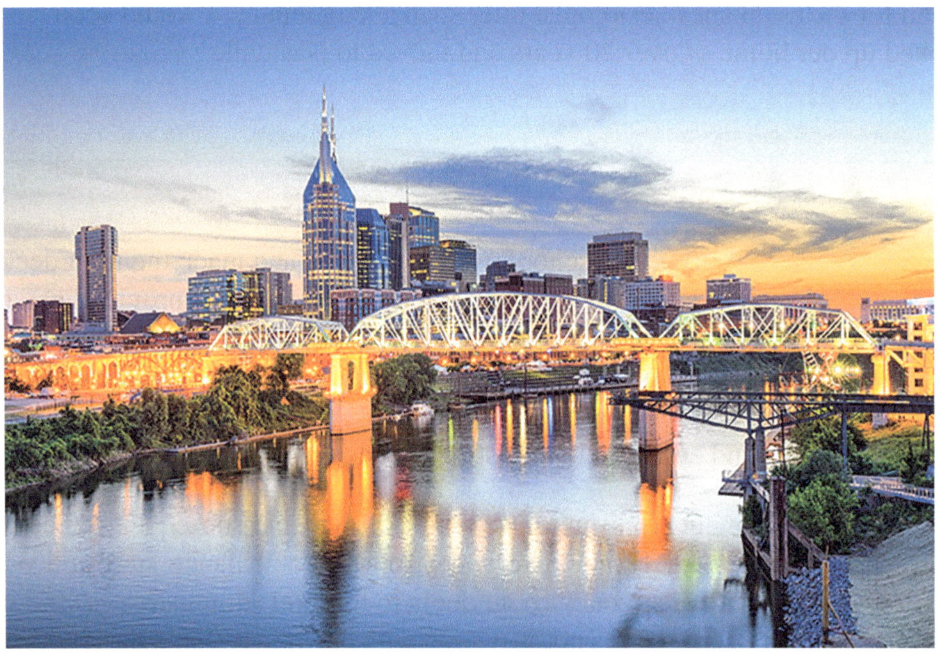

Fig. 24.1 The John Seigenthaler Bridge is also known as the Shelby Street Bridge. It is a truss bridge that spans the Cumberland River. It opened in 1909 and cost $475,000. It was considered cutting edge at the time, as it was the first bridge in the United States to have arched concrete pillars. Although it underwent several major repairs, it was closed to all but pedestrian traffic in 1998, the same year it was listed on the National Register of Historic Places. Photo: Image used under standard license from stock.adobe.com

Getting to Know All About You

Getting to know the nurses and leads on a labor and delivery team is of utmost importance to developing the level of trust needed to be an effective and highly functioning team. This posed quite a challenge for me, however, as I often found myself speaking with the team during high-stress events where little is discussed aside from immediate patient needs. I was having difficulty building relationships, something I truly valued during my career in Cleveland. How could I, as an outsider in this new location, work to build 20 years' worth of rapport in a new place? While I reflected upon this many times myself, I finally realized that I needed to become more intentional as a leader and prioritize development of those relationships.

After a rough start, some soul searching and self-doubt, I remembered a conversation I had with a very special OB nurse in Cleveland who said to me, "just let them get to know you first." I soon learned to purposefully introduce myself to physicians, midwives, OR techs, and nurses. These introductions were extremely important and led to conversations about where we lived, our children, and our work experiences. Such discussions added depth to my relationships, and I became less of a stranger and more of a coworker.

"Cultural" Norms

Furthermore, as conversations progressed, I began to understand how the unit worked and what the department norms were. I realized that if I asked questions about how things functioned, there were opportunities for me to offer alternative methods that may work within the current system and achieve improved outcomes. Understanding the people and the culture has led to a significant improvement in my ability to use my influence as a leader to move our teams forward. It has enabled me to better lead during tough clinical situations and facilitate frank discussions afterward while acknowledging shortfalls in certain situations as well as the great efforts invariably made by our team on a daily basis.

Being intentional is about bringing focus and attention to something that is important to you. By paying particular attention to intentionality in my communications, I was able to more effectively lead. While my integration began with me simply trying to adapt to the new environment, I soon realized that I needed to pivot to a focus on collaboration and the establishment of relationships. This has allowed me to assimilate into and effectively help lead a labor and delivery unit that is very different from the one I was a part of for so long. Though cultures might differ from location to location, the fundamentals stay the same—relationships are the foundation of medical practice.

Lessons Learned

- Making the move to a new position can be stimulating and rewarding, but different cultures, different terminology, and lack of relationships all can make for a difficult transition.
- By focusing on building relationships and learning the culture of your new institution, you will better be able to integrate yourself into the team and become an effective leader.

***Note from the Editors:** We admit that this bridge is an apt metaphor for how transitioning from one job to the next often feels (Fig. 24.2). But always keep in mind that how you progress on the far side can be entirely dependent on how you negotiate the gap.

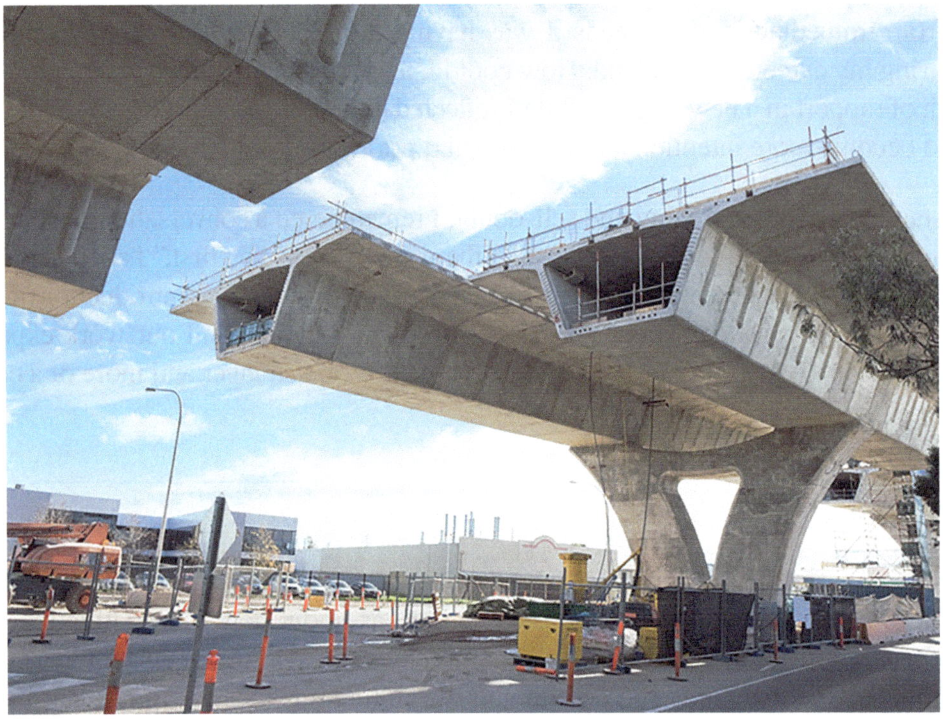

Fig. 24.2 Is this a treacherous, broken bridge or bridge still under construction? It all depends on whether you see a risky leap or an emancipating way to get to the other side and start forward in a new journey. Photo: Image used under standard license from iStock.com

Bonus Content from the Editors! We went straight to the internet when we received the above essay to find more information on starting new jobs. One thing we learned is that, although it seems slow and stressful, anesthesiologists are actually very good at starting and keeping new jobs. In today's employment landscape and across all industries, up to 70% of new hires will quit within a year, with about half of those employees leaving within three months. How often have you seen a new anesthesiologist start and then leave within a year? Not often, we bet.

Experience has taught us that the most important thing you can do in the first 1–2 weeks of a new job is to introduce yourself frequently. And then otherwise mostly keep your mouth shut. In the first days, you need to be seen widely but perhaps not heard widely. Ask the questions that you need to ask—such as log-in information, parking information, how you return drugs to the OR pharmacy or machine, and so forth. Or to clarify a medication, such as Sue Dumas notes above.

Do not ask any questions that are designed to show how much you know and what your plans are to "improve" your new place of employment. Don't talk excessively about the place you came from. If somebody wants to talk about it, just be noncommittal and mention that you are glad to be at your new location. Arrange your face in a neutral expression and disavow any close knowledge of problems or scandals taking place at the place you left. Just make bland, neutral statements, "Well you know, it's a big university hospital with a bunch of suburban satellite locations."

Similarly, do not let yourself get boxed into any "political" positions at the new place of employment or "recruited" to be on a particular side of an issue. You can just say, "I'm just figuring out the culture and way things are done here so I'm not sure." You've got something of a clean slate at your new practice location—don't let anybody else write on it before you do.

Don't be too assertive in trying to mine information from your colleagues in an attempt to gain immediate insider status. That generally has to be earned.

We repeat: Do not go on and on about your previous place of employment and what they did better than the new place. That never goes over well. It's a very short step to somebody thinking or even worse saying, "Yeah, well then, why don't you just go back?"

We were scouting around on the job forums and saw a fun timetable of what to expect when starting a new job (nod to Ian R. on Quora). We added some of our own thoughts, also for fun. So, when starting a new job, expect that it will be:

- **3 days** before your brain stops trying to tell you that you made a terrible mistake. During this time, you might mostly be asking yourself questions such as, "What was I thinking?!"
- **3 weeks** before you start noticing trends and gaining confidence. During this time, ask questions about what you need to know.
- **3 months** before you start feeling comfortable. During this time, ask questions about what it would be nice to know.
- **3 years** before the job starts feeling easy and you start feeling like a long-time member of the team. This is when you can start asking questions to provoke further discussion, or just because.

Remember, both your strategy and your tactics should be heavily based on discretion and professionalism, always! Here's your mantra: "I didn't leave due to problems there, I made the change **because of the opportunities here**."

- Also remember that when you start a new job, leadership is most hoping and looking to see if they have hired someone who conducts themselves in a way to (when and where appropriate) quietly make a meaningful contribution to their new organization.

And finally, it is **always** about the relationships and rapport with your teams. It is easy to lose track of this in a field where the jobs depend heavily on technical knowledge and skills. In some ways, though, establishing and maintaining good relationships is even more important in these situations.

Author

Susan Dumas is currently an associate professor at Vanderbilt University Medical School and medical director of obstetric anesthesiology at Vanderbilt University Medical Center. She and her husband moved to Nashville, Tennessee, from Cleveland, Ohio. They have enjoyed exploring the sights, listening to the sounds, and tasting the cuisine of the Music City.

The Three A's

25

Lee C. Woodson

Introduction

Sometime during my residency, a senior faculty provided a list of qualities required of a competent anesthesiologist. These can be remembered as the three A's: **able**, **affable**, and **available**.

Able

"**Able**" seems self-evident as being the sum of one's fund of knowledge, skills, and judgment, but requires constant career-long striving to improve. During my residency, our chairman, James Arens, valued intellectual curiosity in residents. Our current chairman, Don Prough, has also provided a scholarly example. Continuous reading and consulting with colleagues are essential to maintain and expand one's fund of knowledge. Knowing why as well as how separates doctors from nurse practitioners.

It has been disappointing to me that today, many of our residents seem to use question and answer books instead of textbooks or journal articles as a primary source of information. After residency, it is necessary to continue reading to refresh and keep up. **It has been written that an anesthesiologist's skills peak about 5 years after residency.** This means it is important to continue to focus on those technical skills. Further, judgment comes from clear thinking and experience, and some of the most valuable lessons come from the most stressful experiences.

Affable

"**Affable**" is more than just a smiling face and a fund of amusing stories. In order to be valued by the surgeons and the hospital, anesthesiologists should help make the hospital function better. Rapport with all OR personnel enables everyone involved and fosters teamwork. The nurses and surgical technicians

L. C. Woodson (✉)
Department of Anesthesiology, University of Texas Medical Branch, Galveston, TX, USA

S. Mohamed et al. (eds.), *Anesthesia Bridges*, https://doi.org/10.1007/978-3-032-08294-7_25

are a remarkable resource in so many ways. When treated with the respect they deserve and included in planning, they will give back in many ways. These colleagues helped me out of many jams, enhanced my monitoring during busy times, and made it enjoyable to come to work.

Available

"**Available**" means, in part, accepting that as a perioperative physician, anesthesiologists do not punch a time clock. Residency duty hour restrictions have eroded this sentiment somewhat. Our duty is to our patients whose needs do not punch a time clock either. Anesthesiologists' clinical skills and judgment (airway management, IV access, resuscitation, sedation, and analgesia) are needed outside the operating room and ICU. Being available throughout the hospital not only helps fulfill our duty to patients but also adds value to our specialty within the hospital and enhances one's personal cachet as a capable and caring physician.

One of my favorite professors, **Harry Walfisch**, frequently reminded us that when you are clinically strong, you get clinical prerogatives. That is, when you demonstrate you are able, affable, and available, surgeons and other colleagues will cut you some slack when you inevitably struggle with a procedure or think an unconventional intervention is appropriate.

Lessons Learned

- Lifelong learning and understanding the "whys" and not just the "whats" will help to distinguish you from other practitioners.
- Sometimes, as physicians, we are put in difficult situations wherein our idea of a desired clinical management approach may conflict with that of our peers from other medical specialties. Being affable allows us to work toward a mutually acceptable course of treatment.
- Being available throughout the hospital adds to our value as individuals and as a profession.

Author

Lee Woodson has been retired for several years after 30 years on the anesthesiology faculty at the University of Texas Medical Branch in Galveston. For the last 20 years, he focused on the care of burn patients, especially pediatric patients at the Galveston Shriners Burn Center. Now his time is spent with his wife, Anne, and hobbies: fishing, traveling, cooking, gardening, and grandchildren. Also, he has learned that a professor emeritus has much in common with being a grandparent in that you can show up from time to time and offer unsolicited advice, but not stick around for the consequences.

Dress the Part

26

Ronald L. Harter

Q: "What do you say to an anesthesiologist in a suit and tie?"

A: "Will the defendant please rise?"

Introduction

The above joke was told to me by a non-anesthesiologist professional, in reference to his acknowledgement that—unlike many anesthesiologists he had known over the years—I generally dressed professionally when not in scrubs in the OR. Although I can't say I have worn a suit and tie each day that I come to work, I have always dressed professionally.

Why Bother?

Some may feel this is an unnecessary burden to shoulder. After all, the vast majority of one's day as an anesthesiologist is spent wearing scrubs; why bother with a tie or a jacket that will only be worn from the parking lot to the locker room, and on the reverse path at the end of the day? I will acknowledge that there are days when I literally don't encounter a soul, either walking in or leaving the hospital. However, there certainly have been countless times when I have entered or left with other physicians, nonphysician providers, medical students, and patients and their families. I would contend that at least some of those encounters have created, on some level, an opportunity to build respect—not just for me, but, by extension—our profession.

A common lament of the anesthesiologist concerns the surgeon who refers to one of us as "anesthesia," rather than using our name. Certainly, some of our surgical colleagues have the opportunity to improve in that regard. However, in many cases, we need to accept some ownership of that situation. What have

R. L. Harter (✉)
Department of Anesthesiology, Wexner Medical Center at The Ohio State University, Columbus, OH, USA
e-mail: Ronald.Harter@osumc.edu

S. Mohamed et al. (eds.), *Anesthesia Bridges*, https://doi.org/10.1007/978-3-032-08294-7_26

we done to distinguish ourselves among the other professionals involved in the patient's care? Have we sought out leadership opportunities within the medical staff? Have we sought opportunities to demonstrate that anesthesiologists are indispensable in the perioperative arena? Or are we simply T-shirt-shorts-sandals-wearing, iPhone-obsessed, tuned-out, propofol jockeys? Perception is reality; each of us must ask ourselves, "Am I helping or hurting the image of my specialty?"

The time and effort you spend portraying a professional image, and engaging as a professional in your medical center, will pay dividends not only for you but for our entire specialty.

Lessons Learned

- Just because we are graduates of medical school and residency training programs doesn't mean that our peers and patients will see us as indispensable. Indeed, some of the operating room staff consider the anesthesiologist more like a piece of equipment, rather than a highly trained professional. Respect must be earned.

- Going the extra mile by presenting yourself with both a professional appearance and manner, and getting involved with leadership and academic opportunities, will help you and our specialty to build a strong foundation of respect for anesthesiologists.

***Note from the Editors:** Ron Harter's favorite bridge is the Dublin, Ohio Pedestrian Bridge (Fig. 26.1). He tells us:

> The Dublin, Ohio Pedestrian Bridge spans the Scioto River. It opened early in the pandemic and connects the "old" part of Dublin on the West side of the river with the "new" part of Dublin on the East side. It is located about a mile from my house and is absolutely spectacular, especially when it is lit up at night.

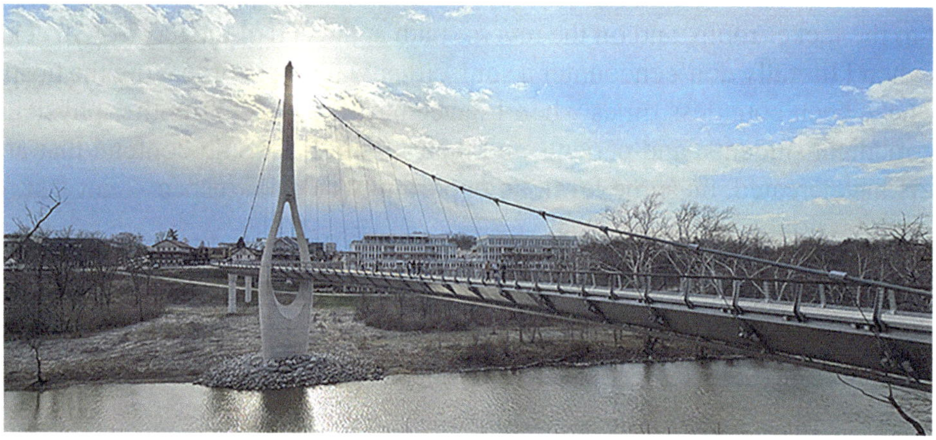

Fig. 26.1 Pedestrian Bridge in Dublin, Ohio. Design for the bridge was initiated in 2013 and the bridge opened in 2020. From the very beginning, a park was planned for beneath the bridge, and the architect was given the unusual challenge of designing a structure that would be iconic and aesthetically pleasing not only from the north and south but also from beneath the bridge. The beautiful, finished bridge is the longest single-tower S-shaped suspension bridge in the world. Photo: Image used under standard license from stock.adobe.com

- **Another Note from the Editors:** When we showed Dr. Harter's essay to a number of the *Anesthesia Bridges* editors and authors, they instantaneously agreed with and wholeheartedly endorsed his position on dressing professionally. **Deb Waterman-Johns** is a highly regarded fashion, textile, and apparel expert and style consultant based in Washington, DC, and she could not agree with Dr. Harter more. Her comment to us was that your apparel presentation will be what somebody sees every single time they interact with you in person—not how good you are clinically or what you've published. And that there is good reason to take care because this sharp sword cuts two ways—it's easy to make a good impression but also easy to make a poor impression.

- Professional dress usually means a coat, tie, jacket, skirt or dress or pantsuit, dress trousers, and dress shoes.

- But there is a caveat for those of us who trained or now work in high-crime urban neighborhoods. When we came up at Temple University in North Philadelphia, we were advised just the opposite our first week on campus—inconspicuous clothes and shoes that you could run in (but no high-end brand sneakers that would make you a target), no professional or business dress, no jewelry, no watches, no large handbag or briefcase, and perhaps not even a wallet. And by the way, don't even leave a pencil on the console of your car and never stand in a lighted window at night, the bulletproof glass in the windows of the medical school and hospital buildings notwithstanding. We are not joking. You had to be careful not to be robbed at gunpoint at the ATM machines *in the hospital*. We agree that it is good to dress for professionalism, but safety considerations must be first and foremost.

- *Anesthesia Bridges* authors **Nee Dalal**, **Carol Bodenheimer**, and **Jeremy Jaffe** were kind enough to preview this essay and send us some additional thoughts. We had an interesting round-robin discussion that really is the whole point of this book—to put some ideas and advice out there and then talk it over amongst ourselves.

- **Nee Dalal** made the point that parking locations are important in how you dress. Are you at a practice location where the early-bird staff park inside and perhaps come straight into the hospital through the ER? Then a pair of leather pumps or dress shoes should be perfectly fine.

- **Carol Bodenheimer** made the interesting point that there has been a bit of dress-code change post-pandemic. She is a rehab medicine physician and never even owned a pair of scrubs until three months into the pandemic. It's all she wears now as the culture has changed for all physician specialties at her hospital. Everybody has personal scrubs with their name and position. Carol makes the additional point that professional attire norms may be different at different institutions, and dressing appropriately and comparably to your colleagues is crucial.

- **Jeremy Jaffe** sent us some interesting and thoughtful comments. First, we must disclose that he was, unfortunately, the victim of a really scary, violent crime one block away from an urban hospital, so he speaks with credibility here. It was after a basketball game, but still light, and he was walking to his car. He was a tall man in his late twenties, wearing sweats and carrying a backpack, and the perpetrator wanted the backpack filled with med student textbooks and clothes. That said, Jeremy tells us that his residency chairman insisted on professional attire for the very reason that Dr. Harter puts forward. It was thought to be important to maintain an appearance on par with the surgeons. This chairman also insisted that his department members wear clean, pressed lab coats with their names and department atall times they left the OR.

- But beyond appearance, which can be professional without being overly conspicuous, is the belief that it is our conduct—be it in the OR during surgery, as a consultant on the floor or in our office, as a schedule runner in the OR, or as a member of a hospital committee—that ultimately earns us the professional respect of our peers. Jeremy agrees that acceptable attire overall has changed, and he often sees defaults to customized scrubs with name, title, and organization.

- Two final thoughts from Jeremy—situational awareness is the unfortunate reality we must navigate, including with our apparel. And you don't often find security and police officer escorts wearing sweats. In other words, these officers show up to work in their professional attire, therefore best enabling them to provide a sense of reassurance and safety, as well as readiness to professionally perform their duties. We think that's really the crux of Dr. Harter's advice.

***Note from the Editors:** Some of the most interesting and innovative bridges in the world are made from a textile-concrete composite. The design paradigm is that textiles don't rust. Of course, the idea of a textile bridge would not be novel to the billions of people who have depended on rope and natural fiber bridges throughout history (Figs. 26.2 and 26.3). And remember that silk has a greater tensile strength, fiber per fiber, than many forms of steel.

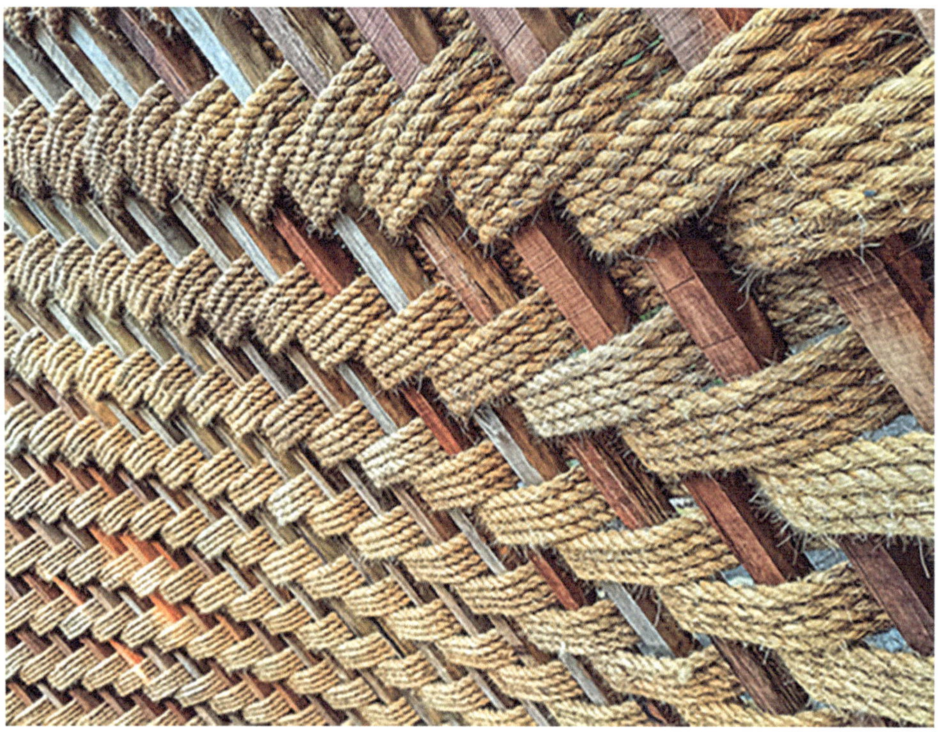

Fig. 26.2 A bridge made of tightly woven coconut fibers. Photo: Muhammad Amin, image used under standard license from iStock.com

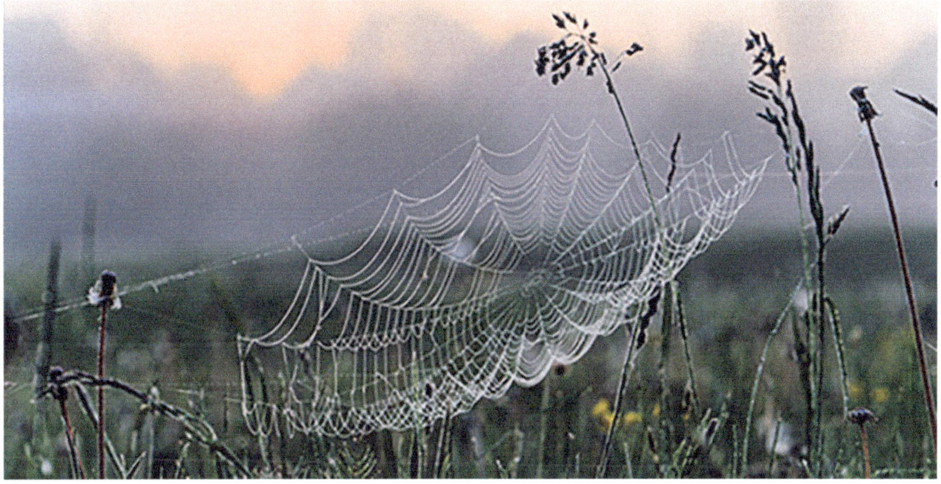

Fig. 26.3 No engineer or architect could do it better. Photo: Image used under standard license from iStock.com

Author

Ron Harter is a native Ohioan, born and raised in western Ohio, and has spent most of his professional career in Columbus. He has served as chair of the department of anesthesiology at Ohio State since 2008. He has served in a number of leadership roles in medical associations, including several leadership roles for the American Society of Anesthesiologists, most notably as an ASA officer since 2012 and ASA president in 2024. He and his wife Kathy have five children.

A "Bridge" Between MGH and Cairo University

27

Ahmed Shash

Introduction

As I reflected on what stories to share, a very defining year in my career came to mind. Although this year did not hold my most significant achievements, it was a year during which I got to observe those around me practice in their specialties. Through this observation, I learned important and impactful lessons that stayed with me throughout my evolving career.

1988

The year I refer to is 1988. I was selected to be a research fellow in the Department of Anesthesia at the Massachusetts General Hospital (MGH). This was after I had finished my residency training program at Cairo University in 1984 and as I was looking for an opportunity to gain some international research experience, I was very grateful to be accepted as a research fellow on the neuromuscular research team headed by Dr. Joan Savarese and Dr. Hassan Ali at the MGH.

So, I moved with my wife and our 2-year-old son to an entirely new country. There was a lot to adapt to and more to observe and learn. At the MGH, I attended a robust clinical practice with a very high patient acuity level and simultaneously worked on high-level neuromuscular research. I was incredibly impressed with the institution's values and ethics.

With each new day's experience, I grew confident that I would soon be able to transfer my growing knowledge to my practice back in Cairo one day. I focused on the interaction between junior and senior physicians. There seemed to be almost no communication barrier, and seniority was not solely linked to age. Senior staff were guiding their juniors by imparting lessons on addressing patient needs and practical elements, such as how to talk to patients. The staff held regular discussions, and everyone could share and talk. It was apparent to me that this teamwork and cohesive dynamic had a significantly positive impact on patient care delivery.

A. Shash (✉)
Department of Anaesthesia and Intensive Care, Cairo University, Cairo, Egypt

S. Mohamed et al. (eds.), *Anesthesia Bridges*, https://doi.org/10.1007/978-3-032-08294-7_27

***Note from the Editors:** The wonderful Longfellow Bridge spans the Charles River about 1.5 miles from the Massachusetts General Hospital (Fig. 27.1).

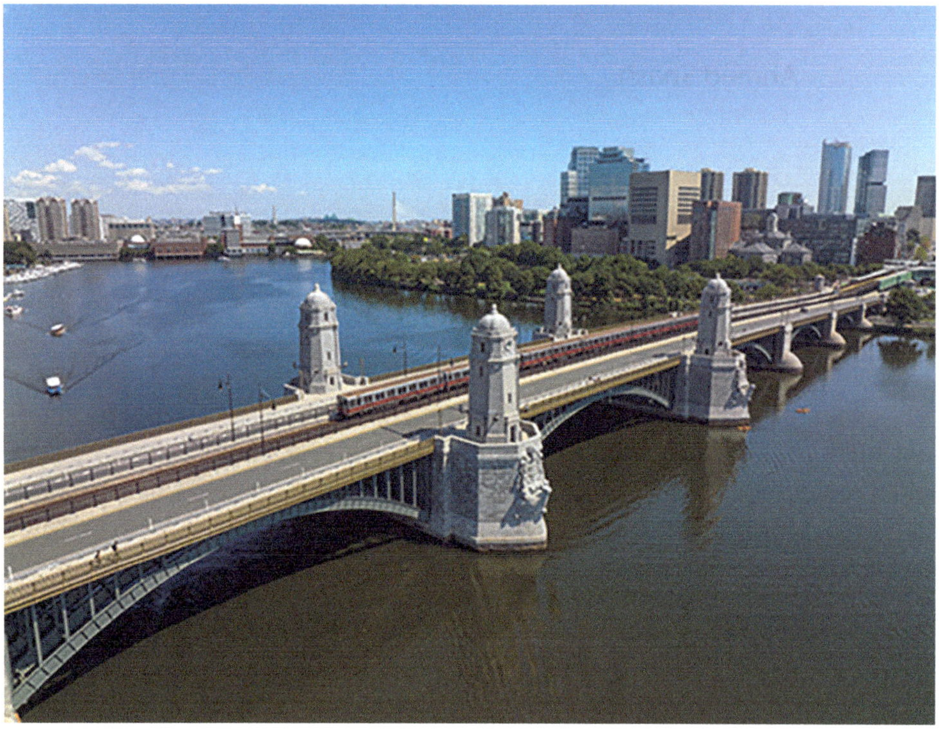

Fig. 27.1 The bridge is also known as the Cambridge Bridge and the Salt-and-Pepper Bridge due to the shape of its towers. It is a steel rib arch bridge that connects Boston's Beacon Hill area with the Kendall Square area in Cambridge. The towers of the bridge are ornamented with replicas of the prows of Viking ships, carved in granite, as legend has it that Leif Erikson sailed up the mouth of the Charles River circa 1000 AD. The bridge carries up to 28,000 cars per day. Photo: Image used under standard license from stock.adobe.com

2011

Many years later, in 2011, we had a revolution in the streets of Egypt, which slowly started affecting other aspects of our lives. Social dynamics were quickly changing, and our society became largely politically polarized. At Cairo University, a new dean was elected. Shortly after that, he appointed me to be the chair of the Anesthesia Department. Grateful for the opportunity, I set out to implement some of what I had learned in 1988 at the MGH. I made efforts to change some of the existing structures and dynamics by empowering junior physicians and staff and ensuring that their voices were heard as well as respected. All staff members of the department became part of the decision-making process.

At that time, people were defined by their political affiliation. The University, like elsewhere, was divided by political tensions. I wanted to give equal opportunity to talent regardless of affiliation. I tried to build trust within our team and create a culture of affiliation to the department and science as our guiding principle, and not our political background. This was not an easy task amidst the country's social and political divides. However, it was the only way I believed we could push forward and build back up to a higher functional level beyond what existed during the slowdown that accompanied the uprising. I was convinced that our focus had to shift entirely to the work we do for our patients and students.

***Note from the Editors:** There is also a similarly memorable bridge near Cairo University (Fig. 27.2). Thousands upon thousands of students have crossed this bridge daily to get to their studies.

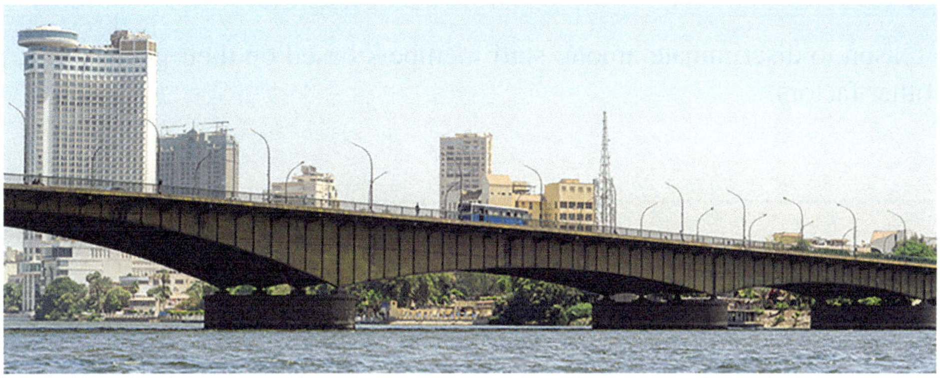

Fig. 27.2 University Bridge, near Cairo University in Cairo, Egypt. It is a steel beam bridge that spans the Nile River. Photo: Image used under standard license from iStock.com

Creating a Clinical Care Culture

I tried to create a culture where we treated each other equally and acknowledged each other's contributions to science and medicine; after all, this was our mission. Our vision did not discriminate based on seniority or political affiliation, and our mission ensured that people should not be penalized or sidelined because of an affiliation. The changes were vividly seen when I started to delegate to younger staff responsibilities such as defining research priorities or distribution of work. Junior faculty members were tasked with managing the daily challenges of running intensive care units or pain clinics as well as other departmental services.

Those were not simple tasks; it is important to note that Cairo University hospitals include four leading referral hospitals, have over 100 operating theaters for elective and emergency surgeries, and function around the clock. Additionally, it was the first time that a committee of younger staff members oversaw the annual educational conference, including resource mobilization, communications, defining the themes, and extending the invitations to participants and speakers.

In closing, my fellowship experience at the MGH provided me with useful tools to slowly redefine the Cairo University Hospitals' mission and develop a new culture of collaboration and respect among all departmental staff, regardless of political affiliations or differences in age.

Lessons Learned

- Transferring the best practices learned from a worldly medical center can enhance the quality of care, intradepartmental rapport, and productivity.
- Invest in and trust the junior staff, as their energy, passion, and dedication are imperative to building a strong department. Teaching and developing junior staff should be of primary importance.
- Junior staff should be treated as equal team members. Seniority is based on knowledge and competence, not on age.
- There is no reason to discriminate among staff members based on their gender, age, position, race, religion, or other factors.

Author

Ahmed Shash graduated with honors from Cairo University, Faculty of Medicine. He joined the Massachusetts General Hospital as a research fellow. His research on neuromuscular blocking drugs was recognized internationally. He went on to become chairman of the Department of Anesthesia and Intensive Care, Cairo University, Cairo, Egypt, until September 2018. During his tenure, he established several committees that advanced the department's reputation on the international scene, particularly the annual conference. He is currently an emeritus professor. Dr. Shash also worked in several prestigious private hospitals in Cairo and volunteered to provide services in remote sub-Saharan African areas. He is married with two children and one grandson.

28 From the Navy to the Island Life: Lessons for the Budding Anesthesiologist

Ali Bilal and Donald S. Prough

Introduction

This piece is an interview with Donald Prough by Ali Bilal, a medical student seeking advice on a potential career.

Foundations

Medicine as a field has one constant axiom—if we see farther than our predecessors, it is neither due to some greater didactic intellect nor a keener clinical acumen, but rather because we stand on and are lifted higher by the sheer height of their achievements. My time as a medical student on anesthesiology services has reminded me time and time again of this sentiment, each instance more humbling than the last. And so, as I waited patiently in a conference room in John Sealy Hospital to meet with Dr. Prough, the gentle breeze of the cool air conditioning on the back of my neck provided a respite both from the sweltering Texas heat and my own growing nervousness.

My trepidation is perhaps best explained by the natural awkwardness of a medical student meeting with a medical school department chair. Dr. Prough had served as professor and chair of the Department of Anesthesiology at the University of Texas Medical Branch at Galveston Island since 1992. His childhood was spent in Pennsylvania in the second half of the twentieth century, a period when the economic boom and technological advances fueled by the dying embers of World War II paved the way for a new and exciting age of discovery in medicine.

Dr. Prough completed his residency training in anesthesiology and his fellowship in critical care medicine at the National Naval Medical Center in Bethesda during his service in the United States Navy, and

A. Bilal
The University of Texas Medical Branch School of Medicine, Galveston, TX, USA

D. S. Prough (✉)
Department of Anesthesiology, The University of Texas Medical Branch at Galveston, Galveston, TX, USA
e-mail: dsprough@utmb.edu

S. Mohamed et al. (eds.), *Anesthesia Bridges*, https://doi.org/10.1007/978-3-032-08294-7_28

then a fellowship in cardiac anesthesia at the University of Alabama. He then went on to practice as a civilian at North Carolina Baptist Hospital and Bowman Gray School of Medicine at Wake Forest University.

Meeting Dr. Prough

Thankfully, Dr. Prough is not intimidating in person. The man who takes a seat in front of me across the table is dressed in a light blue shirt and dark pants, with his history of naval service evident by his straight posture and the matter-of-fact manner by which he crosses his hands. He seems perhaps younger than 74 years of age. As we talk, he is forthright in his singular piece of advice to a budding anesthesiologist.

> "The goal of your training shouldn't be just specialty certification or sub-specialty certification, but to be really really good…and to be very comfortable with your profession by the end of training," he says. "**Just passing boards is not peak performance.** After all, there are a lot of people who make it to the NFL, but they don't score touchdowns." In one of many proverbial hitting-the-nail-on-the-head moments during our time together, Dr. Prough noted, "**The better you are the day when you finish your residency, the better you will be twenty years later**."

How to Train

In his experience, trainees should spend as much time as possible cementing their clinical experiences with their own readings from textbooks and primary source materials while keeping in mind that the true trials of knowledge happen during patient care. "In between intern year and CA-1 year, I literally read the thickest anesthesia textbook available at that time cover to cover…and progressively tried to layer more and more information into my clinical practice," he remarks. "But a lot of my critical care education came when I started to moonlight at a community hospital where the ICU was five or six times larger than the one I did my fellowship in, the patients were sicker, and I was totally on my own. A lot of things that I had read got fleshed out…during practice."

And it is only through repeated applications of physiology and pathophysiology in clinical practice that an anesthesiologist can know when to go off the book and how to do so safely. "I remember a few patients where the protocol wasn't working," he says. "And where it seemed reasonable to do something different that…you could argue was dictated by that patient or was patient-centered but realistically was along the lines of 'Gosh, the protocol isn't working, I need to try something else.'" Dr. Prough smiles and remarks, "Sometimes, but not always, the outcomes were surprisingly favorable."

Of course, this is not to say that mistakes in medicine do not occur. The very nature of our field means that every patient, regardless of whatever rote and established pathophysiology they may present with, is a unique case requiring their own tailored care, with possible unforeseen complications and effects. "Anybody who has practiced anesthesia in the ICU setting will tell you they have made errors." Dr. Prough states soberly. "The main thing that you learn from the rare occasional major error and frequent minor error is that you need to pay as much attention as possible to how well you do your job, taking care of patients, how well you know concepts, and to make sure that the systems you work within make errors as difficult as possible."

***Note from the Editors:** In honor of Dr. Prough, who trained at the US Naval Medical Center Bethesda outside of Washington DC, we went looking for Potomac River Bridges. Instead of the usual standard images of the wide river and tidal basins in the metro DC area, we found this photo of a much more interesting bridge landscape and section of the Potomac River as it flows through Cumberland, MD (Fig. 28.1).

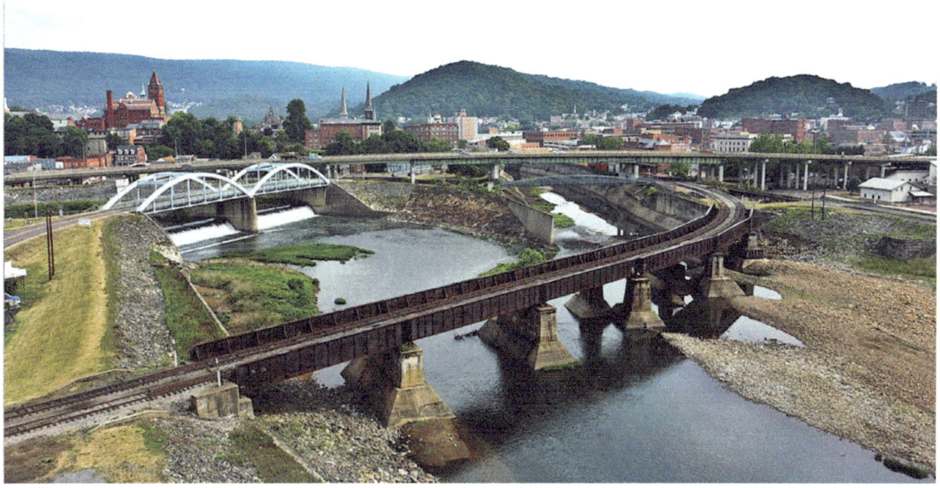

Fig. 28.1 New and old railway and highway bridges over the Potomac River in Cumberland, MD. Photo: Image used under standard license from iStock.com

Work-Life Balance

Inevitably, our conversation meanders to the unavoidable elephant in the room: work-life balance. Though the previously widely accepted reality of 80-hour work weeks is long over in this era of resident duty hour restrictions, the general rule of thumb still stands: the more you work during residency, the more patients you will see and treat, and the more comfortable you will be practicing medicine in the future. But as there are a fixed 24 hours in a day, time spent in the hospital has to be taken from time spent elsewhere. "I know very few people who do [work-life balance] successfully," Dr. Prough wryly admits, "An option would be to wait to get married after residency training, but that isn't possible."

Looking into Your Future

But it is in anticipation of this and other uncomfortable realities of our profession that it is even more important for any anesthesiology trainee to have a clear framework of how they envision their future practice. It is here that the pieces of advice and guidance that mentors offer become doubly valuable. "The first ICU director that I worked with at Bethesda was Mike Rosenthal," Dr. Prough fondly recalls. "From Mike, I learned the politics of critical care medicine at a time when the politics were much more fraught than they are now, the conflict between surgeons and anesthesiologists in the ICU was more intense and frequent, though now it is much better…I saw how Mike handled it, and I decided that it was much too challenging for me to ever do."

In this admission, Dr. Prough lays bare his unspoken philosophy and key to his successful career. Not every obstacle needs to be conquered and mastered. It requires a certain amount of introspection and self-honesty to recognize our strengths and to acknowledge what challenges we as individuals are suited to address. Our time, efforts, and resources are better spent on those passions and pursuits in medicine that invigorate our thirst and zeal for clinical and patient care.

Nevertheless, there are difficulties on the horizon that all new residents and fellows will have to face. "While the political issues in intensive care are much less now, the cognitive basis for critical care is much greater now than it used to be if you go back fifteen or twenty-five years ago," Dr. Prough says. "Concepts were [previously] based on inferences about physiology and pharmacology, while now a great deal of critical care has been subject to clinical trials and evidence-based medicine…A one-year critical care fellowship might not be long enough now. You probably need a substantial interval of practice after that to be facile with the medical aspect of intensive care."

Reflections

Now, days later, as I sit at my desk under the light of a bulb that sorely needs to be replaced and attempt to put the time I shared with Dr. Prough to paper, I cannot help but think that there will always be unforeseen challenges. For the past year, the world has drastically changed as humanity as a whole grapples with a pandemic, and inevitably, there will be events in the future that will leave our best laid plans in disarray. But if we take the advice of senior faculty members like Dr. Prough to heart and to practice, we will be both better prepared and better equipped to handle whatever life tosses our way.

Lessons Learned

- Clinical education cannot be fully encapsulated by board exams, nor should these standards of measure be the limit of your education. Strive to become an extremely competent clinical physician for your patients.

- Errors are unavoidable during your training and subsequent career. Seek to learn the lesson held within these events and improve upon them.

- Challenges are inherent in any clinician's career. Seek to understand, embrace, and cultivate your strengths so as to be best equipped to choose those obstacles that you can realistically address, or put otherwise...sometimes it's okay to finish in second place.

Authors

Ali Bilal was a fourth-year medical student at UTMB Galveston at the time of his meeting with Dr. Prough. Kudos to young Dr. Bilal for undertaking this interview!

Donald Prough is a full professor and the Rebecca Terry White Distinguished Chair of the Department of Anesthesiology at the University of Texas Medical Branch at Galveston.

Mastering the PACU Shuffle

29

Daniel I. Asher and Raymond G. Graber

Introduction

PACU nurses are valuable assets to the anesthesiology community. Work with them to create improved protocols of care, order sets, and methods of communication. Partner with PACU nurses on education, quality improvement, and other projects. This helps build relationships, improves the quality of care, and maybe also the quality of your work environment.

It's Happened to All of Us Before...

You're inducing general anesthesia on a patient whose health is a bit more complicated than can be described as ASA 3, and your pager goes off. You quickly check the return number and, predictably, the PACU needs assistance. The endotracheal tube is safely in, and you quickly place the arterial line... and there goes the pager again. They paged twice... It's probably getting urgent. Instead of calling, you do the smart thing and power walk directly over to the PACU, only to find the nurse sitting at the bedside with no sense of urgency whatsoever. "What's going on? Why'd you page me twice?" Slowly, the nurse looks up from her computer, takes a deep breath, and says, "We need a discharge order."

ASA Standards

The PACU is a fast-paced unit that functions as much as an ICU as it does an outpatient discharge area. The goal is safe and efficient patient throughput to make room for the next patients coming out of the ORs. There is constant turnover of a highly diverse group of patients, who are being managed

D. I. Asher (✉) · R. G. Graber
Department of Anesthesiology and Perioperative Medicine, University Hospitals Cleveland Medical Center, Cleveland, OH, USA
e-mail: Daniel.Asher@uhhospitals.org

S. Mohamed et al. (eds.), *Anesthesia Bridges*, https://doi.org/10.1007/978-3-032-08294-7_29

by different teams, and are all emerging from different levels of anesthesia. This means that acuity is high and, as you know, it can get complicated fast. **You have specific ASA standards to follow in your postanesthesia care:**

- Every patient who has any type of anesthetic, including everything from an "OK Anesthesia" MAC to a general anesthetic, needs to receive appropriate postanesthesia care. It doesn't have to be a PACU, but it usually is.
- Patients actively being transferred from the operating room or from a procedure room need to be continually evaluated and managed by someone who is part of the anesthesia care team.
- Upon transferring the patient to postanesthetic care, whether that be a PACU or anywhere else, there needs to be a verbal report about the patient and their operative and anesthetic course.
- The patient needs to be continually evaluated and monitored in the PACU with a written record of their care.
- And everything from PACU admission to discharge is **your** responsibility as the attending physician. This is your unit. In fact, your department is supposed to approve all policies regarding patient care in the PACU.

The good news is that you don't manage all that by yourself. We have specially trained (and sometimes certified) perianesthesia nurses in the PACU. Having these nurses actively participate on your team will make your life as an attending so much easier. It will allow you to focus on intraoperative management and your more acute patients with the knowledge that your PACU patients are in good hands.

The ability to work well with these nurses rests on understanding what they are capable of, their training and knowledge base, and how to activate them to perform their best at the highest levels of their certification. With the right training and support, your PACU RNs can be the best partners to care for your patients. Here are some pearls of wisdom cultivated on how to ally up with your PACU team.

***Note from the Editors:** The first recorded mention of a type of recovery room was in 1801 and pertained to the Newcastle-on-Tyne Infirmary 1801, predating the first description of anesthesia by 40 years. Five rooms with two beds to a room were described as being adjacent to the operating room theater. To commemorate our historical medical colleagues who were taking care of postsurgical patients over 200 years ago, we went looking for cool bridges in Newcastle and found so many that we couldn't pick just one (Fig. 29.1).

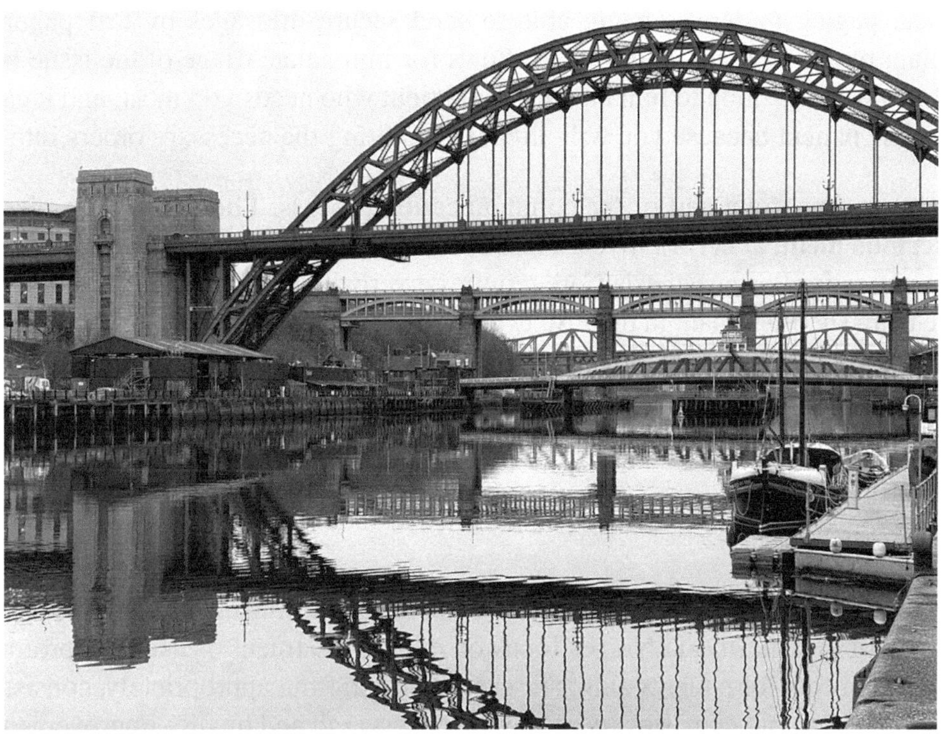

Fig. 29.1 The many bridges over the River Tyne in Newcastle, England create a graphically stunning riverscape. Photo: Mark Duffy, image used under standard license from iStock.adobe.com

Communication

Let's address the vignette above. At first glance, the nurse was getting in your way. You were trying to manage a sick patient, and the nurse double-pages you for a minor issue. There are a few ways that communication breakdown led to this point.

First off, you didn't place the electronic medical record (EMR) order that the nurse needed in order to treat the patient. Almost everything that an RN does for a patient, including admission and discharge, is at the order of a physician. When you put in your orders, it would make sense to include all necessary orders in an order set to allow for expedient PACU management and discharge. Use your orders to decrease phone calls and improve the time to treatment of common PACU issues. As patients recover from anesthesia and surgical procedures, they can suffer from an expected constellation of symptoms. Having PRN orders to treat those symptoms—such as nausea and vomiting, pain, acute postoperative hypertension, etc.—allows for your specially trained nurses to start treatment. It also helps show that you have confidence in the abilities of your nurses to manage basic aftereffects of anesthesia and surgical procedures. If order sets are incomplete or inadequate, get involved and work to evolve them.

Secondly, the traditional practice of paging someone to a PACU phone, especially in a large PACU, generally takes a significant amount of time. By the time the secretary figures out which nurse called for which doctor, the patient's condition could have changed dramatically. A major improvement over a simple numerical paging system is being able to send secure messages by text pager or through a HIPAA-compliant phone messaging app. This allows for immediate triage of the issue by the anesthesiologist. It allows your attention to remain with the patient who needs you most, and it can also shorten the time to treat the patient because you will already be putting the necessary orders into the EMR.

Handoffs are also an important part of the communication process. **The Joint Commission estimates that 80% of serious medical errors involve handoff miscommunications or omissions.** Standard III of the ASA Standards for Postanesthesia Care requires a verbal handoff to the PACU nurse, and that the anesthesia care team should remain in the PACU until the PACU nurse accepts responsibility for care of the patient. When you provide an incomplete handoff, your PACU nurse may be unable to adequately care for the patient, and in addition, this also erodes your relationship with him or her.

Respect

We need to recognize the importance, skills, and goals of PACU nurses. The practice standards of the American Society of Perianesthesia Nurses focus on ethical treatment of patients, promoting safe and comfortable environments for patients and their caregivers, staffing appropriately, consistent evaluation of multidisciplinary care, and consistent contribution to research and quality improvement. You already know by now that not all nurses are the same, but PACU nurses are a different kind of nurse altogether. They are an incredibly valuable resource and deserve respect.

PACU nurses are specialists in emerging patients from anesthesia, managing their acute postoperative care, and getting the patient to where they need to go next. A patient's discharge location could be an ICU, med-surg floor, long-term care facility, or even back home. In this era of Covid-19, PACUs have also had to function as ICUs to manage overflow from other hospital ICUs. Thus, our nurses need to be able to function as ICU nurses and discharge nurses all at the same time. Remember, they don't function without clear direction from their orders and protocols. So, it is up to us to work with them to set expectations and design protocols to help streamline patient care in the PACU.

Our department has gone as far as to create nurse-initiated physician protocols for the PACU to allow RNs to place specific and limited orders that allow them to appropriately admit patients, provide point-of-care testing, start IVs, and measure the patient's height and weight. Yes, everything needs an order! We also educated our nurses to identify patients who may have a considerable risk of obstructive sleep apnea or postoperative respiratory failure and have protocolized their ability to formally consult respiratory therapists to evaluate and treat a patient before he/she has an issue.

Because PACU nurses have expertise and a desire to improve the quality of care they deliver, it makes sense to include them as part of interdisciplinary teams to collaborate on case reviews, quality projects, and other system projects. There is mutual benefit when physician and RN leaders establish a positive working relationship and find better ways to cooperate. This interdepartmental partnership can lead to improvements in our patients' care.

Education

Communication with and respect for our PACU nurses can be further improved by knowledge sharing and interdisciplinary education. In fact, the basis of education is the ability for the student and the teacher to share a mutual respect. Establishing a regular educational series can help cultivate positive relationships among PACU and anesthesia staff. We are continuously evolving our anesthetic management techniques, and also the post-op management of patients, as we try to promote early recovery and discharge. Our PACU nurses are eager to learn about this stuff. So, don't you want your staff to learn about these advances from us, rather than from rumors or off the internet?

Final Thoughts

PACU nurses and anesthesia care teams need to function as a cohesive unit. You might not be critically care trained, but the PACU is **your** ICU. The sooner we take ownership of it and become leaders in postanesthesia care, the better our combined care will be for our patients.

Lessons Learned

- PACU nurses are your allies. Work with them to create improved protocols of care, order sets, and methods of communication.
- Partner with PACU nurses on education, quality improvement, and other projects. including academic and publication initiatives. This helps build relationships, improves the quality of care, and maybe also the quality of your work environment.

Authors

Dan Asher is a cardiac anesthesiologist at University Hospitals in Cleveland who has had the pleasure of being the medical director of the PACU at UHCMC for the past five years. In addition to patient care, he works on various hospital committees to protocolize and improve the quality of care delivered in the hospital system. His four kids (all 6 and under at the time this chapter was written) keep him and his wife busy, but they make time to be active members of their local Jewish community.

Ray Graber is a cardiac anesthesiologist as well as the anesthesiology vice chair for quality and quality initiatives at University Hospitals in Cleveland.

Lawsuits Happen

30

Christopher M. Conley and Mark C. Norris

Introduction

It is a shock to the system when a patient or family initiates a lawsuit against you. The language of a malpractice complaint is often highly stylized, implying you delivered incompetent, negligent, and callous care. What's worse, your legal team quickly reminds you of the "can't confide culture," wherein you can't discuss the case with anyone other than your lawyer or your spouse. In this chapter, we hope to introduce you to some important concepts to help guide you through this difficult and emotional process.

Medical Malpractice Is a Business

Lawsuits are not initiated to make you a better doctor or to "right a wrong." Medical malpractice suits have but one goal: **To get money**. According to a 2016 New England Journal review, among cases that were settled or found in favor of the plaintiff, the average payout was $371,054. The lawyer's take was a little over $120,000. Getting sued is a part of being a physician in the US healthcare system. Understanding this fact is an important part of enduring and surviving the process.

You, the physician, or another insured provider, are an "account holder" of your malpractice coverage. The case you were part of represents an opportunity for the malpractice attorneys to transfer those funds into their own accounts. The lawyers' take is usually 1/3 of the settlement or jury award, but can be up to 40% in some cases. For the lawyers, it is not personal. At best, you, your confidence, family life, and emotional well-being are simply collateral damage. We're bombarded by advertisements from malpractice attorneys on television, the internet, and even on billboards a block away from our medical centers. This targeted advertising seeks to normalize the process of suing doctors.

Patients and families have little or nothing to lose by pursuing malpractice litigation. Most plaintiffs' attorneys do not charge unless they win, and there is no burden of proof to initiate a malpractice lawsuit. Although it has the potential to complicate licensure and credentialing, the medical malpractice suit is not a formal complaint to a medical or licensure board, nor is it a criminal proceeding.

C. M. Conley (✉) · M. C. Norris
Department of Anesthesiology, Boston Medical Center, Boston, MA, USA
e-mail: Christopher.Conley@bmc.org; Mark.Norris@bmc.org

S. Mohamed et al. (eds.), *Anesthesia Bridges*, https://doi.org/10.1007/978-3-032-08294-7_30

What Are the Odds of Getting Sued?

In a 2017 AMA study, across **all** specialties, 34% of physicians had been sued, and 16.8% had been sued two or more times. By the time we're 65 years old, 75% of physicians in low-risk specialties and 99% of those in high-risk specialties will have been sued. Cases that prompt lawsuits often involve unexpected, catastrophic outcomes, especially in neonatal, pediatric, and obstetric anesthesia. Patient dissatisfaction with care, or patient disability after an event, can also lead to a lawsuit. Physician factors may be the best place to channel our efforts, as we may be able to reduce, but not eliminate, our chances of becoming a defendant. A 1992 study in JAMA surveyed plaintiffs who'd pursued lawsuits for perinatal injury. The study showed that 44% of respondents initiated their lawsuit due to either "needing information" or suspicion of a "cover-up" surrounding their child's injury. A recurring theme is the perception by families of poor or dishonest communication by physicians—this can stimulate them to pursue malpractice litigation.

Established, long-standing patient relationships were one of the few protective traits that seemed to decrease patients' tendency to file suit. Physicians with less total, or zero, face time with patients, or lack of an ongoing therapeutic relationship with serial patient encounters—including anesthesiologists, radiologists, and pathologists—are likely at a disadvantage here. While that signature on your informed consent listing various possible complications may seem to be a "legal release," it isn't. However, the absence of a consent discussion and signature may be a fast track to payouts to the plaintiff.

Will a Lawsuit Wipe Out My Savings?

If you are involved in a lawsuit, you will naturally begin to wonder how this is going to affect your professional reputation, your job security, and your family's financial well-being.

What if they win big and the award exceeds my malpractice coverage limits? History is on your side here. It's exquisitely rare that juries award damages above the individual limits of physicians' malpractice policies, which is part of the reason that medical malpractice plaintiff's attorneys are incentivized to name all healthcare workers in the room when filing suit.

While being named in a lawsuit may be out of your control, the choices you make next can define the outcome.

What NOT to Do if You Are Named in a Medical Malpractice Complaint

Do NOT go on a venting spree about the case! You need to be **<u>very</u>** careful who you talk to after being named in a lawsuit. There is a natural, strong initial temptation to "tell your side" to anyone who can listen. At the outset, only your lawyer and your partner/spouse are safe places to discuss the details of the case outside of peer-reviewed conferences. You are permitted to discuss your emotional reaction, but not the specifics of the case. The problem is, as anesthesiologists (and I'm guessing nearly all of medicine's specialties), it's impossible to separate the emotions we have about the case from the details. We need people to know what our thought process was, how we were trying to make choices from a place of reason, a thoughtful plan that addressed both safety and comfort. Our emotions are intertwined with what we did and why we did it.

As the details of the case emerge, and the plaintiff's complaint asserts facts or concerns about the patient's disease state or the "science" of your case, it may be tempting to further your expertise on the topic, collecting papers and evidence that defend the choices and decisions you made during the event. **Please resist this temptation**. Do not go on a "research spree." Your case will not be stronger if you "bone up" on the pathology encountered on the day of the event. Your notes and your understanding of the situation at the time of the event are what matters. Your defense team will independently secure experts of their own who will present evidence in your favor at the time of trial.

At this point, you should not directly access any of the plaintiff's medical records, as you are no longer their healthcare provider, making chart access a HIPAA violation. Your legal team (not you!!!) will obtain the medical records and all the notes surrounding the case that you'll need to reexamine the event and mount your defense.

***Note from the Editors:** This is what being named in a frivolous lawsuit feels like (Fig. 30.1). Ask us how we know.

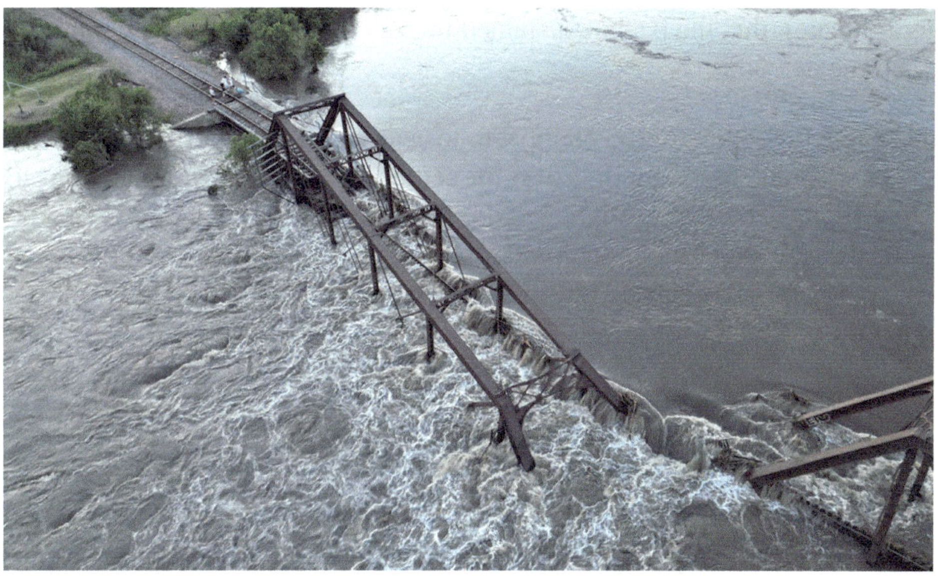

Fig. 30.1 There were no fatalities and no serious injuries in this railroad bridge collapse; it was eventually repaired, just like your career will be after a frivolous lawsuit. But you will feel wrecked for a while, that is for sure. Photo: Image used under standard license from shutterstock.com

What You SHOULD Do if Named in a Medical Malpractice Complaint

Contact your malpractice insurer and get contact info/phone numbers/emails for your legal team. Tell your department chairman you've been named in a suit. You will need time off for meetings, depositions, and so forth. **Finally, breathe.** As anesthesiologists, breathing has a special place in our hearts as it relates to patient outcomes, but this is about a different kind of survival. From the moment you are informed of involvement in a malpractice case, even if the case is dismissed or settled prior to going to trial, this will be a lengthy emotional marathon. Your malpractice insurer will supply you a legal advocate, but **you** need to be your greatest advocate for your physical, emotional, and behavioral health.

Get help early. Find safe spaces and nondiscoverable opportunities to vent. Conversations with your spouse are protected from legal discovery. Yet even the best of life partners often do not have the training or the bandwidth to be your only copilot on this very emotional journey. It is never too early to seek professional counseling following a devastating patient event. Conversations during psychotherapy sessions are protected thanks to the physician-patient privilege. In recent years, most hospitals and healthcare systems have expanded their internal resources in behavioral medicine through low-cost, accessible employee health programs. Private conversations with your clergy or religious leaders are also safe from subpoena and legal discovery.

Despite the emotional toll this process will surely take on you, some things are in your favor when sitting on the defendant side of a medical malpractice lawsuit. While it takes little to no evidence to file a malpractice claim against a physician in the US, winning the case as a plaintiff is an entirely different story. The plaintiff must prove beyond a reasonable doubt that the physician acted negligently (diverting from the standard of care), that the patient sustained harm, and that there was a causative link between the negligence and the outcome.

Any break in this chain is enough for the plaintiff to lose a case. The majority of malpractice claims are dropped by the plaintiff, dismissed by the court, or settled before trial for an amount lower than your malpractice policy limits. The few outright victories for malpractice plaintiffs' attorneys offset their frequent losses. In the rare event that a malpractice case makes it through trial to a jury, the outcome overwhelmingly favors the physicians. Only 2% of anesthesia malpractice suits that go through trial result in a judgment for the plaintiff.

Steps in the Medicolegal Process (and a Few Insights)

Complaint Filing: Each state has its own "discovery" law that determines how long after an event occurs that a medical malpractice complaint can be filed and a lawsuit initiated. This is typically between 2 and 6 years after the incident, but may be up to 18 years in cases involving children.

Discovery Phase: Both teams will secure medical experts to support their case. The plaintiff's team will next send over interrogatories. These are a series of questions about you, the case, and your participation in the event. In a way, this is the "essay contest" portion of your lawsuit. The questions may be framed to make you look bad, callous, and careless. They may also include topics like: Your experience with the patient's disease state, standards of care for treatment of your patient's condition, and your consideration of alternative management of the event may all be called into question. You, your lawyers, and your team's expert witnesses will come together on the answers. This process of combing through and responding to the interrogatories may cause you to reexperience the trauma of the event.

The Depositions: This is a completely separate event and may occur years in advance of the trial. You will likely speak far more during the deposition than you will at the trial. This is arguably the most important, and most stressful, portion of the process for you as a defendant. For the first time, you'll be sitting across from the plaintiff's attorneys, and they are going to take this opportunity to trap you into a misstep that strengthens their case against you and weakens your defense. They are going to try to get under your skin, to wear you down. It's best to take an approach very similar to the oral boards: Prepare, answer questions succinctly and truthfully, and don't guess. For even the shortest, simplest of questions, pause, think, then respond. There is strategy and gamesmanship at play here. Depositions are always transcribed in real-time with a court reporter. Some are also audio- or videorecorded. After the deposition, you will need to review the transcript, both for accuracy, as sometimes the scribe gets it wrong, and for consistency. You may make mistakes in your deposition. It's critical to review your answers with your legal team between the deposition and your time of trial, where some of your responses will be revisited by the plaintiff's attorneys. When you are asked similar questions or confronted with inconsistencies in your response at the time of trial, you don't want to be caught off guard.

Settlement, Trial, or Both: Trials (and juries) are unpredictable, so even as late as the 11th hour, your case is very likely to settle. Depending on your malpractice insurance, you may not get to choose whether to fight the case. Even in cases where physicians have the right to reject a settlement, you may be subject to what's called a "hammer clause." This means if you lose, any rewards to the plaintiff beyond the proposed settlement would come out of your personal assets.

An advantage of settling in advance of a jury verdict may be a more reasonable top end for the payout (thus protecting you from any unprecedented or extreme jury award). Unfortunately, any settlement needs to be reported to the National Practitioner Data Bank and will come up every time you recredential, apply for new jobs, or renew your medical license for the next 10 years. The vast majority of medical malpractice cases never make it to trial, as the cases are either dropped or settled before you have your day in court.

If your case makes it to trial, this certainly is anxiety provoking. However, the good news is that physicians overwhelmingly win the majority of malpractice cases that proceed to trial. Trials typically last 2–4 weeks. Rarely, they can go longer. In most cases, your team will want you to be there every day, as a sign of your personal and emotional investment for the jury to see.

Over the course of a trial, if it appears your side is not going to win, your legal team may still enter into a settlement agreement with the plaintiff's side. This often includes so-called "High/Low Agreements," which create both a basement and a ceiling for what the payout will be to the plaintiff. For the plaintiff, this guarantees they get some minimum payout, even in the event the jury sides with your team/dismisses the case. On your side, this protects you from the jury delivering an "over the top" or "statement" verdict that exceeds the limits of your malpractice coverage.

Conclusion

If and when you're named in a lawsuit, please remember that many of your colleagues either have been or will go through it at least once in their careers. Don't go it alone, seek support, find the safe places and circumstances to talk about it, and don't let this break you.

Lessons Learned

- Medical malpractice is a business. Patients and families have little or nothing to lose by pursuing malpractice litigation.
- Odds are highly likely that you will be sued during the course of your career.
- If you get sued, it is advisable to not share details about the case with friends or colleagues.
- Your legal team will educate you about the process and guide you through it.

***Note from the Editors:** We did an informal survey of the *Anesthesia Bridges* contributors and can validate the advice above. We heard many stories of being sued, but the most remarkable was that one of our contributors was once sued on a frivolous case, along with every anesthesiologist on the case—every single one—including all the residents who had given breaks. It was devastating to the physicians but so impersonal for the plaintiffs that one evening one of the named anesthesiologists was sitting in the cafeteria in street clothes (hospital badge already in the backpack) and the plaintiff and plaintiff's family sat down at the same long cafeteria table and began talking, laughing, and joking about taking the physicians and hospital for a big payout. The plaintiff had no idea who the defendants were, much less that they were sitting next to one. The case was a frivolous one and ended with all physicians being dropped from the case. But the plaintiff's conversation was duly reported to the lawyers representing the anesthesiologists, and certainly didn't hurt the settlement negotiations.

- The photo illustration above was chosen for a reason. Being named in a lawsuit can feel like a devastating smashup of your professional and personal road forward in life, but it **can** be survived without loss of that life or even significant injury, the terror of the moment notwithstanding.

Suggested Readings

1. Jena AB, Seabury S, Lakdawalla D, et al. Malpractice risk according to physician specialty. NEJM. 2011;365(7):629–36.
2. Bondi S, Rusher J, Schuman AJ. You've been served! What to do if you get sued for malpractice. Contemp Pediatr. [Internet] [cited 19 June 2023]. 2019;36(3):47–9. Available from https://www.conteporarypediatrics.com
3. Studdert DM, Bismark MM, Mello MM, et al. Prevalence and characteristics of physicians prone to malpractice claims. NEJM. 2016;374(4):354–62.
4. Hickson GB, Clayton EW, Githens PB, et al. Factors that prompted families to file medical malpractice claims following perinatal injuries. JAMA. 1992;267(10):1359–63.
5. Rice B. Could a malpractice mega-verdict wipe you out? Med Econ. 2003;80:89.

Authors

Christopher Conley is a New England lifer. He completed his anesthesia residency at Brigham and Women's Hospital, followed by a fellowship at Boston Children's. His work passions include feedback systems in graduate medical education, physician wellness, and perioperative optimization in children. He married the love of his life, Anne, and they are the proud parents of Ben and Charlie.

Mark Norris has been practicing anesthesia, in both academic and private settings, for over 40 years. His interests include obstetrical anesthesia, resident education, and expanding the diversity of the medical workforce. Outside of the hospital, he enjoys his family, cycling, and cooking.

Fired? Handwriting on the Wall? Why You Should Lick Your Wounds and Move On

31

Jane B. Jacobs

Introduction

When we accept a new job, we usually are optimistic that we have found a good fit at an institution that provides great care and has excellent management. Unfortunately, sometimes things don't work out. Your relationship with your leadership may sour for any number of reasons. We have also all heard stories of whole groups being discarded by management teams who have succumbed to the lure of a "cheaper" provider. How should one approach these situations? Attorney Jane Jacobs gives us some advice.

Overview

After she lost the Georgia governor's race in 2018, Stacey Abrams famously said, "I sat shiva for 10 days. Then I started plotting."

Perhaps you've been fired. Maybe you've gotten a bad review. Maybe it's obvious that you're not long for your job. Let's assume that you're being treated unfairly. Let's assume that your boss is an inept moron. It's unfair, unjust, and screams for a bloody, public fight.

I've been a management labor and employment attorney for more than 40 years and I'm telling you, be Stacey Abrams. Take a pause to regroup and then start plotting. And, in most cases, your plotting should be plotting a new course, not plotting a legal fight.

Why? First, if your situation is "merely" unfair, it probably is legal. The exceptions are mostly limited to a contract or that your situation is based on a protected class, such as race or sex.

Let's assume that you have some basis to sue—and most people won't—here's what happens when you file with an agency or in court: **almost nothing,** for months on end.

Disclaimer: The views expressed here are for the reader's education and information only and are solely the author's own. Ms. Jacobs provides legal advice only within the attorney-client privilege and based on the specifics of each client's needs and issues. Viewing this content does not establish an attorney-client privilege.

J. B. Jacvobs (✉)
Tarter Krinsky and Drogin LLP, New York, NY, USA
e-mail: jjacobs@tarterkrinsky.com

S. Mohamed et al. (eds.), *Anesthesia Bridges*, https://doi.org/10.1007/978-3-032-08294-7_31

Discovery and Digging for Dirt

If you filed with an agency, chances are that the most it will do is tell you to go to court on your own, and that only after months or even years. If you're in court, eventually, you'll move to discovery, when you have to turn over your texts, your email, your social media posts. Remember that text when you said you may have screwed up? Discoverable. The social media post that you thought was private enough because your account wasn't public? Discoverable. Have you claimed emotional distress (everyone does, that's where the money is)? Then everything relating to your state of mind gets turned over—your therapist's records and testimony, your prescription history, your medical records. Have you had a messy breakup in the past few years? Do you take a lot of Ambien? Do you generally have anxiety? All fair game.

Does your employer claim you weren't very good at what you do? They will do what they can to prove it. They will interview your coworkers, reach out to your prior jobs, and scour your work records.

Eventually you'll be deposed. There's no judge present; it's you and the attorneys in a conference room. You can't refuse to answer. You can be pressed hard to answer uncomfortable questions.

If you sue, that's the next few years of your life, reliving your worst months over and over again. Another unhappy fact: management attorneys are generally better trained, can devote far more time, and have ten times the resources of most plaintiffs' attorneys.

***Note from the Editors:** Jane Jacobs' favorite bridge is "the Brooklyn Bridge, of course." Here it is, in a great aerial view, showing the detail and intricacy of the stonework, with the New York skyline behind (Fig. 31.1).

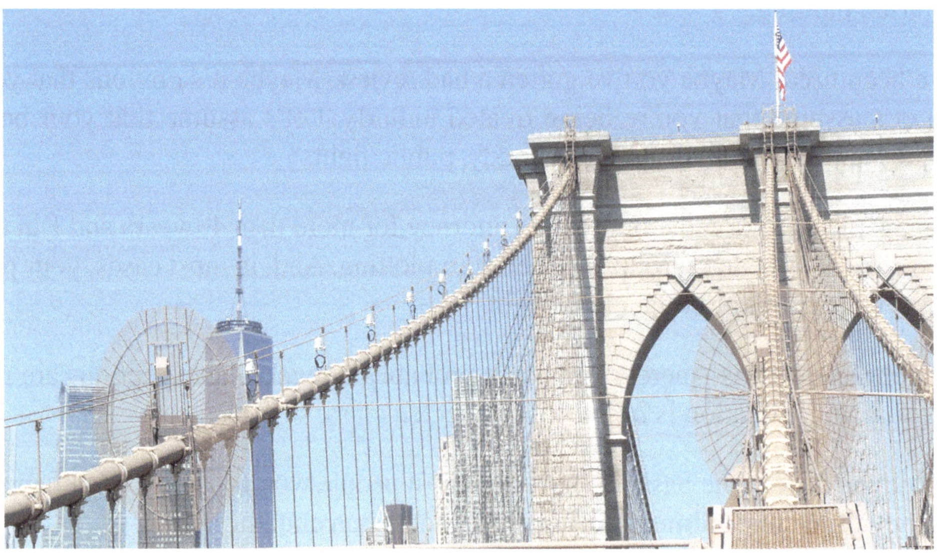

Fig. 31.1 The Brooklyn Bridge is an iconic feature of the New York City skyline and has been a major tourist attraction since it opened. It is a hybrid cable-stayed and suspension bridge. It was the first fixed crossing of the East River and opened in 1883. It was the longest suspension bridge in the world at that time. Only passenger vehicles, pedestrians, and bicycle traffic are permitted today, although both horse-drawn vehicles and elevated railways were a feature of the bridge until 1950. Major refurbishments and repairs were undertaken in the 1950s, the 1980s, and the 2010s. Photo: Image used under standard license from shutterstock.com

The Truth About Trials

But you're thinking that eventually you'll get to trial, and you'll get to show a judge and jury the truth. These cases never go to trial. They always settle. In almost all cases, it makes very little financial sense to try an employment case.

It's said that the best settlements are the ones that leave everyone equally unhappy. You'll wind up with about 40% of whatever the settlement may be. From the gross settlement, a third goes to your attorney, and the expenses are paid, such as transcripts, experts, and filing fees. You get the rest, but it's taxable as ordinary income. If you settle for $250,000, and you'd be doing very well if you did, you'll wind up with less than $100,000. It's not even emotionally satisfying.

Strategies for Survival

So, what should you do? The best thing to do is not to wait until the ball drops. Find an employment lawyer and negotiate the best possible exit, which avoids a termination, preserves your clean record, keeps you insurable, gives you a better story to tell prospective employers, and maybe puts a few dollars in your pocket.

Start working your networks. Let the world know that you're looking for new opportunities. It's immeasurably easier to find a job when you have a job. All of the energy that you'd put into a lawsuit? Use it instead to find a better, happier job.

There will be times when a lawsuit is your best or maybe only option. If you're already fired and your reputation is in ruins, and if you have the intestinal fortitude to do it, make sure you've got someone capable to represent you and try to settle as fast as possible.

Otherwise? It's a lousy thing to go through, but you'll set yourself up for a better comeback if you move on.

Lessons Learned

- Legal and employment issues happen, but they are never a good or positive event in a career. Take every precaution and action to avoid the gravitational pull of this type of professional black hole.

- From the first second of your professional career, be mindful of the written record you are laying down. Watch what you are writing about work, no matter who you are writing it to. **Never** send that pointed memorandum or make any written record of anger on any subject. In an employment action, it's all discoverable, and that anger, no matter how righteous, will be used against you. It is best to close every email, no matter how short, with "Very respectfully, Jane Doe, MD." This might seem artificial or stilted, but it's what they do in the military and for good reason.

Not only is everything discoverable in an employment action, everything is fair game in an employment deposition. You can and will be asked if you passed both parts of your board exams. When you answer yes, you will then be asked if you passed them on the first try.

- If you claim emotional distress in an employment action, expect that your spouse will be deposed, and your relationship will be put under a microscope. Yes, possibly even *that* part of your relationship. The other side might ask for your credit card and bank statements, and your vacation pictures will be picked apart.
- No matter what you are told by allies going into an employment action, **do not** expect any coworkers to put their own reputations, promotions, or jobs on the line for you. Your colleagues may be upset for you, but they can and will find a way not to do much about your sad situation if it involves jeopardizing their own positions with the employer.
- "Winning" an employment action means winning at settlement. The lawyers on both sides understand the dance and have been through it many times.
- **The only real power you have is to vote with your feet**. Put your track shoes on and prepare to keep moving.

Author

Jane Jacobs has been a labor and employment attorney for 40 years. She was formerly the managing partner of Klein Zelman Rothermel Jacobs & Schess LLP and is now a partner at Tarter Krinsky and Drogin in New York City. Jane has two adult daughters, a trained paramedic and a human resources manager. She was also the proud mom to a beautiful greyhound who occasionally saw a squirrel within reach and took the opportunity to demonstrate that she was once a champion athlete. When not working, Jane is a theater buff and gym rat.

32 Preventing Delays of Game: A Systems Management Approach

Charles H. Sandson and Raymond G. Graber

Introduction

Part of being a good anesthesia professional is to work toward getting cases started on time and having a reasonable turnover time between cases. It is tempting to blame delays on individuals, but maybe there are system issues that are the real culprits. So, wouldn't it make sense to evaluate our processes with a systems management approach?

Traditionally, room turnover has been defined as the time from one patient leaving a room till the time the next patient enters the room. It can be broken up into the time it takes to clean the room and the time it takes to set up for the next case. However, there is a relatively new wrinkle—one more thing that needs to be accomplished prior to induction of anesthesia—and that is the preoperative "huddle."

Huddles: Pro and Con

Now that the huddle has been standard practice for a few years, we can begin to analyze it. As with any new innovation, the huddle has solved some problems but created others. The biggest issue with huddles is quite simple—they take time. The actual discussion itself doesn't take long, but rounding up all the necessary stakeholders (who may be scattered across the hospital) can take a significant amount of time. This is especially an issue for second- or third-round starts.

The result? Patients are waiting in a prepped operating room for 20 or 30 minutes. We have now turned our huddle into a "delay of game." This is bad from both a human factors standpoint and for the overall efficiency of the hospital system. Apprehensive patients are endemic to every OR in the

Disclaimer: This information is intended for educational purposes and does not represent the corporate position or business advice of ZS Associates.

C. H. Sandson
ZS Associates, Washington, DC, USA

R. G. Graber (✉)
Department of Anesthesiology and Perioperative Medicine, University Hospitals Cleveland Medical Center, Cleveland, OH, USA
e-mail: raymond.graber@uhhospitals.org

S. Mohamed et al. (eds.), *Anesthesia Bridges*, https://doi.org/10.1007/978-3-032-08294-7_32

world, and making them wait for longer than necessary just makes things worse. For hospital administrators, the further behind the OR runs, the more overtime is necessary, and the lower the efficiency numbers plummet.

Real Issues in a Real Hospital

So how do we reduce turnover time and get our stakeholders to the huddle on time? To answer this question, the application of several industrial engineering principles might be in order. We'll look at the example of a large Midwestern teaching hospital, where one of the authors (Ray) has worked as an anesthesiologist for more than 30 years. His hospital has struggled with both room turnover and huddle delays. In the ideal world, there would be a consistent turnover time, followed by a consistent setup time for any given case—add these together, and you have the expected time for the next huddle.

However, we live in the real world, and there is much uncertainty in these processes. As examples, a joint replacement room may have an average turnover time of 40 minutes, while a cardiac surgical room might turnover in 80 minutes. Of course, these times are averages, and on any given day, they may vary by 15–20 minutes in either direction. So, the range of huddle times might be within a window of 30–40 minutes. This makes it extremely difficult to schedule a huddle while simultaneously finishing up the prior case.

***Note from the Editors:** A bridge to a hospital in Bangkok (Fig. 32.1).

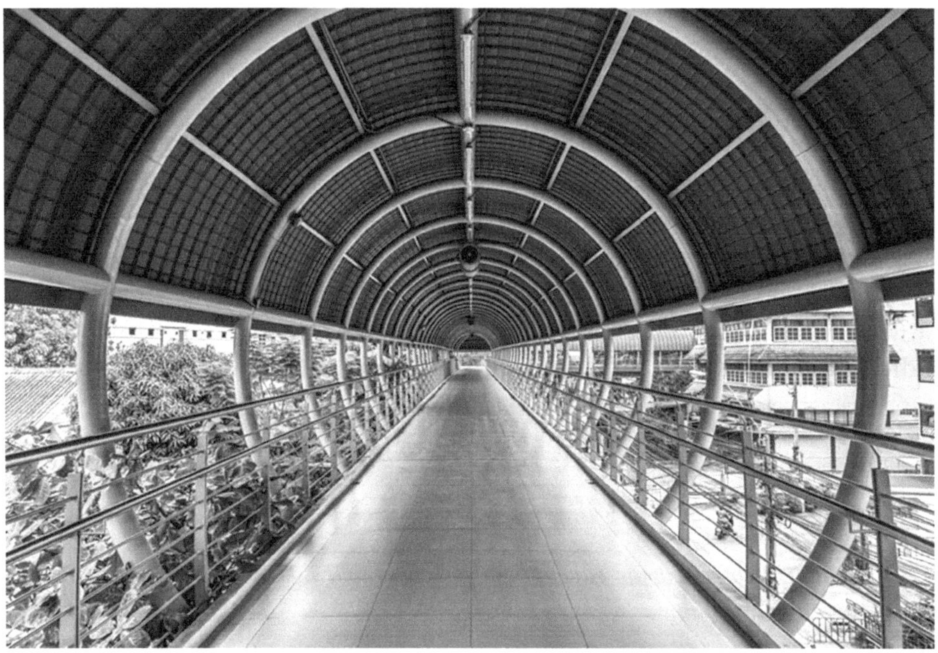

Fig. 32.1 The stunning architecture of a hospital bridge walkway. Photo: Derek Eyre, image used under standard license from iStock.com

Applying Operations Research Principles

To solve Ray's problem, we turn to the operations research methods of measurement, analysis, and standardization. Management consultants call this process the Kaizen approach—the Japanese strategy for continuous improvement where employees at all levels of a company work together proactively to achieve regular, incremental improvements in a system.

The first step is to bring together all involved parties and map out all the steps in a process—all the jobs that need to be completed, and by whom. The next step is to collect data and see if there are any patterns that emerge. Many hospitals have process improvement personnel who can be enlisted to help work on this project. Each step in the process can be timed, and barriers to various task completions can be identified. Reducing barriers reduces variation. The goal is to create order and reduce uncertainty in turnover time.

One can identify many reasons for delays and variations. Room cleanup is slow if there is a delay in calling for room cleanup, or a shortage of cleaning personnel. OR personnel can leave a room tidy or totally trashed. Room setup can be delayed by the need to re-sterilize instrument trays, or the search for missing equipment, or trays that are incomplete or contaminated, etc. Sometimes, instrument trays are overly complicated and are difficult to set up. All these processes are amenable to incremental improvements with resultant reduction in turnover time.

At Ray's institution, they have worked through many of these issues, and the majority of the current variation comes in the time it takes to clean the operating room. Once the room is clean, the amount of time it takes the nurses to set up for the next patient is relatively consistent and predictable. So, the answer to the question of when to set the time for the huddle is clear. The huddle time can be set as soon as the room cleaning has been completed. The nurses will need roughly 15 minutes' head start for a joint replacement, and maybe 30 minutes for a cardiac procedure. The rest of their setup is done concurrently while we are inducing anesthesia, placing lines, and so forth.

Giving the surgeons a planned huddle time that's 15–30 minutes in the future works well—they have time to complete whatever task they are doing and move to the OR. This is a big improvement over "huddle now!" So, you now have a win-win situation. The surgeons can better plan their time, and the huddle will be completed both more quickly and with less variation. Your hospital system may be different from Ray's, and the variation in turnover time may come from a different source. But by analyzing your process, you give yourself the opportunity to inject structure into the system, reduce variability, and improve the whole turnover process.

Communication Counts!

So, to reiterate, once the OR is clean, typically the anesthesia and nursing teams are setting up at the same time, and the two parties can negotiate a huddle time based on the time each group needs for adequate setup. This now needs to be communicated to the surgical team. Who should do that?

It can be done by either the nursing team or the anesthesia team as long as someone takes clear ownership of the task. Ray likes to take the initiative to set the huddle time and text the attending surgeon, but that also depends on his workload and availability. The nurses are setting up one room, whereas the attending anesthesiologist may be supervising two or more rooms. So, although Ray likes to drive the system to improve efficiency, he also realizes he can't always be there to do it. As a result, there is another source of variability and uncertainty in the pre-op system.

What would an industrial engineer think about this communication problem? There are two basic options—a centralized or decentralized system of communication. In a decentralized system, the stakeholder who schedules the huddle (either an anesthesia or nursing team member) would communicate the time and place to all other stakeholders, either directly or through the head of their teams. This could be done over text, pager, or phone. There is no middleman, and the information passed on should be the correct information.

In a centralized system, the OR control desk would be notified, and they would take responsibility for the communication process. The advantage is that they do the work, thus relieving the burden on staff involved in the next procedure, but there's now a middleman and a chance of forgotten calls or misinformation.

Thus, both centralized and decentralized systems have benefits and drawbacks, and ultimately, you will have to analyze your hospital's practices and culture to determine which approach is right for you. This issue could be simplified in the future by the development of some advanced OR management software which would send huddle alerts to all stakeholders.

Summary

In this discussion, we have tried to give an example of a systems management approach to a common operating room problem. In your practices, there are likely other common problems that can be addressed by collecting data and analyzing it. Rather than getting frustrated and pointing fingers at individuals, try to use a data-driven approach to analyze the systems in which you work, and improve them. In Ray's younger days, he worked as a surgical tech at a hospital where his grandfather worked as a general surgeon. His grandfather told him that the key to efficiency was not rushing, but instead to **avoid wasting time**. These words are true to this day.

Lessons Learned

- All complex systems have the ability to break down and come to a halt. The OR is no different. Use hospital process improvement personnel to help model the system so that barriers can be identified and reduced.
- Don't be complacent about slow turnovers—look for ways that you can improve the process.
- Remember these grandfatherly words of advice: "Be efficient not by rushing, but by avoiding wasting time."

Authors

Charlie Sandson holds a degree in industrial and management engineering. He is a consultant for a management consulting firm specializing in the healthcare and pharmaceutical industries. The son of two doctors, he has prior experience working in a mental health institute, applying Lean and Six Sigma techniques to maximize the efficiency of care.

Ray Graber studied engineering as an undergraduate. While in college, he worked vacations and weekends as a surgical tech. Although he really enjoyed the math and science of engineering, after working in the operating room, he decided that medicine was the way to go. It also gave him an appreciation for the jobs that other OR personnel do.

More Wisdom on Professionalism

33

David A. Wallace, Ronald S. Bank, and Catherine Marcucci

Contributors:

Edwin G. Avery IV, MD (EGA)

Andrew B. Barker, MD

Niloofer Dalal, MD

Steven M. Frank, MD (SMF)

William R. Furman, MD (WRF)

Brian T. Gierl, MD

Allan Gottschalk, MD PhD

Daniel M. Joseph, MD (DMJ)

Kirk Lalwani, MD

Mark J. Lema, MD PhD (MJL)

Mark C. Norris, MD

D. A. Wallace
Department of Anesthesiology and Perioperative Medicine, University Hospitals Cleveland Medical Center, Case Western Reserve University School of Medicine, Cleveland, OH, USA

R. S. Bank
Department of Anesthesiology, INOVA Fairfax Hospital, UVA School of Medicine, INOVA Campus, Falls Church, VA, USA

C. Marcucci (✉)
Department of Transfusion Medicine, Clinical Center, National Institutes of Health, Bethesda, MD, USA

S. Mohamed et al. (eds.), *Anesthesia Bridges*, https://doi.org/10.1007/978-3-032-08294-7_33

Steven L. Orebaugh, MD (SLO)

Amy J. Robbins, MD MBA (AJR)

Richard W. Rosenquist, MD

David Sanusi, MD

Neil B. Sandson, MD (NBS)

F. Jacob Seagull, PhD (FJS)

Joseph M. Schwartz, MD (JMS)

Brandon M. Togioka, MD

Toby N. Weingarten, MD

Introduction

Professionalism is defined in the *Oxford* dictionary as "the competence or skill expected of a professional." So that's a completely ridiculous and circular definition—if you are a practicing anesthesiologist, you of course have a certain requisite level of clinical competence. What else makes a physician truly professional? We finish this section with just a few final words of wisdom that we hope, in some way, will help our readers achieve a successful and satisfying career.

In this section, we also honor contributing editor **Ron Bank's** parents—the late Barron "Bunny" and Lois "Cookie" Bank (Fig. 33.5). Ron lost his beloved Mom in October 2021 and Dad in early 2024, and the Bank family misses them terribly. Ron wrote to us that he feels for sure that without his excellent parents, he would not have been able to accomplish what he has.

Thoughts and Advice on Professionalism

- Have one standard: *High!* Strive for excellence every day. Come to work, prepared to work, every day. Take care of yourself first, so that you are prepared to take care of others. Come to work, 100% ready to work.—**DAW**

- Being great is doing a good job *every day*. Anyone can occasionally be extraordinary on any given day. But being great takes time and doing a good job every day, not just some days; with time, this makes you great. It is not hard to do, but it does take effort, persistence, and consistency. It is achievable by all.—**DAW**

- Many people look for reasons not to do something. You should look for reasons to do something, as long as it is appropriate and within the bounds of common sense.—**DAW**

- Professionalism is a packaging of the right physical image, the right presentation, and the right information or "walk the walk, talk the talk, and look the look." —**MJL**

- Professionalism is what you do and how you act. Take care of your actions and your reputation will follow.—**Editors**

- Make every decision as if it will be on the front page of the New York Times the next day.—**JMS**

- Remember that the root of "professionalism" is "profession." It's about your personality, yes, but also hugely about how you do your job. In medicine, professionalism is first and foremost about a deep and abiding concern and care for your patients. The single best thing you can do is to go the extra mile for your patients.—**Editors**

- Unlike many aspects of medical practice, professionalism is something that is completely under your control. You and only you control how you approach situations, your attitude, and how you behave and respond in situations.—**Editors**

- We have this feeling that professionalism is also about punctuality, although we have never formally studied the matter. But we can't think of anybody we know who is a really top-notch professional who constantly runs late. We think that this is because punctuality is largely about respect—respect for the time and priorities of people other than yourself.—**Editors**

- Your patients (and your children!) need you, no matter how you feel. In this context, professionalism means calmness and the ability to cope under stress and fatigue.—**Editors**

- If you're applying for a job, consider the messages that your attire and communication style send. Formal evening wear isn't required, but be careful about overly casual or sloppy dress because it may not communicate respect. In letter writing, business format is your best bet—a formal salutation and complementary close (even via email), direct and to the point, no more than two pages. Business letter? Ask your parents. Or read about it on the internet. Everything is on the internet, pretty much forever. Which brings us to: expect to have been searched online. You searched them, didn't you? Of course you did. Run a search on yourself so you will know what prospective employers have seen. You can figure out what comes next. That feeling when someone else tells you they found your 20-year-old self. —**WRF**

- It is critical to never forget that your behavior can have as much—if not more—impact on your career than your clinical skills. Increasingly, bad behavior of all sorts is not being tolerated. The days of old where the physician could treat other colleagues and staff poorly are long gone. Reports of adverse behavior can very abruptly derail the most brilliant of careers. Don't let this happen to you!!! Be sure that your EQ is at least equal to your IQ. —**RSB**

- To me, professionalism is a matter of diplomacy. So, pick your battles. It's kind of like parenting or dealing with a spousal relationship. You don't need to fight about every little thing. You need to choose the most important aspects of patient care and stand your ground with a surgeon. For things that do not harm the patient and patient care and the outcome—step down, let the surgeon have the bone.—**AJR**

- Speaking of diplomacy and avoiding unnecessary conflict, consider "publication diplomacy" as a matter of both strategy and tactics. What better way to build and strengthen your professional bridges to the other perioperative medical specialties than to look for opportunities for joint publications? Plus, it's hard to ever get into a really vicious conflict with somebody who has the final draft of your joint paper on their desk.—**Editors**

- Professionalism is also about reciprocity. If you get in a bit of a time crunch and somebody does up a chapter for you in zero time, pay back that favor and put the time in on their book or committee, at the earliest opportunity. It's not so much playing well in the sandbox; it's more like, you help me stack my blocks, I'll help you stack yours.—**Editors**

- Professionalism is also not really about playing well in the sandbox, because the anesthesia community is not a sandbox. It's more the size of a shoebox.—**Editors**

- Self-praise isn't much of a recommendation.—**Editors**

- Do not hesitate to offer call coverage for a colleague who has an unexpected situation outside of the hospital. In my experience, you will get paid back when your number comes up and you need help.—**EGA**

- A corollary to that is to be really good to your colleagues who are pregnant. I've worked in departments that routinely held baby showers for the pregnant anesthesiologists. In the pile of baby booties and blankets was always an envelope that held "coupons" for call coverage—including for after the baby had arrived. It's the best present a pregnant colleague or new mom can get—getting to start a call shift a couple of hours late or leave four hours early. And the men in the department participated in this gift coverage as well.—**CM**

- Always realize that anesthesia is a very humbling field. Don't get cocky. Don't get complacent. The risk that you take is not your risk, but that of your patient.—**RSB**

- Don't let your ego get in the way of asking for help with a procedure or any aspect of patient care. It's about the patient, not your ego. We're all type A perfectionists. We lose track of this all too often.—**RSB**

- One of my favorite quotes pertaining to professionalism is by William Osler—"The greater the ignorance, the greater the dogmatism." So, don't do that! Digging in and insisting on something is a tip-off to your colleagues. The most knowledgeable people and physicians are humble and flexible.—**SMF**

***Note from the Editors:** Professionalism is just a process of carefully crossing the tricky areas in your career and getting safely and quietly to the other side of the problems (Fig. 33.1). You don't have to storm through every problem, because careers are more often made up of small moments and small issues that must be dealt with. So, sometimes you just tiptoe across.

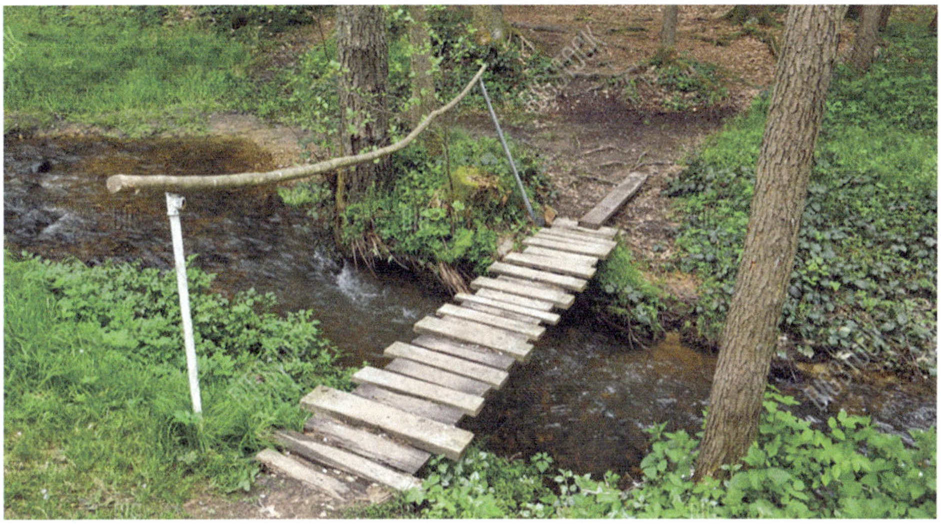

Fig. 33.1 A tiny footbridge across a small stream. No way to drive a tank across this bridge. Photo: Cathy Marcucci

- We were delighted when **Lee Woodson** sent us his essay on the "*Three A's for Anesthesiologists—Able, Affable, and Available*." We've all taught versions of this, as well as personally striving to embody these descriptors. We thought it would be interesting to see what additional "three words" our colleagues might teach and strive to embody, and sent out a quick email survey. We got some fun answers back. Amy's clinical work is in palliative care medicine, so hers make total sense. Nee clarified that hers refer to an anesthesiologist working in a crisis. Cathy's words are for residents who must cope with busy days and also nights on call. Ray's words pertain to being a good anesthesiology colleague. The rest are rather universally applicable, aren't they?—**Editors**

  Amy Robbins: Empathetic, detailed, and attentive

  Rick Rosenquist: Caring, knowledgeable, detailed, and proactive

  Nee Dalal: Confident, intelligent, and calm

  Andrew Barker: Vigilant, flexible, and efficient

  Cathy Marcucci: Fast, friendly, and flexible

  David Sanusi: Early bird, diplomatic, skillful

  Ray Graber: Reliable, cheerful, helpful

Brandon Togioka: Prepared, meticulous, astute

Toby Weingarten: Engaged, anticipatory, adaptable

Brian Gierl: Calm, meticulous, adroit

Ron Bank and **Allan Gottschalk:** Focused, nimble, empathetic, confident

Kirk Lalwani: Details! Deviations! Decisions!

And a final one from **Mark Norris:** I get paid to be paranoid!

What are your personal *three words to live by?* ☺

- I heartily second Nee Dalal's words—to instill trust and confidence in patients and staff, you **MUST** stay calm and in charge in times of crisis. If you cannot do this, you really should not be an anesthesiologist.—**DMJ**
- Don't ever let yourself get pushed into doing something that's unsafe—by a surgeon, patient, or anyone else. This may be especially difficult early in your career when you don't have the "street cred" of your more experienced colleagues or are new to a given location. When possible, enlist the help of a more senior colleague to back you up.—**RSB**
- A corollary to the above—don't permit "anesthesia shopping" by the surgeons. No good can come from it in the long run.—**Editors**
- If you agree to do something that your colleagues would view as questionable, first think hard about doing it in the first place and then, if you still want to proceed, do it yourself. Don't place one of your colleagues in the position of being asked to do something questionable that you agreed to.—**RSB**
- Another "tidbit" for professionalism, which I am borrowing from a patient safety talk I heard: Never do anything that you wouldn't want to explain to your mom.—**FJS**
- The supporting story for the advice above goes like this: two doctors were arguing over how to care for a patient safely—maybe they were both residents. One of them, as part of the argument, goes over to the phone. The other one says, "What? Are you going to call my attending/service chief/chair?" The first one says, "No, I want you to call your mother and explain to her why you are about to do this, instead of doing the right thing?"—**FJS**
- The most professional person I know is a physician who is extremely smart, qualified, and an expert. Yet he is humble, approachable, and accessible. He has the priority of doing the right thing always and putting the patient first always.—**FJS**
- Here's another anecdote: this physician who instituted a new policy of making sure gall bladder surgeries got done in a timely manner said, "if any of you are too busy on a Friday afternoon to start the surgery, call me at home and I will come in and do it." No one ever did. He is the department chair.—**FJS**

- No matter how much things may seem to suck at a given time, always remember that you're in a noble profession and are blessed with the opportunity to have a profound, positive impact on people's lives.—**RSB**

- I am passing along some advice that I was given in the 1990s, when there was a person who died by lethal injection in the Maryland criminal justice system. I was fairly new in training at the time. The case was in the news quite a bit because the condemned prisoner had poor IV access. More recently, cases concerning the "three drug cocktail" and "failed lethal injections" and so forth had been in the news. I was advised to never, ever casually discuss such cases with people in social situations. Of course, we know what we know, and the public can find out what they want to know via the news articles. There is absolutely no need for any anesthesiologist to brief anybody on the insider details. Just say, "You know, I really can't discuss the details of that case, I haven't been following it at all in the news." And then change the subject.—**CM**

- Want some quick lessons in professionalism and decorum? Watch your colleagues who are former or current military. There are exceptions, of course, but we bet that you will see better-than-average punctuality, demeanor, conflict resolution, styles of addressing both subordinates and superiors, cordiality in written communications, neatness of dress, etc. Once, we saw an anesthesiologist who was also an Army reservist get wrongfully creamed on an issue. When asked later how she managed to tolerate the abuse, all she said was, "Well, to be honest, I was in some danger of losing my military bearing. I've been chewed out worse, though, especially when I was stationed at Guantanamo Bay. I think in that case it had to do with the heat. In this case, this person has no excuse, but that's their problem, not mine."—**Editors**

- Professionalism on research and publication teams is a separate skill. Look for teams where there is an opportunity and room for everybody to do well. And where you will learn as much as you teach. On my large collaborative publication projects, my only "rule" is that I want everyone to "know more and know more people" than when we started. If you concentrate on doing that for your collaborators, it's hard to fail.—**CM**

- The only really big mistake you can make while working on a publication team, assuming that whatever you are writing is both relevant, and true, is to disappear. Don't do that. Even if you've promised to have a draft of something done and haven't done it, it's best not to disappear or avoid your colleagues, even for a minute. Just state the situation directly, "I am sorry I don't have the draft done—hit a big boulder."—**Editors.**

- Don't take it personally if somebody doesn't have time or doesn't want to work on your project or team. There are lots of people around who will. And never harangue a co-author, ever. The most effective way to nudge your team is to write and say, "Is there anything I can do to help you?"—**Editors**

- If you have nudged people a couple of times and they are still silent, let them stay silent and go about your to-do list without them. Just assume that there is something big going on, and it may not be any of your business. People will usually get back in touch when they can. We have learned that very often people will drop out of touch due to a serious health issue, often a mental health issue, that they or their family members are working to get through.—**Editors**

- If you are working with junior people, indicate from the get-go that you will provide abundant support. And then provide it. Don't let your junior people fail.—**Editors**

- Once I was working on a book with **Jeff Kirsch**, and when the book was delivered, we realized that there had been a big mistake made in the proofreading stage. There were two authors from his institution who had contributed to the project, and they had the same first name and last names that differed by only one letter. The proofreaders had assumed this was a mistake and "corrected" one of the authors' rights out of the manuscript. Her participation in the project was simply erased with the proofreader's pen. I was completely aghast and flummoxed. Jeff said to me, "Fortunately, this is a really great and professional person, and I know she will understand. She's very calm and will take it in stride." Which she did. She knew that it was unfortunate but completely inadvertent. She was a very junior anesthesiologist at the time, but we both thought she showed great tact and forbearance. I formed an immediate positive impression of this person, and to this day, would take every chance that offered itself to help her in her career. This young person took a circumstance that could have resulted in tension and resentment and turned it into an ongoing plus in her favor. She showed very impressive command of herself and her career.—**CM**

- Have you ever noticed that the people who are most known for their professionalism are rarely known for being loud?—**Editors**

- We cold-call people we don't know all the time if we have an opportunity to work on a book or project. But we rarely cold-call our colleagues; it's so easy to send a text saying, "Okay to call?"—**Editors**

- Don't play hard-to-get with other physicians. Just take their calls. If they are calling, they might need help. I once called **Steve Frank** on New Year's Eve with a pressing clinical problem that somebody had called me about. He said, "Well, given the timing, I figured it must be something important."—**CM**

- Actually, *Steve Frank is an all-around great colleague*. He seems to always have a great talk in his back pocket that, yes indeed, he is available to give this Friday because a scheduled grand rounds speaker canceled. And he is more than happy to share those slides. Back in the day, I mean way back in the day, I had been his fellow. Recently, I called him about a talk that I was giving on a subject of interest to both of us, and he said, "Hey, I think you need my unpublished data to round out this talk. I'll send it to you." Now *that's* a good guy.—**CM**

- So, we advise to do what Steve does. Keep a talk in a fairly current and presentable form and let it be known that you can pinch-hit to give it if a colleague gets into a jam. And be a good anesthesia team member.—**Editors**

*__Note from the Editors:__ Professionalism also means that sometimes you just have to buckle down and get the job done. In June 2023, there was a catastrophic failure of the I-95 highway at the site of a tragic truck explosion in an underpass (Fig. 33.2). State and federal authorities put together and executed a rapid plan to rebuild a temporary roadway in under two weeks so that traffic could flow in this vital transportation corridor (Fig. 33.3). And they were really smart about it. Crews worked 24 hours a day, and authorities also leveraged contacts with private businesses such as the Pocono Speedway to lend needed equipment. They also got the public behind the project with a live cam setup to highlight progress, making what could have been an ongoing disaster into a tale of American can-do spirit.

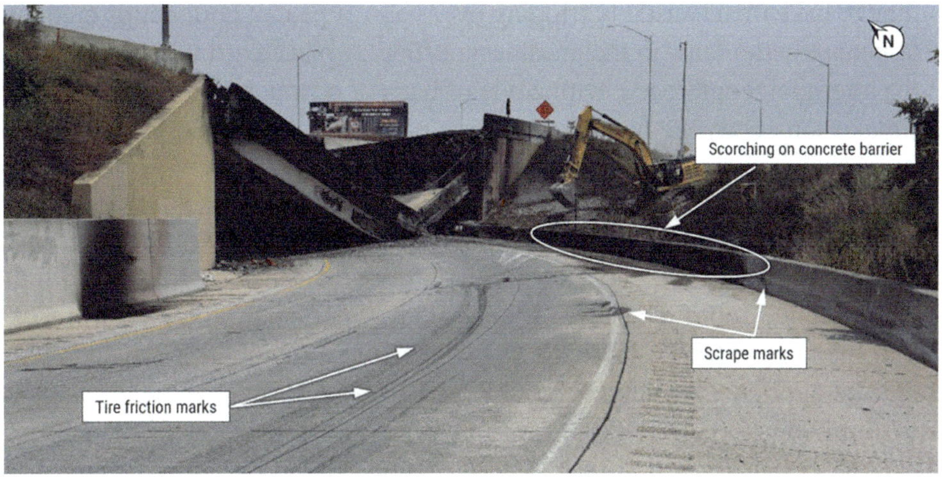

Fig. 33.2 The collapsed roadway of Interstate 95 in the northeast Philadelphia. Photo: ntsb.gov

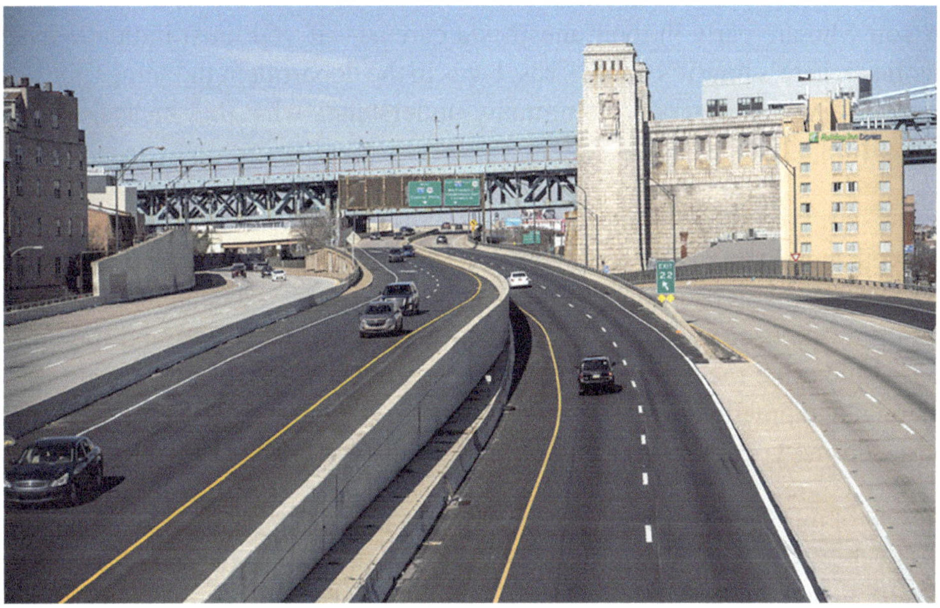

Fig. 33.3 I-95 is the crucial transportation and commercial bridge through and over Philadelphia and multiple other East Coast metropolitan areas. Photo: arlutz73, image used under standard license for editorial use (nonfiction book) from iStock.com

- Be *incredibly careful* about your use of and participation in humor in the workplace. It can have high-magnitude effects in both directions. It can be a bonding experience, but one joke that is in poor taste or bombs can reverberate quickly and widely. You even have to be careful what you laugh *about*.—**NBS**

- That said, a bit of self-deprecating humor is usually not a bad thing, as long as it's not used to deflect a compliment. If you receive a sincere compliment, the only correct response is to say simply, "Thank you, that is so kind of you to mention (or notice) that."—**NBS**

- Similarly, *do not prank people at work*. Unless it is a manifestly supportive and loving "prank." For instance, when someone returns from an active-duty tour and they are known to love peanut butter cups, it is perfectly fine to have them veritably tripping over bags of peanut butter cups on their first day back. Big gift box of peanut butter cups in the anesthesia office. A place card with their name on the conference table at the afternoon conference, with a pile of bags of peanut butter cups, and so forth. But that's it. Never, ever make somebody the butt of a joke or a prank. Nice people don't do it.—**Editors**

- Extend the same professionalism to your applicants that you extend to your colleagues. We know of a situation where one of our anesthesiology colleagues was interviewing for a job and had to do a partly remote panel interview. The interviewing department was having trouble with the audio-visual system in the conference room, so they put somebody's personal laptop in front of the applicant. Unbeknownst to the person whose laptop it was, department members were engaged in a brisk text exchange about the applicant, which she could see as text messages crawled across the top of the screen. Finally, our colleague said, "I just saw a text message that said, 'I like her, but she is kooky.' So, I guess I should let you know that I can see this discussion about me." The take-home lesson? *Do not start the discussion about the applicant until they are out of the building*.—**Editors**

- Gentle, gentle, gentle with the criticism and gossip.—**Editors**

- For those of you who are early in their anesthesia careers—if you must indicate disapproval or disavowal of a college, here's how it's done: "Yes, I was in the department the same time as Dr. So-and-so. *We weren't close*." Everybody in our community understands what that means. No need to say anything else.—**Editors**

- A great place to start your professional program is a thorough review of your hospital's medical staff bylaws. Have you actually read this document carefully and completely? You almost certainly signed something that said that you had been provided a copy, but have you actually read it? We bet not. Pay careful attention to the peer review and disciplinary process procedures and the "professional conduct" sections. Much like the practice statements of the ASA, make sure you do not get outside of these professional and practice parameters. If you think you can't reasonably and reliably stay inside them, start considering your employment options.—**Editors**

- On the other side of this issue, the medical staff bylaws also bind the hospital in any contentious matter between physicians or between physicians and the administration. The hospital is bound by its own documents. In the VA healthcare system, since the physician force was created by Congress under Title 38, VA hospital medical staff bylaws have the force of a federal regulation.—**Editors**

- One of the most difficult aspects of professionalism has to do with the impaired physician. This is a huge issue and subject. We recently did a chapter for Kirk Lalwani's and Jeff Kirsch's new book on it. The book's title is *Professional, Ethical, Legal, and Educational Lessons in Medicine: A Problem-based Learning Approach*, Oxford Press. Keep in mind that Jeff and Kirk are donating all royalties to a social action food group, so we strongly advise that you get yourself a copy of it.—**CM and NBS**

- The definition of an impaired physician is any physician whose distressed personal and/or professional life poses a significant risk of harm to self or patients. Impaired physicians are not new; they have been recognized since the beginning of American medicine. Physician impairment is distributed across the entire demographic and distressingly common, but fortunately, it can often be addressed. Impaired physicians can and do recover and even reacquire or maintain their medical practice.—**CM and NBS**

- However, the most important factor in a successful outcome for an impaired physician is early recognition and treatment. We cannot stress this enough. Do not think that you won't say or do anything to report an impaired physician because you don't want to make any trouble for the person. It's just the opposite—you will make trouble for your colleague if you don't make a report, as impaired physicians very rarely, if ever, can stop their dangerous actions on their own. And if you have to ask yourself whether a physician is impaired, they probably are.—**CM and NBS**

- You have a definite ethical duty to report an impaired physician and possibly a legal one as well. If the physician is engaged in frankly unethical or illegal activity, you have both a definite ethical and legal duty to report. Consult your own legal advisers for help, if necessary, but illegal activity must be reported.—**CM and NBS**

A Collection of Additional Quotes on Professionalism

- Professionalism is nothing more than solving people's problems. And you cannot solve a problem with the same mind that created it. Perspective is as important as patience in solving every problem.

***Note from the Editors:** We think this bridge is a great metaphor for perspective (Fig. 33.4). Always look at all sides of your problem, including where you are starting and where you want to end up. And consider novel approaches and angles, always.

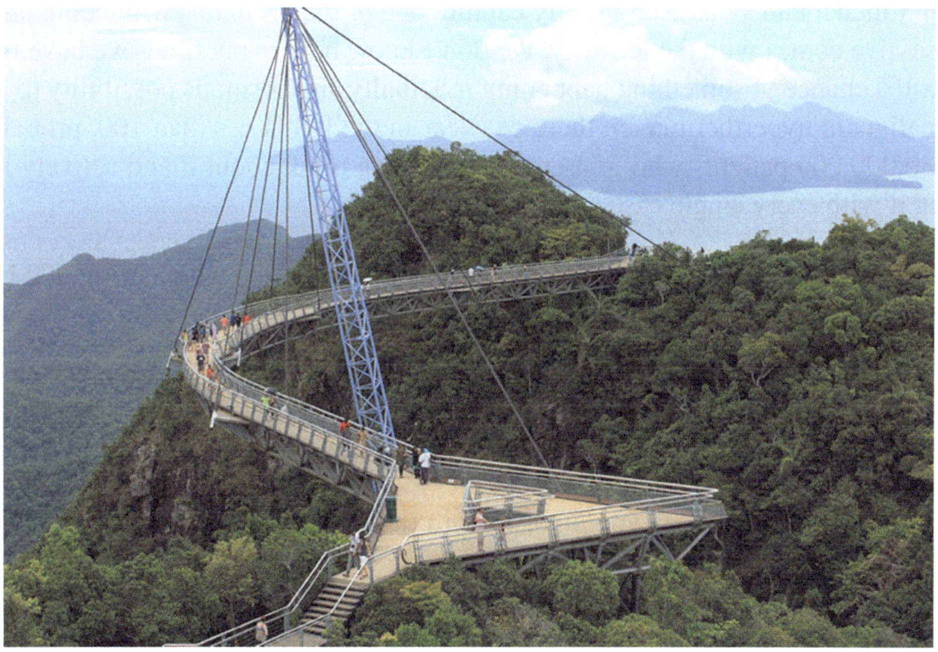

Fig. 33.4 A stunning footbridge in the mountains of Malaysia. Photo: Image used under standard license from iStock.com

- Professional is not a label you give yourself; it's a description you hope others will apply to you.—**David Maister**

- The professional has learned that success, like happiness, comes as a by-product of work.—**Business adage**

- It is good for a professional to be reminded that his professionalism is only a husk, that the real person must remain an amateur, a lover of the work.—**May Sarton**

- Professionalism in art has this difficulty. To be professional is to be dependable, to be dependable is to be predictable, and predictability is aesthetically boring—an antivirtue in a field where we hope to be astonished and startled and at some level refreshed.—**John Updike**

Editor's Note: Okay, if you are an artist, maybe the above is true? But not for us. For us, dependable and predictable *is great*. What we really think is that it is a good thing John Updike never tried to be an anesthesiologist.

- What people don't realize is that professionals are sensational because of the fundamentals.—**Barry Larkin**

- I think professionalism is important, and professionalism means you get paid.—**Erica Jong**

- Ordinary professionalism and 20 years' experience can accomplish a lot, but they can't access the hidden places.—**Jeanette Winterson**

- My idea of professionalism is probably a lot of people's idea of obsessive.—**David Fincher**

- My own position is so far on the obsessive side of preparation and professionalism that I fear my point of view is not going to be shared by anyone.—**Johnny Wilkinson**

Editor's Note: Fincher and Wilkinson exactly capture one of the problems with being an anesthesiologist. Being obsessive comes with the territory. We don't know how many times we have tried to explain to people that a 1% chance of something happening is actually an enormous possibility to us. How many true cases of malignant hyperthermia are there per year in the US? Less than 100, probably. And these occur in over 30,000,000 patients who go to the OR. Yet we think about it and actively look for it and work to prevent it with every single case we do.

- One of the hardest things to learn in life is which bridges to cross and which bridges to burn.—**Oprah Winfrey**

More Advice

- Every day, on the way to work, as you drive in with the looming obstacles and demands in front of you, be grateful for the opportunity to be a physician. It's hard as hell to do it well, in any of our specialties, and to meet the demands of society and individual patients. But there's really nothing better on earth. Wealthy bankers and lawyers, famous singers and actors, powerful bureaucrats and politicians have no idea what it's like to care for ill people for a living—what a gift. And give thanks at the end of your exhausting, demanding day for the same thing.—**SLO**

- Be spiritual. God asks us to create within ourselves the fruits of the spirit: love, peace, joy, goodness, gentleness, kindness, faithfulness, patience, and self-control. Every one of these is difficult in times of stress, but each contributes to a truly professional approach to our role in caring for patients.—**SLO**

- I think people discount how much being nice factors into professionalism. People generally strive for respect and consider this synonymous with professionalism, but I also think there is room for likeability. Why is this? Because "being nice" to people generally involves empathy, kindness, and consideration. So, reach out just for no reason. Go to people's parties, return their calls and emails, and be interested and enthusiastic about their projects and programs.—**NBS**

- Make your professionalism be about progress and productivity, not just platitudes.—**Editors**

- Just be somebody that people can count on.—**Editors**

Note: The editors thank Drs. Schwartz and Sandson for contributing to this chapter.

Authors

David Wallace is the former program director of the University Hospitals of Cleveland anesthesiology residency program. He is now the section head for trauma anesthesia. His colleagues at Case Western tell us that he is truly someone you would like to have at your side during an emergency.

Ron Bank and Cathy Marcucci trained at Hopkins in the 1990s, one year apart. They agree they had the good fortune to be the beneficiaries of outstanding training, including examples of true professionalism. Ron also credits his very special parents for providing a great example of how to do business fairly and with integrity. Barron and Cookie bank are shown below in one of Ron's favorite photos taken at an informal social function (Fig. 33.5).

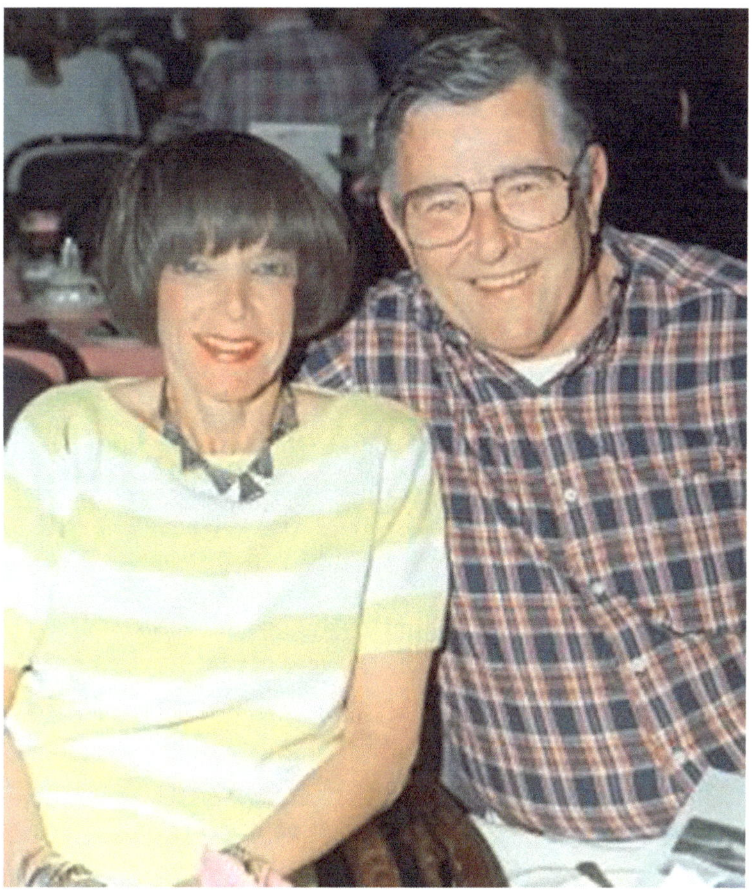

Fig. 33.5 Ron Bank's late parents—Bunny and Cookie Bank. Ron honors his folks as great parents and all-around great people. Photo: Collection of the Bank family

Part III

Leadership

Thurston Avenue Bridge—Cornell University

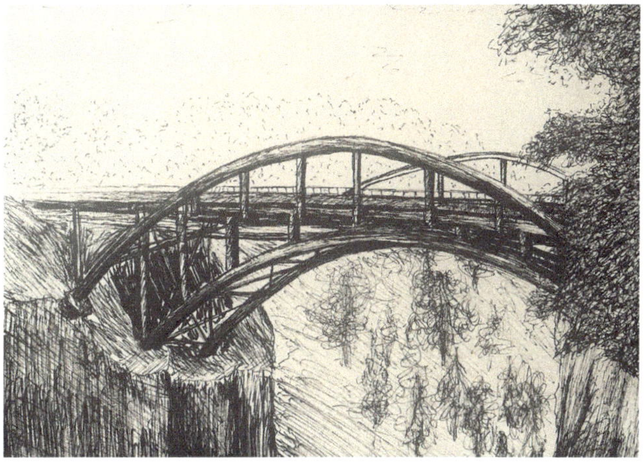

Thurston Avenue Bridge, Ithaca, New York. This bridge is on the campus of Cornell University, the alma mater of authors **Kit Conner**, **Jane Jacobs**, and **Brian Gierl**; and contributors **Mike Graham**, **Deb Waterman Johns**, **Elaine Matte Mut**, **Christie Gilmartin Waters**, and **Michael Liu**. It separates the main campus from the North Campus residential buildings and playing fields. Cornell is noted for its scenic gorges, and this bridge spans the picturesque Fall Creek gorge. It has a steel arch construction and was completed in 1960. Interestingly, it is galvanized rather than painted. It carries vehicular, pedestrian, and bicycle traffic. There is a spectacular view from the bridge, looking east, of the Fall Creek waterfall as it flows out of Beebe Lake.

The entire Cornell Unversity group on the *Anesthesia Bridges* team thank **Craig Riley** of The Architectural Team in Boston, MA, for his beautiful ink drawing of a beautiful bridge in a beautiful place.

Introduction

34

Raymond G. Graber

We recognize great leaders when we see them in action—they make it look easy! Excellent leadership is important to your group's practice and is even more important for us nationwide as a specialty. Most people are not born with these skills—they learn from watching their mentors, and by taking on small leadership roles first. Those who are serious about becoming leaders may want to consider enrolling in a healthcare-focused MBA program. In the end, leadership skills grow by using and polishing them.

In this section, we will hear advice from some well-known leaders in our field. They will tell us how they developed their skills, and how we can work toward developing ours. We hope their experience and wisdom can inspire the next generation of leaders. As a specialty, we need to keep grooming the next generation of leaders, because our specialty is and will be continuously under pressure from multiple directions. As the adage goes—"If you don't know who the fool is in a deal, it's you." We need to continuously be engaged, lead, and prove our value—we have competitors who are doing likewise.

Author

Ray Graber serves as vice chair for quality in the anesthesiology department at University Hospitals Cleveland Medical. He has dual interests in cardiac and orthopedic anesthesia. During his 30+ year career, he has focused on process improvement, reduction of errors, and improving patient outcomes.

R. G. Graber (✉)
Department of Anesthesiology and Perioperative Medicine, University Hospitals Cleveland Medical Center, Cleveland, OH, USA
e-mail: raymond.graber@uhhospitals.org

S. Mohamed et al. (eds.), *Anesthesia Bridges*, https://doi.org/10.1007/978-3-032-08294-7_34

Innovation and Leadership: Our Future Is at the Frontier of Quality, Safety, and Value

35

Daniel J. Cole

Introduction

The origins of anesthesia date back to early civilization and the opium poppy. The first public demonstration of modern anesthesia occurred in 1846 with the successful use of ether, and our specialty is on the brink of another "ether moment."

Last Laugh

Driven by disruptive public policy, medicine is transitioning to a value-based system. In a rapidly changing healthcare landscape, it is critical that our specialty is proactive in demonstrating our relevance over the cycle of care of a patient's condition. Our need to expand our vision and our impact beyond the confines of an induction-to-emergence paradigm is best illustrated by a story Marc Randolph, cofounder of Netflix, tells in his book *That Will Never Work*.

To set the context, it was the year 2000, and Netflix was a startup company seeking a meeting with the entertainment giant Blockbuster, the company whose stores Americans regularly visited to rent their entertainment for the evening. Netflix was financially struggling and seeking to be acquired by Blockbuster for $50 million. The synergies between Blockbuster and Netflix seemed obvious to Netflix leadership.

However, the meeting did not go well, and the Netflix group was literally laughed out of the room. The scenario might have been different. Instead of laughing an industry disrupter out of the room, the Blockbuster group might have seriously listened and embraced the innovation and change they required to better meet a societal need and a secure future. Currently, Netflix is valued at over 200 billion dollars, while Blockbuster filed for bankruptcy in 2010 and its stores no longer dot the strip malls of America.

D. J. Cole (✉)
Department of Anesthesiology, David Geffen School of Medicine at UCLA, Los Angeles, CA, USA
e-mail: djcole@mednet.ucla.edu

S. Mohamed et al. (eds.), *Anesthesia Bridges*, https://doi.org/10.1007/978-3-032-08294-7_35

Change Is the Constant

With an external environment defined by uncertainty, volatility, and complexity, one thing is certain—*change!* Whether we like it or not, change is occurring in healthcare, and we must leverage our strengths against the fulcrum of change. The key to our future starts with a powerful fundamental purpose. Our purpose is best described as "improving health and relieving pain and suffering" with innovation and differentiation supporting strategies. There are four imperatives that are key to creating the change we desire:

- *Primacy of the patient-physician relationship.*
- *Discovery of new knowledge.*
- *Partnering with our stakeholders to provide patient-centric value.*
- *A commitment to do what is necessary to advance our specialty by improving quality and safety.*

The Affordable Care Act laid the framework and provided the impetus to reengineer an intervention-based healthcare system into a system with prevention at the core. Surgery, pain management, and intensive care are indeed inflection points where patients can emerge with better health, and anesthesiologists will have a critical role in caring for the sick. Moreover, our specialty is in a unique position to impact the population health goal of returning patients to better physical, cognitive, and psychological health through a multitude of touchpoints throughout the perioperative episode of care.

Key innovations include engagement of the patient in preoperative risk assessment, optimization, and prehabilitation; care delivery pathways specific to a patient's personal complexity and risk; and data-driven registries that feed improvement information into a learning system. Our specialty needs to learn how to use newer tools such as improvement science, system science, implementation science, and safety science. These can be used to accelerate change and can be integrated into evidence-based pathways of care for medical and surgical conditions. Finally, through collaborative relationships, anesthesiologists should lead in the technology transformation by digital health, which includes artificial intelligence, telemedicine, perioperative genomics, and wearable devices, which will be a driver of value-based care for surgical patients.

***Note from the Editors:** Several of the authors in this section of the book built their careers at UCLA. We went looking for a dramatic Los Angeles bridge and found the Sixth Street Viaduct (Fig. 35.1).

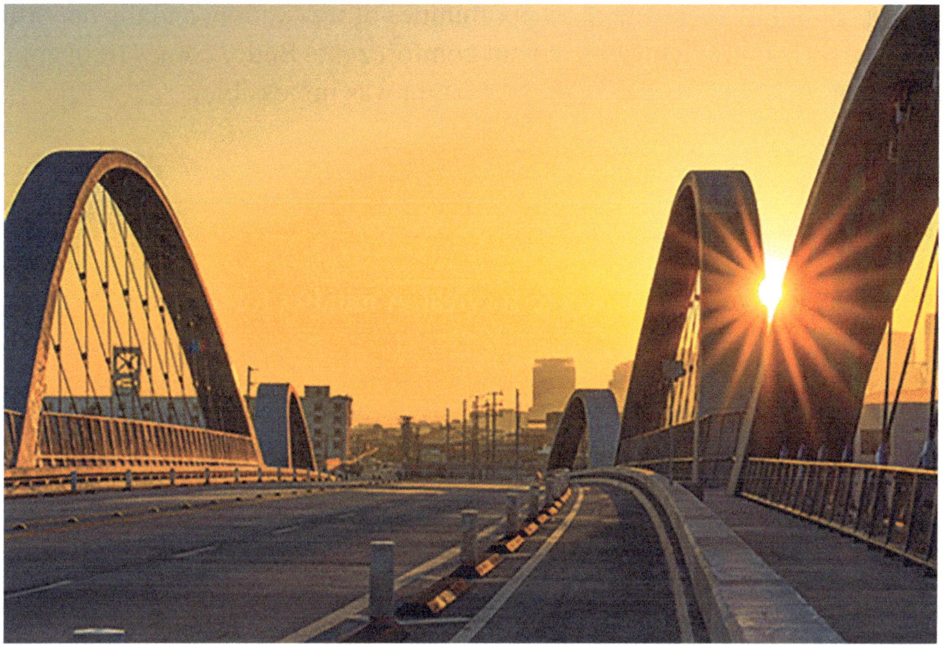

Fig. 35.1 The Sixth Street Viaduct in Los Angeles, CA, crosses the Los Angeles River, two freeways, and several railroad tracks. The current structure cost almost $600 million and opened in 2022. It replaced a structure originally dating from the 1930s. The new bridge incorporates several green spaces both below and around it, although the design was not without some controversy. Photo: Image used under standard license from stock.adobe.com

Why We Work

Let's return to our purpose, which is best illustrated by a personal experience I had.

A few years ago, while on a flight from Chicago to Los Angeles, I heard the call, "Is there a doctor on board?" This has happened about 8–10 times throughout my career, and as usual, I got up to help. I was the first to arrive and saw a man, about 75 years old, sitting beside his wife—he was not breathing. He had a faint pulse and the body habitus of someone with sleep apnea, so I did a jaw thrust, and he lurched out at me. A second responder arrived, and by now, there was no pulse, no respirations, so we placed him on the floor and started chest compressions. Others came to help.

About 10 minutes into the code, the wife became grief-stricken. I later learned that the couple were farmers from Iowa, on their way to Los Angeles for a granddaughter's first birthday. We made an emergency landing in Kansas about 35 minutes later, and that husband, that father, that grandfather left the plane with a rhythm. I will always remember, as the wife walked out with her husband, in a moment that froze in time, tears streaming down her face from a place in her heart we physicians are privileged to connect to, it was all she could do to mouth the words *"THANK YOU."*

America is searching for high-quality, safe, high-value healthcare. Anesthesiology has a rich heritage of innovating at the quality and safety frontier. But our work is not done. We dream big. We seek "better." Because it matters to the thousands of patients who place their lives in our hands.

We embrace the opportunities of change, the opportunities of innovation, and the opportunities of "better." Better does not come from staying within your comfort zone. Better comes from going outside your comfort zone, believing, and achieving what you thought was impossible.

Lessons Learned

- Adaptation to a changing world is the key to survival. A mindset for failure is "we have always done it that way."
- Organizing our culture and processes around a clear purpose, "improving health and relieving pain and suffering," will always meet a clear societal need and secure our future.
- To quote Michael Jordan, "Some people want it to happen, some wish it would happen, others make it happen."

Author

Dan Cole is an anesthesiologist at UCLA with a subspecialty in neuroanesthesia. He is the past president of the American Society of Anesthesiologists, the American Board of Anesthesiology, and has also served as vice president of the Anesthesia Patient Safety Foundation.

36 Get into Your "Discomfort Zone"

Ronald L. Harter

Introduction

We've all heard the expression to "get out of your comfort zone," which can apply to virtually any facet of our lives and careers. However, the expression is used so much that it tends to lose its impact, becoming more cliché than a true plan of action. I suggest intentionally moving toward the things that make you uncomfortable, until you have mastered them and removed them as things to be avoided or that are only accomplished in the face of significant anxiety.

Choose What Makes You Uncomfortable

As an example, in your residency, if you find you are uncomfortable in a particular subspecialty, that should drive you to do more cases in that realm until you attain a reasonable level of comfort. Your goal at the completion of training should be that any case you are asked to perform is in your comfort zone, and your discomfort zone is vacant. In other words, you need to develop the calm confidence to tackle any clinical challenge.

As you progress through your career, this requires continued effort and attention. If you find that performing a specific procedure, such as fiberoptic intubation, is becoming uncomfortable because you haven't had much opportunity to do it in a while, actively seek opportunities to perform it, so you can regain the competence and confidence to perform a fiberoptic intubation whenever it is indicated. Otherwise, the broad skill set you had developed during training will begin to narrow and atrophy, and the corresponding career options open to you will become increasingly limited.

R. L. Harter (✉)
Department of Anesthesiology, Wexner Medical Center at The Ohio State University, Columbus, OH, USA
e-mail: Ronald.Harter@osumc.edu

S. Mohamed et al. (eds.), *Anesthesia Bridges*, https://doi.org/10.1007/978-3-032-08294-7_36

Lean Toward Leadership

In a similar way, many anesthesiologists are uncomfortable pursuing leadership roles at any level. Anesthesiology as a profession tends to attract physicians who may be quite comfortable focusing entirely on their direct clinical role, and may avoid stepping into leadership roles, because they find it uncomfortable relative to the clinical setting.

However, as an anesthesiologist, your training and expertise ideally position you to serve as a leader in a variety of settings. You may certainly explore opportunities to lead within your department, which is important, but I would urge you to ultimately seek opportunities to lead within your hospital, medical staff, and/or local, state, or national medical societies.

Make no mistake, this is an uncomfortable path for many in our specialty to pursue. However, failing to seek such opportunities to lead beyond the clinical care setting represents a missed opportunity for you to develop skills in areas that are outside your comfort zone, and will limit your career options in much the same way that a narrow clinical skill set will. Starting down the leadership path will reduce your discomfort in pursuing subsequent opportunities. It's ok to start small—serving on a medical staff bylaws or credentialing committee, for example. As you become increasingly comfortable in the administrative leadership realm, you will have diminishing discomfort as you seek further opportunities. Your value to your colleagues both inside and outside your department will grow as well, as will your personal satisfaction.

Lessons Learned

- Recognize the facets of your practice and your clinical and nonclinical roles that make you uncomfortable—these are exactly the ones you should move toward—not avoid.
- Look for opportunities for leadership and service at a more local level, then build upon the skills learned there to move to progressively greater leadership opportunities.

Author

Ron Harter is a native Ohioan, born and raised in western Ohio, and has spent most of his professional career in Columbus. He has served as chair of the department of anesthesiology at Ohio State since 2008. He has served in several leadership roles in medical associations, including several leadership roles for the American Society of Anesthesiologists, most notably as an ASA officer since 2012 and president of the ASA in 2024. He and his wife Kathy have five children.

Be Flexible to Achieve Leadership Growth

37

Patricia A. Kapur

Introduction

I was first tapped for leadership duties at an early stage in my career, becoming chief of anesthesiology at our affiliated VA Medical Center four months after my fellowship. I had a steep learning curve and had to handle not only hiring and oversight of physicians, CRNAs, and staff, but also educational responsibilities and institutional oversight for residents, medical students, and student CRNAs. In addition, I was responsible for OR management, equipment and supply decisions, budget management, and interservice politics and relationship building with other leaders in the institution. I moved into the VA chief's office space and never looked back. At that early point, I was not convinced that I would have full opportunities to move up in my academic institution.

Career Progression

Subsequently, I gained progressive leadership experience by establishing a track record that led to further opportunities within my institution. After serving as VA chief of anesthesiology while carrying cardiothoracic (CT) anesthesiology duties there, I next took the role of chief of CT anesthesiology at the university hospital, gaining additional leadership experience and a chance to network with other clinical leaders.

After some years, I pivoted and advanced to become the director of the new outpatient surgery center in a multifunctional ambulatory complex across from the university hospital. This was a fairly sizable location with eight ORs and four procedure rooms. There, I had authority and responsibility for both the surgery center and its personnel, as well as the anesthesiology team with clinical and educational oversight responsibilities.

P. A. Kapur (✉)
Department of Anesthesiology and Critical Care, Perelman School of Medicine, University of Pennsylvania, Philadelphia, PA, USA
e-mail: patricia.kapur@pennmedicine.upenn.edu

S. Mohamed et al. (eds.), *Anesthesia Bridges*, https://doi.org/10.1007/978-3-032-08294-7_37

This directorship made me a member of the hospital leadership structure, with institutional responsibility for the surgery center's budget, HR functions, overseeing the nursing and support staff, QA/QI, and the value proposition for center operations, supplies, equipment, strategy, and in-house marketing. We were able to grow the utilization of the center, for example, by adding 24-hour postoperative stays on-site. This made the surgery center a highly desirable surgical site for the institution. During that period, I did a considerable amount of self-study of business principles and practice, best QI approaches, and so forth.

Department Chair and Additional Leadership Roles

Following those experiences—and as the inside candidate—I became chair of the Department of Anesthesiology. During my tenure, my department team took active leadership roles in managing the health system OR suites and surgery centers, grew the faculty and residency, added fellowships and endowed chairs, expanded our research footprint, increased grants, and expanded clinical coverage to other sites. After these successively increasing leadership responsibilities, I ultimately became president of the faculty practice group. Interestingly, early on, when I was not convinced of opportunities to lead at my institution, I began to pour time and commitment into working for a number of professional organizations, and this was very fulfilling. I rose to leadership positions in the ASA, ABA, IARS, FAER, and my state society of anesthesiologists, and served on the boards or councils of APSF, SAMBA, AUA, and SAAA/AAAC.

Advice on Building Your Career

I encourage those who aspire to leadership to pursue opportunities, whatever your institution or practice setting. There is no shortcut for hard work, but plan to build upon each level of experience. Find good mentors—including "nontraditional" mentors—inside and outside of your environment. Hire, nurture, and empower a great team to work together for the best outcomes. Be open to pivoting to the next opportunity for further leadership responsibility. I undertook a self-study of business principles and had a number of opportunities along the way to learn fiscal and organizational operating principles. However, for those not in similar situations, I recommend considering formal business training, through a "business for healthcare" program or an MBA program, to be prepared to seriously and credibly engage in the important responsibilities you will have.

Lessons Learned

- If you are interested in becoming a leader, be open to opportunities, work hard, find good mentors, and consider formal business training.

Author

Patricia Kapur spent her career at UCLA in anesthesiology and health system administration, education, and clinical care. She is now sharing the pearls from that experience with her current colleagues at Penn. Patricia's involvement with state and national professional organizations is another career highlight that she recommends to others.

Reflections on Communications and Negotiations in Anesthesiology

38

Mark V. Boswell

Introduction

Early in my anesthesiology career, clinical care was the focus of my practice. After several years, I became a service chief of a hospital-based pain service and later became chair of an anesthesiology department. With each change, my job required more administrative work. As I moved up the administrative ladder, I began to think about getting some formal business training.

MBA

At the suggestion of a friend and colleague, I enrolled in a healthcare-focused MBA program. At the outset, I knew that business involved communication (emails and phone calls) and negotiations (doing deals). But what I came to see is that healthcare requires communication and negotiation with colleagues, supervisors, and patients.

Although I knew that taking care of patients didn't provide much insight into how to be an administrator, I began to see that being a better administrator improved my clinical care and my relationships with colleagues. Communication style and negotiation strategies can make or break a relationship.

In the following vignettes, I share two personal experiences and some suggestions for additional reading that illustrate these concepts.

M. V. Boswell (✉)
Department of Anesthesiology, University of Toledo College of Medicine, Toledo, OH, USA
e-mail: mark.boswell2@utoledo.edu

S. Mohamed et al. (eds.), *Anesthesia Bridges*, https://doi.org/10.1007/978-3-032-08294-7_38

Dealing with a "Difficult" Patient

Please take a moment to ponder the simple sentences below.

"You are right." "You have a good point." "Thank you." These are phrases that I added to my conversation during my MBA training. *So, What's Your Point? A Practical Guide for Learning and Applying Effective Interpersonal Communication Techniques* is one of my favorite books from MBA School [1]. It changed the way I approach challenging conversations. The focus of the book is on learning how to discern important information using nonthreatening questions, making adjustments when there is doubt or conflict, and building rapport. With practice, small changes in the way we communicate can have dramatic effects on our professional relationships, whether dealing with patients or administrators.

I recall a conversation I had a number of years ago during a difficult patient encounter on rounds at a hospital. The specifics about the patient have been changed to preserve confidentiality, but the essence of the conversation remains. My fellow had seen a "difficult" patient who was having severe headaches. The patient had suffered a closed head injury in a motor vehicle crash several months previously and had been readmitted for pain management. The fellow informed me that the patient had been unpleasant and warned me that the patient's partner had a shady background and did not trust doctors. He noted that they both appeared to be angry. The fellow was not sure how to proceed with making recommendations.

Despite what we may have learned in medical school about using open-ended questions, the patient encounter typically is a physician-directed interview, not a conversation. Rather than asking the usual medical questions, I asked the patient and partner if we could talk. I took a relaxed, nondefensive pos-ture. The conversation started something like this:

Me: "Hello, I am Dr. B. Is it OK if we talk? Can we sit down?"

The Patient: "Yes."

Me to the Partner: "Hello, I'm Dr. B," and looked the partner in the eye and shook the partner's hand. Then, addressing both of them, I simply said, **"How are things going?"**

The response proved to be quite unexpected. They both began to talk. With only a few open-ended questions, I had a large part of the story about the accident, and some insight into what was bothering the couple.

One of my initial objectives was to evaluate the veracity of the patient and exclude potential complicating conditions, such as drug abuse and possible malingering. The patient's account was coherent and agreed with the points noted by the resident. There were some concerning "social" issues. However, there was more to the story. The MVA was not simply a rollover. The crash happened at the end of a high-speed chase. These details were not in the medical record.

Within 15 minutes, the couple told me much of what I needed to know. A few additional follow-up medical questions, including where it hurt and what the pain was like, filled in the details. A focused examination confirmed several impressions. We were able to proceed with writing orders with reasonable confidence. I did not find the patient difficult.

As the fellow noted, the couple was upset, and now I appreciated several of their concerns. They did not understand the nature of the injury or what to expect with recovery. I also learned that they had a lingering suspicion that the patient's former partner, who was in the pursuit vehicle, inflicted the head injury with a screwdriver at the accident scene. This misconception was not supported by the CT scan. It was easy to dispel their concern. This appeared to be an important breakthrough.

Establishing rapport and trust are some of the most challenging goals in clinical medicine. They are particularly difficult to achieve in the short time available during the typical anesthesiology visit. In this case, investing a small amount of time upfront was a good choice. Sitting down and using "openness" gestures and letting the patient and partner talk helped develop a therapeutic relationship that led to an effective treatment plan.

A Notable Negotiation

Getting to Yes—Negotiating Agreement without Giving In is a classic business book that advocates a principled approach to negotiations, by separating people from problems and interests from positions [2]. It also emphasizes looking at multiple options, controlling emotions, and building rapport. It is my other favorite book from MBA School.

I recall an important negotiation I had with a key faculty member in my department. The scenario was more or less as follows. The program director of our anesthesiology residency program came to me with an ultimatum. Unless I hired more CRNAs to cover resident lectures at 3 PM on Mondays, we would receive an adverse judgment from the Review Committee of the Accreditation Council on Graduate Medical Education. Recalling previous discussions that were quite unpleasant, I was worried that the conversation would not go well. The stakes were high. I certainly didn't want the residency program to get a citation.

With my new MBA negotiating skills, I decided to change my usual approach. Our meeting went something like this: I said, "Would it be possible for us to talk in your office today?" While sitting across from the program director, I thanked him for pointing out the urgent problem he had identified. I was concerned that my choices were limited, as we had no hiring budget and very little time. However, as we examined our options, it became clear that there were possibilities that did not involve hiring more CRNAs. We noted that several surgical departments had their teaching conferences on Friday mornings. We soon concluded that we should move our lectures to Friday mornings. With a reduced OR schedule on Friday mornings, we could cover the schedule with our current CRNAs. Why hadn't we thought of that solution before?

Several points are worth mentioning. The principled negotiation approach led to a solution that addressed the needs of the residency program, not the personalities and positions of the program director and chair. Moving our lectures to Friday mornings also allowed anesthesia faculty and residents to attend an important monthly Friday morning Trauma Service conference that we were previously unable to attend. While solving our lecture problem, we improved our rapport with our surgical colleagues—and my working relationship with the program director. The results were unanticipated and quite pleasant.

Lessons Learned

- Communication and negotiating skills are important in everyday life, clinical care, and hospital management.
- As many realize sooner or later, medical training and residency do not provide all the tools we need to be successful in our profession, particularly when it comes to working as a team.
- For me, repeating the same management mistakes was just not an option. Like playing golf—or flying an airplane—sometimes it's a good idea to take lessons. The references for my two favorite MBA books are listed below.

References

1. Wetherbe J, Wetherbe B. So, what's your point? A practical guide for learning and applying effective interpersonal communication techniques. Stevens Point (WI): Mead Publishing; 2012.
2. Fisher R, Ury WL, Patton B. Getting to yes: negotiating agreement without giving in. New York: Penguin Group (USA) Inc.; 2011.

Author

Mark Boswell attended medical school at Case Western Reserve University and did his residency at the University Hospitals of Cleveland. His interests in academic medicine and healthcare administration have provided opportunities to work with wonderful people at many great locations around the country.

39 Transparency, Science, and Healthcare Policies

Marc Leib

Introduction

After practicing medicine for almost a quarter of a century in Arizona, I decided to concentrate my efforts on formulating healthcare policy. I eventually became the chief medical officer (CMO) for Arizona's Medicaid program, where I spent the next 10 years drafting policies for a program that provides health care to over 1.5 million people.

Policy Professional

As Medicaid CMO, I learned important skills that helped me provide the leadership necessary to achieve my policy goals. One of the more important skills was being transparent. The term "transparency" has multiple definitions, but when I use that term, I am referring to being open and honest in communications in order to build trust between all parties. One example illustrates how I used transparency to formulate healthcare policy in that program.

Arizona Medicaid provides healthcare services almost entirely through contracted managed care organizations (MCOs), each of which conducts its own prior authorization program. The MCOs required physicians to provide detailed information about patients when requesting prior authorization for procedures or treatments.

However, the MCOs were far less forthcoming with details when they denied those prior authorization requests. Frustrated physicians often contacted me because they had no idea why the requested services were denied. When I contacted the MCOs to inquire about the "why" behind their denials, I would often receive vague answers that the requested service "did not meet medical necessity requirements," which is like saying "because we said so." That was the antithesis of transparency.

M. Leib (✉)
Health Care Consultant, Phoenix, AZ, USA

S. Mohamed et al. (eds.), *Anesthesia Bridges*, https://doi.org/10.1007/978-3-032-08294-7_39

Requiring Transparency

Finding those answers unsatisfactory because they provided no information that requesting physicians could refute, I instituted a new policy that required the MCOs to be transparent when they denied requested services. This policy required MCOs to provide details regarding specific medical reasons for their denials, including explanations of the criteria necessary to meet the plan's medical necessity requirements.

The plans complained that this policy required them to provide a road map to help physicians and patients appeal request denials, which was exactly my intention. The new policy required that denials be made on the basis of the facts regarding the patient's medical condition and scientific evidence regarding the requested treatment. It was anticipated that once physicians understood specific medical necessity requirements, they would not submit prior authorization requests for services that did not meet those requirements.

***Note from the Editors:** Speaking of transparency, this is the perfect place to feature the dramatic Grand Canyon Skywalk, a glass bridge over the West Rim of the Canyon near Meadview, AZ (Fig. 39.1), and the glass canopy over the pedestrian bridge over the Kura Mtkvari River in Tbilisi, Georgia (Fig. 39.2).

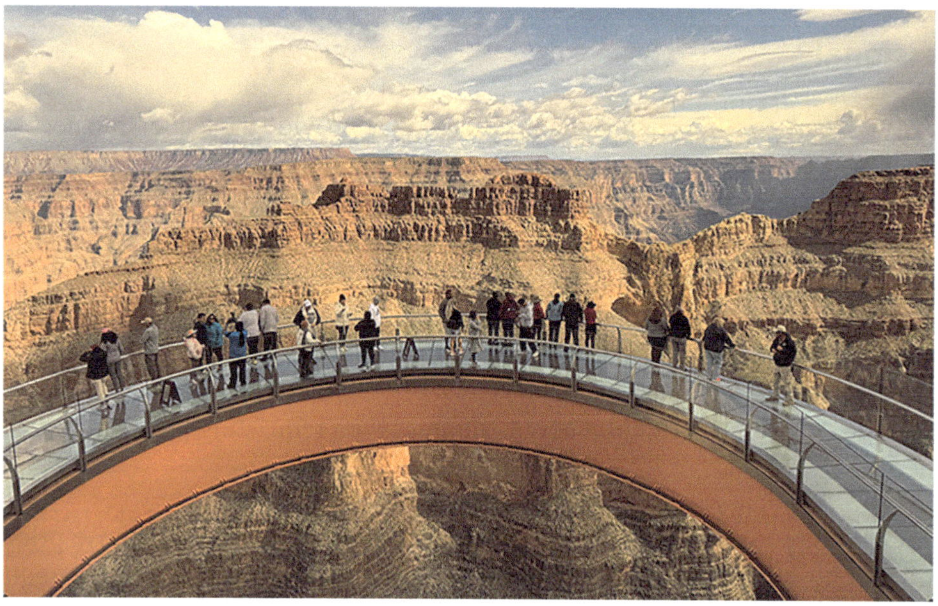

Fig. 39.1 The dramatic Grand Canyon Skywalk in Arizona. Skywalk is located at Eagle Point on a side canyon in the Grand Canyon West area and is not affiliated with the National Park Service. It was commissioned and is owned by the Hualapai Indian Tribe and was opened to the public in 2007. It is highly engineered and can withstand an 8.0 magnitude earthquake within 50 miles. The design also underwent an extensive wind loading and pedestrian vibration analysis. The Skywalk receives over 300,000 visitors per year. The project and subsequent proposed development around the Skywalk have generated considerable controversy. Photo: Image used for editorial purposes (nonfiction book) under license from shutterstock.com

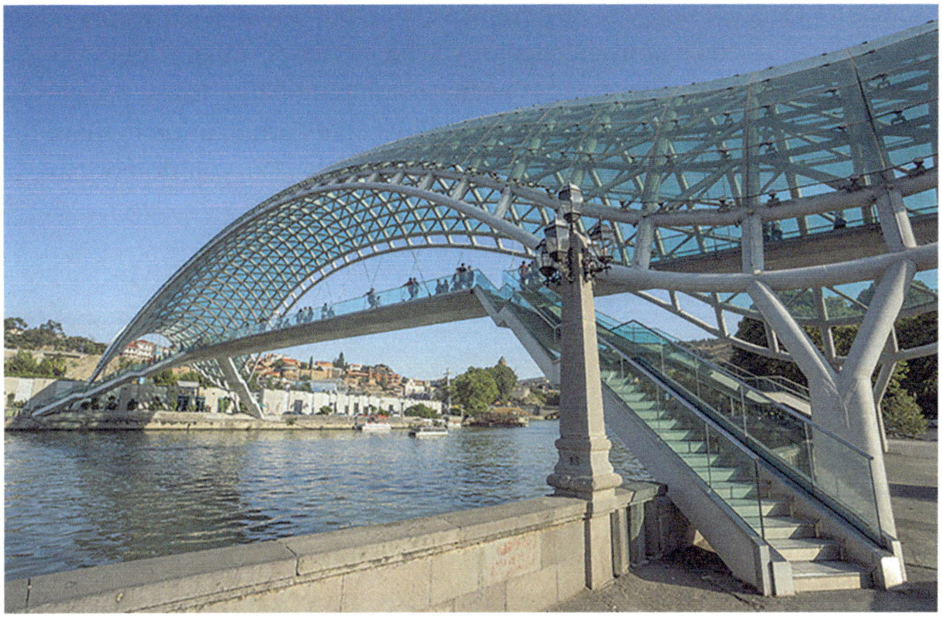

Fig. 39.2 This steel and glass bridge is known as the Peace Bridge. Photo: Image used for editorial purposes (nonfiction book) under standard license from adobe.com

Transparency Works!

Two years later, the MCOs reported that the number of prior authorization denials had declined significantly due to fewer requests that did not meet medical necessity requirements. Similarly, the number of complaints from physicians and patients had also decreased. Providing information to physicians reduced inefficiencies generated by their ignorance of the metrics by which prior authorization requests would be measured. Transparency—open and honest communications that result in trust—was beneficial to all program participants.

Transparency is also critical when healthcare policies are debated and implemented. When communicating with policy makers, such as legislators or CMS, I stated the facts as best I knew them, whether helpful or not. It was then up to the policy makers to draw their own conclusions from those facts. When I presented evidence clearly, honestly, and objectively, the results may not have been perfect, but they were almost always acceptable.

Developing Policy: Science Versus Ideology

As physicians, it is incumbent on us to be transparent about scientific facts when we participate in policy discussions, honestly presenting the facts as they are known at the time. Those facts may change over time, but that is the nature of science. We must use science to guide public health policies. To do otherwise results in increased morbidity and mortality from the very diseases that public health systems seek to eradicate.

Policies based on scientific facts are not typically controversial, but not all healthcare policies are based on science. Some policies are based on political ideology, which often result in widely varying responses among physicians. It is important for us to express positions on politically driven policies because they may have profound effects on our practices and patients. Physician participation in those discussions is essential because failure to participate may prove the old adage that "if you do not have a seat at the table, you are likely to find yourself on the menu."

Lessons Learned

- Being transparent (open and honest) in communications allows one to build trust.
- The best policies are based on scientific facts, not political ideology.

Author

Marc Leib practiced anesthesia for over 20 years, serving as president of the Arizona Society of Anesthesiologists and the Arizona Medical Association. Later, he attended the University of Arizona College of Law while continuing his anesthesia practice. He later served as the CMO for Arizona's Medicaid Program, a position he held for over 10 years. Since his retirement from Medicaid, Marc provides consulting services mostly involving Medicare and Medicaid issues. He continues to serve the American Society of Anesthesiologists and the Arizona Society of Anesthesiologists.

Why Leadership Training Matters

40

Jay Mesrobian

Introduction

When I finished residency and fellowship, I joined a midsize practice in Columbia, South Carolina. The practice was well established within a large county hospital with all the "fixins"—Level I Trauma, Level III NICU, high-risk labor and delivery, and a children's hospital, all in a great diverse clinical practice. I gradually took on responsibilities for the group and committee work within the hospital, primarily in the pediatric anesthesia arenas, and eventually served on the practice's management committee. I had developed a reputation as a reliable manager who could deliver results, and the hospital was comfortable with my performance in nonclinical areas.

New Position!

About five years into practice, the hospital suggested a new position, Professional Director for Anesthesia Services. This new position, funded by the hospital, would primarily be a liaison between the group and hospital (which also employed the CRNAs), and create alignment in clinical, operational, and financial performance.

But Then...

Not even two years later, the hospital and practice jointly decided to eliminate the position due to a lack of efficacy and deliverable benefits.

What Happened?

While there may have been some lack of clarity and purpose around this new position, the majority of the responsibility for its failure lies at my feet. I did not recognize that this new position likely made many people, both within the practice and hospital administration, uncomfortable. Despite a large port-

J. Mesrobian (✉)
TeamHealth Anesthesia, Milwaukee, WI, USA
e-mail: jay_mesrobian@teamhealth.com

S. Mohamed et al. (eds.), *Anesthesia Bridges*, https://doi.org/10.1007/978-3-032-08294-7_40

folio of successful committee work, I still did not understand the different motivations across the practice and administration. I did not really understand how decisions were made within the organization. As a result, I foundered, trying to navigate poorly defined relationships with the practice, the management committee, the existing department chief, and the hospital administration. Frankly, I failed because I did not take time to listen to and understand each stakeholder's perspective, prioritize areas of common interest, and communicate in a way that would motivate all parties and create consensus.

***Note from the Editors:** Speaking of failure followed by recovery, we think that the Daniel Hoan Bridge is the most stunning bridge in Milwaukee. It looks like a seagull to us, and we love the way the sky blends into the water. And that little red lighthouse just really makes the whole visual experience work! (Fig. 40.1).

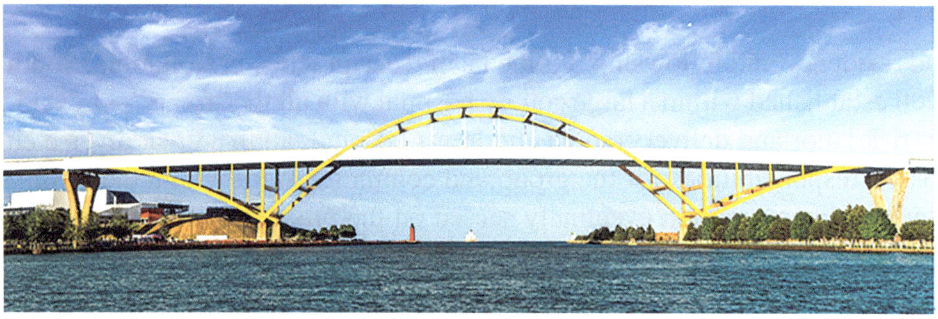

Fig. 40.1 The Daniel Hoan Bridge in Milwaukee, originally called the Harbor Bridge. It is a tiered arch bridge. It was constructed between 1970 and 1972, but did not open until 1977 due to protests over the construction of the connecting highways. The bridge required extensive rehabilitation and reconstruction after several sections failed, but is now considered to be in a sound structural status for the next 40–50 years. A capital campaign was undertaken to light the bridge at night; this was inaugurated in late 2020. Photo: Image used under standard license from adobe.stock.com

Lessons Learned

What "lessons learned" would I tell my 35-year-old self now? When you are offered a new position in leadership, think about the following:

- *Define clearly* the purpose and goals of the position. How will success be measured?
- Understand the governance structure around the position. How does this new position interact with the existing leadership and management structure?
- Before accepting, speak with key stakeholders to understand their perspectives and concerns about the position.
- The title does not give you instant credibility and, in fact, may limit your ability to influence. Above all, spend the majority of your time listening to your colleagues, other clinicians, and administration, so that you understand their perspectives, develop trust, and establish a foundation for ongoing communication. *It is all about the relationships.*

- Understand that much of your medical training has little to do with leadership, team building, and effective communication skills. Ask for coaching and/or formal training, as everyone has an interest in your success.

Unlike 25 years ago, there are multiple options for emerging and established physician leaders to develop their leadership skill set. The ASA certainly has developed a strong portfolio of options through its Conference on Practice Management, partnerships with both ACHE and the Kellogg School of Management, and the new Committee on Professional Development. We highly advise that entry and mid-level leaderships take advantage of these resources.

Author

Jay Mesrobian is a native of Chicago but has spent the past 20+ years living behind the "cheddar curtain" in Milwaukee, Wisconsin, and the prior nine years in Columbia, South Carolina. He is passionate about patient experience, the development of young physician leaders, and defining ways anesthesiologists can drive improvements in patient care. He has advocated in both state and national organizations, including serving as ASA Treasurer, and is eternally thankful to the mentors and partners who encouraged him along that path. He and his wife Beth have two adult daughters and an adult Newfoundland, Dilly.

41 Be the Best You Can Be

Michael A. Ramsay

Introduction

There are a few key concepts to consider that will greatly help you have a successful and satisfying career.

- *Be the best you can be*. Always lead by example, which leads to respect gained.
- **Keep anesthesia off the administration radar screen!** Deal with issues before they escalate, as you may not be able to control the outcome if they do escalate.
- *Embrace new programs and lead them into your facility*. The natural reaction for members of your department is to resist anything that takes them out of their comfort zone. The development of a liver transplant program was met with much resistance from the anesthesia staff, who had heard stories of "blood baths" with these cases. I was able to lead a small number of colleagues in starting the program and providing anesthesia for the first liver transplant in Texas. We developed a clinical research team around these patients and published numerous papers in peer-reviewed journals. Our program became known as a center of excellence for patients with porto-pulmonary hypertension. This resulted in invitations to present at major meetings around the world. This also culminated in my being elected president of the International Liver Transplant Society and invitations to author chapters in major anesthesia textbooks on the liver and transplantation.

Lessons Learned

- When you are leading, strive to lead by example, deal with issues early, and learn to embrace change.
- The best decision of my career was actually a strong decision by my wife Zoe, and that was our move to Baylor. I am not sure where my accent has landed. In London, they are critical and call it Yankee, and in Texas, most say I am Australian!?

M. A. Ramsay (✉)
Department of Anesthesiology and Pain Management, Baylor University Medical Center, Dallas, TX, USA
e-mail: michael.ramsay@bswhealth.org

S. Mohamed et al. (eds.), *Anesthesia Bridges*, https://doi.org/10.1007/978-3-032-08294-7_41

- The move to Baylor has allowed us both to travel together around the globe on lecture tours. This has resulted in many international friends as well as local friends, and also great memories. Along the way, we have managed a few influences on medicine and providers as well. What an exhilarating and fun career!"

- The editors wholeheartedly agree with Mike's advice to keep anesthesia off the administration's radar. Sometimes, if you let issues get away from you, they take on a life of their own and really are never put back in the bottle. We've seen situations where certain issues have surfaced years later to everybody's detriment.

- The editors also urge junior people to borrow from Mike's example and try to develop programs and centers of excellence whenever and however you can. There is more advice about this elsewhere in the book. But since you are doing the work and developing the expertise anyway, why not do the publications and develop a reputation?

Author

Michael Ramsay was born in Dublin, went to medical school in London, and after two years on the faculty of the London Hospital, he moved to Baylor University Medical Center in Dallas, a move he credits with great things happening in his career.

42 Be (A) Ware of Leadership

Frank Rosinia

Introduction

You just matched in a great residency program. The patient is at the center of your thoughts and motivation to become a great anesthesiologist. And then what?

Trust

You begin to realize that trust is essential for the care of your patient. You trust the team in the operating room. You trust the colleague who provides relief during a long case. Trust is foundational for this clinical mission. A great outcome for the patient is what connects everyone to a thick band of trust. You press on even to gain greater knowledge and clinical expertise. Soon, you are recognized for your commitment to patient care and leadership. The title and position of chief resident feel good. The younger residents ask for advice on the best technique for an arterial line, a central line, and managing a difficult airway. During downtime, there are lots of great discussions on tricky clinical scenarios. This is good stuff.

All your hard work pays off. You land a great job with a solid group. Your motivation continues to serve you well. Soon, people at work will request you to care for their family members for an upcoming surgery. They trust your commitment to ensure the best outcome for their loved one. They trust your clinical skill and intrinsic motivation to always do what is best for the patient. Your ability and work ethic begin to pay dividends. You are offered leadership opportunities because you are a great and trusted clinician. These leadership roles begin in your department and over time, evolve into the larger organization. Things now begin to change.

F. Rosinia (✉)
Department of Anesthesiology, UT Health San Antonio, San Antonio, TX, USA
e-mail: rosinia@uthscsa.edu

S. Mohamed et al. (eds.), *Anesthesia Bridges*, https://doi.org/10.1007/978-3-032-08294-7_42

Transitions

You are wearing scrubs and a lab coat in a conference room, while others have coats and ties. Many of the people in the room have never delivered clinical care. They have not experienced the responsibility that direct clinical care demands. The discussions are different from the involved conversations about patient care and outcomes. Administrators are focused on the budget, the Joint Commission, Leapfrog scores, and contract terms. You continue to work hard and recognize that a different skill set is required for your evolving leadership responsibilities. Success and opportunity are available in a new venue. You are motivated to develop this administrative skill set alongside your clinical expertise. You begin to think, what makes these administrators tick? Can I trust them? Are they ethical?

One day, you meet the CEO and other executives. What an experience. These are exciting people. They are energetic, motivating, and even charismatic. This is a whole new experience that requires a new skill set. You think, "I never got taught this stuff in medical school or residency!" You begin to read books on leadership. Ethical leadership. Resonant leadership. Adaptive leadership. Level 5 leadership. How to build great teams. You find out that trust is the foundation of Patrick Lencioni's model of teamwork. This is a whole new world.

Takeaways

The scenario above is an accurate representation of a professional transition in my career. The lessons I share below are a distillation of my experience as a clinical physician, evolution into formal physician leadership roles, and work as a physician executive in the C-suite. I hope that these life lessons will improve your chance for success in an administrative work environment. Below, I will discuss three important takeaways that will serve you well during your administrative development.

The first lesson is to understand that humans, including you, have a default for the truth. This is well discussed in Malcom Gladwell's book, *Talking to Strangers,* and in this short article by Levine [1, 2]. The key point to understand is that we are social creatures who tend to believe that others are telling us the truth. This is overall a good thing, much better than assuming people are not telling us the truth.

With that understanding, be aware (and beware!) in administrative settings, especially at the senior executive level. **Go on high alert** if you are told, "Let me be honest with you about this issue." That is a sure sign there is another side to this issue that is worth knowing. Enjoy the fact that we believe in the overall honesty of our fellow humans, but think differently in an administrative and senior executive environment.

The second lesson is to be aware of narcissism in executive-level leaders. We like to think that our senior administrative leaders are collaborative, modest, and generous. Jim Collins studied over 1400 companies in his popular book, *Good to Great.* He found only 11 modest and humble leaders. You are much more likely to have a narcissist sitting in the C-suite. The traits assigned to narcissists are self-importance, arrogance, a lack of empathy, and a belief that they are special and unique. They very often seek the admiration of others. They also commonly use the first-person singular, "I" in conversations and interviews, for example, "I did such a great job last year with this organization." The takeaway here is to study and understand the tendencies and behaviors of narcissists. Jeffrey Pfeffer provides a thorough, evidence-based discussion in his recent book, *Leadership BS* [3]. There is a good chance they are at the top of your organization.

The third and final lesson is that the higher you go in an organization, the thinner the trust. The definition we will use for trust is that it requires people to keep their commitments [3]. This makes sense. As an example, if I commit to "have your back" during a politically charged project you are working on, that should give you comfort and courage. All is good until my commitment to you creates a restriction for me. What happens next is all too common. I will decide to do what is best for me and not honor my commitment to have your back. Commitments present restrictions for administrative leaders.

There is rarely a consequence for organizational leaders when they break trust. "There are scores, if not hundreds, of examples in companies big and small of individuals often losing political battles and getting deposed by the very same people that they had themselves promoted." [3] Leaders typically do not break trust out of malice but are forced to choose between competing priorities–and you may not be their highest priority. This comes as a shock to physicians who, with rare exception, honor commitments for clinical care. This is counter to the books you have read about trust being the bedrock of great teams. My closing advice is to honor your commitments, make trust a part of your team, but be aware that the organizational leadership values trust very differently.

The three big takeaways—my own *personal* "lessons learned" are below.

Lessons Learned

- As human beings, we have a default to believe others are telling us the truth. This is a good thing, but be aware when you are in or dealing with the executive suite.
- Many of our organizations are run by narcissists. Make sure you understand this personality type. It is essential.
- Trust gets thin in the executive suite. Be aware.

References

1. Gladwell M. Talking to strangers. New York: Little, Brown and Company; 2019.
2. Levine TR. Truth-Default Theory (TDT): a theory of human deception and deception detection. J Lang Soc Psychol. 2014;33(4):378–92.
3. Pfeffer J. Leadership BS. New York: HarperCollins; 2015.

Author

Frank Rosinia's career has involved academic and private practice anesthesiology as well as work as a physician executive in health care. He is married to Ninfa, and they raised three daughters in New Orleans. Frank is now pursuing certification in executive coaching.

Developing Good Judgment: The Basics

43

Catherine Marcucci, Christopher C. Conner, Jennifer P. Wilson, Neil B. Sandson, and David A. Zvara

Introduction

This topic was suggested by several authors who have sought and relied on the judgment of a few key colleagues, **Jeff Kirsch** among them. The authors decided to talk over the subject and try to put together some advice and wisdom for junior anesthesiologists. A long and interesting conference call ensued. And, as it so happens, Cathy's childhood friend (same kindergarten) is the **Hon. Christopher Conner**, federal district judge of the Middle District of Pennsylvania, and the group decided that it would be fun and intriguing to see if their conclusions were shared by the "pros." Judge Conner's colleague, the **Hon. Jennifer P. Wilson**, was kind enough to also join him in reviewing our conclusions and giving us some additional thoughts and advice. There are additional thoughts on developing good judgment in Chaps. 44 and 122.

Here are the questions we discussed.

What Is the Definition of Good Judgment?

All the physicians and the judges agreed on this—good judgment is the objective application of existing facts and personal expertise to resolve problems in an appropriate and effective manner.

C. Marcucci (✉)
Department of Transfusion Medicine, Clinical Center, National Institutes of Health, Bethesda, MD, USA

C. C. Conner · J. P. Wilson
Middle District of Pennsylvania, Harrisburg, PA, USA

N. B. Sandson
Department of Psychiatry, VA Maryland Health Care System, Baltimore, MD, USA

University of Maryland, Baltimore, MD, USA

D. A. Zvara
Department of Anesthesiology, The University of North Carolina at Chapel Hill, Chapel Hill, NC, USA

S. Mohamed et al. (eds.), *Anesthesia Bridges*, https://doi.org/10.1007/978-3-032-08294-7_43

Is It Possible to Learn Good Judgment or Is This Some Sort of Innate Character Trait?

Although Cathy wasn't sure about this one, Dr. Zvara stated his conviction that good judgment can absolutely be learned. We asked the judges to do a tie-break, and they both sided resoundingly with David.

Judge Wilson sent us these thoughts:

Fear not, it is entirely possible to learn good judgment! The whole concept of experience teaches us that we can learn from historical events, and we can apply those lessons to future events. The key is identifying precisely what information to extract from prior experiences and how to apply those information bites to the next problem event.

In federal judge orientation (aka "baby judge school"), we receive a presentation on the concept of procedural due process, which is the judiciary's rough equivalent of a differential diagnosis, albeit in an adversarial system. The key is to develop a complete factual record—not simply one side—on the issue at hand. Like the differential diagnosis, presentations from all sides allow judges to consider alternative findings based upon each party's view of the evidence presented. Then, and only then, can we weigh the evidence and decide the matter at bar. For physicians, this would be to make the diagnosis or other final determination.

Where Can You Look to Learn the Qualities of Good Judgment?

For the authors, it really has been an amalgamation of exposure to people we respected and trusted and people we observed in the act of exercising good judgment, namely our parents, siblings, teachers, and professors, but also our colleagues and mentors.

Equally important are the lessons learned from those who have exercised bad judgment in our presence. Everybody has often heard about learning from your own mistakes, but of course, learning from the mistakes and misjudgments of others is critical in developing good judgment, especially clinical judgment. We advise our junior colleagues to attend every morbidity and mortality conference, every quality assurance meeting, every formal or informal staff debriefing that they can. Not to gloat over others' misfortunes, but because there will be a wealth of information wherever and whenever mistakes and mishaps are honestly presented. Truthfully, it's sometimes so much easier and more efficient to process and absorb the lessons to be learned from other people's experiences without the psychological and emotional burden and barriers of personal involvement.

***Note from the Editors:** David Zvara is from Toledo, OH, and we just couldn't make up our minds about which Toledo bridge we wanted to feature, so we decided to include two—the old and the new—the Veterans City Glass Skyway and the old Cherry St. Bridge (Figs. 43.1 and 43.2).

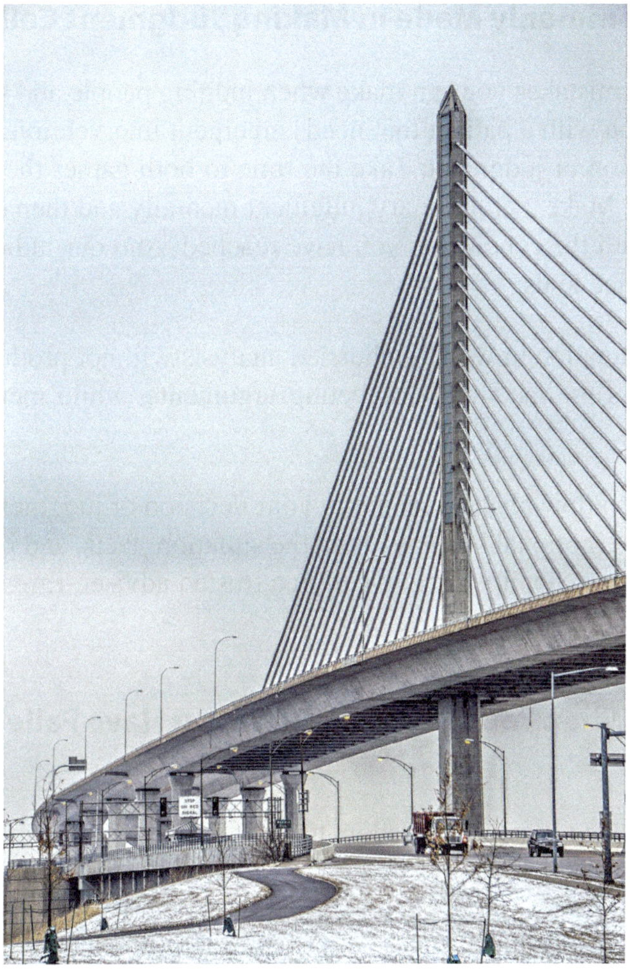

Fig. 43.1 The beautiful and dramatic Veterans' Glass City Skyway in Toledo, OH, is commonly called the Toledo Skyway. It is a cable-stayed bridge that opened in 2007. It spans the Maumee River and low-lying land on either side of the river and is dramatically lit at night. Photo: Image used under standard license from adobe.stock.com

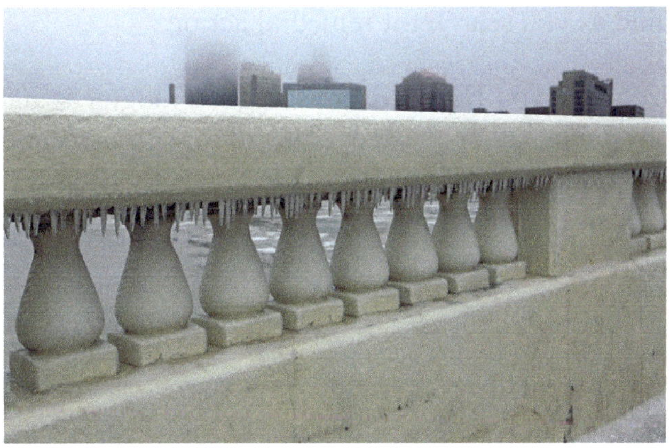

Fig. 43.2 Architectural detail from the Old Cherry St. Bridge across the Maumee River in Toledo, OH, on an icy day. It is a double-leaf bascule bridge near downtown Toledo. The structure opened in 1914 and has been extensively rebuilt. It is now officially known as the Martin Luther King Memorial Bridge. Photo: Image used under standard license from adobe.stock.com

What Mistakes Are Commonly Made in Making Judgment Calls?

We think there are two big mistakes you can make when judging people and situations. First, unless you are facing an acute situation with a patient that needs emergent intervention, the biggest mistake by far is to make a hurried decision or judgment. Take the time to both gather the facts and to analyze them carefully and thoughtfully. Make a preliminary judgment mentally and then evaluate whether emerging facts are still consistent with the conclusion you have reached. And our judicial colleagues agree completely. Their succinct advice to us:

- It is hard to imagine a situation in which unhurried analysis will not produce a more thoughtful conclusion. Carefully assess the facts and competing arguments, while methodically eliminating any irrelevant considerations.

- The second mistake is to allow bias to creep into your decision or judgment. It is imperative that you exercise intellectual and emotional honesty about the situation, facts, and people you may be judging. If you find this is difficult to do, it is time to call in a trusted adviser. Emphasis on trusted.

What Should You Do When You Recognize That You Have Failed to Exercise Good Judgment?

Justice Felix Frankfurter once observed: "Wisdom too often never comes, and so one ought not to reject it merely because it comes late."

Obviously, those in a position to judge must understand that they also have the responsibility to unjudge, or rather, re-judge. In the medical profession, some matters simply do not permit corrective action, and we must live with the result. Often, however, there is the opportunity for an improved resolution of the issue at hand. Maya Angelou once said that the goal is to do the best you know. But when you know better, you must do better. And we agree. If you have made a serious error in judgment, start making amends. Be honest and communicate openly regarding the erroneous judgment within ethical boundaries. Use an open mind as you search for remedial action.

On the other hand, recognize when you **HAVE** exercised good judgment and stand by yourself. One of the coolest things that the physician authors have ever heard in their careers happened when a colleague was being pushed a little on a judgment call she had made—a really tricky combination clinical-personnel issue, if memory serves correctly. She said simply, "I had a difficult decision to make, and I made it." And that shut the second-guessing down immediately.

How Do You Teach Good Judgment?

Obviously, by being a good example. But how else? We asked the judges for the basic principles they use when instructing juries on how to weigh evidence. They shared an excerpt from an actual trial court's instruction to a jury:

There is nothing particularly different in the way that a juror should consider the evidence in a trial from that in which any reasonable and careful person would deal with any very important question that must be resolved by examining facts, opinions, and credible testimony. You are expected to use your good sense in considering and evaluating the evidence in the case. Give the record evidence a reasonable and fair construction in light of your common knowledge of the natural tendencies and inclinations of human beings.

In other words—think about what is reasonable and maintain a healthy dose of reality about human nature. We think these watchwords have applicability to judgment in the medical sphere as well. When asked, the authors have always encouraged junior people who have to make judgments to draw on their experience and common sense, and give.

Lessons Learned

- Good judgment is really just common sense, experience, and the careful analysis of facts.
- Good judgment can be learned!
- We just don't believe in snap judgments, and neither do the pros we consulted. Federal judges are taught in their orientation symposium that one of the biggest mistakes that can be made is to judge too quickly.
- If you realize that you have made an error in judgment, work as quickly and completely as the boundaries of ethics allow to remediate your decision or the effects of your decision.
- Study, study, study the bad judgments of yourself and others. Review every root cause analysis that you can find information on. What exactly went wrong? What exactly were the untoward or deleterious results? How did the system compensate?

When you feel you have made a good decision or the best decision that could be made in the circumstances, stand by it and yourself. Feel free to borrow this line, "I had a difficult decision to make, and I made it."

Acknowledgment: The physician authors thank the Hon. Jennifer P. Wilson and the Hon. Christopher C. Conner for generously sharing their time and thoughts with us.

Authors

Cathy Marcucci grew up in Mechanicsburg, PA, an incorporated borough on the West Shore of the Susquehanna, near Harrisburg. She had the great good fortune to train at Hopkins in the 1990s where she acquired her clinical judgment by watching the best—Tommy Toung, Dr. Raja, Chas Emala, Dave Lange, Ed Norris, Brett Simon, Fritz Sieber, Mark Mirski, Genie Heitmiller, Lynne Maxwell, Steve Frank, Steve Parker, Bill Merritt, Rose Christopherson, and many others. She is also grateful to Jeff Kirsch for the opportunity down through the years to discuss her decisions and dilemmas and to have the ongoing benefit of his advice.

Christopher Conner is a federal judge who was appointed in 2002 after practicing commercial litigation for 20 years. He is the proud father of four accomplished children, one of whom is a resident in physical medicine and rehabilitation at Spaulding (and also an *Anesthesia Bridges* contributor). His best judgment was timely in recognizing his inability to sing, dance, or become a professional golfer, although he still enjoys all three activities.

Jennifer Wilson was appointed to the federal bench in November 2019, leaving her practice as a trial lawyer after nearly two decades. She is working hard to raise three wonderful children with her husband, while doing her part to keep the wheels of justice rolling. She frequently feels that her experience in resolving sibling squabbles has provided her with the best training as a trial judge.

Neil Sandson is a psychiatrist in Baltimore, Maryland. He is the proud father of two young adult children. His outstanding judgment is evidenced by having married Cathy Marcucci, his wife of 30+ years. Less astute was his decision to become a mesomorphic squash player.

David Zvara was born and raised in Toledo, Ohio. His father and mother both worked for the labor unions at the height of their influence in the 1950s and 1960s. This exposure to understanding the power of the common good has influenced his thinking greatly. David accepted a military scholarship for medical school and subsequently served in Operation Desert Storm. He has chaired at both Ohio State University and the University of North Carolina at Chapel Hill and is now CMO of UNC Hospitals while remaining a professor of anesthesiology.

Developing Good Judgment: Be Careful Who and How You Judge

44

Jennifer P. Wilson, Christopher C. Conner, Neil B. Sandson, and Catherine Marcucci

Introduction

Whether for purposes of hiring professional staff, determining whether and how to mobilize disciplinary procedures, choosing who to trust and depend upon, or a host of other issues, becoming an accurate judge of our peers' character and capabilities is a critical part of thriving in a medical system. We have to provisionally judge others on a nearly constant basis. It is important to understand that such provisional judgments are superficial and should evolve, hopefully in a positive direction, as we come to better know our colleagues over time.

What Is the Best Way to Do This?

First and foremost, acknowledge that judging people is inherently stressful. There is an inevitable tension between empathy, sympathy, and equity.

Second, we recommend that you understand the nature of subjective versus objective judging. And that judging people is often really about judging their honesty and credibility. Naturally, our judicial colleagues had a lot to say on this subject. Their advice, when considering the general question of "Do I believe this person?" is to analyze the following:

- The quality of the person's knowledge, understanding, and memory of a specific event or set of circumstances.
- The person's appearance, behavior, and manner.
- The person's relationship with others with whom you are interacting on the question at hand.
- Whether the person previously said or wrote anything different from the current presentation.

J. P. Wilson · C. C. Conner
Middle District of Pennsylvania, Harrisburg, PA, USA

N. B. Sandson
Department of Psychiatry, VA Maryland Health Care System, Baltimore, MD, USA

University of Maryland, Baltimore, MD, USA

C. Marcucci (✉)
Department of Transfusion Medicine, Clinical Center, National Institutes of Health, Bethesda, MD, USA

S. Mohamed et al. (eds.), *Anesthesia Bridges*, https://doi.org/10.1007/978-3-032-08294-7_44

- Whether the person has an interest in the outcome of the issue or any motive, bias, or prejudice.
- Whether you yourself have a particular interest in the outcome or any motive, bias, or prejudice in the question at hand.

A forthright and honest evaluation of these factors will help build a factual or objective framework to a subjective decision. Transparency in the exercise of subjective judgment is really important because it promotes confidence in the ultimate conclusion.

A third point is that sometimes it is easier to frame a disbelief rather than a belief. In other words, why do I disbelieve this person? Or alternately, why should I pass on hiring this person?

Fourth, while our work lives and our personal lives are often quite separate, the qualities that should concern us in judging others are mostly the same. What do you value in your personal and family relationships? Most likely, you value and count on honesty, consideration, reliability, and competence. How does the person you are evaluating do with this type of analysis?

Fifth, **be very careful who you judge**. It's only human nature to have opinions on people and personnel matters, but we have found that it is wisest to stay at a sufficient distance from issues that don't require your actual input, involvement, and judgment. In order to be truly confident in judging another's character, you need to have access to an extensive and accurate understanding of the contributory background elements and all pertinent facts that inform why they make the choices that they make and to discern intentions from others' actions. This level of understanding is hard to come by, and we should thus be reluctant to make fixed and immutable judgments of others based on incomplete information.

And Lastly....

It also bears mentioning that as we judge, so shall we be judged. That is why the authors regard honesty, kindness, and reliability as the most important personal qualities to embrace and model, regardless of what specific medical specialty, or for that matter, walk of life, one pursues. As reasonable as it might be to concern oneself with the judgment of others, it is also true that the world is full of mirrors, and we would like to be able to look into them comfortably.

Lessons Learned

- Judging people is stressful. People and their motivations are complex, and therefore so is the process of judging them. Be wary of situations where your conclusions or decisions seem too easy. There may be an opportunity to explore the facts more thoroughly.
- Try to build an objective framework for subjective decisions.
- If you are having difficulty evaluating or judging a person, mentally place them in the context of a friend or family member and then reanalyze the issue.
- Judge carefully, kindly, and sparingly. Remember, there are mirrors everywhere.

Acknowledgment The physician authors once again thank Judge Jennifer P. Wilson and Judge Christopher C. Conner for their time and thoughts.

Authors

Jennifer Wilson graduated from high school in central Pennsylvania and told her parents she would never move back home. She kept that commitment through college near Philadelphia, law school in New York, clerkships in Memphis and Newark, New Jersey, and working in New York and Washington, D.C. But then—in a move that has proved to be her best judgment call to date—she decided to come back home to central Pennsylvania when she was expecting her second child.

Christopher Conner has exercised judgment in many different capacities—spouse, parent, church trustee, professor, lawyer, and federal judge—but he still has no dietary judgment when it comes to chocolate chip cookies or carrot cake. He has wisely accepted that for now (and possibly always) dessert is his judgment-free zone.

Neil Sandson a psychiatrist who helped raise two children, has thus developed a nearly foolproof ability to spot lies of both omission and commission. This has become known in both his professional and personal circles as his "spidey sense."

Cathy Marcucci considers that her best decision in life, hands down, was having the above mentioned children with Neil Sandson. Her second-best decision was trusting his wise ways of parenting. Although she is constantly resolving to think a bit more carefully at the bridge table—especially when declaring a game contract—her judgment about when to draw trump and which finesses to take often leaves her wide open to comment and correction.

On Leadership: Lessons Learned

45

Zeyd Ebrahim

Introduction

Over the years, I have had the opportunity to serve in many leadership roles at the Cleveland Clinic. Fortunately, and more importantly, I have had the opportunity to work with, observe, and learn from many outstanding leaders. Below are some observations that I have made on being a successful, respected, and serving leader.

- Be a good listener. This is so important. In order to be a good listener, you have to be a sincere and honest listener and be open to someone else's ideas and thoughts.
- There is this great quote by Maya Angelou: "I've learned that people will forget what you said, people will forget what you did, but people will never forget how you made them feel." I strongly believe that this quote (along with an attitude of treating people the way you would like to be treated) personifies the essence of being a great leader.
- Too often in academic medicine, we equate managerial skills with leadership skills. I would recommend all potential leaders review the "list of differences between a manager and a leader" written by Warren Bennis in his book *On Becoming a Leader*, written in 1989.
- Be wary of those who take themselves too seriously. Take your patients and your work seriously. Always have a sense of humor; it will help in interpersonal relationships and conflicts. Always be transparent in dealing with others and matters of policy.
- If an anesthesiologist is lucky, they will have the good fortune of working in an anesthetic practice where there is mutual respect and collegiality within the group, the anesthesia trainees, and with all OR personnel. In this environment, going to the hospital every day is not going to work!

Lessons Learned

- When leading, strive to be a good listener, treat people right, and have a sense of humor!

Z. Ebrahim (✉)
Anesthesiology Institute, Cleveland Clinic, Cleveland, OH, USA
e-mail: EBRAHIZ@ccf.org

S. Mohamed et al. (eds.), *Anesthesia Bridges*, https://doi.org/10.1007/978-3-032-08294-7_45

Which of the figures in the illustration below is in the leadership position (Fig. 45.1)? The answer is all of them, depending on your viewpoint. Sometimes leaders are in front, sometimes they are sweeping up at the back, and sometimes true leaders are providing momentum and support from the middle of the pack.

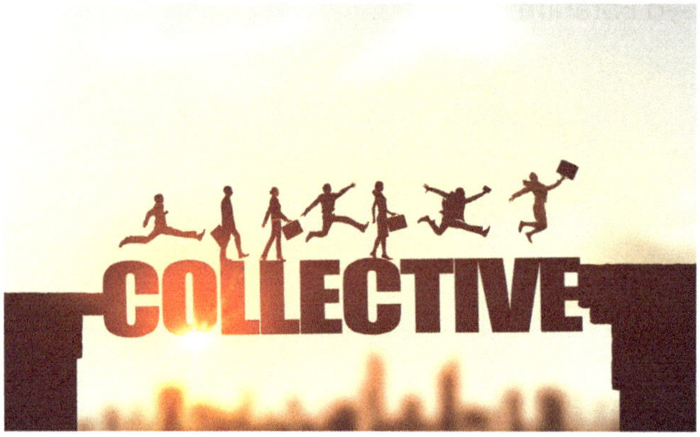

Fig. 45.1 Leaders lead, but they also create and support situations for others to forge ahead. A team knows who its leaders are, but sometimes it's not completely obvious from the outside. Photo: Image used under standard license from shutterstock.com

Bonus Content!

The editors must confess that Dr. Ebrahim's excellent wisdom sent us straight online to continue reading about leadership, especially as it contrasts with managing. We agree with the recommendation of *On Becoming a Leader*, but if you have only a bit of time, there are lots of fun, short articles and summaries to think about and discuss. Here's one from Forbes [1]:

- Leaders create a vision, managers create goals.
- Leaders are change agents, managers maintain the status quo.
- Leaders are unique, managers copy.
- Leaders take risks, managers control risk.
- Leaders are in it for the long haul, managers think short-term.
- Leaders grow personally, managers rely on existing, proven skills.
- Leaders build relationships, managers build systems and processes.
- Leaders coach, managers direct.

We are not recommending that our readers just accept these points uncritically. Strategy is not the same as tactics! And management skills have their appropriate place. If the task of the day is to complete the changeover of anesthesia machines or to get the anesthesia carts stocked more effectively, you don't need to invoke the oratory of Winston Churchill or the brilliance of Marcus Aurelius. We also stress elsewhere in this book that building safety into processes means building safety *systems* and not relying on the individual excellence of the people concerned. In truth, anesthesiologists need both leadership *and* management skills and expertise in where, when, and how to deploy them.

Reference

1. Arruda W. 9 differences between being a leader and a manager [Internet]. Forbes; 2016 Nov 15 [cited 2022 Sep 30]. Available from: https://www.forbes.com/sites/williamarruda/2016/11/15/9-differences-between-being-a-leader-and-a-manager/.

Author

Zeyd Ebrahim and his wife Lilian did their respective residencies at the Cleveland Clinic, and upon completing their training, joined the professional staff. Residents of Cleveland since 1977, they consider themselves fortunate to have had professionally satisfying careers at the Cleveland Clinic.

46 Lessons Learned from Leading a Large Academic Practice

Charles Whitten

Introduction

In holding multiple leadership positions during my 33-year career as a member of a large, multihospital, academic practice, I have learned many things. Some of my best lessons learned include:

- Be sensitive to the different work motivations of the respective generations. Also, be aware that the different generations expect different things from their leaders. We are at an interesting point in our history as we have five generations within our population and/or workforce—the Greatest Generation, Baby Boomers, Generation X, Millennials, and Homelanders.
- Be sensitive to the demands and stressors individuals have outside the workplace.
- Foster teams. The junior members of the specialty enjoy functioning on teams that can achieve mutually agreed-upon goals.
- Develop and mentor leaders. Leadership development is not a linear process.
- Allow individuals to identify their passion at work. Dr. Jenkins had a famous saying: "Let faculty find their bliss and get out of their way!" This philosophy will allow individuals to reach their full potential.
- Foster shared governance. Individuals are more likely to meet expectations and follow rules that they have had a role in creating. Secondary leaders can help "sell" change to the "slow adapters."
- Find a true north. You need an individual to help make sure you don't stray from what you need to be mindful of as you make difficult decisions. This person needs to know you and understand your motivations at the deepest level.

C. Whitten (✉)
Department of Anesthesiology and Pain Management, University of Texas Southwestern Medical Center, Dallas, TX, USA
e-mail: charles.whitten@utsouthwestern.edu

S. Mohamed et al. (eds.), *Anesthesia Bridges*, https://doi.org/10.1007/978-3-032-08294-7_46

- Have an overarching guiding principle to drive your leadership decisions. I had a sincere desire to maintain a sense of "family" within the workplace. I was attracted to the specialty as a medical student because I felt individuals were concerned about me as a "real person."

- As you assume larger leadership positions, it's important to utilize an executive coach to help you navigate complexities related to matrix-driven organizations.

Leadership is doing what needs to be done, on the day it needs to be done.—Chuck Whitten

Lessons Learned

- The editors have a few favorites among Dr. Whitten's lessons. First, we think the advice to let people find their passion and then get out of that way is great wisdom that executives don't always follow. It's easy when trying to make the system work and the wheels turn to expect and ask that everybody essentially do the same thing—but this is not always the wisest. Second, shared governance is hard to do, but great when it happens.

- The advice on hiring an executive coach is really fascinating, and Dr. Fleisher also discusses the benefits of this in his chapter (Chap. 71). It might seem like a big and unnecessary expense, but you must ask yourself if you are in a leadership position if you can afford *not* to do it, in the bigger scheme of things.

Author

Charles Whitten is a native of Missouri but considers himself a Texan. Following receipt of his BSEE at SMU, he has spent the last 41 years at UT Southwestern in a multiplicity of capacities. His wife Cheri is the strongest positive in his life. His current professional passions include physician leadership development and collaborative projects related to the economics of academic anesthesiology practice. If you play golf, you are his friend!

47 If You Don't Have Budget Authority, You Are Just a Cheerleader

Amr E. Abouleish

Introduction

When I decided to proceed with an executive MBA degree (from 1996 to 1998), I sought out and took positions with my university's health system to learn about the business of health care. These positions included utilization management and provider relations for our own insurance product, utilization management, and care management in our hospitals, and then, in late 2000, I took on the position of medical director and/or chief medical officer in one of our hospitals. In this role as medical director, I was in charge of utilization management, care management, and medical policy.

What Have I Signed Up For?

I communicated with our physicians daily. In addition, it became clear that we would be better financially if we created a lower level of care within the hospital (equivalent to a skilled nursing facility—"SNF") to manage patients who could be discharged but an outside SNF would not accept.

I presented a business plan with projected savings and reduced costs to the vice president, who was the CEO of the hospital, and the chief nursing officer (CNO). Without any feedback to me, the proposal was not approved. Furthermore, I found that I was not included in meetings that involved medical policy. It was then that I realized I had no authority over the hospital budget and, in reality, no one actually reported to me. All the nonphysician colleagues I worked with reported another person, usually the CNO.

That is when it dawned on me that "if you don't have budget authority, you are just a cheerleader." That is, my role was simply to communicate medical issues to the physicians rather than have a nonphysician do this messaging. Now, I do strongly believe that to have effective communication with physicians, it is a good strategy to have physician communication champions. On the other hand, I wish that I had known that I needed to negotiate for involvement in policy making and budget decisions prior to taking on the position.

A. E. Abouleish (✉)
Department of Anesthesiology, The University of Texas Medical Branch, Galveston, TX, USA
e-mail: aaboulei@UTMB.EDU

S. Mohamed et al. (eds.), *Anesthesia Bridges*, https://doi.org/10.1007/978-3-032-08294-7_47

So, this is the most common advice I give to colleagues when they take on a hospital administrative job: Make sure you know what authority and decision-making capability you actually have! Otherwise, you are accepting a job as a cheerleader.

Lessons Learned

- When taking on a leadership role, be sure to understand what responsibilities and decision-making capability you are signing up for.

Author

Amr Abouleish joined UTMB Galveston in 1993 as the first chief of pediatric anesthesiology. His motto for teaching pediatric anesthesia to residents is "every month is July!" He is also a national speaker on economics in healthcare, especially for anesthesiology departments.

The First Chairwoman at Cairo University

48

Inas Kamel and Hanan Mohamed Mostafa

Introduction

For this chapter, Inas Kamel was interviewed by Hanan Mohamed Mostafa.

The Interview

From Dr. Kamel: I have been working in the field of anesthesia for 40 years, more than 20 years of which were in leadership positions at Kasr Al Aini University Hospitals. My roles varied from heading an operating theater team, then being in charge of all the specialty theaters, and finally being responsible for all the operating theaters in our university hospitals. I also helped establish the surgical theaters at Kasr Al Aini Specialized Hospital (The French hospital).

When I was first appointed professor, I became director of the anesthesia training program, and in addition, overlooked the daily scheduling of assignments to our anesthesiologists—I did this until becoming the chair of the anesthesiology department. I was the first woman in the Middle East and Africa to chair such a critical university post. Later, I also helped to establish and chair the Egyptian Fellowship in Anesthesiology, which is a four-year-long graduate medical education program aimed at upgrading the experience and knowledge of the anesthesiologist workforce in Egypt.

Chairperson

As a chairperson of the Department of Anesthesiology at Cairo University, I was always mindful of the challenge and the responsibility I was carrying. I was committed to showing endurance, perseverance, and vision. One of the ways that I demonstrated that commitment was my presence—I was the first to arrive at the operating theater and would not leave until the last patient on the schedule was recovering.

I. Kamel
Department of Anaesthesia and Intensive Care, Cairo University, Cairo, Egypt

H. M. Mostafa (✉)
Anesthesia, Surgical Intensive Care, Pain Medicine, Cairo University, Cairo, Egypt
e-mail: Hanan.mostafa@kasralainy.edu.eg

S. Mohamed et al. (eds.), *Anesthesia Bridges*, https://doi.org/10.1007/978-3-032-08294-7_48

Another sign of that commitment was showing respect to everyone and communicating with everyone in a way they would understand. I learned this during my time as the leader of the whole theater. When working with my team, I always expected the best performance from everyone without accepting a half-done job or unreasonable excuses. On the other hand, I have always shown kindness when there existed a situation that was out of my team's hands. I always tried to be logical and asked for doable and not impossible targets. I always gave a second chance (and even a third) when I believed it was necessary.

Disciplinary Duties

When discipline was due, I was always objective, fair, and still showed respect. I would close a door and ask all my questions, and say all my comments behind the closed door, but after that, I would let the person step outside with dignity in front of colleagues. I was always patient and fair when disagreements occurred among my anesthetic staff. If a member of my anesthetic staff was involved in a dispute, I would always support them, be there for them, comfort the young anxious ones, preserve their respect, and solve the issue immediately. I believe that the dignity of a doctor is the most valuable asset—this helps build a responsible character and ensure good practice ethics.

One of the main obstacles I faced was learning how to create a balance between my work and my family. Truly, I delayed having those commitments till after my residency, but still, I had to make a constant effort not to jeopardize either one of them. Having good time management skills is very important to be able to do all duties, whether at work or at home. Prioritizing tasks, keeping lists of duties, and maintaining records of useful contacts can help one avoid missing an important family event. I believe this should be easier nowadays with all our current methods of communication!

Lessons Learned

- Spend more time thinking about career options and never rush into decisions, whatever specialty you choose.
- Strive for excellence, and be meticulous, dedicated, and respectful.
- Be respectful to everyone without differentiation, and more importantly, respect yourselves.
- Remember to be grateful and be appreciative of your seniors, even those who taught you the least.
- Always try to keep your dignity and ambition. I understand there are a lot of societal pressures and challenges, now more than ever, but never compromise on dignity and ambition.

Authors

Inas Kamel is a retired professor of anesthesiology and former chairperson of the Anesthesia Department at Cairo University. She received her medical degree from Cairo University and completed her training at Kasr Al Aini, Cairo University Hospital. She served in a number of leadership roles at Cairo University as well as the Egyptian Fellowship of Anesthesia—with a focus on anesthesia education and training. She is a mother of two girls—one is a professor of chemical pathology, and the other is a professor of ophthalmology.

Hanan Mohamed Mostafa is an anesthesiologist and intensivist at Cairo University. She also has additional qualifications in healthcare management and spent time at Cincinnati Children's and Shriners to build her skills in PICU and burn critical care. She and her husband (an interventional radiologist) are the busy parents of two adolescent boys. In her spare time, she learned to play the flute and is a proud bookworm in all topics.

49 Leaders Speak and Speakers Lead

Berend Mets

Introduction

I provide this as good advice for all who wish to live dangerously as leaders.

- To stand up and be counted, to speak your mind clearly and concisely, without "fear or favor," is hard-earned and not easily come by.
- Practice what you are going to say fervently, in your mind, or out loud and on your own. Never stand up and speak out, before rehearsing in some fashion what you are about to say—write it down on a napkin if you must. To do so is foolhardy and fraught with failure.
- Be brief. Be concise. Make at most three points. And make them again. For as **Oscar Wilde** has said:

  "I would have made it shorter, but I did not have enough time."
- And **Sir Winston Churchill**:

  "If you have an important point to make, don't try to be subtle or clever. Use a pile driver. Hit the point once. Then come back and hit it again. Then hit it a third time—a tremendous whack."
- It requires energy and gumption to speak up, and that is the work of leadership. A false position not challenged is a point made; while an occasion not taken to speak when that is called for, is an opportunity to lead, lost.
- Professor **Warren Bennis** has defined leadership as "the art of communication and the management of meaning."
- Work at it, because: **Leaders speak, and speakers lead.**

B. Mets (✉)
Department of Anesthesiology and Perioperative Medicine, Penn State College of Medicine, Penn State Milton S. Hershey Medical Center, Hershey, PA, USA
e-mail: bmets@pennstatehealth.psu.edu

S. Mohamed et al. (eds.), *Anesthesia Bridges*, https://doi.org/10.1007/978-3-032-08294-7_49

Lessons Learned

- Dr. Mets' advice is concise and meaningful. We recommend you go back and read it again. And a third time. He includes a point that is especially important to our profession—"A false position not challenged is a point made." This piece is a fitting conclusion to this section.

Author

Berend Mets was born in Indonesia to Dutch parents and lived on three continents before settling in South Africa, where he studied medicine and anesthesia. He served as the anesthesia residency director at Columbia University in the 1990s before becoming chairman of Anesthesiology & Perioperative Medicine at Penn State University.

More Wisdom on Leadership

50

David A. Zvara, James K. Gilman, Ronald S. Bank,
Joseph M. Schwartz, and Catherine Marcucci

Contributors:

Edwin G. Avery IV, MD (EGA)

Charles W. Emala, MD (CWE)

Lee A. Fleisher, MD (LAF)

Evan J. Kharasch, MD (EJK)

Mark J. Lema, MD PhD (MJL)

Amy J. Robbins, MD (AJR)

Neil B. Sandson, MD (NBS)

Toby N. Weingarten, MD (TNW)

Introduction

The best leaders never stop learning and thinking about how they can be better and do better for their teams. We are fortunate to have so many experienced and top-notch leaders collaborating on this project. We are grateful to these experts for taking the time to pass on some final wisdom on leadership as follows:

D. A. Zvara
(Emeritus) Department of Anesthesiology, The University of North Carolina at Chapel Hill School of Medicine, Chapel Hill, NC, USA

J. K. Gilman
Office of the Director, Clinical Center, National Institutes of Health (Retired), Adjunct Professor of Medicine, Uniformed Services University of the Health Sciences, Bethesda, MD, USA

R. S. Bank
Department of Anesthesiology, INOVA Fairfax Hospital, UVA School of Medicine, INOVA Campus, Falls Church, VA, USA

J. M. Schwartz
VA Maryland Health Care System,Baltimore, MD, USA

C. Marcucci (✉)
Department of Transfusion Medicine, Clinical Center, National Institutes of Health, Bethesda, MD, USA

S. Mohamed et al. (eds.), *Anesthesia Bridges*, https://doi.org/10.1007/978-3-032-08294-7_50

- The personality of the department takes on the personality of its leader. An open, caring, and supportive chair breeds the same type of department. A selfish, demeaning, and distrusting chair also breeds the same type of department.—**MJL**

- As a corollary to Mark Lema's advice above. There are no perfect leaders, just as there are no perfect subordinates. You don't have to be without faults to be a strong leader; you get to have strengths and weaknesses just like everybody else. But don't make the mistake of thinking that your weaknesses won't become known to your team, just as you will come to know their weaknesses. And just as you evaluate and act with those weaknesses in mind, so too will your team.—**Editors**

- Solving problems is never as good as preventing them.—**JKG**

- So much of medical training requires superior individual effort, but all the best outcomes in the practice of medicine accrue from efforts of large groups. Teamwork should be taught in all medical schools.—**JKG**

- Most people in senior positions get fired by the people who work for them, not by the people they work for.—**JKG**

- Leadership is not just about being the boss. It's as much or more about service. In academic medicine, one job of leaders is getting their people promoted.—**Editors**

- Earning and holding respect is an absolute essential to being a good leader. Being liked is a close second and will allow you to perhaps accomplish a bit more, but do not plan or try to substitute popularity for respect.—**Editors**

- Leadership can be both taught and learned—there are a variety of ways to accomplish this, but we think the best way is by example.—**Editors**

- When we were getting this topic together, I thought it was important to delve into the natural personality characteristics that make a good leader. What I read is that leadership skills can certainly be taught, but that innate leadership is a lot like height. You can line up a bunch of small children, and they will all get taller with proper nutrition and medical care. But the tallest small children have the greatest chance of being the tallest adults. So, it is with leadership. You can line up people and train them all, and they will all increase in leadership skills. But certain people probably started with extra personality gifts and so will advance to greater leadership heights. What are those natural-born personality traits that predispose for leadership? We think the two most important are *curiosity and empathy***.** These are both hard to teach. You can instruct people how to be inquisitive with checklists and structured questions. But inborn curiosity—a true zest and delight in exploring and learning—is much harder to teach. The same is true with empathy because it requires a certain emotional and situational sensitivity that is hard to superimpose on somebody who is a different personality type.—**AJR**

- A good leader does not tell their team what to do when there is a challenge, conflict, or bobble. A good leader helps those teammates figure out how to solve the situation. When somebody brings you a problem, as the leader, it is always appropriate to say, "What are your ideas?"—**AJR**

- Leadership is about finding out what motivates people, both positive and negative motivators. The best way to find out is just to ask. "What motivates you? Is it more money, more flexibility, promotion, or more responsibility? Are you more motivated to move toward positive aspects of the job, or is your primary motivation to distance yourself from difficult and unpleasant aspects?"— **Editors**

- Don't just complain about things—get involved, take charge, take a leadership role!! Taking a leadership role in solving an issue gives you an opportunity to meet and interact with members of other departments, support staff, administrators, etc. These connections can lead to larger leadership roles and opportunities to effect change, which benefits more than just the patients under your direct clinical care.—**RSB**

- It is said in politics that if you're not at the table, you're on the menu. Nothing could be truer. Get involved in legislative advocacy early in your career—ideally as a resident. Attend the ASA Legislative Conference. Legislative advocacy from the local to the national level allows you to safeguard patient care and the specialty that you worked so hard to be a part of on a far larger scale than direct patient care. You may find that you want to run for office yourself!—**RSB**

- Thinking about a move to the executive levels? Remember the old saying—"administration never sleeps."—**Editors**

- You can be in a leadership role and not be a leader, and the reverse is true as well.—**Editors**

- A leadership role is defined by the position, not the person in it. A true leader will shine whether or not they are in a specified executive position, even if it is only leading morale and a sense of *esprit de corps.*—**Editors**

- Leaders do not have to be all things to all people, either on or outside their teams. Leadership is about focused progress toward goals, not schmoozy salesmanship and empty promises.—**Editors**

- An antecedent principle of leadership is to identify 2–3 overarching goals. Approach every ensuing "issue" through the filter of achieving these goals and goodwill, and the establishment of credibility will flow as a natural consequence.—**Editors**

- As we thought about the best advice we could provide on leadership, we read an interesting article on the nine types of leadership styles [1].

  1. Autocratic leadership: Leader retains strict control, good for urgent decision-making.

  2. Bureaucratic leadership: Enforcement of regulations and status of hierarchy.

  3. Charismatic leadership: Infectious presence that motivates the team to emulate.

  4. Democratic leadership: Welcomes participation, not advantageous when quick action is needed.

  5. Laissez-Faire leadership: Hands off approach, good with highly motivated staff.

  6. Servant leadership: Power and decision-making is shared.

7. Situational leadership: Leadership strategies and tactics are based on individual events and needs.

8. Transactional leadership: Based on rewards/consequences.

9. Transformational leadership: Seeks to create an engaged workplace.

There is a lot of debate in the business and psychology literature about which leadership styles are the most desirable and favorable. The answer, of course, is No. 7—situational leadership. The other good leadership styles for physician teams are democratic, laissez-faire, and transformational. Which style of leader are you? Can you change styles if necessary? The leadership style that is required for nonphysician healthcare teams is important, but a subject for a different day. These issues are something we all probably already have some ideas about.—**Editors**

***Note from the Editors:** There was no greater leader than Winston Churchill who was by all accounts a complicated and fascinating man. He started painting in the years after WWI as an emotional and psychological escape from the aftermath of those turbulent times and loved to paint bridges (Fig. 50.1).

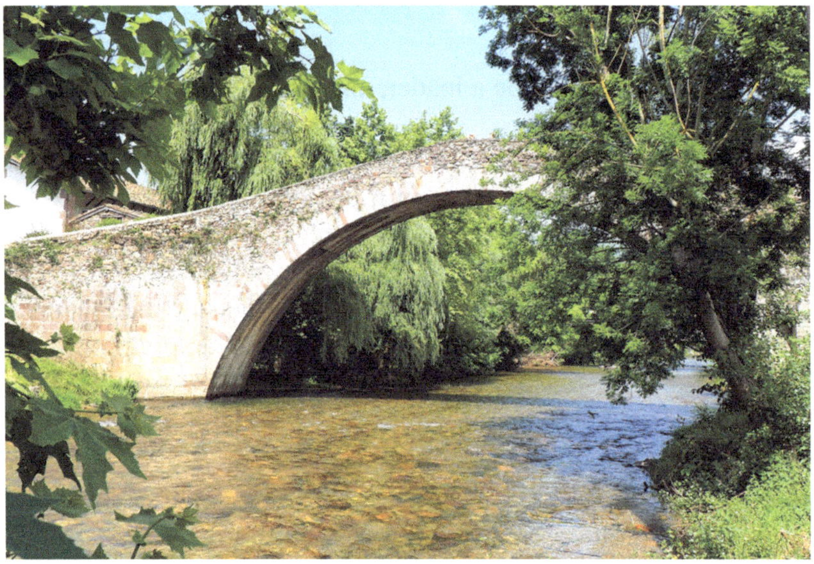

Fig. 50.1 This bridge over the River Arc was painted by Winston Churchill in 1948. The bridge was also featured in two watercolors by postimpressionist French artist Paul Cézanne, who was an inspiration to Churchill. Photo: Image used under standard license from iStock.com

- I worked in a hospital system where affecting meaningful change was referred to as trying to make an aircraft carrier do a sharp 90-degree turn. My supervisor told each person on the team that they could pick one issue to try to make progress on and have the assurance of his steady support. He was very upfront and honest about this with each new physician. But this also meant that the group in aggregate was actively working within the system to improve care and safety on a half-dozen issues at all times, which ended up being pretty effective over time.—**CM**

- The best leaders know how to deal effectively with interpersonal conflict. You will not be a really good leader if you try to cope with conflict on your team by avoiding. We feel it is best to have a light touch but to know when to weigh in when necessary. It takes a while to learn how to do this.—**Editors**

- The best job in the world is the one in which you get to help develop the future.—**EJK**

- Skim the contents of *Anesthesiology* and *Anesthesia & Analgesia* the day it hits your email inbox. If you are short on time, go back and at least read the abstracts of the main articles later. But you can't be (or consider yourself to be) a leader in the field of anesthesiology if you don't know what's in the leading journals.—**Editors**

- Ask your family to get you one good biography of a historically great leader every year for your birthday or the holidays. There are many "leadership manuals" out there—especially for the business school people, but it's much more fun to read about leadership in its historical context. You can start with the standards—the Roman emperors, Napoleon Bonaparte, George Washington, Harriet Tubman, Queen Victoria, and Dick Winters.—**Editors**

- And there are entire interesting lists of other great women leaders in history, as well! [2] One of the most fascinating (and complicated) leaders in US history was Mary G. Harris Jones, known commonly as Mother Jones. She was a schoolteacher and dressmaker who lost her family and livelihood in a series of tragedies. She became an enormously successful and influential, although controversial, union organizer, labor leader, and activist, who could negotiate with John D. Rockefeller without batting an eye. At one point, she was known as "the most dangerous woman in America." She was revered by her constituents, and 50,000 people attended the dedication of her gravesite memorial in 1936. Another fascinating area of history is the timeline of female religious leaders in the US. Our point is that there are countless interesting leaders to learn about and from, in addition to the ones in the high school history books.—**Editors**

- Practice thinking, speaking, and reading about leaders who were not and are not men. Work actively to expand the images that jump into your mind when you hear the word "leader."—**Editors**

- Good leaders are almost always long on humor and short on anger.—**Editors**

- The questions you ask as a leader are much more important than the answers you provide. And the answers your team provides are also better than the answers that you provide.—**Editors**

- "There is no us, but us." I say this all the time when looking to solve a problem. No one is magically going to appear to solve our problems.—**DAZ**

- "Sin Boldly." Attributed to Martin Luther and a beacon of my leadership orientation. In other words, if you are going to do something, do it completely and without hesitation.—**DAZ**

- Trust is everything. The trait I value most is trust in a leader. I assume they have the skills, and if they lack the skills, they will learn them. But trust must be unshaken, completely solid. When I tell you something, you may not like it, but you can trust that it is the truth to the best of my understanding at the time. You expect this of me, and I depend on it from you.—**DAZ**

- Be wary of accepting "leadership roles" that involve coming into a system to be a change agent. Make sure you understand the terms and consequences of undertaking such a position. It hasn't worked out very well for a whole lot of people we know—**Editors**

- If you do find yourself considering a change agent position, make sure you will be bringing something new and valuable to your new team, above and beyond "you're not going to be able to do things the same way."—**Editors**

- Try not to be interim anything. Interim positions have all the disadvantages of the position and none of the advantages. If you are interested in the permanent position, an interim is not always a great way to get a feel for what the position is like. Rather, "assistant program director" or "vice chair" is a better way to evaluate what the position entails. Also, if you are interested in the position, being in the interim position is just an extended job interview. Who wants to be in an interview that's six months long?—**Editors**

- Not everybody is dealt the same leadership hand. Don't waste time wishing for different cards.—**Editors**

- Think carefully about taking a job if you have ascertained or been told that the boss's leadership style is based on the same attributes that you disliked the most about your parents. Or interpersonal skills that are similar to what's currently frustrating you the most about your partner. Nobody wants to feel like they are working for their father when they have specifically chosen **not** to work with their father.—**Editors**

- There is a strong tendency to imbue leaders with transference-based projections, especially leaders who are new to you. So, it is important to be aware of this and remember that even the best of the best of the leaders are real human beings with flaws and limitations. And give your assessment of the new leader time to settle in. You may find it going both up and down.—**NBS**

- Your accomplishments are amplified if you mentor others.—**CWE**

- Understand that when you step into a leadership role that there will be at least one person who is unhappy with you at all times.—**NBS**

- If any responsibility of your leadership role involves promotions for the people on your team, recognize that and apply consistent efforts to make them happy. It's an important metric that you yourself will be judged on.—**Editors**

- Accessibility is an easy thing you can do to establish leadership. We've never heard a leader criticized for being too accessible to his team.—**Editors**

- The late James Schauble, MD was a senior anesthesiologist at Hopkins, and he was also the senior quality assurance officer for the hospital, if memory serves correctly. One thing he taught the junior people was to never bluff. He also didn't take on issues he couldn't win. Or rather, as a safety officer and leader, he made sure he had the conflict won before he engaged the other side.—**Editors**

- Make all the introductions you can. I still remember Lee Fleisher's thoughtfulness when he asked if I would walk the lobby with him at a national meeting. I was a complete nobody—a clinical fellow who was churning out the cases and not much else that year. By the time the meeting was over, I had met Dr. Barash and Dr. Stoelting. I remind Lee of this at least once every five years. He then reminds me that it was his job to further the careers of the people junior to him, and part of that was making introductions whenever he could.—**CM**

- One other admirable thing about Lee Fleisher is that, even as a young faculty member at Hopkins, he was constantly on the lookout to include the really junior people on whatever publishing opportunities came his way. He wasn't my supervisor after I finished training and joined the faculty; we were both youngish faculty in the same division of the department, although he was one rank ahead of me on the promotion curve. I doubt he remembers it, but he passed on a first-author spot for a piece on perioperative hypertension for one of the anesthesia review yearbooks. I still have it (Fig. 50.2).—**CM**

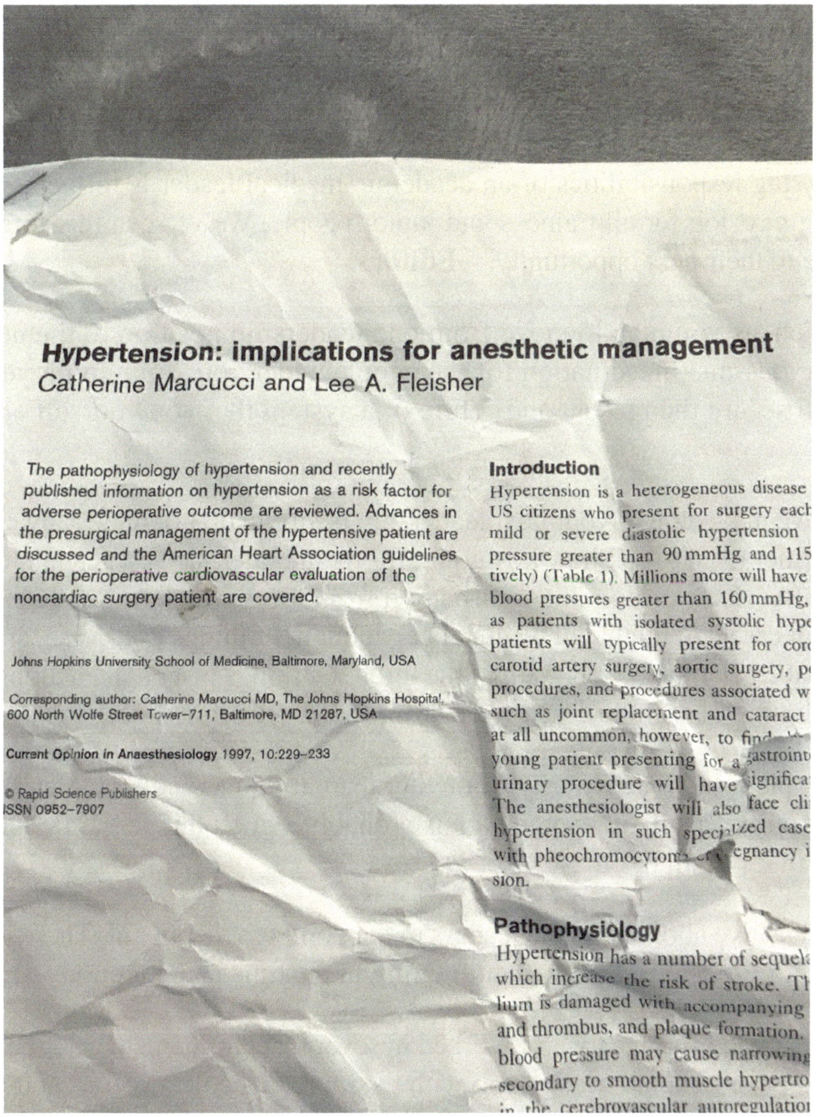

Hypertension: implications for anesthetic management
Catherine Marcucci and Lee A. Fleisher

The pathophysiology of hypertension and recently published information on hypertension as a risk factor for adverse perioperative outcome are reviewed. Advances in the presurgical management of the hypertensive patient are discussed and the American Heart Association guidelines for the perioperative cardiovascular evaluation of the noncardiac surgery patient are covered.

Johns Hopkins University School of Medicine, Baltimore, Maryland, USA

Corresponding author: Catherine Marcucci MD, The Johns Hopkins Hospital, 600 North Wolfe Street Tower-711, Baltimore, MD 21287, USA

Current Opinion in Anaesthesiology 1997, 10:229–233

© Rapid Science Publishers
ISSN 0952–7907

Introduction
Hypertension is a heterogeneous disease
US citizens who present for surgery each
mild or severe diastolic hypertension
pressure greater than 90 mmHg and 115
tively) (Table 1). Millions more will have
blood pressures greater than 160 mmHg,
as patients with isolated systolic hyp
patients will typically present for cor
carotid artery surgery, aortic surgery, p
procedures, and procedures associated w
such as joint replacement and cataract
at all uncommon, however, to fin
young patient presenting for a gastroint
urinary procedure will have significa
The anesthesiologist will also face cli
hypertension in such specialized case
with pheochromocytoma egnancy i
sion.

Pathophysiology
Hypertension has a number of sequel
which increase the risk of stroke. Th
lium is damaged with accompanying
and thrombus, and plaque formation.
blood pressure may cause narrowing
secondary to smooth muscle hypertro
in the cerebrovascular autoregulation

Fig. 50.2 The article on hypertension that Cathy Marcucci wrote with Lee Fleisher for *Current Opinion in Anesthesiology* in 1997. A little the worse for wear, but it is almost 30 years old and has been in numerous filing cabinets and moving boxes. Photo: Catherine Marcucci

- In order to improve collaboration between the anesthesiology and surgery residents, we instituted several strategies. We had joint grand rounds in which a surgical and an anesthesiology attending oversaw several case presentations in which both resident groups jointly presented. We also ensured that during our newly instituted base year, the anesthesiology residents rotated on surgery. Finally, we integrated the surgery and anesthesiology residents on the SICU teams and made sure they alternated between a surgical and anesthesia attending.—**LAF**

- Seek out leadership training throughout your career. It is generally not taught in med school or residency, so learning by watching as much as you can early in your career, but also recognizing the utility of formal instruction.—**RSB**

- Beyond that, behaving well and treating all colleagues, peers, and patients respectfully and well is the right thing to do; it also goes a long way toward building loyalty, trust, and effective teams. Further, having good people skills is critical to today's aspiring physician leaders achieving their leadership goals.—**RSB**

- One of the really big responsibilities of an academic medical leader is to facilitate and sponsor the acquisition of the next job for all trainees and junior people. We've seen this forgotten as the leader prepares to move to their next opportunity.—**Editors**

- Speaking of which, as you plan to move from one leadership position to the next, remember that this is a very nervous-making situation for the people under you. Your employees are being asked to work hard and secure the present and future of a system that you yourself are looking to move past.—**Editors**

- And once you have moved on to your next leadership position, do not under any circumstances, "call back" to your former team to ask how it is going for them under the new leadership. If they call you, that's one thing. But don't try to mine information from former underlings. Things either got better for them, in which case you might not want to hear about it, or things got worse, and they're not going to want to talk to the person who left them in the lurch. Or things just creaked along pretty in the same way, in which case it will seem like you were never there.—**Editors**

- Don't expect complete and total honesty from your team if you are not completely and totally honest with them. And you're most likely not, which is probably a good thing. A little bit of radical honesty goes a long way in a system or on a team.—**Editors**

- Teams are very sensitive about absentee leaders to the point of resentment. There just doesn't seem to be any other way to "do leadership" without putting in the time and attention.—**Editors**

- I have had the great good fortune to have worked in several departments where the leaders did not shy away from clinical work, including working with the more difficult surgeons and doing the more difficult cases. And I once worked for somebody who took in-house overnight call every single Friday night and most of the holidays that nobody wanted to work. This had the result of engendering a lot of loyalty from his "troops."—**CM**

- Remember that leadership can happen outside the employment realm. There are lots of leadership opportunities available in our anesthesia community, and the national leadership group gets credit for that across the decades. We've never heard of anybody wanting to get into a leadership role and not being able to do that. But you have to step up and speak up and make your availability known.—**Editors**

- One of the most important types of leadership is mentoring.—**Editors**

- Mentoring is a really interesting endeavor, especially person-to-person mentoring. There are all different styles and ways to do it, and many ways to be mentored. Mentoring should not be about hearing complaints and grievances. Or trying to coax and motivate people into doing things they are really not interested in doing. It should be about providing an example, opening doors, and problem-solving. It can also evolve into a partnership between peers over time.—**Editors**

- We think that mentoring works best if there are some temperament and personality similarities between the mentor and mentee. And the mentoring relationship should be enjoyable and enriching for the mentor as well.—**Editors**

- I agree with the editors! When I started as a resident, I would spend hours after call nights going over charts and climbing around the Mayo library attic, printing off papers on carcinoid from the 1950s to 1960s. I met this Croatian guy ϑ with a similar work ethic, and we still work on papers all the time. Today, I find that mentoring is easiest for me and most productive for my mentees if they have a motivational level and work style that matches mine somewhat.—**TNW**

- *Note* that "Croatian guy" is **Juraj Sprung, MD, PhD,** a truly great colleague. A more brilliant, astonishingly productive, kinder, and generous anesthesiologist cannot be found on several continents. Several of the editors of this book are honored to have collaborated with him on numerous previous projects.—**Editors**

- The best leader I ever worked for was great because of the range of his leadership efforts and activities. This person could be down in Washington DC, working on a national panel, but also once walked through the snow in a blizzard to visit me when I was in the hospital with pneumonia. A different way to say it is that this leader moved effortlessly from the policy to the personal level.—**NBS**

- This has been said for a long time in a bunch of different ways, but you, as a leader, are only as strong as your weakest team member.—**Editors**

- But do yourself a favor and never tell that weakest team member that they are your biggest problem. For one thing, it's demoralizing, and they will resent it and you, and won't forget it for the rest of their career. But the more important reason is that you don't want to tip your hand that you view your supervisees or team members in rank order. The correct approach is to create a grid of your employees' strengths and weaknesses, not a pecking order of good people and problem people.—**Editors**

- Similarly, we don't advise that you tell anybody they are the "best" employee. It's hard for the person hearing that to be unaffected by such information. Overconfidence or a sense of superiority sometimes creeps in a bit. A better way to frame it is to let the person know that their contributions are noticed and valued.—**Editors**

- The very best leaders know when and why to say no. But much more importantly, they know **how** to say no. "No" should never be a dead-end for your team. It should be an indication that there is a fascinating alternate detour or solution to be explored.—**Editors**

- Leaders really prefer not to lead the loud and dramatic people. Especially the drama part. You don't have to be a sheep, but make it easy for your team leader to advocate for you by maintaining a modicum of decorum in your personal presentation. If you want to really make a loud and bold splash, publish some landmark research.—**Editors**

- Don't set up "tests" of your team. You'll have to figure out how honest and/or loyal they are some other way.—**Editors**

- Let your leader say what needs to be said. It's really not your job to do that.—**Editors**

- Think carefully about whether your leadership style is to push or pull. Can you switch back and forth as the situation dictates?—**Editors**

- We've noticed how easy it is for leaders to forget the golden rule of punctuality once they are in a leadership position. Yes, you have additional responsibilities and are now answering to emergencies as well as the people above and below you, but if you have a meeting or a telephone conference scheduled and are running late—that's what text messages are for. Be respectful of your team's time and schedule as you want them to be of yours.—**Editors**

***Note from the Editors:** Another favorite bridge of Winston Churchill's—the Palladian Bridge at Wilton House. He painted the bridge several times (Fig. 50.3).

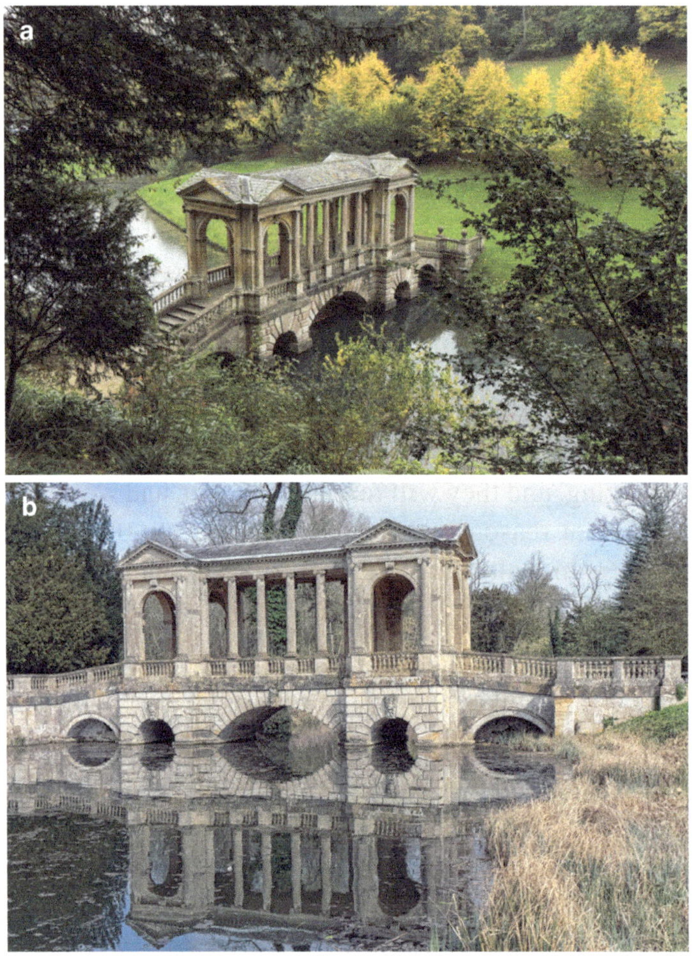

Fig. 50.3 **a**, **b** The Palladian Bridge at Wilton House in Wiltshire, UK. It has been said that he was more interested in capturing the reflection of the bridge in the lake than a mechanical rendering of the structure. Photos: Images used under standard license from iStock.com

- It is sometimes said to be a huge mistake to be on a personal friendly basis with people on the teams you lead. In fact, the military forbids it. But we are of two minds about this. We've seen it and we've done it and it's worked out just fine. We've been friends with people who then became our supervisors, and had supervisors who then became our personal friends. So, it can be done.— **Editors**

- That said, it can be discouraging and demoralizing to be the person on the team who doesn't have a personal relationship with the supervisor. You will usually feel like you can't get on the right side of the triangle.—**Editors**

- Don't get in the habit of referring to the people you supervise as "the children" or "a bunch of kindergarteners." Sooner or later, somebody is going to overhear you saying that and resent it.—**Editors**

- We think resentment is the hardest emotion to deal with in supervisees. A leader can overcome anger, laziness, and ineptitude. But resentment is very hard to eradicate and very hard to overcome when trying to motivate.—**Editors**

- An employee's job is to become indispensable. A supervisor's job is to make sure no employee becomes indispensable. All parties should keep this in mind at all times.—**JMS**

- To truly supervise a person, you need to be able to step into his/her role if he/she is absent. If you don't know how to do his/her job, you aren't really supervising.—**JMS**

- You can't order (nonmilitary) employees to do a task. You either explain and convince them to do it, or they will do just enough to comply but not enough for it to matter.—**JMS**

- Pleasantness is much more important in a work setting than excellence. Eventually, almost any employee can master the basic skills of the job. A toxic employee will poison the work environment for everyone, no matter how exceptional he/she is.—**JMS**

- Bad hires are worse than unfilled positions.—**JMS**

- Not mine, but one that I follow is below.—**JMS**

  > In looking for people to hire, you look for three qualities: integrity, intelligence, and energy. And if you don't get the first, the other two will set you and the team back. You think about it; it's true. If you hire somebody without [integrity], you really want them to be dumb and lazy.

- If you have the obligation or responsibility to be a change agent or to choose a change agent, think about that very carefully. Outsiders can be reformers and change can be compelled or coerced, BUT it is more readily and genuinely adopted if it is done by winning hearts and minds from within. People don't like to be told "you haven't been doing this right."—**JMS**

- People are always going to be afraid to some extent of the devil they don't know. If you want to motivate and lead people, you must keep this in mind.—**NBS**

- And you must understand that emotion drives action, just as much as the reverse. Marketing people know this, of course.—**Editors**
- The quickest way for a leader to lose effectiveness is to start to scrimp on time for your team members and involvement in their issues and to let personal prejudices, issues, and agendas creep into decisions.—**Editors**
- Good leaders don't make their issues more important than their team's issues.—**Editors**
- A senior OR nurse once confided in us that OR nurses generally look to the anesthesiologist to "run the room," not the surgeons. She mentioned that OR nurses tend to see the surgeons as the VIP guest experts and consultants, but the anesthesiologists as the working executives of the OR, charged with the responsibility of getting the day's cases done and the patients safely through the surgery.—**Editors**
- Remember that even supervising one resident is leading a team, even if the team is just two anesthesiologists. Every basic leadership principle applies.—**Editors**

Some Additional Quotes on Leadership

- To handle yourself, use your head; to handle others, use your heart.—**Eleanor Roosevelt**
- Before you are a leader, success is all about growing yourself.—**Neil Sandson**
- When you become a leader, success is all about growing others.—**Jack Welch**
- A leader is a dealer in hope.—**Napoleon Bonaparte**
- Always do right. It will gratify some people and astonish the rest.—**Mark Twain**
- Great leaders are almost always great simplifiers who can cut through argument, debate, and doubt to offer a solution everybody can understand.—**Gen. Colin Powell**
- If your actions inspire others to dream more, learn more, do more, and become more, you are a leader.—**John Quincy Adams**
- Leadership is a combination of strategy and character. If you must be without one, be without the strategy.—**Gen. H. Norman Schwarzkopf**
- To lead people, walk beside them. As for the best leaders, the people do not notice their existence … When the best leader's work is done, the people say, "We did it ourselves!"—**Lao Tzu**
- Good leaders take a little more than their share of the blame, a little less than their share of the credit.—**Arnold Glasow**

- Leadership is not an expertise; it is a constant education.—**Unknown**
- Leadership is action, not position.—**Unknown**
- Great leaders don't need to act tough. Their confidence and humility serve to underscore their toughness.—**Unknown**
- He who cannot be a good follower cannot be a good leader.—**Aristotle**
- Finally, whichever of the nine leadership styles you use, do not try to substitute leadership for clinical skill and acumen. You have to up your clinical skills and practice if you want to lead a team of clinicians, not start to relax and let things go. In other words, you must become more of a physician as you become more of a physician leader.—**Editors**

Acknowledgment: The editors thank Drs. Gilman, Schwartz, and Sandson for contributing to this chapter.

Disclaimer: Several of the contributors to this chapter are federal employees. The views expressed herein are solely the authors' own and do not represent the positions, official or otherwise, of the United States of America, the Department of the Army, the Department of Veterans Affairs, the Department of Health and Human Services, or the National Institutes of Health.

References

1. Femtech Leaders The top 10 famous female leaders in history [Internet]. Femtech Leaders; [date unknown] [cited 2022 Jul 5]. Available from: https://www.femtechleaders.com/the-top-10-famous-female-leaders-in-history/
2. Schooley S. What kind of leader are you? 9 leadership types and their strengths [Internet]. Business News Daily; 2023 Oct [cited 2023 Jul 5]. Available from: https://www.businessnewsdaily.com/9789-leadership-types.html

Authors

David Zvara is a full professor and past chair of anesthesiology at the University of North Carolina at Chapel Hill. David's personal goal as the leader of his department was to provide inspiration and a worthy example to his group with a sizable dose of common sense and humor. He is now the CMO of UNC Hospitals.

Jim Gilman was the CEO of the Clinical Center of the National Institutes of Health. He retired as a Major General from the Army in 2013. During his military career, Dr. Gilman held leadership posts ranging from chief resident in internal medicine at Brooke Army Medical Center (BAMC) to chief of cardiology and cardiology fellowship director at BAMC to senior executive positions, including Commander of BAMC and Commander of the Walter Reed Health Care System. He is a graduate of the Command and General Staff College and the Army War College. Just prior to joining the National Institutes of Health, Dr. Gilman was executive director of the Johns Hopkins Military and Veterans Institute. His leadership style is based on approachability, straightforward communication, and humor. In addition to his successful military and civilian careers, he is a devoted family man.

Ron Bank is a senior anesthesiologist and assistant professor of anesthesiology in the Inova Health Care System. In addition to his regular in-hospital work, Ron Bank has found interesting and rewarding ways to apply his trauma anesthesia skills outside of work in the field of tactical medicine since the early 2000s. In this capacity, he has worked with and trained law enforcement, federal, and military personnel. Ron has been a sworn reserve deputy sheriff since 2002.

Joe Schwartz is a senior psychiatrist and service line chief in Maryland. He grew up on Long Island before relocating to Baltimore to train at Hopkins. He is the proud father of five children and therefore beyond busy. In addition to his family, he loves science fiction, baking, and tinkering with electronics and gadgets of all kinds.

Cathy Marcucci is a senior anesthesiologist who has worked on thousands of anesthesia care teams and provided leadership for several large book and publishing projects. She would characterize her leadership style as "intuitive leadership" if there is such a thing.

Part IV

Academic Promotion and Career Development

Ambassador Bridge—Detroit, MI

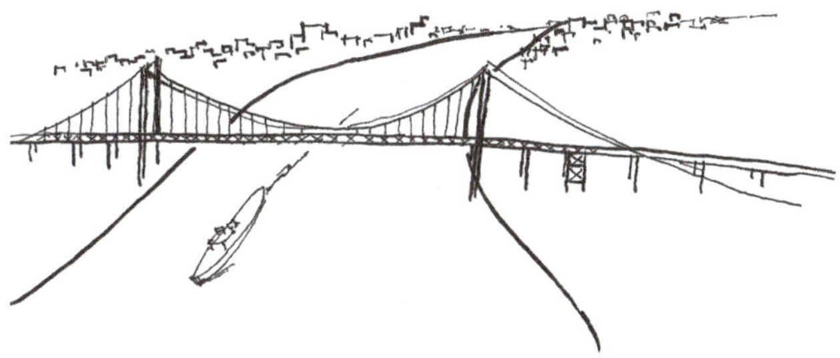

Editor **Jeff Kirsch** selected the Ambassador Bridge as his favorite bridge. It is a tolled international suspension bridge across the Detroit River, connecting Detroit, MI, to Windsor, Ontario. The bridge opened in 1929 and is the busiest bridge in terms of trade value between the US and Canada, carrying 25% of all merchandise trade between the two countries. The bridge also acts as a prime driver of the local economy (on both sides of the river) as up to 150,000 jobs and $13 billion in annual production depend on this border crossing. Only the central span is suspended, and the approaches are supported by steel cantilever truss structures. The bridge underwent an extensive refurbishment from 1995 to 2000, which included changing the color from the original glossy black to teal. Interestingly, this is one of the few privately owned US–Canada crossings. Previous owners placed shares of the bridge on the New York Stock Exchange, and a private owner acquired enough shares to take the bridge private under the auspices of two different transit companies.

Jeff Kirsch and the *Anesthesia Bridges* editors and authors thank design student **Mark Liu** for his lovely drawing capturing the elemental lines and elegant architecture of this beautiful and important bridge.

51 Introduction

Jeffrey R. Kirsch

The common denominator in many of the pieces in this section is that the authors describe how they identified what brought them joy in their professional life that allowed them to sustain their effort to develop a successful career. From these stories it is clear that "success" as an anesthesiologist comes in many different shapes and colors.

Indeed, the term "success" includes many shades of gray. There are certainly many people who hold impressive positions and look to be "successful" from external optics, but do not feel successful. We hope that these stories help the reader find a path of professional joy and sustained feeling of contentment, achievement, and satisfaction. The common denominator for sustained joy relates to having a positive impact on our specialty, medicine as a whole, or an individual patient/colleague.

I would like to give special mention to my late mentor, colleague, and friend Richard J. Traystman, PhD.* Dick guided the careers of over 100 academic anesthesiology physicians and scientists.

***Note from the Editors:** Dick Traytsman was a great scientist and great friend and supporter of the national and internal anesthesiology and critical care medicine communities (Fig. 51.1).

J. R. Kirsch (✉)
Department of Anesthesiology and Pain Medicine, University of Washington School of Medicine, Seattle, WA, USA

(Emeritus) Anesthesiology and Perioperative Medicine, School of Medicine, Oregon Health & Science University, Portland, OR, USA

S. Mohamed et al. (eds.), *Anesthesia Bridges*, https://doi.org/10.1007/978-3-032-08294-7_51

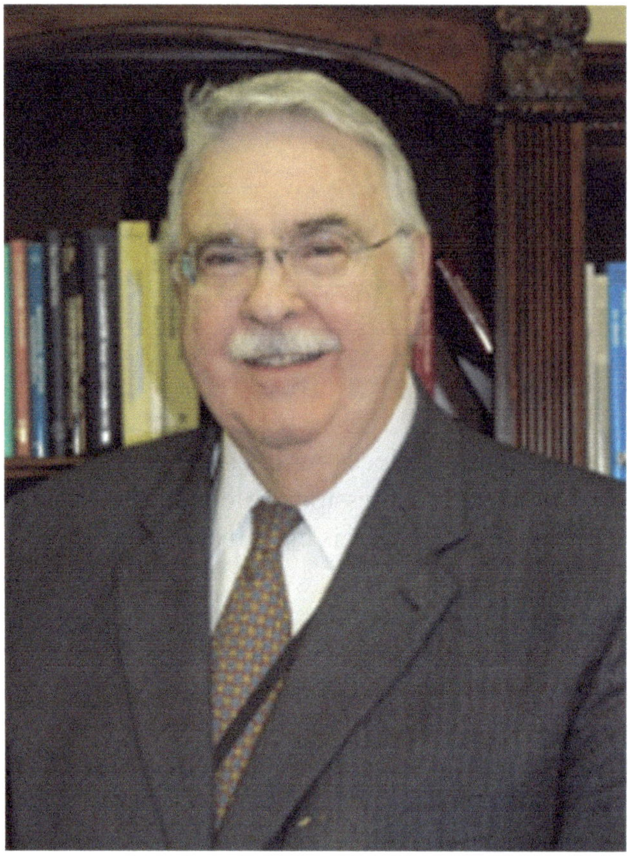

Fig. 51.1 Richard J. Traytsman, PhD. His CV included 475 publications, and he did foundational work in the areas of collateral ventilation, control of cerebral circulation, cardiopulmonary resuscitation, and cerebral ischemia. Photo: Courtesy of Traytsman family

Author

Jeff Kirsch is the chair emeritus of the OHSU Department of Anesthesiology and Perioperative Medicine and formerly associate dean of Faculty Affairs and professor of anesthesiology at the Medical College of Wisconsin. He is currently a professor and the department head of Anesthesiology and Pain at the University of Washington's Harborview Medical Center.

Graceful Self-Promotion: Noticing, Documenting, and Sharing Your Accomplishments

52

Harriet W. Hopf

People don't get promoted for doing their jobs really well. They get promoted by demonstrating their potential to do more.—Tara Jaye Frank

"Wow, I would have loved to do that! Why wasn't I asked?" Early in my career, that happened to me a lot. I thought my work would speak for itself, but being great at what you do is not always enough to get you noticed, especially if you are from a group of underrepresented in medicine. Plus, talking about your accomplishments and asking for resources or opportunities is uncomfortable: what if you are seen as a braggart or greedy? Besides, is the work you are doing even worthy of credit? The culture of medicine often makes individuals feel they are "not enough." How can you *notice* and *acknowledge* the great work you are doing, and then document it so that you have it handy for *sharing* when the opportunity arises? Graceful self-promotion is the art of talking about your strengths and accomplishments with tact, humility, and authentic confidence.

Over the past fifteen years, I have held senior leadership roles in my department and the school of medicine, at the university level, and in national organizations, all focused on faculty development and promotion. Using the expertise I developed in those roles, I now co-lead a year-long curriculum, *Building Your Career Infrastructure*, for the Executive Leadership in Academic Medicine (ELAM) program at Drexel University. In this essay, I will describe a framework for capturing your accomplishments in a way that helps prepare you to share them when you have an opportunity to gracefully promote yourself.

Noticing Your Achievements

In our goal-oriented professional culture, we often neglect to celebrate achievements—unless you consider checking something of your to-do list a celebration. Your achievements are often driven by your strengths, that is, the things you naturally do best. Strengths are often invisible to you because they just feel *normal*. Taking the time to recognize your strengths and how they have contributed to the successful completion of a goal is a good way to notice your achievements.

H. W. Hopf (✉)
Utah Coaching and Advancement Network (U-CAN), Department of Anesthesiology, University of Utah, Salt Lake City, UT, USA
e-mail: Harriet.Hopf@hsc.utah.edu

S. Mohamed et al. (eds.), *Anesthesia Bridges*, https://doi.org/10.1007/978-3-032-08294-7_52

But how do you notice the invisible? A number of tools identify your strengths, including the widely used Clifton Strengths Finder and free online tools. One of these tools can be found at https://high5test.com/strengthsfinder-free/. You can also ask friends, family, and colleagues; your strengths are almost certainly not invisible to them!

My Clifton strengths are ideation, strategy, future, relator, and activator. When I consider the work that brings me joy, such as creating better policies, coaching faculty, and strategic planning for the future of organizations, it makes sense. But my strengths were not obvious to me until I completed the Clifton Strengths Finder, discussed them with colleagues, and recognized how they drove my choices and actions.

Documenting Your Achievements

The STAR technique is an established approach to answering questions in an interview [1].

- S: What was the **Situation**?
- T: What was the **Task** you identified to address the situation?
- A: What specific **Action(s)** did you take to achieve the target or complete the task?
- R: What was the **Result?**

The **STAR** technique works for capturing accomplishments for purposes beyond interviewing, including for reports, applications, proposals, formal presentations, and elevator pitches. Identifying the strengths you used to complete the task and achieve the result facilitates describing how you contributed and allows leaders to envision giving you future opportunities.

Strengths you identify using a tool are only a starting point—the words you use to describe your strengths should be more specific and tied to the accomplishment. Here is how I, with input from a colleague, have reenvisioned my strengths for a **STAR**:

- Expertise (ideation)
- Boundary-spanning connections (strategic, futuristic, and relator)
- Collaboration (relator, activator)
- Coordination (strategic, relator, and activator)
- Continually update (ideation, strategic, and futuristic)

To create a **STAR** think of an accomplishment you want to be ready to share. On a piece of paper or on your computer, capture the *Situation*, *Task*, Action, and *Result*. How did your strengths contribute? Add them to the **STAR**. Do not worry about elegance—just get it written down, to start.

Figure 52.1 is an example of a **STAR I** created to describe my work in the provost's office during the COVID-19 pandemic. Note that my strengths are incorporated into the *Task* and *Action* sections. This is not the first draft—I spent several hours polishing it! Usually, I do the refining on walks with my husband, recording the conversation on my smart phone.

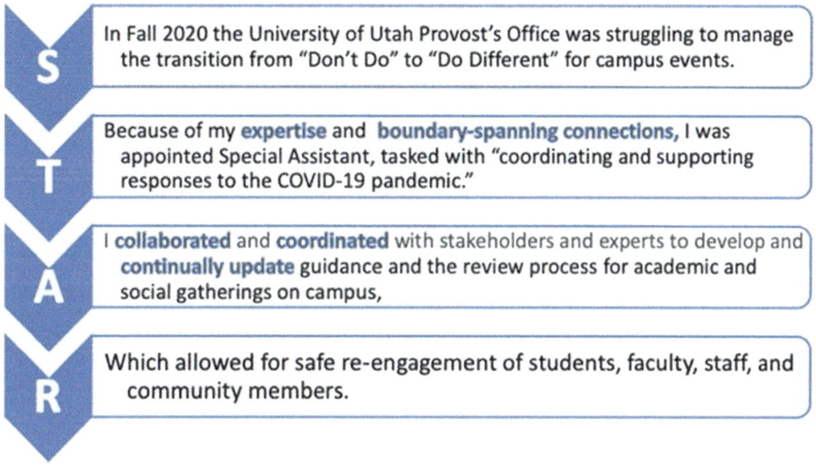

Fig. 52.1 Basic linear **STAR**. Illustration: Harriet Hopf

You can collect your accomplishments as a database of **STARs** (ideally searchable!) that includes the strengths you demonstrated. Then, when you want to highlight an accomplishment in a promotion file, cover letter, interview, or proposal, you have the information right at hand.

Sharing Your Achievements

STARs capture and organize information; they are building blocks for sharing your accomplishments. You can change the order and emphasis of each component to adapt them for different contexts and purposes, depending on where you are sharing and how long you want to take.

The basic **STAR** you have already created is linear and is especially well-suited for interviews—for which it was designed. For example, an interviewer may ask, "Give me an example of a difficult problem you solved. How did you solve this problem?" A linear **STAR** provides context for the situation or difficult problem and then allows you to highlight the strengths and competencies that allowed you to solve the problem.

In an interview, you might want to tell more of a story about your **STAR**. The "And, But Therefore" framework created by Randy Olson is a good way to add tension and interest to your story [2]. Describe the situation using "and" (context) and "but" (the problem), then describe the task, action, and results using "therefore." Figure 52.2 is an example of my **STAR** in this format.

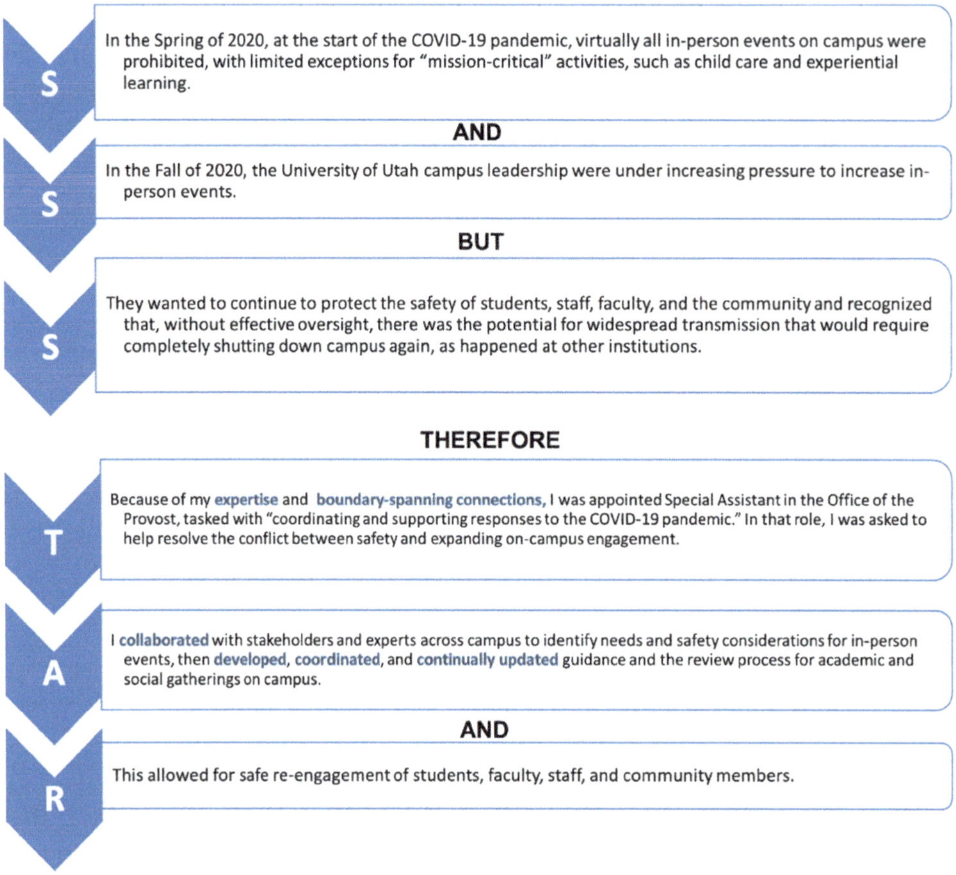
S
In the Spring of 2020, at the start of the COVID-19 pandemic, virtually all in-person events on campus were prohibited, with limited exceptions for "mission-critical" activities, such as child care and experiential learning.
AND
S
In the Fall of 2020, the University of Utah campus leadership were under increasing pressure to increase in-person events.
BUT
S
They wanted to continue to protect the safety of students, staff, faculty, and the community and recognized that, without effective oversight, there was the potential for widespread transmission that would require completely shutting down campus again, as happened at other institutions.
THEREFORE
T
Because of my expertise and boundary-spanning connections, I was appointed Special Assistant in the Office of the Provost, tasked with "coordinating and supporting responses to the COVID-19 pandemic." In that role, I was asked to help resolve the conflict between safety and expanding on-campus engagement.
A
I collaborated with stakeholders and experts across campus to identify needs and safety considerations for in-person events, then developed, coordinated, and continually updated guidance and the review process for academic and social gatherings on campus.
AND
R
This allowed for safe re-engagement of students, faculty, staff, and community members.

Fig. 52.2 And/but/therefore linear **STAR**. Illustration: Harriet Hopf

In a *cover letter or executive summary*, you can abbreviate the **STAR** by condensing the situation and task and focusing on your actions, the results, and highlighting strengths specific to the opportunity description (Fig. 52.3).

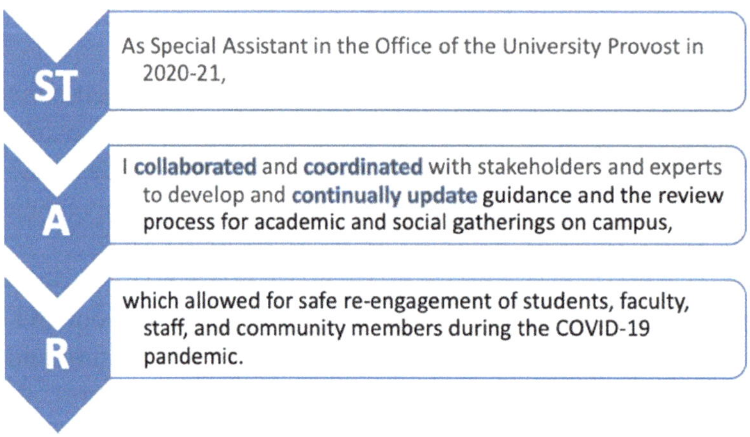

Fig. 52.3 Abbreviated **STAR**. Illustration: Harriet Hopf

Linear **STARs** work well for interviews. When *presenting* an accomplishment to an executive audience, on the other hand, reversing the order (Fig. 52.4) focuses on your key message, which is ideal for capturing and holding the audience's interest, and preparing them to move forward on a further action, for example, giving you and opportunity or resources! In this context, the situation and task are usually known, implied, or incorporated in some way. Make sure you still include the *strengths* you demonstrated!

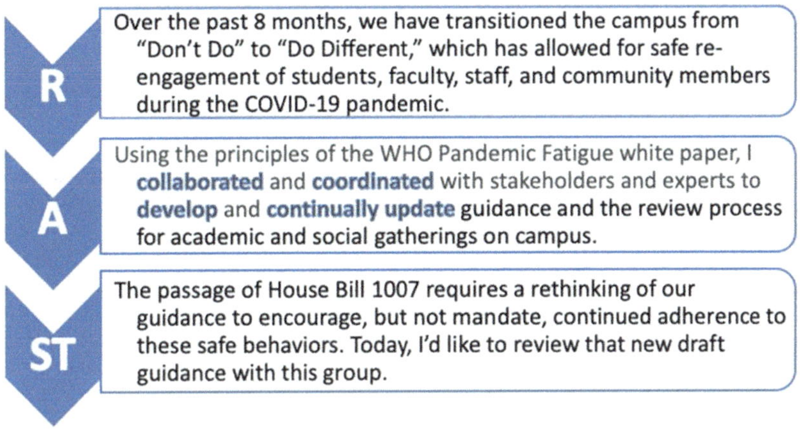

Fig. 52.4 Lead with conclusions flipped **STAR**. The context is a presentation to the Council of Deans, one of many. Illustration: Harriet Hopf

- *Results*: Focus on what you accomplished; this can be most effective when tied to purpose or a story.
- *Actions*: Brief description of what you did and how you did it.
- *Situation/Task*: It is useful to end with a focus on next steps, which could be a call to action—here is what we should do next—or call for input–what should the next steps be? One approach to the focus on *next* steps is to describe the new *Situation and Task* that arise from the *Results and Actions* you have just presented. For example: what is the situation given the current status of your accomplishment? What discussions, input, and/or decisions do you want to elicit from your audience?

Practice

The **STAR** format is a useful tool for capturing and organizing your achievements in a way that allows you to access them for the purpose of graceful self-promotion. Getting good at graceful self-promotion takes *practice*, both polishing various ways to present your achievements and taking advantage of opportunities to do so. A great strategy is to work on with a group of peers for input and practice. Then you will be ready to highlight each other's accomplishments, too.

Now, it is time to go out and practice!

Lessons Learned

- No, your accomplishments will not just "get noticed." Learn the art of graceful self-promotion!
- Tying your accomplishments to your strengths makes them easier to organize and share.
- Capture your accomplishments using the **STAR** (Situation, Task, Action, and Result) format and collect them in a journal or database for easy reference.

References

1. Doyle A. How to use the Star interview response method. The Balance Careers. https://www.thebalancecareers.com/what-is-the-star-interview-response-technique-2061629. Accessed 18 June 2025.
2. Olson R. The ABT Framework. http://abtframework.com/. Accessed 17 June 2025.

Author

Harriet Hopf held senior leadership roles at the medical school, university, and national level that positioned her for her current focus on nurturing career and leadership success in the next generation. As a three-sport college athlete she learned leadership, persistence, and how to get things done. Her husband Leo, whom she met playing volleyball, is an expert in strategy and decision-making and a peerless peer mentor. Their offspring, McKinley, is a grad student busy reinventing the way history is told. Harriet is content never to have learned to say "No."

Seize the Moment

53

Saundra E. Curry and Catherine Marcucci

- The editors of *Anesthesia Bridges* are honored to posthumously publish the following essay by the late Dr. Curry, an esteemed author, teacher, mentor, and clinician.

Introduction

Saundra Curry was a determined and disciplined person, the daughter of missionaries. She was originally from Forest Hills, New York, but was also raised in Paris and Cameroon. Early in her anesthesiology career, she was approached by a publisher to write a question-and-answer book for residents. At that time there were many similar books available. Therefore, she wondered how they were going to break into such a competitive market. She asked, and they said that that was their problem! So, she looked around at the available books and decided that indeed there was room for a better book with more in-depth questions that could be used as a real study guide. Below is Saundra's personal account of how she got it done.

Starting the Book

I enlisted the aid of four colleagues, and we set to work. It was one of the hardest projects I have undertaken. Dividing the work out was easy. Getting them to do the work was a trick, which I as an editor, found most stressful. However, we got it done and ended up with two successful editions. That book, with my name on it, helped me get promoted from assistant to associate professor. But for that to happen, I had to seize the moment with no clear view of where it might go.

***Note from the Editors:** Saundra Curry was originally from the Forest Hills section of Queens (Fig. 53.1).

S. E. Curry
Department of Anesthesiology, Columbia University, New York, NY, USA

C. Marcucci (✉)
Department of Transfusion Medicine, Clinical Center, National Institutes of Health, Bethesda, MD, USA

S. Mohamed et al. (eds.), *Anesthesia Bridges*, https://doi.org/10.1007/978-3-032-08294-7_53

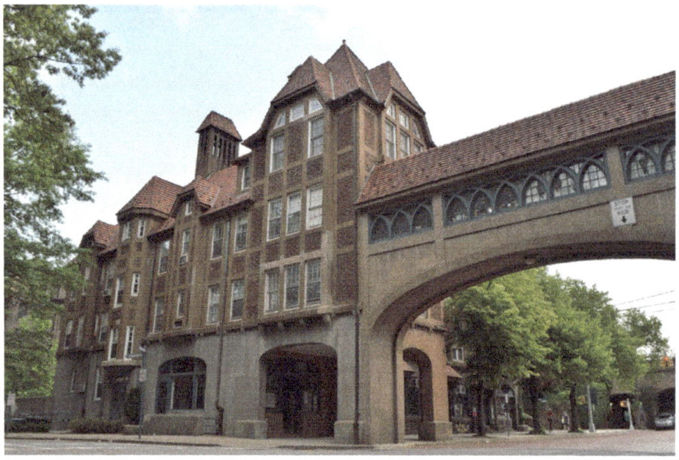

Fig. 53.1 Historic architecture and bridge walkway in Forest Hills. Photo: Image used under standard license from stock.adobe.com

Again, early in my career, I volunteered to take over the medical student teaching program in our department. The students seemed to be getting short shrift by the person who was previously serving as the medical student director. The chair gave it to me, and I went with it. What had originally been just lessons in ACLS became a real course in anesthetic management that was based on a strong curriculum. It was a required course and ended up being very popular among the students. I seized the moment.

Educational Efforts

The same chair, when he offered me the students, showed me a brochure about the Society for Education in Anesthesia (SEA). It was fledgling at the time. "If you're interested in education you should belong to this group," he said. As it turned out, one of my colleagues' brother-in-law was the founder, so I hung on to her coattails and started to go to meetings. I was primarily interested in the medical student initiatives that were going on. However, just by being present at the two annual meetings I got to be known and recognized for my expertise as an educator.

I ended up successfully running for president and ran the organization, with great help from the board of directors. I was also able to mentor other members of our faculty, who ultimately also became members of the Board and eventually became leaders in SEA. My success as a leader of SEA was very helpful in my subsequent application for promotion to full professor. I seized the moments.

Board Examiner

Becoming an oral board examiner used to be a very elusive proposition. It really was an old boys' network with all that implies. One day a senior colleague of mine, who was an examiner, said to me "I'm going to put your name in to be an examiner." I had never approached him. To this day, I have no idea why he said this. I, however, went with the flow and just said "Sure, thanks."

At that time, one bided one's time writing questions for the written board before getting the call. When the call came, I was ready, and I spent nearly 20 years contributing to the board certification process of our specialty. I enjoyed it immensely. I seized the moment. Today the process is more transparent, and I have supported a number of my colleagues to become examiners. Just the other day a junior faculty member said to me "I'm taking your advice and seizing the moment. Will you support me to become a board examiner?" Of course, I said "Yes!" It is nice to know that someone listens.

Lessons Learned

- Even if you cannot tell where something is going to lead, seize the moment. It may end up being a game changer for your career.
- People are always listening; so be careful about what you say.
- Be supportive of those trying to seize their moments.

Authors

Saundra Curry: trained at Columbia and never left the mother ship. She was a clinician and so wisely used her time teaching residents and medical students about anesthesia and medical professionalism. She was an active member of The Society for Education in Anesthesia (past president) and the ASA, serving on national committees and giving talks on education and professionalism nationally and internationally. Her early childhood was spent in Paris and Cameroon, and we went looking for the most beautiful bridges in those places in her honor (Figs. 53.2 and 53.3).

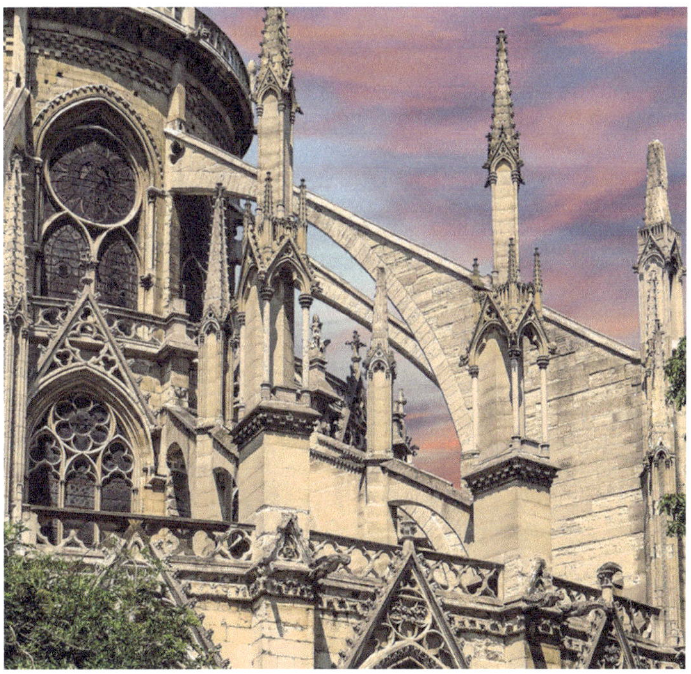

Fig. 53.2 The famous flying buttresses of Notre Dame cathedral. The arguably most famous bridges in Paris are on a building, not over water. Photo: Image used under standard license from iStock.com)

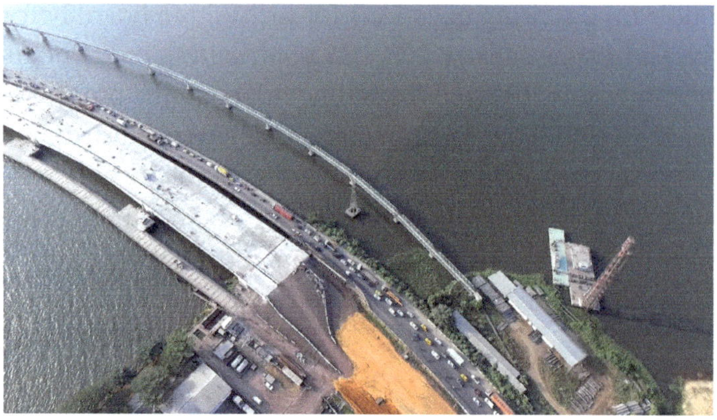

Fig. 53.3 A dramatic aerial shot of the Bessengue Bridge in Cameroon. Photo: Image used under standard license from adobe.stock.com

Cathy Marcucci is a senior academic anesthesiologist and inveterate anesthesiology educator. She is also fellowship-trained in transfusion medicine. When not taking care of patients and/or putting the latest book together, she dedicates her time to mentoring junior colleagues, writing copy for animal rescues, and travel.

Mentors: Lifelong Learning and the Master Clinicians

54

Saundra E. Curry and Catherine Marcucci

The editors of *Anesthesia Bridges* are honored to posthumously publish the following essay by the late Dr. Curry, an esteemed author, teacher, mentor, and clinician.

The induction sequence and airway management techniques described are from Dr. Curry's own experience and teaching and we must respectfully make the point that they do not necessarily represent the views and/or typical clinical practices of the authors and editors at large.

Introduction by Dr. Curry

Like most people, I have had many mentors over the years. Mentors are useful for specific or general purposes and it is rare for one person to fulfill all one's needs across the spectrum of personal and work lives.

An Early Mentor

My first mentor was my one-to-one attending when I became an anesthesia resident. Because I never left my training institute, I was fortunate to be able to keep her for a long time. I remember during those first terrifying weeks she taught me to never give a muscle relaxant, including succinylcholine, until I had established that I could ventilate the patient. That was the rule I followed for years.

One day when we were both on faculty, I happened to be in her room for something and I noticed that she gave succinylcholine right after the thiopental, then ventilated. Here was a law being broken, so I asked her about it. She said "Well, over time I've noticed that what we really want is maximum optimal conditions for intubating and if you get into trouble, you're going to give sux anyway. May as well give it up front." She changed her practice for patient safety, well into her career. (*See Editor's Notes above and below*).

She became the airway maven for the department. Any new gadget that came out, she was the one to try it. She would say to the surgeons "We're learning how to use the light-wand today, so you'll just have to

S. E. Curry
Department of Anesthesiology, Columbia University, New York, NY, USA

C. Marcucci (✉)
Department of Transfusion Medicine, Clinical Center, National Institutes of Health, Bethesda, MD, USA

S. Mohamed et al. (eds.), *Anesthesia Bridges*, https://doi.org/10.1007/978-3-032-08294-7_54

wait." And they would! When fiberoptic intubation became popular, on her own, she bought a model for the resident to practice on. She would also occasionally anesthetize her own airway so residents could practice.

She pushed for the use of laryngeal mask airways when they were first introduced for clinical use and I am sure that, had she still been alive, she would have spearheaded the drive for video laryngoscopy. It is easy to rest on your laurels once you have them. She was the ideal mentor, in that she was never satisfied with what was, if something better was coming along. Lifelong learning was her credo and I hope I have been able to do the same. The department teaching award is named for her.

So, never be totally satisfied. There is always another way that can be assessed and tried. It keeps things fresh, interesting, and often better for the patient.

Finding a Mentor

Mentors are often foisted upon one—someone in your area of hoped-for expertise. That does not mean they are always the right person. And, sometimes no one exists within your own department, in your area of interest.

I was the expert in medical student education in my department. I had run our clerkship for many years and was known nationally for the curriculum that we built, the experiences that we provided, and the residents we produced. I decided I wanted to write about what we did and get it published. I decided it would be more interesting if the paper discussed what was being done nationally so on my own, perhaps not wisely, I devised a national survey of student clerkships, got IRB approval, and gathered data. Now what? I realized that to publish I needed the ear of a journal, and I did not speak journalese. Nor did I know whom to turn to as a mentor for this subject.

But I then thought of someone. This faculty member was our head of research and certainly knew how to get it published. Fortunately, as an engaged member of our teaching faculty, he had direct experience with our efforts to excel at teaching medical students. I presented him with my paper and asked if he could help. He was sure he could and with a lot of tweaking and rewording the paper was accepted for publication. I had found the right mentor for my project! I learned to explore until I found the right person.

So, if you think you have a good idea do not give up until you get it handled. The path may not be the one you first think of.

Reaching Far Away

One expert bit of mentoring I received from my chair was to reach out away from my institution. He asked me whom I admired, and I gave him a few names from the department. He agreed that those were good people, but said that if I wanted to go anywhere in academics, I had to reach out nationally and internationally to get known. That of course required support from the chair to go to meetings of interest, such as the ASA, IARS, and others – to get known through my presentations at these meetings and through networking.

So many young faculty do not get this advice and thus go nowhere. It can start as simply as presenting abstracts for research, PBLDs for education, and getting involved with subspecialty meetings. One does have to show interest and prepare to get that support. Presenting medically challenging cases is another route on which to start. Presenting a case with a senior member helps get started as well. These paths served me well as I started in my career.

Lessons Learned

- Reach out to those more experienced, both in and out of your department, to get the support you need.
- The mentor you find may not have been the original one you sought.
- Use your imagination to get the mentoring you need.

A Second Editor's Note: Readers should keep in mind that the *2022 Difficult Airway Algorithm and Guidelines* can be found at https://pubs.asahq.org. With the accompanying discussion and appendices, it is over 50 pages long and everybody should read every line of it. It is interesting that the evidence model for the basis of the new guidelines includes, "Administration of neuromuscular blockade to improve mask ventilation." However, the guidelines also state, "Upon encountering an unanticipated difficult airway, determine the benefit of waking/restoring spontaneous ventilation." It is almost certainly more difficult to do this if the patient has received "upfront" neuromuscular blockade including succinylcholine. In recent years, there has been quite a bit of discussion on the issue regarding administration of succinylcholine or rocuronium with sugammadex rescue before mask ventilation is established. *For starters*, we recommend several editorials and articles for review.

- Patel A. Facemask ventilation before or after neuromuscular blocking drugs: where are we now? *Anaesthesia*, 2014, 69:811–15.
- Soltesz S, Alm P, Mathes A, et al. The effect of neuromuscular blockade on the efficiency of mask ventilation in patients difficult to ventilate: a prospective trial. *Anaesthesia*. 2017, 72:1484–90.
- Shetty N, Rao S, Vijayakumar V. Questioning succinylcholine usage in grade IV (difficult) mask ventilation. *Anesthesiology*. 2011;115(2):444–7.

There is quite a bit to consider with this issue, for both the anticipated and unanticipated difficult airway, and the stakes for the patients are high. We must always remember that the *ultimate* goal is not to ensure that the patients are intubated but rather that they remain oxygenated.

Authors

Saundra Curry trained at Columbia and never left the mother ship. She was a clinician and spent her time teaching residents and medical students about anesthesia and medical professionalism. She was an active member of The Society for Education in Anesthesia (past president) and the ASA, serving on national committees and giving talks on education and professionalism nationally and internationally.

Cathy Marcucci is a senior academic anesthesiologist and inveterate anesthesiology educator. She is also fellowship-trained in transfusion medicine. She herself relies on the ability to wake up a patient when she has encountered an unexpected difficulty airway and so is very careful about giving neuromuscular blockade.

Anesthesiologists "Out of the OR": Are There Opportunities?

55

Neal Cohen

Introduction

The practice of anesthesia and perioperative care continues to evolve. As it does, the concept of the anesthesiologist "hidden" behind the ether screen (if that term is relevant to current practice) is not consistent with the diverse roles and responsibilities anesthesiologists have in the healthcare environment. Not only has perioperative care been transformed by anesthesiologists, but anesthesiologists have also been able to assume leadership roles in intensive care units, pain medicine, palliative care, sleep medicine, and other related services. Many anesthesiologists have also sought additional training in business and healthcare administration so that they can assume leadership roles in anesthesia practices, as medical directors of perioperative care, or chief medical officers.

Other Opportunities

In addition to these "obvious" roles for anesthesiologists, many other opportunities arise for which an anesthesiologist may offer value. The key to identifying these roles and being considered requires a "presence" in the healthcare environment, organizational leadership, and a "volunteer" attitude. My career has changed in ways I never would have imagined. My goal was to train in anesthesia and critical care medicine and to hopefully advance into a leadership role of an intensive care unit. Fortunately, I was provided opportunities to pursue my goal—but also given the chance to assume other interesting, challenging and rewarding roles never imagined earlier in my career.

Beginning with Billing

As a junior faculty member in the Department of Anesthesia, I was asked to take over responsibility for anesthesia billing from a senior faculty member who had been managing the billing for many years. While I was not sure what I had "agreed" to do, I was able to put a structure in place to optimize anes-

N. Cohen (✉)
Department of Anesthesiology, University of California, San Francisco School of Medicine, San Francisco, CA, USA
e-mail: CohenN@ucsf.edu

S. Mohamed et al. (eds.), *Anesthesia Bridges*, https://doi.org/10.1007/978-3-032-08294-7_55

thesia billing and collections. To do so required coordination with the surgical departments and medical center at a time when each department managed its own finances. The experience allowed me to meet and work with a group of people I would otherwise have probably never known.

The experience opened doors for me that transformed my professional career.Based on my experiences with anesthesia billing, I was asked by the dean to lead a team that was managing a CMS audit of teaching hospital billing. I would not describe the experience as "rewarding", though we were successful in challenging some claims by CMS regarding our billing practices. Most interesting was our "exit" meeting with CMS and the US Attorney in San Francisco whose name may sound familiar—Robert Mueller. His participation brought logic to the discussion and subsequent decisions.

***Note from the Editors:** Neal Cohen is at UCSF, so we decided to look for a San Francisco bridge other than you-know-what. We found this dramatic picture of the Richmond-San Rafael Bridge (Fig. 55.1).

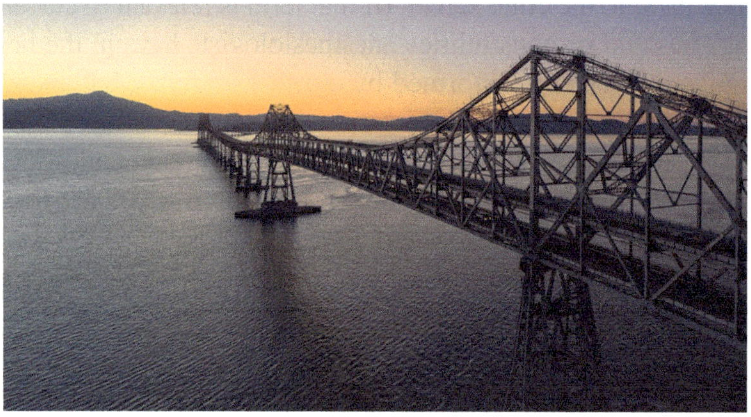

Fig. 55.1 The Richmond–San Rafael Bridge spans San Francisco Bay, connecting Richmond in the east to San Rafael on the west. It opened in 1956, although planning had begun in the late 1920s, before plans for the Golden Gate bridge were initiated. It crosses two shipping channels and has an unusual, depressed center truss section, which gives the bridge a roller coaster appearance. Photo: Image used under standard license from stock.adobe.com

Career Development

From that experience, doors opened for me that I would not have anticipated, including an offer to serve as vice dean for academic affairs and my roles as CEO for the UCSF Medical Group and president of the medical staff. I also served as medical director for the International Medical Service, building collaborative relationships with other health systems and academic institutions, particularly in the Pacific Rim. This opportunity allowed me to experience different cultures and health care systems. I cherish the friendships developed as a result of these experiences.

I reflect on these opportunities to emphasize that each of us has the ability to pursue opportunities both within and beyond the operating room, when given the chance to do so. As anesthesiologists, we have an understanding of hospital medicine in particular better than most other physicians, including surgeons. We also have the ability to manage complex situations in a logical and evidence-based way—independent of whether we are managing a clinical problem or other challenging issues. Team and crisis management skills can also be transferred to other settings—if we are open to new challenges, accept, and are willing to assume roles that might seem inconsequential, but can open new doors.

Lessons Learned

- To advance your career, have a "presence" in the healthcare environment, take on a role in organizational leadership, and have a "volunteer" attitude.
- Each of us has the ability to pursue opportunities both within and beyond the operating room, when given the chance to do so.

Author

Neal Cohen has been a member of the faculty at the University of California San Francisco for the majority of his career. During his tenure, he has been fortunate to participate in the care of patients in the operating room and both pediatric and adult ICUs. In addition to his clinical opportunities, he has extensive experience in building relationships with other health systems and academic institutions internationally, primarily in the Pacific Rim. His current role is vice dean for the Stanford school of medicine providing oversight of professional service relationships and affiliations as well as compliance, risk management, and regulatory affairs.

56 Say "Yes" to Quality Improvement

David P. Martin and Raymond G. Graber

Open advice to our former selves: Why you should say "*yes*" to the opportunity to join your group's quality improvement activities!

First, Let Us Talk About Why Quality Improvement Is Important

Think of the many frustrating problems at work that you do not know how to solve. Your hospital administration has policies and rules that seem to be a tangled mess that prevents you from implementing "obvious" solutions. However, by engaging yourself in the process of becoming an expert in quality improvement, not only will you gain personal satisfaction, but you will increase the satisfaction of your colleagues, and you will facilitate improved patient care.

We all take pride in the quality of care we provide for our patients. However, to really make a difference in outcomes, you will find that you need to look at the systems in which patients are taken care of. Making a change in group practice has the potential to have more benefit than changing one person's practice. You will be able to touch far more patients by extension of your improvement efforts than you could with personal patient care alone.

So, What Do I Need to Know?

Starting the process of quality improvement requires a little bit of education and necessitates getting to know people outside of your comfort zone. This includes surgeons, nurses, administrators, pharmacists, and other colleagues throughout your healthcare organization. Your focus on quality improvement will open doors, and you will discover that many others in your institution share the same passion.

D. P. Martin
Department of Anesthesiology and Perioperative Medicine, Mayo Clinic, Rochester, MN, USA

R. G. Graber (✉)
Department of Anesthesiology and Perioperative Medicine, University Hospitals Cleveland Medical Center, Cleveland, OH, USA
e-mail: Raymond.graber@uhhospitals.org

S. Mohamed et al. (eds.), *Anesthesia Bridges*, https://doi.org/10.1007/978-3-032-08294-7_56

You will come to understand why so many rules seem to be fixed and immovable.But when you learn the background behind rules and policies, you will gain the insight you need to modify them in adaptive and improved ways. You will also become a resource to your fellow colleagues, who will turn to you when they have problems. You will learn to think about the concepts of structure and process, and how they affect outcomes.

- *Structure* refers to the organization of your department and hospital. Does your department have adequate equipment and the training to use it? Are there sufficient staff to handle the caseload, and are shifts organized in a way to match the expected caseload at different times of the workday and day of the week? Does your staff in the OR have easy access to information such as departmental clinical guidelines for case management—either printed or on departmental websites? Is there continuing education that matches the needs of the department?

- *Process* refers to how things are done. Does your department use and develop clinical guidelines and policies? Our national organizations are useful resources. The American Society of Anesthesiologists actively publishes practice parameters such as "Practice Guidelines for Management of the Difficult Airway" and "Practice Guidelines for the Perioperative Management of Patients with Obstructive Sleep Apnea." The American Society of Regional Anesthesia has developed a number of useful guidelines such as "Regional Anesthesia in the Patient Receiving Antithrombotic or Thrombolytic Therapy." The Anesthesia Patient Safety Foundation is another great source for education and ideas.

- In addition, enlist your local department experts to write in-house guidelines for their areas of expertise. In academic programs, there is a constant stream of students and residents who are new to clinical subspecialties, and who can benefit from written guidelines to supplement their discussions with attending staff. However, you will find that this useful information will not be of much impact if it not easily accessible to students, residents, and staff—preferably on the department's intranet.

- *Outcomes* refer to the results of your department's efforts. Most departments and hospitals have some mechanism by which problems with process or outcome are collected for review—hospital incident reports, departmental quality improvement reports, and departmental databases. Incident reviews can be funneled into morbidity and mortality conferences, improvement projects, departmental education, or peer review.

***Note from the Editors:** To remind Dr. Martin of his time in St. Louis, we are featuring the old Chain of Rocks Bridge (Fig. 56.1). The bridge spans the Mississippi River with the east end being on Chouteau Island (part of Madison, IL) and the west end being on the Missouri shore of the river. The bridge is noted for a 22-degree bend in the middle of the span, which was necessitated by the non-uniform geographical location of the bedrock at the river bottom.At one time, the bridge carried vehicular traffic from Rte. 66. Today it carries only pedestrian and bicycle traffic.

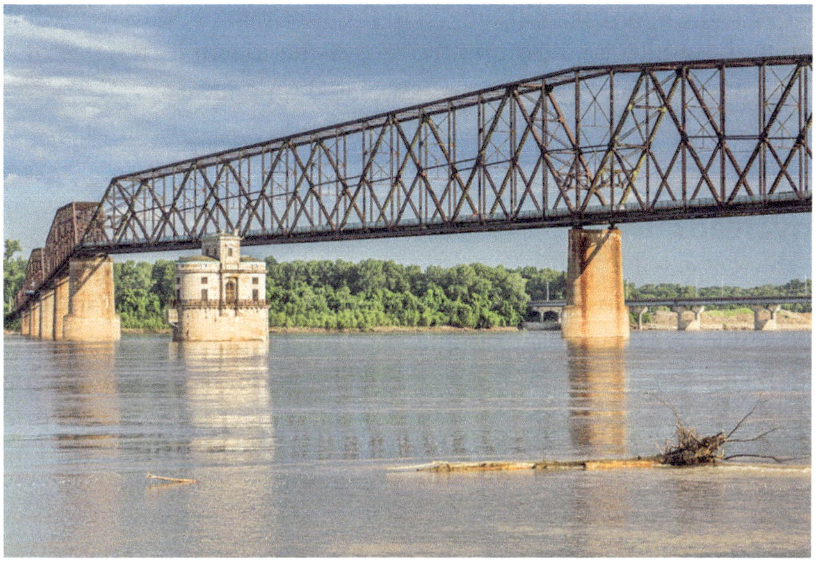

Fig. 56.1 The old Chain of Rocks Bridge in St. Louis, MI is now owned by the city of Madison, IL. This point in the river was previously notable for the water intake plant for the city of St. Louis and a series of rock ledges that made navigation of this portion of the river extremely treacherous. You can see the "corner" in the bridge span center left in this view of the bridge. Photo: Image used under standard license from iStock.com

Can You Give Me Examples of Projects?

You will find that if your department has excellent people, structure, and processes, then you will have the foundation for good outcomes. However, medicine is in a constant state of evolution, and new procedures, processes and expectations will inevitably lead to the need for ongoing redesigning of how you will deliver care. Ideas for quality improvement projects will come to you from a variety of sources.

Incident reports and other quality data will lead to ideas for projects. For example, cases of corneal abrasions after general anesthesia lead us to work with our ophthalmology colleagues to develop protocols to reduce incidence and also to manage and treat these ourselves in the PACU.

National guidelines can be interpreted and adapted to satisfy the needs of your local practice. To illustrate, we have worked with our infectious disease and pharmacy colleagues to write protocols for perioperative antibiotic prophylaxis, including alternative regimens for patients with significant beta lactam allergy or who are colonized with MRSA. We also developed redosing guidelines based on creatinine clearance.

Changing practice patterns can lead to a need to develop new strategies for care. For instance, patients undergoing total joint replacement used to have a hospital stay of around four days. It is now commonplace for these patients to be discharged on the day of surgery or the next day. We have worked with our surgeons to develop early recovery after surgery (ERAS) protocols that feature multimodal analgesia, liberal use of regional anesthesia techniques, and early physical therapy and ambulation.

In addition, keep an eye out for new developments in the literature, and assess whether there is enough evidence to incorporate these into your group practice. As an example–the use of lower tidal volumes may be associated with a lower risk of ventilator associated lung injury.

How Can I Get Involved?

There are numerous ways to get involved with quality improvement. You can work with your service line to develop better protocols of care, for example, total joint replacement or colorectal ERAS.You can volunteer to work on your departmental or hospital quality committees. You can look for opportunities to try to incorporate lessons learned from case reviews into teaching activities, orientations, and other department education. You can expand your horizons and get involved with committee work at the state and national levels.

What Are the Benefits?

Quality improvement work can be personally rewarding, and it will help build your reputation and relationships with surgeons and other staff throughout the hospital.It is possible to tie a theme of patient safety and quality improvement to almost any pursuit related to the practice of anesthesiology. In doing so, you will gain essential administrative and educational credit for academic promotion and leadership appointments.Even non-clinicians will recognize your achievements in improving patient safety, eliminating waste, and increasing efficiency.

Lessons Learned

- Quality improvement provides an opportunity to help more patients in your practice than you could touch personally.
- Quality improvement offers a meaningful and interesting way to expand your professional career and help your colleagues.
- Quality improvement serves as an excellent theme to augment your leadership, academic promotion, and administrative goals.

Authors

Dave Martin has survived *approximately* 30 Minnesota winters since coming to Mayo Clinic upon completion of his MD and PhD training in balmy St. Louis. His early anesthesiology career focused on pain medicine, but more recently has shifted to an OR practice where he works in most all clinical areas. The broad clinical exposure helps maintain perspective in his role as vice chair for safety and quality in the Department of Anesthesiology and Perioperative Medicine. He has been married to his best friend, Laura, for 35+ years and they have two grown children.

Ray Graber started working on quality issues in 1990 when his chairman said, "I have a committee I want you to run." Dave and Ray first met when they did visiting professorships at each other's institution. Dave lectured on corneal abrasions, and Ray talked about medication errors. He now also serves as a vice chair in the Department of Anesthesiology and Perioperative Medicine at his institution.

57 Practicing Anesthesia in an Era of "Cost Containment"

Brian C. Fitzsimons and Raymond G. Graber

Introduction

Practicing medicine in an era of "cost containment" presents both unique challenges and new opportunities in anesthesia practice. As conversations regarding increasing national health care expenditures have become more prevalent, the age of practicing medicine regardless of cost has rightfully drawn to a close. In the United States today, we have an opportunity to provide the type of medical care that our population has come to expect, but in a way that limits how much of our gross domestic product we spend providing it.

Considering Costs

One may ask, "Why should I care about cost when that was not what I was trained to do?" No matter what type of practice you're in—academic, a mixed academic/private model, or a private group or solo practice, your relationship with the hospital and its administration is critical to your group and personal income. You need to consider your hospital's administration as one of your "customers," since they sign your contract to provide anesthesia services at your institution.

Being aligned with your administration's goals significantly improves goodwill in that regard and helps your hospital gain patients and health insurance contracts in your larger market. Health insurers do not want to send their patients to hospitals where the cost of care is higher than other hospitals in your market that provide the same quality of care. Also, the reality is that the frequent excuse, "We provide better care, which is more expensive!" does not end up holding true when actual quality measures are examined and published. Your focus should be to improve value: improved measurable outcomes at decreased cost.

B. C. Fitzsimons (✉) · R. G. Graber
Department of Anesthesiology and Perioperative Medicine, University Hospitals Cleveland Medical Center, Cleveland, OH, USA
e-mail: Brian.Fitzsimons@uhhospitals.org

S. Mohamed et al. (eds.), *Anesthesia Bridges*, https://doi.org/10.1007/978-3-032-08294-7_57

Reducing Costs

Now that you are interested, you might ask yourself, "But how do I actually go about reducing costs?" You can start out by thinking about supply costs. Practically speaking, you can divide supply costs into two "buckets"—supplies that are purchased with capital dollars (think, expensive durable equipment), and supplies that are disposable, which are purchased with operations dollars.

Anesthesia practice requires some expensive capital outlays; anesthesia gas machines with monitors typically list for $80,000 to $100,000 each. When you add additional devices such as cerebral oximeters, ultrasounds, video laryngoscopes, and fiberoptic airway equipment, the equipment cost to provide anesthesia services can soar. Your involvement in picking equipment that meets your practice's and your hospital's needs without "overdoing it" can help contain costs. Buy what you actually need instead of what you want.

When you discuss your equipment needs with industry reps, make it known to them that cost is a factor in your decision making—both purchase price and service contract cost, that is, the ongoing cost of ownership. Treat your practice's requests for capital equipment similar to your shopping for a new car. Would you pay the list price? Would you try to get a better deal? Would you buy the most expensive model when the midrange model will do the job? Taking ownership of the process in terms of cost helps improve the financial standing of your institution overall, and the goodwill of your hospital's administration will extend to you when your practice contract comes up for renewal.

***Note from the Editors:** Ohio has many charming and historic covered bridges. One of the most picturesque is the Kidwell covered bridge is in Athens County, OH where Brian Fitzsimons spends time with his family (Fig. 57.1).

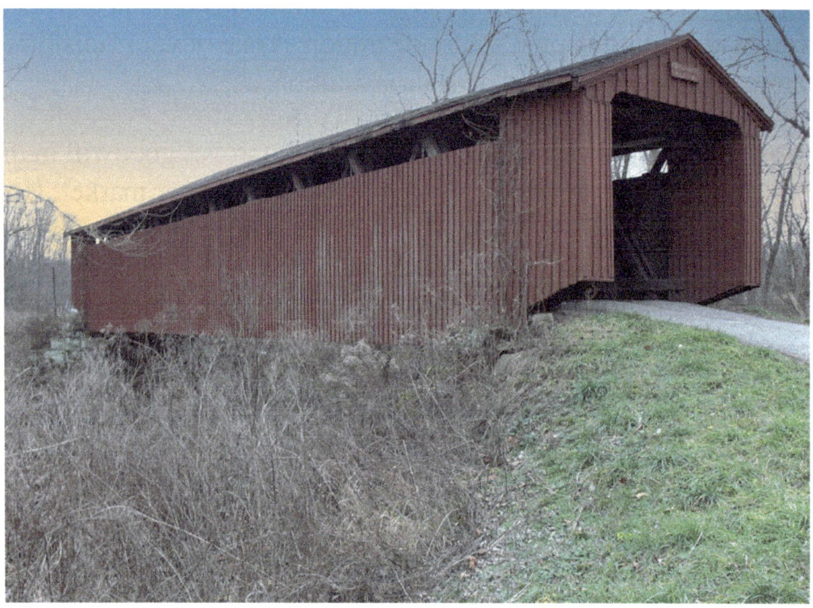

Fig. 57.1 The picture-perfect Kidwell bridge spans Sunday creek. It is a covered Howe truss bridge constructed in 1880 by the Hocking Valley Bridge Works. It was closed in 1978 due to damage by an overweight truck but was fortunately later repaired and reopened. Photo credit: Image used under standard license from stock.adobe.com

Pharmacy Costs

Pharmaceutical usage is another area of practice that is ripe for cost containment opportunities. Some of the commonly used drugs in our anesthesia armamentarium have undergone significant price changes over time. Changes occur because of things like corporate consolidation and lack of competition, the use of brand name versus generic drugs, and the supplier your pharmacy uses. Incorporating pricing into your drug selection strategy can have a significant impact on the overall cost of care.

It is worth developing a relationship with a hospital pharmacist who can help you navigate drug cost/charge information. For instance, intravenous vasodilator and vasoconstrictor drug prices have a wide variance. At the time of this writing (early 2020s) our standard norepinephrine (8 mg/250 ml) drip costs about $5, while vasopressin (20 units/100 ml) costs about $180. Looking at vasodilators—nitroglycerine (50 mg/250 ml) runs $10, while clevidipine (50 mL single use vial with 0.5 mg/mL) costs about $70. A sodium nitroprusside drip (50 mg/250 ml) currently costs about $40, but several years ago it was over $800!

By the way, hospitals will typically charge patients about 5 times the procurement cost—so that $800 drug cost becomes a $4000 charge on the patient's bill! Another case in point—the elimination of inhaled nitric oxide from our institution, and replacing it with inhaled epoprostenol, created savings that totaled in the millions of dollars annually. Here are some more examples of drug choices with financial implications: isoflurane vs. sevoflurane vs. desflurane, oral vs. intravenous acetaminophen, neostigmine vs. sugammadex, bupivacaine vs. the liposomal encapsulated form. In your practice, you will have to decide whether the potential advantages of one drug over another outweigh the extra costs involved. There is some additional information on this below.

Equipment Costs

Let us get back to supply costs—specifically, disposable equipment. One area of "low hanging fruit" that any interested physician can pursue is to look at procedure kits. Kit consolidation can reap significant rewards in terms of cost savings. If you tally the number of different types of kits that perform the same function at your institution, you will find that maybe 10 or 20 different types of kits are ordered that essentially serve the same purpose. Do you really need 20 different central line kits? Is there a way to reduce the number of kits down to 5 or less? Often, when the origins of these kits are traced, these kits had their contents specified by physicians who are no longer practicing at your institution.

By spending some time and energy on disposable procedure kits, you afford yourself the opportunity to modernize the kit with appropriate equipment and reduce the overall different types of kits ordered, thereby gaining a volume discount price on your new kit. On the back end of this exercise, you can also save the institution money because frequently the kits that are ordered to satisfy the needs of an individual physician will expire before they are all used. By limiting the total number of kits, you increase utilization of each kit and reduce the chances that kits will need to be thrown away because they expire. When you consolidate your kits, you may also find that you are less affected by backorders, since manufacturers will tend to prioritize their higher volume kits.

Another strategy to consider is the outright elimination of disposable equipment that is sporadically used, if at all. Is there a capital equipment (non-disposable) item that may be able to be used for the same purpose, but at a cheaper cost? A perfect example of this is investing in a new noninvasive cardiac output monitor for use during cardiac, vascular, or transplant cases versus continuing to use continuous cardiac output pulmonary artery catheters.

This achieves a few advantages. For one, your institution is able to depreciate the value of the monitor over successive years on their taxes. Secondly, you will reduce costly waste as you eliminate the possibility of expensive disposables expiring in a storeroom because of low utilization. Thirdly, you eliminate the loss of expensive disposable equipment that occurs at the hands of personnel from other departments like the ICUs and step-down units who, despite having the best intentions, come and "borrow" a disposable from you without charging the patient for it. You do not want your budget to supply other parts of the hospital! The conversion from single-patient-use disposable to multiple-patient-use capital items may help save significant amounts of money in the long run.

Conclusion

In conclusion, we hope we have opened your eyes to some opportunities for you to reduce costs and improve the value of care you and your department provide for your hospital. In doing so, your personal value to your department and hospital will also rise.

Lessons Learned

- There are ample opportunities to reduce the costs of care in medicine—from equipment to supplies and drugs.
- You increase your personal value and the value of your department when you are a good citizen with the budget supplied to you.

***Note from the Editors:** Speaking of costs, the most expensive bridge ever built is the eastern span of the San Francisco–Oakland Bay Bridge (Fig. 57.2). A significant portion of the total bill was due to the engineering costs.

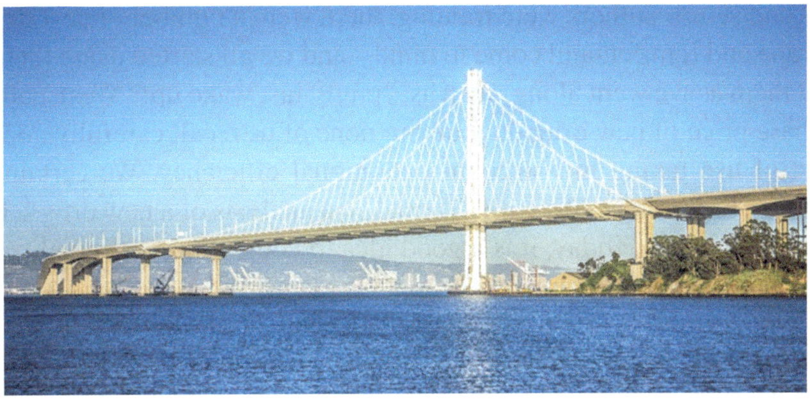

Fig. 57.2 The new and replaced East Span of the Oakland Bay Bridge was completed at a cost of around $6.4 billion dollars. The cost of the gargantuan design-build project largely accrued in response to the need to make the structure earthquake proof. It was designed to withstand the largest ground motions predicted for the next 1500 years. It employs seismic energy-absorbing shear link beams in the tower of a cable-supported bridge. It is the world's longest single-tower, self-anchored suspension bridge and the largest public works project in California's history. Photo: Image used under standard license from stock.adobe.com

Bonus Content!

- Remember as stated above that the total or "true" cost of a drug is not just the purchase cost. The overall cost of using the drug in the actual clinical setting is what really counts and this almost always dependent on the length of time under anesthesia care.

- Let us take the neostigmine vs. sugammadex question that Brian and Ray mention above. Is sugammadex a "better" drug than neostigmine and what does that even mean? Better might mean safer in any number of ways, such as fewer side effects or less potential for drug errors. *but* it might also mean faster and cheaper. But what is the definition of faster and cheaper?

- There is quite a bit of research on this. Moss et al did a retrospective review and looked at sugammadex vs. neostigmine for routine reversal of neuromuscular block and the effect on perioperative efficiency [1]. They concluded, "For 8,120 patients, sugammadex use was associated with shorter operating room and surgical durations as well as shorter postanesthesia care unit stay. The favorable pharmacodynamic profile of sugammadex may improve surgical and perioperative efficiency and offset higher medication cost."

- Interestingly, a study was done in Taiwan that showed the opposite—the purchase cost in sugammadex was not offset by increased operational efficiency but the authors concluded that this might be due to the relatively lower labor costs there [2].

- One of our contributors remarked that there is quite a bit of sugammadex controversy at his hospital—they are increasingly using it, and the new ASA guidelines will lead to heavier use. However, their pharmacy does not care about room turnover or reintubation issues—all they care about is their silo of costs—and have been trying to find ways to restrict use.

- When the editors and senior authors were training, there were a number of new drugs introduced into practice—desflurane and remifentanil come to mind—and we all started using them and decided what we thought about them as we went along, such as, "pretty fast wake up!" We usually had some knowledge of the purchase price of new drug du jour, but none of us recall carefully considering or reviewing the total cost of use taking into account operational efficiency. We certainly can't recall any conferences, lectures, or journal clubs with a formal cost analysis of a new drugs. This was something we could have done better on. Today, it is a good idea to consider overall total from the get-go or as the cost analysis studies become available.

- Keep in mind, however, that if you ever do any overseas or medical mission work, you will almost certainly be faced with using the older, cheaper drugs—isoflurane and succinylcholine and neostigmine are still the staples in many places of the world.

- If a new drug is really better in every way, then adopt its use and let the old drug go. But if there is a lot of gray area as to whether it is truly cheaper and you are interested in providing anesthesia care in developing countries, at least retain a passable knowledge of the older drugs, because they will almost certainly be what you are using.

References

1. Moss AP, Powell MF, Morgan CJ, et al. Sugammadex versus neostigmine for routine reversal of neuromuscular blockade and the effect on perioperative efficiency. Proc (Bayl Univ Med Cent). 2022;35(5):599–603.
2. Lan W, Tam KW, Chen JT, et al. Cost-effectiveness of sugammadex versus neostigmine to reverse neuromuscular blockade in a university hospital in Taiwan: a propensity score-matched analysis. Healthcare (Basel). 2023;11(2):240.

Authors

Brian Fitzsimons is a cardiac anesthesiologist who trained at the Cleveland Clinic. He currently serves as the chief of the cardiac anesthesia service at University Hospitals Cleveland Medical Center. He, his wife, and their two teenage/young adult sons are avid outdoors people. When not in Cleveland, they are usually at their farm near Athens Ohio, enjoying fishing, canoeing, hiking, and riding ATVs.

Ray Graber splits his time between cardiac and orthopedic anesthesia. He believes it is important for young physicians to learn all they can about the costs of care they deliver. Correct billing is important, too!

58 The IT Expert in Me, Could This Really Be?

Katya H. Chiong and Raymond G. Graber

Introduction

Ever wonder what the information technology (IT) department at your institution does? Most people think of the IT department only when computer programs or systems go awry and work comes to a screeching halt.However, the IT department is always working in the background, and they are tasked with establishing, monitoring, and maintaining information technology services, which includes everything from physical electronic equipment, network access and security, system redundancy, technical support, and software applications for the electronic medical record systems.

What? How?……Me?

How about us physicians, why should we get involved with IT? Well, we are the *end users*—we can assess what works and does not work. Do we have the equipment we need? Is it functional? Do the programs we have help workflow? Are they readily accessible? Can we obtain the information we need? Is the system reliable? Can it change with us?There are many computer-related issues that a clinician with IT interest can help assess. In short, if you do not have someone representing your group, your needs may be overlooked and wrong decisions can become a big headache for your department and/or institution, costing more in the long run.

So, now that you know that you need someone with an interest in IT issues in your department, you may be wondering if that person could, or should, be *you*? If we could give one piece of advice to physicians everywhere—please, **be a part of the solution.** We all know when something is not working, and some of us have "obvious" solutions. The problem is, you have to be in the correct setting and have the right contacts to make the changes needed possible. If not, one is often "preaching to the choir" about what is wrong.

K. H. Chiong (✉) · R. G. Graber
Department of Anesthesiology and Perioperative Medicine, University Hospitals Cleveland Medical Center, Cleveland, OH, USA
e-mail: katya.chiong@uhhospitals.org; Raymond.graber@uhhospitals.org

S. Mohamed et al. (eds.), *Anesthesia Bridges*, https://doi.org/10.1007/978-3-032-08294-7_58

If you are *that* person who has ideas about how to make improvements, or you notice all the work-arounds everyone creates just to make workflow bearable, you are the right person for the job! Now imagine, if you had a seat at the table, where decisions were being made about equipment, software, logistics, applications, including customization opportunities for **YOUR** own work environment! The potential to improve workflow directly seems downright enticing, does not it?

Let us now discuss some common information and IT issues that most of us are likely to run in to.

Did Someone Order New Equipment?

We have seen the installation of "great computer systems" that were not functional for the end user or the application of barriers that impeded workflow. Years ago, we had new computer workstations installed and attached to our anesthesia machines—for the purpose of charting on our electronic anesthesia records and accessing the hospital electronic medical record (EMR). However, the system was programmed to go to a lock screen after a relatively short period of inactivity. We had to constantly log back in to access our computer screen. Why did this happen? The problem was that there had previously been a generic login used for the OR computers, and these remained unlocked indefinitely. This was a huge security issue, and while the new system immediately solved the main issue of security, it overlooked the workflow needs of its end users. Ultimately, we were able to work with our IT group to come up with reasonable lock screen settings that considered the end user workflow and addressed everyone's concern.

Your IT people will periodically upgrade the computer hardware throughout the hospital. They may have the best intentions but may not realize that if something works great for one group, it does not mean it works for yours. As an example, our PACU needed more functioning computer workstations, not computers on wheels as was initially planned. In fact, what was needed was an overhaul of outdated equipment and restructuring of the location of workstations, including adding more units in different locations throughout our operating rooms. In addition, our anesthesia department moved to the use of tablets, which worked well with our mobile workflow, improving efficiency in our preop evaluations and postop hand-offs in the PACU.

Remember, an IT liaison with your background and experience brings valuable information from your specialty and the physician community at large that is often lacking. You have expertise in function and the use of hospital systems, and your perspective is invaluable. This could be *you*!

Did Someone Just Say They Are Going to Get Rid of That?

Years ago, our hospital system embarked on a goal of building a unified, hospital-system wide electronic medical record. Of course, that also led to plans to discontinue older legacy applications. This sounded reasonable, until we all discovered that there were plans to abolish the only application that easily linked the community outpatient record to the inpatient world. From IT's viewpoint, they were trying to streamline software and support, thus making the system more cost effective.

In their defense, any IT department is used to getting pushback regarding any change, regardless of the expected benefit. They expect that there will be complaining and growing pains until end users get acclimated to the new technology and learn to love all the new available features. We get it, but this time workflow was going to be significantly impacted, and end users were going to lose easy access to the information they needed. Physician liaisons were able to contest this planned change and preserve the essential software.

Your departmental IT liaison, someone who both understands the overall institutional goals as well as the impact these plans make "on the ground", can help steer plans forward while maintaining system integrity. This person could definitely be *you*!

***Note from the Editors:** Katya Chiong and Ray Graber are both tech people; so will appreciate this bridge (Figs. 58.1 and 58.2). They may have even built ones like it in college; most engineering students have. The loading requirements vary—sometimes you get extra points for every brick you can pile on top. When Cathy Marcucci built hers as a freshman engineering student a thousand years ago, it had to hold a Western Electric model 500 desk telephone with a rotary dial that weighed five pounds. That bridge is long gone, unfortunately, so Neil Sandson rebuilt one for her from her description.

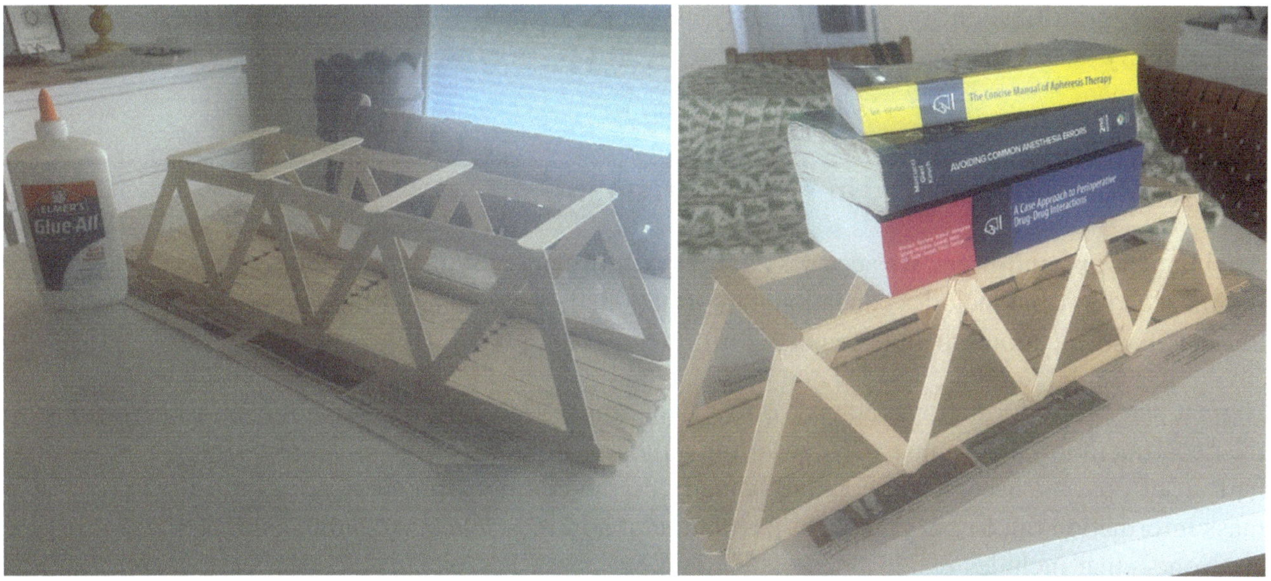

Fig. 58.1 and 58.2 A classic stick bridge holding at least five pounds of books. Sometimes the requirement is for students to use toothpicks instead popsicle sticks. What type did you build? Photo: Neil Sandson

That Generic Chart and Order Set Is Not Going to Work for Us

So now you have got a new hospital EMR program and it is time to customize notes and orders. If you do not have a person or committee that works on order set issues, you have got a problem. Your department needs to have input on design of initial order sets—examples would include for PACU or ICU care, and epidural infusions—but the list goes on and on. We are also currently working on our third completely different electronic anesthesia record—that again requires attention to multiple details to get it right.

Do not miss the chance to build things how you want and need them to be. For example, our cardiac anesthesia group built a custom template in the echocardiography report system to streamline the writing of intraoperative echocardiography reports. No one else knows your workflow the way you do. If you are at all interested, we encourage you to be a part of the process. It is both personally and professionally rewarding to have an impact in optimizing workflow, utilization of resources, and quality patient care across an entire enterprise.

Why Is Everything So Difficult to Change?!

When tailored to your practice, order sets can enhance safety, efficiency, and help drive standard of care across the entire system. They must however, reflect a consensus among the group and be able to be modified as necessary. Order sets need to evolve over time as drugs get added to the formulary, and as care guidelines evolve, for instance think of ERAS protocols.

When there is no departmental point of contact, multiple requests without vetting and prioritization remain idle in the queue. A department committee that screens and evaluates requests for order set changes is an effective way to help ensure good working relationships with the IT department. The truth is that while writing the code for these requests does not actually take the months allotted, the number of requests, prioritization levels, and quality assurance reviews to make sure the requests have been appropriately vetted take considerable time.

How Is Information Stored in Your Department?

As clinicians and end-users, we need easy access to information. What kinds of information? The answer is almost endless, but includes educational information, department and hospital policies, clinical guidelines, call and vacation schedules, and so forth.

A great place for information storage is on the department's site on your hospital's intranet. Working on the department intranet can be very rewarding although at times may seem more restricting with a limited set of options, access, or people to actually do the editing. Nonetheless, making the effort to get mass information out to the group and maintain it at an accessible and centralized location is great for everyone—that includes residents and attending, but also CRNAs and AAs. We have spent countless hours developing clinical guidelines and protocols, in an effort to improve and standardize care. But if no one can find these easily, then that work will have little impact.

We have guidelines posted by clinical section for specific types of cases—such as orthopedics, cardiac, and obstetrics. We have a perioperative antibiotic section, which includes antibiotic selection by type of case, MRSA status, beta lactam allergy; and redosing schedules based on creatinine clearance. A quality and best practices section includes guidelines like how to manage corneal abrasions, dental injuries, and anaphylaxis. An equipment section includes manuals for new equipment. Do you have any sites on your hospital intranet that are difficult to get to? Make a direct link from your departmental intranet. Honestly, you'll find that what is helpful to you, most likely will be helpful to many others.

Alternatively, you can house information on an external website. This will entail some cost to build and maintain, so you will have to go to your chairperson for funding. On the other hand, you will not be constrained by the design limitations of your hospital intranet. It is likely that someone in your department has experience and interest in website design and will be glad to use their skills to help with this project.

An education website can be an excellent resource for all trainees. This site can include faculty handouts and rotation guides, rotation goals and objectives, program policies, as well as rotation and call schedules. It is also helpful to include quick links to case logs, evaluation systems, library resources, and the hospital or departmental intranet. Information and available resources are now easily accessible whenever needed. An education website can be a potential game-changer for your residency program. Don't underestimate its impact on your trainees and graduate medical program in general. Its plethora of information and clearly outlined expectations for trainees can be made readily accessible to program evaluators as well.

In closing, these are only a handful of examples of how information technology impacts us on a daily basis. No question, we need to be involved in the development and evolution of IT systems in our hospitals. Every anesthesia department needs a champion to represent their interests. If you have interest or expertise in these matters, this person could be *you*!

Lessons Learned

- Bring valuable information from your specialty and the physician community at large when you work with the IT department. You are the experts in function and use of hospital systems.
- Work with your IT people to develop order sets and assist them in setting relative priorities for work efforts.
- Provide feedback as electronic medical records grow and evolve.
- Work to identify content that your department needs easy access to and develop a site where it can be posted.

Authors

Katya Chiong left a partnership in website design and hosting to pursue a career in medicine. She never imagined she would serve as a physician informaticist, integrating her interest in IT and medicine together.

Ray Graber serves as the vice chair for quality at University Hospitals Cleveland Medical. He is a believer that easy access to information improves quality of care.

Working as a Medical Legal Expert

59

Jeffrey A. Grass and Raymond G. Graber

Introduction

In this subsection, Jeff Grass shares his experiences working as an expert medical witness.

How Did You First Get Involved Working as a Medical Legal Expert?

My mentor at Johns Hopkins, where I trained and was on faculty for four years, began referring legal cases to me as soon as I finished residency—because he had more cases than he had time to review.

What Kind of Training or Education Did You Do or Continue to Do to Prepare for This Work?

Again, my mentor at Johns Hopkins was U.S. Congressman Dr. Andrew Harris. He was the director of OB anesthesia at Johns Hopkins and a tremendous resource in guiding me through my initial experiences in reviewing lawsuits. There are multiple educational platforms for training to be a legal expert. I have attended multiple symposia offered by a group of lawyers known as SEAK, Inc. These symposia are typically of two eight-hour days and include CME credits. SEAK, Inc. was founded in 1980, and they have trained over 40,000 expert witnesses, physicians being only a small fraction of them—as basically all civil litigation relies on expert witnesses.

Are There Any Organizations That Certify One to Be a Good Expert Witness?

I am not aware of any. However, there are legal registries that lawyers subscribe to that share depositions and court testimony of legal experts along with evaluations of their performance. The network of lawyers is very swift in weeding out ineffective expert witnesses.

J. A. Grass · R. G. Graber (✉)
Department of Anesthesiology and Perioperative Medicine, University Hospitals Cleveland Medical Center, Cleveland, OH, USA
e-mail: jeffrey.grass@uhhospitals.org; Raymond.graber@uhhospitals.org

S. Mohamed et al. (eds.), *Anesthesia Bridges*, https://doi.org/10.1007/978-3-032-08294-7_59

Is There a Mechanism to Screen Out Hired Guns Who Will Say Anything for Money?

The first tenet of being a legal expert is to tell the truth. Engaging in junk science or false testimony can result in a Daubert motion to exclude one's testimony. If this occurs, you are done as a legal expert. You will never be asked to review another case. There are many times upon reviewing a case when I have told an attorney that the case was indefensible. They respect this opinion, when properly explained to them, and continue to employ as they will still need guidance in settling the case. It has not been my experience at all that attorneys doctor shop until they get the answer they like best.

Do You Work for Both Plaintiffs and Defense? Why?

Historically I have been on the plaintiff's side 32% of the time and on the defense side 68% of the time. This breakdown is not necessarily by choice but rather represents the frequency with which I am contacted by plaintiff's vs. defense attorneys. I think it is extremely important to be unbiased in representing both sides. Nonetheless, there are data to suggest that 70% of physicians who engage in medical legal expert work will only defend other physicians. I think this is completely biased and wrong and will not present well to a jury.

Do You Ever Turn Cases Down, and Why?

First and foremost, I would never take a case that is outside my area of expertise. For example, I do not practice cardiac nor pediatric anesthesia. Thus, I would never review a case in either of those two sub-specialties. However, I will do my best to refer the lawyer to an experienced medical expert in the sub-specialty. If a plaintiff's attorney describes a case to me or sends the records to me for initial review, and I find the case has no merit I will tell them so and turn the case down. But this is extremely rare as every plaintiff's attorney I have ever worked with has told me that for every hundred cases they are contacted by patients to potentially represent, they only take one—1% of plaintiff's cases are accepted by the attorneys. Otherwise, they would be out of business because virtually every case on the plaintiff's side is done on contingency—if the patient does not collect money, the attorney does not get paid, after incurring significant costs.

Tell Me About the Process You Go Through for a Given Case: Detail the Steps from First Contact Through Court Proceedings

I am initially contacted by email or telephone call. We have a brief telephone discussion about the case and if it fits my area of expertise they will send me the medical records to review. After my review we will discuss the case in detail. The next step in many cases is to write a detailed medical expert review that has a specific format expressing my opinions on the case, and is ultimately sent to the opposing side's attorneys. Often a deposition ensues during which I am interrogated under oath regarding my opinions on the case. Depositions from all parties are involved, including the patient, family members, all physicians deposed, and other medical experts are sent to me to read and review.

Rarely, the case may ultimately go to trial wherein I have to travel to the jurisdiction where the case is being tried and testify in court before a jury. To put these various tasks in perspective, over my thirty-two plus years as a medical legal expert I reviewed approximately 400–425 cases. I have written about 150 expert reports. I have given about 80–100 depositions. I have testified at trial only four times. Nearly all cases resolve or settle prior to going to trial. The number of hours one puts into an individual case can vary from 3 hours to as many as 140 hours, depending on the amount of medical records involved, the number of depositions to review, and how long the case lasts over time.

How Do Lawyers Find You? How Do You Get Your Referrals?

Much of my work is repeat business from lawyers I have worked with before. Early on in my career, lawyers often found me from looking up a topic related to their case and finding a publication I had written, or a related lecture I had given at a national meeting. Other medical legal experts who have different areas of expertise also often refer lawyers to me. For those interested in getting involved in medical legal expert review, it is best to establish a niche for which you are known to attract cases. For example, a regional anesthesiologist who is expert in peripheral nerve block injuries.

***Note from the Editors:** *Jeff Grass is from* Vermont and that beautiful state is full of covered and other rustic bridges but also at this stunning walkway/bridge installation in Montpelier (Fig. 59.1).

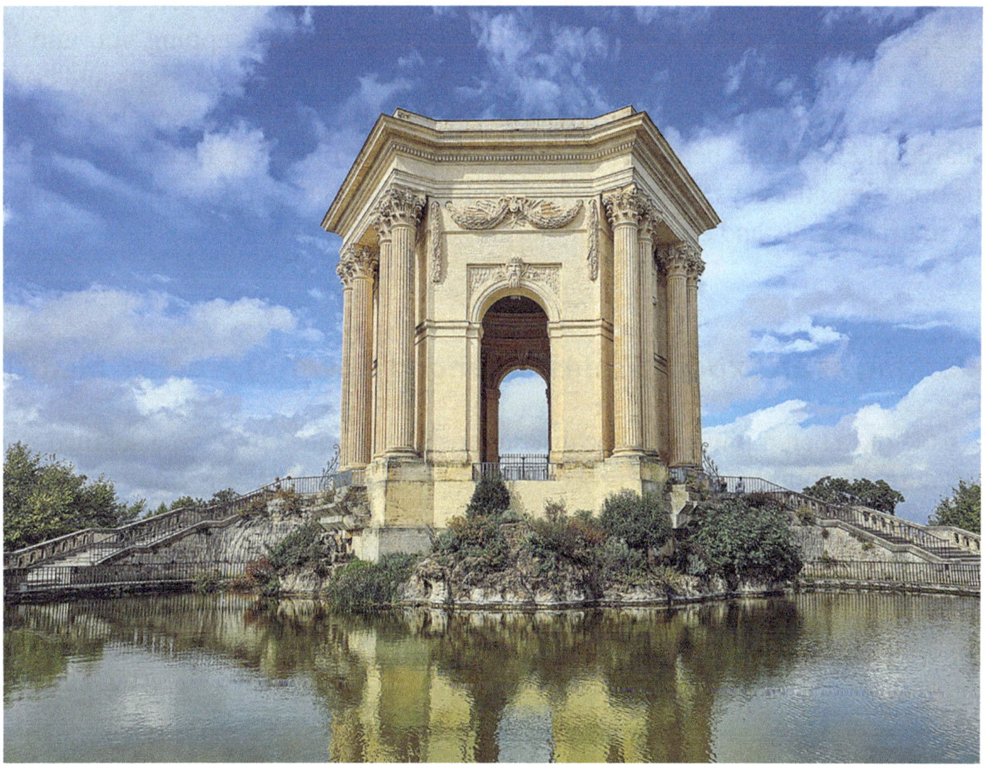

Fig. 59.1 The Water Castle in the Promenade du Peyrou in Montpelier, VT. (Photo: jaouad.K, image used under license from iStock.com)

Do You Agree with Malpractice Lawyers That a Faulty Consent Can Sink a Defense?

I have never had a case wherein the consent came into play in the outcome of the case.

Do All of the Cases You Review Involve Anesthesia Medical Malpractice Litigation?

The vast majority yes, but not all. Because of my extensive background in the early implementation of IV-PCA, I am often asked to review IV-PCA mishaps that do not involve anesthesiologists at all, but rather surgeons and hospital nurses. I have done a number of product litigation cases wherein a medical device or pharmaceutical delivery system was accused of malfunctioning. I have also been involved in patent litigation, wherein a generic drug maker is challenging the legitimacy of the patent of a drug before its patent has expired.

What Do You Like About This Work? What Do You Dislike?

First of all, being a medical legal expert is certainly not for everyone. One must always be well prepared and put sufficient time in to know the details of the case. Insist that the attorney you are working with adequately prepares and practices with you for any deposition or court testimony. It helps to be an experienced public speaker. Opposing attorneys are very adept and coy at trapping you into saying things they want you to say that may contradict your actual opinions during depositions and court testimony. They can also be very aggressive and intimidating. Nonetheless, with a reasonable amount of experience, a medical legal expert can be ironclad in defending their opinions, recognize the trap questions, and outwit the opposing attorneys. Oftentimes there are deadlines to get the work done and one must be very timely in returning calls and emails from attorneys.

How Has Working as an Expert Witness Changed How You Practice Medicine?

I think it has made me a better physician because in most cases I need to review detailed minutiae about a specific procedure, anatomy, or disease process, to be prepared to write a review, and to be interrogated at deposition about the case. Working as an expert witness has made me take better care of my own patients because I learn from the mistakes that other doctors make.

Lessons Learned

- If you would like to work as an expert medical witness, there are educational sources and meetings that can be attended to train you for this endeavor.
- It is best to take on cases in which you have a specific interest based on your training, research, or practice.
- The workload will vary from case to case, and extensive preparation may be involved.

Authors

Jeff Grass is a native Vermonter who trained at Johns Hopkins, then spent four years on faculty there. He later became chairman of the anesthesiology department at the Western Pennsylvania Hospital and Allegheny General in Pittsburgh for six years. He spent the next fifteen years at University Hospitals Cleveland Medical Center and is in the interesting process of moving to the next meaningful phase of his life. He enjoys traveling with his wife to go whale watching out of Gloucester, MA and to visit their two sons who both live in the state of New York.

Ray Graber serves as vice chair for quality in the anesthesiology department at University Hospitals Cleveland Medical. He has dual interests in cardiac and orthopedic anesthesia. During his 30+ year career, he has focused on process improvement, reduction of errors, and improving patient outcomes.

The Importance of a First Impression: Believe in Yourself!

60

Vesna Jevtovic-Todorovic

Our greatest weakness lies in giving up. The most certain way to succeed is always to try just one more time.—Thomas Edison

First, Shocked and Overwhelmed

It was getting late, and long shadows were crisscrossing the walkway leading to the hospital parking lot. My steps were hurried and uncoordinated. All I could think of was getting to my car before I could let myself be overtaken by emotions. A few more minutes, I kept telling myself. Just a few more minutes! Once I got in my car, I let the tears overcome me. I sat there for a while sobbing and contemplating the next steps, but mainly just feeling sorry for myself. What am I to do next? This is an impossible situation! My career is over! Oblivious to my surroundings, I just sat there completely unaware that it got pitch black while one thing became very clear—I was the main star in this pity party!

A couple of hours earlier, I sat in my chief's office and was told that my plan for the next step in my career was poorly laid out and without any merit in particular, my research direction was considered weak, my choice of mentor questionable, and the research technology I was to employ and master in order to conduct my research projects was referred to as dubious at best and obsolete at worst. As I kept sinking deeper and deeper into my chair, his voice got more and more distant, and all I could hear was his reference to my research plans as "clueless." The punchline was that if I was to pursue this research path, I was not to be paid and supported for my research endeavors and could be considered for a very part-time clinical pay upon finishing my residency training that was only a couple of months away.

Next, Discouraged and a Little Despondent

When I arrived home that night, my husband thought that someone really dear to me had just died. This is indeed how I felt. Once we put the children to sleep, I quietly sat in the family room slumped on the sofa as if the whole world was on my shoulders. He sat next to me and did not know how to begin. We

V. Jevtovic-Todorovic (✉)
Department of Anesthesiology, University of Colorado Anschutz Medical Campus, Aurora, Colorado, USA
e-mail: vesna.jevtovic-todorovic@cuanschutz.edu

S. Mohamed et al. (eds.), *Anesthesia Bridges*, https://doi.org/10.1007/978-3-032-08294-7_60

spent a long time in quiet contemplation and an even longer time talking it over. It was indeed a long night!

In desperation, I started to haggle with myself and question my career choices. Should I look for a different mentor who would be more agreeable to my chief? Should I consider a different line of research? What should I do to make my ideas more exciting and avant-garde? Am I a loser? What am I missing? Was all that I had done until that point meaningless? My husband just sat there growing more and more troubled.

All of a sudden, something hit me and got my undivided attention. I had been told that I could not accomplish something that I had set out to do! Something I believed in! Something that was important to me! I thought to myself, "This is my research, this is my passion! Is it worth it? Is it important? Do I want to live a life of quiet desperation, or do I want to follow my dreams?" I got off the sofa and, in a passionate voice, said to my husband, "I am going to do it despite all the hardships I will face! We will continue living the lifestyle of two residents in-training. We will make it financially and I will do what I set out to do!" There was a mischievous smile on his face as if it said, "I got my wife back!"

Onward

And so, the story goes. I met with my chosen mentor the next day and informed him that I would be happy to join his research team and that I would do it without being personally reimbursed as long as he was willing to support my research needs and provide me with the necessary resources in the lab. Once he agreed, I spoke to my chief and informed him that I would be glad to accept part-time clinical work so that I could maintain my clinical skills as an anesthesiologist. Then, I set out to do the work. Day in and day out, I worked in the lab, dropping off my younger son at daycare and my older son at school in the morning to begin my day working for free doing what I believed in and enjoyed so much! I was growing as a researcher every day learning massive amounts of information.

I cannot count how many times I was told by my colleagues that what I was doing was stupid. As a board-certified anesthesiologist, I was substantially underpaid and greatly overworked. But I had a plan and a goal—I set out to be a well-regarded and extramurally-funded clinician scientist and was willing to pay the price. And, surely, I did—for three long years until the first substantial funding came my way. Somehow, after so many months of pushing against all odds and seemingly getting nowhere, new avenues opened up for me.

Preparation and Presentation

So, what would I say to my younger self? More importantly, what would I say to my young colleagues? Although it sounds like a cliché, it is true today as it ever was – believe in yourself. After all these years of living an academic life, as I analyze what happened to me very early in my career, I realize how important it is to always be prepared to present yourself in the best possible light. Do not assume that someone will be able or willing to read between the lines and guess your true passion!

We live very hurried lives in a sound-bite culture; we may have only a couple of minutes to tell our story and grab someone's attention or even more importantly, impress them. It was not until I was in business school many years later that I learned the importance of a two minute elevator speech marketing what was referred to as the "Me, Inc." The main take-away—do not ever come across as "Clueless."

I close with a seemingly simple quote by Craig D. Lounsbrough:

> **In time, we become who we believe ourselves to be. And, if who we believe ourselves to be is less than who we are, we will live a life that is less than what it was supposed to be.**

So, keep on dreaming and do not let anyone tell you otherwise! Always be prepared and on top of your game! As the old adage goes, "You never get a second chance to make a good first impression." Indeed, it has been shown that first impressions are formed within the first few seconds, and these impressions, either positive or negative, will likely never change.

Lessons Learned

- Believe in yourself!
- Always be prepared to present yourself in the best possible light.
- You never get a second chance to make a good first impression.
- One last note from the editors—we do not know who the person was, who was so negative to the young Dr. Jevtovic-Todorovic and, frankly, we do not want to know. All we can say is what a terrible way to mentor. The take home message—*do not trash the young people*!

Author

Vesna Jevtovic-Todorovic has passion for her life and her career, as demonstrated by the events of her story. With the support of her loving husband, Slobo, she has three beautiful and accomplished children who look to both their parents as tremendous role models and great inspirations. Vesna continues to aspire to the next level. She is an accomplished and renowned clinician–scientist, educator, and mentor, patent holder, and chair of the Department of Anesthesiology at the University of Colorado Hospital.

Boundaries Should Not Define Us

61

Marc Leib

Introduction

Boundaries separate the known from the unknown, the possible from the impossible, and the likely from the improbable. Flat world maps of the ancient world sometimes labeled lands and oceans beyond charted regions as terra *incognita* or unknown lands, warning that "Beyond here there be monsters" Over hundreds of years, explorers pushed back these boundaries, proving the world is round not flat, exploring the unknown lands and gradually filling in the maps of previously uncharted territories.

Limitations and Life Choices

As young children we push back on our boundaries and explore our world with its almost limitless possibilities for our futures. As we age, however, we accept increasing limitations on our activities and our futures. Some of these limitations are of our own making through life choices while others are imposed by the outside world and its expectations of us. The decision to become a physician, knowing the hard work and self-sacrifice that it entails is one of those life choices. It creates boundaries that limit our fields of study, the amount of free time in our lives, and years of delayed gratification. These are boundaries we willingly accept to achieve our goals.

What Defines a Boundary?

Boundaries are what we make of them. We can choose to see them as walls that block out the light and keep us from seeing what lies beyond our current world. After all, we know that "Beyond here there be monsters." I prefer to view boundaries as sheer fabrics with openings I can step through any time I choose. Those boundaries allow me to see what lies on the other side and access terra incognita beyond the operating room and anesthesia.

I choose to define the boundaries that limit me rather than let others do so based on their own preconceived notions of what physicians should or should not do. We are often told that we should "stay in our

M. Leib (✉)
Health Care Consultant, Phoenix, AZ, USA

S. Mohamed et al. (eds.), *Anesthesia Bridges*, https://doi.org/10.1007/978-3-032-08294-7_61

lane" and practice medicine while leaving policy and business decisions to those who are "trained" to make them. I do not accept such limitations. Rather, I seek to expand my horizons, push back on artificially imposed boundaries and take some control over my professional life.

Early in my professional career I chose to push beyond the boundaries typically surrounding young physicians. My initial steps were relatively safe ones, including being elected as chair of the Department of Anesthesia within two years after beginning my career. I also got involved with the Arizona Society of Anesthesiologists and the Arizona Medical Association, beginning a lifelong involvement in organized medicine. After serving as president of the Arizona Society of Anesthesiologists and as only the second anesthesiologist to serve as president of the Arizona Medical Association in its more than 100-year history, I decided to pursue activities related to healthcare policy. That's when my sheer boundary turned into a slightly more imposing barrier.

***Note from the Editors:** Arizona has many notable bridges, but we think the historic Navajo Bridge is one of the most stunning (Fig. 61.1). The Bridge is a set of twin steel spandrel arch bridges that cross the Colorado River in the Grand Canyon. The first bridge opened in 1929 and the matching bridge was opened for vehicular traffic in 1995.

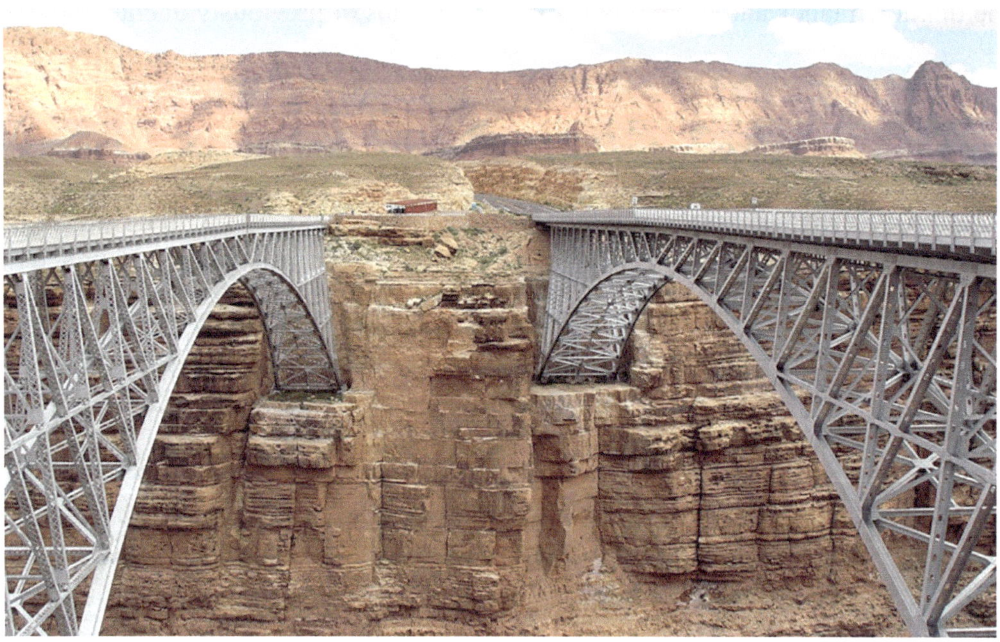

Fig. 61.1 The Navajo Bridge in Grand Canyon National Park. The original bridge is to the left and carries only pedestrian and bicycle traffic today. Photo: nps.gov

Healthcare Policy Boundaries

Although physicians are acknowledged as being experts in the science of medicine, we are not generally thought of as having any expertise in terms of healthcare policy. Policy makers are typically politicians, lawyers, lobbyists, and others with no medical training. To influence healthcare policy, my mentors recommended that I gain knowledge of how healthcare policy is made at the federal and state levels.

This could be accomplished in a number of ways, ranging from a weekend seminar to obtaining an advanced degree such as an MBA or JD degree.

Although certainly not necessary, I decided to go all out in this endeavor, so I cut my practice to half time and attended law school full time, graduating with a J.D. degree three years later. I joined a law firm in Washington, D.C. and helped represent its clients' interests to CMS, the 800-pound gorilla of healthcare policy. My medical knowledge was a definite plus. After three years in D.C., I was recruited back to Arizona to become the chief medical officer for the state Medicaid program that provides healthcare to over 1.5 million people. For me, this was a perfect combination of medicine, law, and healthcare policy. During the more than ten years as CMO for the State of Arizona, I continued to serve on the boards and committees of a number of medical organizations, including the American Society of Anesthesiologists, the Arizona Society of Anesthesiologists, the American Medical Association, and the Arizona Medical Association. I continue to do so to this day.

Not all of us need to get a formal degree or are in a position to do so, but any of us can learn the basic principles of business and policy decision-making. Young physicians should do this to protect themselves over the next 30–40 years of their practice careers instead of being at the mercy of others. Older physicians can apply their years of accumulated experience to help guide policy makers to make decisions that benefit physicians, our patients, and the Healthcare System.

Let Go of Excuses

After years of urging physicians to take some control over their professional environment, I believe I have heard almost every possible excuse justifying their desire to stay safely in their more limited worlds. They are too busy, have family obligations, do not want to make waves, or any number of other reasons for not engaging in activities that others may not appreciate or may even oppose. They confine themselves to going to the operating room, performing anesthesia, then going home without challenging the boundaries that define their professional environments.They never challenge those exercising control over our profession because we have collectively acceded that control to them.

But these are the same physicians who complain the loudest about government interference in their practices, unreasonable insurance rules, unnecessary prior authorization requirements, inadequate payments, and all the other complaints we hear every day. They expect others to bring about the desired changes but resent any suggestion that they have any responsibility for doing so themselves.

It is up to all of us to bring about the changes we desire. Not all of us can lead efforts to change our environment, but we can all participate in processes designed to bring about those changes. Join state and national organizations working on our behalf, get involved in political activities that promote changes that benefit our specialty and our patients, donate to candidates that support medicine, and donate to national and state PACs. These are activities that every physician can do to promote changes that benefit our profession and patients. We should not fear pushing beyond the boundaries of our safe worlds, either professionally or personally. We should take on the monsters that lie beyond the borders of the known, fill in blank spaces with new knowledge, and lead explorations into unknown territories. The alternative is stagnation, or worse, increasing encroachments on our profession by others.

Lessons Learned

- Choose to define your own boundaries and limits, rather than let others do so.
- Remember, a boundary is not an impenetrable wall, it is a transparent delineation that you can step through.
- It is up to all of us to bring about the changes we desire.

Author

Marc Leib practiced anesthesia for over twenty years, serving as president of the Arizona Society of Anesthesiologists and the Arizona Medical Association. Later he attended the University of Arizona College of Law while continuing his anesthesia practice. He later served as the chief medical officer for Arizona's Medicaid Program, a position he held for over ten years. Since his retirement from Medicaid, Marc provides consulting services mostly involving Medicare and Medicaid issues. He continues to serve the American Society of Anesthesiologists and the Arizona Society of Anesthesiologists.

An Englishman Abroad: Professional Tales and Travels of an Imported Anesthesiologist

62

Michael C. Lewis

Introduction

While career plans are unquestionably made in advance, progress can often be shaped by small inconsequential and possibly random events. Many of these experiences may be classified as "chance" recognition of *opportunity*. These events can also be a result of interaction with *mentors*; or the result of the recognition of *talent* by external entities. Regardless, in my case they sometimes led me a long way from where I intended.

Launch Pad: Family and Medical School

I grew up in the latter part of the twentieth century and was captured by the spirit of the times, seeing myself becoming an historian. This frightened my parents who thought the chance their child would become an underpaid historian merited intervention. Together, we struggled with this important question. Since their will was stronger than mine, I found myself applying to medical school.

In the UK, medical education was divided into distinct periods. The first two years focused on "preclinical" studies. One then had a choice: proceed directly to clinical studies (3 years); or take an additional year, obtain a bachelor's degree, and then proceed to clinical studies. I chose the latter. It was the start of an exciting adventure. Some of the highlights I will describe below.

Stepping Out of One's Comfort Zone: Professional Training

I was slated to immigrate to Israel. There I obtained a residency spot in oncology. However, it was not long before I learned that this was not for me. I applied and was offered an anesthesiology position in a small training program. At that time Israel was in the midst of a recession. The hospital where I was training was at risk of closing. I sought a more stable environment and obtained a position at a larger urban teaching hospital.

M. C. Lewis (✉)
Department of Anesthesiology, Pain Management, & Perioperative Medicine, Henry Ford Hospital, Detroit, MI, USA
e-mail: MLewis2@hfhs.org

S. Mohamed et al. (eds.), *Anesthesia Bridges*, https://doi.org/10.1007/978-3-032-08294-7_62

The chair of anesthesiology at that hospital became one of my first formal mentors. Through him I learned the *great power of mentorship*, the value of which cannot be emphasized enough. During my career I have had positive mentors from whom I have incorporated portions of their repertoires into my style. On the other hand, there were negative mentors whom I can point to and say I never want to behave like them—recognizing and learning from both is essential. In 1989, I moved back to the UK for what I thought was a temporary sabbatical. Now, the adventure took another strange turn, the impact of which was not obvious at the time.

***Note from the Editors:** Because bridges are about where you have been as you get to where you are going, we wanted to feature a beautiful bridge in Israel in honor of Mike's journey. We were delighted to find the pedestrian walkway of the Rabin Medical Center. The official name is the Petah Tikva Bridge of Strings. Interestingly, there is no intended symbolism to the bridge—the architect's main focus was only to "lend a bit more beauty to the important and moving project of the hospitals." (Fig. 62.1).

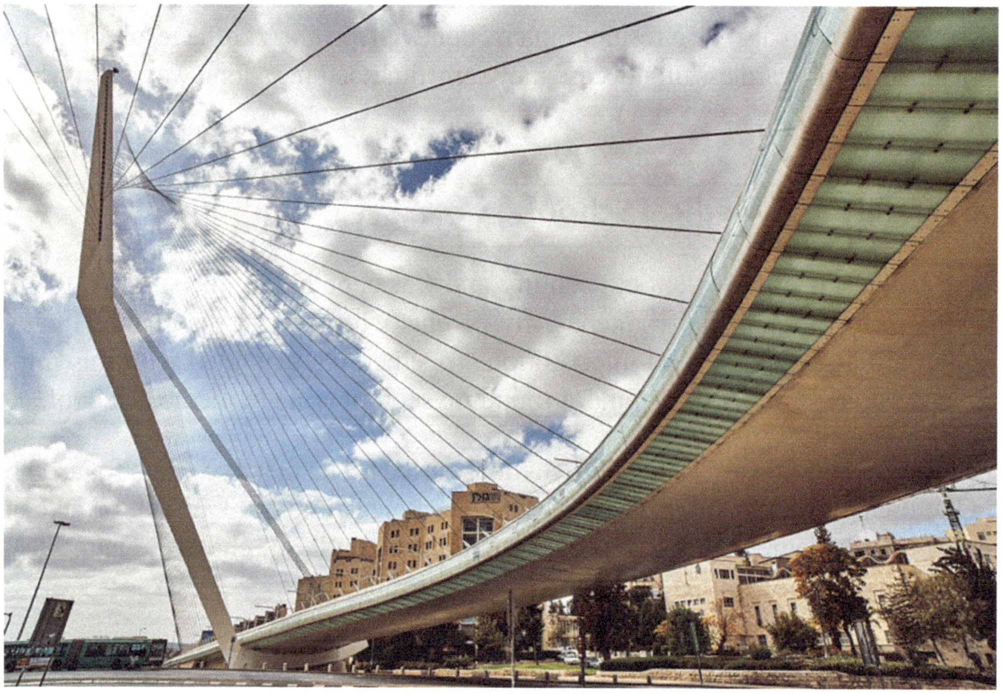

Fig. 62.1 A dramatic view of the Bridges of Strings in Petah Tikva. There is a larger bridge of the same name, designed by the same architect, in Jerusalem. Photo: Image used under standard license from stock.adobe.com

Back to My Roots—Never Let a Setback Hold You Up

In London, I had to restart my postgraduate training. My teachers encouraged me to sit for anesthesia boards. My fear was that taking the exam so early was a mistake.They reassured me, telling me with three years of training under my belt there was no way I would not pass. However, I failed. It was an emotional blow having never failed an exam. I seriously thought about giving up anesthesia. However, even a single disappointing failure cannot undermine dedication and resilience; my story was far from over. We decided the best way forward was to move to the USA.

Rites of Passage

I spent six months successfully studying for the required US licensing exams. The self-doubts were conquered, and the focus shifted firmly to the future. I secured an internship in Philadelphia. The focus continued firmly on the future. My next step was to find a residency program. I was offered a position in Miami by Manny Papper, which I accepted. Prior to his passing, Dr. Papper and I had many extended conversations, ranging from clinical anesthesiology, to professionalism, geopolitical issues, and theology. His mentorship and role modeling was invaluable to the development of my career and is something I have tried diligently to emulate.

Life as a Faculty Member

On graduating from residency my first job was at the Miami VA. I took my first tentative steps into the world of education, overseeing the anesthesia medical student program. Here I introduced one reform that had a significant impact. At that time, medical students at the University of Miami were exposed to anesthesiology only as part of a fourth year surgical clerkship almost always after residency application. As a member of the school curriculum committee, I was able to get the timing of the clerkship changed to a third year experience. This change resulted in a significant increase in University of Miami medical students applying for anesthesiology. *Engagement, no matter your experience level, is an opportunity to enact meaningful change in your surroundings.*

Eventually I became the service chief. The VA chief of staff requested that I become a full time VA employee with a secondary University of Miami faculty position. The process for the change was put in motion, but the department chair informed me that the University might not continue with the VA affiliation because of contractual issues. This obviously concerned me because my university appointment was important to my academic goals. I proceeded to discuss my concerns with the VA chief of staff, who curtly said "I accept your resignation."

For years I have reflected on those words and have tried to discern what to learn from the situation. First, I am a person of faith and believe, perhaps naively, that things happen for a reason and there is direction to the universe. Usually, I interpret the world using the construct of Most Respectful Interpretation (MRI); however, occasionally one encounters those whose motives are neither positive nor transparent. In this instance I appear to have been caught in a power entanglement. I transferred from the VA to Jackson Memorial Hospital, where I worked for over a decade.

New Adventure: Fulbright

At Jackson I joined the solid organ transplant team. I enthusiastically jumped into my new clinical role and also took my first foray into university governance. I served as the speaker of the medical school's faculty council and was elected to the university senate and served as its vice chair.

At that time, I applied for a Fulbright Scholarship. Before submitting I went to speak to my chair, David Lubarsky, about the idea. He was very supportive. Given the competitiveness we agreed that the chances of acceptance were low, but risk was worth it. However, he let me know, if I was successful, he would support me all the way. There are two lessons here; *if you do not ask, you do not get, and leadership is about supporting your team as fully as possible.*

The application process for a Fulbright is arduous and competitive. It is a long form-based process that has to undergo local review, then review in the host country. I was not successful. Although I was disappointed, it was kind of expected. This is where the story gets interesting. About a week after getting the rejection I received a letter at my office. The note was from the US State Department informing me that I had been accepted. You cannot imagine how much I was elated.

Later that day I received a phone call from the State Department telling me that the letter had been a mistake! I was devastated. It was a Tuesday afternoon. The next day the University Senate met, and I was an officer. Let me introduce Donna Shalala. She was the President of the University of Miami, and she attended every Senate meeting. Among a long line of leadership roles, she had served as Health and Human Secretary all eight years of the Clinton administration. I gave her the letter, and she congratulated me. Then I told her about the phone call. She asked me to leave the letter with her.

That Friday afternoon, at home, the phone rang. It was the State Department. A voice said, "Professor Lewis, I am honored to tell you that you have been accepted as a Fulbright Scholar." I was elated. Immediately, I sent an email of thanks to President Shalala thanking her. Not long after that I received a reply, saying it was her pleasure. She said that she had spoken to Condoleezza Rice's office, and it was taken care of. There are a few principles to be highlighted here.

- *First*, get involved, it is always better to have a seat at the table, if not, sometimes you can be the meal.
- *Second*, be ambitious, even if it feels out of reach.
- *Third*, and not so easily controllable, it is good to have an ally in leadership.

I completed my Fulbright, became the program director and senior associate dean for graduate medical education, and eventually left Miami for my first chair at the University of Florida. From there I was recruited to be chair here in Detroit. There are a lot of lessons along the way. However, these will have to wait for another time. Good luck!

Lessons Learned

- Always be present. Opportunity is a fleeting event. Unless one is at hand you may miss it.
- Lead one's team from the front. One's motto should not be 'charge'—rather it should be 'follow me.

Author

Michael Lewis is an "Englishman abroad." Following medical school graduation, he relocated to Israel where he met his wife, Judy. He followed her and their growing family to the USA, where they moved gradually northward to Detroit. Centrally located—they as parents can now easily visit their family on the East and West coasts.

Make All Your Good Ideas Happen

63

Berend Mets

It's not how many ideas you have. It's how many you make happen.

That is what I would have told my 30-year-old self, looking back three decades later. And "take the time to smell the roses" on the way up. It is the only career and life you have got; you might as well enjoy the journey.

Why do I give you this advice? Well, it is (relatively) easy to have ideas, but whether they are feasible in the context within which you find yourself, and so can be executed upon, is quite another matter.

Figuring this out takes work. A great deal of work. I always keep the words of Steven Covey close to hand. "Keep the End in Mind."

Let me give you an example to explain what I mean. Let us say you have an idea for a clinical research study. Can it be done in your institution: Enough Patients? Right Equipment? Analysis Expertise? And so forth.

But, more importantly, and this must be your ultimate goal, is *to publish the work, otherwise the idea did not happen*. So to achieve this goal find a model, a role-model if you will, in an already published paper that you can copy the structure for your research from; its statistics, its graph's and table's design, and then *imagine* the data that will be generated by your study and populate your planned paper with it, so you have a very good idea—before you ever start the actual study—what the effort of your work will translate to, and hence, whether it would look like something that the Journal you have in mind might be willing to publish.

Do not say. "Oh. I will see how it works out." "I do not have time for that now." No. Sit down, and pencil it out on paper. Predicting the likely outcome of your research so that you know in advance whether it will tell "the story" that is likely to lead to publication. Then you will know if your idea has at least a chance of being published, and you can make it happen.

B. Mets (✉)
Department of Anesthesiology and Perioperative Medicine, Penn State College of Medicine, Penn State Milton S. Hershey Medical Center, Hershey, PA, USA
e-mail: bmets@pennstatehealth.psu.edu

S. Mohamed et al. (eds.), *Anesthesia Bridges*, https://doi.org/10.1007/978-3-032-08294-7_63

And then be efficient. Always start one project at a time, and only when it is securely under way, can you start another. *Never leave an unfinished project to die*. You wasted time that you will never get back: a research abstract must be written as a full paper, submitted and if rejected, another journal must be found for its publication. Over and over, till you made all your good ideas, happen

Lessons Learned

- To be successful, finish what you start, and take it all the way to publication.
- An already published paper can serve as a good model as you plan a potential research project.
- If you plan well before you start a project, you increase the chance that publication will be the end result.

Author

Berend Mets was born in Indonesia of Dutch parents and lived on three continents before settling in South Africa, where he studied medicine and anesthesiology. He served as the residency director at Columbia University in the 1990s before becoming chairman of Anesthesiology & Perioperative Medicine at Penn State University.

An Airway Book for Acute Care Practitioners: From Conception to Reality

64

Steven L. Orebaugh

Introduction

Long ago, when I was a resident, I became interested in airway management. Not just providing it, since all anesthesiologists are interested in airway management, but also teaching it.

Early Days

I remember that we would have an occasional "airway lab" with a dedicated faculty member, on Friday afternoons, after the cases were finished. This was before the times of simulation centers. I liked playing with, and learning about, the various implements, and discovering how they could be used in patients. There was no internet then, just books, and I was disappointed at the available texts. While informative, they were not well-illustrated, in my opinion. Even the laudable "Bible" of airway management in anesthesia, the Benumof text, was largely illustrated with cartoons and black-and-white photographs that did not do justice to the devices and techniques.

Got the Plan on a Plane

A few years later, I was splitting my life between anesthesiology and emergency medicine—I had previously been an emergency physician. I attended my first ASA meeting, on the West coast, and began to imagine, on the long plane ride home, how I might design an airway atlas. Text would be secondary to the figures and pictures that would be lavish and explanatory. For each technique, I envisioned describing the practicality, affordability, portability, and evidence in favor of the implement or practice. It seemed like a good idea, and I resolved to call a publishing company about it.

Soon after I returned, I made a few phone calls, and one editor, at Lippincott Williams and Wilkins, expressed a degree of interest, soliciting my proposal for the book. I typed it up quickly and mailed it to him as we still did "formal" things by snail-mail in the 1990s. We talked on the phone, and he suggested

S. L. Orebaugh (✉)
Department of Anesthesiology, University of Pittsburgh School of Medicine, Pittsburgh, PA, USA
e-mail: orebaughsl@anes.upmc.edu

S. Mohamed et al. (eds.), *Anesthesia Bridges*, https://doi.org/10.1007/978-3-032-08294-7_64

that he would take it to his editorial board and see if they were interested. Unfortunately, that is where the idea met a dead-end. I never heard from him again. So, I shelved the proposal and went on about my business.

Proposal Redux

Several years later, I found myself in Portsmouth, Virginia, working at the Navy Hospital. As a reservist, I was called up to help the staff cope with a planned influx of casualties from the Iraq war. Fortunately, the number of casualties were comparatively few, but I spent a year there, which I enjoyed, as an opportunity to serve service members and their families. A few months before I was destined to leave, I received a letter. Shockingly, a new editor at LWW had found my proposal letter (the old editor had moved to a new position) amongst some other papers as he was becoming oriented with his position. He was interested! He contacted me, and after a phone conversation, gave me the go-ahead to develop the book.

One of the perks of my year with the Navy in Portsmouth was an opportunity to spend a couple of weeks aboard the aircraft carrier *USS. Harry S. Truman*, as "ship's anesthesiologist." It was not a taxing post—we had a few minor traumas and a number of dental cases under sedation. But it gave me some free time to explore the book concept—after I spent three days lying in my bunk, seasick!

Up until that time, I was spending half my life in anesthesiology and half in emergency medicine. An interesting job description, but logistically challenging. It worked well enough for a few years when I was single, but when I met my wife, we were somewhat older and brought things together in just over a year: engagement, new home, marriage, puppy, pregnancy…then a baby. Spending nights at the hospital between the end of the evening ER shift at 01:00 AM and the 06:30 AM OR the next day just did not work out with the obligations of a new family. I moved to full time anesthesiology just before I was called up by the Navy, which turned out to be a very satisfactory choice. But my interest in airway management straddled both professions.

A certain degree of credibility comes with anesthesia training when it comes to airways, and there was a hunger to do airway management consistently well in emergency medicine, as I learned when I would speak annually at a national EM meeting for the American Academy of Emergency Medicine. I wanted to take advantage of this and put out a quality atlas for practitioners and trainees in EM, internal medicine, perhaps even anesthesiology and nurse anesthesia. While I was bobbing about on the high seas in the Truman, I spent my spare time writing the short text chapters for the book. I also envisioned what photographs I would have to set up, and how I would capture them.

Putting the Project Together

When I disembarked, and soon thereafter was released back to my home institution, I had a pretty good idea of what I wanted to do. I set about obtaining permission from the administrators to take the appropriate photos (as well as the patients, of course), and turned everyone I could find, who was willing, into a model. It was surprising to see how eager people were to be part of the process. I spent a number of evenings in my office, trying to numb myself sufficiently to insert an LMA, so I could use an old bronchoscope to take photos of my glottis to illustrate just what happens when the device is in place (Fig. 64.1). It did not work—I just could not suppress my gag reflex sufficiently, so I had to obtain those photos on patients. But I did learn just how bad the "Lidocaine Lollipop" actually tastes!

After a year of writing, editing, and taking photographs, I finally finished working on the atlas. In 2006, Lippincott Williams and Wilkins published the *Atlas of Airway Management: Tools and Techniques*. In the book, I tried to carefully weigh the pros and cons of each of the available airway management techniques, devoting a chapter to each, and including a discussion of the prevailing evidence. I was very pleased with the way the publisher produced the book, and the illustrative emphasis was very clear. I received some complimentary critical review, which was very satisfying.

***Note from the Editors:** We went looking for built bridge structures that mimic what we see in our airway scopes every day and think the Golden Gate Bridge (from the air) comes close (Figure 64.1).

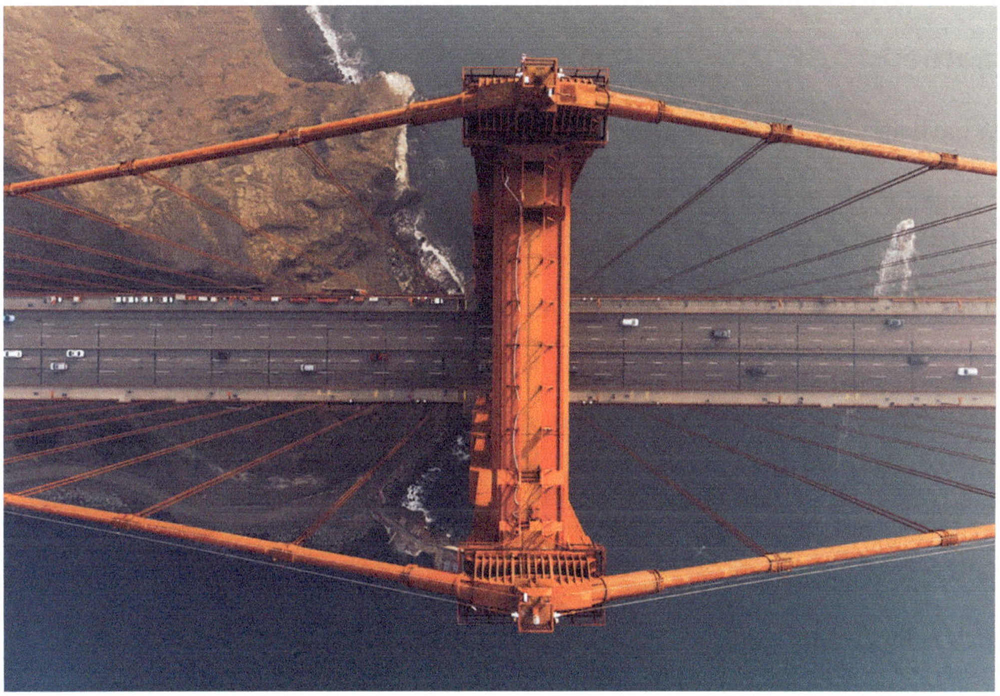

Fig. 64.1 From the air, the Golden Gate Bridge sort of looks like a sideways vocal aperture, wouldn't you say? Photo: Image used under standard license from shutterstock.com

Second Edition

What was very exciting was to be asked to develop a second edition in 2010. In the short five years between the development of the first book and this request, much had transpired: electronic texts, websites for airway management, and the pre-eminence of the video-laryngoscope. The project felt too big for a single author, and I reached out to others, both within and outside my department, to assist with the writing and the editing.

It was again a multi-year process, but in 2012, we put the second edition out. This was a much more comprehensive and more visually appealing atlas. Our sales were much more robust, and a Polish-language edition was created—since my mother is Polish, this was particularly gratifying to me, though I could not translate the text! This book included an e-version, in keeping with the times, and I was asked to provide videos of the various techniques, which I developed at my hospital, after obtaining consent from administration and patients. Unfortunately, the video editors that the publisher hired were unwilling to mask the patients' faces, and I eventually had to exclude these from the electronic version of the book.

By the early 20-teens, the availability of a nearly endless array of websites and online photos and videos of airway techniques rendered the utility of hard-copy books far less useful and desirable. There was no real market for a third edition of the airway atlas. But I had a wonderful adventure developing, writing, and then editing these two books. For that time period, I believe these atlases served a niche in acute care medicine, and the opportunity to help educate other practitioners and trainees was very gratifying.

Lessons Learned

- When you have an idea that really makes sense to you, pursue it.
- Do not be daunted by the system—it may appear impenetrable or unresponsive, but the people within it are not.
- Be persistent. Projects have inertia—if you let them sit, they do just that, but once you get them in motion, they take on an energy that will get you across the finish line.

The airway is an anatomic and engineering marvel. Respect it *every second* of your working life.

Author

Steve Orebaugh enjoys teaching regional anesthesia skills and other aspects of anesthesiology to residents and students. In his spare time, he enjoys running, swimming, woodworking, and gardening. He claims that he aspires to be a writer when he retires from medicine, but we happen to that he already is! Steve published his novel *The Stairs on Billy Buck Hill* in early 2022 to great reader reviews. It is available on Amazon and a great read!

Mentorship and Sponsorship

65

Vilma A. Joseph

Introduction

Mentorship and sponsorship have played major roles in the development of my career. The encouragement by others to achieve my goals is what I deem to be *mentorship*. It includes supporting my progress and being my advisor. On the other hand, *sponsorship* entails the opening of doors towards additional opportunities by those with the power or position to do so. Sponsorship includes all the characteristics of being a mentor and adds a few more things like advocating on one's behalf and influencing decision makers. *In other words, a mentor gives you perspective, while a sponsor gives you opportunities.*

Home and Early Life

A strong foundation at home is necessary for one to become successful in the world. I have been blessed to have a loving family who fostered a strong work ethic and a love of education. They were my first mentors and sponsors. My father is a civil engineer, and my mother is a homemaker and concert pianist. They encouraged my siblings (older sister and two brothers) and me to embrace education. Whenever there was an opportunity for enrichment activities, for example, math clubs, summer science programs, and the Westinghouse Talent Competition, they made sure that we were front and center.

College was a pivotal period for me since I originally was intent on a career in math and engineering. Allowing myself to be exposed to minority summer enrichment programs geared towards those interested in the health field helped me make the switch. Due to the influence of my family and my guidance counselor, I redirected my interests to medicine and excelled in college and the MCATs, thereby achieving acceptance into the world of medicine. My advice is to realize that parents and some guidance counselors truly have a young person's best interest at heart and may understand us better than we think.

V. A. Joseph (✉)
Department of Anesthesiology, Montefiore Medical Center, New York, NY, USA

S. Mohamed et al. (eds.), *Anesthesia Bridges*, https://doi.org/10.1007/978-3-032-08294-7_65

Beginning My Anesthesiology Career and Building Skills

As a junior anesthesiologist, I realized that I needed to find my niche in my field. I had a mentor and sponsor in my first supervisor. He sat me down and told me it was time to find an area of interest, start speaking publicly at meetings, apply for a grant, and begin writing papers. *I firmly believe that if you have any area of weakness, you must face it head on.*

As a naturally quiet person, I dreaded public speaking. Repetition is the key to becoming comfortable with public speaking. My interest in quality improvement allowed me to start practicing public speaking while providing resident lectures on that topic. I moved on to speaking at departmental grand rounds, interdepartmental grand rounds, state component society district meetings, state society meetings, national meetings, and international meetings.

A good way of figuring out how you are perceived is to listen to an audiotape or review a videotape of yourself. Have a trusted person, be it family member or colleague, critique your performance. It is essential to have a dry run of your talk so you can eliminate the pauses and glitches in one's presentation. In order to retain your audience's attention, stay current with the latest and greatest techniques of keeping adult learners engaged. This includes but is not limited to using different colors to emphasize a point, adding animation, inserting relevant clipart, showing figures and graphs from the journal article by using some type of snipping tool, or making your presentation look like a movie. It may be a challenge but try to show a video clip and use the audience response program to enhance participation.

Grants

Grant writing and creating publications are things that may require more expertise. It is a skill that must be developed. Ask for help at your academic center for grant writing techniques. There may be people within your department who can be your mentor and help you through the process. Try to get a grant within the first five years post residency when the reviewers are more lenient.

There are several places to seek a grant including your own academic institution, the American Society of Anesthesiologists, subspecialty societies, and the National Institutes of Health. Writing is something that can also be mastered. I have heard of people taking noncredit college writing courses. Often your job will reimburse you for your efforts. Fortunately, I worked with people and have a husband who loves to write, is patient, and does not mind revising my articles. *Remember, if you worked hard on a research project, it is an injustice to the medical community for you to not share your new findings.*

Branching Out

At some point it may be necessary to try something completely different in one's career. Through sponsorship, I was offered the opportunity to become involved in my state component society. I realized later that the invitation to attend a state district meeting that was having an election was really an opportunity for me to branch into another aspect of anesthesiology.

I started as the secretary for the district and over the course of the years became president of the New York State Society of Anesthesiologists. It was awkward being the only African American woman in the boardroom, but over time I became more comfortable. It is an honor to interact with colleagues and understand the issues anesthesiologists face and then bring it to the boardroom where decisions can be made to effect change. It also introduced me to the world of advocacy and interacting with state and federal legislators about anesthesiology. I would recommend taking a few hours out of the year to talk, text, email, or visit these legislators, since they have a major impact on our world.

Remember that all advocacy is local, so take time and visit a state or federal legislator pre- or post-call and tell them what issues are important to the specialty of anesthesiology. At first it may seem scary, but your state anesthesiology society and the American Society of Anesthesiologists are very willing to walk you through the issues. They even have classes on how to speak to legislators and the press.

Overall, mentors and sponsors may come in different genders and races/ethnicities. The key is to be receptive and be willing to walk through the door that someone is opening for you. A mentor will support you face-to-face while a sponsor will advocate for you behind closed doors. Remember to keep that door open for the next person and to move forward.

Lessons Learned

- Finding good mentors and sponsors can be key to developing your career.
- A mentor will support you face-to-face while a sponsor will advocate for you behind closed doors.
- Repetition is the key to becoming comfortable with public speaking. Practice your talks and get feedback from colleagues.

Author

Vilma Joseph is a professor of anesthesiology at Albert Einstein College of Medicine/Montefiore Medical Center. Her area of interest is quality improvement/patient safety, and she has worked at the state and national level on this issue. She is a past president of the New York State Society of Anesthesiologists. Vilma credits her success to her loving family that includes her husband and daughter.

66 Just Finished My Anesthesia Training and Now It Is Official, I Am an Attending Anesthesiologist. But Is It Enough? No!

Edwin Tavarez and Vilma A. Joseph

Introduction

There is so much to learn after you finish residency that cannot be taught in three years. You are constantly learning new things everyday clinically, but also on an interpersonal level there is so much growth to be had. If you are lucky, you will find someone to guide you through your journey, but most of us will find out the hard way what lies ahead.

From Vilma: Launching My Career

As an anesthesiologist we have minimal contact with patients. We see them a few minutes before they are anesthetized and a few minutes after they emerge, most of which they will not remember. Our largest interaction is with nursing staff and surgeons. Many times, throughout your career, we will not all be on the same page. The key to one's survival in this profession is how to deal with those times. The main concern is to do the best and safest anesthetic for our patients, but you will find that can sometimes be an inconvenience for a surgeon. At times this will create conflict and tension which can be difficult to manage. You will find yourself in situations where the safest thing to do for a patient is to cancel a case. Canceling a case can be a bigger hassle than just doing it. The big question is how we deal with all these obstacles. How do we maintain our role as a physician anesthesiologist, who is acting as a respected consultant and member of the perioperative team?

When I finished my residency, my first job was in a small community hospital in Texas. I was about to do a carotid endarterectomy on a 65-year-old male patient. He had a past medical history of coronary heart disease, hypertension, and type I diabetes. While taking his history, we learned that a month ago he went to the emergency room complaining of chest pain. He ruled in for myocardial infarction, was treated medically, and was supposed to follow up with a cardiologist. Unfortunately, he arrived for his elective surgery without a preoperative medical evaluation or tests.

E. Tavarez · V. A. Joseph (✉)
Department of Anesthesiology, Montefiore Medical Center, New York, NY, USA

S. Mohamed et al. (eds.), *Anesthesia Bridges*, https://doi.org/10.1007/978-3-032-08294-7_66

What did I do? I discussed my concerns with the surgeon and said that it was not safe to proceed with the case until the patient was deemed medically optimized by his cardiologist and had all appropriate preoperative tests. As it turns out, this surgeon was not accustomed to having an anesthesiologist contradict him and we ended up getting into a screaming match in front of the patient. Ultimately, the case was cancelled and was done a month later after a proper work up. Could I have handled that situation better? Yes.

Courtesy and Collegiality

As an attending anesthesiologist you must also learn to get along with your colleagues. I have, on many occasions, had arguments with fellow anesthesiologists over a variety of issues. One time, I remember having a major conflict with someone for showing up 15 minutes late to relieve me from call. To this day, I think about how I overacted over something so trivial that could happen to anyone.

Someone once gave me a piece of advice that I practice to this day. When you feel frustrated and angry over something, you do not have to necessarily respond to it at that moment in time. Take a minute, cool down, and think it over. You will find that you will look at a situation from a different perspective and a calmer approach.

You will meet people throughout your career who have different coping skills during stressful situations. Nothing beats the stress of taking care of someone else's life. This stressful work life is further complicated by whatever "drama" they may be having in their personal life. Often one needs to take a step back and look at the big picture and not get caught up in someone else's drama. The old adage is true: do not let your problem become my problem.

The lessons I have learned throughout my career have not only made me a better anesthesiologist, but also a better person. Peaceful discussion and expression of empathy will go a longer way in getting a point across. When we argue and become confrontational, the focus will always be about the nuances of the battle rather than the point we are trying to get across. Tackle the delicate balance of being firm but reasonable. These are skills that make one a good leader and can be used as a stepping stone in life. There is a lot to be said about learning the art of negotiation.

This can be clearly seen in our current fight for social justice and equality for all Americans. Peaceful demonstrations have gone a long way whereas violence has only taken the focus away from the issue that started the debate. Learning these lessons can be difficult at times, but in the long run, will get you further in life.

Nothing gives one person so much advantage over another as to remain always cool and unruffled under all circumstances.—*Thomas Jefferson*

Lessons Learned

- There will be times during your career when you will find that you are not on the same page with nursing or surgical staff. The key to one's survival in this profession is how to deal with those times.
- When you feel frustrated and angry over something, you do not have to necessarily respond to it at that moment in time. Take a minute, cool down, and think it over.
- Do not get caught up in someone else's drama.

The editors thank *Edwin Tavarez* for his assistance with this subsection.

Author

Vilma Joseph is a professor of anesthesiology at Albert Einstein College of Medicine/Montefiore Medical Center. Her area of interest is quality improvement/patient safety, and she has worked at the state and national level on this issue. She is a past president of the New York State Society of Anesthesiologists. Vilma credits her success to her loving family that includes her husband and daughter.

67 Always Say Yes

Charles Whitten

Introduction

In 1988, when I joined the faculty, I specifically remember sitting in A.H. "Buddy" Giesecke Jr.'s office. At the time, Dr. Giesecke was my chairman. Also present on that fateful day was M.T. "Pepper" Jenkins MD, the founding chair of our department. They were reminiscing about their careers as I intently listened to gain wisdom. What I heard that day has influenced me throughout my career.

Always Say "Yes!"

They encouraged me that when opportunities are provided, you should always say "yes." Saying yes provided you the chance to pursue an opportunity. You could always determine later that it was not the best path for you. If you said no, you were not giving yourself the chance to determine for yourself if it was the correct path.

Write It Down!

What was insinuated is that you should keep accurate records about positions held, responsibilities, and accomplishments. They encouraged me to maintain an accurate CV, to memorialize my progress. They also encouraged me to "write it down." This meant sharing the knowledge you have gained, via publications, regarding your observations and activities within the multiple realms of medicine.

If you follow these two principles, you will be well on your way to achieving academic promotion. It will also be important to be an excellent clinician, a skilled bedside teacher, and a subject matter expert within the topic of your choosing.

C. Whitten (✉)
Department of Anesthesiology and Pain Management, University of Texas Southwestern Medical Center, Dallas, TX, USA
e-mail: charles.whitten@utsouthwestern.edu

S. Mohamed et al. (eds.), *Anesthesia Bridges*, https://doi.org/10.1007/978-3-032-08294-7_67

Based on the discussion that day, *I have always said yes*. It has led me on a career that has included performing research on coagulation, the inflammatory response, and issues related to the economics of academic anesthesia practice. It has led to an in-depth study of the generations and the implications to medicine, in general, and our specialty in particular. This study of the generations has greatly influenced my leadership style. Saying yes has propelled me down a leadership path involving OR management, responsibilities as a cardiovascular anesthesia chief, educational leadership, interim chair, and chair responsibilities. I look back and truly appreciate the gift I was given on that fateful day. *Always say yes*!

Lessons Learned

- Always say yes to opportunities.
- Maintain an accurate CV to record continuously what you have accomplished.

Author

Charles Whitten is a native of Missouri but considers himself a Texan. Following receipt of his BSEE at SMU, he has spent the last 41 years at UT Southwestern in a multiplicity of capacities. His wife Cheri is his greatest advantage in life. His current professional passions include physician leadership development and collaborative projects related to the economics of academic anesthesiology practice. If you play golf, you are his friend!

Sometimes You Have to Say No

68

Judith Hellman

Introduction

This is some advice I want to share with my 30-year-old self, my present self, and others in our field, who are pursuing high-intensity academic anesthesiology careers.It is an issue that I keep revisiting at each new stage of my career. It is so that, at the same time as you stretch the boundaries of science, medicine, and health care, *understand your limits*. Fiercely protect yourself from becoming overextended.

Valuable Wisdom Then…

Five or so years ago, I was speaking with a mid-career successful anesthesiologist-intensivist-researcher. She brought up a conversation that we had fifteen years ago, when she was a resident and I was a junior ICU attending. At the time, I was getting some real traction in research. To paraphrase, I told her: "It's so important to know your limits and keep your eye on your professional goals. Establish your research program, stay clinically excellent. Do good but do it in areas that synergize with your expertise and professional goals. Sometimes you have to say 'no' to a request, an opportunity to serve on a committee, or an invitation to do a presentation on a topic that's outside your area of expertise."

And Later…..

At the time that she reminded me of this long-ago conversation, I had just hit a new stage of my career. It was an exciting and expansive phase. It was also a very stressful phase. I found myself at the boundary of what I could manage in the short-term and was starting to worry about how I would sustain this in the long haul. Worse, I was seeing some of the negative results of being oversubscribed. In particular, I was

J. Hellman (✉)
Department of Anesthesiology, University of California, San Francisco School of Medicine, San Francisco, CA, USA
e-mail: judith.hellman@ucsf.edu

S. Mohamed et al. (eds.), *Anesthesia Bridges*, https://doi.org/10.1007/978-3-032-08294-7_68

not finding time to write quality grant applications. In short, I was struggling. It was an interesting moment to have a former mentee remind me of my lesson to her some 10 years earlier. I had to face the reality that this would be a career-long issue, and that long-term strategies and vigilance would be needed to keep the right balance in my life through the different career phases.

While you are all on your individual journey, you will face this issue. If your career is going well, you will be recognized. That recognition, and the appreciation of your abilities will manifest in requests for you to take on leadership positions, join committees, editorial panels, and boards, and contribute to educational initiatives.

The tricky part is figuring out which and how many of these opportunities and responsibilities to add to your already busy schedule, which of them to decline, and how to gracefully decline. Please remember that nobody has unlimited reserves. Being oversubscribed or in perpetual sprint mode leads to reduced resiliency, lack of balance between work and other parts of your life, suboptimal performance in the areas that are of greatest importance to you, frustration, dissatisfaction, and can lead to professional burnout.

Suggestions

Although I cannot advise you on your individual limits, I have some general suggestions.

- *First*, pause before you take on a new responsibility. You do not need to immediately respond to requests to be on a committee, to do a presentation, or to organize a major event. If it is a large responsibility and/or you are uncertain, give yourself a few days to find out more. Make an informed decision. Talk to people, who can give you a sense of time requirements. Decide if the new commitment aligns with your professional goals and expertise.

- *Second*, stay vigilant for signs of being overextended, such as being slow to answer important time-sensitive emails, rushing to finish grant proposals without sufficient time to edit or to get critical input from others, working on slides late into the night or the wee hours of the morning of a presentation, being slow to write papers that are critical to grant submissions, and complaints from friends and family that you are stressed and overworked.

- *Third*, come up with some gracious ways of declining offers or of deferring an offer to a future date. It is okay to say that you are not able to take on another commitment for now due to time constraints, but that you do hope they will consider you in the future.

A high-powered academic career is a long-term endurance event, not a sprint. It is important to maintain reserves, to nurture yourself, and to organize your career so that you can achieve your professional goals.

Lessons Learned

- Fiercely protect yourself from becoming overextended.
- During your career you will be offered opportunities to take on new jobs and responsibilities. The tricky part is figuring out which to add to your already busy schedule, which of them to decline, and how to gracefully decline.

Author

Judith Hellman grew up in New York City and Vermont. She has also lived in Portland (Oregon), Boston, and San Francisco. She trained clinically in internal medicine, anesthesia, and critical care medicine, then did extensive research training. After completing her training, she wove together a career involving clinical work in the ICU, basic-translational research on the immunology of sepsis and critical illness, and the research training and development of physicians and scientists, in particular anesthesiologist–scientists.

The Sea of Faceless Bodies

69

David J. Ninan

Introduction

When you finish residency training you will be dumped out into a "sea of faceless graduates" vying for similar positions with nearly identical credentials. You will even compete directly with more experienced providers. The challenge is deeper than just getting a good job, it includes negotiating the best possible pay, benefits, and the type of work you will have the opportunity to do.

Employment Whys and Wherefores

Why would someone want to interview you, let alone work with you for years to come? How would they determine where you should start on their salary scale? What would make you stand out from the crowd?

A "value proposition" is a business concept describing a product's unique qualities that customers perceive as monetarily valuable. The more a person thinks it will meet a need, the more they will be willing to pay for it. This same principle applies to a career as a physician. The more value you bring to the table relative to your competitors, the more likely you are to land your dream job or negotiate the best possible compensation package. The concept is universal. The more value you bring to any setting in life the more power you can wield personally and professionally.

Be Aware of Your Unique Value

In the context of a career as a physician, a value proposition is a direct reflection of what you bring to your role that others do not. In other words, the more valuable you are to a person or organization the more power and authority you will be able to exert. Your curriculum vitae (CV) is essentially your first impression when applying for a position. Employers critique it to separate impressive candidates from

D. J. Ninan (✉)
Kansas College of Osteopathic Medicine, Wichita, KS, USA

S. Mohamed et al. (eds.), *Anesthesia Bridges*, https://doi.org/10.1007/978-3-032-08294-7_69

the rest of the pack. Thus, it is vitally important your value proposition is readily apparent on your CV, and you treat it as your primary marketing document.

Individuals can bring extrinsic and intrinsic values to their career. Extrinsic value refers to external components such as specialized areas of knowledge and expertise. In anesthesia, these can be formal things like fellowships, degrees, or certifications. They can also be less formal distinctions like being a subject matter expert in an area your employer values. For example, an employer concerned with accrediting body site visits may value someone with a deep understanding of regulatory compliance. It is wise to take an inventory of your areas of strength and passion to learn what may be valuable to an employer. On your CV, the informal attributes can be presented in the form of work projects, task forces, committees, papers, and lectures.

You can also tout intrinsic values that are personal traits or characteristics. For example, many anesthesia groups want attendings who are solution-oriented and possess a great work ethic. These characteristics are harder to quantify on your CV than extrinsic distinctions. One way to objectively demonstrate intrinsic values is to consistently update your CV. For example, imagine you are selecting one individual to interview, and the first CV has medical school, residency, and one poster presentation at a national meeting. A second CV has six posters spread out throughout the years in residency. All things being equal, this second CV demonstrates a more consistent willingness to go above and beyond minimum requirements.

***Note from the Editors:** David Ninan is from and practices in California and there is no more beautiful place in that beautiful state than Muir Woods National Monument. This little bridge spans Redwood Creek in the Woods (Fig. 69.1).

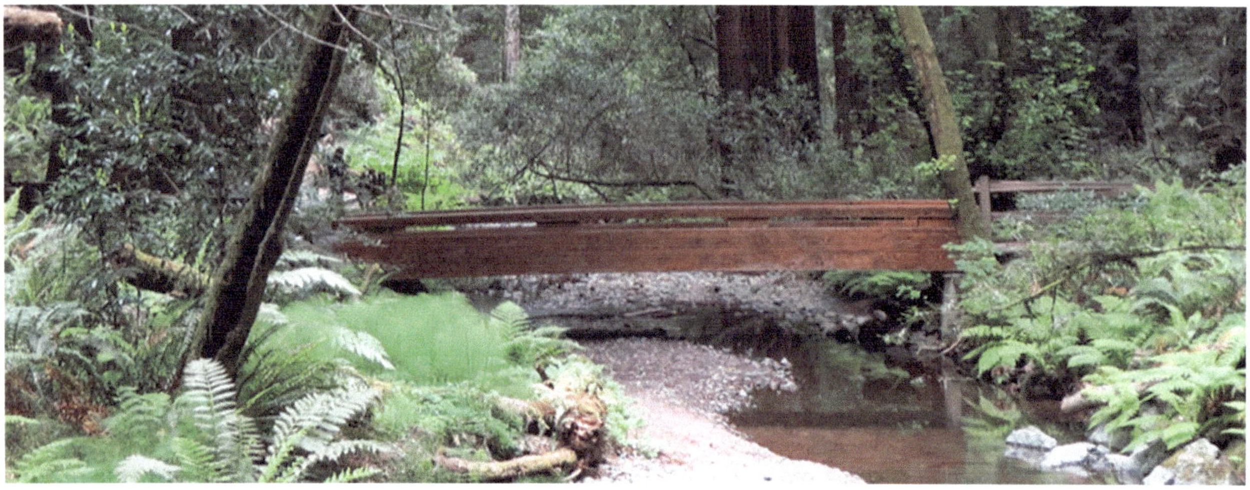

Fig. 69.1 The bridge over Redwood Creek at Muir Woods National Monument. It is a breathtaking and awe-inspiring place. *If you have never been, put it on your bucket list near the top and try to get* there. Photo: nps.gov

Is There a Fit with What the Employer Is Seeking?

After taking a personal inventory of your unique areas of value, you need to assess what your customer or future employer is seeking. You can often spot extrinsic areas of need in the form of their employment posts looking for physicians, for example, looking for a specific fellowship or subject matter expertise. Learning the intrinsic values that they are seeking generally requires learning about the job environment and its culture by tapping your network.

In addition to your existing network, you can use professional networking websites like LinkedIn, Sermo, or Doximity to gain valuable information as to what their needs may be. If you do not have anyone in your sphere with internal knowledge of the organization, find ways to talk to current employees for an informational interview and ask them what they are looking for, what their challenges are, and so forth.

I recommend if you are in training (or in practice) that you pick a few employers that you may like to work for and research what areas they seem to need help in. This can provide clues as to what areas are more in demand in your specific market and allow you to develop the areas that overlap with your own interests and passions. For example, if quality improvement is a concern, you can take on a few quality projects each year and add them to your CV. Three years later you could have six items on your CV that are specific to one of their pain points. Not only is this work relatively easily spread out over the course of your studies; it objectively demonstrates to the outside observer that you have a longstanding interest in quality.

Lessons Learned

- As I reflect back on my own career, the most important thing I have learned is to always seek ways to create value.
- Ultimately, a strong value proposition gives one a powerful voice that will directly translate into better care for our patients.

Author

David Ninan is a California native with a mission to support physicians along their career journey to create meaningful lives. Life is too short to leave your career up to chance. Live your passion.

70 My Part-Time Career as a Military Anesthesiologist

Gregory K. Applegate and Raymond G. Graber

Introduction

For this chapter, Ray interviewed his colleague Greg Applegate about his career in the military. The information below describes Greg's personal experiences.

My Army Background

My father went to Vietnam as an Army veterinarian and then joined the Reserves and subsequently the National Guard after he returned. So, the military was always a part of my family life as I grew up. When I was accepted into medical school, I decided to apply for the Army's Health Professions Scholarship Program (HPSP) to help offset the cost of school. The benefits included a full tuition scholarship, health insurance, books, a stethoscope, and a monthly stipend. This would be in exchange for a few years of active-duty service. Reassurances were provided that medical school and residency would not be interrupted in the event of an international conflict, and my assignment was to complete my education. I chose the Army specifically because of its robust graduate medical education (GME) programs.

Combining Training and Medical Education

During the summer between my first and second year of medical school, I went to San Antonio for the Army's officer basic course – which was a requirement for all medical and dental students who were in the program. Military "boot camp" for medical students sounded like intense training; however, I would volunteer that my fellow two hundred medical students enjoyed this time away from medical school lectures.

Disclaimer: The views expressed in this presentation are those of the author and do not reflect the official policy of the Department of the Army, Department of the Air Force, the National Guard Bureau, the Department of Defense, or the United States Government.

G. K. Applegate (✉) · R. G. Graber
Department of Anesthesiology and Perioperative Medicine, University Hospitals Cleveland Medical Center, Cleveland, OH, USA
e-mail: Gregory.Applegate@UHhospitals.org; Raymond.graber@uhhospitals.org

S. Mohamed et al. (eds.), *Anesthesia Bridges*, https://doi.org/10.1007/978-3-032-08294-7_70

During my third and fourth years of medical school, my military obligation was to participate in two four-week elective medical school rotations at military hospitals. These clerkships would be influential in helping to choose a specialty as well as an opportunity to network with residency directors. With so many clinical rotations and locations to choose from, I selected an anesthesiology rotation in Washington, DC, for my third year and then a surgical intensive care unit (SICU) rotation in San Antonio, TX, for my fourth year clerkship.

Both of those rotations were excellent and instrumental in helping me to decide on my future career. Medical students interested in anesthesiology were required to apply to at least five military transitional year internships. However, the Army's GME department approved my request to enter into the civilian match for my anesthesiology residency – I had a goal to try to be closer to home. I completed my internship at Tripler Army Medical Center in Honolulu, Hawaii, where there are beautiful beaches! I then returned home to Ohio to do my residency at University Hospitals of Cleveland.

On the Job

After finishing residency, I was stationed at Walter Reed Army Medical Center in Washington, DC, as an anesthesiologist and started my medical school payback. A majority of my mentors from residency volunteered that I would learn a ton about anesthesiology during my first six months as an attending anesthesiologist, and they were correct. Eight months after finishing residency, I was deployed to Iraq as a combat anesthesiologist for six months. The deployment was challenging; however, I was thankful to be surrounded by a "Band of Doctors" who were colleagues, mentors, and friends.

After deployment, my military obligation was half complete, and I was starting to think about where I wanted to work and move to. Although very tempting to separate from the military, I realized I wanted more experience in regional anesthesia. A large population of patients at Walter Reed were wounded in combat and benefited from continuous peripheral nerve blocks which helped reduce opioid consumption.

During my last year of active-duty payback, I applied for the acute pain and regional anesthesia fellowship at Walter Reed Army Medical Center. Many of my colleagues advised me that I could learn regional anesthesia on my own; however, I sensed that this would be a great learning opportunity with a short payback of two years.

The fellowship was a unique year that was loaded with clinical training, cadaver dissection, and a humanitarian trip to the Republic of Vietnam to teach ultrasound-guided regional anesthesia. Completing a fellowship after working as an attending anesthesiologist was also an interesting experience. With ultrasound not readily available during my residency, the residents at Walter Reed had more regional anesthesia ultrasound experience than I did when I started my fellowship. Immediately after fellowship, I was relocated to Womack Army Medical Center in Fayetteville, NC, for two years – which fulfilled my active-duty service obligation.

After seven years of active duty, I decided to voluntarily separate from the Army and accepted my first civilian job back at University Hospitals (UH) in Cleveland, where I had trained. Active-duty life provided many unique opportunities to travel and relocate, but I wanted to be closer to family.

Return to Civilian Life

About three years after returning to Cleveland, my hospital decided to open Level I trauma services to Northeast Ohio. To be honest, I transfused more blood in Iraq than during my entire residency and was not really interested in trauma anesthesia. With my previous combat medical deployment, I was approached and asked if I would participate in the trauma schedule. As a new trauma hospital, my anesthesiology colleagues and I embraced this new service to make sure that our patients were receiving the best care that we could deliver.

One of our trauma initiatives involved having an anesthesiologist and mid-level anesthesiology provider paged to the emergency room for full activations. Multiple trips to the emergency room for trauma activations triggered a lot of memories from my deployment. During those early months of providing trauma services, I was appreciative that the military provided me the experience to expeditiously set up the Belmont Rapid Blood infuser in the operating room. I suppose you can say that things happen for a reason, but the implementation of a new Level I trauma hospital, combined with my prior military service, spiked my interest in pursuing a military career in the National Guard.

***Note from the Editors:** Did somebody say something about *THE* Ohio State University in his bio? It just so happens that while we were editing the first draft of this chapter, we were in Columbus for the first round of the NCAA basketball and made a visit to the OSU campus. In Greg's honor, we snapped this picture of a small but dramatic bridge over the Olentangy River (Fig. 70.1).

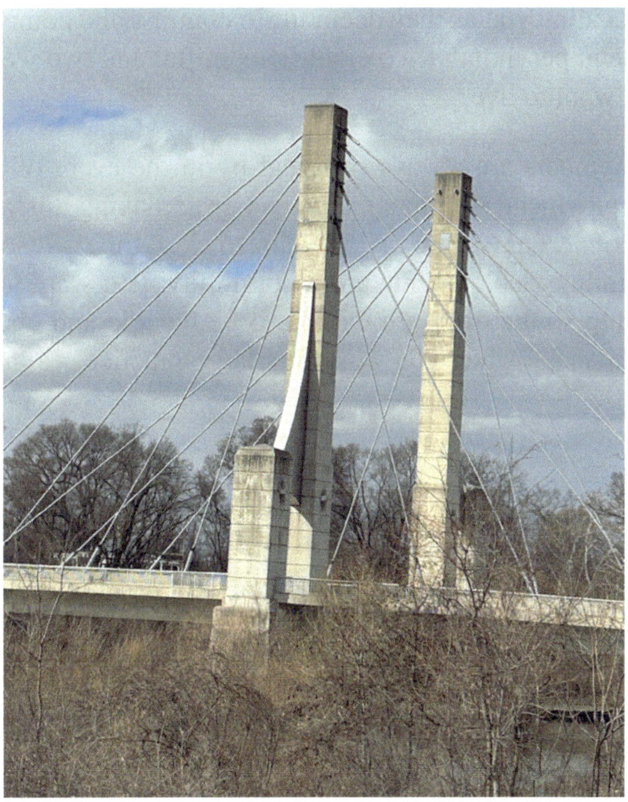

Fig. 70.1 Bridge over the Olentangy River in Columbus, Ohio, just northwest of the Ohio State stadium. Photo: Catherine Marcucci

Working as a Reservist

The Reserves and the National Guard are both reserve components of the US military; however, they are separate military organizations. The National Guard is a state-based military force that can transition to the reserve components when activated for federal deployments. Each of the 50 states and four territories of Guam, the Virgin Islands, Puerto Rico, and the District of Columbia maintains a National Guard which is under both state and federal government. Reserve soldiers do not have a state mission and fall under the federal government. The Reserves and National Guard are available for national defense, and both contribute to humanitarian missions at the state (Guard), federal, and international levels.

I was always interested in aviation during my childhood but never pursued flying lessons. One of the surgeons I worked with at UH was a flight surgeon for the Air National Guard and advised me to pursue the Guard, given my prior active-duty service. These two factors led me to take advantage of an opportunity to join the Air National Guard medical unit in my hometown. It has been interesting to learn about the aeromedical considerations of flight. My anesthesiology background would also allow me to work with surgical teams as well as transport patients in the "Flying ICU" of military airplanes.

Integrating Civilian and Reserve Jobs

The decision to join the National Guard while also working full-time for an academic medical center did require some careful thought. Specifically, I wanted to make sure that I would still fulfill my civilian in-house call and weekend obligations. Active-duty military service is 24-7 and 365 days a year combined with the military relocating you as they deem fit. In contrast, the commitment to National Guard/Reserves duty is one weekend per month (two eight-hour shifts) and two weeks a year for training and you can choose where you want to live.

National Guard/Reserve members are always on stand-by in the event of a national or international emergency that requires deployment. Communication is key to making this work. I always try to update my civilian employer as soon as I am aware that I will need extra time off, so that my shifts can be covered. Although rare, last-minute deployments are a possibility, you want to have a good relationship with your hospital leadership so that they are willing to be flexible and understanding of this issue. I think that this is easier to manage when you work in a large practice – a larger group will have more manpower to cover for you.

Benefits

The benefits of being a reservist are as follows. Reservists and National Guard members receive compensation for working weekend drill duty or any days spent on active duty. Reservists and Guardsmen have access to TRICARE health and dental insurance at an affordable cost. Depending on how many years of service, a Reservist or Guardsman can retire and earn partial retirement compensation after 60 years of age. The true reward of the Reserves/Guard is that they both provide the opportunity to serve the Nation and help provide medical care for our military.

Duty Experience

What is my duty like? When on weekend duty, one day consists of training and reviewing policies on various military topics. The goal of training is to optimize readiness in case of a deployment. The other day involves patient care; however, our medical clinic functions as an occupational medicine clinic and I review medical documentation from service member's civilian health care providers. Medical record review is very important in establishing that Reservist/Guard members are medically qualified for deployment. Although easy to assume that military personnel are physically fit, medical conditions do arise that are not compatible with military service. As previously stated, in the event of an overseas deployment, I would work as an anesthesiologist with a surgery team or participate in aeromedical evacuation.

Equipment

The anesthesia equipment for a deployment or humanitarian mission would be comparable to hospital-based setting with the exception of size and portability. Drager manufactures the Fabius Tiro M, which is an anesthesia machine on the smaller side with the ability to deliver volatile anesthetic gas. Familiarization with assembly/disassembly and establishing safe volatile anesthetic gas scavenging are important considerations.

For more austere environments, portable transport mechanical ventilators are available which require TIVA instead of volatile anesthetic gas. Portable transport monitors permit ASA standard monitors to include pulse oximetry, heart rate, blood pressure (non-invasive or arterial), end-total carbon dioxide, and temperature for surgery and/or medical evacuation. Humanitarian medical missions and military anesthesia are similar as both have unique considerations for the austere medical environment.

Time Commitment

If you were to ask me how long the time commitment is, the answer would be – it depends. Some medical specialties in the Reserves or Guard may be eligible for a bonus that requires a multiyear obligation; however, it is always changing depending on the Defense budget. If one decides to decline the bonus or one is not available, you can serve just one year at a time. The process to separate or retire usually takes anywhere from 6 to 12 months.

Closing Comments

Looking back on my time as a military medical physician, I am appreciative that my experiences in trauma, blood resuscitation, regional anesthesia, total intravenous anesthesia (TIVA), and acute pain ketamine infusions have provided a positive influence on my career and practice as an anesthesiologist.

You only get one or two chances to plan out your career, and sometimes we do not necessarily appreciate how those decisions will play out. I am proud to have chosen this path of military anesthesiology, or perhaps it chose me. My best advice for any professional is to promote the Air Force's core values:

Integrity First

Service Before Self

Excellence in All We Do

These are a great beacon for today's practicing physician.

Lessons Learned

- Working as a reservist or Guard member offers financial incentives as well as the chance to serve your country.
- The key to making it work is having a good relationship with your civilian colleagues and leadership.
- My career as a military anesthesiologist has enriched my civilian career and I would say the reverse is true, as well.

Authors

Greg Applegate is an anesthesiologist who trained at University Hospitals-Case Western Reserve University and Walter Reed Army Medical Center. He has practiced in both military and civilian healthcare systems. Teaching regional anesthesia with ultrasound-cadaver workshops is a passion and he loves to ask residents to draw the brachial plexus. An enthusiastic Ohio State alumnus, you will find him spending his autumn Saturdays in Columbus at the "Horseshoe!"

Ray Graber serves as vice chair for quality in the anesthesiology department at University Hospitals Cleveland Medical. He has dual interests in cardiac and orthopedic anesthesia. During his 30+ year career, he has focused on process improvement, reduction of errors, and improving patient outcomes.

71 My Journey from Surgical Resident to Anesthesia Chair to CMS Chief Medical Officer

Lee A. Fleisher

Introduction

When I finished medical school, I thought I would be a physician-scientist in the field of transplant surgery. I entered a residency at the University of Minnesota, where you could obtain a PhD during training. Having always lived in the New York–Philadelphia area, I was excited to explore a new part of the country. However, being far from home, especially when you felt you had chosen the wrong specialty, was not easy. I made the very hard decision to change specialties—I still remember the call to my parents—and was fortunate enough to obtain an anesthesiology residency closer to home at Yale University.

Another Difficult But Great Decision

The next major difficult decision occurred when I finished my residency. I met a fantastic woman at Club Med in Mexico, but she was from Baltimore while I had just joined the faculty at Yale. Once again, I had to make a difficult decision about where I would work and live and, in the end, I felt it was best to move to Baltimore to marry that woman, now my wife of 30+ years.

However, I still remember the difficult conversation of talking with my mentor and the chair of the department, Paul Barash. Paul thought I was making a mistake in moving to Baltimore since it would negatively impact my career. However, it was clear that both my wife and I would have good jobs in Baltimore, while the job climate in Connecticut was extremely difficult for my wife due to a major economic downturn in the state. Important life lessons – focus on what is best for the team and it is important to start a life together.

L. A. Fleisher (✉)
Center for Clinical Standards and Quality (former CEO and Director), Center for Medicare and Medicaid Services, Baltimore, MD, USA

Departments of Anesthesiology and Critical Care and Medicine (Emeritus), Perelman School of Medicine of the University of Pennsylvania, Philadelphia, PA, USA
e-mail: Lee.Fleisher@pennmedicine.upenn.edu

S. Mohamed et al. (eds.), *Anesthesia Bridges*, https://doi.org/10.1007/978-3-032-08294-7_71

What I Would Tell My 30-Year-Old Self

Despite the move, I was able to quickly re-establish my academic career at Johns Hopkins. I was very focused on my career and traveled frequently despite having two young children. I would clearly tell my 30-year-old self that it is okay to work hard and enjoy the benefits of academia, but it is important to integrate it with your personal life. Most importantly, when at home, it is critical to be present for your family. I may have been home but was frequently distracted, especially once I became a chair, and I would do it differently now. I would carve out special time for my children and not allow calls to interrupt. I would not bring my phone to the dinner table and no longer do.

Here's a Mistake I Once Made, and What I Learned from It

"*What got you there does not always keep you there.*" After six years as chairman, I thought I was doing extremely well and felt that I was an excellent leader. Fortunately, Penn reviews its chairs every six years, both by an internal and external committee. The internal review was chaired by a former chair of surgery and included representatives from outside of the department. Despite receiving favorable reviews from the dean and the department, the health system felt that I was not supportive of their mission and the director of perioperative services (a surgeon) painted the department as the reason for the slow turnover. The external reviewers (fellow anesthesia chairs) were very supportive of the department and openly disagreed with the hospital and health system leadership. Unfortunately, this made the situation worse because the health system viewed the external reviewers as biased toward the department.

In analyzing the situation, it became clear that my leverage to achieve the goal of leading and negotiating on behalf of the department had been compromised. On the positive side, I still had the support of the dean/executive vice president for health affairs, who was technically over the health system and my department. However, the day-to-day negotiations to obtain more support, such as additional faculty/CRNAs and anesthesia technicians, were limited and they were clearly accepting the surgeon's narrative. My analysis of the situation was that my current approach of "fighting" with the system to make them understand our needs was not effective, but resigning would be worse, given my continued support by the dean. It became clear that the current approach was not working but how would I learn a new one?

***Note from the Editors:** One of Lee Fleisher's favorite bridges is the Hertford College Bridge in Oxford, England (Fig. 71.1). The Bridge is actually a skyway that connects two parts of Hertford College—the administrative offices with the student lodging areas. The legend that it was once closed so that students would be forced to take extra flights of stairs and lose weight is false—the bridge has always been open at all times to students at the College, who are frequently seen in silhouette crossing it. The skyway is closed to the public.

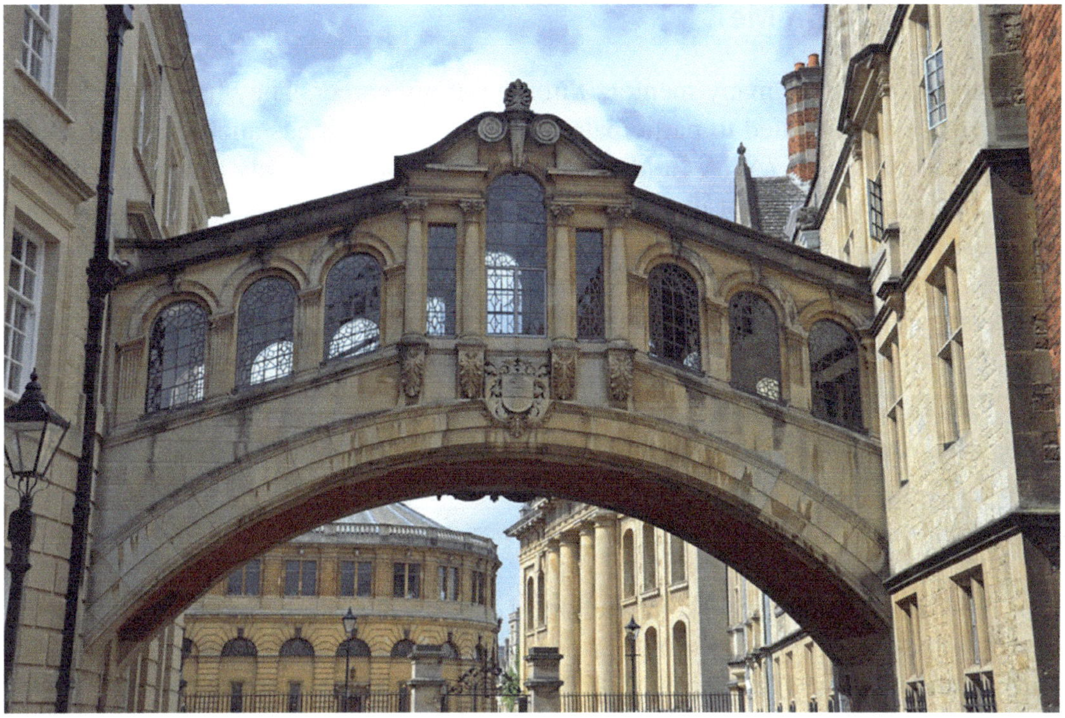

Fig. 71.1 Hertford College Bridge, in Oxford, England. The bridge is also known as the Oxford Bridge of Sighs due to its similarity to the better-known Bridge of Sighs in Venice. Photo: Image used under standard license from stock.adobe.com

Coaching

One of the health system leaders suggested an executive coach. I interviewed several and found one whose style I liked—blunt and no nonsense. After she completed a 360-degree review, she came back and started teaching me new skills to not get hijacked by the director of perioperative services and take up my "role" as the chair of the Department of Anesthesiology and Critical Care in all situations. By the time I was reviewed at the end of my second six-year term, I had the full support of the system and was able to get substantially more financial support from the hospitals and an unconditional and rare third term as chairman. When it came time for the director of perioperative services to retire within the past year, the new hospital CEO appointed my clinical director to the open position despite the surgeon's desire to have another surgeon.

My key learning was that sometimes you need help to get to the next level. Additionally, skills such as staying in role and responding unemotionally are critical to achieving one's goal. Finally, my coach taught me that if you do not control the narrative, then someone else will. The Director of Perioperative Services controlled the narrative that long turnover times were an anesthesia issue, and we were always looking for more financial support. I had to learn how to reframe the narrative in such a manner that the hospital and health system leadership could understand that it was multi-factorial and the Department would work to be part of the solution.

What My Mentors Taught Me

I have been very lucky to have many mentors throughout my career. They have frequently told me to choose wisely. I have been invited to participate in multiple committees and opportunities ever since I was invited to serve on the ACC/AHA Guideline Committee approximately four years after completing my residency. However, you cannot do everything and being too diffuse, especially at a more junior stage of one's career, can be detrimental to long-term goals. Personally, I reviewed each new opportunity along a few dimensions: potential to advance my primary research and career agenda, potential to advance my personal interests, and the amount of effort or the opportunity costs. So, if an opportunity had a low potential to advance my career or was not of major personal interest during a period in which my time was limited, I frequently declined the offer.

Other Lessons

There will be multiple opportunities throughout one's career when offers for advancement will be made and decisions will be needed. Interviewing for new positions takes an emotional toll and interviewing too frequently can lead to less support at your home institution. One of my mentors advised against interviewing for positions that you would never accept. If you interview for a position that you might accept, make sure you do not go for a second interview unless you are prepared to accept, since the process can snowball quickly.

Additionally, you should think hard about whether a position will advance both your professional and personal goals. For example, I never interviewed for positions that were greater than 2–3 hours of total travel time away from the northeast corridor since it was unlikely that my family would move (until recently) or that my wife would be willing to be further away from our children. These are important considerations *since a happy life is critical.*

Also, remember that it is not always about the money, and you never know when a unique opportunity will be offered. For example, I had been looking for dean positions as I was completing my third term as chair but given my geographic and personal constraints, I had yet to find a position. I had decided to finish my term and take a sabbatical at CMS in order to decide on the next phase of my career. I was busy overseeing the department's response to the COVID-19 public health emergency and the dean had notified me that he was starting the search for my successor when the CMS Administrator's Chief Operating Officer called me and asked me to apply to be the CMS CMO and Center Director. This was not in my career plans but the opportunity to do something important and help lead during a time of crisis in the healthcare system was too important to pass up. Opportunities occur when you least expect it and you need to take advantage.

Lessons Learned

- When looking at jobs, focus on what is best for your family.
- Work can be time-consuming and intense. However, when at home, it is critical to be present for your family.
- Sometimes you need help to get to the next level—such as executive coaching or an MBA. Do not hesitate to get that assistance.
- If you do not control the narrative, then someone else will.

Author

Lee Fleisher is a native Philadelphian who has trained and been on the faculties at Yale and Hopkins before returning as chair to his undergraduate alma mater, the University of Pennsylvania. He was then the senior career (non-political) policy Center Director at CMS and worked remotely from his home in the suburbs of Philadelphia while spending several days a month in his offices in Washington at the Health and Human Services headquarters and in Baltimore at the CMS headquarters. During this interval, Lee also continued to provide anesthesia services including teaching residents twice a month at the Hospital of the University of Pennsylvania. His more recent professional activities include joining the Duke Margolis Institute for Health Policy as a visiting fellow, acting as a senior advisor to the Bipartisan Policy Center's Health Program, and working with Leonard Davis Institute of Health Economics to advise and teach on the development of novel ideas and technologies to drive quality and value in the Penn Masters in Healthcare Innovation. He remains professor emeritus in the Department of Anesthesiology and Critical Care Medicine at the University of Pennsylvania.

What a Great Choice Anesthesia Is

72

Jeanine Wiener-Kronish

Introduction

Work for bosses who want to support you. Learn techniques and strategies that make you effective in your efforts. Learn skills that are important for patient care. Continuous learning is part of our commitment to our patients.

My Background Led Me to Medical School and Fellowship Training

My grandparents were immigrants, and in particular my maternal grandfather had worked his way through pharmacy school and then medical school (Fig. 72.1). His message was clear, one or more of the grandchildren were to become physicians, and three out of seven did so.

My mother had been a war widow and then remarried, and she worked evenings so she could get her graduate degree in education during the day (Fig. 72.2). My mother made it clear that education was everything, and her three children would all go to college and graduate school. So, it was no surprise that I was the oldest of my two siblings to go to college at 16 years of age and then to medical school at 20 years of age. I was lucky; 50+ years ago, I married my college sweetheart, and my personal life has been wonderful. My career has been an ever-changing lesson – exciting and rewarding, but at times taxing and difficult.

***Note from the Editors:** Jeanine Wiener-Kronish's hardworking and prosperous family, starting with her grandfather, built an incredible educational legacy for her and then insisted that she travel on that bridge to her own successful future and career (Fig. 72.1).

J. Wiener-Kronish (✉)
Department of Anesthesia & Critical Care & Pain Medicine, Massachusetts General Hospital, Boston, MA, USA
e-mail: jwiener-kronish@mgh.harvard.edu

S. Mohamed et al. (eds.), *Anesthesia Bridges*, https://doi.org/10.1007/978-3-032-08294-7_72

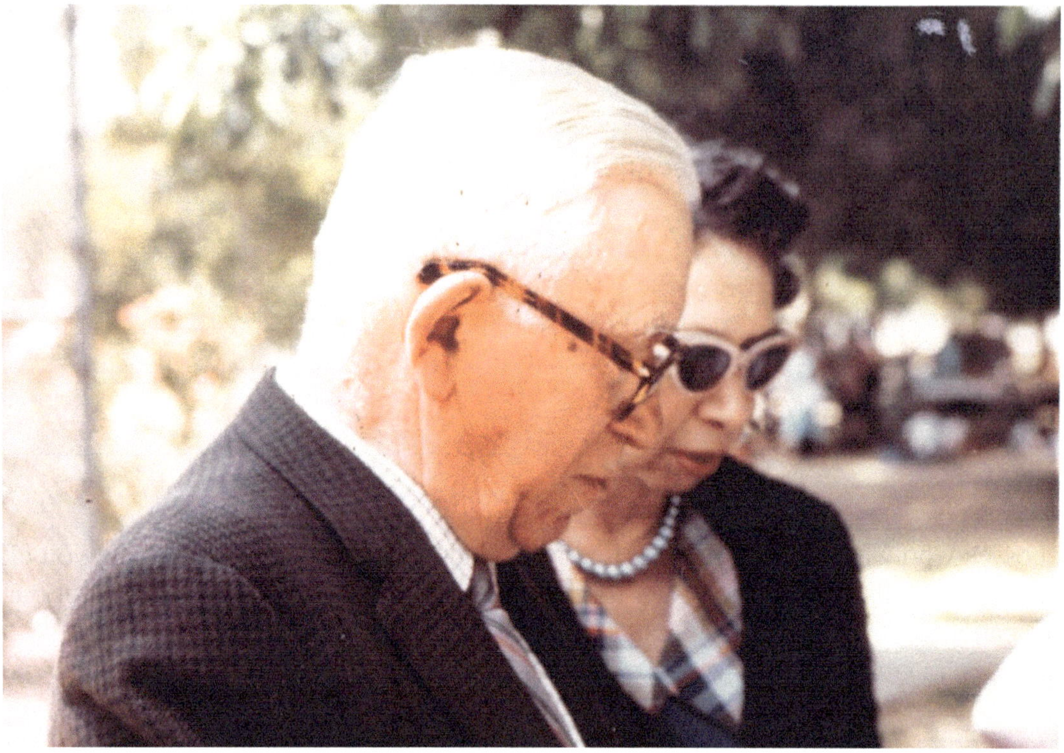

Fig. 72.1 Jeanine's brilliant maternal grandfather, Samuel Lessinger MD, and aunt, Esther Kline, in December 1965. Samuel was an immigrant from Ukraine and arrived in NYC with no family and speaking only Yiddish and Russian. He taught himself English, went to pharmacy school, and *then* went to the Flower and 5th Medical School, later New York Medical College. Esther attended Julliard and was a pianist. Photo: Collection of the Lessinger-Wiener family

I went into internal medicine because I wanted to become an intensive care physician. My rotations at UCSF placed me first at the county hospital, where pulmonologists ran the ICU. I became the second woman pulmonologist to be produced at UCSF in 1979. I spent 4 years in Norman Staub's laboratory and had some great publications and learned to love medical research. Nonetheless, when it was time to look for a job, the division chief made his displeasure clear that my research had not been with his lab and that since I was married, I really did not need a salary. Needless to say, I did not see a lack of salary as a viable option for a career.

I had several wonderful mentors who suggested I retrain as an anesthesiologist, as anesthesia leaders were in the ICU at Moffitt Hospital. I met with the new UCSF chair, Ronald Miller, who promised me that if I retrained, he would support my academic career. It was my best career decision and Dr. Miller was true to his word. I am forever grateful for entering a field where I could succeed and work in a multidisciplinary intensive care unit of the highest caliber.

My Research Work Helped Me Start to Learn About Administration

I spent about 35 years in research, running a laboratory. It helped create relationships with wonderful researchers and teachers around the world. It increased my insight into the problems and solutions in medicine beyond the location I worked in. Running a laboratory introduced me to personnel issues, choosing collaborators and employees, and keeping to a strict budget. I also helped my department with administrative tasks and learned about the politics, traditions, and economics of hospitals and medical schools.

Aspiring to higher administrative posts meant I needed to learn different skills to succeed and different approaches to be effective. I took courses, including ELAM (Executive Leadership in Academic Medicine), and at the AAMC and learned that becoming a chair is not an award but another kind of job. Chairs have to advocate for their faculty, but they also have to be effective negotiators with their bosses, the hospital leadership, and the medical school leadership.

***Note from the Editors:** Jeanine's equally inspiring parents, Paul Wiener and Jeanette Lessinger Wiener, continued the family's educational legacy. Here they are in 1994 (Fig. 72.2).

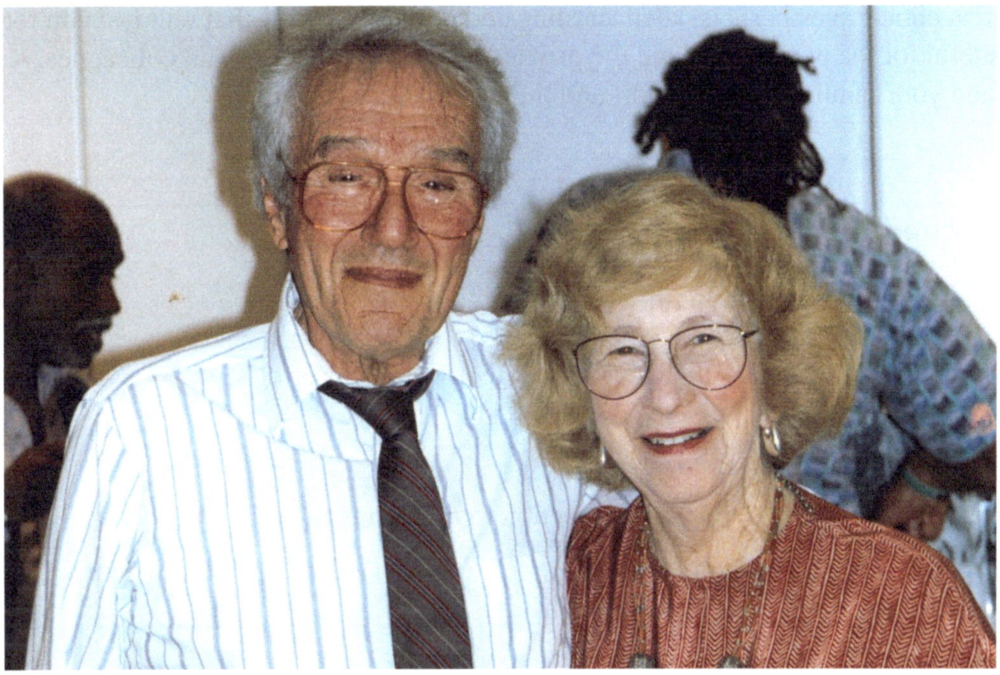

Fig. 72.2 Jeanine's father Paul was an electrical engineer for Los Angeles Power and Water. Her mother Jeanette could be a role model for all of us – she worked nights so she could go to grad school during the day, ultimately obtaining her doctoral degree in education from UCLA when Jeanine was around five years old – this was at a time when only 5% of women in the United States had any type of education after high school, much less an advanced degree. Photo: Collection of the Wiener family

Jeanette Wiener was then a successful career woman and was the assistant superintendent and second-in-command of Los Angeles County Schools as well as the wife of a busy professional and the mother of three children. Paul and Jeanette passed on their belief in education as well as their drive and discipline. Jeanette, in particular, insisted that each of her children receive a top education, including a graduate degree. And they did – Jeanine's sister Diane is a lawyer and juvenile law expert for children in the foster care system and her brother Gerry is a theoretical mathematician who predicted wind patterns for the National Weather Service.

What I Am Grateful For and What I Wish I Had Done Differently

As an intensivist, I am grateful for my health and my time with my family. Working in the ICU was humbling and a constant reminder not to take things for granted. I am grateful for a career that made me want to go to work, made me want to continuously learn, and gave me the privilege of trying to help others.

I have some minor regrets. I wish I had also trained in cardiac anesthesia, as I never became as good at echocardiography as I wanted to be. This skill is really important for modern intensive care physicians, and I admire our new double-boarded intensivists. I regret I did not learn to be more effective in communication and negotiation and have better emotional intelligence. This would have been helpful with patients, with hospital leaders, and maybe even my children.

But my regrets are minor compared to my joy in my career and with my life. What I would say to myself is "what a great choice anesthesia is, keep learning and perfecting skills that will last you for 40 or more years, be grateful for the opportunity and the privilege of helping patients and colleagues. And take care of yourself and your family, as life is short and they are so very important.

Lessons Learned

- Work for bosses who want to support you.
- Learn techniques and strategies that make you effective in your efforts.
- Learn skills that are important for patient care.
- Continuous learning is part of our commitment to our patients.

Author

Jeanine Wiener-Kronish graduated from UCLA with a BA in psychology and then received her MD from UCSF in 1976. She completed an internal medicine residency at an affiliate hospital of UCSF and a pulmonary fellowship at UCSF in 1979. She then completed an anesthesia residency at UCSF after four years of research in the Cardiovascular Research Institute. She became chair of Anesthesia at MGH in 2008 and has loved being on the East Coast for now, closing in on 20 years. She and her husband of 50+ years walk, do Pilates, and also do high-intensity exercise to keep up with their children and grandchildren.

73 Try to Find At Least One Big Way to Expand Your Practice: Mine Was Acupuncture

Rose Christopherson

Introduction

I am retired from a 35-year clinical practice, thanks to the coronavirus pandemic. For the last third of my career, I incorporated acupuncture into the treatment of my anesthesia patients as often as possible. I have often been asked how I accomplished this.

Initiation and Acupuncture Training

My initiation to acupuncture was a fortuitous one. In 2004, I was working in the Veterans Affairs health care system and was sitting in my office at the Portland VA Medical Center when Laura, one of my anesthesiologist colleagues, walked in with two needles sticking out of her head. She had to go to run the preop clinic, so I helped her hide the needles, which had been placed by Diane, another anesthesiologist in our group. Diane was studying acupuncture in the Helms Medical Institute, which is a branch of UCLA. She needed to practice on her colleagues and soon she was regularly treating me for my GERD. The GERD disappeared and I became fascinated with acupuncture. The following year, Laura studied acupuncture at a different acupuncture school.

In 2006, I myself studied medical acupuncture at the Helms Medical Institute. I became a medical acupuncturist in less than a year of very hard work. This is quite different from non-physician licensed acupuncturists who study acupuncture for three years, but as allopathic physicians, our study of acupuncture is placed upon the mountain of knowledge about anatomy, physiology, and disease states that comes with our previous medical training.

R. Christopherson (✉)
Department of Anesthesiology (retired), Portland VA Medical Center, Portland, OR, USA

S. Mohamed et al. (eds.), *Anesthesia Bridges*, https://doi.org/10.1007/978-3-032-08294-7_73

Acupuncture and Anesthesia

For several years, Diane, Laura, and I all practiced anesthesiology with adjunctive acupuncture therapy at the Portland VA under our medical licenses. We were the only three physicians on staff at the hospital who undertook acupuncture training and provided acupuncture care. At that time, there were no separate credentialing processes or consent forms in the VA health care system for acupuncture care. We did discuss the risks and benefits of adjunctive acupuncture treatment for patients undergoing anesthesia and annotated our standard anesthesia consent procedures and records accordingly.

I offered acupuncture to patients I was preparing to anesthetize as a supplement to their anesthesia in several ways. Sometimes, when I was covering two rooms with nurse anesthetists, I simply placed one needle in the top of the patient's head in the preop area, then removed it just before induction of anesthesia, so as not to interfere with intubation. Acupuncture was used as a supplement to the anesthetic, never as a substitute for it. It could be given to reduce postoperative nausea, to reduce postoperative pain, and to enhance cardiac or pulmonary function.

In the postoperative area, nurses often decide on indications for acupuncture. I would sometimes be called by a nurse to give acupuncture for postoperative nausea only after the nurse had given all the antiemetic drugs available. Acupuncture works well for nausea, and patients would respond well to this particular acupuncture treatment. Some nurses tended to call me earlier, before giving all the drugs, and again, the acupuncture worked well. Nurses were also helpful in setting up spaces where I could spend more time with a patient and give them a more aggressive acupuncture treatment for postoperative pain, anxiety, nausea, and/or cardiac or pulmonary function. A single acupuncture treatment can help with several of these goals.

Acupuncture Practice in "Retirement"

I continued my acupuncture practice even after I had retired from my work in clinical anesthesia. My VA anesthesia colleagues had established a community acupuncture clinic that was often attended by VA patients and their families. A group of us, both medical acupuncturists and licensed acupuncturists, provided acupuncture therapy for a variety of clinical conditions and needs. We maintained formal written charts for patients and covered our own malpractice insurance. Our patients were encouraged to donate small amounts of money to the clinic.

What little funds the clinic generated were used to purchase needles and other acupuncture supplies and were donated to the church that provided the space to the clinic. I found this continuation and extension of my traditional anesthesiology practice to be deeply rewarding. Unfortunately, the coronavirus pandemic rendered direct patient care and required cleaning and isolation too problematic for us to continue.

I slowly resumed giving acupuncture treatments once the coronavirus was under better control and will continue my acupuncture practice as long as I feel I can benefit the patients.

Lessons Learned

- There will be multiple opportunities for you to expand and build on your basic medical and anesthesia training—lean into this as it can result in manifestly better care for your patients at all points in your career.
- Although the practice of anesthesia has become continually safer across the decades, we must remember and always be vigilant that individual treatments, procedures, and drugs can pose a significant risk to the patient. If acupuncture can reduce the need for a medication that, if doubled, would kill the patient, then acupuncture is very attractive!

Author

Rose Christopherson studied philosophy in college and was madly in love with Immanuel Kant. She wrote a dissertation on Kant's influence on Charles Pierce and received a PhD from Penn State. She couldn't find a job teaching philosophy, met the love of her life who was teaching at Hershey Medical School, and eventually went to medical school there. She went to Johns Hopkins for her residency and fellowship. She was on the hospital ethics committee and taught in the Physician and Society course for first-year medical students. After 15 years at Hopkins, she transferred to the VA hospital in Portland, Oregon. Only very late in her career did she discover acupuncture.

Success in Medicine Takes a Village

74

Kathryn K. Lauer

Contributors:

Catherine Marcucci, MD

Neil B. Sandson, MD

Things I Would Tell My 30-Year-Old Self

There are so many things that I would love to share with my 30-year-old self. Try to enjoy both work and your personal life, especially your family, and try your best not to stress about everything. You will waste energy aiming for perfection, and it won't matter. Trying too hard to be the perfect anything is counterproductive. Also, please take care of yourself, just as you take care of others. Get rest, exercise, take some time for yourself, and understand that barriers and self-care are not selfish—they are healthy.

Here's a Mistake I Once Made, and What I Learned From It

The first research project I did as a young attending was something that one of my senior colleagues asked me to do. However, at the time, I did, not understand how much mentorship and guidance was missing from my colleague's request. It was a miserable process, met with eventual publication, but it took far longer than it should have. I was also trying to do this work while juggling care for my small children, passing my exams, and I felt overwhelmed. I transformed the anxiety and incompetence that I

K. K. Lauer (✉)
Department of Anesthesiology, Medical College of Wisconsin, Milwaukee, WI, USA
e-mail: klauer@mcw.edu

S. Mohamed et al. (eds.), *Anesthesia Bridges*, https://doi.org/10.1007/978-3-032-08294-7_74

felt going through this into a feeling of personal failure. Eventually, I was able to experience working in a more supportive, collaborative environment in another research lab, and only then did I understand what I had previously missed.

Dissecting this, there were a number of trouble spots:

- A lack of formal research training
- Work overload, leading to chronic exhaustion and fatigue
- The challenge of balancing personal and professional responsibilities
- A lack of mentorship
- Self-consciousness and imposter syndrome
- Inability to ask for the right help.

In 1989, Neinstein evaluated the role of formal research training on success. They surveyed half of the first authors of 18 journals over a six-month period and asked about their research training. They found that 87% of first authors reported having had only informal training, but 57% had statistical training during their residency or fellowship [1]. Since then, there have been a myriad of studies chronicling the relative advantages of formal research training in success and retention [2–4]. Missing this background can create challenges for aspiring academicians unless resources and mentorship help fill gaps along the way.

Furthermore, work overload has been shown to lead to a lack of success in academics as well as to burnout. In a recent study by Ellinas et al., work overload, especially in women, was a factor in the inability to progress. It fostered the sense that one would have to self-promote for others to appreciate their work, and an overall lack of recognition [5]. There are several gender-neutral issues that contributed to burnout, including a lack of support and role conflict [6]. This is a universal challenge. However, as work overload includes both professional and domestic work, societal imbalances may still put a unique strain on women.

***Note from the Editors:** Kathy Lauer built her career at the Medical College of Wisconsin. We went looking for some beautiful Wisconsin bridges and found a bunch (Figs. 74.1 and 74.2). Makes sense because of all the Wisconsin water.

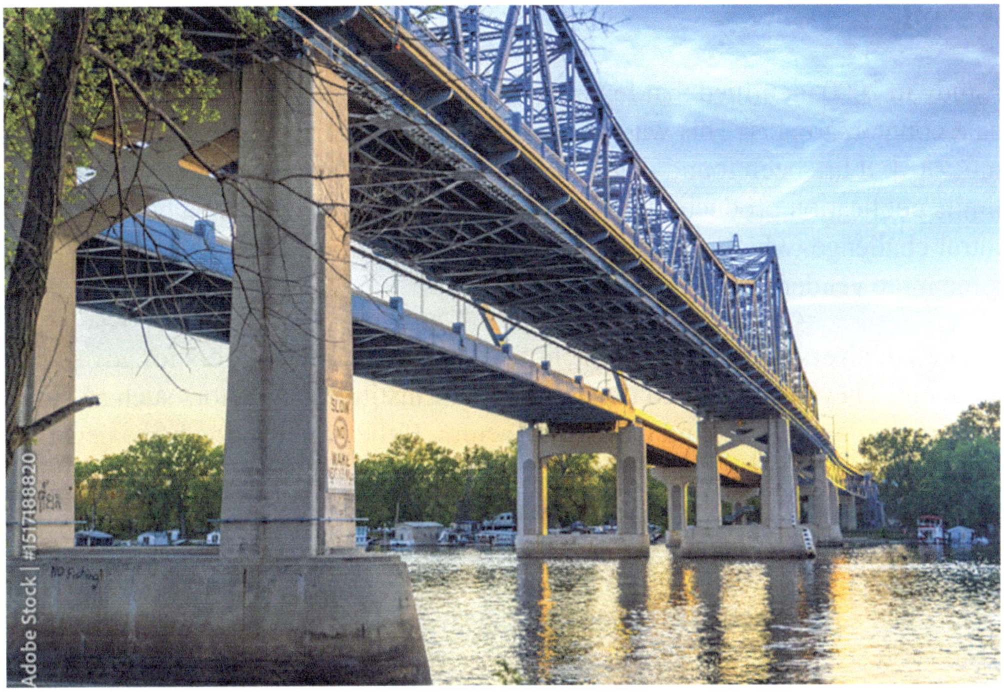

Fig. 74.1 A dramatic view of the beautiful Cass Street bridge in La Crosse, Wisconsin. Photo: Image used under standard license from stock.adobe.com

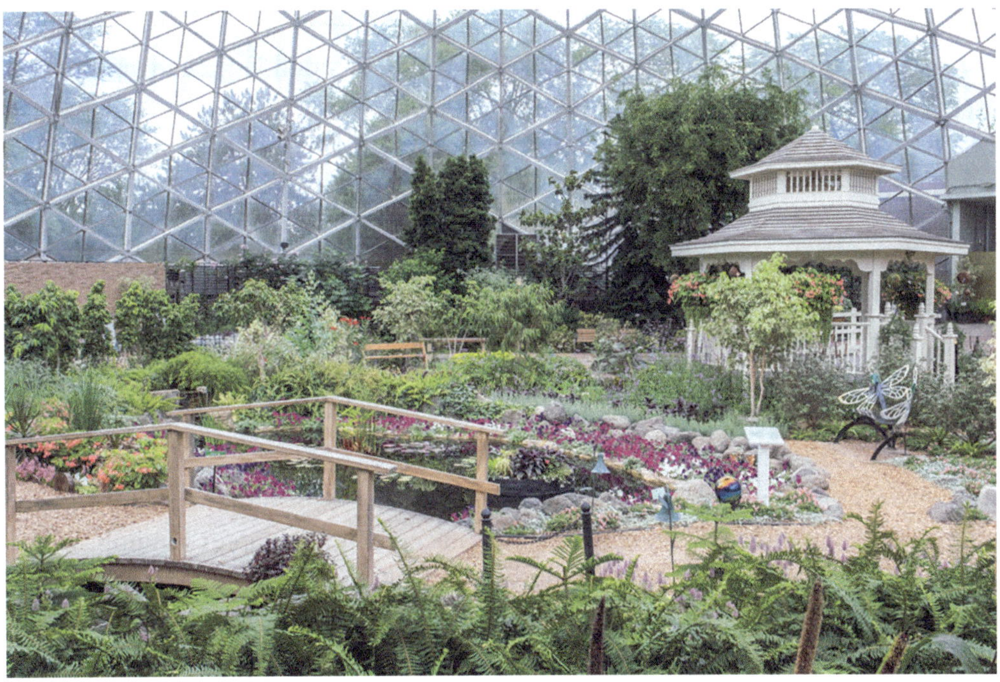

Fig. 74.2 Mitchell Park Horticultural Conservatory Dome housing the Spring Show in Milwaukee, Wisconsin on July 20, 2022. Photo: Image used for editorial use non-fiction book from stock.adobe.com

Important Studies

A landmark study in 2000 identified that female faculty were at a disadvantage for promotion compared with their male counterparts [7]. This was reviewed 20 years later and unfortunately the needle has not moved too much [8]. It has been found that in early-career physicians, struggling with child rearing and caregiving limits publication productivity. This is most pronounced in women but has been identified as a gender-neutral challenge, which may only progress as domestic and caregiving responsibilities continue to become more gender neutral [9].

A study done at the University of Michigan identified barriers and facilitators for advancement within a surgical department. They characterized the categories of institutional factors such as culture and institutional policies, relational factors, and individual factors. If the organization had a negative culture that was highly political and there was a lack of attention to diversity and inclusion and unaligned incentives, the challenges were higher. If there were negative relationships without positive mentoring or collegiality or family support, again, the challenges for an individual were greater.

Individual factors had an impact as well including the ability to self-advocate, be able to balance work-life priorities and perceive growth and reputation. These predicted positive outcomes [10]. Naiveté, lack of confidence, and behavior based on perceived expectations can be barriers, and these are common in an early faculty experience.

These concepts were expanded upon in an article in BMJ in 2020. The authors identified 13 different areas that need to be addressed to ensure an equitable environment for women in academics [11]. This included personal factors, such as financial considerations like level of debt, confidence and ambition, orientation to the roles and appropriate onboarding, competing demand as well as ability to garner support.

More Studies

There was also a cadre of interpersonal factors, like support from mentors, receiving practical support, discrimination, or compensatory behaviors for the discrimination. The organization and society play a role as well. If the academic or clinical workplace culture is supportive vs. hierarchical and transparent, this impacts the retention and success of faculty.

In addition, society and national policies play a role in setting expectations as well as things such as research funding. It is a challenge that an emphasis is placed on early career funding, when often this is the peak of childbearing years for women. Similarly, a recent study looking at barriers to academic success in anesthesiologists, similar themes arose including work overload, lack of training and mentoring as well as lack of confidence [12].

So, how does one overcome these barriers? In the Michigan study, there were several institutional factors that helped facilitate advancement, such as the presence of positive mentors, and having access to advancement opportunities. Important personal factors identified included having adequate family support, the ability to prioritize, being resilient, and having the ability to self-advocate.

Imposter syndrome is defined as an inability to internalize success and the tendency to attribute success to external causes such as luck, error, or knowing the appropriate individuals [13]. This is increasingly being recognized as a source of anxiety and burnout among physicians at all levels. The sense of support, personal affirmation, and validation as well as personal and shared reflections were protective [14]. Again, what I felt at that time was representative of common experience; however, I did not realize it at the time. There are continued structural and cultural changes that will need to be addressed to fully ensure the holistic development of faculty.

What My Mentor Taught Me

Despite this rocky start, I look back on a day when Dr. John Kampine, my former chair, came to the lab when I was working and mapped it out for me. He shared that from his vantage point, there are many paths to success in medicine. On the basic level, one becomes proficient at their craft and develops a reputation and brand based on this. This can be very fulfilling. On the next level, one can teach the craft. At an even higher level, one can ask questions and add to the knowledge base of medicine—and in all these different methods of contributing, there is inherent value and joy. He also created the sense that we were all family to an extent and valued for who we were.

Other Lessons

The last observation is one that I believe we have all learned in the pandemic—the values that ring truest are those closest to our hearts. This includes working with compassion, spending time on the things that renew us, and cherishing the moments in which we give ourselves to others.

Lessons Learned

- We must take time to keep ourselves renewed throughout the hard work that we do. Staying connected to the people who really know us is one route and another is being present to those whom we help, especially in a challenging time.

- Saying no is often a good answer, but you have to say yes sometimes. It seems that more people get stuck by never saying yes and wonder why they feel passed by.

***Note from the Editors:** We so wanted to include a cheese bridge to honor Kathy and our other Wisconsin authors, but all the online photos of such bridges were under copyright. So, we made one for her. ☺ We think it turned out okay (Fig. 74.3)! A different friend from Wisconsin said, "Make sure you say the state correctly."

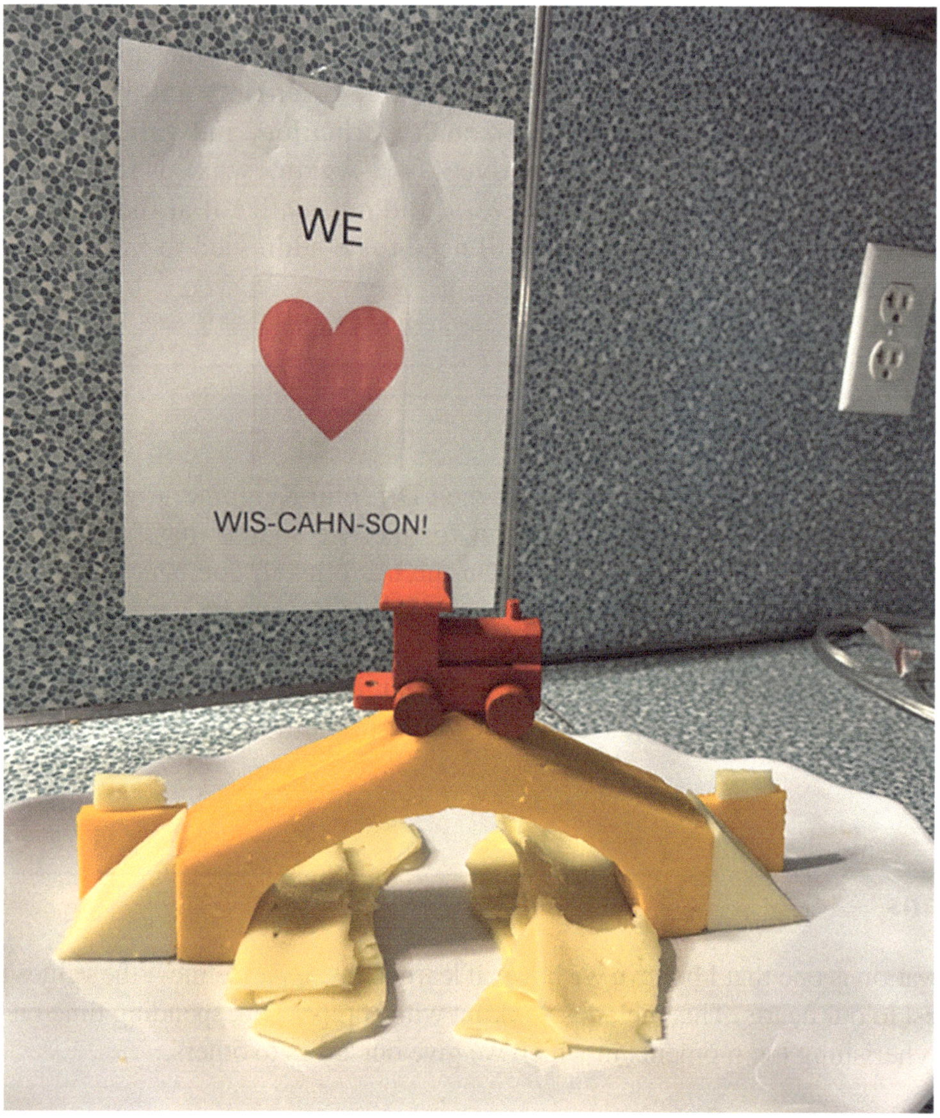

Fig. 74.3 A cheese bridge for our Wisconsin colleagues. Bridge design, purchasing, construction, and kitchen cleanup by Neil Sandson. Photo: Cathy Marcucci

References

1. Neinstein L, MacKenzie RG. Prior training and recommendations for future training of clinical research faculty members. Acad Med. 1989;64(1):32–5.
2. Tsen LC, Borus JF, Nadelson CC, et al. The development, implementation, and assessment of an innovative faculty mentoring leadership program. Acad Med. 2012;87(12):1757–61.
3. Bobian MR, Shah N, Svider PF, et al. Does formal research training lead to academic success in otolaryngology? Laryngoscope. 2017;127(1):E15–21.
4. Wilson TA, Langston RG, Wong KH, et al. Characteristics and career outcomes of Neurosurgery Research and Education Foundation research fellowship recipients. J Neurosurg. 2019;132(3):802–8.
5. Ellinas EH, Kaljo K, Patitucci TN, et al. No room to "lean in": a qualitative study on gendered barriers to promotion and leadership. J Women Health (Larchmt). 2019;28(3):393–402.
6. Ellinas EH, Fouad N, Byars-Winston A. Women and the decision to leave, linger, or lean in: predictors of intent to leave and aspirations to leadership and advancement in academic medicine. J Womens Health (Larchmt). 2018;27(3):324–32.

7. Nonnemaker L. Women physicians in academic medicine: new insights from cohort studies. N Engl J Med. 2000;342(6):399–405.
8. Richter KP, Clark L, Wick JA, et al. Women physicians and promotion in academic medicine. N Engl J Med. 2020;383(22):2148–57.
9. King AA, Vesely SK, Vettese E, et al. Impact of gender and caregiving responsibilities on academic success in hematology. Blood Adv. 2020;4(4):755–61.
10. Thompson-Burdine JA, Telem DA, Waljee JF, et al. Defining barriers and facilitators to advancement for women in academic surgery. JAMA Netw Open. 2019;2(8):e1910228.
11. Vassie C, Smith S, Leedham-Green K. Factors impacting on retention, success and equitable participation in clinical academic careers: a scoping review and meta-thematic synthesis. BMJ Open. 2020;10(3):e033480.
12. Matot I, De Hert S, Cohen B, et al. Women anaesthesiologists' attitudes and reported barriers to career advancement in anaesthesia: a survey of the European Society of Anaesthesiology. Br J Anaesth. 2020;124(3):e171–7.
13. Clance PR, Imes SA. The imposter phenomenon in high achieving women: dynamics and therapeutic intervention. Psychother: Theor Res Prac. 1978;15(3):241–7.
14. Gottlieb M, Chung A, Battaglioli N, et al. Impostor syndrome among physicians and physicians in training: a scoping review. Med Educ. 2020;54(2):116–24.

Author

Kathryn Lauer has spent her career in Milwaukee at the Medical College of Wisconsin. She feels fortunate to have experienced a diverse career, though working in the same institution. With her husband, she also raised a large family. She feels that this period of her career has been most gratifying: developing the next generation of colleagues and enjoying the next generation of family.

Life Lessons From a Mentor

75

Maya Jalbout Hastie

Introduction

In *Mentor,* Laurent Daloz views education as a developmental process which means "successively asking broader and deeper questions of the relationship between oneself and the world." On this transformational journey, mentors "provide support, challenge, and vision" to their mentees [1]. A mentor's ultimate goal is to guide you on your journey, to inspire you, and to ignite ideas and interests. Effective mentors have the credibility that one only gets from being a recognized expert in their field. They also have the ability to "hear" you and "see" you: it's the ability to understand human motivation, what drives you, and what prevents you from engaging.

Dr. Baraka

A good mentor is hard to find. I had a great mentor in Dr. Anis Baraka.

Dr. Anis Baraka was the chair of the department of anesthesiology at the American University of Beirut, and he held that position for over 30 years. He led the department through a vicious war, despite threats of violence, and at significant personal cost. When I met Dr. Baraka as a medical student on my anesthesia rotation, I was planning to apply for a residency in pediatrics. By the end of that rotation, I had found a home in the operating room and realized that I had just discovered my future career.

You learn a lot by observing your mentor. I was inspired by his passion for the science of anesthesiology, intrigued by its practice as a minimalist art, and awed by his ability to control the operating room with his mere presence. Our mentoring sessions were informal, unplanned, thought-provoking, and always rewarding. It's been 20 years since and not a week passes, where I don't recall his advice and his teachings. I share my favorite five lessons learned.

M. J. Hastie (✉)
Department of Anesthesiology, Columbia University, New York, NY, USA
e-mail: mj2081@cumc.columbia.edu

S. Mohamed et al. (eds.), *Anesthesia Bridges*, https://doi.org/10.1007/978-3-032-08294-7_75

1. “**Learn something new every day**”

   For years, Dr. Baraka would lead daily morning reports, gathering all members of the department, to discuss clinical management or research updates. Residents and medical students often led the presentations. The best presentations were those that taught him something new. Your reward was seeing him taking notes, with a smile on his face. Despite a brain foggy with sleep, I learned more during those mornings than from any other opportunity. He had the thirst for knowledge, and the humility to admit he can learn from everyone and anyone.

2. **“There’s more to life than a career”**

   On one of the days that we worked together, and during a quiet phase of the procedure, he asked me what I wanted for my career. I shared my fascination with clinical research and with academic writing. He smiled, paused, and said: “This is all good. Don’t forget, there is more to life than a career. If you decide to get married one day, find someone who is willing to support your aspirations.”

3. **“Write concisely and clearly”**

   When I’d struggle with putting ideas onto paper, he’d ask me, “Talk to me - tell me what you’re trying to say.” When I’d finish expressing my idea, he’d say: “Ok, write that down.” He practiced parsimony of words—only use the words you need to express your idea in the simplest way for the reader. Authors often struggle to let go of carefully crafted sentences. He was never reluctant to edit out paragraphs that were not serving the message.

4. **“Less is more”**

   When high-ranking government officials presented for surgical procedures, he’d remind everyone on the team to treat them like they did the last patient. He believed in the elegance of a simple, straightforward anesthetic, where less often meant more.

5. **“In the OR, you are alone with your conscience”**

   Of all his advice, this one I carry the closest to my heart in the OR and in life. I believe this goes beyond doing the right thing. It means doing the right thing even when no one is watching, even when it won’t matter to others, and it won’t change outcomes. Do what’s right for right’s sake, not for fear of punishment or for the promise of a reward.

How do you thank a mentor? You pay it forward by becoming a patient, compassionate mentor to the next generation.

Lessons Learned

- Learn something new every day.
- Find a partner in life who is willing to support your aspirations.
- Write concisely and clearly.
- Do the right thing, even when no one is watching.

Reference

1. Daloz LA. Mentor: guiding the journey of adult learners. 2nd ed. San Francisco: Jossey-Bass; 2012.

Author

Maya Jalbout Hastie started her career in anesthesiology at the American University of Beirut, on a beautiful campus overlooking the Mediterranean Sea. Coincidence has led her to New York City, to Columbia University, to starting a family, to meeting mentors and friends, to building relationships, to establishing a career path, and to dedicating her work to eliminating health care disparities. It has been said that "A coincidence is nothing but a destiny that we ignore" (Mohamed Mbougar Sarr 2021). Sometimes it's best not to ignore one's destiny, but to embrace it and enjoy the journey.

76 Bridges That Shaped a Career

Christopher A. Troianos

Introduction

For those that do not know, Pittsburgh has more bridges than any other city in the world—446 to be exact. In this "City of Bridges," I attended college, medical school, and then was lucky to match with the anesthesia residency at Mercy Hospital, which is currently known as UPMC Mercy. There, I formed bridges with individuals who would become my mentors and help shape my career.

Ephraim S. Siker, MD

My first mentor was the late Ephraim S. (Rick) Siker (1926–2013), who served as my chair and residency program director at Mercy. Dr. Siker had trained under one of the early pioneers of the specialty, Francis Foldes, who was also the previous chair at Mercy. I admired Dr. Siker as one of the few individuals who became a leader of both our national specialty society, the American Society of Anesthesiologists or ASA, and our specialty certification Board of Directors, the American Board of Anesthesiology or ABA.

Rick served as president of the ASA in 1973. At the time, he was one of the youngest ASA presidents ever elected. He was president of the ABA in 1983. He delivered the ASA's highly prestigious Rovenstine lecture in 1981 and received the ASA's highest honor, the Distinguished Service Award, in 1983. He also served as a member of the American Board of Medical Specialties Executive Committee 1987–1989.

While observing Dr. Siker, I came to realize that it takes a very special and unique set of character traits to succeed within the realms of both a specialty society and a board certification organization. Dr. Siker was also a strong advocate for patient safety at a time when anesthesiology needed to become a leader in this area. He was a founding member of the Anesthesia Patient Safety Foundation (APSF), mixing his own passion for the foundation's mission—that *"no patient shall be harmed by anesthesia"*—with the wit and wisdom that was so characteristic of his personality. In fact, the APSF executive office was at one time physically located at the Mercy Hospital of Pittsburgh.

C. A. Troianos (✉)
Anesthesiology Institute, Cleveland Clinic, Cleveland, OH, USA
e-mail: TROIANC@ccf.org

S. Mohamed et al. (eds.), *Anesthesia Bridges*, https://doi.org/10.1007/978-3-032-08294-7_76

I met Dr. Siker as a medical student in 1983, while I attended the University of Pittsburgh School of Medicine. Although I didn't quite know why, Dr. Siker identified me as one of the first medical students to match into the specialty's new 4-year integrated curriculum, which was previously a 3-year continuum of internship plus 2 years of anesthesiology. One of the traits I admired most about Dr. Siker was his seemingly natural ability to get his point across with a very calm but convincing demeanor that integrated his wit, wisdom, and conviction.

One vivid example was reading a medical consultant's evaluation of one of our patients, which stated that the patient was "cleared for spinal, but not for general anesthesia." Dr. Siker summoned the consultant to the perioperative holding area *before* surgery, and had him add an addendum to his consult, which read "My recommendation for the type of anesthesia this patient should have, is based upon the two weeks of anesthesia training I had in medical school." Needless to say, that same internist never again recommended a certain type of anesthesia within any future medical consults. Dr. Siker had a profound impact upon me and sparked within me the desire to emulate his career with the personality traits that he so eloquently displayed.

***Note from the Editors:** One of Chris's favorite Pittsburgh bridges is the Roberto Clemente Bridge, formerly the Sixth Street Bridge (Fig. 76.1). He told us why:

> Roberto Clemente was my favorite player when I was growing up. He played third base, which is the same position I played in T-shirt league baseball. More recently, I bike across that bridge all the time when I am bicycling in Pittsburgh with my cycling club, the Pittsburgh Major Taylor Cycling Club. Besides the sentimental reasons, the bridge is very aesthetically pleasing to my eye, especially the perspective views and when the bridge is lit at night.

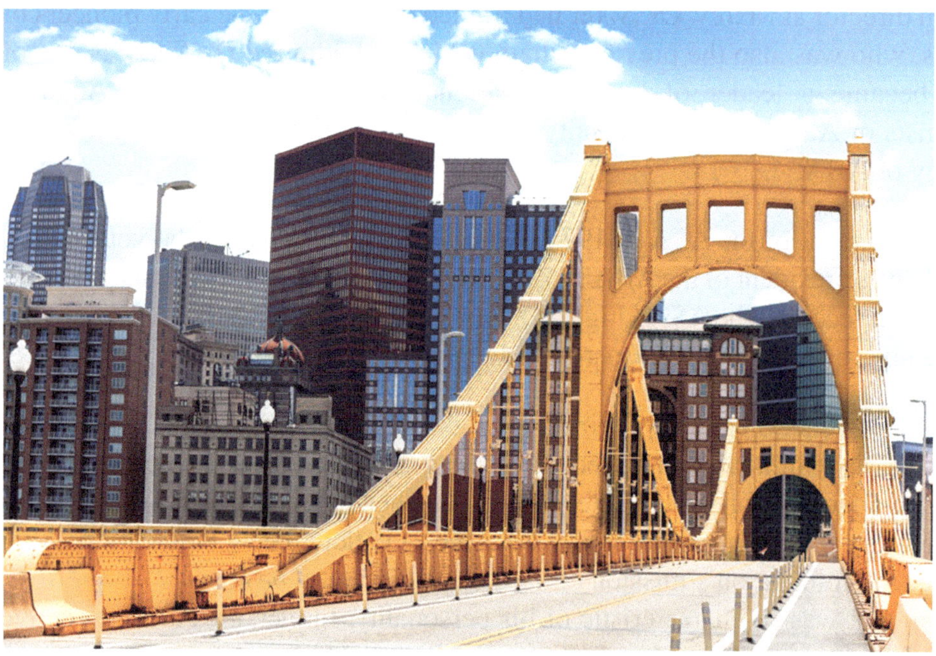

Fig. 76.1 The Roberto Clemente Bridge in Pittsburgh, PA, formerly known as the Sixth Street Bridge. It spans the Allegheny River in the downtown area. The bridge was completed in 1928 and is the fourth bridge at this location. It is one of the Three Sisters bridges that lie parallel to each other on Sixth, Seventh, and Ninth Street. It is closed to vehicular traffic on home game days of the Pittsburgh Pirates and the Pittsburgh Steelers. Photo: Image used under standard license from stock.adobe.com

John Ammon, MD

Early after beginning my anesthesiology residency in 1985, I realized that I had a calling to become a cardiac anesthesiologist. This occurred as a result of my careful observation and admiration of another early mentor, John Ammon, who had trained under Ed Lowenstein in the early days of cardiac anesthesia at Massachusetts General Hospital (MGH).

Dr. Ammon often relayed to me the debate over whether the best cardiac anesthetic was an opioid-based technique, promoted at MGH, versus an inhalational-based technique as had been promoted at the University of Pennsylvania, where I ultimately trained to become a cardiac anesthesiologist. Dr. Ammon always had a calm demeanor in dealing with challenging cardiac patients who were very sick and never displayed the tension he must have felt when rescuing patients from hemodynamic collapse.

One of the most memorable words of wisdom I gained from Dr. Ammon was that *"a good cardiac anesthesiologist under-reacts, aggressively,"* meaning that you must always anticipate, and be on top of the patients' clinical condition, but not to overreact in treating either hypertension or hypotension. Dr. Ammon was also a "master" oral board examiner, and I tried to emulate his style when I became an ABA oral board examiner. He had a calm, yet probing style of examination that was fair and comprehensive. He made me realize the critical importance and obligation we have as board examiners to the public and to patients, to accurately identify candidates who are deserving of the designation "Diplomat of the American Board of Anesthesiology."

Ronald Pellegrini, MD

Before I left Mercy Hospital to pursue my training as a cardiac anesthesiologist at the University of Pennsylvania, I asked another mentor, Dr. Ron Pellegrini, for his advice on what area of cardiac anesthesia that I should focus my attention. Dr. Pellegrini was the chief of cardiac surgery at Mercy Hospital and was always ahead of his time in treating his patients.

He had great insights into the future, as evidenced by his performance of mitral valve repairs in the 1980s. He assessed the success of his repairs by initially using a sterilized stethoscope placed epicardially within the patient's open chest to listen for murmurs! He told me "Son—you learn as much as you can about transesophageal echocardiography and bring that unique skill set back to Mercy!"

And the rest is history. It was indeed an honor to teach countless others this special skill over the years through direct patient care, lectures, as a course director for my own TEE courses through Mercy Hospital, and ultimately as a program director for the Society of Cardiovascular Anesthesiologists' week-long course on Comprehensive Review of Perioperative Echocardiography.

And Others…

I have certainly benefited from the words of several other important mentors during my career, and they deserve mention by name. August Mantia introduced me to anesthesia through a medical student anesthesia technician program. Joseph Savino was my cardiac anesthesia program director at U Penn. Norig (Skip) Ellison was acting chair of the Department of Anesthesiology at U Penn and a past ASA President. They have all provided me with countless words of wisdom and career guidance throughout the years.

Dr. Ellison encouraged us to find a better and safer way to access the internal jugular vein using ultrasound nearly 30 years ago, and this has now become the standard of care. He was also a strong supporter of the APSF. It is my hope that these experiences with my mentors convey how their simple, yet profound, words of wisdom shaped my future and guided my career path to become the cardiac anesthesiologist, colleague, chair, society president, and board certification leader that I have become.

I encourage all who read this to be extremely aware of the words we use and the advice we give, often seemingly without much thought or consideration. Our words of wisdom have the potential to make a significant impact upon those around us and affect their future. Thank you for the honor of allowing me to share these few thoughts and experiences as bridges to my past, which will hopefully bring more awareness to the impact we may have upon the careers of those around us.

Lessons Learned

- Our words and behaviors are constantly on display and can have profound and career altering impact on everyone with whom we interact with on a daily basis.
- Follow your passions and be strong in your conviction, sharing them through venues beyond your immediate circle of friends and colleagues. The establishment of the Anesthesia Patient Safety Foundation, echocardiography training, and ultrasound guided vascular access are examples that I have personally observed or received encouragement to pursue from my mentors.
- Leaders who encourage and foster the ideas and aspirations of junior colleagues, can have long and extended impact beyond their own career, extending the impact of their approach and encouragement to future generations of leaders.

Author

Chris Troianos is a cardiac anesthesiologist at the Cleveland Clinic and serves as chair of the Anesthesiology Institute. He was an early adopter of intraoperative transesophageal echocardiography and use of ultrasound for vascular access. His passion for these skills led him to become an avid educator and author of practice guidelines that supported their daily clinical use. He notes that his marriage to his wife Barbara is the best thing that has happened to him, along with raising their three grown children Rachael, Andrew, and Rebecca. Chris loves cycling outdoors when weather permits, having biked the 340 miles both ways (different years) between Pittsburgh and Washington, DC. He also did a great bike trip from Florence to Venice (in the Dolomites of Italy) with his son. If you do not find him on a bicycle, you will likely find him attending a local car show on weekend summer days or watching the sunset over Lake Erie on a lovely summer weekday evening in Cleveland.

From Telemachus' Perspective: Lessons Learned from My Mentor

77

M. Christine Stock

Introduction

I learned to do clinical research working with John B. Downs, MD during my first year after medical school, a fortuitous and incredibly lucky consequence of my wanting to live with my new husband, who was a PhD student at University of Illinois, Champaign-Urbana, and John's recent move back to his hometown Urbana, Illinois. That was 1981.

John B. Downs, MD

John took me on as a clinical research "fellow"—for lack of better description—in a community hospital in Urbana, IL just after I graduated from medical school. I was the only learner. John provided one-to-one daily lectures for the initial several months, first on pulmonary physiology, which he observed medical schools taught poorly. Later, lectures were on support of ventilation and support of oxygenation—and distinguishing these different beasts. I took copious notes and used those same presentations for the entire 35 years I was a medical school faculty member. John was correct—the many residents and fellows I taught over the years, who were graduates from many august medical schools, rarely had been provided with a substantive working knowledge of pulmonary physiology.

My time working with John as a clinical research fellow in 1981–82 was extremely productive and provided a huge kick-start to my academic career. From our work during those 16 months in a community hospital with no research infrastructure, we published five peer-reviewed original research manuscripts.

M. C. Stock (✉)
Department of Anesthesiology, Northwestern University Feinberg School of Medicine, Chicago, IL, USA
e-mail: c-stock@northwestern.edu

S. Mohamed et al. (eds.), *Anesthesia Bridges*, https://doi.org/10.1007/978-3-032-08294-7_77

Lesson No. 1A

Start with the basics

Provide your students/trainees with sound knowledge of basic physiology and the experimental basis for current medical practice so they can ask the right questions to advance medicine—and so they can make rational decisions regarding patient care.

Lesson No. 1B

Embrace your learning environment as an opportunity rather than as an obstruction.

I did my first OR/clinical anesthesia case with John. After the induction of anesthesia, John asked me, "If I told you that there was no attending anesthesiologist available to help you finish this case, how would you feel?" I could not exhale. I replied that just thinking about finishing the case without supervision made me sufficiently anxious that I could barely speak. John said, "Remember that feeling for the rest of your career and you'll likely be a safe anesthesiologist."

***Note from the Editors:** We think the most beautiful Northwestern University bridge is the arch over the entrance to campus (Fig. 77.1).

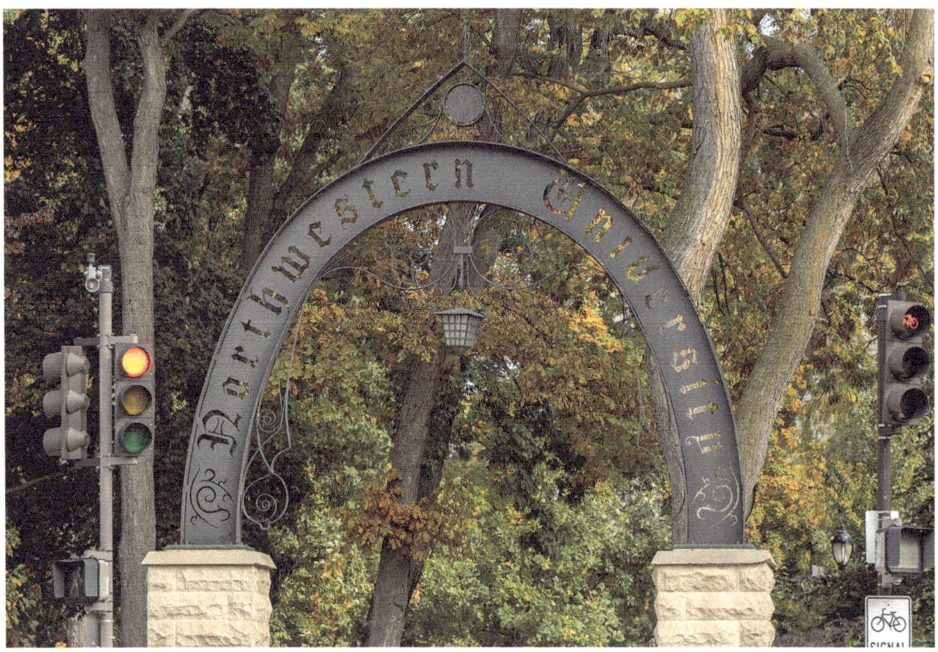

Fig. 77.1 The lovely arch at the entrance to the main campus of Northwestern University in Evanston IL. Photo: Image used under standard license from stock.adobe.com

Lesson No. 2

Remember the anxiety and terror you felt the first time you were left alone and responsible for an anesthetized patient, and you will likely continue to be a safe anesthesiologist.

When I first worked with John, he said that he would never ask me to do anything he would not do/had not done himself—at least in the professional environment. This statement came from the person who, in the early 1970s, developed intermittent mandatory ventilatory (IMV) for adults at a time when the current ventilators did not have a setting of less than 6 breaths/minute. John described sitting at the bedside of his study patients, pressing the "sigh" button on the Puritan-Bennett ventilator every 15 seconds for an IMV rate of 4 breaths/minute, every 20 seconds for an IMV rate of 3 breaths/minute and so on until the patient (study subject) reached no mechanical breaths/minute and was weaned from mechanical ventilation.

Sometimes this weaning process took many hours to days. Nevertheless, determined to demonstrate what he knew was right, John performed this exercise for every patient enrolled in the study, sometimes sitting at the patient's bedside for 2 days. John went on to develop IMV, not just as a method of weaning from mechanical ventilatory support, but also as a way to administer partial ventilatory support and to allow unrestricted spontaneous ventilation. Until then, adult ventilatory support was all or nothing, with no opportunity for the patient to breathe spontaneously.

I had the opportunity to work with John again in 1985 when I was a real fellow (after residency) in a whole animal research laboratory. John had just moved to *The* Ohio State University where he was vice chair of anesthesiology, and I followed to work in his lab. In addition to my own ideas that he allowed me to pursue, he charged me to build a ventilator that would supply a "high" level of continuous positive airway (CPAP) and allow unrestricted spontaneous ventilation, then drop to a "low" level of CPAP briefly—very briefly, perhaps 2 seconds. This change in CPAP level would allow the lungs to passively empty and then refill when the higher level of CPAP was reinstituted.

Thus, the fundamental premise for airway pressure release ventilation (APRV—now often called "BiPAP") began. None of the available respiratory therapy equipment in 1985 would function as needed: the switches were too slow, and the resistance in the CPAP valve and switching mechanisms was too high. So, I went to the hardware store, studied the specifications on plumbing equipment—gas is a compressible liquid, after all—and purchased what I hoped would work. The Ohio State University engineers built the ultra-rapid response switch required to quickly open and close the valve that would allow the change in CPAP level. Of note, the development of this switch preceded the era of microprocessors.

I built the first APRV ventilator in my apartment. John and I used it first to ventilate each other and then performed a more appropriate proof of concept experiment on anesthetized, paralyzed dogs. John always jokes that we got the phylogenetic hierarchy right by starting with ourselves.

Soon thereafter, my fellowship ended. Homemade ventilator in hand, I moved to Atlanta and joined the faculty at Emory University. APRV needed a first human trial. I gained IRB approval to use this homemade device in the Grady Hospital Surgical and Trauma ICU on postop cardiac patients—provided that there was a back-up conventional ventilator at the bedside, and provided that a clinical member of the research team was at the bedside the entire time our experimental ventilator was in use. These were understandable provisions, considering that the prototype ventilator was devoid of a disconnect alarm, a high-pressure alarm, a continuous pressure alarm—basically any alarm other than that provided by the oxygen analyzer.

And so, I found myself sitting at the bedside of my patients and study subjects for 24–36 h during the prototype ventilator's use. This was following in my mentor's footsteps—doing nothing he had not done himself.

Lesson No. 3

Be prepared to do what is necessary. Work hard. Keep an open mind.

John B. Downs is one of the most innovative and creative thinkers in anesthesiology and critical care medicine (CCM). His ideas changed the practice of CCM and anesthesiology, although they were often contrary to "current thought." As a result, throughout his entire career, John constantly battled against mainstream thinking when he introduced new ideas or alternative ways of thinking about patient care—including through the COVID pandemic in the spring of 2020 when he opined for the use of mask CPAP rather than intubation/ventilation for COVID patients, most of whom could breathe well (they did not have ventilatory failure) but were hypoxemic [1]. His persistent, unrelenting pursuit of better patient care through data-driven change in medicine is a lesson for all.

Lesson No. 4

Be persistent and unrelenting in the pursuit of data-driven, physiologically based improved patient care, even if you are David facing a Goliath of "current thought."

John has remained my mentor and confidant for nearly 40 years; I have learned many lessons from him, some of which I related above. John and his delightful wife, Lori, have remained close friends and confidants with me and Stuart, that PhD student I married in 1980.

Lesson No. 5

Nurture and cherish friendships.

Enduring friendships are one of the joys of life and some of the fabric of society.

Lessons Learned

- The editors concur with every single one of the lessons discussed above. If we could distill and summarize even further, we would say that the keys to this very important life and career advice are to master the physiology at the deepest and most profound level possible, go where it takes you and *do NOT let go of your friends*.
- Chris still has those notes! They even made the big move that she and Stu undertook several years ago, although they are now in semi-retirement.

Reference

1. Downs JB, Weled B, Räsänen J, et al. Proposal for coronavirus disease 2019 management (commentary). Crit Care Explor. 2020;2:e0127.

Author

Chris Stock a native of Chicago's South Side, and met her husband of 40 years while both were Northwestern undergraduates. Both is had academic careers—Stu in materials science, Chris in anesthesiology/CCM. Together they raised three children, which provided Chris exquisite preparation for chairing an academic department. Chris enjoys photography and is relearning to play the piano. Together Chris and Stu enjoy ballroom dance—both performing solos and social dancing.

When Things Don't Go As Expected

78

Brenda G. Fahy

Introduction

As a junior attending at the assistant professor rank, I applied to become a member of the American Society of Anesthesiologists (ASA) Committee on Critical Care. I received a letter (snail mail then) that my application for this committee was not accepted but that they would appoint me to the Committee on Surgical Anesthesia. This group is now the Committee on Surgical and Procedural Anesthesia. My initial reaction upon opening that letter was incredible disappointment. I remember thinking this was *not* the committee nor even close to the committee I had sought with my application.

A (Committee) Bird in Hand

Well, I decided it was a committee appointment with a prestigious organization that operated at a national level but also had international reach, and that I should join and try it. The year was 1999, and I received an official appointment to that ASA committee. Little did I know where that would lead. That ASA Committee on Surgical Anesthesia appointment—whose invitation I had greeted with initial disappointment—provided me numerous opportunities during my service. Fundamentally, I believe many of those opportunities would not have been available to me had I received the committee appointment I originally requested.

As I began serving on this committee, I participated in the group discussions, and there was one I remember vividly. It dealt with requirements for compounding medications under a hood and impacts on operating room medication administration. This was a topic on which I did not have expertise. I approached an institutional pharmacist who was a recognized expert on this issue and who had just returned from a meeting where she garnered additional and timely information on this particular issue.

B. G. Fahy (✉)
Department of Anesthesiology, University of Florida College of Medicine, Gainesville, FL, USA
e-mail: bfahy@anest.ufl.edu

S. Mohamed et al. (eds.), *Anesthesia Bridges*, https://doi.org/10.1007/978-3-032-08294-7_78

Orin "Fred" Guidry MD and the ABA

I posted that information on the committee discussion board and, unbeknownst to me, it came under the eye of the individual who was responsible for oversight of this committee for the ASA, Dr. Orin "Fred" Guidry. Dr. Guidry subsequently served as president of both the ASA and the American Board of Anesthesiology (ABA). At the time, I thought this distribution list only consisted of committee members, but Dr. Guidry was behind the scenes and not actively participating in the discussions. *My lesson*: contribute actively to ASA committee discussions, as they are monitored by leaders other than the committee chair and members.

I found out later that this particular post of mine and my activities on this committee impressed him. I believe his support led to my nomination and subsequent selection for his spot as a director for the ABA upon his completion of service. This appointment ultimately allowed me to follow in his footsteps, serving as president of the ABA from 2018 to 2019; the fifth woman to serve in this role since the board's creation in 1938.

New Committees

Four years after joining the Committee on Surgical Anesthesia, I was asked to serve as the ASA liaison to the American College of Surgeons (ACS), as this committee sends one representative to serve on the ACS Committee on Perioperative Care. The physician whose service immediately preceded mine described the role as attending a meeting during the ACS Clinical Congress, providing feedback on behalf of the ASA when attending those meetings, and writing a liaison report on the proceedings to the ASA Committee. This report served as part of the annual ASA committee report, with its inclusion in committee reports to the ASA House of Delegates.

At the time I assumed this role, I discovered there was a new group forming known as the Council on Surgical and Perioperative Safety. Representatives from the ASA and the ACS would serve on this council. Since I would soon be attending my first ACS Committee on Perioperative Care, I reached out to the administrative staff at the ASA to ask who would be attending this new group as the ASA representatives and requested their contact information. My request was denied, with the response that I did not need that information in my role. Clearly, from my perspective, the system was changing around me as I was trying to understand my new role.

I attended my first meeting of the ACS Committee on Perioperative Care, and it was clear—the system had changed since the last liaison's service. The ACS planned to use this committee to vet any ACS initiatives that would ultimately be presented to the Council on Surgical Safety. I again approached the ASA, detailing this information, and stated that it would be helpful if I could communicate with the ASA representatives to the Council. I received an email with their names and email addresses. Both were prominent leaders in the field of anesthesiology who had made significant contributions to the ASA and other outside organizations. They were Drs. Joseph Annis and Robert Stoelting. To provide context, I will only provide a brief synopsis of some of their accomplishments and contributions for those who may be unfamiliar; one cannot do these gentlemen justice within the space constraints of this chapter.

***Note from the Editors:** Brenda Fahy lives and works in Florida. We think the Bridge of Lions in St. Augustine FL is among the most spectacular in the state (Figs. 78.1 and 78.2). It was completed in 1927 and spans the Intercoastal Waterway. It is a double leaf bascule bridge that connects St. Augustine on the mainland with Anacostia Island.

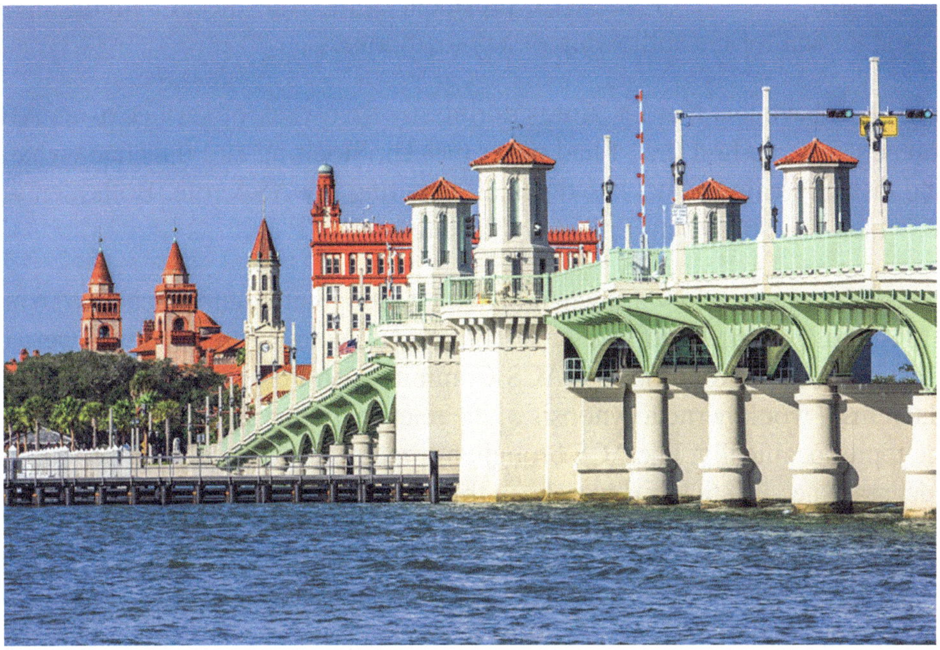

Fig. 78.1. A perspective of the stunning Bridge of Lions with the beautiful buildings of St. Augustine, FL in the background. It was added to the National Register of Historic Places in 1982. Photo: Image used under standard license from shutterstock.com

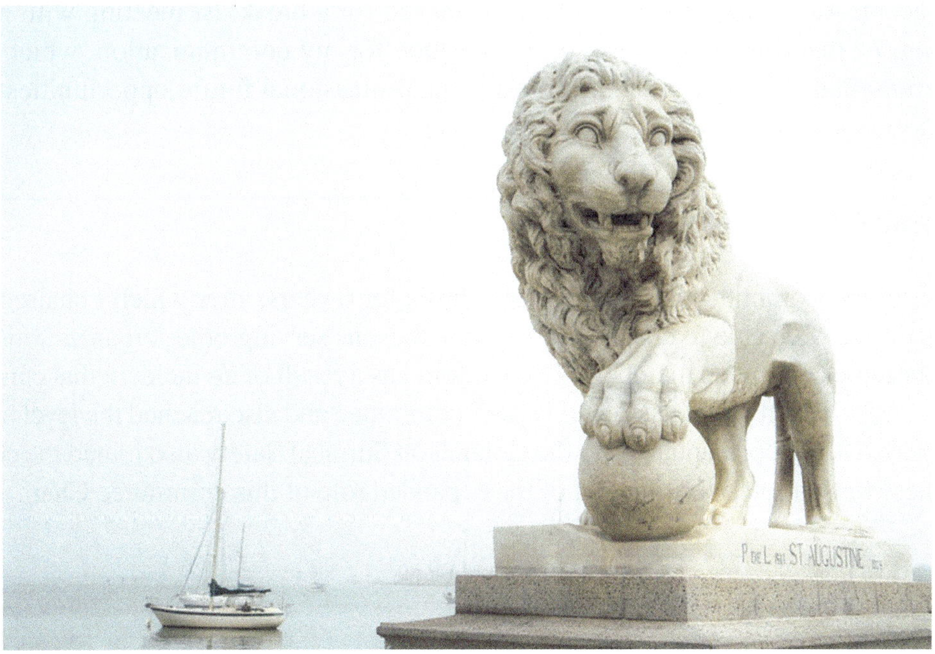

Fig. 78.2. A closeup view of one of the lions who stand guard on the Bridge of Lions in St. Augustine, FL. Photo: dosecreative, image used under standard license from iStock.com

Joseph Annis, MD and Robert Stoelting, MD

Dr. Annis served many roles with the ASA and on the Board of Directors for the Foundation for Anesthesia Research and Education (FAER) and was subsequently elected to serve on the American Medical Association Board of Trustees. Dr. Stoelting received the ASA Distinguished Service Award, served as a director and president of the ABA, president of the Anesthesia Patient Safety Foundation, and is perhaps best known for his authorship of key textbooks.

I was lucky enough to have just met Dr. Annis during my first week of service as an ABA oral boards examiner, so I reached out to him first. I had never met Dr. Stoelting and thus had (what I perceived to be) the daunting task of writing him a "cold" email detailing my ASA role. Both men were incredibly gracious to me, which was something I much appreciated.

I have tried to carry this practice forward when I am interacting with junior faculty who are trying to get involved. One of my roles involved ensuring that both ASA Council representatives were informed early of any topics that were covered during the ACS Committee on Perioperative Care that could become Council agenda items. I would write a synopsis of the relevant topics and send any supporting materials. I remember one topic specifically. The ACS brought a surgeon from Japan to present on the use of blunt tip needles to decrease needle stick injury risks in the operating room.

I figured if the ACS brought this surgeon to their meeting, it would probably be a future Council topic. The presented materials were all paper-based and I recall copying and posting them to Drs. Annis and Stoelting. I remember thinking it might be a while before this topic appeared at a Council meeting, and I wrote a cover note to that effect. Later, when attending a meeting, one of my fellow attendees walked over to me with Dr. Stoelting, stating, "He wanted to meet you in person." Dr. Stoelting then went on to express his appreciation for the information I had been sending and mentioned specifically the blunt tip needles and how well prepared he felt based on my supplied materials, mentioning it was his first exposure to this concept. Along the same line, Dr. Annis asked for a breakfast meeting with me at the ASA Annual Meeting. At that time, he expressed his gratitude for my communication, which prepared him for his ASA representation role, and he discussed some professional future opportunities for me.

Evolving Committee Roles

I was a member of the Committee on Surgical Anesthesia for 6 years, after which I chaired it for 8 years. While I was chair, we were able to ensure that all ASA liaisons serving other organizations with Council representation became committee members. This occurred as a result of an incident that came to my attention while in my ASA liaison role outside of this ASA committee and also reached the level of the President of the ASA. The two ASA representatives to the Council on Surgical Safety also joined the committee. The oversight for these liaison roles became part of the expanded role of this committee Chair.

So, I think back to that original ASA committee application and the rejection for my requested committee appointment. Interestingly enough, I did have a future opportunity to serve on the ASA Committee on Critical Care when I served as president of the Society of Critical Care Anesthesiologists. Luckily for me, the ASA provided me another committee opportunity that most likely offered me opportunities that I would not have received had my initial committee request been honored.

Final Thoughts

When I accepted the alternate committee appointment that was offered by the ASA, I had no idea where that would lead, and the high-quality leaders I would have the opportunity to interact with, and the learning experiences offered. I shudder to think what I would have missed had I, in a moment of disappointment, turned down that opportunity! Sometimes, when things do not go the way you expect them to, they can lead to something even better. Be open to those opportunities!

Lessons Learned

- As they say, sometimes a door closes, but a window opens somewhere else.
- Take advantage of any opportunities offered, even if it is not exactly what you wanted, you may be surprised where they lead. In Brenda Fahy's case, they led to her being the president of the ABA. ☺
- Follow the lead of Drs. Annis and Stoelting (and Dr. Fahy!) and practice welcoming inclusiveness to the junior people and a willingness to listen and learn from them.
- Committee work, while it can be time-intensive and labor-intensive, it a great way to build a career and a national reputation. It does not always have to be through RO1's and a gazillion hours in the lab.
- Earlier in this book, we made the point that most positive things in a career flow from something that is written. Note what happened when Dr. Fahy put the information that she was collecting into memoranda. You can't just know new things and talk about them; you have to write them up!

Author

Brenda Fahy spent her career in academic medicine serving in various roles spanning the clinical, educational, quality, and administrative arenas. Participation in National/International activities have provided career opportunities. Some of what she viewed as disappointment yielded better experiences than if she had received her requested assignments.

From Clinical Anesthesia to the Biotech Boardroom: Wendye Robbins Shares Her Journey

79

Lindsey N. Gouker, Wendye Robbins, Bryant A. Murphy, and Catherine Marcucci

Introduction

Wendye Robbins is an anesthesiologist, serial biotech CEO, and board member for several corporate and industry groups. She has dedicated her career to discovering and shepherding development of therapeutics for grievous diseases. While incubating nascent drug development technology for investors, she also practiced anesthesiology and taught at UCSF School of Medicine (1995–2000) and the Stanford University School of Medicine (2002–2016).

Because Wendye has had such an interesting career—from full-time anesthesia practice to a hybrid career as both an anesthesiologist and a biotech physician-scientist to a full-time biotech CEO—we thought it would be fun and informative to do a full-length interview. She was gracious enough to take time from her busy schedule to have several conversations with Lindsey Gouker and Bryant Murphy. In the next two chapters, she reflects on her professional and personal journeys and shares her best advice for junior anesthesiologists who may be considering widening the boundaries of their careers.

The Interview

Lindsey Gouker: Let's start at the very beginning of your career journey—when did you recognize your interest in medicine?

Wendye Robbins: Until I graduated from college, I didn't consider exploring medicine as a career. You could say medicine was in my DNA, nonetheless. I'm a third or fourth generation physician, depending on how you count. I liked school and found many subjects interesting. I did my undergraduate work at Berkeley. I saw that the theoretical

L. N. Gouker · B. A. Murphy
Department of Anesthesiology, The University of North Carolina at Chapel Hill, Chapel Hill, NC, USA

W. Robbins
Blade Therapeutics, Inc. (former), South San Francisco, CA, USA

Incendia Therapeutics, Inc. (at present), Boston, MA, USA

C. Marcucci (✉)
Department of Transfusion Medicine, Clinical Center, National Institutes of Health, Bethesda, MD, USA

S. Mohamed et al. (eds.), *Anesthesia Bridges*, https://doi.org/10.1007/978-3-032-08294-7_79

finance program was a center of excellence there. I applied to the Haas School of Business and was accepted into the program at the start of my junior year. I imagined that I would work in international economic forecasting or something like that after graduation.

I couldn't quite make the leap into this industry after college—too tedious. I traveled for several months and pondered my future. I realized that my education had prepared me to work in what I saw as an uninspiring area, for example, corporate revenue forecasting. At the same time, there was this burgeoning tragedy of HIV. You would see patients with facial Kaposi's Sarcoma lesions and lipodystrophy everywhere. I found that to be a compelling social problem and something that I was interested to work on. I decided to learn more about the science of virology. But I had no training whatsoever and this was a highly infectious disease—not an ideal place for a science newbie.

I mapped out a path for developing expertise. I enrolled in the Mills College post-baccalaureate program and held a series of part-time jobs at the same time. When I finished the post-bac, I went to Baylor Medical College to do a year of research in the Department of Virology. That program was chaired by one of the greats in the field of virology, a virologist by the name of Dr. Joe Melnick. I spent that year learning from outstanding virologists and molecular biologists in his department. Additionally, I was intellectually nurtured by the faculty there. My lab was led by a brilliant and wonderfully inclusive couple, Dr. James Smith and Dr. Olivia Pereira Smith. It was a big lab full of all kinds of bright grad students. Jim and Olivia were terrific leaders and teachers. I realized I was on the right track. I was falling in love with science. And I realized that by completing a medical degree, I could continue to develop tools to tackle many diverse human afflictions. I was hooked.

Lindsey: Where did you go to med school and were you able to continue to do research?

Wendye: I applied to several medical schools that year while I was in the lab. And I was grateful that I had a handful of acceptances. I ended up choosing to go to Medical College of Pennsylvania (MCP), a formerly all-women's free standing medical college in Philadelphia. It was a lovely place, and for various personal reasons, I picked that one and I went. And it was a very happy decision. I had a great experience, and they let me have a mentor and work in the lab while I was a med student. I got a grant funded and met some phenomenal classmates who are still close friends today. Importantly, I also met my husband during my second year. He was not in the medical field. He was a wonderful supporter during my medical training, and he has been a great life partner. I could not have succeeded in this process without the strong support and care of my husband, Craig.

***Note from the Editors:** Photos of this solid bridge across the Schuylkill River in Philadelphia, PA have often been in the yearbooks of the Philadelphia medical schools, including the Medical College of Pennsylvania, Wendye's alma mater (Fig. 79.1). It has been there forever and is imprinted in the memories of anybody who ever travelled up and down Kelly Drive.

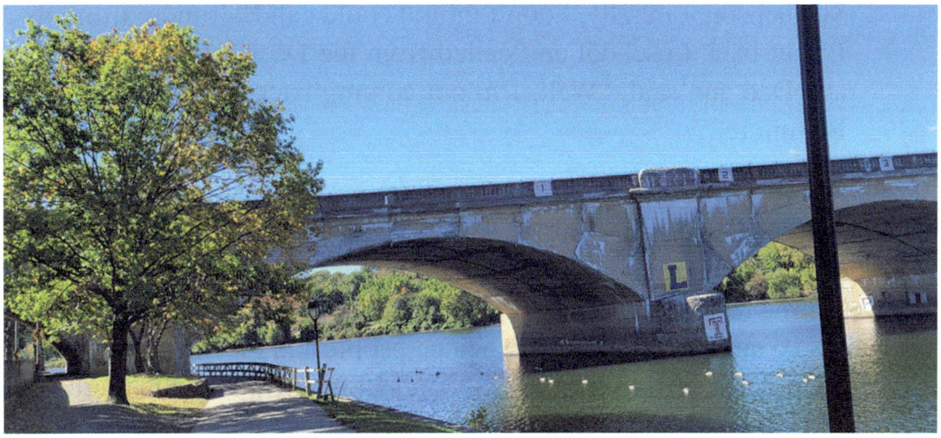

Fig. 79.1 Bridge spanning the Schuylkill River in Philadelphia, PA. It is near the old MCP campus but we spot the Temple "T" and maybe an "L" for Lasalle? Photo: Kama Linden, image used for editorial (non-fiction book) purposes from iStock.com

Lindsey: How did you choose your anesthesia residency program?

Wendye: In my third year and fourth year, I did several away rotations in academic anesthesia departments. These experiences proved to be very important in setting up my internship and residency opportunities. I particularly liked my month in the MGH RICU. I had applied to anesthesia programs through the MATCH. I had my heart set on matching at either MGH, the Brigham, or Stanford. Surprisingly, in October of 1989, I was called to the Dean's Office at my medical school. Bob Stephenson, the Johns Hopkins Anesthesia residency director, was on the line. "We want to offer you a spot and you have 24 hours to give an answer." My instincts were to decline although I was honored that they had offered me the spot. And I felt like it's a great, great institution and the people were phenomenal, but Baltimore…why would I want to go there?

Craig came home that night and I said, "I got this surprising call from the Hopkins residency director today. It was an amazing offer—they would commit to giving me a spot, but I have to let them know by tomorrow. And I'm not going to do it, I'm going to do the MATCH and the reality is, I hopefully will place at either Mass General or Stanford. That's what I want and I'm just going to trust that the MATCH is going to work out."

And Craig said, "Look, I've got to tell you that I've been really worried about your choices. The economy is not good in the area of real estate that I'm in, in either Boston or San Francisco. If you took this spot at Hopkins, I could keep my partnership in my firm." He was working for a real estate consulting firm outside of Radnor, Pennsylvania. He said, "We could get married." And I said, "We've never talked about getting married." He said "No, no, no, if you take Hopkins, we'll get married and we'll move to Baltimore, I'll commute back to Philadelphia." So, we spent all night talking about it. The next morning, I went back to school to call Bob

Stephenson. Literally, I don't think I could call Baltimore from my apartment, and I went back to school and called from the Dean's office. Then I called my Mom and Dad and said, "Well, I'm not coming back to California, I'm going to go to Baltimore."

Lindsey: And how was your residency at Hopkins?

Wendye: After spending my intern year in internal medicine at Penn, I went to Hopkins. It was the best decision. It was an amazing place and such a privilege to train there. I met so many brilliant and dedicated people and I learned a lot. I also really enjoyed the city and getting to know more about the Mid-Atlantic region. And, but for that funny call from the residency director, that wouldn't have happened. So that's the story.

We had this amazing scientific mentor named Dick Traystman as head of research in the department. He helped me find a lab. He supported me and all interested house staff with research ideas and funding and mentoring. That was, for me, tremendous. Also, the department was very welcoming. I remember on many Thursdays or Fridays; I would receive a page that an attending I hadn't yet met would like to invite Craig and me to their home for dinner. That's what would happen for a CA-1, you would just get invited to someone's home.

Lindsey: That is so interesting. I don't think many programs are like that.

Wendye: I've always tried to model that with my Stanford house staff. Our guestroom was frequently full. In fact, one couple got together and eventually got married after hanging out at my house at Thanksgiving. They had my kids as attendants in their wedding. It was very cute.

Lindsey: That is awesome.

Wendye: That was Hopkins. They just took care of you. And they cared. My classmates and I would just say to each other, "Ok, it's Friday night, whose house are you going to?" We loved it.

Lindsey: You've chosen a path not taken by many—you've chosen to leave clinical medicine after so much learning, training, and sacrifice. Was there a specific moment that prompted this transition away from clinical medicine?

Wendye: There was not one moment—it was more a series of events. I finished my pain fellowship in June 1995. I arrived in San Francisco with a six-month-old baby, a husband, a nanny, and a dog, and moved into a tiny row house in San Francisco (Fig. 79.2). I was thrilled to be joining the faculty as Assistant Professor in Residence at the prestigious University of California, San Francisco, School of Medicine, Department of Anesthesia.

Barely three months into my UCSF tenure, I found myself pregnant again. I felt fine and managed to continue to meet my clinical, administrative, teaching, and research obligations. I was warned that "two pregnancies in the same decade" was not done in this department. I was advised to use vacation time to cover the maternity leave. My middle daughter was born 4 weeks before my anesthesia oral board exam (Thankfully, I somehow passed).

By then, the department was clearly signaling that I should not have more children. Eighteen months later I became pregnant with our son.* The departmental body language was no longer low pitched. I was a pariah because of my growing family. It was clear that I should move on. I had remained productive, met deadlines, got funded, published, kept my patients safe, mentored house staff, and remained engaged. The department and I were not synchronized about priorities and what I would need to do for a really thriving career at UCSF.

I had been working in research on topical transient receptor potential (TRP) channel agonists for neuropathic pain. The University of California - San Francisco (UCSF) patent office had begun filing patent applications on this work. In 1999, I was approached by venture investors with interest in the technology. They suggested that they might create a company. It felt like an interesting opportunity. I didn't see a reason not to go. I didn't want to spend more years in my current situation. It's not that there weren't good people there—there were lots of brilliant people with noble purposes. But I had antagonized the departmental leadership. There would be no growth for me there.

***Note from the Editors:** Wendye's greatest loves and pride have always been the family she built with Craig McGahey (Fig. 79.2).

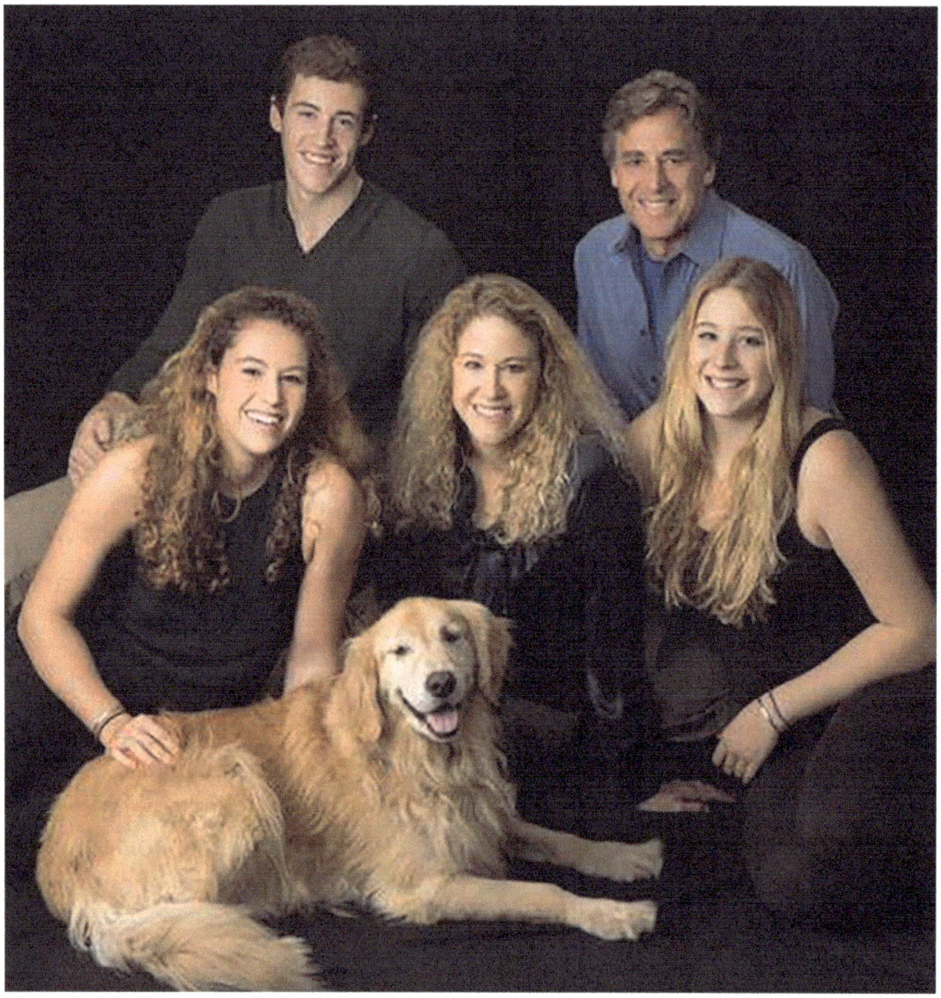

Fig. 79.2 The gorgeous Robbins—McGahey family. Simon is in the back row with his father and sisters Elena and Robin are next to Mom. Wendye and Craig see the kids as often as possible but it is harder to get everybody together now, of course. Photo: Collection of the Robbins-McGahey family

I would be untruthful if I didn't admit that I was relieved to leave full time academic medicine. I didn't miss the endless committee and departmental meetings or being relegated to working so many days without house staff. I disliked being sent to one of many different operating theater sites outside my skill set on short notice when needed.

On the other hand, I knew absolutely nothing about drug development. In my new role, I became an instant chief medical officer. I was tasked with being both the chief clinical strategist and the operational executive (designing clinical trials), something I knew nothing about. But I found great mentors and was lucky to have some great board members. We were able to create a drug from the early technology (later called Qutenza). That drug eventually got approved in the US and the EU. Eventually, we hired a real chief medical officer. I was able to learn from him. At that point, I pivoted to working on the corporate side. I left that company in late 2003.

I accepted a faculty position at Stanford University School of Medicine. I chose to be part-time faculty. On my nonclinical days, I worked with investors and collaborated with other scientists to develop technology around untreated diseases. By staying under 50% full-time equivalent (FTE), I was able to keep the intellectual property separate. I had no office, no phone, no administrative or secretarial support, but I owned my own brain. This meant that I was able to work with a series of talented people focused on developing therapeutics for patients in need. That's what I've been doing ever since. I'm on my fifth or sixth company, depending on how you count them.

Lindsey: Was there any guilt or sadness when you decided to leave? Do you have a sense of wasted time or effort?

Wendye: I really enjoyed my time in the OR and the opportunity to collaborate with surgeons, house staff, and nursing in the mission of making surgery safe for patients. The lessons in basic pharmacology and the requirement for second-to-second decision making was tremendous, tremendous training.

I have absolutely no regrets. Life moves in different stages. I was absolutely committed to anesthesia and pain management during my postgraduate training and in my years at UCSF and Stanford. I still rely on that training to lead my company. In drug development, we rapidly interpret complex and often incomplete data to make critical decisions. Sometimes we see results that surprise us. This may force us to pivot our development plans. This is when anesthesia training really helps me. On more than one occasion my board has commented on how quickly I was able to react to data and make changes in the plan. My response is—yep, that's anesthesia training.

Lindsey: Can you speak to the aspects of biotech at the time that made you excited to make that transition?

Wendye: It's all the unknowns of drug development. You come to the office and every day it is different. It's the challenge of recruiting the team, raising the money, telling the story, and advancing the science. In biotech, you sometimes operate in a bit of a vacuum—you don't always know what the next biotech company is doing or what will happen in the regulatory space. You make decisions with limited information and with great speed and you commit large sums of money without certainty of the outcome. At the same time, it feels great to be on a learning curve all the time. It's one of the best things about working in the drug development/pharmacology world. I get to meet people who are very passionate about what they do.

Life Lessons

- After reading over Wendye's early professional and medical education, it is clear that her eventual careers did not just come out of nowhere. The building blocks were put in place from her earliest undergraduate days. As you go through your career, think carefully about your own building blocks, where you will get them, and how you will stack them.

- It is also notable that Wendye was willing to go where the opportunities were, including prime consideration of the opportunities that were meaningful for her partner. Her journey around the country and through different institutions eventually landed her back "home" in California, where she made her life, built her career, and raised her family.

- In revising and editing this chapter we had a lot of fun reminiscing about the Hopkins days. Wendye's recounting of the support and camaraderie there in the 1990s is correct! It was a remarkable place to train.

- If you must face the facts that an employment situation is not working in your best interests, face them. Be clear about your priorities and what you are and are not willing to do. When you leave, leave only to the degree that is needed to give yourself room to change directions and go forward. For instance, Wendye did not leave clinical anesthesia all at once and continued to practice part-time at Stanford for many years while she built her biotech career.

Authors

Lindsey Gouker is an assistant professor of anesthesiology at the University of North Carolina Chapel Hill, but the journey there was a bit… winding. After med school, she first completed a pediatrics residency and fellowship in hematology/oncology. After 4 years as a pediatric hematologist/oncologist, she made the very difficult, but ultimately very rewarding, decision to return to training and completed a second residency in anesthesiology at the University of North Carolina in 2019. She has also obtained a Master of Healthcare Administration from the Gillings School of Public Health at the University of North Carolina in 2020. She has been on faculty at the University of North Carolina since 2020.

Wendye Robbins at the time of this interview, lived in California, she has recently become the CEO of Incendia Therapeutics in Cambridge, MA. She is very passionate about her husband Craig and three young adult children, her community, and fitness. Wendye and Craig were frequently found in the stands cheering for Bay Area sports team including the Warriors, Giants, 49'ers, and the Stanford Cardinals and Cal Bears football teams. She encourages aspiring entrepreneurs to build their foundations with diligence and advises that clinicians interested in biotech stay in medicine at least long enough to understand their constituencies and systemic inefficiencies. She believes that the rigor of her Johns Hopkins anesthesia training prepared her well for the minute-to-minute challenges of running venture-backed startups.

Bryant Murphy is a professor of anesthesiology and the associate dean for leadership development within the UNC School of Medicine's Office of Faculty Affairs and Leadership Development. In this role, he leads efforts to ensure comprehensive and coordinated leadership development and training opportunities for faculty, staff, and learners across the UNC School of Medicine. Bryant Murphy did medical school, anesthesiology residency, and cardiothoracic anesthesiology fellowship at Wake Forest University. Prior to returning to academic practice at UNC, he was a partner in a private practice in Fayetteville, NC. He also obtained an MBA degree from George Washington University in 2012.

Cathy Marcucci was one year behind Wendye Robbins in residency training at Hopkins in the early 1990s. She also received one of those calls from Bob Stephenson but hers was to the Dean's Office at Temple University School of Medicine. She and Wendye recalled, without difficulty, dozens of dinners, holiday parties, barbecues, baby showers, brunches, and oral boards study sessions they attended at the homes of faculty members.

From Clinical Anesthesia to the Biotech Boardroom: Advice on Mentoring and Making the Leap

80

Lindsey N. Gouker, Bryant A. Murphy, Wendye Robbins, and Catherine Marcucci

Introduction

In the previous chapter, Wendye Robbins shared the stages she traveled in her journey from practicing anesthesiologist to CEO of a biotech company seeking novel therapies for incurable diseases. In this chapter, she talks further with Lindsey Gouker about mentoring and managing a major life and career transition.

The Interview, Part 2

Lindsey Gouker: How did you prepare for that transition? That first leap into the biotech world.

Wendye Robbins: It really was just jumping off the cliff with a dose of high self-confidence and a crazy but rational passion for solving critical diseases. You never know exactly what all is coming your way in biotech. You trust your instincts and trust that you are well-trained. And you must above all be rational and faithful to the data. I remind myself that it's all about creating tools for patients. If what we're doing makes sense for patients, we should do it. But the second it doesn't, we stop. I think about that all the time. For my first leap, I focused on the treatment of complex neuropathic pain. There would be bigger leaps to take in other disease areas as my career progressed.

L. N. Gouker · B. A. Murphy
Department of Anesthesiology, The University of North Carolina at Chapel Hill, Chapel Hill, NC, USA
e-mail: bryant_murphy@med.unc.edu

W. Robbins
Blade Therapeutics, Inc. (former), South San Francisco, CA, USA

Incendia Therapeutics, Inc. (at present), Boston, MA, USA

C. Marcucci (✉)
Department of Transfusion Medicine, Clinical Center, National Institutes of Health, Bethesda, MD, USA

S. Mohamed et al. (eds.), *Anesthesia Bridges*, https://doi.org/10.1007/978-3-032-08294-7_80

Lindsey: As you made your transition, who was mentoring you both inside and outside your department?

Wendye: I talked to Jeff Kirsch and Dick Traystman at Hopkins. I also talked to my physician family members (my uncle, my Dad, and my cousin), and of course my husband. Everybody said the same thing to me, "You have your boards, you're well-trained. You can try biotech and see if it works and if it doesn't you can just go to another academic institution or to private practice. There are options." The wide range of potential outcomes did not scare me. I hadn't been someone who wanted to be an anesthesiologist since the age of two years old. I have always had a passion to be part of a profound solution for patients. What that looked like was something I found I could be very flexible about. And going back and talking to Hopkins colleagues really helped clarify that. I am grateful that I received support from people that I cared about.

At the same time, I felt it was incumbent on me to leave UCSF as honorably as I could. I wanted to leave from a position of strength. I gave 3 months' notice, and I got through it. I worked every call that I was scheduled for after I gave notice and took the best possible care of my patients. I didn't feel that I had the right institutional and departmental support to stay. But I do feel that most of the department members that I worked with were good people. And resolving that tension is something that only you can work out for yourself.

Lindsey: What do you recommend as a good first step to take as you begin to consider or even plan to transition away from clinical anesthesia practice?

Wendye: Get your personal and financial house in order. That is so important. You can't take risks with your career if you have big debt obligations. Also, marry or partner well. Choose someone who supports what you want to do and believes in you and also carries their own weight. I look at partnership/marriage like being doubles tennis partners. You've got to know that your partner can cover the back court. And you've got to trust them. And the reason it all worked in my situation is because I married a terrific guy who was very supportive of me doing what I wanted to do (Fig. 80.1). He had known that I had many interests and a background in business. So, when he saw me unhappy, he just said, "There are other areas for you, don't forget that. You have other skills." And I am so grateful that he always encouraged me.

So, if you have chosen well and have your financial house in order and your primary relationships are in good shape, don't be afraid to take risks. That's the key—don't be afraid! Just try it. Also, I moved forward but I didn't leave everything and everyone behind. I still have a great peer-group from Hopkins and several physician friends from San Francisco, Stanford, and UCSF. I cherish them. I see my doctor friends all the time.

***Note from the Editors:** Wendye advises that it is incredibly important to put a lot of thought into your choices of a life partner—who you marry or partner with can make a huge difference in how your life goes (Fig. 80.1).

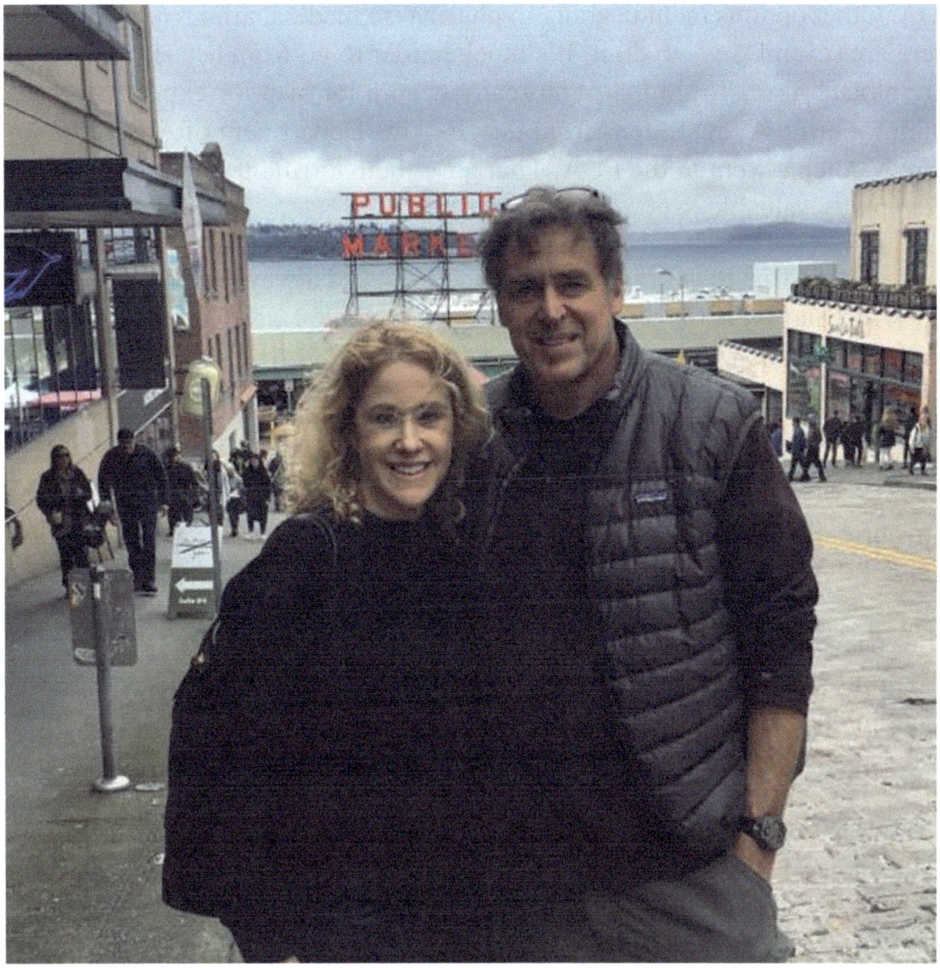

Fig. 80.1 Wendye with her husband Craig McGahey. She credits Craig with providing steadfast support through her entire busy and fascinating career. Photo: Collection of Wendye Robbins

Lindsey: As a CEO, is there any specific training that you would recommend? If there is time to prepare for a transition from clinical medicine into the biotech world, would an MBA help or a master's in healthcare administration be advisable?

Wendye: First and foremost, find a mentor who's taken a range of risks to build a company or significant organization. Find somebody who has done what you want to do and get them to talk to honestly about what's missing in your background and on your resume. Next, if you can't take the time to get an MBA, go to an executive education program at a top university. Stanford has one. Harvard has one. Hopkins has one. So does Wharton. It costs a lot and it's a few weeks away from your family and your work. These programs provide great introductions to business.

Develop a sense of whether your interests are in administration or hospital management, drug development, devices, public health or regulatory science. Consider working for the

FDA. Other options include going to pharma (in medical affairs or as a research scientist)—there are several ways to do it. It's much harder to go from academic clinical medicine to a tiny biotech firm. To do that, you really need a lot of prior experience because there's no room for error. A few friends from the Hopkins Department of Anesthesiology and Critical Care Medicine went to the FDA. That gave them terrific training and experience and made them really valuable to companies.

Above all, be true to your ideals and principles, and always remember to take time for yourself. Trust and value the opinions of your inner circle … rarely can you embark on high-risk ventures like this without your support team.

Lindsey: Where do you see yourself going from here? Do you serve on boards? Do you see yourself advising the government? Are you heavily recruited by Big Pharma?

Wendye: I am currently the CEO of Blade Therapeutics. **Editor's note: After this interview was completed, Wendye went on to be the CEO of Incendia Therapeutics.*

After 6+ years, we are in the process of taking the company public. This is an exciting process. I also serve on the board of a clinical stage company focused on drugging targets in inflammation and oncology (Rapt Therapeutics). I'm on the board of the California Life Sciences Association and a new trustee at the Buck Institute for Research in Aging. I also spend a fair amount of time mentoring junior colleagues and former residents.

At this point, I don't really see myself going into Big Pharma. I love what I am doing today. So long as I have the excitement and energy and interest, I'll keep trying to develop tools for patients. That's what really matters.

Lindsey: What is your work/life balance?

Wendye: I try to keep a rational and balanced lifestyle. I have a wonderful husband, and I adore my kids. I also love my friends, especially my doctor pals. We hike together. For fitness and mental clarity, I try to run about 75 miles a month. I do Pilates. I also love to swim. Keeping fitness in my life is important to me and keeps me energized. If I miss a few days of running, I'm just not as focused. My husband and I see our kids a lot as well as friends.

Overall, I would say I lead a quiet life—my family and friends and work. I probably work 75–80 h per week. There are times that I work weekends. As the CEO, I cannot ever really turn it off. But it's such a privilege, it really is great work. I'm just inspired to advance these drugs to help patients.

***Note from the Editors:** Speaking of work-life balance, we happen to know that Wendye gets to Paris as often as she can. The Pont Alexandre III connects the Left Bank and Right Bank of the Seine River and has been called "the most beautiful bridge in the world" (Fig. 80.2). We are inclined to agree. The bridge was inaugurated in 1900 and named for Tsar Alexandre III.

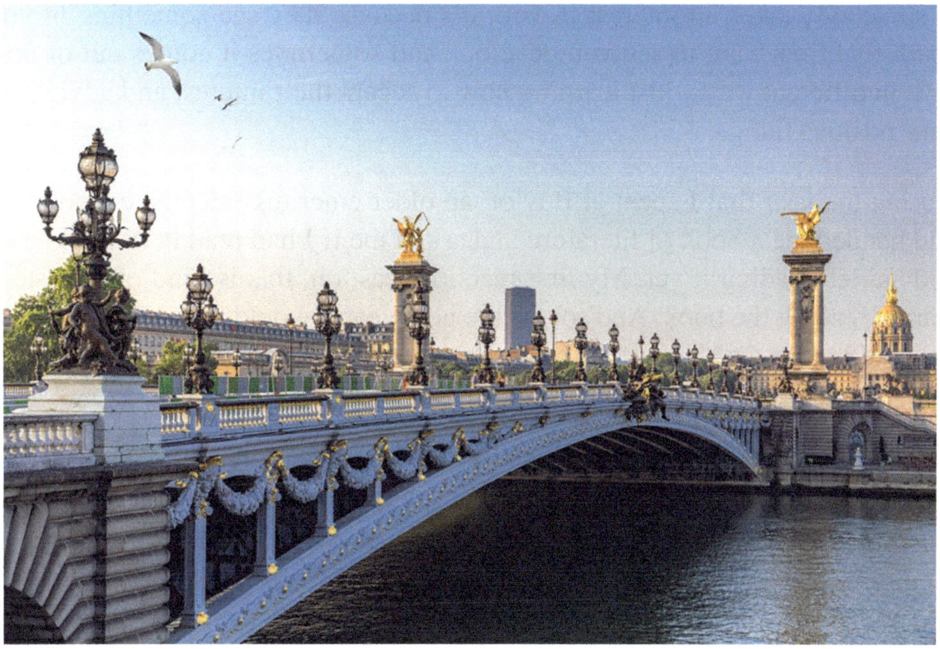

Fig. 80.2 The Pont Alexandre in Paris spans the Seine River and is famous for its spectacular Art Nouveau lamps and statuary. Photo: Image used under standard license from stock.adobe.com

Lindsey: Young people are always advised, "Find a mentor." But how do we find that person? How do you know that someone that you reach out to will be a good mentor? And how do you personally get hooked up with your mentees?

Wendye: Let's explore that. When someone asks you how you are doing, accept their query as sincere interest. I made a practice at Stanford of connecting with every resident or medical student that was on my service. I would try to understand their personal situation and goals and follow-up with them. For instance, if they had a baby, I would send a card or present. Some people don't know how to take that. Some trainees withdraw if you ask them a personal question, as if you are invading their private space. That's fine—I get it. And I don't bother them. But those residents and students who respond well to the genuine interest, I stay in touch.

Social media is a great tool for this. I follow several of my former house staff this way—I wish them happy birthday and follow their growth. They know that I care about them. When I see that something is going on in their life, I'll send them a note asking them if they want to talk about that and then we'll have a phone call. There are probably a couple of dozen former trainees—I call them my bonus kids—that I keep up with. It just makes me happy to see them advancing their lives and figuring things out. And if it's not a positive situation, say a divorce, they still know that I care.

So, from your side, I would just say, if you see a faculty member or former faculty member reach out to you with a question—how are you, what's going on?—just take it for what it is, sincere interest. You've impressed them in your training years and they care about you.

If somebody takes an interest in you, it's because they see something in you—they see a spark that they want to see you develop. And sometimes it comes out of nowhere. People give in different ways. Just learning how to accept their interest and advice and support is a very positive thing.

During the year that I spent at Baylor, an older emeritus scientist called me into his office and handed me a book of literature and asked me if I had read it. A week later he asked if I had started reading it yet. My first reaction was, oh, this is kind of a waste of time. But I started reading the book. And so, for the next year, I would visit him every week or two and he would make me a cup of tea and we would talk about literature. It was the most wonderful and unexpected mentoring relationship.

If I can just make one point for this book—just listen to the great minds around you. Don't always think you have to direct the conversation. Let them explain things to you. I remember in my residency how much I enjoyed hearing stories from the great senior anesthesia faculty in our department—Tommy Tung, Scott Eleff, Jim Schauble and Bob Donham—and also from distinguished surgeons whom I worked with. I loved hearing their stories about the early days of anesthesia or the early days of neuroimaging. When senior leaders want to talk to you, take the time to listen. Because they are giving you something. It might not always be obvious, you might be tempted to think, oh this guy just likes to talk. But, more likely they are offering you some valuable life or professional lessons.

Lindsey: Can you share a mistake that you made and what you learned?

Wendye: Hiring well is critical. Hire people smarter than you. Hire the best. Do your diligence. Talk to their former bosses and colleagues. Meet their partners/spouses. At my first company, I took guidance on hiring from the venture investors. I didn't do enough diligence. Some of those early hires were the wrong people. The culture at my first company became toxic very quickly. I left within 3 years when I was fed up. That was a disappointment. Since then, I have taken pains to recruit people who excel at their work and are positive team contributors. It makes all the difference in one's work experience.

Lindsey: If you had only four sentences to summarize your personal and professional journey and advise junior people, what would you say?

Wendye: I would say that:

1. *Yes, I took big career risks by stepping away from precedent—many times.*

2. *But I believed in the mission, and I trusted my instincts.*

3. *Listen to your heart.*

4. *Believe in yourself and don't be afraid of risk.*

Lessons Learned

- If you think you might want to make a major change in your professional life, get your personal and financial affairs in order. Remember, you land farther out if you jump off a platform than if you try to jump out of a ditch, so try to get a financial berm together to launch from. Also, do the people in your life support you and are they available to help cover all the things that are important outside of work?
- Finding mentors can be as simple as not brushing off people who express interest in you. If you do find someone who is interested in you and wants to share their wisdom, by all means, *LISTEN!*
- Leaving an employment situation doesn't mean, and shouldn't mean, leaving all the people behind. Value the relationships that were a positive factor in your life and take the time to maintain them.
- When you are in the position to do so, hire the best people you can find. The time and diligence you put into your hiring decisions is well worth it.
- Believe in your mission and believe in yourself!

Authors

Lindsey Gouker was raised in Michigan and attended the University of Michigan for undergrad (Go Blue!), ultimately attending medical school in New York. Outside of the OR, Lindsey enjoys working on QI and patient safety initiatives and spending time with her two sons and husband on the North Carolina beaches.

Bryant Murphy is an avid college basketball fan, and longs for the days when the conference tournaments were big events, and the teachers would cancel classes for the first day of the ACC tournament. He also enjoys Disney and makes multiple trips (sometimes even without his kids) to discover new hidden Mickey Mouse icons throughout the resort. He believes in mentorship and leadership for the next generation and will always make time for a student or resident that needs assistance along the way.

Wendye Robbins has dedicated her career to discovering and shepherding development of therapeutics for grievous diseases. She is convinced that her work-life balance keeps her energized and focused. She sees her family and friends as often as possible, spends date nights at lap swim facilities (Stanford's Avery Aquatic Center has been a favorite), and enjoys paddling rivers in the western U.S. (most recently on the Middle Fork of the Salmon). Wendye remains a frequent mentor to medical students and house staff.

Cathy Marcucci did her anesthesia training at Hopkins and was mentored by the best. She is grateful to still be in contact with a lot of her Hopkins colleagues. She has made several leaps in her career, although not as big as the ones that Wendye took.

More Wisdom on Career Advancement and Development and Promotion

81

Kirk Lalwani, Harriet W. Hopf, Evan D. Kharasch, and Catherine Marcucci

Contributors:

Ronald S. Bank, MD (RSB)

Dawn Dillman, MD (DD)

Brian T. Gierl, MD (BTG)

Vincent L. Hoellerich, MD (VLH)

Michael P. Hutchens, MD, MPH (MPH)

Julia K. Labovsky, MD (JKL)

Michael A. Ramsay, MD (MAR)

Neil B. Sandson, MD (NBS)

Amy J. Robbins, MD (AJR)

Richard W. Rosenquist, MD (RWR)

Joseph M. Schwartz, MD (JMS)

Toby N. Weingarten, MD* (TNW)

K. Lalwani
Department of Anesthesiology and Perioperative Medicine, Oregon Health and Science University, Portland, OR, USA

H. W. Hopf
Utah Coaching and Advancement Network (U-CAN), Department of Anesthesiology, University of Utah, Salt Lake City, UT, USA

E. D. Kharasch
Department of Anesthesiology, Duke University, Durham, NC, USA

C. Marcucci (✉)
Department of Transfusion Medicine, Clinical Center, National Institutes of Health, Bethesda, MD, USA

S. Mohamed et al. (eds.), *Anesthesia Bridges*, https://doi.org/10.1007/978-3-032-08294-7_81

Introduction

Career development starts the minute you begin anesthesia residency training. The development of a vision for your career is something that really should not be far from your mind at all times, except maybe when you are on maternity or parental leave. It's generally not a good idea to be a ruthless climber of the career ladder—that type of strategy often backfires—but you must be the prime force looking out for your own career development and satisfaction. An anesthesiologist's career is both long and short, and there are many ways to do well and even have fun doing it.

General Wisdom

- No matter how much things may seem to suck at a given time, always remember that you're in a noble profession and are blessed with the opportunity to have a profound, positive impact on people's lives.—**RSB**

- Take your time. You'll have a long career and plenty of time to achieve your goals. Definitely plan 4 to 5 years into the future, but allow for 6 to 7 years to get there.—**AJR**

- I wish I had listened more and talked less in the early to mid-years of my career. When those in leadership roles and with many years of experience want or need your input, they'll ask. *Until then, keep your eyes and ears open, and your opinions to yourself.* Take it all in.—**AJR**

- Be open to hearing about new opportunities but extremely deliberate in making career changes.—**AJR**

- My most meaningful advice came from Mike Cahalan. As my mentor (at UCSF) and as my chair (at Utah), whenever I proposed taking on something new, he would ask me what I was going to give up. And then held me to it.—**HWH**

- In every presentation on career development, I use this wisdom from Jack Michenfelder. It is from his 27th Rovenstine Lecture [1]. He warned about "hangers-on," pseudo-academicians, and "self-appointed so-called experts" who promote the unimportant to the status of importance, as a means of gaining self-importance. Boom. Said another way, do not confuse notoriety with respect.—**EDK**

- Words from my graduate school thesis advisor: Do not promote yourself; let your science speak for itself.—**EDK**

- More words from my graduate advisor: It is more important to learn how to think than to learn techniques.—**EDK**

- Always work on the basics and build your foundations with great energy and attention (Fig. 81.1). You advance your career by deepening your understanding of the foundations of anesthesiology and professional life to a profound level. The fancy and showy stuff should not play an oversized role—**Editors**

- Best job in the world is one in which you get to help invent the future.—**EDK**

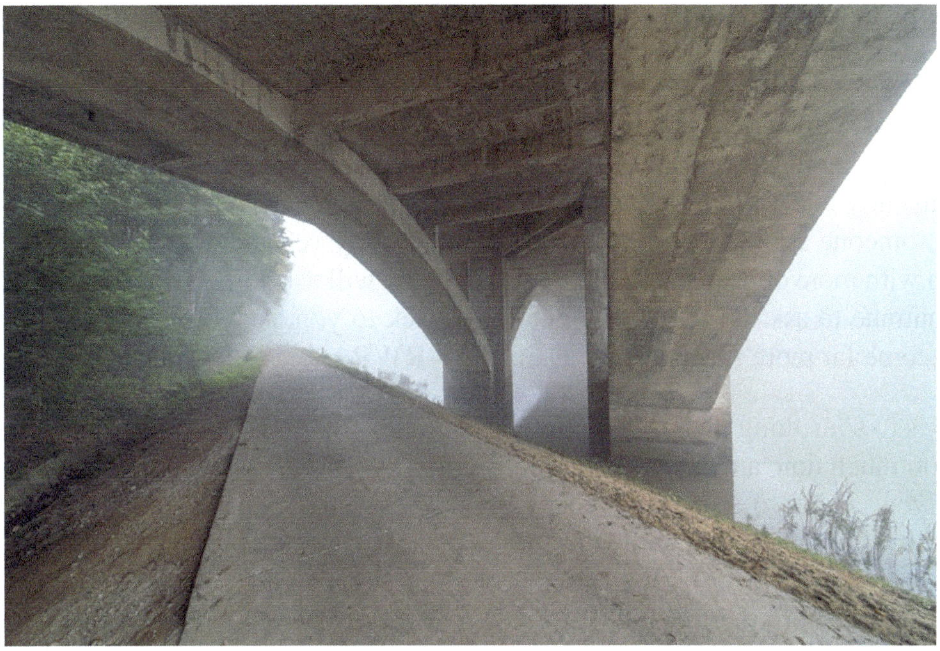

Fig. 81.1 This is an apt metaphor for what you are aiming for as the basis of your career. Make it rock solid!. Photograph: Image used under standard license from shutterstock.com

- It was during my first year of medical school that I received the best single piece of advice of my career. At this point in time, in the late 1990s, the consolidation of hospitals into health care organizations was taking place, and there was a big push for medical graduates to enter primary care fields of medicine. Medical schools were incorporating new curricula, mentoring opportunities, and loan forgiveness programs for students planning to practice primary care medicine. At the beginning of a class in neuroanatomy, the neurosurgeon who was giving the lecture stated that as he noticed this new trend, his advice to my medical school class was this: "Look at what everyone else is doing and do the opposite." He urged us not to pass up a medical specialty for which we had a passion, because times change. In his opinion, the profession of medicine can be challenging for any number of reasons, so it's best to be doing something that you love. At the time, my passion was for anesthesiology, and jobs after residency were scarce. As a result, residencies in anesthesiology were difficult to fill for some programs. On the bright side, there were opportunities to enter the best training programs. So, I did the opposite of what everyone else was doing. I went into the field that everyone said would have no future, and I have been happy with my choice ever since.—**JKL**

- Advice from a patient who was a previous Archbishop of Canterbury when I was trying to decide whether to go to the USA or stay in a great practice in London. "Mike, you are not going to like what I am going to tell you as I sense that you want to stay in the UK. You must go to the USA otherwise you will regret it the rest of your life. We hope that you will come back but probably you will not!" Best advice I ever had.—**MAR**

- We are all on the same train. All of us will be a young, relatively inexperienced anesthesiologist, then a too-busy mid-career person, then a senior doc who is somewhat astonished to find that retirement is not so far in the future. Have as much empathy as you can for the people ahead of you and behind you. You were once there. And you will be there soon enough.—**Editors**

- Although there is a great deal of wisdom regarding the need to focus and have a life balance, in the beginning of a career that is not always possible or even the best choice with regard to creating opportunity. I frequently told various mentees that it was important early on to "Say yes, when it is inconvenient." If someone asks you to do something and you say yes and do it well, they will come back to you again with more opportunities. If you say no, they will ask someone else, and if they do it well, they will continue to ask them and may not come back to you. As your career advances, focus and selection become far more practical and available.—**RWR**

- If you say yes to something that does not interest you, it is likely you will find it an onerous task that takes way too much time and gives little satisfaction. It's unlikely you will do your best work in that situation. If you say yes to everything, you won't have time to do any of them well. Say yes to things that align with your goals, align with your interests, and matter to *you*. And to things that no one else wants to do (be a good citizen), especially if you think you can do them well. Say yes to things that make no sense in the big picture, but that you are drawn to. Doing great work is a powerful way to create a reputation and open opportunities. Saying yes too often is a recipe for frustration, overextension, missed deadlines, and burnout. When someone asks you to do something, get in the habit of asking for time to consider. Then consult with people you trust before making a decision. William Ury's *The Power of a Positive No* is a great resource for saying no without burning bridges—you should say yes to reading it!—**HWH**

- Pay close attention to what type of anesthesia cases are the most natural fit for you. Let's say you are sitting in the anesthesia break room, and an emergency case comes up from the ER so fast that the rails on the stretcher are smoking. As you stand up, do you think, "okay, let's see if we can help this person" or do you think, "I hate this type of case," and you mean it? Conversely, does the prospect of 20 or more patients having outpatient surgery make your eyes glaze over—nothing but a blur of consents and sign-outs? Or are you excited by the challenge of having an entire schedule of patients who find themselves back home so smoothly that they have trouble believing they even had surgery that day? Our point is that not every type of anesthetic practice is for everybody, and that's okay. There probably isn't a bigger split than the question of doing OB anesthesia. Many of us would prefer not to work in the OB suite. Kudos to the people who will do it.—**Editors**

- If you are *not* in the OR 5 days a week, try not to feel superior, career-wise, to the people who are. Their careers are going to look a little different than yours. Perhaps they give anesthesia care at a VA hospital, which can mean little or no possibility for protected non-clinical time and hence less chance for promotion. So, they end their careers as an assistant professor. So what? Or perhaps they have taken another detour, for whatever reason. At any rate, the clinical-five-day-a-week people deserve a nod; it's not always an easy way to be an anesthesiologist. Don't believe us? Try it for 6 months and see what you think.—**Editors**

- I agree with the points above. I was repeatedly urged to do cardiac/echo when I was a resident at UCSF. The idea made my eyes glaze over. I do not find the heart interesting beyond its capacity to deliver perfusion (molecular oxygen! and cefazolin!) to the skin and subcutaneous tissue (weird, I know). The physiology and potential for anesthetic management to affect the outcomes of abdominal, orthopedic, and plastic surgery cases have always fascinated me.—**HWH**

- I'm really a born generalist, and I am happy that I realized that and did not do what it was assumed I would do. I did a research fellowship in wound healing and surgical site infection prevention, so it made sense for my work, and as noted above, I love the general OR cases. I enjoy having a variety of levels of acuity, and the mix of cases and anesthetic techniques always kept it interesting for me. The last 6 or 7 years at UCSF, I was a (non-fellowship trained) OB anesthesiologist. I was also "OB Wound Kenobi"—managing their complicated wounds. And I ran a wound clinic (one day a week) for 12 years, nine at UCSF and three in Utah, which I also enjoyed. Lately, I mostly work at the eye center, supervising CRNAs in 4 rooms, as I work through the rehab on my hands. I've also never done more than two clinical days a week. This required a commitment to obtaining grant funding, publishing, mentoring, and taking on administrative roles, but it supported work I love and has enabled me to grow into leadership roles (within and outside of anesthesiology) at the institutional and national levels. Which would not have been possible without my phenomenal colleagues who want to be in the OR four or five days a week.—**HWH**

***Note from the Editors:** We asked Harriet Hopf about her favorite bridge, and she sent us the following thoughts:

> There are lots of spectacular bridges in this world. We walked across the Golden Gate many times when we lived in the Bay Area, and it is a favorite. But I always prefer roads 'less traveled by,' so I'm picking a bridge with personal meaning rather than awe-inspiring beauty.
>
> My favorite bridge was one we called the 'rickety-rackety bridge' when I was a kid—a very old wooden surface railroad bridge on Summit Avenue in Kensington, MD. It has been replaced (probably a good thing!) and I can't find an old photo.
>
> Instead, I have chosen a photograph of a pedestrian suspension bridge we crossed on the Heaphy Track in New Zealand (Fig. 81.2). It gives me the same feeling of challenging footing and uncertain destination-- which is what I most enjoy in life.

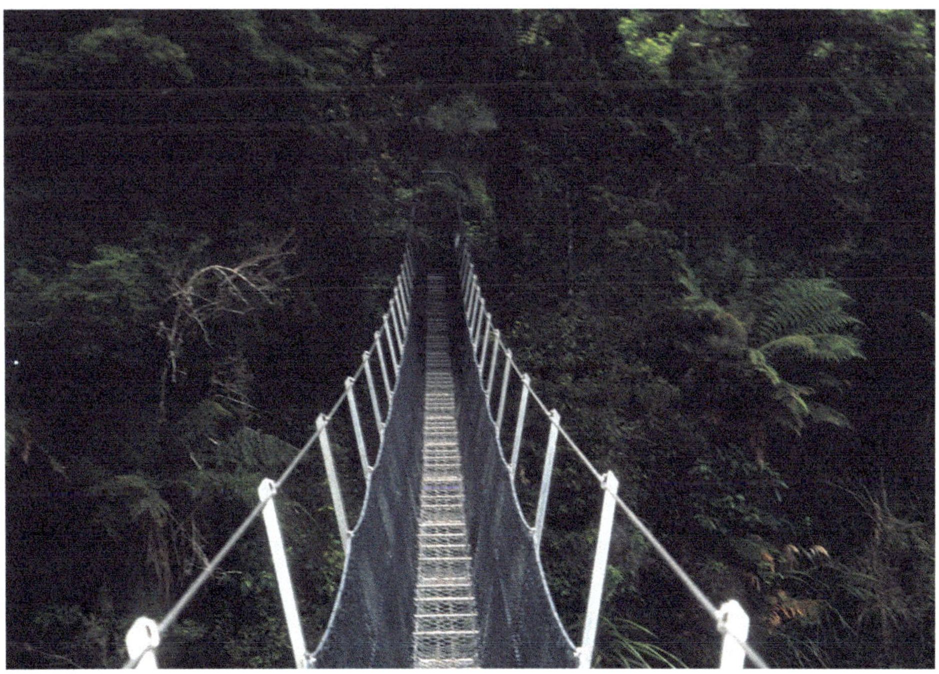

Fig. 81.2 Stunning pedestrian suspension bridge on the Heaphy Track in New Zealand. Photograph: Harriet Hopf

- As a vice-chair for faculty development and fellowship program director, I look for the extras on the CV of a job applicant. Meaning engagement in learning opportunities and publication, and departmental activities. Is there participation in QI? If a resident, did the person seek out research, chapters, or leadership roles? I don't look for any one particular thing. But I do want to see *something* above and beyond a blank slate—as in, "I come to work and look after patients."—**KL**

- Remember that developing your career should *always* include space for the people to whom you have made commitments to develop *their* careers. And this includes your children and other young people in your life. Their schooling efforts and their outside activities *are* their careers, in a sense. They are engaged in the business of growing up.—**Editors**

- Part of developing an academic career is writing and publishing. Part of writing and publishing is getting the reviews back on submitted articles. Don't waste time on complaining and being upset that the reviewers "didn't get" your data or your article. Just buckle down and deal with the suggested revisions or edits as requested. Yes, you might feel like just chucking the whole thing in the trash for a brief instant. But we have found, if being honest with ourselves, it's usually a better paper (and sometimes a really better paper) after the revisions are made.—**Editors**

- Grieving is a part of life and is necessary to process loss. Reviews represent loss: of the time and effort you poured into that manuscript, of ideas and work you loved that have been criticized, and, sometimes, of your confidence. Not all reviews are kindly and non-judgmentally delivered (looking at you, reviewer #2). It's okay to take the time to grieve. I find it therapeutic to write a brief and NSFW response, making sure it never sees the light of day. Once I release that anger, sadness, frustration, irritation, and affront, I can go back to the review with an open mind, curious about what I didn't communicate successfully and what constructive comments I can incorporate to make my manuscript better.—**HWH**

- A corollary to the above is that working on the journals, even if you review papers, is a great way to develop your career and give back to our specialty. It's a lot of time and hard work, but it's so important.—**Editors**

- And it's a great way to keep up with the literature!—**HWH**

- Keep in mind that you have to be invited to review for a journal. That happens after you write papers and are invited to review similar papers that are submitted. Writing papers is the currency for everything. How to start writing papers? Hooking up with an "old" person (mentor) who needs help is usually the best way that I know of.—**TNW**

- Also keep in mind that "career development" means many things—developing what's on your CV, developing your contacts and network, and developing your clinical skills. Unfortunately, there is no way to put on paper how good you are clinically, which is really what counts the most, of course. Strive to make sure that every career step you make helps you to be, in some small way, a better clinician.—**Editors**

- Don't be a publication snob! Yes, it's nice to publish in *Anesthesiology* and *Anesthesia and Analgesia*. But there are actually more than 30 recognized anesthesia journals[1]. And this doesn't count the critical care journals. You build your academic publishing muscles the same way you build any type of muscle—start with low-intensity work as tolerated and repeat.—**Editors**

- The worst way to mess up your own career and career development is to screw over other people. Not only is it not nice in and of itself, but it will also hurt you in the long run. Remember, people have very long memories! You don't want to have a single person in the professional world who is dedicated to or even interested in seeing you not do well. We know of a few people in both Neil Sandson's professional community and the anesthesia community who didn't mind stepping on people and screwing people over a bit. Ultimately, things didn't quite work out for them, and/or they didn't quite have the careers they thought they would. And nobody is too upset about it, either.—**NBS and Editors**

- Be particularly conscious of this if you hold many types of privilege because bullying has traditionally been an effective tool for climbing the career ladder for some—albeit one that is both unethical and harms the institution and discipline. Bullying behaviors silence and sideline individuals who otherwise might have made enormous contributions. If this chapter prompts you to read one thing, please read the article cited below.—**HWH**

  https://www.nature.com/articles/s41562-022-01311-z.epdf

- The other really sure way you can mess up your career is to seriously misrepresent yourself in some way, especially during the hiring or credentialing process. *Do not do this.* Generally, it always comes out sooner or later, and you will be in a much worse position than if you had faced the issue head-on. Careers get dinged from time to time—it happens. You'd be surprised what can and has been overcome if you are a good clinician and a good person—meaning ethical, law-abiding, and professional. Be honest and forthright about whatever it is.—**Editors**

- Remember that every single person you meet, or even interact with, in a job application process is interviewing you. The stories about the hiring authority watching you walk across the parking lot on your way in are true. Same with these people talking to the secretarial and administrative staff.—**JMS and Editors**

- Every person with hiring authority has what we call the "No, No, Never!" list. This is a mental list of people they have come across or dealt with that they are just never going to hire. At least not if they can help it. Make sure that you do everything you can to not get on those lists.—**JMS and Editors**

- A corollary to the No, No, Never list that you don't want to get on is the "Yes, Can Do It and Will Do It Well" list that you *do* want to be on. Does your department need somebody to give a talk? Interface

[1]Don't believe us about the number of anesthesiology journals? This is a list we saw online:

British Journal Of Anaesthesia, *Anesthesiology*, Pain, Anaesthesia, *Anesthesia & Analgesia*, Journal Of Neurosurgical Anesthesiology, European Journal Of Anaesthesiology, Regional Anesthesia And Pain Medicine, Clinical, Journal Of Pain, European Journal Of Pain, Pain Physician, Minerva Anestesiologica, Pain Practice, Acta Anaesthesiologica Scandinavica, Current Opinion In Anesthesiology, *Canadian Journal Of Anesthesia*, Pediatric Anesthesia, Anasthesiologie & Intensivmedizin, Journal Of Clinical Monitoring And Computing, International Journal Of Obstetric Anesthesia, Journal Of Cardiothoracic And Vascular Anesthesia, Anaesthesia And Intensive Care, Journal Of Clinical Anesthesia, Anaesthesia Critical Care & Pain Medicine, BMC Anesthesiology, Journal Of Anesthesia, Schmerz, Annales Francaises D Anesthesie Et De Reanimation, Anaesthesist, Revista Brasileira De Anestesiologia, Anasthesiologie Intensivmedizin, Notfallmedizin Schmerztherapie

with the front office? Interview an applicant? Organize the company party? You want to give the people who hire you maximum flexibility in how they can deploy your talents.—**Editors**

- So, about locum tenens. How you feel about it might signify which "generation" of anesthesiologists you are in. Previously, a lot of *locum* work wasn't a mark of distinction on a CV. It might not have been fatal, but hiring authorities weren't looking for it unless it was a hiring authority for another *locums* position. Generally, let's say, you had a job lined up in North Carolina and had already bought a house there, and the job had fallen through, some locums work might be something you did to temporize those circumstances for a couple of months. And that's how you would explain it in interviews. People who did only locum work were sometimes not considered to be the best clinically. You may still run into a decent proportion of senior people in the anesthesia community who have the same viewpoint.—**Editors**

- I have held a number of leadership and hiring positions in the anesthesia community, and I generally agree with the advice just above. However, I am starting to see younger anesthesiologists who seem more focused on "work-life balance" who are either doing locums or part-time work. They are basically able to self-schedule and allow for extended periods of time off for other recreational activities. They are not interested in commitment for full-time work in a practice but may be excellent clinicians.—**VLH**

- We have also known junior people who have done locum work on their vacation to generate funds to help with loan repayment.—**Editors**

- That said, we can't give a lot of advice on doing locum tenens work because we don't have a huge amount of experience with it. Some people do it and make it work, at least from time to time. But we also know people who have been involved in really unsafe situations, especially in the smaller or very rural hospitals, and have sworn to never do it again. Proceed very, very carefully, is all we can say.—**Editors**

- Locum tenens opportunities in other countries, for example, Australia or New Zealand, can be an outstanding way to expand your network and learn new ways to approach anesthesia.—**HWH**

- You might find that you are going to need a little something in the way of a secondary credential if you are just starting your career. A lot of us in the "older generation" have only a plain old MD. And we will finish our careers strong and proud with just that. There were only two ABA subspecialty exams if you trained in the 1980s or 1990s—critical care medicine and pain medicine, and pain medicine didn't require a fellowship. Today, there are seven—critical care medicine, pain medicine, hospice and palliative care medicine, sleep medicine, pediatric anesthesiology, and neurocritical care. And the ABA began offering a subspecialty exam in adult cardiac anesthesiology in 2023. Everybody's time availability is different, but subspecialty certification merits consideration. Everything pertaining to the subspecialty exams (and sample questions) is organized at the link below.—**Editors**

  https://www.theaba.org/subspecialty%20certification%20exams.html

- I concur with the above. I did a fellowship in vascular, thoracic, and transplant anesthesiology back in the day. Loved it and loved those cases. But, if I had to do it again today, I'd probably pick fellowship training in something with a subspecialty exam.—**CM**

- The other thing I would do is take a formal ECG interpretation certificate course. There are a whole bunch online. I'd do the most advanced course for physicians that I could find, such as one that awards 30 CME hours.—**CM**

- For people just starting out in anesthesiology, make up your mind that using echocardiography and ultrasound-guided techniques in your clinical practice means a lifetime of workshops, coursework, and certificates. There just isn't any way around it. The education center tab on the ASA website is a great place to get an overview of what's available and when.—**Editors**

- Also, someone might say that it is easy for me to advise this, as my children are grown, and my house is once again very quiet—but try not to do just do the minimum in terms of professional development and especially maintenance of proficiencies. It was a bit different back then in terms of the professional requirements, but I did take the voluntary recertification board exam in 2009. I have a non-time-limited board certification but just decided to do it. My practice at that time was all general adult anesthesia—bread and butter cases - and I was starting to have a little trouble answering people's questions about other areas of anesthesia at parties. As I recall, this was the last time you could just sign up for the exam and go in and take it without a lot of MOCA hours and such. So, I thought, okay, I better do this.—**CM**

- I had to study quite a bit—pain, pediatric anesthesia, etc.—and I remember that a ferocious storm came up the night before and blew the roof off my house. Literally. I thought, well, I certainly hope this isn't some sort of omen. The last thing I did before going out of the house to take the exam was look up through the gaping hole and talk to the guys on the roof who were trying to put down a gigantic blue tarp to keep the rain from flooding my living room below. I did pass it and have always been glad I did it. It was somewhat difficult to gather the motivation to do it, I will admit it. And it wasn't cheap. But I needed a mid-career refresher on the basics in some of the practice areas where I was getting a bit rusty, and I thought, well, if I'm not willing to invest a little extra in my anesthesiology credentials, what should I invest in? Plus, I had the satisfaction of being able to own just the tiniest bit of professional excellence.—**CM**

- Early in my career, when I knew I was interested in education, I was actively exploring what might be avenues for further development of my career. I was course co-director for one of the first-year medical student courses, as well as the medical student coordinator for the department. I also still loved working with the residents, though, and held the role of the associate program director. My chair, Jeff Kirsch, gave me the advice that I would eventually need to choose to focus on undergraduate medical education or graduate medical education. It surprised me at the time because it seemed like I was getting to work in both areas, but of course, he was right. They each had their own nuances and definitely their own networking circles. In order to devote enough time and energy to do a great job in an area, I would need to focus on that niche. I ended up choosing undergraduate medical education because I loved the enthusiasm of the students, as well as being able to make a broader impact. In fact, refining down even further from med student education in general to student affairs or education was another decision I eventually had to make. That being said, I now have my fingers back in both pots (and CME!) as the vice-chair for education, so I advise that it's always good to keep doors open.—**DD**

- There are interesting certificate programs available from the AAMC (Association of American Medical Colleges). They offer three certificates for medical educators: Leadership Education and Development *(LEAD)* Certificate Program, Medical Education Research Certificate *(MERC)* Program, and Teaching for Quality *(Te4Q)*. Information about all courses is online at: https://www.aamc.org/career-development. The price for the courses is very reasonable.—**Editors**

- The LEAD certificate program is a one-year cohort-based national leadership development program that focuses on: strategic vision and setting direction, developing people, developing organizations, and managing effectively.—**Editors**

- The AAMC defines the content for eight workshops that comprise the AAMC Medical Education Certificate Program. The workshops are Data Management and Preparing for Statistical Consultation, Formulating Research Questions and Designing Studies, Hypothesis-driven Research, Measuring Educational Outcomes with Reliability and Validity, Qualitative Data Collection Methods, Program Evaluation and Evaluation Research, Questionnaire Design and Survey Research, Searching and Evaluating the Medical Education Literature, and Publishing Medical Education Research. Each participant had their own survey that they developed through the different steps of the workshop, but survey completion and publication were not required.—**BTG**

- If doing your job for more than 8 hours a day is a waste of time, you are probably wasting the first 8 hours as well.—**BTG**

- Better to retire 5 years too early than 5 minutes too late. Get out of the OR before the first coworker, or worse yet, the first patient, remarks sadly that you are no longer in your prime. You will miss it—sure. But there are lots of other interesting things to do.—**Editors**

- The time to start thinking about retirement is when you take your first job out of residency. What are your goals? What legacy do you want to leave? How do you want to spend your time after retirement? What other parts of your life do you need to keep developing so you have something to look forward to? Don't get in the position of clinging to clinical work because you can't think of anything else to do.—**HWH**

- No less a person than Benjamin Franklin believed that business lives and personal lives can and should be mixed and that nobody should be afraid of individuals higher than themselves on the social or wealth ladders. Especially "working" people. He started as a tradesman and remained so at heart for the rest of his life. Of course, he was born with that famous personality and sense of humor, and he decided that the new country was going to be very different than the old European society. He was one of the first Americans to see his patrons socially, and he ran in diverse social groups his entire life. So perhaps the good doctor figured out something for the rest of us.—**Editors**

- Being a Mayo doctor, I have always taken Dr. Will Mayo's famous quote to heart: "The best interest of the patient is the only interest to be considered, and in order that the sick may have the benefit of advancing knowledge, union of forces is necessary." I am fortunate to work at an academic institution and consider "advancing knowledge" as integral to my career. Whether just writing a simple letter to the editor, working with a medical student on a poster, or conducting complex clinical-based research, this is how I can better the lives of patients to come.—**TNW**

***Note from the Editors:** Toby Weingarten is a fly fisherman, and his first favorite bridge is the Minnesota State Highway 60 bridge over Cold Creek in Zumbro Falls, MN (Fig. 81.3). His second favorite bridge is in the Florida Keys. His description of why they appeal to him:

> The MN-60 Cold Creek bridge has three big culverts that spill cold, clear, pure water into a big hole full of trout. I like to go there after call and go fly fishing for a couple of hours.
>
> Second favorite bridge is the Seven Mile Bridge to Key West. Many good fishing spots. Also, it's a pretty cool engineering feat.

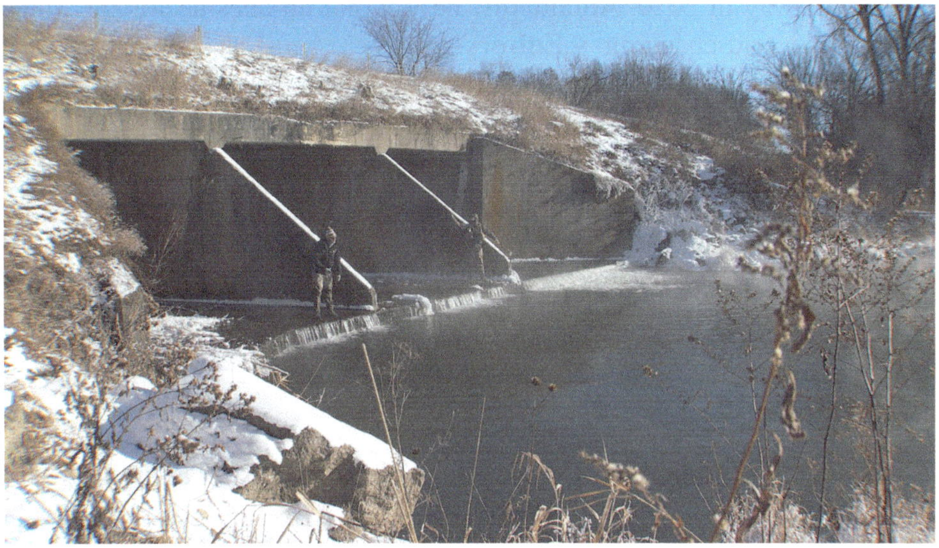

Fig. 81.3 MN-60 highway bridge over Cold Creek in Zumbro Falls, MN. Toby Weingarten reports that it is a great place to fish for trout. Photograph: Toby Weingarten

- Lean into each phase of your career, no matter how brief, starting when you are in training. When I was in training, I remember that I had an attending on my neuro-anesthesia rotation who asked me to look at, just look at, the neuro-anesthesia articles in the previous 12 months in both *Anesthesiology* and *Anesthesia & Analgesia.* I've always remembered that he said, "You probably aren't going into neuro-anesthesia as a career concentration, most people don't. But you've got this rotation, your neuro-critical care rotation, and then neuro cases to do on call. But why don't you just assume that you are a neuro-anesthesiologist for these months and approach your cases with the eye of a developing expert. This will serve you in good stead for the rest of your career when the occasional neuro case comes your way. You will think, okay, cool, I'm happy to do this case, I have a special interest in neuro-anesthesia." This was great advice for that rotation and others.—**CM**

- Cruise the "big four" anesthesiology websites at least monthly—of course, we are referring to the websites of the ASA, ABA, APSF, and FAER. At least monthly. There is a lot of good information on the sites—clinical information, legal news, research updates, and news and updates about what is going on with our specialty and the people in it.—**Editors**

- In our previous books, we wanted to do some content on the historical figures in anesthesia but didn't have the manuscript space. Now we do. ☺ Here are a few fun reads.

- There's an interesting 2017 blog post at theanesthesiaconsultant.com on William New, MD, PhD. The blogger (a Stanford and private practice anesthesiologist) makes the claim that Dr. New is arguably the most important anesthesiologist of the last hundred years. Bill New was a Stanford anesthesiologist and engineer who developed the prototype of the pulse oximeter and was the first president of Nellcor. The blogger states his opinion that, "Bill New changed the world with the pulse oximeter. No single device in the 20th century changed medical care more than the oximeter."—**Editors**

- Harriet Hopf also notes that the recognized "parent of pulse oximetry" is Takuo Aoyagi, a Japanese engineer who received the Gravenstein Award in 2013 from the Society for Technology in Anesthesia and, sadly, passed away in 2020. Admittedly, he was not an anesthesiologist, but his impact on anesthesiology was world-changing.—**Editors**

  (https://www.ncbi.nlm.nih.gov/pmc/articles/PMC7237228/)

  The same blogger a really interesting piece on 01-12-2022, "The Top 10 Living Anesthesiologists." He lists the major accomplishments of each. You can guess them, most probably:

  *__Ron Miller__—*The Book* and building his UCSF department. Not mentioned in the blog but equally important was his work in trauma transfusion and resuscitation in Vietnam.

  *__Archie Brain__—the LMA

  *__Dan Sessler__—most cited anesthesiologist (and an *Anesthesia Bridges* author)

  *__Lee Fleisher__—preop testing (another *Anesthesia Bridges* author)

  *__Steve Shafer__—pharmacology of IV anesthetics

  *__John Benumof__—difficult airway algorithm

  *__Richard Jaffe__—*Manual of Surgical Procedures* (*Anesthesia Bridges* author!)

  *__Robert Stoelting__—the textbooks and APSF work

  *__Jim Eisenach__—editor of *Anesthesiology*

  *__David Gaba__—simulation work and *Crisis Management in Anesthesiology*

- Our personal list of anesthesiologists who have made seminal contributions to the field of anesthesiology also includes *Evan Kharasch*, for his ground-breaking work on the metabolism of anesthetics and drug-drug interactions involving the cytochrome P450 enzyme system. As far as we can tell, he was way far out in front of everybody else in the anesthesia community with his work, and we review and refer to his papers frequently, more than 25 years after publication. And proud to say—an *Anesthesia Bridges* contributor.

- It is also fun to read about the late, great giants of anesthesia. How they developed their landmark research and what made them tick. First among these has to be Sir Robert Macintosh of the eponymous blade fame. He was born in 1901 and lived to the late 1980s, so he was still alive when some of the editors and authors were beginning training and anesthesia practice. A lot of us are engineers and interested in gases, so we have always been fascinated by how Edmond (Ted) Eger and John Severinghaus discovered the principles of uptake and distribution of inhalational anesthesia, including the concept of minimum alveolar concentration. There's a great "Classic Papers Revisited" in *Anesthesiology* that tells the story and great short bios of Dr. Severinghaus (who died in 2021) and Dr. Eger on the UCSF Department of Anesthesia and Perioperative Care website. Here are the links.

1. https://pubs.asahq.org/anesthesiology/article/96/1/238/39788/A-Brief-History-of-the-Origin-of-Minimum-Alveolar
2. https://anesthesia.ucsf.edu/news/john-severinghaus-pioneer-anesthesia-and-medicine-has-passed-away-may-6-1922-june-2-2021
3. https://anesthesia.ucsf.edu/giant-anesthesia-dr-ted-eger

– What is so inspiring about these pioneers of anesthesia is that they weren't careerists. They didn't seem to be all that interested in how brilliant they were or how their careers were developing. Severinghaus was a physicist, and Eger was a chemist, and they both worked tirelessly to solve what to them were absolutely burning questions. But they also led full lives. The bio of Ted Eger contains an astonishing list of the dozens of leaders in anesthesia that he trained—and we mean dozens as the list includes 24 anesthesiology department chairs—but also shows him attending resident conferences until the end of his life. And it gives a wonderful account of his large family—13 grandchildren—and the fact that he climbed Half Dome in Yosemite when he was 75 years old. If you have a few minutes of extra time, read about these anesthesia visionaries, and be thankful that you are not doing anesthesia in the days before the pulse oximeter was developed, and nobody really knew how much inhalational agent it took to do a general anesthetic.—**Editors**

– It's disappointing, but not surprising that the list above contains no women or (as far as we are aware) people of color. The editorial group concurred that we certainly aren't going to publish this list without the appropriate editorial amendments. The notable physicians below belong every bit as much.—**HWH and Editors**

- **Emory Brown**: ground-breaking work on the nature of consciousness and the mystery of general anesthesia.
- **Selma Harrison Calmes**: pioneer, leader, and co-founder of the Anesthesia History Association in 1982.
- **Cynthia Wong**: debunked multiple myths about epidurals in labor using randomized controlled trials, including the NEJM article that demonstrated early epidurals did not increase the risk of C-section; chair at Iowa
- **Patricia Kapur**: former chair at UCLA and executive vice president of UCLA Health System, former president of ABA and FAER, and received the 2019 ASA Distinguished Service Award, and a *Bridges* contributor.

  - **Monica Vavilala**: ground-breaking work in TBI and patient and community-centered research, and is the only anesthesiologist to lead an NIH-funded Injury Prevention and Research Center

  - **Jeanine Wiener-Kronish**: understanding ARDS and pulmonary infections in critical care; former chair at MGH—and thanks for your contributions to *Anesthesia Bridges,* Dr. W-K.

- A great resource is *A History of Women in American Anesthesiology,* by Selma Harrison Calmes in Ted Eger and Larry Saidman, and Rod Westhorpe's book *The Wondrous Story of Anesthesia.* If you haven't read it, it's time to get a copy! And don't miss the ongoing podcast *Women of Impact in Anesthesiology.*—**HWH**

  https://www.asahq.org/education-and-career/women-of-impact.

- We also give a shout-out to author Harriet Hopf herself for her leadership (chair, board of directors) of FAER and advocacy work, and Karen Domino and Lorri Lee for their hugely influential work with the Anesthesia Closed Claims Project.—**CM and Editors**

- So, as mentioned elsewhere in this book, I trained at Hopkins in the early 1990s. This came with the good fortune of joining a department with a number of really great role models. Carol Hirshman, Rose Christopherson, Lynne Maxwell, Genie Heitmiller, Laurel Moore, and Karen Lindeman come to mind. These women had trained in the 1970s and 1980s. They were great clinicians and researchers. Lynne and Genie were double boarded. Carol and Karen had serious research careers. Carol was a full professor with tenure and had a national reputation. She had robust, ongoing NIH funding, if memory serves correctly. Rose did a lot of vascular cases and was in the select group of go-to people for the big cases. Laurel Moore did the single most complicated case I ever saw as a resident—a circulatory arrest case that was complicated by serious blood loss very late in the case. I remember her talking to one of the esteemed neurosurgeons once about an aspect of an anesthetic plan and the surgeon taking notes.—**CM**

- Then there was yet another group of faculty women who were strong examples—Deb Schwengel did pediatric anesthesia and pediatric critical care, and Lynette Mark did cardiac anesthesia and also managed the difficult airway service. All these women had families and/or busy husbands and/or kids and houses and dogs and never even bothered to pretend they didn't. Jane Matjasko was the chairperson across town at the University of Maryland while serving on the ABA board. So, I always knew that it was possible to have a full-time anesthesia career and a meaningful personal life, and it was right in front of me. And I saw a lot of support among these women and for the junior women in the department. If you are training or working where this is not the case, maybe make haste to find a new practice location.—**CM**

- We've mentioned this elsewhere in this book, but as your career develops, be humble about what you don't know, and areas that you are not an expert in. You will be an expert in some areas of anesthesia but not in all. For instance, when I was first attending at Hopkins, the attending covering the general ORs also covered peds cases over the age of two years if the patient wasn't a PICU patient, either pre- or post-op. I got in the habit of calling the peds anesthesia attending on call, just to review my plan with them and make sure I wasn't missing anything, for anybody who was younger than a teenager. Similarly, once when I was a fellow, I got a question from a cardiac anesthesiologist and intensivist who, for some reason, was doing a thoracic anesthesia case. Did we put central lines in for routine thoracic anesthesia cases? This was an experienced person, but he still wanted to quickly review our standard of care at that time. I was junior to him, still a fellow, but he had no hesitation or chagrin about asking.—**CM**

- Your career is going to occur in sections and segments and intervals, and like the image below, they are now going to be all the same dimensions. First, there are the short periods of training, and then perhaps more training. Then, like the center span of a bridge, a longer interval in the middle of your career where perhaps what you see as the highlight of your career occurs. But every bit of progress you make in your career has a reflection associated with it—perhaps it's less time at home or less time for your hobbies.—**Editors**

- For a lot of anesthesiologists, there are shorter intervals toward the latter part of their career, and they are part and part of their journey of taking care of patients, as well.—**Editors**

***Note from the Editors:** This multi-span over Lake Champlain is one of the best visual metaphors for an anesthesia career that we saw (Fig. 81.4). A bridge span is the horizontal distance between two supports and also can refer to the structure itself. What in your career represents the center span or arch—was it a leadership position you held or a single case you did? It's different for everybody. And look at the supports again—you are going to need complex support both on your way up and your way down.

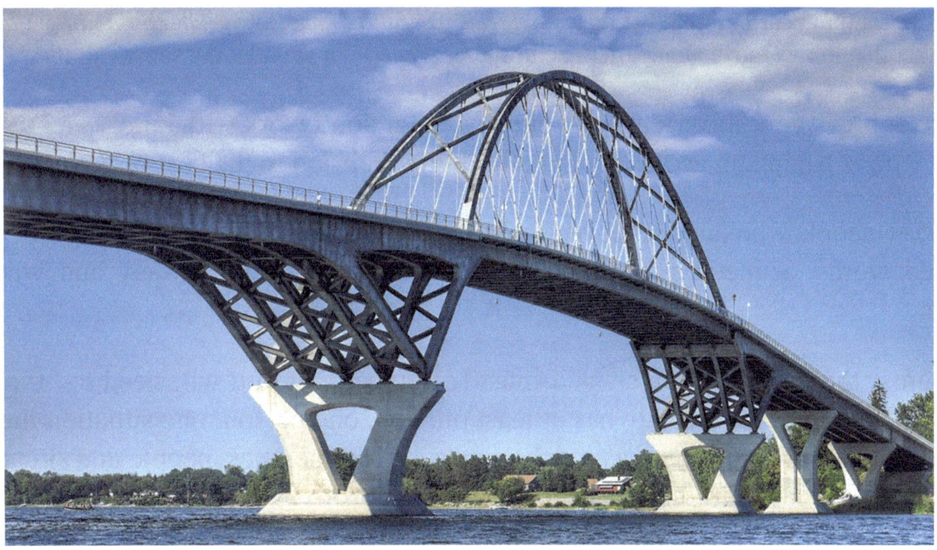

Fig. 81.4 Beautiful image of a Vermont bridge. Photograph: Image used under standard license from stock.adobe.com

- Take joy in the ability to declare failure and retreat from a plan that is not succeeding. This is what creates a new path.—**MPH**

- Think carefully from the start of your career about what type of situation and practice you want to age into. As you become an older working anesthesiologist, what will you want and what can you let go? Will you need a professional position that doesn't have as many calls? Doesn't have as many procedures? Where is there less patient contact or tort exposure? As crazy as it seems when you are young, you will age, and you will need to retailor your job. As you think about this, start early in building the bridges you will need to get you there. Will you need an MBA? An informatics degree? A master's degree in education? A podcast or website? Certification in one of the anesthesia subspecialties? Lay the keystone of those professional bridges as early in your career as you can.—**AJR**

- A corollary to Amy Robbins' advice above is to think about the bricks you will use to strengthen the *current* stage of your career. Are those brick publications? Administrative service? Committee work at the regional or national level. Don't just haphazardly try to build a career by throwing straw at it—set it in concrete, brick by brick.—**Editors**

- Anesthesia training teaches a risk-reduction approach to patient management, which is lifesaving, but is a very poor approach to discovery; in science, fortune favors the bold. So, when you are approaching a scientific problem, ask whether you are taking enough risk. Is it big enough? Are you going far enough? If it's terrifying, you might be on the right track.—**MPH**

- You may love your job, but your job does not love you back. As important as your roles may seem, if you leave tomorrow, you'll be replaced quickly and forgotten even more quickly. Remember, we are all just cogs in a giant wheel.—**KL**

- Or, as was published in the Abilene Reporter way back in 1909:

  Young man, as you perambulate down the pathway of life toward an unavoidable bald head bordered with gray hairs it would be well to bear in mind that the *cemeteries are full of men this world could not get along without*, and note the fact that things move along after each funeral procession at about the same gait they went before.

- People make or break your job. Treat everyone you do or don't work with kindly and respectfully. You never know who is having an awful day but still doing their job to the best of their ability.—**KL**

- There are a few people who are so beloved that they are immune to the weapons formed by their own ill-considered words. Sometimes, you just have to know what not to say and when not to say it.—**Editors**

- As you progress through your career, you must remember that you will need to "forget bigly"—at least once in your career. Everybody has at least one job, one person, one situation that just must be moved on from and put out of mind as much as possible. Sometimes, people and situations and even feelings and emotions are part of your history but not part of your destiny. And if you can't let it go, then let it be.—**Editors**

- Raise a career as you would raise a child. Early on, the career will occasionally/often require unconditional attention and nurturance, and later on, it will need to fend for itself as you focus on other matters. As with any "child," your personal investment and care will play a very large role in how it develops. And no one else will care about its welfare more than you will, so act accordingly. That being said, when the needs of your real children and your metaphoric child (career) come into conflict, prioritize your real children. You are the bridge to their future, and they are the bridge to your future. Your career is what you use to buy that future.—**NBS**

***Note from the Editors:** It's really interesting how many bridge logos are available to purchase for use in promotional materials (Fig. 81.5).

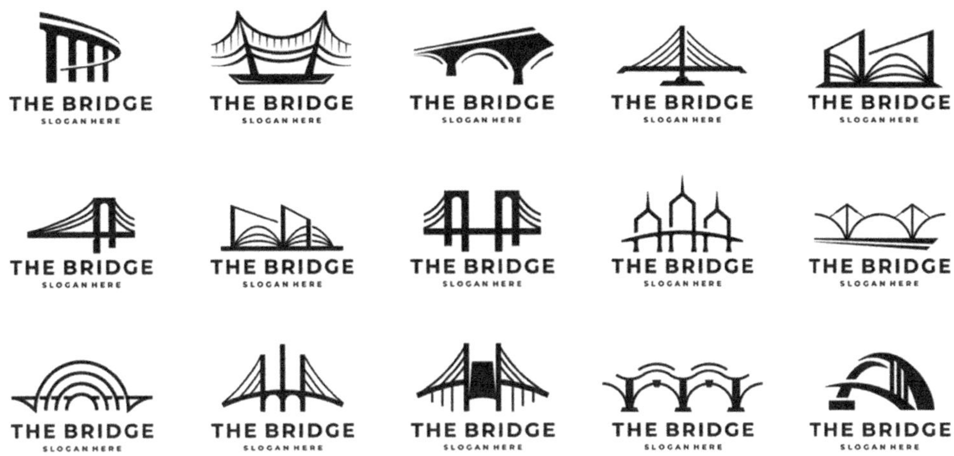

Fig. 81.5 Bridge graphics available for purchase on the internet for use in advertising and promotional materials. Illustration: Image used under standard license from shutterstock.com

Promotions

- On promotion: *Decide if this is important to you.* It may be because at your institution it is elective and you value it, or because it is mandatory—the proverbial "up or out."—**EDK**

- Understand that promotion is institution-specific. Know your institution's promotion criteria, policies, and processes. Know your institution's culture, what it values, and what it will recognize and reward.—**EDK**

- Consult and discuss with your department chair and the departmental promotions committee chair. Honestly assess your own progress, accomplishments, deficits, and gaps between where you are and where you want and need to be. Get a forthright colleague to do the same—you want an honest opinion.—**EDK**

- You will know you're ready for promotion when your department suggests it to you. It is better to sail through than fight through the process.—**EDK**

We wholeheartedly second Evan Kharasch's excellent advice. We want to reinforce it by including the information from a feature "One-Pager" that **Kirk Lalwani did for the Society of Pediatric Anesthesia (SPA). We got permission from **Jim Fehr**, who is the president of the SPA board of directors and who was in Amy Robbins' and Cathy Marcucci's residency class at Hopkins, to include for our readers.

- Academic promotion and tenure are formal recognition of your expertise, effort, and reputation in the areas of *service*, *scholarship*, and *education*.

- Every institution has unique criteria that need to be fulfilled to be considered for promotion, typically in these three areas of achievement.

- Promotion usually results in higher compensation and is often viewed as a prerequisite for some leadership roles in the department or institution.

- Some institutions have a minimum number of years in rank as a prerequisite to applying. Applying early is unlikely to be successful, so be patient and be ready when the time is right.
- Decide which faculty track you are most suited for at the time of appointment, if you have a choice, and if the institution has multiple tracks.
- Realistically assess your inclination and likely productivity for clinical or basic science research. Determine the productivity and collaborative strength of the research faculty to gauge whether you will be able to achieve the benchmark necessary for promotion. *Above all, follow your passion.*
- Get involved at the institutional level and in your national society.
- Educational presentations like PBLDs, scientific posters, and committee work prioritize your attendance at national meetings, giving you more opportunities to get involved and build a network.
- Find a mentor who has a good track record with junior faculty and with whom you have a good rapport. Ask your chair about mentorship if it's not a part of the department's faculty development plan.
- Meet with the department promotion and tenure leader 1–2 years *before* the cycle in which you plan to apply to assess your readiness. This gives you time to work on areas you need to strengthen in order to meet promotion criteria in each area.
- When the time comes, give yourself plenty of time (2–3 months) to prepare your application, so it is practically perfect when you submit it.
- Your personal statement will need to be in line with institutional style. Plan on multiple drafts, no typos, excellent grammar, and a modest tone without underselling yourself.
- If external referee letters need to be unbiased, make sure they are! Ask your department chair for help.
- If the tenure track is an option, review the requirements and timeline carefully.

Kirk Lalwani's professional promotions summary for the SPA also included the FOCUS-POCUS mnemonic. It is reproduced below, again with Kirk's permission and permission of the SPA.—**Editors**

F: Find your passion.

O: Organize your professional activities and develop skills to highlight and align with your chosen passion/s.

C: Channel your energies into working smart. Develop a plan and ask for guidance.

U: Understand that academic promotion is a process—it takes time, dedication, and a strategic plan of action.

S: Simply the process of keeping your CV and teaching portfolio updated regularly—it is never too early to start.

P: Review promotion and tenure policy and process.

O: Outline 2–3 objectives for the following year at your annual chairperson meeting.

C: Collaborate with others for projects, research, and other clinical or QI initiatives.

U: Resources like the promotion and tenure chair, your faculty development champion, and your department chair.

S: Save all raw teaching evaluation data, QI project details, and complimentary emails, with backup paper copies.

Finally, remember that sometimes baby steps are in order, especially when you hit rough spots in your career. It is rare these days for anybody to have a career that is a smooth, unbroken arc of always-upward career progress. It is much more likely that your career will have stops and starts and rough spots, not to mention downright quagmires. Despite these tough times, *you can still get to where you want to go, but not if you stop moving*.—**Editors**

Note: The editors thank Drs. Schwartz and Sandson for contributing to this chapter.

Reference

1. Michenfelder JD. The 27th Rovenstine lecture: Neuroanesthesia and the achievement of professional respect. Anesthesiology. 1989;70(4):695–701.

Authors

Kirk Lalwani is a professor of anesthesiology and pediatrics at the Oregon Health and Science University. He is also the director of the pediatric anesthesiology fellowship program and vice-chair for faculty development at OHSU.

Harriet Hopf is a true expert in career development. She is a professor of anesthesiology and adjunct professor of biomedical engineering at the University of Utah. Her clinical research interests center around surgical site healing and the role of oxygen delivery in wound healing. A second major focus of her work has been sponsoring, mentoring, and coaching trainees and early career faculty in research and other career development. She is a co-director of the Utah Coaching and Advancement Network (U-CAN).

Evan Kharasch is the Merle H. Harmel Distinguished Professor of Anesthesiology and vice-chair for innovation in the Department of Anesthesiology at Duke University. He was also the editor-in-chief of *Anesthesiology*, the leading journal in our specialty. He is an elected member of the National Academy of Medicine. Prior to joining Duke University, he was the Russell D. and Mary B. Shelden Professor of Anesthesiology, director of the division of clinical and translational research, and vice chancellor for research at Washington University in St. Louis, and co-founder and founding director of the Center for Clinical Pharmacology at Washington University in St. Louis and St. Louis College of Pharmacy. Earlier in his career, he was a professor of anesthesiology, vice-chair for research, and assistant dean for clinical research in the School of Medicine at the University of Washington, Seattle. He is a basic, translational, and clinical investigator with an interest in pharmacology, optimizing care, and medical policy, has been federally funded for three decades, and has published more than 320 peer-reviewed articles. Evan is an inveterate fan of minor league baseball. But not the designated hitter.

Cathy Marcucci holds no formal administrative position or credentials with respect to faculty or career development. She doesn't even have a PhD. However, she decided early on that she could best develop her own career by doing book projects that would include a large number of people in the anesthesia community and contribute in whatever small way to their careers. She's been told that participation in the book projects has helped some of her colleagues a tiny bit with their promotion committees.

Part V

Education and Training

Stari Most—Mostar, Bosnia and Herzegovina

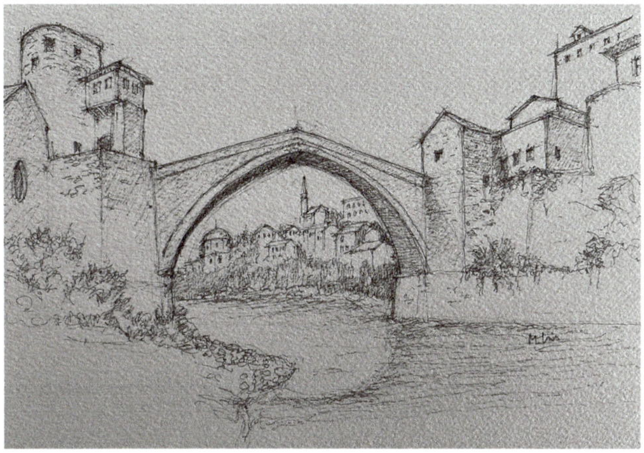

Michael Liu was Senior Partner and Design Principal of The Architectural Team (TAT) in Boston, MA. We asked him if he would be kind enough to draw a bridge of choice for us, and he sent us this exquisite and evocative drawing of the Stari Most in Bosnia and Herzegovina. He is especially appreciative of the peaked archway that has made this bridge so famous in Europe and across the world.

Stari Most is also known as the Mostar Bridge and spans the Neretva River. It is a rebuilt 16th Ottoman bridge that is considered an exemplary piece of Balkan Islamic architecture and was commissioned by Suleiman the Magnificent in 1557. Instead of foundations, the bridge has wing walls made of limestone—legend has it that the original mortar for the bridge was made with egg white. The bridge was destroyed in 1993 in the military conflict that enveloped the region. By report, more than 60 shells hit the bridge before it collapsed. Reconstruction was an international effort involving multiple European countries, the World Bank, the United Nations, UNESCO, and the World Monuments Fund. The bridge was rededicated in 2004.

The editors, authors, and contributors of *Anesthesia Bridges* thank Michael for his great generosity in taking time from his specialty to contribute to ours and arranging for his busy design staff to donate their beautiful original drawings to the anesthesia community.

82 Introduction

Amr E. Abouleish

Although one might think this section is meant only for academic anesthesiologists, many of the lessons learned apply to private practice clinicians as well. As Dr. Kapur starts one of her stories, "The transition from resident to junior faculty can be a daunting and even scary transition—even if new faculty members do not verbalize it." The same can also be said for the transition from resident to private practice anesthesiologist.

We hope that the new anesthesiologist will learn some lessons from the following stories. But more importantly, we hope you, as a new or young anesthesiologist, will feel able to ask for advice from senior anesthesiologists in your own department or group. That is creating bridges at your own institution. Someday, it will be your turn to share your hard-earned wisdom with anesthesiologists who are junior to you.

Author

Amr Abouleish joined UTMB Galveston in 1993 as the first chief of pediatric anesthesiology. His motto for teaching pediatric anesthesia to residents is "every month is July!" He is also a national speaker on economics in healthcare, especially for anesthesiology departments.

A. E. Abouleish (✉)
Department of Anesthesiology, John Sealy School of Medicine, The University of Texas Medical Branch, Galveston, TX, USA
e-mail: Aaboulei@utmb.edu

S. Mohamed et al. (eds.), *Anesthesia Bridges*, https://doi.org/10.1007/978-3-032-08294-7_82

83 When Supervising a Resident, and the Resident Is Not Able to Complete a Skill, You Should Stop and Ask Yourself What You Are Not Communicating to the Resident

Amr E. Abouleish

Introduction

After finishing my residency, I returned to Texas and became a new faculty pediatric anesthesiologist in September of 1993. For my first month as a faculty, the resident who was on the pediatric anesthesia rotation was a chief resident who was in her last month of residency. She was finishing late because she had taken maternity leave during her training. During this first month, I thought I was the best faculty member. All the cases went smoothly. We had no airway issues or any other anesthetic complications.

And then, for my second month as faculty, the resident assigned to pediatric anesthesia rotation was a CA-2 (second year anesthesiology) resident who had never taken care of a pediatric patient or performed an inhalational induction. In the first week of the month, we had 3–4 patients who had laryngospasm during inhalational induction.

My first thought was that I had a "bad" resident since last month, I had no issues. While talking to a senior faculty member, the faculty member suggested I try to figure out what the resident was doing or not doing that was different than if I were doing the mask inhalational induction. So, I spent time in my office visualizing the induction process with the resident and came to realize that the resident was "squeezing the bag" during induction without timing it with the patient's breaths.

What I realized is that I had not communicated this critical step in inhalational inductions. It was second nature to me, but it was not obvious to a resident. On that day, I came up with the analogy that masking a patient during inhalational induction was like pushing someone on a swing. You push the swing as it goes away from you. You want to squeeze the bag as the patient takes a breath in.

I met with the resident. I apologized for not explaining inhalational induction well and went on to talk about how to do it better.

A. E. Abouleish (✉)
Department of Anesthesiology, The University of Texas Medical Branch, Galveston, TX, USA
e-mail: aaboulei@UTMB.EDU

S. Mohamed et al. (eds.), *Anesthesia Bridges*, https://doi.org/10.1007/978-3-032-08294-7_83

Lessons Learned

- When things are not going well, don't look to the resident to blame, but stop and think about what you might do as second nature and need to verbalize to your resident.

Author

Amr Abouleish joined UTMB Galveston in 1993 as the first chief of pediatric anesthesiology. His motto for teaching pediatric anesthesia to residents is "every month is July!" He is also a national speaker on economics in healthcare, especially for anesthesiology departments.

84 Criticism in the Moment Does Not Facilitate an Emergency Response

Patricia A. Kapur

Introduction

I was working with a CA-2 (second-year anesthesiology) resident caring for a healthy 8-year-old boy for a forearm orthopedic procedure. In the midst of the mask inhalation induction, the over-eager junior orthopedic surgery resident jerked up the child's operative arm for the surgical prep, prompting severe laryngospasm.

My resident froze and totally stopped engaging in the patient's care. I did not want to criticize or shame the resident into action by saying, "Why aren't you doing something—you know what to do for laryngospasm!" At the same time, I was very curious and concerned why a good resident was paralyzed into inaction. So, I started to calmly say the emergency action steps for laryngospasm, that is: do "A," do "B," do "C," and so forth. The resident complied with the rote instructions in a somewhat robotic manner. Once the laryngospasm broke and the airway was secured, the surgery was carried out, albeit with an educational moment for the orthopedic surgery residents.

After the case, I asked my resident what was going through his head, and heard the astonishing reply that with the laryngospasm-induced drop in SpO2, the resident was imagining in full detail the patient dying and having to tell the devastated parents, so he could not muster the attention to deal with the emergency itself. At that later time, we discussed how to overcome such feelings in order to rise to the occasion to treat emergent situations. The resident successfully completed the residency.

P. A. Kapur (✉)
Department of Anesthesiology and Critical Care, Perelman School of Medicine, University of Pennsylvania, Philadelphia, PA, USA
e-mail: patricia.kapur@pennmedicine.upenn.edu

S. Mohamed et al. (eds.), *Anesthesia Bridges*, https://doi.org/10.1007/978-3-032-08294-7_84

Lessons Learned

- Never raise your voice in frustration or anger, ever, when teaching—it does not make a trainee perform better. For the patient's best outcome as well as the resident's learning, deal with the situation calmly, and discuss teaching points and implications later.

***Note from the Editors:** We typed "angry bridge" into a search window and danged if something didn't pop up in the results (Figs. 84.1 and 84.2). This unusual hotel walkway was installed at 13th and Cuthbert Streets in Philadelphia, PA. Are the large figures angry or fearful, or both, as they struggle to keep the building and themselves upright?

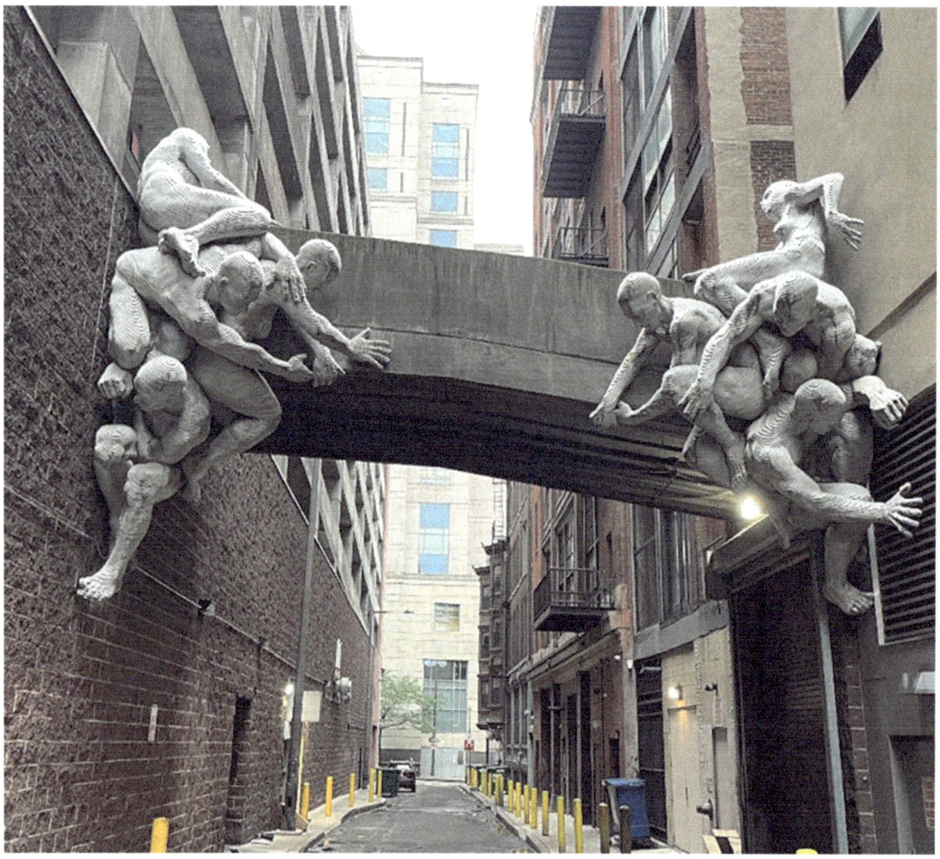

Fig. 84.1 Public view of the hotel walkway bridge from the street. Photograph: James Nguyen

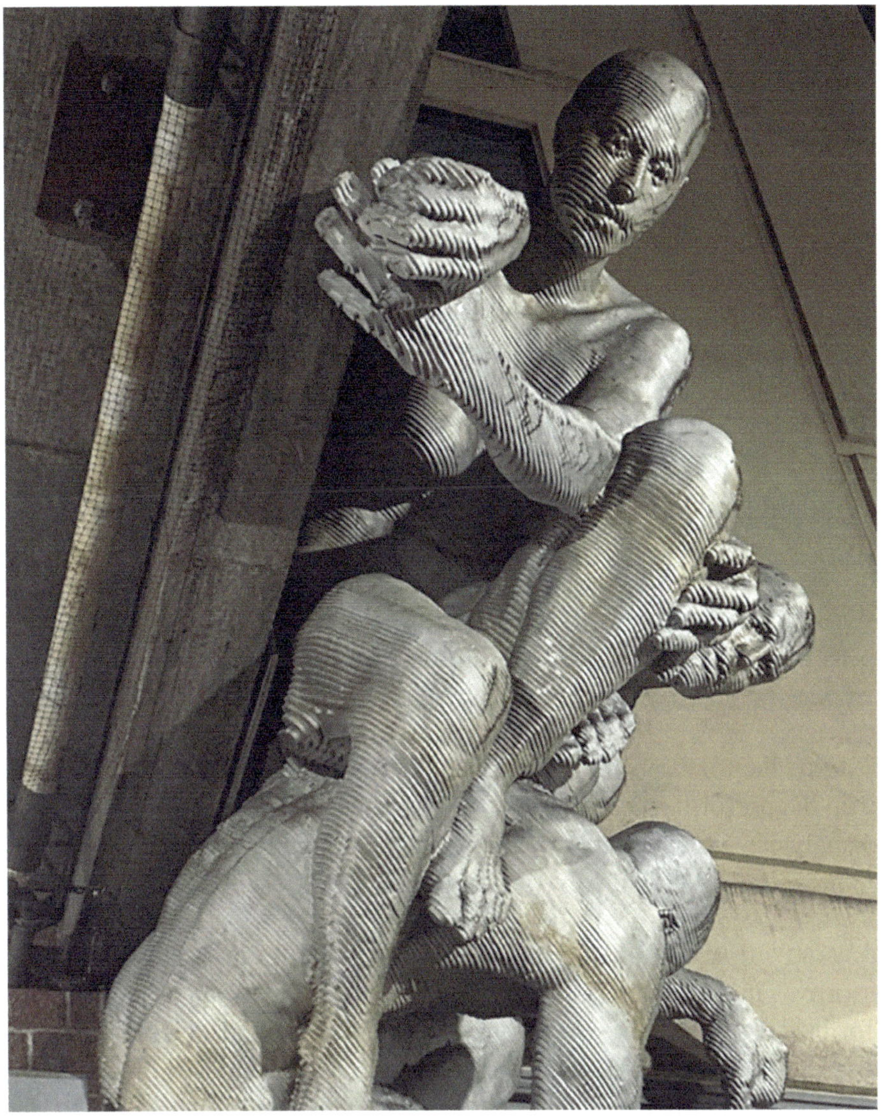

Fig. 84.2 View of the building from the pavement underneath—equally fascinating and dramatic. Photograph: Isabella Giglio

Bonus Content from the Editors

Dr. Kapur is completely correct that you should never raise your voice or display anger when teaching or supervising. But why is this so?

- First, *anger is very personal.* It is a complex product of a person's fear, anxieties, needs, insecurities, and negative memories. It is so individual and multi-factorial that it is one of the most valuable tools that mental health professionals have in treating patients. Because it's such a vivid snapshot of an individual's mental health composite, they are always looking for what makes a patient angry.

- You can use your own anger to motivate and effect change in yourself, but recognize that your anger will not necessarily be very motivating to those who don't share your emotional, psychological, and experiential background. In fact, it usually won't. Put simply, it is a mistake to assume that others share your triggers and are concerned about them. It's one thing to say, "I am angry, and *I need* to do something about it," but entirely another thing to say, "I am angry, and *you need* to do something about it."

- There are tiny positive effects of anger as a motivational tool for others. For one, it can establish a degree of power and authority, and this *sometimes* has a benefit in a chaotic situation with poorly defined team roles. But have you ever noticed that the privilege of being angry is usually not granted to every person in every position in a team? Anger is usually only tolerated from those who possess some degree of leadership.

- There are some intriguing psychology studies that seem to indicate that subjects will work harder to obtain neutral objects (like a pen) when simultaneously being shown angry faces on a screen, but these studies require a nuanced analysis. And remember that the research lab of a psychology grad student is not the same as an OR. Even the experts are still debating these results, with the current consensus being that anger *might* have *limited* benefits in motivating a low-performing team but not a high-performing team. We'll just go there and suggest that you assume your anesthesia care team to be of the higher-performing caliber, and that viewing your angry face isn't going to have any sort of positive effect on somebody you are trying to supervise.

- After decades of study, the relationship between anger and performance remains unclear. It seems to transiently speed up the performance of manual tasks but has a deleterious effect on tasks that require mental effort and analysis. You can yell at someone to throw something on the back of a truck, but you can't yell at someone to hurry up and solve a problem and expect reliable results

- The downside of using anger to motivate is that it creates and reinforces a sense of entitlement and false moral superiority. Think about it—displays of anger are often seen as people indulging their hot tempers and so forth, when we rarely speak of people indulging in bravery or honesty or calmness. Teams or individuals under duress will quickly discern arrogance and dishonesty in their leaders. and motivation will quickly extinguish.

- Displaying anger is closely related to motivating by fear—which is also not an effective long-term strategy. Using fear to motivate behavior and change is a large and complex field of study. Everybody, from pediatricians to the corporate world to the military, has studied these issues.

- Fear is one of the most powerful and primal motivators. It's what gets people out of burning buildings. Advertisers use it constantly—for brakes, tires, alarm systems, and anti-bacterial soaps, as just a couple of examples.

- However, we know from the psychology and human factors communities that constant fear leads to discouragement and demoralization, which will ultimately lead to poorer performance.

- Fear has also been shown to lead to chronic stress and burnout, and it kills innovation and initiation.

- To avoid making your OR and ICU into a fear-based culture, be on the lookout for the following negative occurrences in yourself or others [1]:

- Excessive blame
- Emotional outbursts
- Expressing irritation when asked for assistance or guidance
- Ridicule
- Micromanaging
- Inappropriate conduct—especially by team leaders
- One-way communications—especially from the top down
- Core values that are not clearly understood or articulated

- Instead of trying to lead and motivate by fear (which serves to increase doubt and confusion in the moment concerning complex tasks), perhaps leading by *eliminating doubt* might be an approach.
- There is a lot of interesting and common-sense information online pertaining to these issues, and a quick review would be worthwhile. For example, one business website discusses several other positive motivation strategies as detailed below [2].
- *Protection motivation theory* is based on people having the tools and being able to accomplish both threat appraisal and coping appraisal
- *Affiliation motivation* refers to the fact that most people want to belong to a group. It tries to harness needs for affiliation, power, and achievement
- *Expectancy theory of motivation* is based on the theory that people will choose behavior that they expect will lead to the best outcome and greatest reward. It is deployed by establishing clear connections between effort and performance and resulting "rewards."
- *Power motivation* is based on the theory that some people seem to be motivated by the acquisition of power and prestige. This won't be true for every member of your team, but some people will welcome the opportunity to increase the morale and motivation of the group.

Conclusion

Motivating and correcting your team members is just about courtesy and common sense. And always keep in mind that people detest being lied to and will remember how you made them feel.

References

1. Methods. Fear is not the best motivator [internet]. Methods. 2021 [cited 2025 Jul 27]. Available from: https://methodsof.com/blog/fear-is-not-the-best-motivator.
2. What is fear motivation? And 4 positive motivational techniques to use instead [Internet]. Indeed Career Guide. [cited 2025 Jul 27] Available from: https://www.indeed.com/career-advice/career-development/fear-motivation.

Author

Patricia Kapur spent her career at UCLA in anesthesiology and health system administration, education, and clinical care. She is now sharing the pearls from that experience with her current colleagues at Penn. Patricia's involvement with state and national professional organizations is another career highlight that she recommends to others.

85 Make Sure That the Trainee Knows More at the End of the Day Than When They Came in That Morning

Patricia A. Kapur

Introduction

I spent a number of years as both an adult and pediatric cardiothoracic (CT) anesthesiologist. After several years in the CT operating rooms, I could see that the period of time the patient was on cardiopulmonary bypass (CPB) was a golden teaching opportunity that was not always fully utilized.

Teaching Time

So, although I taught throughout each case, I determined to use that CPB time period to systematically teach the principles of cardiopulmonary bypass to every resident with whom I worked. This teaching included principles of gas exchange on bypass and impact of cooling, types of circuits and oxygenators, pump parameters as a pseudo cardiac output, the relationship of the CPB reservoir volume to the patient's vascular capacity, and so forth. I wanted the residents to be able to stay engaged with their patients' progress during CPB, since there were implications as to how the patients' physiology may respond post-bypass.

I also wanted them to understand what the CPB tech was doing and to interact meaningfully to help manage the patient during CPB. I did not realize how much the residents appreciated that effort until the year following initiating that commitment, when the residents voted me to be Teacher of the Year. I was told by senior residents that they had effectively lobbied their junior colleagues who had not had a CT rotation prior to the vote.

My conclusion for young faculty is not that everyone will be named Teacher of the Year, but everyone who, every day, gives their trainees some new insights or clarity into how or what we do, will be greatly appreciated. No matter what the circumstances, we all should make sure that trainees know more or have greater knowledge and insight at the end of each day than when they walked in that morning.

P. A. Kapur (✉)
Department of Anesthesiology and Critical Care, Perelman School of Medicine, University of Pennsylvania, Philadelphia, PA, USA
e-mail: patricia.kapur@pennmedicine.upenn.edu

S. Mohamed et al. (eds.), *Anesthesia Bridges*, https://doi.org/10.1007/978-3-032-08294-7_85

Lessons Learned

- There is almost always "downtime" during a case that can be utilized for teaching. An educator should strive to accomplish the following goal: His or her students should have greater knowledge and insight by the end of each day.

Author

Patricia Kapur spent her career at UCLA in anesthesiology and health system administration, education, and clinical care. She is now sharing the pearls from that experience with her current colleagues at Penn. Patricia's involvement with state and national professional organizations is another career highlight that she recommends to others.

86 When Can You "Relax" and Enjoy Being a Faculty Member?

Patricia A. Kapur

Introduction

The transition from resident to junior faculty can be daunting and even scary transition—even if new faculty members do not verbalize it.

New Attending Nerves

One of the most nerve-racking aspects of this transition is that new faculty members must now provide care through the residents' hands and minds, especially in high-stakes situations. Some of the anxiety is that the faculty have very high standards for themselves and feel the responsibility keenly to their patients and the patients' families to see that care is delivered to that standard for each patient. But that is not the only reason for the junior faculty's anxiety.

From my own early experience and observing this transition among many faculty, the transition from new faculty to "seasoned" faculty member occurs when the faculty member becomes confident in their own abilities to be able to "get the resident out of whatever they have gotten themselves into." The faculty member is then able to allow residents to have the educational opportunities needed to make forward progress toward independent practice.

One example is to allow residents to place an invasive line—share the technique pearls, but don't let them take all of the viable arteries or central veins—save at least one for you. Another is to allow residents to try new-to-them regional or airway techniques, or to obtain an ultrasound image—give them a reasonable chance(s) and make a thorough effort to talk them through it before taking over. A third is to try a new-to-them anesthetic pharmacologic combination—know the pharmacology thoroughly to assist/counteract if results are not as expected.

P. A. Kapur (✉)
Department of Anesthesiology and Critical Care, Perelman School of Medicine, University of Pennsylvania, Philadelphia, PA, USA
e-mail: patricia.kapur@pennmedicine.upenn.edu

S. Mohamed et al. (eds.), *Anesthesia Bridges*, https://doi.org/10.1007/978-3-032-08294-7_86

Unfortunately, in many departments, this message—that we know it will be challenging for new faculty members to learn how to provide safe care while teaching residents—is not communicated to the new faculty. By acknowledging this challenge, new faculty are given permission to ask for advice from "seasoned" faculty members.

In addition, because faculty benefit now in many institutions from the opportunity to take their fair share of "personally provided" cases, even seasoned faculty members can better understand what the residents must accomplish on a daily basis. The faculty members providing personal or direct care are reminded of how their OR and procedural suites work and to keep current on all aspects of the processes of anesthesiology care in their institution. This includes preoperative evaluation, room set-up, holding area issues, OR interactions, PACU/ICU transfer, and so forth, without the buffer of a supervised resident or CRNA. Residents benefit from faculty who have not only the factual knowledge and experience with anesthesia care *per se* but also are confident enough from first-hand institutional operational experience to have the comprehensive insights to facilitate a great learning experience for others.

Lessons Learned

- One of the largest challenges facing a new faculty member is to learn how to provide safe care while teaching residents.

Author

Patricia Kapur spent her career at UCLA in anesthesiology and health system administration, education, and clinical care. She is now sharing the pearls from that experience with her current colleagues at Penn. Patricia's involvement with state and national professional organizations is another career highlight that she recommends to others.

Mistakes Past and Present

87

Saundra E. Curry and Catherine Marcucci

The editors of *Anesthesia Bridges* are honored to posthumously publish the following essay by the late Dr. Curry, an esteemed author, teacher, mentor, and clinician.

Introduction from Dr. Curry

Everyone makes mistakes. We're human, and the key thing is to make sure our patients don't suffer for them. Maturity in handling these situations is one of the hallmarks of successful senior clinicians. I have made several drug mistakes over the years, either giving the wrong medication or the wrong dose. Sometimes I think eyesight is to blame; usually it's just a momentary lapse.

Face Up, Don't Double Down

Years ago, while my resident was on break, I gave a dose of what I thought was ondansetron. When he came back, the blood pressure was hovering in the low 200 s, where it had never been. He was concerned, and we discovered that I had actually given phenylephrine 10 mg. I had just picked up the wrong vial and carelessly did not double-check it. This was potentially serious for the patient, and we watched his ECG anxiously. Fortunately, the patient was an otherwise healthy patient and tolerated the lapse well.

But did I have to tell the patient? "Can I avoid this?" I said to myself. "Nothing actually happened." I did tell the surgeon, who was quick to say he believed in full disclosure. So, I went to recovery with the patient, and when he was awake with his wife present, I told him what had happened and the signs he should look for in the next day or so for a possible MI. He was relaxed about it, but his wife was furious.

S. E. Curry
Department of Anesthesiology, Columbia University, New York, NY, USA

C. Marcucci (✉)
Department of Transfusion Medicine, Clinical Center, National Institutes of Health, Bethesda, MD, USA

S. Mohamed et al. (eds.), *Anesthesia Bridges*, https://doi.org/10.1007/978-3-032-08294-7_87

I stayed until all questions were answered and finally left with my tail definitely between my legs. This was me, the boss, not my resident who had made the error. A month or so later, the patient returned for follow-up surgery. "Remember me?" he said. I didn't, but when he reminded me of the incident, it loomed large. "Oh yes," I said. "Don't worry, I have learned my lesson, and it won't happen again." Again, he was relaxed. It was his wife who raised the concern. All went well.

There Is Teaching Everywhere

More recently, with the new prefab syringes, I found myself pushing fentanyl 250 mcg instead of lidocaine. This in itself was not a big deal, but it was the wrong drug in an outpatient setting. I was kicking myself about it, furious with my lapse. But instead of running to hide, I used it as a teaching moment for the resident. What actually happens when you push that much at once, not on cardiac? We watched the ventilation (LMA) slowly make its way back. We watched as the blood pressure dipped, but not too low, and then slowly made its way back. Fear and anger at myself had turned into an educational tool. That patient suffered no ill effects, and there was no need for disclosure. But he was very comfortable when woke up!

Lessons Learned

- What's the point of making mistakes if you don't learn from them?
- As faculty, the mistakes you make are an eye-opener for residents since they think you're infallible. It's good for them to know that they can make mistakes but must learn how to fix them without harm.
- Make mistakes into teaching moments, particularly for residents.
- From the Editors: Remember that lying by omission, as opposed to commission, is still dishonesty. And you can't falsify the anesthesia record—*you cannot falsify the anesthesia record*—so it is likely that your patient will see the mistake recorded there anyway, especially if there was a perturbation in vital signs. They might not understand the anesthesia charting, but rest assured, they will have a medical family member or friend look it over for them if they can.

Authors

Saundra Curry trained at Columbia and never left the mother ship. She was a clinician and spent her time teaching residents and medical students about anesthesia and medical professionalism. She was an active member of The Society for Education in Anesthesia (past president) and the ASA, serving on national committees and giving talks on education and professionalism nationally and internationally.

Cathy Marcucci is a senior academic anesthesiologist and inveterate anesthesiology educator. She is also fellowship-trained in transfusion medicine. She was taught early in her career not to ever push a full syringe of medication into a patient who was not in arrest.

John Williams, MD: A Mentor

88

James Berry

Introduction

As a resident in Houston in 1988, I remember one morning attending a lecture/demonstration by a junior faculty member named John Williams. He had a nerve stimulator and a quantitative TOF monitor displayed on an oscilloscope, and he seemed prepared to demonstrate neuromuscular monitoring on himself. Strangely, he also had a tourniquet on his arm and a heplock IV in his hand.

Teacher As Subject

He explained that he wanted to demonstrate a non-depolarizing blockade and would isolate his arm before injecting a small dose of curare. We were fascinated as he also explained the presence of a blade, tube, and AMBU bag "just in case." The demonstration commenced with a baseline example of train-of-four and tetanus. Amazingly, he never flinched as his hand cramped up from a 50 Hz tetanic stimulation. After inflating the tourniquet and injecting his arm, he did briefly note that he had a bit of double vision; we argued as to who would intubate him.

Overall, we were in awe of an amazing demonstration and of the faculty who would put themselves at risk for the sake of education. Only later did we discover the secret to his stoicism in the face of a tetanic shock. A colleague had consented to place an ulnar block at the elbow prior to our demonstration. He never felt a thing. Dr. Williams, as many know, went on to great things as a cardiac anesthesiologist/intensivist and as the longstanding (now retired) department chair at Pittsburgh.

Tradition of Teaching

I later incorporated some of John's flair for the dramatic into my own demonstration, this time in the area of electrical safety. I was the new program director in Houston, not that long out of training, after Dr. Jeff Katz had taken over the chairmanship of the department from Dr. Joe Gabel.

J. Berry (✉)
Department of Anesthesiology and Pain Management, UT Southwestern Medical Center, Dallas, TX, USA
e-mail: James.Berry@UTSouthwestern.edu

S. Mohamed et al. (eds.), *Anesthesia Bridges*, https://doi.org/10.1007/978-3-032-08294-7_88

My residents showed up one morning to find me with a 10-gallon aquarium full of water and a 120 V electrical cord. One end was plugged into the wall, and the other had two bare wires. I explained the principles of electrical circuits and safety, emphasizing that electricity always takes the path of least resistance and that pure water is non-conductive. They seemed to understand, but reacted when I placed the bare wires into the tank.

Nothing happened, of course, and I explained that the TV depictions of death from toasters in the bathtub were not really an accurate reflection of reality. Sadly, no one volunteered to place their hand into the tank, so I did, noting that I was not elsewhere grounded. I hope I made an impression.

> **"The first job of a leader is to allay anxiety"**
>
> *and*
>
> **"...Better never than late."**
>
> *—Joseph Gabel, MD*

Lessons Learned

- Although we are unlikely to do anything as dramatic as John Williams did in this story, it is a good practice to think of a lecture as a form of entertainment. How can you tell your story in a way that keeps your audience's attention?

Bonus Content!

We were discussing an early draft of this chapter with Denny Bourke, when Denny chuckled and said, "John Williams lived in my garage apartment when he was a second-year anesthesia resident and fellow."

Denny remembers John as very bright and extremely careful and conscientious in his anesthesia practice and research. Dr. Bourke recounted how his own mentor was Ted Smith, who did early clinical research into neuromuscular blockade, and how Denny and other faculty would be their own guinea pigs for experiments on the different effects of succinylcholine on respiratory and peripheral muscle strength, so he believes every word of the anecdote above. Evidently, back in the day, it's what they did in that department. ☺

And speaking of dramatic, it appears that everything in Texas makes an impression (Fig. 88.1).

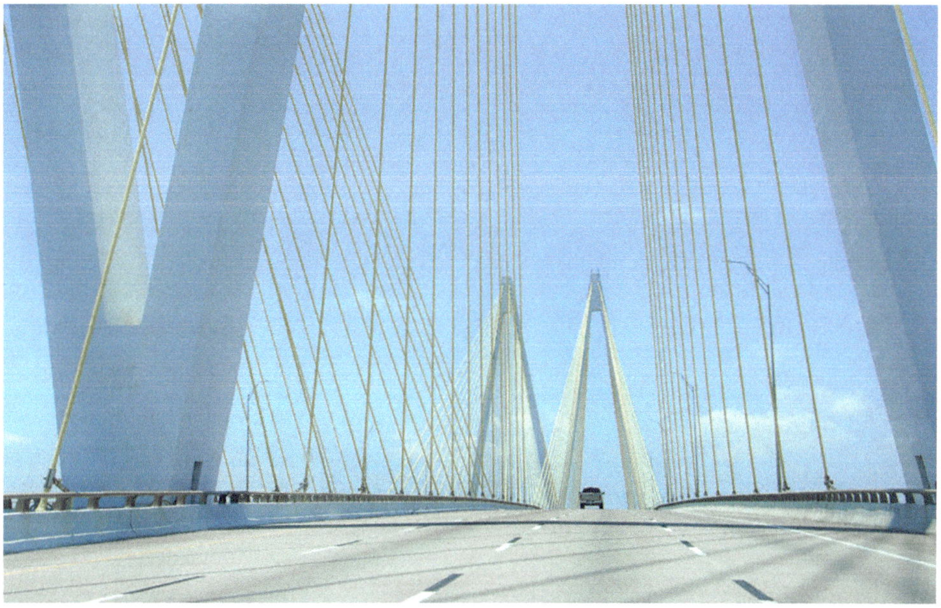

Fig. 88.1 Fred Hartman Bridge is a cable-stayed bridge that spans the Houston Ship Channel. It replaced the tunnel under the channel when the depth of the shipping lane was increased. It's beautiful, but the contracting and construction were not without considerable controversy. Photograph: Image used under standard license from stock.adobe.com

Author

James Berry has a sense of accomplishment and enjoyment for the 35+ years spent in academic medicine, gaining perspective in four very different institutions: University of Texas—Houston, University of Mississippi, Vanderbilt, and now University of Texas—Southwestern. He also leads a busy non-academic life, with interests in aviation, radio/electronics, history, and home/auto repair. His life goal is to have some common ground with everyone he meets.

I've Been a Student Forever and Haven't Yet Applied for an Actual Job: What I Would Tell My 30-Year-old Self About Applying and Interviewing for an Early Career Job

89

William R. Furman

Introduction

For the first 29 years, it was so simple: high school led to college; college begat medical school; residency training and fellowship followed. Each step positioned you for the next one, but none of them prepared you to apply for and interview for a job. Now, more than three decades on, and having interviewed countless applicants myself, here's my advice.

The Task at Hand

Information asymmetry is inherent in every hiring process, and the applicant is usually the disadvantaged party. There's nothing immoral about it. It just comes with the territory. The situation is that they know what they're looking for and what they're really offering, and you have yet to figure that out. From your perspective, interviewing is mostly about convincing prospective employers that they are eager to hire you, and that's where you should expend most of your energy. But be sure to reserve some intellectual bandwidth for the equally important task of learning about and evaluating the opportunity and the people offering it. Think of it as a puzzle to be solved. Try to enjoy the challenge.

How To Begin a Job Search

Consider: What am I looking for? How do I want to spend my work life? Clinical patient care? Research and scholarship? Teaching, with or without research and scholarship? And what are my personal goals for work/life balance? As in, we spend half our waking hours at work, so how much of me do I want to invest in the job, and how much do I want to reserve for myself, my family, and friends? Even if the answers to all these questions are not clear at the start of the process, keep the questions in mind. Answers will come to you. Only pursue positions that are in line with what you are looking for.

W. R. Furman (Retired) (✉)
Department of Anesthesiology, Vanderbilt University Medical Center, Nashville, TN, USA

Physician Hospital Surveyor, The Joint Commission, Boston, MA, USA

S. Mohamed et al. (eds.), *Anesthesia Bridges*, https://doi.org/10.1007/978-3-032-08294-7_89

As you learn about each opportunity, ask yourself: What are they looking for, and do I have that? What situation are they offering, and what qualifications do they require? For a clinical patient care role, applicants need to show themselves to be clinically excellent and fully committed to patient care. For an academic position involving research and scholarship, applicants should have a research track record or, at a minimum, should have impressed someone with their potential (which usually means completion of a project). For a primary teaching role, applicants should be clinically excellent, empathic, have strong communication skills, and be willing to focus on educational technique.

Identify opportunities using any online and networking resources available to you. If a position you seek is highly sought-after, your elegant introductory letter and outstanding CV might not distinguish you from 5 other applicants. But a personal message from someone who taught or worked with you may be what gets you an interview.

About Your Letter: Business format with a formal salutation and complimentary close (even via email), direct and to the point, no more than two pages. Communicate respect but not sycophancy. Introduce yourself, express interest in the position, highlight things that show that you have what they are looking for—do as much homework as you can on this in advance—say thank you. Get an experienced person to review your CV to make sure it follows a standard format and doesn't contain unnecessary filler.

Expect to have been searched online. You searched them, didn't you? Of course, you did. Run a search on yourself so you will know what prospective employers have seen. If you do not get an acknowledgment of your letter, follow up by email or by phone, just to confirm receipt. If the answer is "No, thank you," be gracious about having been considered and move on.

During the Interview

Consider: Do I fit what they're looking for? Be honest with yourself. Keep listening for clues about the social aspects of the culture, the unspoken behavioral expectations that everyone is expected to meet. There's an adage that employers should screen for skills and then interview and hire for culture. You'll be happiest and most successful where you are a good match.

Some FAQs About Interviewing

Q: I have several invitations for job interviews. Which do I schedule first? Do I rank them and start with my top choice?

A: Quite the opposite. The "pearl" is to interview somewhere low on your list first and save the ones you most desire for a little later.

Q: What will they ask me?

A: It may not be obvious, but the true meaning of nearly every question is probably going to be who you are and you are a good fit. The workplace is a family. Do they want you to be part of it?

Q: What do I say?

A: Tell the truth—it's what you remember best. Be ready to be asked at least one question that stimulates introspection and reveals something you haven't fully considered and maybe don't completely understand about yourself. That's why it's a good idea not to interview first at your top choice. After one or two interviews, you'll be better at explaining and revealing yourself through clearer verbal communication.

Q: What do I not say?

A: You do not have to tell all the truth, but you should tell nothing but the truth. It's okay to feature the narrative about your strengths and why you would be a desirable hire (a continuation of your introductory letter) without communicating the extent of your self-doubts. No need to over-share. Be very careful about the unguarded use of humor.

Q: Are there things they are not supposed to ask me?

A: *Yes.* There are questions that should not be asked but might be raised, nonetheless. Let's be gracious and say this is because interviewers aren't perfect. For example, questions about family (marriage, children, family members with special needs) or your own health history would be out of bounds. Asking questions about your ethnicity and religious or political views for the purpose of qualifying you would be off-limits as well. However, if you bring any of these up, the topic could be considered open for discussion.

Think in advance about how you would respond to an improper question. Will you be offended and unable to control your emotional response? Will you be troubled, but able to say something like: "Gosh, I don't know if HR would be comfortable with this being an official part of a job interview." Or something to that effect? Finally, consider what it may mean about this employer if the interviewer steps over that line. Is there systematic disregard for social equity, or was that merely a mistake by an interviewer who should have known better?

Q: How do I say it?

A: We only get one chance to make a first impression. Be respectful and concise, but not abrupt. Don't speak for too long in answer to a question without pausing. Let the interviewer check in or redirect you. Make sure you are answering what was asked. A recruiter once told me that no matter how uniquely fascinating you are, there is a limit to how much continuous content anyone wants to hear.

***Note from the Editors:** To commemorate Bill Furman's time in New Hampshire, we found the Portsmouth Memorial Living Bridge (Fig. 89.1).

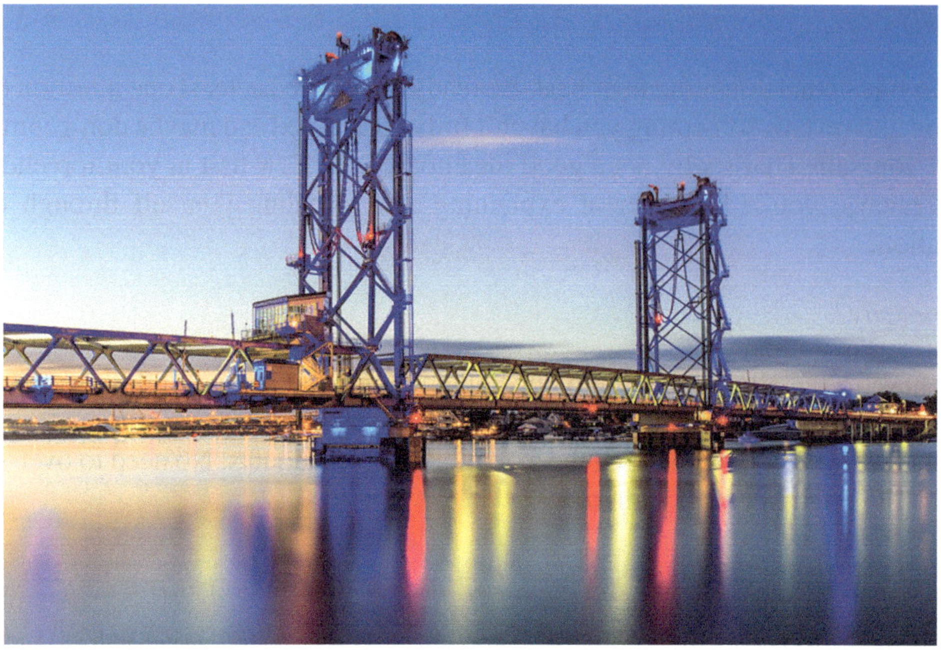

Fig. 89.1 Portsmouth Memorial Bridge spans a tidal estuary between New Hampshire and Maine. The bridge acts as a living laboratory for scientists and engineers, the bridge owner, municipal authorities, University of New Hampshire engineering students, and even K-12 students. It is outfitted with sensors that capture structural performance, traffic patterns, performance patterns of specific bridge elements, weather fluctuations, and tidal patterns. It also seeks to maximize the social impact of the engineering environment of the bridge itself and the surrounding area. Photograph: Image used under standard license from stock.adobe.com

After the Interview

Many jobs look very enticing at first. The interviewers present their best face, just as you do. It's polite to send a brief thank-you note for the time and the enjoyable conversations, but don't make or communicate a decision right away. Let a few days elapse, and think about what was and wasn't said. Sometimes we only become cognizant of "red flags" after we've replayed the events of the day once or twice. Other times, it takes a while for what's truly important to become clear.

If You Get an Offer

Offers are typically communicated verbally first, with a written contract to follow. Some thoughts about the contract:

- The written contract should faithfully match what you thought you were told. If it doesn't, this might be a "red flag."
- One of the most important relationships in your work life is the one with your boss (or bosses). Who is that? Is it a good fit?

- Are you and the culture a good fit? The adage is that we choose to leave jobs because of the people more than because of pay or other employment aspects.
- Can you access anyone who has worked there in the past and left? A friend of a friend, maybe?
- Employment contracts are 15% about the marriage and 85% about the divorce. Don't be offended or surprised by this when you see it in writing. We avoid thinking about worst-case scenarios, but at contract time need to consider: What could go wrong? Under what conditions can they fire me? What are the severance terms and obligations?
- If there's a financial impasse, decide whether the issue has enough zeroes in the number to be worth digging in. You might not want to allow a 3- or 4-figure issue to drive you away from a good 6-figure job.
- The contract negotiation is the beginning of your employment relationship. Your conduct reveals what you might be like to work with and can reverse the offer decision. Ask for things that are important to you, but be polite. Stand for principle but remain respectful.
- It is also true that your prospective employer's conduct tells you something about the culture and signals what it might be like to work there.
- The contract negotiation is the beginning of your employment relationship. Your conduct reveals what you might be like to work with and can reverse the offer decision. Ask for things that are important to you, but be polite. Stand for principle but remain respectful.

Turning Down an Offer

If you tend to be conflict-avoidant by nature, you will need to recognize and deal with that. Saying no is an important skill. Whether you have received multiple offers or simply have decided that a specific opportunity just is not right for you, you'll need to communicate your decision. An email is sufficient, and written communication is appreciated.

While not every interaction follows us for our entire career, it's generally best to be gracious and respectful whenever possible. You do not have to express the reason why you have chosen to decline an offer. However, if you find the urge to provide an explanation irresistible, something about family (as opposed to the job or the compensation) offends nobody, diminishes nobody, and tends to leave all parties in good humor.

Remember for the future that information asymmetry can work both ways and can be to your advantage. This probably is not going to be the last time you interview. The next time you apply for a job, prospective employers will have limited knowledge about you until they meet you, unless your internet presence has told them too much already. Online reviews by former employees and applicants may have helped make your decision to decline an offer, and you may be motivated to post your own comments, especially if you feel you have had a negative experience. Be careful about that, choose your words with great care, and don't be in a hurry. Because: The Internet. Flame is forever.

Lessons Learned

- Be polite.
- Listen carefully.
- Tell your truth.
- Learn from every experience.

Author

Bill Furman retired in 2017 after a 35-year career in academic anesthesiology, critical care, and medical leadership. He was born in New York, trained at Hopkins in internal medicine, pulmonary medicine, and anesthesiology and critical care, and worked in Baltimore, Chicago, Chapel Hill, NC, Nashville, TN, and New Hampshire before retiring to Cambridge MA, to be near the grandchildren. He can do most of the regional accents of all those places, but his favorite is Balmer, Hon. He was pretty sure he'd flunk retirement, so he works part-time in accreditation and consulting, which allows him to see health care delivery literally everywhere in the USA and its territories.

Always Ask a Senior and Respected Peer for Advice Before Making a Life-Changing Decision

90

Michael A. Ramsay

Introduction

As a junior consultant (faculty) at The London Hospital, London University, after two years as the youngest physician appointed to that position—and this is important as the UK was full of tradition and this was expected to be a lifetime career appointment—I received an offer of a staff position in Dallas, Texas.

What I Had

The anesthesia practice I had was full-time employment at The London Hospital, but if I took a one-eighth cut in salary, I would be allowed to do private practice in my spare time. The surgeons I worked with had taken this option, so I did as well. This meant that I began to work 24/7 every week. This is not a family pleaser, especially when you have four small children at home. However, the full-time job was very fulfilling with academia, teaching, research, and exciting clinical work in a tertiary referral unit.

The "Private Practice" included many of London's elite—Royals, noblemen and noble ladies, actors and actresses, so it was not something I was ready to give up, plus I knew I was a young consultant and if I left I would hurt the chances of other young physicians, as my elders were sure to say "There I told you so, we never should have appointed a young consultant." The pressure from home increased as did the timeframe to make a decision decreased. I needed advice—but where to get it?

Where I Was Going

One of my patients was the Archbishop of Canterbury—the head of the Church of England, could I discuss this with him? I summoned courage, and after his surgery was over and he was recovering well, I made another postoperative visit and brought up the topic of leaving England for the USA with him. I

M. A. Ramsay (✉)
Department of Anesthesiology and Pain Management, Baylor University Medical Center, Dallas, TX, USA
e-mail: michael.ramsay@bswhealth.org

S. Mohamed et al. (eds.), *Anesthesia Bridges*, https://doi.org/10.1007/978-3-032-08294-7_90

must say that I felt sure he would talk me out of going, and I would be able to go home and tell my wife that the Archbishop said that I must stay.

How wrong could I be! He graciously took four hours to discuss my life, my ambitions, and my family, and he got to know me. He told me that he had spent some time in the United States and that it had been very worthwhile. He concluded by saying, "Mike, you are not going to like what I am about to tell you. You must go to the United States and Dallas, or you will regret it the rest of your life. I hope that, like me, you will come back, but realistically this is unlikely. Your family needs to see more of you, that is most important, and the opportunities that will come along, you cannot imagine."

So, I went home and told my wife that we were going to Dallas, she was delighted. I went to the US Embassy in Grosvenor Square, London, and was told that there was a small window of time that they were processing papers for physicians, as the requirements were about to change. So, in four weeks we were on our way to Chicago and down to Dallas. My children were nervous as they had not been on a plane before and clung to their mother. I knew then that this was the right decision and the Archbishop had advised me well.

Lessons Learned

- Always put family first.
- Don't be afraid to seek advice from the most knowledgeable person you know.

Editor's note: We were really fascinated when Mike sent us this essay. Such a distinguished person as the Right Reverend Archbishop of Canterbury Emeritus must have been very busy with a full calendar and many people to speak to, but this senior person took the time to listen carefully and speak with a junior physician and a young family man. Use this as an example. Be accessible, take the phone call or meeting, and be willing to share your own experiences. And if somebody asks you for advice—that is, if your opinion is actually solicited—*give it.*

Author

Mike Ramsay was born in Dublin, went to medical school in London, and after two years on the faculty of the London Hospital, he moved to Baylor University Medical Center in Dallas. He tells us, "This was a strong decision of my wife Zoe, and the best decision in my career. I am not sure where my accent has landed. In London, they are critical and call it Yankee and in Texas most say I am Australian!? The move has allowed us both to travel together around the globe on lecture tours. This has resulted in many international friends as well as local friends and also great memories. Along the way we have managed a few influences on medicine and providers as well. What an exhilarating and fun career!"

Passing the Torch

91

Mada F. Helou, Nicholas L. Pesa, Matthew P. Norcia, and David A. Wallace

Introduction

There have been substantial changes in the administration and education of anesthesia residency programs over the course of the years, certainly accelerated in the last decade or so. In this chapter, we overhear a conversation between Drs. Matt Norcia and Dave Wallace, our elder statesmen who ran the anesthesia residency program at University Hospitals Cleveland Medical Center from 2001–2012, and Drs. Mada Helou and Nick Pesa, our "juniors," who have run the same residency program from 2018 until the present day.

The Interview

Mada and Nick: Technology seems to have driven a lot of changes in the expected skillset of an anesthesiologist. Although ultrasound has been around for some time, increased accessibility (with reduced cost) and improvements in the quality of images/loops took place during your tenure. How did you strategically integrate a newer technology like this into resident education? What obstacles did you meet and how did you overcome them?

Dave and Matt: One of the hardest parts of teaching the residents newer technologies, like ultrasound, was getting a critical mass of our core faculty comfortable and competent enough with it to properly teach it to our trainees. In addition, it was challenging to gain approval from finance for costly equipment. Once secured, making sure that such a scarce resource was available for teaching was another barrier. Luckily, we had a very supportive chairman who preemptively budgeted for educational initiatives and equipment, and who supported faculty development programs.

M. F. Helou (✉) · N. L. Pesa · M. P. Norcia · D. A. Wallace
Department of Anesthesiology and Perioperative Medicine, University Hospitals Cleveland Medical Center, Cleveland, OH, USA
e-mail: Mada.Helou@uhhospitals.org

S. Mohamed et al. (eds.), *Anesthesia Bridges*, https://doi.org/10.1007/978-3-032-08294-7_91

Mada and Nick: So, what strategies do you advise us to employ in order to succeed in integrating newer educational initiatives?

Dave and Matt: It must come from the top down in the department—the chairperson needs to be fully supportive, or the initiative is at risk for failing. A cultural change needs to be driven by the chair—he/she must set expectations regarding how new technology will be implemented. This can help get buy-in from the older core teaching faculty so that they can begin to pursue competency in the area. Utilizing "fresh" out-of-training junior attendings is paramount as they will really help push forward the newest techniques of care. They are also a resource for older core faculty who wish to learn new skills.

Mada and Nick: Leveraging the unique skill set that anesthesiologists achieve to expand the scope of the anesthesiologists' practice into a perioperative surgical home (PSH) model has been a challenge for the specialty as a whole. How did you help prepare your residents for a future that includes more than intraoperative care?

Dave and Matt: We spent a lot of resources expanding the curriculum into the areas of pre- and post-operative care. Adding rotations like PACU, perioperative medicine, pre-admission clinic, and expanding our critical care rotations were some of the main objectives. Integrating a hospitalist into our department who was fellowship-trained in perioperative care was vital to the expansion of this curriculum. Adding a primarily internal medicine-trained physician to our teaching faculty added a breadth of knowledge and training that extended trainee insight past the end of the PACU stay.

Mada and Nick: How would you advise us in terms of further expanding our anesthesia residents' education to prepare them for PSH and beyond?

Dave and Matt: Unfortunately, the time residents have to learn everything they need to learn is limited. As you add more experiences and rotations that involve learning outside of the OR, you decrease their intraoperative exposure and reduce their experience there. It's a very careful balance that requires constant follow-up regarding milestones and the core competencies. Either adding more time to residency, requiring fellowship training, or completely revamping medical education might be necessary if this balance is too disrupted or if the additional areas of training expand too rapidly.

***Note from the Editors:** To honor the authors for their diligent efforts to impart flexibility and adaptability in today's junior anesthesiologists, we are including the following cool bridges from the new and old adaptable bridge movements (Figs. 91.1 and 91.2).

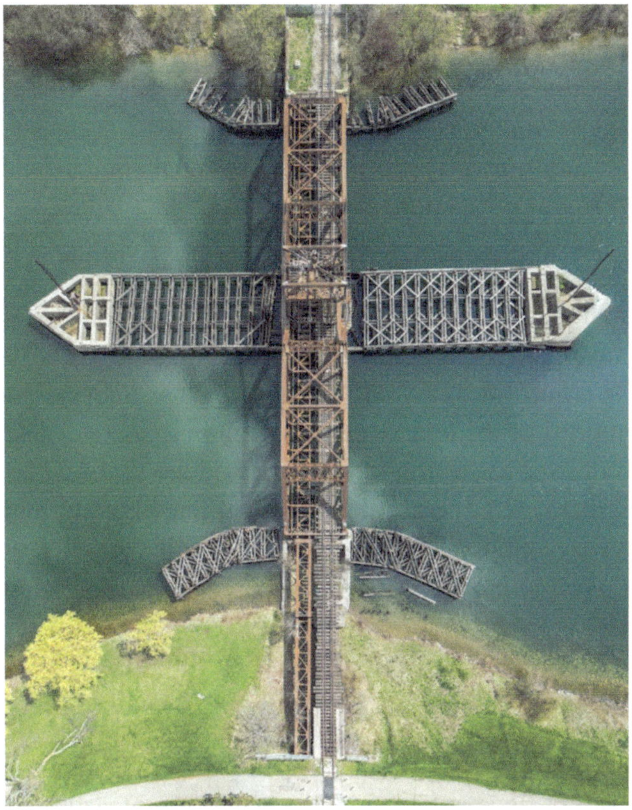

Fig. 91.1 The present-day adaptable bridge movement is admirable, but the principles of adaptability are universal and timeless. The bed of a bridge can either be retracted, raised and lowered, or turned, as with this old iron railway bridge. Photograph: Katie Bernaski, image used under standard license from iStock.com

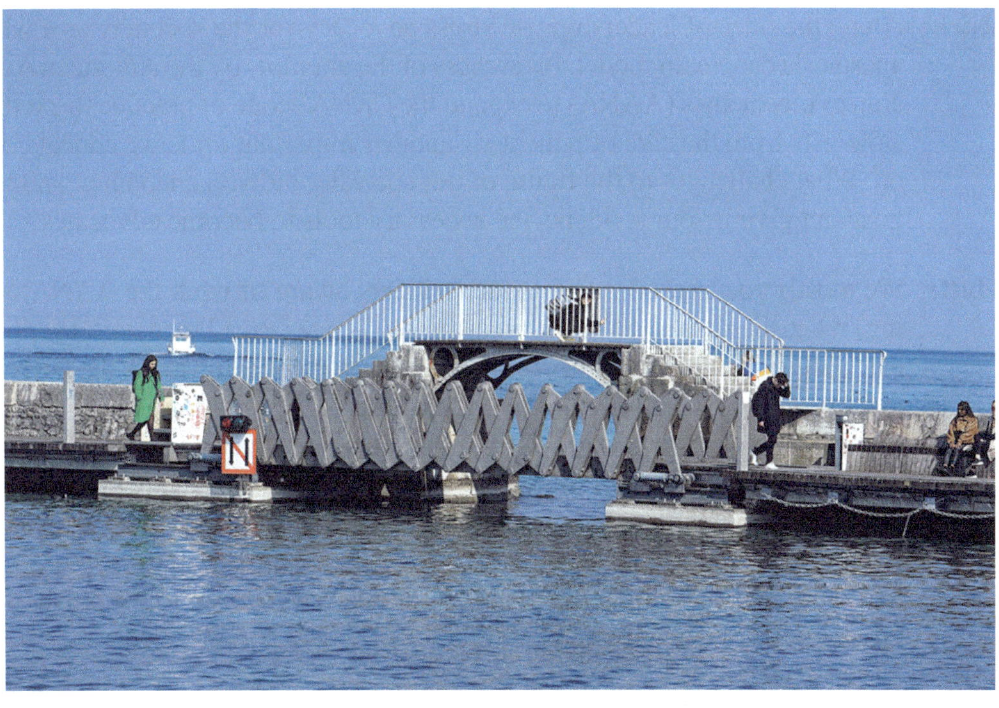

Fig. 91.2 Small metal bridge in Geneva, Switzerland, can be scissored open in about 90 seconds to allow the passage of boats out to the main portion of the lake. Photograph: Michael Derrer Fuchs, image for editorial use non-fiction book from iStock.com

Mada and Nick: An ever-changing healthcare landscape in the USA has driven us to focus more on producing residents equipped with the tools to become healthcare leaders. We have discovered that teaching leadership qualities and skills outside of the OR isn't necessarily easy to integrate into a heavily clinically focused educational program. Was this a focus during your administration? What educational initiatives did you have in regard to teaching "leadership?"

Dave and Matt: We started by integrating our chief residents into more of our departmental meetings and committees. Having them involved in decision-making at a departmental level, and at a hospital level when able, was important to us. We also had our residents rotate at the OR control desk, where our group of anesthesia coordinators runs the day-to-day operations of the operating rooms and organizes anesthesia, nursing, and surgery teams to deliver care. In addition, we believe that resident involvement in research, academic presentations at all levels, and teaching students from a broad set of programs, for example, anesthesia assistant students, SRNAs, medical students, and PA students, is an important part of developing leadership and communication skills.

Mada and Nick: If you could have your druthers, what would you have us do with our current residents to impress upon them leadership qualities?

Dave and Matt: If we had our way, every resident would need to be a chief resident. This would make every resident be involved in the operations of a department/residency, personnel decisions, and the logistics of running an anesthesia department. Getting them involved in the ASA and their grassroots advocacy efforts and showing them how our national organization works should be a priority as well.

Mada and Nick: Along the lines of leadership, we stress advocacy for the specialty as a whole and the anesthesia care team model. Awareness of the attempts by the American Association of Nurse Anesthetists (AANA) to expand the CRNA scope of practice to exclude anesthesiologists from the care of patients is another important topic we educate our residents on. What challenges to the future of our specialty did you encounter, and how did you go about giving your residents the necessary tools to become advocates?

Dave and Matt: We mostly focused on making our residents aware of what the AANA was purporting, what the data show, and what the challenges are. Journal clubs examining the evidence regarding the safety of the anesthesia care team versus the CRNA-only care models were a yearly event. We encouraged fellowship-based subspecialty training in the fields of critical care, pediatric anesthesia, and cardiac anesthesia to elevate the physician's skill set from the basics of general anesthesia care. We also encouraged donations and involvement with the ASA-PAC and our state chapter's efforts as well. In our program, residents also work side by side with Anesthesia Assistants and learn that these anesthesia professionals are closely aligned with physician anesthesiologists and the care team model.

Mada and Nick: If we had unlimited resources and financing, what would be on your wish list for the residency in the arena of advocacy?

Dave and Matt: At the top of the list would be paying for all of them to attend the major conferences throughout the year, especially the ASA Legislative Conference held in our nation's capital. Exposing them to our anesthesia leadership at the national level and the federal politics surrounding our specialty is a good place to get them started on advocacy. Also, paying for their memberships in advocacy groups like Physicians for Patient Protection and by making donations in their names to the ASA-PAC would hopefully set a lifelong pattern for them.

Lessons Learned

Adaptability is a key component of working in residency education; new tools are constantly becoming available in the world of anesthesiology education, but the basic principles are still basic (Fig. 91.3).

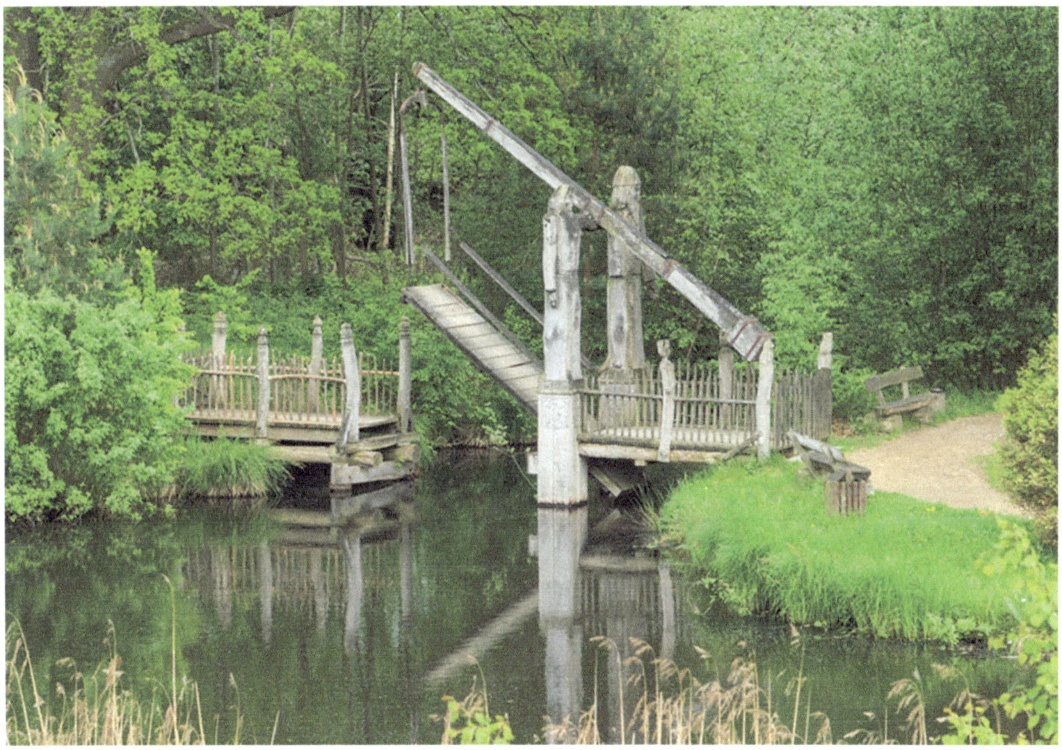

Fig. 91.3 Our favorite adaptable bridge. Photograph: Image used under standard license from iStock.com

- Understanding the history of a residency program/department and "why things are the way they are" can help guide change and progress in a meaningful way.
- Making "every resident a chief resident" encourages teamwork and empowers residents to drive their program forward. Leadership is expected of every physician.

Authors

Mada Helou completed her training in anesthesiology and critical care medicine at the Cleveland Clinic. She joined the faculty at University Hospitals Cleveland Medical Center and is now Program Director. She enjoys time with family and friends and traveling!

Nick Pesa trained at the University Hospitals Cleveland with Drs. Norcia and Wallace as his program directors. Following residency, he completed a fellowship in critical care medicine and then stayed at UHCMC as an attending physician. He has three young children who make his life outside the hospital busy and fun!

Matt Norcia is a former program director and vice-chair for education at University Hospitals Cleveland Medical Center. At present, he remains a senior staff member, is the medical director of the Anesthesiologist Assistant training program at CWRU, and an airway management professional for the Cleveland Browns football team.

Dave Wallace did his training in anesthesiology and pain management at the Cleveland Clinic Foundation. He is a former program director and vice-chair for education and has been at University Hospitals Cleveland Medical Center for 25+ years. He is the director of trauma anesthesia and supports residents and faculty in the area of wealth building and financial risk management to allow them to focus on career building and patient care.

A FAER e-Tale

92

Richard A. Jaffe and Catherine Marcucci

The editors of *Anesthesia Bridges* are honored to posthumously publish the following essay by the late, great Dr. Jaffe. He was so full of life and wisdom and so highly regarded. He was also known for his love of chocolate (Figs. 92.1 and 92.2).

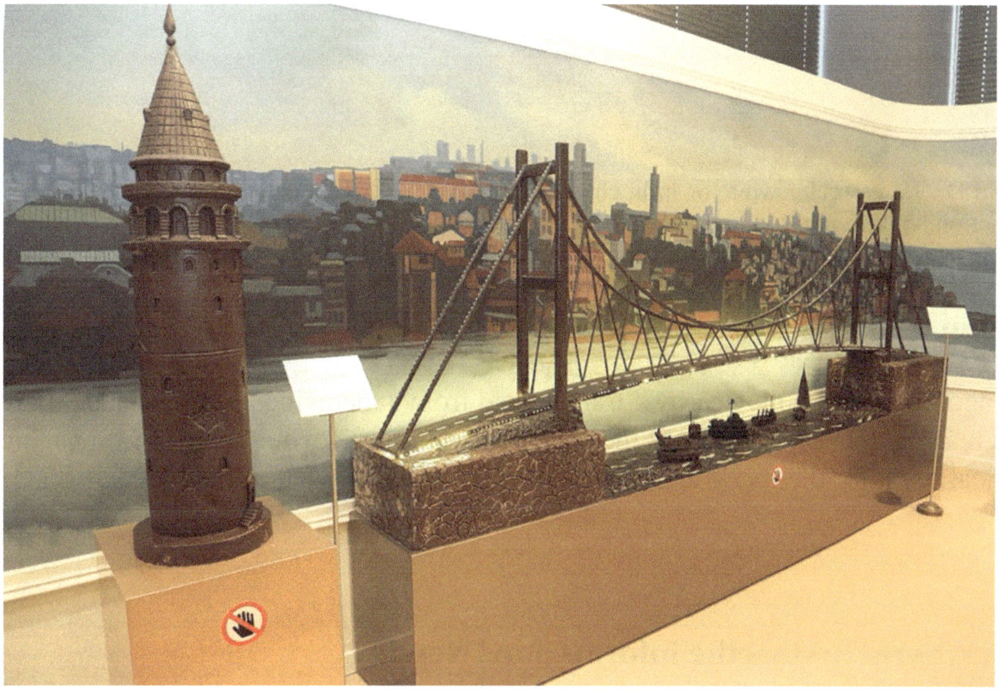

Fig. 92.1 Being from the Bay Area and a lover of chocolate, we thought this confectionery suspension bridge would be the perfect way to honor Dr. Jaffee. Photo: Image used under standard license from shutterstock.com

R. A. Jaffe
Department of Anesthesiology, Perioperative and Pain Medicine, Stanford University School of Medicine, Stanford, CA, USA

C. Marcucci (✉)
Department of Transfusion Medicine, Clinical Center, National Institutes of Health, Bethesda, MD, USA

S. Mohamed et al. (eds.), *Anesthesia Bridges*, https://doi.org/10.1007/978-3-032-08294-7_92

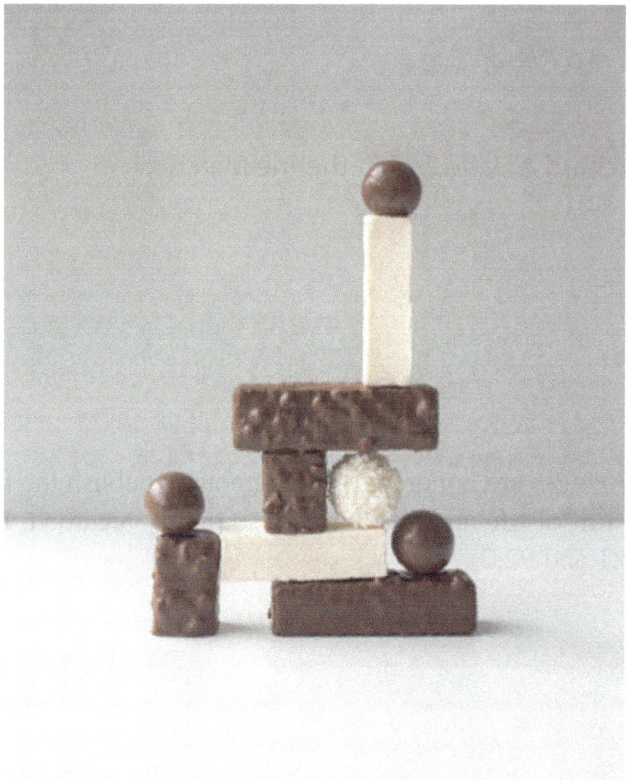

Fig. 92.2 Did Dr. Jaffee prefer white or milk chocolate? Maybe both! Photo: Anatolii Frolov, used under editorial license non-fiction book from iStock.com

Introduction

Long, long ago, in a place quite nearby, I transitioned from a medicine intern to an anesthesiology resident. I soon realized that my mastery of the dark art of anesthesia would benefit from an understanding of any medical basis for the many apparent idiosyncrasies of my anesthesia and surgical attendings. I was naïve.

Why? And Where Do I Get the Information I Need?

In response to my CA-1 questions, I was told too often "just do it" or "that's the way I was taught to do it" or "great question, why don't you do some research and report back to me." The only way of knowing your attending's special needs often required last-minute consultation with a more experienced resident, not a very efficient form of information transfer.

I also realized that my medical student surgery clerkship didn't give me much insight into aspects of the surgery that would be particularly relevant to an anesthesiologist. For example, surgical vs. gross anatomy, structures at risk during surgery, potential complications, expected blood loss, pathophysiology, etiology, associated conditions, and the reason for special anesthetic requests would be useful to know but difficult to assemble the night before surgery. By the second year of my residency, I became convinced that an anesthesia textbook with a primary surgical focus would be useful. That was the inspiration for *The Anesthesiologist's Manual of Surgical Procedures,* now out in the 6th edition and into the 7th [1].

Getting the Book Together

The book concept and its unique format were well received by the publisher, and we began actively recruiting authors. Somewhat later, I was fortunate enough to be awarded a FAER grant to support my research on the role of primary sensory ganglia in the modulation of sensory input to the spinal cord. In theory, the grant provided me with financial support, academic time, and research space to set up my laboratory. In practice, laboratory space could not be created instantly, and the acquisition of equipment and the training of a research assistant were sources of further delay. This downtime seemed to be the perfect opportunity to work on my Anesthesia textbook.

In concept (and eventually in practice), *The Anesthesiologist's Manual of Surgical Procedures* would rely on both surgeons and anesthesiologists as contributors. To ensure author uniformity, I created what I thought were simple word processing templates for each section of the textbook. Working from detailed examples, a surgeon or anesthesia author would only need to type within the template to ensure that the complex format of the text would be consistent and include all the pertinent information. I was so naïve.

Although I had identified 150+ Stanford contributors, I realized that I was a relatively unknown commodity to them, and their willingness to contribute to my textbook might be limited. I decided I needed a senior faculty coeditor who was well known and liked by both my anesthesia and surgical colleagues. Dr. Stanley Samuels, a charming Irish anesthesiologist, fit the bill perfectly. He thought the book concept was good, and he proved to be extremely helpful in recruiting authors. So, with detailed text examples, word processor templates, an administrative assistant with a strong editorial background, and a charming coeditor, I believed that we could pull off this whole project in 6 months. Two and a half years later, with lots of handholding, editing, formatting, and rewriting, we finally reached our content goal, and the manuscript was published.

Today

The textbook was pleasantly well received and new editions have appeared at approximately five-year intervals. As I write this, it is time to start work on the seventh edition. I have come to realize (and recently told my publisher) that textbooks have become simply the fossilized remains of tree-eating dinosaurs and should be abandoned in favor of an UpToDate © style digital information transfer format, where contributors are paid to keep their sections current. I thought that transitioning the print format to an UpToDate-style e-text would be simple to produce and offer significant advantages over a conventional textbook. I am so naïve.

Lessons Learned

So, what have I learned?

- FAER grants are incredibly valuable for early-career research anesthesiologists.
- Multi-author textbook projects can be extremely difficult to produce unless you have some leverage with the contributors, for example, being their department chair.
- Balancing the setup of a research lab, applying for an NIH grant, completing a major textbook project, and working in the OR while trying to maintain some vestige of work–life balance was more difficult than I thought.
- Although I really am naïve, that proved to be quite useful.

Reference

1. Jaffee RA, Schmiesing CA, Golianu B, editors. Anesthesiologist's manual of surgical procedures. 6th ed. Philadelphia: Lippincott Williams & Wilkins (Wolters Kluwer); 2019.

Authors

Richard Jaffe was a professor of anesthesiology and, by courtesy, a professor of neurosurgery at Stanford University School of Medicine. He also served as chief of the neurosurgical anesthesia service and director of the neuroanesthesia fellowship. He was a proud parent who admitted to too many hobbies, and he always maintained a special interest in promoting organized labor for faculty physicians as a counter force to the (often) misplaced priorities of the ever-expanding bureaucracy. Many thanks to Dr. Jaffee for providing a compilation of the facts involved in understanding surgical procedures for decades of anesthesiologists.

Cathy Marcucci is a senior academic anesthesiologist and inveterate anesthesiology educator. She is also fellowship-trained in transfusion medicine. When she is not taking care of patients and/or putting the latest book together, she dedicates her time to mentoring junior colleagues, writing copy for animal rescues, and travelling.

Simulation in Anesthesia

93

Michael D. Altose and Edwin G. Avery IV

Introduction

In this chapter, **Mike Altose** (interviewed by **Ed Avery**) shares his experiences in utilizing simulation in anesthesiology training.

What Does "Simulation" Mean: What Does It Include?

Many people equate "simulation" with managing a cardiac arrest in a robotic patient at a high-fidelity simulation center. But, in fact, simulation encompasses many different technologies and can take place in a variety of settings. In general, medical simulation involves imitating or representing real-world situations so that healthcare providers can learn, practice, and assess their medical knowledge, skills, or behaviors in a safe environment. Simulation can be accomplished with high-fidelity whole-body manikins; task trainers that are designed to teach procedures on a specific part of the body; standardized actors who portray patients; simulated medical scenarios using virtual reality; computer-based role-playing software; or even verbal questioning, like oral boards. To take a classic example—when a student practices intramuscular injections on an orange, that's also simulation! And therefore, simulation can occur in a simulation center, a skills lab, in situ (in a clinical space), or even at home.

How Did You Come to Be Involved In the Use of Anesthesia Simulator Training?

During my residency, I always looked for opportunities to teach. I even set up a 1-month elective at a nearby simulation center to explore simulation-based teaching. When I graduated and was recruited to stay on as faculty, my department chair knew I was interested in teaching, and he encouraged me to get involved with our department's very small simulation program. I'll admit, I was really more interested

M. D. Altose (✉) · E. G. Avery IV
Department of Anesthesiology and Perioperative Medicine, University Hospitals Cleveland Medical Center, Cleveland, OH, USA
e-mail: Michael.Altose@UHhospitals.org

S. Mohamed et al. (eds.), *Anesthesia Bridges*, https://doi.org/10.1007/978-3-032-08294-7_93

in other aspects of education like didactic teaching and curriculum development, but before long, I was running our department simulation lab, created a new weekly simulation-based curriculum for residents, including developing a host of new scenarios, and designed a simulation component for our new intern orientation curriculum.

How Common Is It For Anesthesia Training Programs To Employ the Use of a Simulator To Train Residents?

The ACGME expects that residents will participate in at least one simulated intra-operative clinical experience each year of training. But they do not require programs to use a simulator or have a simulation center. As a result, simulation-based education varies widely among training programs. Some programs may only bring residents to the simulation lab once a year for an event in which some learners participate in the scenario while others observe and participate in the debrief. Other programs have a much more robust simulation component to their curriculum, with residents using the simulation center regularly for hi-fidelity simulation, skills workshops, and even independent self-study.

Is the Presence of a Biomedical Engineer Required to Run Most Simulations?

As I described above, there are many different types of simulations that would not require any advanced engineering abilities. Focusing specifically on high-fidelity scenarios, it can be difficult to implement effective scenarios without a dedicated technician who can focus solely on the technological component of the scenario, making sure the scenario is running smoothly and behaving in a realistic fashion. This person does not need to have a degree in biomedical engineering, although it may be helpful in a large simulation center.

There is also a certification called Certified Healthcare Simulation Operations Specialist (CHSOS). But any technologically minded clinician could learn to operate a high-fidelity manikin, and many resources are available from the manufacturers including technical support, maintenance agreements, and pre-programmed scenarios. There is also a robust community of healthcare "simulationists" who are eager to share ideas and scenarios.

Is There Evidence In the Peer-Reviewed Literature That Use of an Anesthesia Simulator Affects Resident Performance or ABA Board Scores/Passing Rates?

I am not aware of any data showing that simulation-based education directly affects resident performance on knowledge exams like the ABA BASIC or ADVANCED written exams. One would expect a well-designed curriculum to improve the performance on the APPLIED exam, which includes the Standardized Oral Examination (SOE) and the Objective Structured Clinical Examination (OSCE). Similarly, there is a large body of literature describing improved clinical performance when learners have simulation-based instruction.

These studies are published in general medical and nursing journals, specialty-specific journals, and in *Simulation in Healthcare*, the journal of the Society for Simulation in Healthcare. There are countries that require applicants to complete high-fidelity simulation scenarios successfully in order to obtain certification in anesthesiology.

***Note from the Editors:** Are there simulators for bridge design? Of course there are! And lots of them, too. Bridge Up! is one of our favorites (Fig. 93.1). The interactive curriculum provides free classroom resources and instruction for Minnesota school children based on bridge design and construction to assist in teaching math and science (see Disclaimer below).

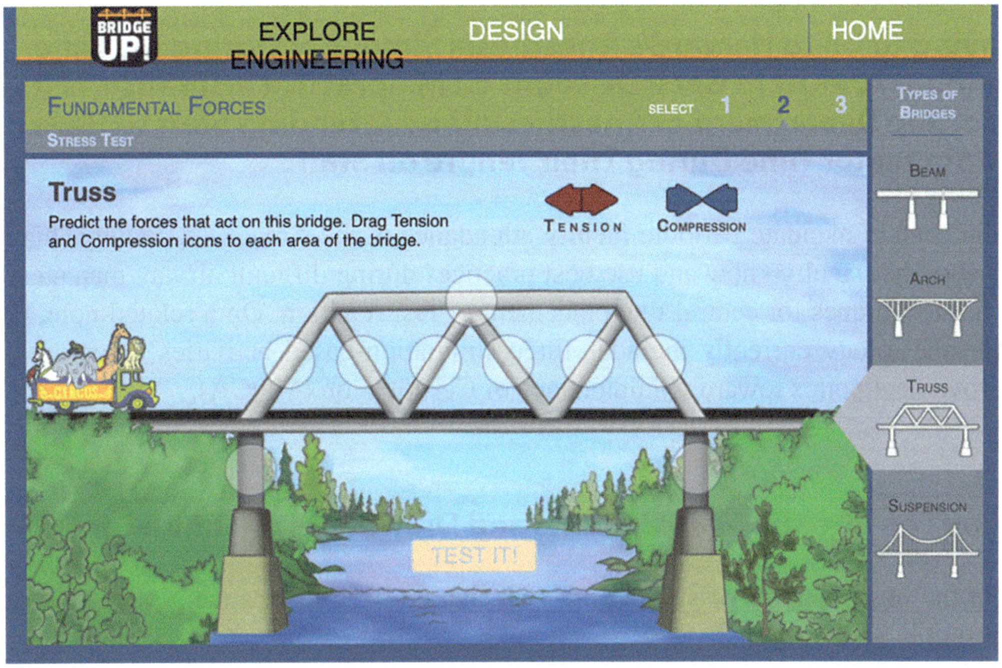

Fig. 93.1 Bridge Up! Allows you to drag tension and compression icons to each area of the bridge and then test to see whether the structure will support a wagon of circus animals that want to cross. Illustration: Image from Bridge Up! curriculum website—dot.state.mn.us, disclaimer below

What Kind of Monetary Investment Is Needed to Acquire a Simulator and Get One Up and Running?

Again, the financial commitment will depend largely on the type of simulation one hopes to implement. Focusing on high-fidelity simulation, this is a complicated question to answer. You need to consider what type of scenarios you intend to develop, and your learners' needs. Anesthesia-specific considerations that I feel are important include, first and foremost, realistic airway situations for bag-mask ventilation, laryngoscopy, laryngeal mask airway replacement, one-lung ventilation, bronchoscopy, invasive/surgical airway, and difficult airway conditions. Also important are credible interactions with mechanical ventilators and accurate physiologic responses to pathologic conditions, anesthetic agents, and other medications. There are many cool features out there, but if they are not the features that keep your learners engaged with the scenario, then you're just paying for things you don't need.

To answer your question, very basic whole patient simulators can start at under $10,000, but very high-end manikins sell for more than $250,000. That is separate from any maintenance, accessories, extended warranty, computer hardware, software, and training costs. One would also need to consider the physical space simulated operating room, a control room, audio-visual hardware, and an anesthesia machine may all be necessary to create realistic scenarios.

But don't be discouraged, much can be accomplished on a budget! In fact, the Society for Simulation in Healthcare has a "low-cost & low-resource affinity group," with lots of tips on how to achieve your educational goals when money is tight.

I Recall Having to Go to Harvard's Anesthesia Simulator During My Time as an Attending at MGH to Get a Discount on Malpractice Insurance. Is It Common for the Department of Anesthesiology Attending Staff to Have Mandated Simulator Time During Their Tenure on Staff?

Some medical centers mandate periodic faculty attendance at the simulation center. This requirement may be to ensure that faculty know and use best practices during difficult airway management or demonstrate proper techniques for central line placement or resuscitation. On a related note, the American Board of Anesthesiology currently includes three simulation-based activities as options for earning Quality Improvement points towards Maintenance of Certification (MOCA).

What Do You Feel Are the Main Benefits and Drawbacks of Simulator Training?

To appreciate the main benefits of simulation, I always go back to Issenberg's list of key features of high-fidelity simulation. They include:

- *Hands-on or interactive learning experience*
- *Repetitive practice*
- *Feedback (debrief) during the experience*
- *Controlled and safe environment*
- *Adaptable, individualized learning*
- *Validity (realism)*
- *Integration into curriculum*

Who wouldn't want to learn under those conditions? Who wouldn't want to be cared for by a clinician who learned under those conditions?

As for the drawbacks, I would mention two issues from two very different domains. From the learner's standpoint, one needs to know the limitations of the simulation. Realism is never 100%, and therefore, excellent performance in simulation does not mean excellent performance in a real clinical situation. Identifying these limitations is a key part of simulation-based education.

From the educator's standpoint, simulation can demand significant resources such as faculty time, learner time, space, and money. Therefore, it is important to design a curriculum that utilizes these limited resources most effectively. To conclude, I often remind people that simulation is not an end unto itself; it is only a tool. If you use this very powerful tool to further your educational goals, then you can see much success.

Lessons Learned

- There are many different types of simulation.
- Simulation may be required during training, for certification, and in clinical practice.
- Although simulation can require significant resources, there are also ways of implementing effective, low-cost simulation.
- Simulation is a powerful and effective educational tool.
- Always think carefully about your learners' needs before you invest time and money in developing a simulation-based curriculum.

****Disclaimer** *The Bridge Up website states, "Parents, substitute teachers, after school program administrators, students, or anyone else interested in science and math can use and modify these resources from anywhere!" The learning modules use bridge design and construction to cover geometry, materials science, statics of mechanics, concrete manufacture, and bridge runoff management. The curriculum is offered in English, Spanish, Hmong, and Somali.*

The State of Minnesota Bridge Up! modeling and educational programs and the data they contain are provided for informational purposes only. The Minnesota Department of Transportation (MnDOT) does not guarantee the accuracy or quality of the data or predictions contained in the educational and/or modeling programs and makes no warranty—express or implied—with respect to the data or predictions contained in the model. All end users of the modeling program, its data, and its predictions assume all risk associated with use.

Authors

Mike Altose grew up in the Cleveland, Ohio area. After 4 years away from home studying chemistry at Brandeis University, he returned to his hometown, where he joined the MD PhD program at Case Western Reserve University, followed by residency in anesthesiology at University Hospitals of Cleveland, where he is now on faculty and serves as the section head for neurosurgical anesthesia. He is thrilled to be fulfilling his lifelong interest in teaching: he teaches both pharmacology and physiology to the Anesthesiology Assistant students at CWRU, coordinates the orientation boot camp for anesthesia interns, runs the department simulation center, serves as chair of the Program Evaluation Committee, and teaches residents regularly in the classroom and clinical setting. He especially credits Helmut Cascorbi MD, Howard Nearman MD, and Murray Altose MD (Fig. 93.2—his father!) for their support and mentorship in guiding him toward a career in education and academic medicine.

Ed Avery is a New Englander who trained and worked at the Massachusetts General Hospital for over a decade before being recruited to Cleveland. He is a cardiac anesthesiologist with multiple areas of interest—including blood pressure control, the coagulation system, and improving patient outcomes. He has served as chief of cardiac anesthesia, vice chair for research, and chair of the transfusion committee during his time at University Hospitals Cleveland Medical Center.

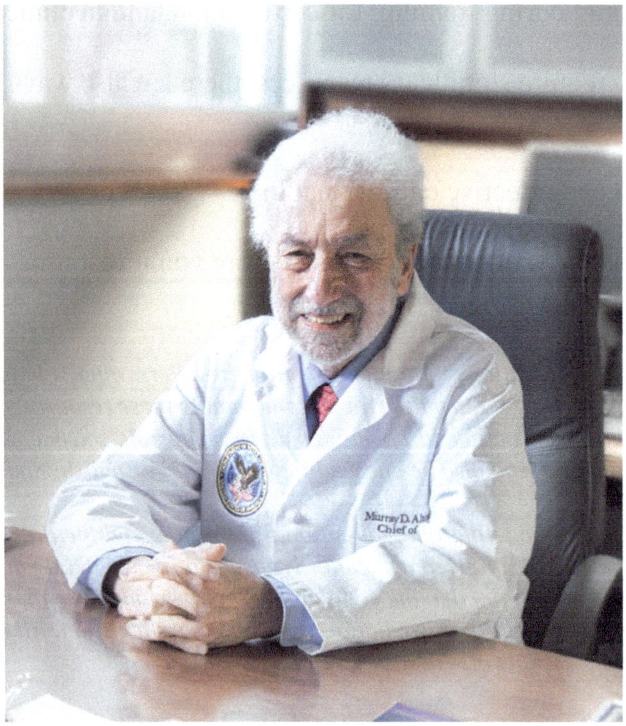

Fig. 93.2 Dr. Murray Altose was born in Winnipeg, where he attended medical school. He was chief of the pulmonary division at Cleveland Metropolitan General Hospital and then moved to the VA, where he was the longest-serving chief medical officer/chief of staff in the entire VA health care system 30 years. He was also associate dean and professor of medicine at CWRU School of Medicine. He has more than 200 publications on the topic of respiratory physiology. A proud father of 3 Eagle Scouts, in retirement he remains a loving and generous father/grandfather and still encourages us to be the best we can be. Photo: Collection of the Altose family

94 Don't Forget About the Med Students! It's a Great Opportunity to Teach and Mentor

Sarah K. Lee, Niloofer F. Dalal, and Catherine Marcucci

Introduction

Every medical specialty is only as strong as the young people entering it. As such, The American Society of Anesthesiologists (ASA) closely tracks the metrics pertaining to anesthesiology residency applications and fill rates of available residency slots. The ASA's Center for Anesthesia Workforce Studies (CAWS) reports the trends in anesthesiology resident matches after the release of the National Resident Matching Program (NRMP) Results and Data is published in May each year. The latest numbers are strong for the specialty. The ASA Monitor reports, "In 2022, a total of **4,861** candidates applied to 1,980 anesthesiology positions and filled all but seven available positions. The number of anesthesiology positions offered increased 7% between 2018 and 2022." [1]

This is great news, especially since the interest in anesthesiology has waxed and waned over the decades. The reasons for the recent increase in applicants and the competitive nature of residency slots are multifactorial, of course, but suffice it to say that medical students are working hard to find the anesthesiology careers they want. An interesting reverse question is whether we are working hard to find the medical students we want?

When **Nee Dalal** and **Cathy Marcucci** were classmates at Temple Med, back in the day, exposure to anesthesiology wasn't built into the curriculum for third year med students. There was sometimes no available time to do even a two-week rotation during the basic surgical rotation, which was only six weeks long. There was a 4-week elective during the fourth year, and based on those 20 days of clinical work, they threw their hat in the residency application pool and made a life-long commitment to a medical specialty.

S. K. Lee
Department of Anesthesiology, Lewis Katz School of Medicine, Temple University, Philadelphia, PA, USA

N. F. Dalal
Emory Clinic, School of Medicine Faculty, Emory Health Care, Atlanta, GA, USA

C. Marcucci (✉)
Department of Transfusion Medicine, Clinical Center, National Institutes of Health, Bethesda, MD, USA
e-mail: Sandson.marcucci@comcast.met

S. Mohamed et al. (eds.), *Anesthesia Bridges*, https://doi.org/10.1007/978-3-032-08294-7_94

Anesthesia Rotations for Medical Students

It seems the situation is quite different today. Many students are offered a two-week anesthesia rotation as part of their surgical rotation. Some medical schools, such as UCLA, offer a 3-week sub-internship in anesthesia, which was unheard of in the 1980s and 1990s. UCLA even has an Anesthesia Student Interest Group (ASIG). The ASIG website mission states the following [2]:

> The Anesthesiology Student Interest Group (ASIG) at UCLA is dedicated to introducing and educating medical students about the field of anesthesiology through a variety of meetings and activities, where students have opportunities to learn clinical skills and explore their interests by shadowing in an OR. Clinical skills workshops are held to introduce students to airway management, including techniques such as bag-valve mask and intubations.
>
> Students are also encouraged to participate in the shadowing program to follow residents and faculty in the OR, allowing them to experience directly what it is like to work in this rapidly growing and exciting field. Meetings focus on the general practice of anesthesiology as well as an in-depth exploration of several subspecialities within the field.

The Medical Students on How and Why They Chose Anesthesiology Careers

Is this outreach and mentoring of med students who are in the early phases of their clinical rotations effective in fostering and maintaining interest in anesthesiology? Coauthor **Sarah Lee** shares her experience:

> I decided to do an anesthesiology elective on my 3rd-year surgery rotation. I knew a little bit about the field from my future mother-in-law, Nee Dalal, but was curious about what it entailed day-to-day. It was a stark contrast from surgery, where my only role was to use the Army-Navy retractor during a 6-hour open abdominal case.
>
> The first day I was inducted into the anesthesiology side of the OR when the attending handed me a Macintosh blade for intubation and asked, "have you done this before?" I clearly stated said "No." I anticipated him taking the blade away from me but instead, he said "Great! I'll teach you, then." That day was filled with many firsts – first IV, first Glidescope, first LMA.
>
> Once the drapes went up and the patient was stabilized, the head of the bed transformed into a makeshift classroom where the attendings used the back of a 4x4 gauze wrapper to teach me about airway management and dilution calculations. They were able to teach a course without taking one eye off the patient, making that left-to-right sweep every so often. It was during this elective that I decided on anesthesiology.
>
> While there are many reasons why I chose anesthesia, the main reason was how much mentorship is an integral part of training. We build our foundation by learning from experienced physicians, so we are well-equipped to respond to a crisis and manage the most unstable patients on our own. I have always put mentorship at the forefront of my medical career and owe a lot of my success to the incredible mentors in my life. It seemed only natural that I pursue a field in medicine that puts an extraordinary emphasis on teaching and mentoring.

Other medical students that we have talked to have expressed the same sentiments. One mentioned to us his appreciation that the students received the same level and priority of teaching that the residents did. Another mentioned that it was great and unusual to have a rotation where the students got to do the most important elements of the case—intubations, lines, and spinals, for example. They would never get to do this on, say, a neurosurgery rotation—"No med students putting the aneurysm clip on, that's for sure!" was a facetious description we heard. And finally, a third student said to us once, "Med students go into anesthesiology *because* of the attendings they have had on the rotation, not in spite of them."

It can sometimes be a bit tricky to have a med student early in the academic year due to perceived competition with residents. The solution to this is to post the med students with senior residents and make your resident part of the mentoring and outreach program—we have found that most residents will readily embrace this and enjoy the opportunity to begin to learn to teach. It's also important to make sure that the students have ample time in the simulator setting.

Lessons Learned

- Interest in our specialty is currently strong!
- Teaching and mentoring of medical students is not wasted time or effort. It's a great opportunity to find the students who are a great fit for anesthesiology.
- We've noticed that a second cohort of students who do anesthesia rotations are headed towards the surgical specialties. These young people are interested in learning a bit about what goes on "on the other side of the drapes." This is altogether a good thing, we think.
- Medical students appreciate the fact that they get to do way more than just observe during rotations with us. Being taught the basic anesthesia procedures is especially fun and meaningful for them.

References

1. Rock-Klotz JA, Miller TR. Anesthesiology programs continue record-setting matches in 2020. ASA Monit. 2020;84(9):41–3.
2. UCLA Health. Anesthesia Student Interest Group (ASIG) [Internet]. UCLA Department of Anesthesiology and Perioperative Medicine; [cited 2022 Oct 15]. Available from: https://www.uclahealth.org/departments/anes/education/medical-students/anesthesia-student-interest-group-asig.

Authors

Sarah Lee is originally from Seattle, graduated from Drexel Med, and is doing her anesthesiology residency at Temple University. When she isn't busy launching her career in anesthesiology, she is an avid biker and hiker. Her favorite travel destinations are the US national parks and any cool SCUBA diving spot. She loves to cook and is learning her family's favorite Korean dishes from her mom.

Nee Dalal is an anesthesiologist in the Emory University system. She enjoys teaching and mentoring junior anesthesiologists at all levels of training. When not working, she loves spending quality time with her family, especially biking and traveling to international destinations.

Cathy Marcucci graduated from Temple Med in 1991 and was one of 18 graduates from that class to go into anesthesiology (along with Nee Dalal). She still remembers that *Anesthesia Bridges* author Rodger Barnette helped her put her first arterial line in when she was a fourth-year medical student and he was a young attending. She then had the good fortune to land at Hopkins for residency and fellowship, where she found life-long mentors and made life-long friends.

"Good to Go": How I Learned About Mitral Valve Repair

95

Raymond G. Graber

Introduction

Back when I started my career, almost all the mitral valve surgery I saw was replacement surgery, with either a mechanical or prosthetic valve. Meanwhile, repair techniques were being developed and were gradually being introduced in cardiac centers across the world. Here is my story about how I first learned about mitral valve repairs. But for me to learn, I had to get sick first…

Night Shift

I was working a night shift in our labor and delivery unit when I started to develop crampy abdominal pain. It was diffuse and generalized, and I self-diagnosed myself with gastroenteritis. Luckily, I was on call with our chief resident Dave, who was very good. He handled most of the issues that night, and we didn't get any more cases, so I was able to finish my shift uneventfully and head home. It was a Thursday call, so I had a 3-day weekend to recover.

Over the next 3 days, the pain waxed and waned. I had periods where I was feeling reasonably well, and in fact managed to cut our grass with my gasoline push mower. I tried to rest and hydrate, assuming my condition would recover soon. On Monday morning, I felt not great, but not excessively bad either. I decided I was in good enough shape to go to work. So, I got dressed, and headed in.

Couldn't "Shake" It Off

My only assignment was a CABG, working with the same resident on Thursday night. We induced and started lining the patient, and while Dave was working on placing a right IJ central line, I started getting shakes and chills. At this point, it was clear to me that my condition was worsening. I called the OR desk

R. G. Graber (✉)
Department of Anesthesiology and Perioperative Medicine, School of Medicine, Oregon Health & Science University, Portland, OR, USA
e-mail: raymond.graber@uhhospitals.org

S. Mohamed et al. (eds.), *Anesthesia Bridges*, https://doi.org/10.1007/978-3-032-08294-7_95

and talked to the anesthesia coordinator—who promised to relieve me, but it would take some time to shuffle people around. About the time that we got the patient on bypass, one of my senior partners came in and relieved me.

I paged a GI doc friend, and he started the evaluation process. The workup revealed that I had a ruptured appendix and a pelvic abscess. I was admitted to the surgical service, with a treatment plan of CT-guided trans-rectal drainage, IV antibiotics, and appendectomy down the road once the infection cleared. The drain was successfully placed the next day (under propofol sedation), and in the meantime, I had developed an ileus. Thankfully, over the course of several days, the antibiotics kicked in, the ileus resolved, and I started feeling better.

On Saturday morning, I was feeling reasonably good. I was eating again, and I was able to get out of bed and walk. I heard there was a visiting professor scheduled to come give a talk to the cardiac surgeons that morning, so I thought why not go and check it out? My IV was capped, my drain was inside my pajama pants leg, I had on my hospital slippers along with my long white coat—I was good to go!

Visiting Professor

It turned out that this wasn't just any visiting professor. This was Alain Carpentier, who was a true pioneer in his field. He was one of the innovators who developed the first bioprosthetic mitral valves and then went on to develop our current techniques of mitral valve repair. He had come all the way from France—he was a friend of our cardiac surgical chair. This was the early 1990s, and our surgeons were still generally replacing mitral valves.

Those of us who do cardiac anesthesia and echocardiography will recognize the Carpentier name from his nomenclature for mitral valve anatomy and his classification of types of regurgitant lesions, along with the various valve prostheses with his name attached to them. Of course, at the time, I didn't know what I had stumbled upon. To me, it was just a Saturday morning conference I had decided to attend to pass the time.

Mitral Valve Repair

I walked in just before the lecture started and was able to grab a seat near the back. I was sitting there in my hospital pajamas and my white coat, but no one seemed to notice. One of our surgeons proceeded to present a case in which a mitral prosthesis was placed. Dr. Carpentier then did a presentation and showed how he would have repaired the valve instead. This was educational and eye-opening to me and also the rest of the assembled crowd. Afterwards, I returned to my room with the satisfied feeling that I had learned something new. My medical status continued to improve, and I was discharged home a day or two later.

Years later, as I was attending TEE review courses to prepare for the TEE boards, I learned more about mitral valve evaluation and repair techniques and realized I had had the good fortune to hear one of the cardiac surgery world's living legends speak on these subjects. All because I ruptured my appendix.

So, I am not sure what my "lessons learned" are here. The lesson probably is not, "If you are going to get sick, make sure there is a great grand rounds speaker scheduled." I was just lucky, in the right place at the right time. So maybe that is the lesson—you never know when the next learning opportunity will arise, so be ready for it when it comes.

***Note from the Editors:** Ray Graber is from the Albany, NY area, so we decided to feature the charming Park Lake Bridge (Figs. 95.1 and 95.2). Ray ran cross country in high school, and apparently, the home races started and finished right there at this bridge.

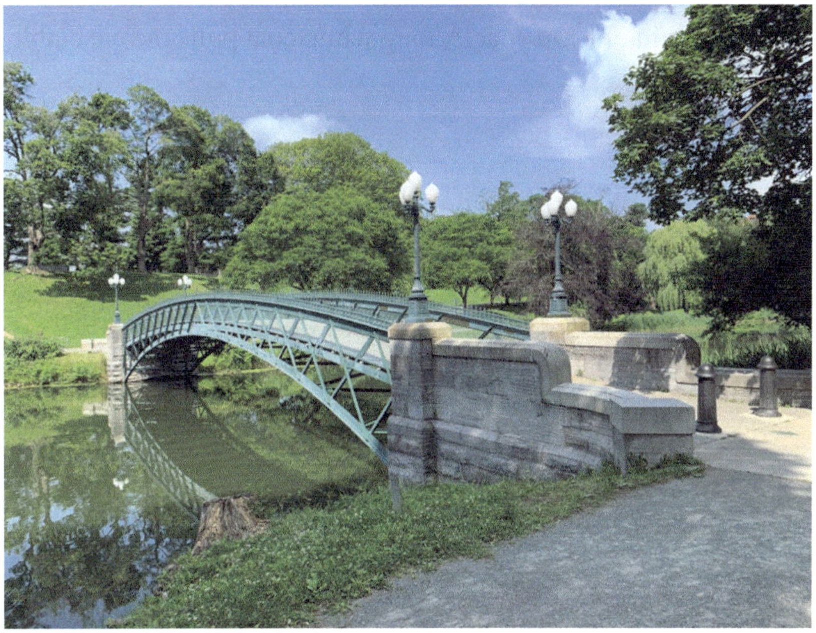

Fig. 95.1 The Park Lake Bridge in central Albany, NY. This beautiful, small pedestrian bridge has wonderfully detailed ornamental iron and crosses the Lake in Washington Park. It was built around 1875 and is one of the oldest riveted bridges in the country. It is not a true arch bridge as half of the arched construction is below the pedestrian deck of the bridge. Photo: Kathleen Naughter

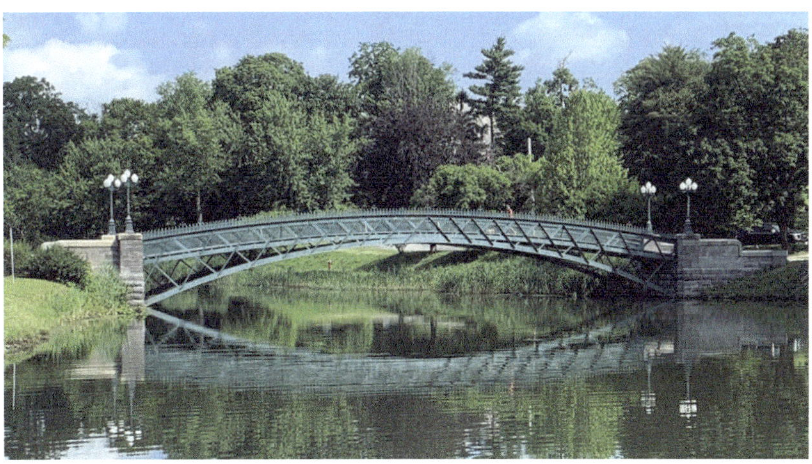

Fig. 95.2 The lake view of the Washington Park Lake bridge. Photo: Kathleen Naughter

We couldn't decide which view of this sentimental and great bridge we liked the best, so we decided to feature them both.

Lessons Learned

- There are many education opportunities when you work at an academic medical center. If you keep your eyes open, you may stumble across the chance to see a true medical luminary speak.
- If you do plan on attending grand rounds in hospital pajamas, try to do it as an attending or at the very least when you are past your internship year. A long white coat pulls the ensemble together much better than the hip-length jacket.

Author

Ray Graber serves as the anesthesia department vice chair for quality issues at University Hospitals Cleveland Medical. He has served there for 30+ years, and for about 25+ years without his appendix!

Wisdom on Teaching and Education

96

Brandon M. Togioka, Ronald S. Bank, Mark Nelson,
Asad Mansoor, and Catherine Marcucci

Contributors:

Abdullah Alswied, MD (AA)

Edwin G. Avery IV, MD (EGA)

Jordan W. Bank

Michelle Capdeville, MD (MC)

Niloofer Dalal, MD (ND)

Dawn Dillman, MD

Raymond G. Graber, MD (RGG)

Ronald Harter, MD (RH)

Ziyad O. Knio, MD (ZOK)

Mark J. Lema, MD PhD (MJL)

Kirk Lalwani, MD (KL)

M. Concetta Lupa, MD (MCL)

B. M. Togioka
Department of Anesthesiology and Perioperative Medicine, School of Medicine, OregonOregon Health & Science University, Portland, OR, USA

R. S. Bank
Department of Anesthesiology, INOVA Fairfax Hospital, UVA School of Medicine, INOVA Campus, Falls Church, VA, USA

M. Nelson
Department of Anesthesiology, Virginia Commonwealth University, Richmond, VA, USA

A. Mansoor
Department of Anesthesia, University of Iowa, Iowa City, IA, USA

C. Marcucci (✉)
Department of Transfusion Medicine, Clinical Center, National Institutes of Health, Bethesda, MD, USA

S. Mohamed et al. (eds.), *Anesthesia Bridges*, https://doi.org/10.1007/978-3-032-08294-7_96

Carolyn B. Metzler, PhD (CBM)

Lucas Meuchel, MD

Amy J. Robbins, MD (AJR)

Neil B. Sandson, MD (NBS)

Mark Nelson, MD MEd (MN)

Maria K. Orlic, MD (MKO)

Richard Sheffield, BA MS (RS)

Robert D. Togioka, MA (RDT)

Jennifer N. Tripi, MD

Bradford Winters, MD PhD

Brant M. Wagener, MD PhD

Introduction

The practice of anesthesiology continues to grow and evolve, and thus education in the art and science of our specialty must be a lifelong process. There is an ongoing tension between wanting to make the case go as perfectly as humanly possible and allowing trainees to learn. The authors have compiled just a few additional bits of wisdom to help both the student and the teacher.

Wisdom for Trainees

- For anesthesiology, Dr. Jared Barlow said it best, and I've used it over the decades. Show up on time and have your room ready. Read about the case the night before to anticipate the pitfalls. Ask a few questions to show that you are engaged. When I was a resident, I set a goal (before computers!) to read 10 pertinent articles each week and a chapter from Miller on the rotation in which I was currently training. I seldom if ever achieved that goal but it kept me focused on prioritizing clinical education as a weekly obligation.—**MJL**

- A piece of advice I give to all my trainees is, "Solicit feedback, and don't take it personally if it is not what you want to hear. Feedback is meant to be constructive—not destructive. That being said, it is better to learn from others' mistakes than your own."—**MC**

- Several major failings of medical education are the lack of teaching of health care law, the business of medicine, leadership training, and strategies to maintain effectiveness under stress. Seek out knowledge of all of these.—**RSB**

- Never say "no" to an OR break that is offered by your attending as you never know when your next break might be.—**EGA**

- Here is a trick I picked up when I was training in transfusion medicine with the pathologists. When they are studying or doing clinical work, they usually have their attention and eyes focused on their scopes and don't like to have to hold books open. If they are forced to work with an actual softcover textbook or manual, they take them to any neighborhood copy center and have them spiral-bound so that they lie flat on the table next to the microscope (Fig. 96.1). It costs about ten dollars to do this and makes everything so much easier. If it's a review book, you can move the answers up with the questions or ask to have the chapters rebound in whatever order works best for you.—**AA and CM**

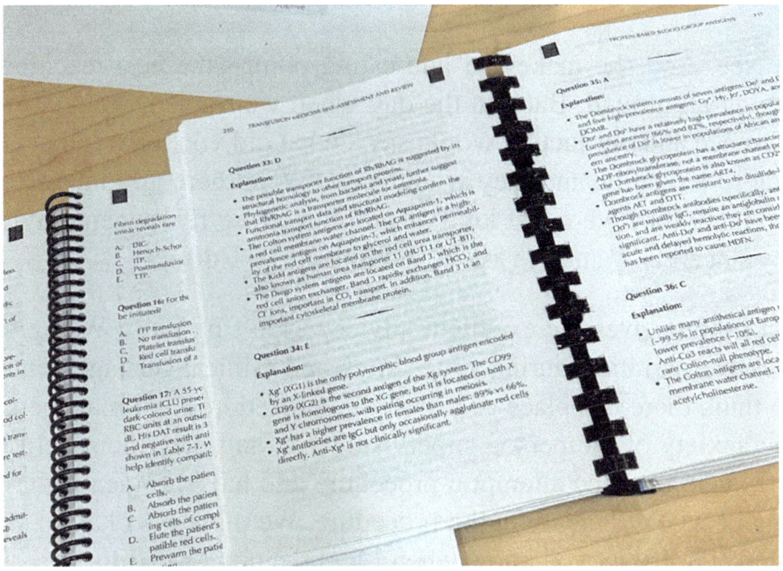

Fig. 96.1 Abdullah Alswied's rebound transfusion medicine study manuals. Photo: Catherine Marcucci

- Knock yourself out to maintain a good rapport with your program director (PD). Because, really, this is the last person you want to tangle with. Your PD is hopefully one of your first and longest-lasting mentors. Mine was—I had the good fortune to have had Jeff Kirsch as my program director, and he has been nothing but supportive throughout my entire career.—**CM**

- We can say categorically that your PD wants you to do well. He/she may be worried that a trainee won't do well but they are never looking to reinforce that. They want nothing more than for everybody to be flying high on all cylinders. Seriously. A PD doesn't want or need a metaphorical fall person. They are not looking to do paybacks or sabotage people. You must believe us on this point.—**Editors**

- The worst thing you can do, as far as your PD is concerned, is to do something unethical with respect to patient care. Because there is no way to defend that. The next worst thing you can do is to be dishonest. There is no way to defend that, either. If your clinical care leaves something to be desired and you are motivated to do better, that can be remediated. Characterological issues can't be remediated; most other things can.—**Editors**

- But what is going to get you a glowing reputation with your faculty and glowing recommendation from your program is your good citizenship in the program and your friendly and flexible personality. Assuming that you have adequate clinical skills. That's just the way it is.—**Editors**

- The best residents are prepared by knowing about the case and patient and they have thought of all possible scenarios and have the drugs and lines ready…They are engaging and have an intellectual curiosity and ask questions that allow for meaningful discussions that help us both become better physicians.—**ND**

- We so agree with Nee. And she makes an interesting point—the best teaching relationships work when there is learning all around. Back in the day when we trained, we'd come back to our rooms after resident conference and our faculty would say, "what did you learn today at conference today?" Or you'd be talking to a faculty, and they would say, "Were there any interesting cases on call last night?" We used to think they were just kind of probing to see if we were paying attention but then we figured out they sincerely wanted to know and to learn.—**Editors**

- In Chap. 181, Lisa Leffert gives the excellent advice: "don't narrate." We agree with her with one caveat. Avoid excessive narration during procedures and clinical management to soothe your own anxiety, but we do think there is a place to narrate the procedures and management you are doing in order to soothe the anxiety of the person supervising you and help them help you. It can really be nerve-wracking to watch a trainee attempt a procedure and have no idea if they have a firm idea of what they are doing or where they are in the procedure. We think it's okay to say, "I'm going to use the paramedian approach. I'll let you know when I feel the pop."—**Editors**

- Don't be afraid to ask questions in lectures and conferences and grand rounds. Trust us, they are more welcome than you might think. Sometimes there is a tendency for the trainees to not say very much in a conference, especially if there is an outside speaker. You don't want to monopolize the discussion or ask questions that are intended to show how much you know, but everybody benefits if the junior people speak up and ask sincerely motivated questions. The person who arranged the speaker is happy because the interest and engagement is respectful of the expert's time. The program director is happy to have his smart, attentive trainees showcased. The faculty gets to listen to somebody else's questions for a change.—**Editors**

- The best grand rounds are the ones where there are a lot of discussions and questions, right up to the second the conference has to end. Several good questions to ask are, "If you could change one thing about where the FDA (or whomever) is with respect to this issue, what would you change?" And "Where do you think we will be on this issue in five years?" If the topic is a clinical one, ask about whether the researchers have considered the ramifications in septic, transplant, and pediatric patients, or what the plans are for the next clinical trial.—**Editors**

- Whatever you do, don't be disrespectful and sleep through conferences and never log onto an online lecture or conference and then leave your computer, except for a few seconds. Sooner or later, someone is going to ask you a question or to make comment and it is beyond embarrassing to get busted as somebody who "logs on and leaves."—**Editors**

- In the end, your in-service exams are for you to gauge how you are doing. Really. Yes, the metrics are tracked, and you might have a discussion with your program director if you seem to be way under the curve, but you're the one who has to pass the dang thing in a year or two.—**Editors**

- Give your board exams the serious attention to which they are due. You shouldn't trash your life preparing for them or miss a family funeral but perhaps you can divert an extra measure of discretionary time towards them. It's not necessarily devastating to your career if you fail one part or the other, quite a few people have, but it's also not nothing—it's a lot of time and expense and aggravation to redo them, if nothing else. *Really focus* on both parts of your anesthesia board exams, nobody has ever said they regret the time spent getting ready to pass.—**Editors**

- I spent quite a lot of money on review materials and exam courses, especially for my oral boards. At the time, this felt like it was helpful in passing, although I can't say for sure all these years later. Somebody at my program said I was wasting money and the best prep for oral boards is actually to be working full-time in the OR and asking my own faculty to give me mock orals. They might have been right.—**CM**

- I have never been a board examiner, so I can only pass along what I was told by people who are/were. And that is to try to just relax and "talk it over" with the examiners. Say what you know how to do and don't offer to do something in the oral board exam that you wouldn't or couldn't do in real life. I remember that I had a question about whether I would do a spinal anesthetic for a cholecystectomy. I said no and was asked why not. I said, "Because I wouldn't even know how to do that. I've never even seen one done with a spinal." However, there was a Hopkins faculty who claimed to know an anesthesiologist who got a similar question and said, "Yes, I would do that. I just got out the Navy. Of the 200 cases I did like this in the Navy, I did at least 150 of them under spinal."—**CM**

- Boards are headachy and a hurdle to get over, no doubt about it. But there's no way around them, you just have to buckle down and do it. I took my written boards on July 8, 1995, and it was my birthday. I certainly felt quite sorry for myself. Until sometime later, I was at a party talking to a Jesuit priest (not joking) about when he went off to the Vatican to get his PhD in something or other. He said, "Hey, the same thing happened to me! It was my birthday, and I had to appear before committee of cardinals to defend my doctoral thesis. In Latin."—**CM**

- We know a lot of oral boards examiners, of course, and asked a number of them for advice. They requested anonymity but sent the essential message that, above all, what the examiners are looking for is a knowledge of safe practice. Their job is certify people who will be safe anesthesiologists and in doing so, effective representatives and ambassadors for our specialty. It's a simple as that. They are not looking to be gratuitously nasty or harsh or punitive—they are truly hoping each and every person taking the boards passes.—**Editors**

- When you encounter a faculty member who has knowledge you want, relentlessly pelt them with questions and let nothing stop you.—**NBS**

- Ask your faculty how their research is going. People like to talk about their research. Read the most recent publications by your three favorite attendings. Then do the same for your least favorite attendings.—**Editors**

- Keep in contact with your faculty after you've finished training. Drop them a text or email if you can, to let them know how and what you are doing. And what about your training has been helpful. They will be more than happy to hear from you.—**Editors**

- You will find as you complete your training and start your career that not every teaching point needed to be transcendental to be valuable and not every case you did needed to be a landmark one. You will put your practice together based on something that somebody told you here and something that somebody else told you there. You will have your favorite faculty and your less favorite faculty. But you may be surprised some day to do something or use something that somebody told you or showed you that you weren't particularly close to.—**Editors**

- It's stressful to teach in more than one room. You'll see. If there is a break in your schedule during the day or you finish for the day, it's a nice idea to ask your attending if they need any help or breaks in their other room(s).—**Editors**

- Remember that your attending carries the medical and legal responsibility for the case. If things don't go as planned, they are going to have to answer for what they did AND what you did. So, always leave them a way forward. Don't blow every vein before you call them. Maybe leave them the radial artery on the other side for the art line in case you can't get it.—**Editors**

- If your attending asks you to take so many tries at something and then stop, do that many tries and *THEN STOP!* Once I was at a departmental QA review (not Hopkins) and the hospital malpractice attorney appeared unexpectedly. Apparently, the trainee had wanted to get the spinal in no matter what. Dozens of passes of the needle had ensued. On the first day POD, an enraged family came to the administration with the following question, "Based on the marks on our father's back, are we to understand that somebody stuck him *seventeen* times?"—**CM**

- Don't argue with your attending about whether the patient should be extubated. You might think your faculty is being overly conservative, but they have their reasons. Besides, if the extubation fails, it's not going to be you that the burden of reintubation falls on.—**Editors**

- I remember tripping over my words while attempting to describe my anesthetic plan to a senior attending during my first week of residency. I was overcomplicating the plan. They asked me, "what is your goal?" I thought about it. They said, "it's simple, figure out what the surgeon needs and provide it in the simplest manner possible."—**BMT**

- Remember that there is no such thing as a non-educational case. Every hour matters. Malcolm Gladwell popularized the idea of the 10,000-hour rule—that it takes at least 10,000 hours of purposeful practice to become an expert. In order for an anesthesiology resident to reach 10,000 hours during their 3 years of clinical training, they need to be in the operating room 70 hours a week. Very few anesthesiology residents reach that threshold these days.—**BMT**

- How would I describe the qualities of some of my favorite residents? Punctuality, manual dexterity, work ethic, "teachability."—**RH**

- The best resident that comes to mind is a great resident who made a substantial error. He took immediate responsibility, owned it, and told me immediately. He was harder on himself then anyone was on him. In the end, the experience made him better and was quite the learning experience. The story is below.—**RSB**

  **We had a fantastic military CA3 a few years back in hearts. He was, to my memory, intending to go into cardiac anesthesiology. He and I had a very large, very complex case with one of our aortic specialists. The surgeon was even tense about the case. Very shortly after induction, the resident called me urgently. He told me that he had inadvertently given an entire bag of IV insulin instead of the intended bag of tranexamic acid or Amicar (whichever we had at the time). I told the surgeon. He was a very intense and blunt surgeon—one that I like working with very much but one who is not so tolerant of errors. The only reason that I did the case with a resident at all was because he was so strong. I remember the surgeon's reply: "Can you fix it?" I said yes, but we need a little time. In the end, we managed it, and the case went well.

  The resident took it extremely, extremely hard. He was far harder on himself than was anyone else on him. It really got him down to the point that he was questioning his very ability to do complex cases. I talked to him about this at length. I was impressed at how he took responsibility, that he called me immediately, and that he stayed focused and finished the case. Perhaps I should have switched him out but he wanted to stay and seemed focused so he did. He had not thought of the implications of the insulin overdose on serum potassium. Had he not told me until later if at all this could have been a disaster. I told him that we are human. We will all, unfortunately, make medication errors. The key is to catch them ASAP and to treat them immediately and correctly. I also told him that when such an adverse event happens it's best to consult a colleague as they are emotionally detached and might think of things that we missed.

  We also discussed how to avoid med errors—especially in big cases with many IV push meds and infusions. The human factors component of what we do is so important. I always stress this to students, residents, and fellows. I've seen other residents conceal errors. I've seen other residents make substantial errors and essentially blow them off—not giving them the serious attention that they deserve. This resident did neither. He was a star. I remember this incident to this day because of that.

***Note from the Editors:** Unfortunately, there aren't many bridges named for women in this world. But there is a little gem of one near Ron Bank's home in the northern VA/metro Washington DC area—the Betty Cooke Memorial Bridge in Fairfax, VA. Jordan Bank, Ron's son, took time out of his busy schedule recently to get us this wonderful original picture of the bridge as it crosses Scott's Run (Fig. 96.2).

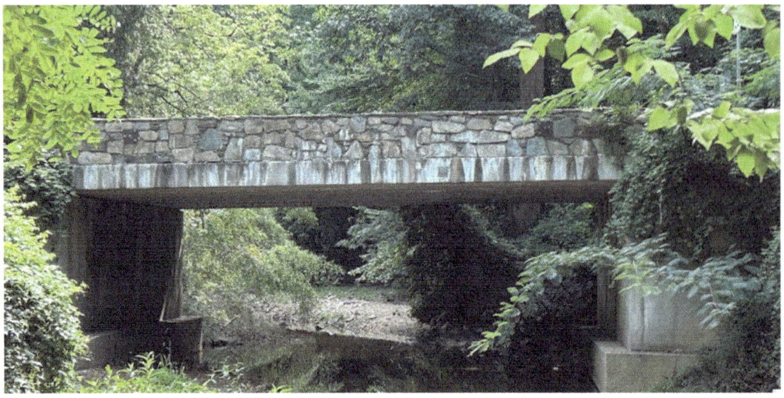

Fig. 96.2 The Memorial bridge was renamed for Betty Cooke, shortly after her death in 1999. Betty was an historian, artist, and nature lover who was instrumental in the creation of the Scott's Run Nature Preserve. The stream passes through a forest of hemlocks, beeches, and maples. Photo and caption: Jordan Bank

- There is a high likelihood that one day all this training and education will allow you to save the life of someone in your family. Ask us how we know. And when that happens whatever residual negative feelings you might have about the labor and tedium of anesthesia training as evaporates.—**AJR and CM**
- The safest medical students are the ones who state their limitations, ask for help, and demonstrate some level of anxiety about doing something new or unfamiliar. I would choose to work with a safe medical student over one that is overly confident any day of the week. I'll allow the safe medical student to struggle, and even fail, at new procedures whereas I would not give the careless student that opportunity.—**ZOK**

For Faculty

- As a teacher of 47 years who has taught students from elementary age through college, I find that the most important thing I can do to have a productive communication atmosphere is to bond with the students in the first few days of school. Making that all important connection is Job #1. Work to have a true understanding of each persons' thoughts, feelings, and activities. Knowing that someone loves sports, music, or has a special pet creates a feeling of caring between persons.—**BDT**
- "The mediocre teacher tells. The good teacher explains. The superior teacher demonstrates. The great teacher inspires."—**William Arthur Ward**
- If you observe a trainee making a clinical mistake do your best to offer them a better way to have handled the situation and hence avoid direct criticism which shouldn't be necessary.—**EGA**
- If you teach residents and fellows, the highest compliment you can get is to be told that when a former trainee was faced with a difficult clinical situation, they thought about what you would do in the same situation.—**Editors**

- You can't make a trainee want to learn. You can only show them what they need to learn and why they need to learn it.—**Editors**

- Once a resident was trying to think of something that would be a slow burn to say about me on an evaluation. So, he wrote, "Does the same simple anesthetic over and over." I read it and thought, "Ha! He thinks he's dissing me. I don't think he realizes that he's actually dissing Sir Robert Reynolds Macintosh." Of the eponymous laryngoscope fame. Sir Robert lectured and taught constantly that anesthetics should be "safe and simple" above all else. The other thing I thought was "I hope he remembers this simple anesthetic plan the first time he's on call by himself and gets into a jam." I got a call several months after this resident had gone into private practice, telling me just that.—**CM**

- Don't rush through the preop discussion. The key is to help the residents sketch out a case in their minds where all parts match each other and matches what you are reading in the chart. Plus, the preop discussion with your resident sets up the preop discussion with the patient. For instance, once a resident reported that the patient was on beta-blockers without any cardiac or psych history. Okay, that doesn't make any sense. Also pay attention in the preop discussion to whether the psych meds might also be for chronic pain or seizures.—**RGG and Editors**

- If you plan to teach on a specific topic in the OR, pick one and let the resident know what it is beforehand. You don't want to get to the OR and start the case and say, "What do you want to talk about today?" That's not efficient of everybody's teaching time.—**Editors**

- We put together *Avoiding Common Anesthesia Errors, 2nd Edition* specifically to teach from ourselves and think about errors (Fig. 96.3). It's not a comprehensive clinical anesthesia handbook but has lots of the basic and some not-so-basic topics that are short and easy to review. We aren't a bit bashful about boosting the book because all proceeds, every single penny, are pledged in perpetuity to FAER.—**Editors**

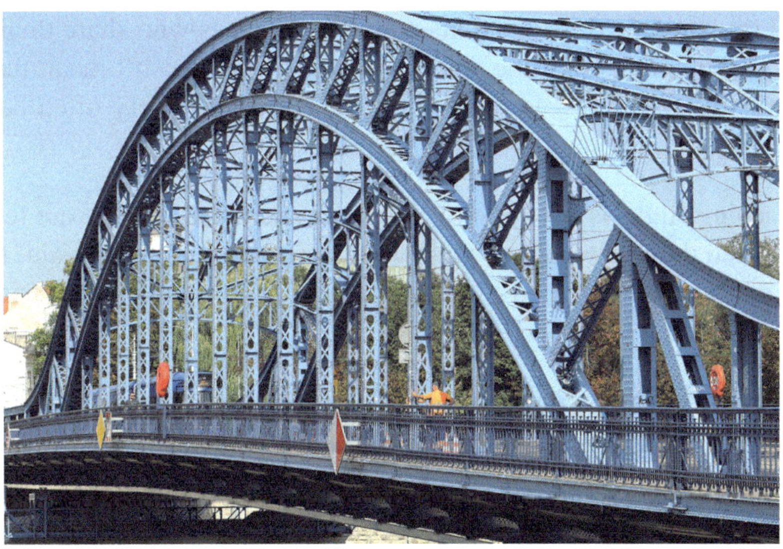

Fig. 96.3 Speaking of errors, one of the *Anesthesia Bridges* authors once took a wrong turn and ended up crossing this bridge in Poland. Image: Pawel Kot, used under license from iStock.com

- Get involved in teaching pre-hospital providers. It's fun, rewarding, and helps you to think outside of the usual OR/hospital box. We're the airway experts. We should be teaching them. They appreciate it very much when we do. It is a great service to the community. Also, it could you be your family's airways that they will someday manage.—**RSB**

- People that I've trained know that they are welcome to ask me questions for the rest of their careers.—**NBS**

- Remember that evaluations should be 360 degrees—mentors have as much to gain from feedback as mentees.—**BMT**

- Don't play favorites with the residents. They will be at different levels of skill acquisition but assume that each trainee is doing their best until you have proof otherwise. Plus, Brant Wagener sent us some great thoughts about this: "I don't really have a favorite resident. At least not without thinking about it for too long. I tend to like them all."—**BMW and Editors**

- It is now well-recognized that no one becomes a successful researcher without a strong mentorship team. The role of mentorship in medical education has received less attention, but it is no less important.—**BMT**

- Anesthesia and non-anesthesia practitioners often get nervous when they encounter pregnant patients. This is unnecessary. I teach my residents to think of pregnancy as a syndrome that affects multiple organ systems. Create an anesthetic plan by systematically thinking through each organ system while keeping in mind how the physiological changes of pregnancy affect each one.—**BMT**

- Something the faculty should hear themselves saying every single clinical day: "Thank you for your hard work today."—**Editors**

- This is for faculty and residents: My personal opinion is that medical students are hungry for feedback. The medical students' favorite residents are often the ones who share their written evaluations or complete them in the company of the student rotators. This doesn't mean that students won't be receptive to constructive criticism—in fact I find that criticism is very often better received in real time, without anonymity or ambiguity.—**ZOK**

- Remember that teaching adults is not the same as teaching children! There are few groups of learners where the powerful and durable words of Malcolm Knowles are more relevant, needed, and applicable. The learning of adults is governed by the following six principles and therefore makes them a separate entity from children.—**MN**

    1. **Adults need to know why they need to learn something**. Adults are not motivated to learn something without a good reason to do so.

    2. **Adult learning builds on previous experiences**. This must be taken into account when teaching. Adults are not empty vessels that we pour in knowledge. They have rich and formative pasts which must be taken into account.

3. **Adults must own or feel responsible for their learning**. Depriving them of this is a serious handicap for their effective learning and implementation. They must have a substantial hand in the formation of goals and objectives as well as the curricula.

4. **Adults are ready to learn if the material solves a near or immediate problem**. This *immediacy* raises their motivation. They are "ready" to learn. A desire to learn alone is not enough; they must be ready and desire to take action.

5. **Adults prefer training that is problem focused**. Not only must the "problem" be in the immediacy, but it should also be important. Adults have little motivation to solve problems that are unimportant to them, *personally*.

6. **Adults are internally motivated to learn**. External coercion or reward are minimally effective and can even undermine internal (lifelong) motivations to learn. Best to avoid "patting them on the head" for learning.—**Malcolm Knowles, 1980.**

Favorite Faculty

We asked our authors and editors to tell us a bit about the anesthesiologists who provided the most impactful teaching and why this teaching was so memorable. We must start out by saying that virtually every person who was ever at Johns Hopkins for a minute gave a shout-out to the late, great **Tommy Tung (Thomas J.K Tung, MD)**. Tommy, who sadly left us late in 2022, was Socrates, Plato, Aristotle, Yoda, *and* Obi Wan Kenobi all rolled into one brilliant and legendary clinical and academic anesthesiologist. He was universally revered and was the person that even the most senior faculty called when they needed advice on a patient or help with a clinical situation, especially if it was an emergency. Literally, no anesthesiologist at Hopkins was too proud to say, "Get Tommy!"

Tommy would then proceed to make the most fantastic saves and later chuckle and deny that he had even been in the room. I was told that no matter how much he shook his head no, it was true that he had once run into a room, climbed under the table, and reintubated a prone patient in pins and with an open cranium with just his fingers.

Another time, Cathy Marcucci was working with Dr. Tung in the ECT suite and somehow there was an airway emergency, and the patient was both seizing *and* vomiting, you know, like at the same time. As luck would have, the panicked psychiatry resident pulled out the IV accidentally at that precise moment. Cathy remembers Tommy's lightning responses in securing IV access and the airway and managing the seizure. The first thing he did was whip in an IV and dose a barbiturate through the needle to stop the seizure—no time for a tourniquet or bag of IV fluid. Then he intubated the patient nasally, without any visualization of the airway—and the patient was still seizing a bit! She has never seen anything like it to this day. When the case was over and the patient was stable, Dr. Tung disappeared for a moment and came back with doughnuts.

Tommy was totally humble, always kind, incredibly hardworking, and was seldom seen without the exact twinkle in his eye and smile in this picture (Fig. 96.4). There are literally hundreds of anesthesiologists who are better and safer clinicians because of him.

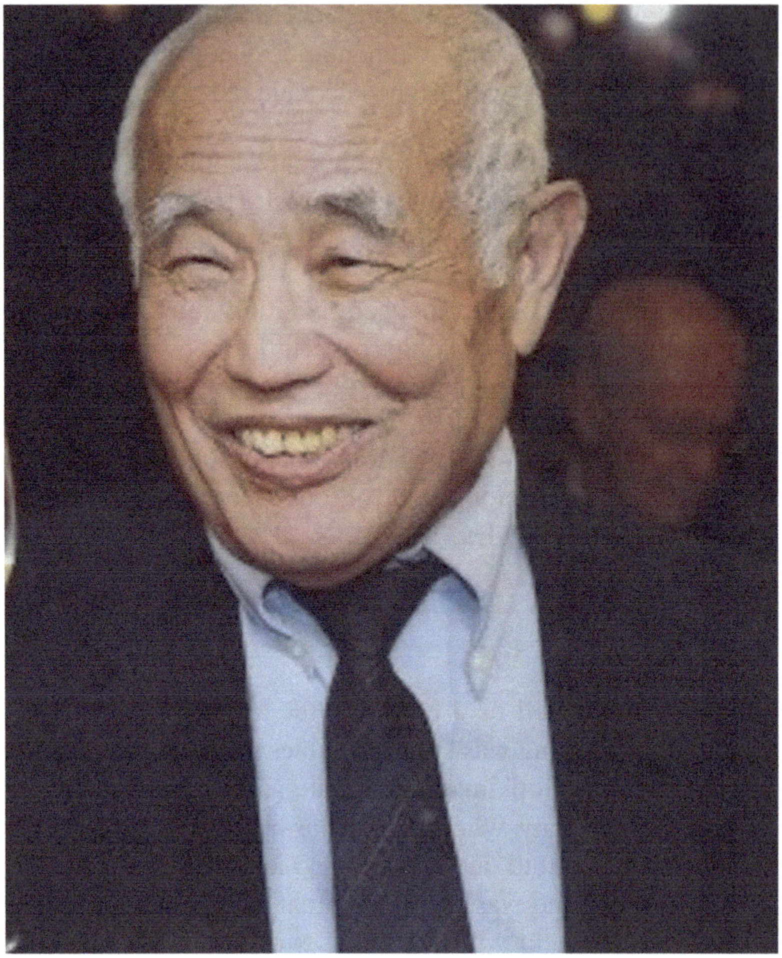

Fig. 96.4 The late great Thomas J.K. Tung, MD. Legendary Hopkins anesthesiologist and mentor. Photo: Collection of the Tung family, used with permission by Jeany Lundberg, MD.

Here are several other anesthesiologists who are especially remembered for their great teaching.

From Amy Robbins:

- Reuven Pasternak: Reuven really set a superb example of professionalism and career development for me as a young trainee. He was trained in pediatrics, preventive medicine, anesthesiology, and pediatric critical care. He also has both an MPH and an MBA. He was so knowledgeable in so many areas and had such excellent relationships and rapport with everybody in the perioperative arena that he provided this terrific, calm, and safe space to learn the practice of anesthesiology in. He was the role model who inspired me to become triple-boarded and recently complete an MBA program.

Note: Reuven was at Hopkins during the early and early middle years of his career. He then spent a number of years at Stonybrook. The astonishing roster of his leadership roles includes chairman, vice dean, system chief medical officer, president, hospital chief executive officer, system executive vice president, and consultant. His most recent credential is advisor on federal policy for the Department of Homeland Security.

- Pete Rock: I always loved working with Pete. He had this in-depth command of every aspect of whatever case we were doing. Somebody told me, "Pete Rock knows how to make a good anesthesia resident into a great anesthesiologist." And that was true! He really was the person who taught me the importance of taking care of the "details" in a successful anesthetic. I also remember calling him after I had been out of residency for a couple of years, and he was very generous with his time and advice in helping me figure out my career direction.

Note: Pete is an internist and anesthesiologist who trained and was first on faculty at Hopkins. He then moved to Washington University and was chief of the Barnes Hospital division. A leadership position as vice chair of the Department of Anesthesiology at UNC-Chapel Hill followed before he was appointed as the Dr. Martin A. Helrich Chair of Anesthesiology at the University of Maryland. He chose to step down from his administrative duties in August 2023 to return to the full-time faculty as professor of anesthesiology. Pete has always been known for his wry sense of humor (but with a twinkle in his eyes), calmness in any clinical situation, and as somebody you could just call and talk over your problems with.

From Steve Orebaugh:

- Jan Smith: Jan was a gentle and kind man, an excellent clinician with an insightful mind. He provided capable leadership for our department and was a joy to work with in the OR. He was one of several who worked with Peter Safar to establish critical care as a discipline in our institution.

Note: The late Jan D. Smith was a legendary and beloved clinician and faculty member at UPMC. He was trained in pediatrics, internal medicine, anesthesiology, and critical care medicine. He was from South Africa and his obituary mentioned that he simply ignored the hateful racial segregation policies of that era and was the only white trainee in his internship class of 10. He did his anesthesiology training at Peter Bent Brigham under Dr. Vandam and then found his way to UPMC. He then held leadership and/or chairman positions at UT-San Antonio, University of Iowa, and the University of Nebraska before finally heading home to Pittsburgh. He also continued to maintain credentials and do volunteer medical work all over the world. At the end of his UPMC anesthesiology career, he even headed alumni outreach efforts and researched and wrote the history of the department.

From Chetta Lupa:

- Ann Bailey: Ann was one of the founding pediatric anesthesiologists of the pediatric anesthesia division at UNC. She has been an amazing mentor and, while working with her, both as a resident and later as a co-faculty member, I learned the art of pediatric anesthesiology. She had a subtle but efficient command of the room. She gained trust from families and surgeons quickly and had a Spidey-sense like no other. And she had a really amazing way of helping me as a resident to believe in myself and my potential. As a mother to six children, Ann brought her maternal instincts of raising independent anesthesiologists to the operating room. I vividly remember her giving me just enough latitude to feel myself grow in my capabilities, entrusting me with big cases, and giving gentle feedback to help shape me into a strong clinician. She was an amazing teacher and continues to be a role model for me as a woman in medicine and in leadership. I think of Ann as a fantastic example of a woman lifting other people up—and for being a great mother and wife within her own family, often giving sage advice to many of her protege' on how to "do it all." She's just one of those people who you hope to be half as good as in every way when you grow up.

Note: Ann Bailey retired from clinical practice several years ago. She was a professor of anesthesiology and pediatrics at UNC-Chapel Hill. She also served as an Associate Medical Officer of UNC Hospitals. She was universally admired by her colleagues and trainees.

- Franklyn Cladis: Franklyn was my fellowship program director at UPMC. In addition to being one of the best-dressed people I know, he remains one of the kindest. He has such a way about him that I can't imagine anyone who knows him does not immediately respect him or like him. He is brilliant but humble. Franklyn believed in me and saw something in me when I was a fellow that forever shaped the trajectory of my career. I was considering a career of mixed pediatrics and adults in private practice. He looked at me during a case when I was discussing my options with him and said: "You have to do academics—you just have to." He pushed me to see myself in a different way, as a teacher. Eventually, he also encouraged me to become more involved in leadership and was a pivotal mentor for me as I ran for a leadership position in the Pediatric Anesthesiology Program Director's Association. I will forever be grateful for the guidance given to me and the opportunity to have trained with him.

Note: Franklyn Cladis trained at the University of Rochester and at The Children's Hospital in Boston for pediatric anesthesiology. He is a professor and the chief anesthesiologist at UPMC Children's Hospital, as well as the clinical director of perioperative medicine and the fellowship director of the pediatric anesthesiology fellowship.

From Brandon Togioka:

- Jeff Kirsch: The model of servant leadership and hard work. He was always ready to help, and he put in more than twice as much clinical work as anyone else in the department—while serving as chair. I remember one of our first late nights together. He said, "Please call me anytime if you need help. I live very close, and I don't sleep much." I thought this was more of a hypothetical statement, but he was serious. "Here is my cell phone number, call me anytime." Sadly, I had to take him up on this offer a few times, and he arrived in the middle of the night with a smile. All members of our department felt that continual support. Conversely, he would let us go home early when he was the overnight attending. I realized that his experience and clinical acumen allowed him to handle more than the rest of us because he was able to predict upcoming clinical challenges and staffing needs.

Note: Jeff trained and was first on the faculty at Hopkins. He was known for his prodigious work ethic as an academic neuro-anesthesiologist and his advocacy for the residents as program director. He was universally respected and admired as chair at OHSU as he built that department into a true academic center of excellence. He remains chair emeritus at OHSU while moving on to accept leadership positions at Medical College of Wisconsin and Harborview Medical Center-UW Medicine. He has held numerous positions in the national anesthesiology community and has published eleven highly regarded textbooks.

- Miriam Treggiari: A brilliant researcher and extraordinarily gifted writer. Miriam has this amazing ability to turn clinicians into clinician scientists. Manuscripts that sit as works in progress quickly become published articles under her tutelage. She is a selfless leader who is always willing to help with manuscripts and research protocols—even if she is not a co-investigator or author. Her abilities were widely known within our department. Miriam would have back-to-back 30-minute sessions with faculty for eight straight hours. We joked that we needed to install a conveyor belt to efficiently move faculty through her office. The most influential researchers are strong mentors. Miriam has developed clinician-scientists who are currently working in every corner of the country. I am one of these researchers, and I am eternally grateful for the amazing mentorship that she has provided.

Note: Miriam Treggiari trained in Europe before moving to the University of Washington. She then joined OHSU, where she was director and then vice-chair of clinical research. After several years at Yale, she accepted a position at Duke as professor of anesthesiology and vice chair for research. She is known for her scholarly, yet pragmatic ability to shape and direct large clinical outcome studies and her work in developing national and international clinical guidelines.

From Brant Wagener:

- My best faculty was a guy who at the time of my training, worked at nights and was the "Trauma Guy." He was great. One time, when I asked, he and I took apart the rapid transfuser and we looked at every component so that I understood completely how it worked—then we put it back together. He could teach and take your brain from the smallest detail to a good 30K foot view of a patient in no time. Taught me to appreciate details and the bigger picture.

From Dawn Dillman:

- Jeff Kirsch: As a program director, I knew he would always try to do what was right and fair, while wanting people to be happy and successful. He was a talented clinician who worked in the OR enough, so you knew he knew who the surgeons and nurses were and what the culture and system issues were. He was in it for the growth of the residents, not for the growth of himself or his ego.

- Valerie Sera: A talented clinician who could take care of the sickest patients and an educator who took personal interest in the residents. She was invested in our success in our personal and professional lives. She modeled professionalism and grace in her interactions with everyone in the OR, balancing advocacy for the patients with respect for the other team members perfectly.

Note: Val Sera did her residency and fellowship training in cardiac anesthesiology at Hopkins before heading out to OHSU, where she is the medical director of the adult cardiovascular anesthesia service and the program director of the adult cardiothoracic anesthesiology fellowship. She has always been known for her professionalism, superb hand skills, and being calm and effective in emergencies.

From Brad Winters:

- I don't recall who it was, but when I was a resident, one faculty member (it was one of the pediatric anesthesiologists) told me that, "Heroics are bullcrap. People love to save the situation after it has already gone sideways, but the best doctors rarely let themselves get into that situation very often. Planning and preparation to avoid needing to 'pull it out of the fire' is the sign of excellence. I've made it my focus to make cardiorespiratory arrests a zero event rather than focus on CPR and ACLS like others. Once it has gone sideways or downhill, the opportunity was already missed." His/her advice stuck with me all these years.

From Cathy Marcucci:

- The single best 30 minutes of teaching I ever had in all of my training years was by Chas Emala. And this is saying something because I was the beneficiary of some pretty outstanding teaching. But I remember being on OB call one night back in the early 1990s in the old Nelson 2 Labor and Delivery suite at Hopkins. There was an epidural that "wasn't working" and the L&D nurses called me to come deal with it. I got to the labor room and the patient was screaming hysterically. The father of the baby was yelling mightily. I had this overwhelming desire to just put my hands over my ears and walk away. Instead, I redosed the epidural—I still couldn't tell what was going on. She seemed somewhat numb but was still crying. At this point, I couldn't even tell if the IV was working. Chas was right down the hall, it was the middle of the night and I hated to, but I had to call him. I guess he could tell by the sound of my voice because he said, "I'll be right over." I still remember him walking down the Nelson 2 hallway, just as calm as could be.

- He went into the room, and I'll always remember that the very first thing he did was look at the fetal tracing. Next, he assessed the block, or actually the lack thereof. Then, he went through this amazing algorithm, saying, "Okay, here's what I think is going on. I think she is going to need a section and here's why. With that in mind, here's what we can tolerate and here's what situation we don't want to get into, and what we don't want the patient to get into." He then talked through the various scenarios, "Let's think about this—what will happen if the epidural isn't in the right place, and we dose it vs if it is the right place and we don't dose it?"

- He proceeded to review the literature for me as to the minimum dose of intravascular injection of local anesthesia that had ever been known to cause significant neurological sequelae. We were still below that. So, he helped me develop a plan—we redosed the epidural without good labor analgesia, then quickly took it out, and did a combined spinal/epidural technique with a new catheter with great results. Somewhere in there, Chas also put a new, larger IV in. Before he left to go back to the call room, the patient and her partner had calmed down enough that they actually asked him to take pictures with them. I called him again several hours later to go back to the OR for the predicted section and we were all set with our nice, new working epidural and nice new IV.

- What impressed me was that there was no guessing. Chas knew how to read the fetal tracing. He knew all the possible clinical scenarios. He knew the literature. He knew how to assess his labor epidural and when and how to redo it. He knew how to mitigate the fact that we were behind with our labor analgesia and do the combined technique. He knew how to calm the patient and her partner down, as well. The patient eventually needed a sort of slightly urgent operative delivery, just as Chas predicted, and she went to the OR in the best possible position, anesthesia-wise. The coolest part of the story is when I sent him the draft of this chapter and asked if we could use this anecdote, he didn't remember it. And that's the point about the best of the best. They are quietly that way every single day. What was a memorable case for me was just another day covering OB call for him.

Note: Chas did his residency and fellowship at Hopkins and was first on faculty there. He then moved to Columbia, where he is now the Henrik H. Bendixen Professor of Anesthesiology and vice chair for research. He has always combined superb clinical and research skills with unfailing kindness.

- Tied with Chas Emala is Dr. Raja (Srinivasa Raja, MD). Dr. Raja (or "Raj" as he was called by the other faculty) was a regional, pain, and obstetrical anesthesiologist and my advisor during residency. His clinical skills were legendary, and I can remember him telling me, "The anatomy is fixed and static and beyond correctly positioning the patient you can't do anything about what's there. You have to accept that don't control it. So, regional anesthesia is about what you can control—what's in the syringe, what's not in the syringe, and what your hands are doing with the needle."

- I can remember as a young attending calling Dr. Raja when I *had* to get a thoracic epidural in a patient (it was a lung volume reduction) and I just could not do it. I called him for help, and he came up to my OR from several floors away and said quietly, "I think the paramedian approach is the correct one here." He had that perfectly placed and perfectly working thoracic epidural in within a matter of seconds, it seemed and saved me from having to postpone the case. Plus, he was the best resident advisor ever and helped me understand and set my career priorities in the kindest and most insightful way! I feel lucky to have been trained by him.

Note: Dr. Raja trained at the University of Washington and the University of Virginia. At Hopkins, he was a professor of anesthesiology and critical care medicine and neurology, as well as the director of pain research. He was a superbly talented clinician who could do any block as well as a prodigious researcher who led a team that had almost 30 years of continuous NIH funding. He held numerous national and international leadership positions and among his many awards was the 2011 John J. Bonica Award from ASRA and the John J. Bonica Distinguished Lecture Award at the IASP 2021 World Congress. Despite these accolades, he was known for his quiet and calm demeanor and kindness.

From Ziyad Knio:

- The best educators are those who find teachable moments in otherwise routine cases. I am a current CA-3. Early in my residency, I had one attending task me with drawing an ABG and a mixed venous gas to estimate cardiac output during a chest closure. When I asked if he was proposing I use the Fick equation, he peppered me with additional questions, eventually asking if I could state Fick's first name (I was unsuccessful in answering that one). When I asked if we could simply use the thermodilution function of our PA catheter, I was asked if the patient's recently implanted LVAD would have an impact on this method of cardiac output estimation. I was not given the opportunity to respond before he left the room, forcing me to reason through the patient's hemodynamics and circulatory course (and do some independent reading). This was all during a one-hour Saturday morning add-on case, one that I did not expect to come with so much teaching. Thanks, Keith Littlewood, for that one.

Note: Keith Littlewood trained at Virginia Commonwealth University and is now a cardiac anesthesiologist, the assistant dean for clinical skills education, and the vice chair for education at the University of Virginia. Besides education, he is also known for his commitment to social justice.

- There have been many other impactful faculty in my learning journey. One introduced me to the concept of a fragility index, and now I include it in all of my current research studies. It was not at all related to our case or any assigned reading, just a fun topic for us to discuss. I'm not sure that I would have come across it in my own reading, even today.

- My favorite faculty are the ones who take the time to get to know me personally. They ask about my personal life, weigh in with opinions on where I should take my career, and look to me for clinical knowledge when we (the *team*) are faced with uncertainty.

- I also appreciate it when faculty share practice guidelines—articles that I can store in a folder for future reference. This has also motivated me to search for literature when I don't have a quick reference on hand. The articles I find can then be discussed with both my medical students and my attendings.

From Ron Bank:

- I was extremely fortunate to have several great faculty members during my training. If I had to pick my "three best" it would be Cathy Marcucci, Steve Frank, and Dan Nyhan.

Cathy Marcucci's focus on avoiding errors even small ones, so they don't become big issues (like correctly securing IV's/lines) and her overall compulsion and attention to details and ability to see priorities in a case—and her "knowledge is power" mantra profoundly shaped my thinking early on. These concepts have, in fact, shaped and guided my practice for my entire career. They have also shaped my mentoring of students, residents, and fellows. Reflecting back on 25 years of routinely doing very complex, high-risk cases, her teaching has made me better than I otherwise would have been, has saved lives, prevented morbidity, and I have paid it forward by passing these concepts on to a great many trainees over the years. In fact, to this day, I often mention Cathy by name!

Note: Cathy trained at Hopkins and was first on the faculty there. When raising her family, she held academic appointments at the University of Maryland and the University of Pennsylvania while concentrating her clinical work in the Veterans health care system. She just recently completed her second fellowship in transfusion medicine. She is known for her extensive personal and professional network and her inclusive team building. *Anesthesia Bridges* is her fourth major book project.

Steve Frank taught me how to approach and love big, complex cases. I have focused on just such cases throughout my entire career. I try to pass on my enthusiasm for such cases to residents and fellows—and to demonstrate to medical students how much more that we do than the public and, sadly, many physicians understand.

Note: Steve trained at Hopkins for residency and fellowship and has been on faculty there since, with an interim stint in private practice. He is a professor of anesthesiology and the medical director of the Bloodless Medicine and Surgery Program. He is known for his clinical acumen, robust and clinically relevant academic output, and his professional courtesy and collegiality.

Dan Nyhan instilled in me a love and appreciation for cardiac anesthesia. He is largely responsible for my staying on and doing a cardiac anesthesia fellowship. I'm now the longest-serving cardiac anesthesiologist in a very large, quaternary system flagship hospital. How time flies!

Note: Dan trained at Hopkins and has been on faculty there in cardiac anesthesiology since the 1980s. His leadership positions have included professor of anesthesiology and critical care medicine, director of the cardiac anesthesia division, and interim chair.

I am so grateful for the wonderful faculty that I was blessed to have. I have tried to honor them by passing on their lessons to future generations so that their contributions live on long after they (and I) have finished practicing.

***Note from the Editors:** Cathy Marcucci is beyond honored to receive such a gracious acknowledgment from Ron Bank. She was trying to teach all those years, but she was never quite sure anybody was listening, so Ron's words mean a lot to her. She, in turn, acknowledges her family, who built a strong legacy and bridge of education and lifelong learning for her and were on the right side of history in educating their girls. That leggy teenager below is Cathy's mom, the late Nancy Jordan Marcucci, who went to Miami of Ohio. She is with Cathy's great-grandparents Charles and Sue Jordan, sometime in the very early 1950s (Figs. 96.5 and 96.6).

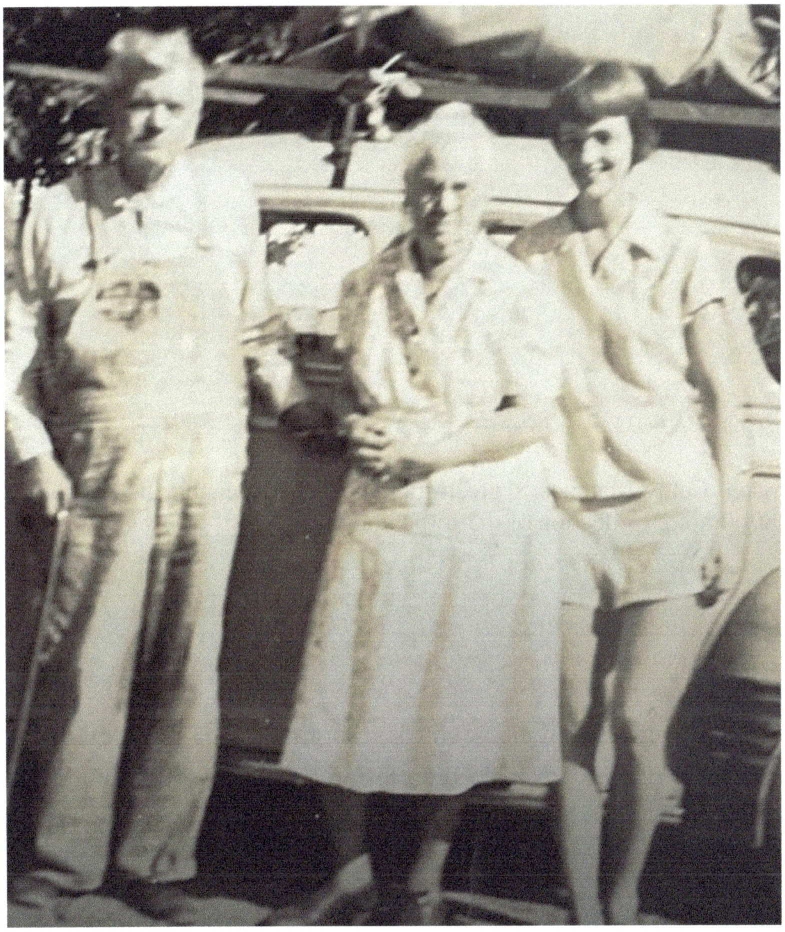

Fig. 96.5 Think those old folks were simple, unsophisticated country people? They were actually among the most educated people in the country, for that time. The gentleman in the denim overalls was actually Dr. Charles H. Jordan, who graduated in the first dental class of Northwestern University in 1896. The elderly lady with the white bun and the (literal) granny glasses is Sue Harrison Jordan, and she graduated with an AB from Ohio Wesleyan in the Class of 1891, when less than 1% of girls in the US went to college. She was a teacher and later school principal of the Oak Harbor School in Oak Harbor, OH, in the mid and late 1890s. The family still has her brass school teacher's bell. Photo: Collection of the Jordan family

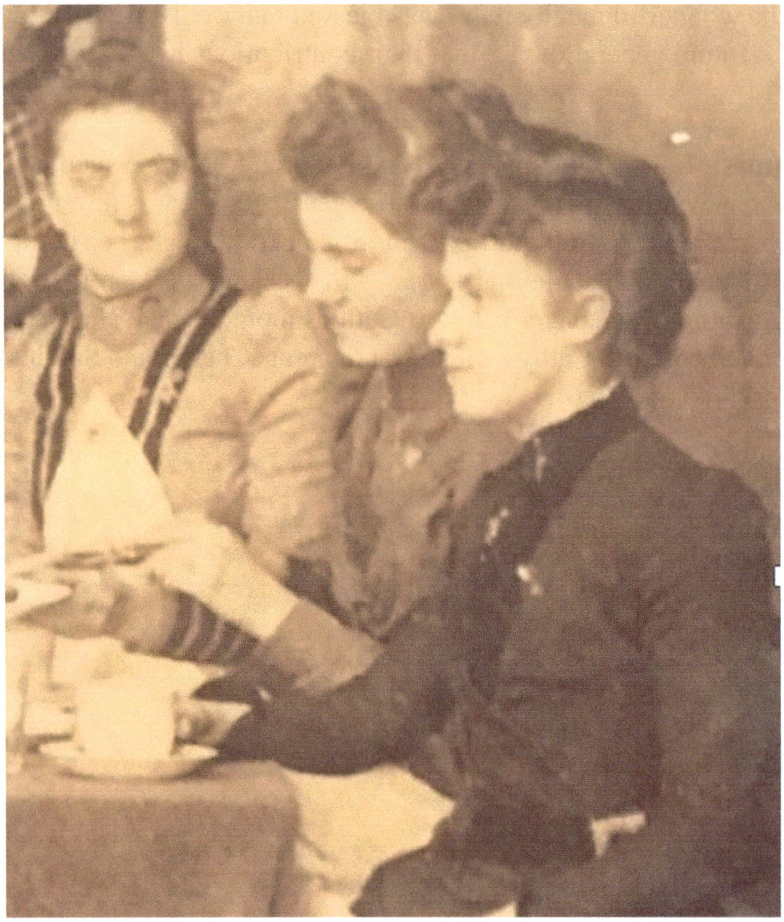

Fig. 96.6 Sue E. Harrison, Cathy Marcucci's great-grandmother, center, having tea with her classmates at Ohio Wesleyan in the late 1880s. Photo: Collection of the Jordan family

Research = Education!

- Research is as much about education as career development. The best research occurs when you are working hard to *educate yourself* as well as the journal readers. Think about what you have a burning desire to know and what questions you would like to have answered for yourself (and your patients)—that's the direction you should go in when developing a research career.—**Editors**

- Remember also that we still don't even definitely know how general anesthesia works and the longitudinal effects on the brain! And there are also still a great many areas in the practice of anesthesiology that need investigation, especially in the anesthesiology subspecialties.—**Editors**

- There are also great research opportunities anytime a new drug or piece of equipment comes into widespread clinical use at any point in the perioperative period.—**Editors**

- Other areas of research involve health disparities, sustainability and energy conservation in the OR and ICU, and the preop optimization, and enhanced recovery protocols. And every study that is done for adult patients needs to be done for pediatric patients as well. The research fields are pretty much wide open.—**Editors**

- We asked our senior authors and editors to give us just a few specific ideas out of the literally thousands of research topics that are out there.—**BMT, KL, RGG, AJR, and CM**

1. Should we be giving oxytocin for known cesarean hysterectomy procedures for known placenta accreta?
2. What is the reason for the large variance in incidence of GETA for cesarean delivery?
3. What is the optimal postoperative analgesic regimen for parturients on buprenorphine or methadone?
4. When is the last time your institution's Maximum Surgical Blood Order Schedule (MS-BOS) was reviewed and revised? Hint: this might be a good opportunity for a QI project if it's been a while.
5. How effective is your institution's Massive Transfusion Protocol in terms of clinical outcomes? In terms of inventory and costs in the blood bank?
6. What is the role of complementary medicine in any and all aspects of the perioperative period?
7. What regional anesthesia techniques (fascial plane blocks) improve postoperative pain after cardiac surgery, and do they change the length of stay?
8. What monitoring, hemodynamic, transfusion, and medication strategies reduce the risk of organ (kidney, brain, and so forth) dysfunction after cardiac surgery?
9. What strategies reduce the inflammatory effects of cardiopulmonary bypass?
10. What are the effects of artificial feeding in patients with cancer and dementia?
11. What are the appropriate indications, efficacy, and outcomes for the use of appetite stimulants in palliative care?
12. Do we understand the PEG tube spiral in the palliative care patient?
13. How do we best implement and assess competency-based residency and fellowship training?
14. How can we identify and close gaps in professionalism during training?
15. Are we ensuring a selection process for residents that is free of unconscious bias?
16. How do we select residents with the new Pass/Fail USMLE Step 1?
17. Etc., etc., etc.!

Artificial Intelligence in Perioperative Medicine

It goes without saying that artificial intelligence (AI) applications are going to have a gigantic effect on clinical medicine. We asked applied mathematician **Carolyn Burr Metzler, PhD**, for just a few of her thoughts on AI. Dr. Metzler has been thinking about these issues for some time and sent us the following advice:

- First of all, non-mathematicians should realize that "artificial intelligence" is a broad term that encompasses many different technologies. Asking whether AI is "bad" or "scary" is like asking whether the internet is bad or scary.—**CBM**

- In general, the math and computing pros are not afraid of the technical applications for AI, but we are concerned about the social and political misuses, particularly when AI can be used to mislead the general population.—**CBM**

- The editors asked me for the simplest definition of AI that I could come up with for non-professionals. Basically, it's just the graduated allowance of computers making decisions that historically have been made only by the human brain.—**CBM**

- The concepts of AI, such as neural networks and language processing, have been researched as early as the 1950s, but it wasn't until the era of big data in the early 2000s that AI began to advance more quickly. With cheaper data storage and faster processors, AI models can ingest more data and be used in a wider array of applications.—**CBM**

- Remember that AI is built on data sets. The AI application can only be as good as the data that it is trained on.—**CBM**

- If the data sets are somehow biased, then the conclusions that the AI application is making can also be biased. For example, in a medical application, if the model is trained on data of mostly white males in their 40s, the AI application may not properly work for a Hispanic woman in her 60s. There was a highly publicized case for facial recognition software whose training set was built on a majority white population and would incorrectly identify people with darker complexions.—**CBM**

- AI will have a long runway. However, it is going to be ubiquitous. The trick will be in creating trust in the applications that are beneficial while controlling the deleterious effects, just as with the internet. The ethics and technical aspects of applying and the maximizing medical AI applications would be a s great field of research to get into. Personally, if I was a physician, I would go to every course and conference on "medical AI" that I could.—**CBM**

- AI in everyday life and perhaps (probably) in everyday medicine will be something of an equalizer for the digital divide. Think about it. It doesn't really require any coding knowledge or tech literacy or skills in search It doesn't even require a password. You don't have to watch any YouTube videos and then watch them again. It is being designed so that all it really requires is a question. Every generation thinks it owns the future. With AI, people on the wrong side of the digital divide are going to be able to achieve a speedy catchup. Figure out how to do the most good with this, especially for your patients.—**RS and Editors**

- "Safety" in AI will eventually come to be dependent on things like the validity and integrity of digital watermarking. If you want to follow anything in the safety of AI industry, these and similar developments would be the ones to watch.—**CBM**

Educational Outreach

- Every training program should have at least one lecture, from the psychiatry consultation and liaison team, on the consent process. Competency to consent is not the same as capacity to consent. And consenting to surgery is not the same as consenting to anesthesia—you cannot assume there is an ironclad implication that one guarantees the other. Another area of educational outreach that the psychiatrists can help us with is the confusion over delirium—what it is, what it isn't, and what to do.—**CM and NBS**

- And don't forget educational opportunities with the physiatrists! Once, when I was on call, a patient pulled out her trach and promptly coded. We did not have anesthesia support at that particular hospital. I looked at my colleague to ask if I should try replacing the trach, he said, "Well, right now she's dead." We did get the trach back in and successfully resuscitated the patient. But I tell this story to illustrate that the rehab medicine docs and services would welcome educational outreach from our anesthesiology colleagues on basic airway skills and management of the complicated airway. We also should collaborate and create joint educational and professional conferences on regional blocks and pain management. Anesthesiologists and physiatrists bring different backgrounds to similar patient problems; willingness to learn from each other would make all of us better physicians.—**CFB**

- As we have stressed elsewhere in this book, there are tons of opportunities for educational outreach and cross-pollination with the blood bank. I am trained in both anesthesiology and transfusion medicine, and it is really surprising how little the specialties know about each other. I really feel that trainees should have multiple teaching conferences in the other specialty and there should be clinical review conferences, at the attending level, as interesting situations arise.—**CM**

***Note from the Editors:** The wonderful detail of the Bow Bridge in Central Park is a great metaphor for the complexity and variety of medical education—both what you teach and what you learn (Fig. 96.7).

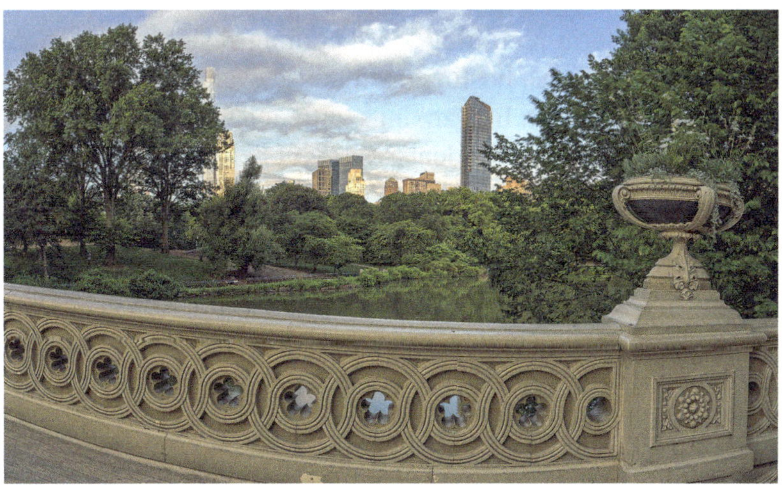

Fig. 96.7 A detail of the Bow Bridge in Central Park, New York City. Photo: Image used under standard license from shutterstock.com

Considerations for Chief Residents—Asad Mansoor, Lucas Meuchel, Ziyad Knio, and Jen Tripi

Congratulations! You have been named chief resident for the upcoming academic year. Up to this point, you have likely excelled throughout your residency training at the clinical, academic, and professional levels. As chief resident, you are now tasked with the privilege to serve as a leader amongst your peers, acting as a liaison between department administration and your residency program. While this is no simple task, we highlight the pros, the cons, and key qualities required to thrive (or at least survive) in this role.

Why Be a Chief Resident?

From Asad Mansoor:

- The most obvious benefit of serving as chief resident is the opportunity to hone your leadership skills. In this role, you now have the chance to represent your peers and serve as a "voice" to help advocate for and hopefully enact positive change within your department. As the "voice of the residents" you inherently become heavily involved in important administrative discussions and serve as an asset to the department leadership, providing a resident's perspective which administrators and executives in the department may not otherwise appreciate.

- Engagement with department executives "pulls back the curtain" on the inner workings of your department and hospital system at large. These interactions provide a crash course in the complex interplay between patient care, residency and fellow training, and the business of healthcare. This interplay also includes the various rules and regulations put in place by accrediting agencies, such as ACGME and Joint Commission. Ultimately, a greater appreciation for these details and this complexity provides context for policies and decisions that are made at an administrative level.

- While chief residency provides a deep dive into the inner workings of the department, with a chance to represent your peers, it also affords you the opportunity to leave a lasting impression on the future of your residency program in the form of resident recruitment and educational endeavors.

- Chief residents play a vital role in recruiting the incoming residency class. As chief, you may be responsible for screening applications, hosting open house events (virtually or in-person), interviewing applicants, and determining match list rankings with department administration. Ultimately, this is your opportunity to find prospective residents who you believe can help the department and residency program continue to move in the direction you envision.

- Chief residents are also heavily involved in the educational component of the residency program. As Chief resident, you may be responsible for the evaluation and improvement of the existing residency curriculum or even tasked with organizing and implementing new educational endeavors, which could range from starting a resident journal club to negotiating for department support of a Resident Wellness Retreat. The possibilities are almost endless.

- In summary, chief residency opens the door to help leave a lasting impact on your program, all while providing high-quality leadership experience required for those interested in an executive or administrative role within a hospital system in the future.

From Lucas Meuchel:

- Advocacy for your colleagues and the chance to lead by example—you will never know how lucky you are to have the colleagues you do until you are asked to lead them. Rarely during training do we have the opportunity to direct change, serving as chief allows one to be directly involved in multiple areas affecting the day-to-day lives of residents.

From Ziyad Knio:

- This is a question I've gotten several times before, from both medical and non-medical personnel. After all, it means taking on extra work for essentially no extra pay. I surveyed several former chief residents before agreeing to keep my name in consideration for the position. Most valued their experience, at least in part. One candidly told me that he would under no circumstances do the role again, if given the opportunity.

- The chief resident role is an opportunity for personal growth. Keeping this in mind, even the "bad" days have a lot of value. They are few and far between, however. I'm much more likely to have a good day—one in which my impact on the residency program is tangible.

- The chief resident role is also an opportunity to work with your peers. I find that anesthesiology residency is lacking in teaching this skill—most often we are learning how to staff our own cases, often viewing independence as the end-goal. Rarely are we leading rounds or taking on supervisory roles like our medical and surgical senior-resident counterparts. I'm envious of my partner (a chief resident in internal medicine) for mastering these skills. This is also particularly important to me, as I prepare for critical care fellowship training.

- Participating in recruiting is fun and enlightening—an inside look into the medical education, residency, and faculty selection processes that have honestly been kept secret from us until now.

- When things get rough, I remind myself that the operating room is where we as anesthesiologists are faced with life-or-death decisions. The mountain of emails related to chiefly administrative duties are at worst an inconvenience, at best an opportunity to help others, but never a threat to someone's health or safety.

From Jen Tripi:

- It is an excellent opportunity to build your leadership skills.

- It provides experience that opens doors for an academic career or administrative role.

- It allows for building professional relationships both within and outside of your department. I am truly amazed at the number of people I have met and connected with since becoming a chief resident!

- With dedication and perseverance, it serves as a pathway to make a change within the residency.

Reasons NOT to Be a Chief Resident

From Asad Mansoor:

- With great privilege comes great responsibility. While chief residents can make a large impact on their program and department, actually making said impact requires sacrifice. Frankly, the role of chief resident involves an added workload of primarily administrative duties on top of pre-existing, and in many cases, more demanding clinical duties.
- Before, you had the luxury of focusing primarily on your own personal development and your own challenges, but as chief resident, you will quickly learn that your peers' challenges and concerns now become your challenges and concerns as well. While this is a great opportunity to act as a resource to your peers, understand that nearly every time you walk into a room, someone will bring their concerns to your attention. Whether it be an error in their vacation schedule, a grievance about a staff member or a concern that the refrigerator in the resident lounge is broken; you are now the first person your peers come to with their problems. What may have previously been a chance to go home after clinical responsibilities were complete can sometimes turn into evenings in the hospital or at home addressing the administrative issues surrounding your program or department.
- Another major challenge of being a chief resident is balancing the role of an administrator and a friend to your peers. This can usually be done effortlessly, but challenges can arise when attempting to remain neutral and fair if forced to make decisions that impact your peers. Chief residency is a balancing act that pushes you in and out of the roles of "friend" and "administrator" almost instantaneously. Part of being a fair leader may require you to set boundaries even with your closest colleagues, which can strain friendships and relationships that existed before assuming the role of chief resident.
- While balancing relationships amongst peers in the role of chief resident can be challenging, balancing the competing interests of the residency and the department administration is another obstacle. Amongst peers, chief residents are atop of the chain of command, but amongst department administration, the chief residents end up on the completely opposite end. Therefore, while discussions and negotiations are possible, the final decision will generally be that of the administration. As a result, chief residents will need to deliver unpopular news to their stakeholders, and regardless of opinion, must defend those decisions for the best interest of the department.
- The greatest challenges chief residents face are the personal sacrifice of time and energy and the balancing act between stakeholders, primarily the residents and department administration.

From Lucas Meuchel:

- Time. Serving as a chief comes with increased responsibility toward your fellow residents, and you must become more available than you might otherwise have been. Make no mistake, it is a rewarding experience but comes at a cost.
- Responsibility. Ultimately, a lot of the decisions come down to you and while that is empowering, you answer directly to your closest colleagues, and if you are lucky, your friends—good, bad, or neutral they will look to you and hold you accountable for things even beyond your control.

From Ziyad Knio:

- This is not a role to be used to "pad" one's CV. I think the motivation for this role needs to be intrinsic and not extrinsic.
- Additionally, the timeline for fellowship applications in many cases precedes chief resident elections. I know that my fellowship rank list was submitted prior to my accepting the chief resident role.
- Making & approving schedules, while appearing like the bulk of the job, is in fact a small fraction of the responsibilities.

From Jen Tripi:

- To build your CV. Being a chief resident is no easy task. It is hard work, and all extracurricular activities from your already demanding clinical duties.
- To say you were a chief resident.
- To become a better clinician. Remember, the role of chief resident is mostly administrative.

Qualities of a Good Chief Resident

From Asad Mansoor:

- While people differ in leadership styles, being a strong chief resident starts with being a strong resident. Chief residents must lead by example and be willing to set the standard for what their peers should strive for as trainees, budding clinicians, and professionals. This does not imply that chief residents must have the best clinical skills or the highest exam scores in their residency class, but instead suggests that they make a consistent and genuine effort in their practice, all while exemplifying professionalism and respect in the workplace. In addition to being a strong resident, excellent Chief Residents tend to be collaborative, empathetic, and fair-minded.
- Chief residents will face the challenge of making decisions to resolve conflict, which will inevitably lead to dissatisfaction at some point. While it is difficult to create a situation that provides complete satisfaction to everyone every step of the way, remaining empathetic and being conscientious of personal bias is critical to helping validate the concerns of involved parties as it pertains to disagreement. A focus on collaboration instead of competition can help ensure that reasonable decisions are made with all stakeholders in mind.

From Lucas Meuchel:

- Be available, be approachable, be fair. Be willing to do any shift, any assignment, any case you would consider asking your residents to do—and ultimately be humble and ask for help.

From Ziyad Knio:

- Chief residents should be advocates for their co-residents.
- It is easy to follow the status quo, but challenging systems may be necessary to impart some positive change.
- The importance of communication cannot be overstated. When I have to deny a request, including the "why" makes delivering the "no" so much more effective.

From Jen Tripi:

- Approachable
- Receptive to feedback
- A good listener
- An advocate
- Dedicated to the residency
- Honest
- Friendly
- Organized

How to Be a Chief Resident

From Asad Mansoor:

- There is no protocol that can prepare someone to be a great chief resident. Many of the challenges chief residents will face are often unpredictable and out of their control. The best way to be a chief resident is to fail quickly and learn from the consequences of each decision. While it is tempting to brainstorm ideas and come up with the perfect plan to address issues that arise, nothing can be achieved unless there is execution. Most people are unaware of their personal blind spots until they get exposed, so ultimately, the best way to grow as a leader is to make mistakes and learn from them. While there will always be criticism, it is important for chiefs to be patient with themselves and with others, as this is a challenging but incredibly rewarding experience that will serve you well in the future.
- Seek the opinions of those who aren't complaining while still listening to those who are. Not every resident will bring their concerns or needs to your attention, so you may have to ask others to cover the full spectrum of your cohort.

- Never assume that any issue has only one side. Be patient and willing to gather the supporting evidence.

- Be willing to extend yourself on behalf of your colleagues, but not at the expense of your own self.

- *Ask for help.*

From Ziyad Knio:

- Time, like money, is a limited resource and needs to be budgeted appropriately. If you're assessing whether an additional monthly expense is in your budget, it would be prudent to move that dollar amount to savings for several months and assess the impact that it has on your finances. Similarly, if you anticipate needing 5–10h per week to devote to a new work role, such as chief resident, you either need to carve out that 5–10 h before accepting or drop an existing activity that's occupying 5–10 h of your time.

- I politely made it clear to my research mentors that I would need to put a pause on my research pursuits during my chief year. I thought out my conversation. In doing so, I made the time for this role without taking away from my already limited free time.

- Also: checklists, calendar reminders, and scheduled email responses. I don't think I could do this job without them.

From Jen Tripi:

- Being a chief resident is hard, but one of the most rewarding jobs I have had to date. As a current chief resident, I will say you must have great time management skills. This truly is one of the keys to success. It will take time to figure this out, but I recommend dedicating one hour each day during the week to complete chief duties. This way, you don't fall behind, which will only lead to undue stress.

- Stay organized. As a chief resident of medical education, I created multiple folders in OneDrive and used the Outlook calendar to accomplish this.

- Ask for help when you need it. Do not be ashamed of this. Remember, you are human too.

- Check in on your residents frequently. It can be a quick run by the operating room with a few simple questions: "How are you doing? How is your family doing?" It is amazing how far these simple gestures can carry you.

- Do not let emails overwhelm you. Set a specific time of day and amount of time to read them and respond in an appropriate time frame.

- Use checklists. This keeps your tasks accounted for and allows you to sleep well at night.

- When you are on vacation, completely disconnect from work. Create an automatic email response, and do not look at your email. It is important for your well-being and ability to continue to be a great chief resident.

- Organize social events outside of the workplace. Building community is a key component of creating a supportive and collegial work environment.

- Maintain a positive attitude. Your attitude has a large impact on the entire residency.

A Few Final Words of Wisdom from Junior Anesthesiologist Maria Orlic

- As a new resident, there's a lot of pressure in the OR to move quickly and keep things on schedule, but that's when mistakes happen. I've promised myself that I am always going to teach trainees to take the time you need and do things right, even if that means keeping people waiting a few extra minutes.—**MKO**

- At the beginning, everything is scary to trainees. The faculty know this but perhaps do not recall so vividly what it is like to feel so scared. To the people coming up behind me—remember to breathe and call for help earlier than later. It's better to have extra hands and feel embarrassed than to face a scary situation all by yourself.—**MKO**

- I've been taught to welcome help from others, but also to always personally verify that an important task was done, even if it's something as simple as supposedly turning on the Bair Hugger. I would say that being taught to be vigilant always, literally and figuratively has been the most important lesson I've learned. I will always be grateful for this.—**MKO**

Bonus Content! Don't Forget Books!—by Raymond G. Graber, MD

Somehow through the years, I have collected a wide assortment of anesthesia textbooks, and in effect they also show the history and evolution of anesthesia practice. These textbooks are "bridges" that link me to the authors—past and present. My favorites are my regional anesthesia books. I did not set out to collect these—I just sort of accumulated them and am guilty of not throwing anything away, much to my wife's chagrin.

My grandfather (Raymond Leddy) was a general surgeon, and from him I inherited a second edition copy of Gaston Labat's *Regional Anesthesia*, published in 1930. This was the first major textbook of regional anesthesia techniques published in the United States. It includes excellent anatomic drawings and diagrams of local anesthetic injection techniques for surgeons but also includes a nice chapter on spinal anesthesia (Fig. 96.8). Labat founded the first American Society of Regional Anesthesia (ASRA) in 1923, which dissolved in 1939 after merger with the ASA. Nowadays, the Gaston Labat Award is annually given at the annual ASRA Regional Anesthesiology and Acute Pain Medicine Meeting to an individual who has demonstrated outstanding contributions to the development, teaching, and practice of regional anesthesia.

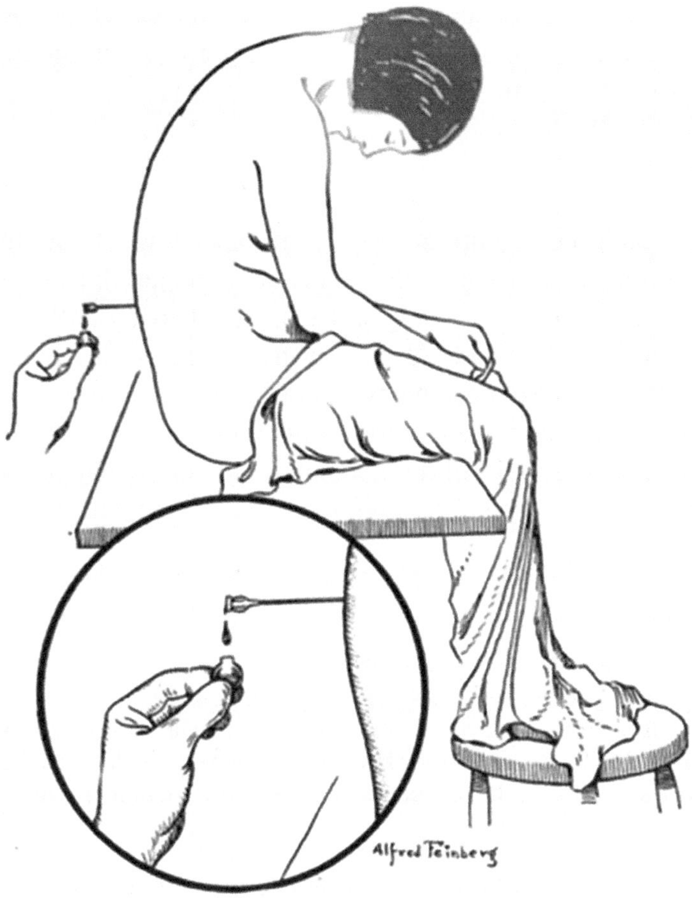

Fig. 96.8 From Labat, demonstration of the technique of adding cerebrospinal fluid to a vial of local anesthetic crystals. Photo: Aubrie R. Graber

My father, James Graber MD, was an anesthesiologist. From him, I inherited books such as *Epidural Analgesia* by Phillip Bromage, *Physiology of Spinal Anesthesia* by Nicholas Greene, and *Plexus Anesthesia* by Alon Winnie. These books were like bibles to me when I was a resident and young attending, and the authors were my personal heroes.

Of these, my personal favorite was Alon Winnie's book, which had excellent artwork and descriptions of his techniques and theories. Winnie's story is fascinating—he contracted polio as a resident, required tracheostomy and mechanical ventilation, and eventually recovered but remained paraplegic and was wheelchair bound for the rest of his life. This did not stop him from completing an anesthesia residency, becoming an expert in regional anesthesia, and becoming a founding father and first president of the reborn ASRA in 1975. I bought a second copy of that book, and at one point in my career had the honor of introducing Dr. Winnie as a speaker—and had the foresight to bring that book with me. Dr. Winnie graciously signed the book for me and added the following sly comment:

> Hoping this will bring your success rate to 100%—at least with brachial plexus anesthesia!

During my career, the practice of regional anesthesia has moved away from the paresthesia technique to use of nerve stimulation, and now the use of ultrasound. I got to meet and correspond with some my generation's superstars and book authors/editors—like Admir Hadzic (who both wrote an excellent textbook and founded the NYSORA website), and Vincent Chan—who was a pioneer in ultrasound guided techniques.

It is with some regret I watch the evolution away from paper towards digital content. Don't get me wrong, I'm a big user of online journals and other educational material. But I have always loved books, dating back to my childhood—I was the nerdy kid who spent many an hour browsing the stacks of libraries. There is a pleasure in holding a book in your hands and paging through it that you just don't get with a digital reader. Paper is easier on the eyes, doesn't depend on battery power, and looks good on your bookshelf. I can't tell you how many interesting articles I have discovered by browsing through books or journals, whereas with digital I find this much less likely to happen. And of course, you can't someday meet a personal hero and get a digital book signed by the author!

Authors

Brandon Togioka is an associate professor of anesthesiology and perioperative medicine at OHSU. He has a wide range of clinical and research interests, especially obstetrical anesthesia. Besides teaching and educating trainees and students at all levels, Brandon is recognized for his outreach work in underserved communities and communities with healthcare disparities—showing that educational interventions can increase epidural use among Hispanic women.

Ron Bank is a cardiac anesthesiologist and assistant professor in the INOVA/UVA health care system and campus. He has wide-ranging clinical interests and has been active in the regional and national anesthesiology communities. He enjoys teaching a wide range of anesthesia topics to students and trainees at all levels. While we were getting this chapter together, we had a wonderful conversation with him about his fascinating Nana, the beautiful Bernice Bank Altshul, who was born in 1909 and also had a college education (Fig. 96.9). We agreed that one way for a family to thrive is to prioritize education for their girls. The pictures below show Bernice Jacobson Bank Altshul at Farmville State Teachers College in 1929 and Ron and Jordan Bank posing in front of the same building almost 95 years later (Fig. 96.10).

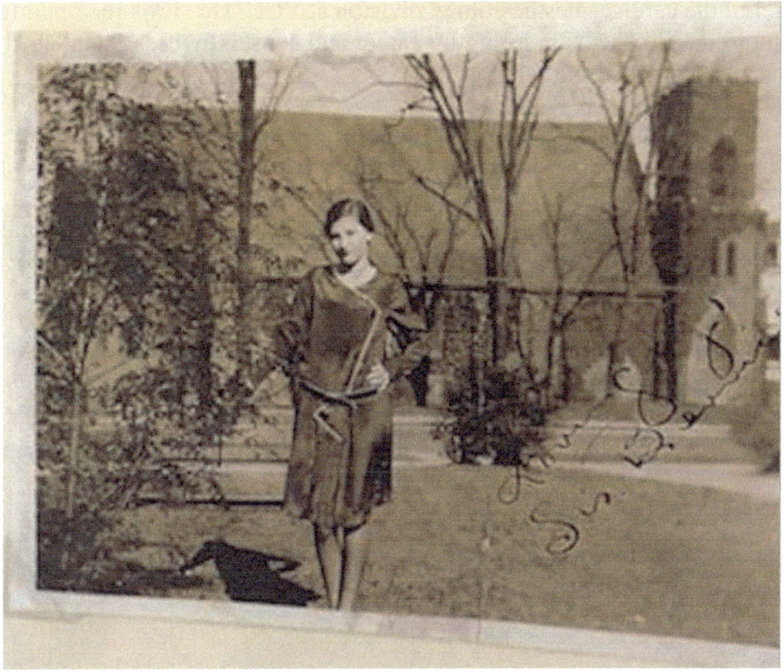

Fig. 96.9 Bernice was born in Portsmouth, VA into a large, upwardly mobile, observant Jewish family. Although she grew up in racially integrated neighborhoods, at college she was one of only six Jewish students in the entire student body. Bernice was strongly supported in college, especially by her mother, and she received money to take a trip to Baltimore as a graduation present. She steamed up the Chesapeake Bay in the Old Bayline steamship and was introduced to Simon Bank. She and Si were married and settled in Baltimore to raise their family, including Barron Bank, Ron's dad. She was widowed in 1974, remarried to Jack Altshul, then widowed again. She lived to age 100 and always spoke of how absurd it was and how much society missed out in the past by not having girls educated. Photo: Collection of the Bank family

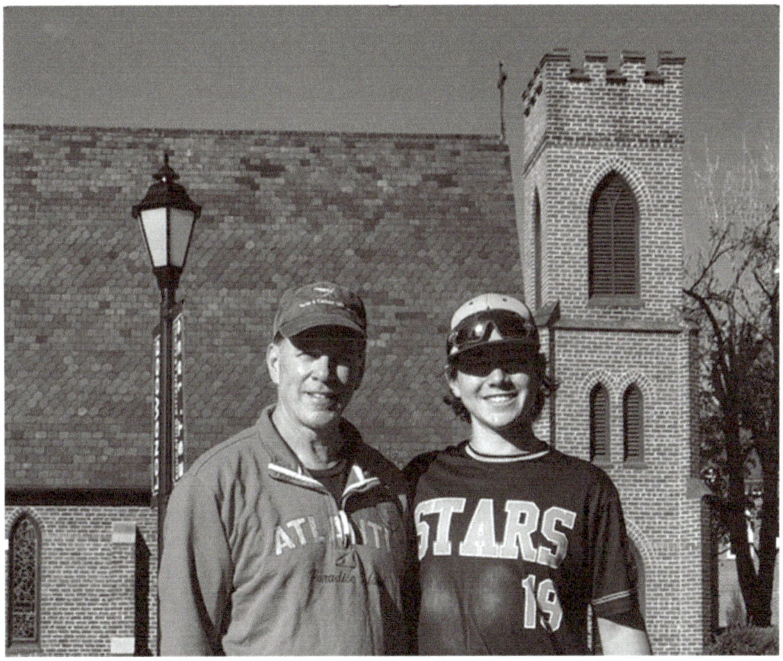

Fig. 96.10 Ron and Jordan Bank are Bernice's grandson and great-grandson. Jordan had an away baseball game near Farmville State Teacher's College, now Longwood University, and he and Ron found the exact spot where Bernice posed in the 1920s. Photo: Collection of the Bank family

Mark Nelson is the chief of the cardiac anesthesiology division at VCU. He views the opportunity to obtain his MEd as one of the most fortuitous developments in his entire career and constantly uses established educational theories in his daily teaching of students, residents, and fellows.

Asad Mansoor was a chief resident within the Department of Anesthesia at the University of Iowa Hospitals and Clinics (UIHC). He then completed fellowship training in adult cardiothoracic anesthesiology at the University of Michigan in 2024–2025. Asad enjoys spending his free time with his wife, Mahsaw Mansoor, MD, who did her residency training in ophthalmology at UIHC as well. They both plan to pursue careers in academic medicine with particular interests in political advocacy, graduate medical education, and enhancing access to medically underserved populations.

Cathy Marcucci is a senior anesthesiologist who found her life's work and educational career mission when she was asked to put together a team to do a "new kind" of anesthesia handbook. That book, *Avoiding Common Anesthesia Errors*, was eventually translated into six languages and is in its second edition. She was also the lead editor of *A Case Approach to Perioperative Drug-Drug Interactions*, which she considers to be her magnum opus.

Part VI

Doctor-Patient Relations

Tiny Bridge in the Yellow Mountains, China

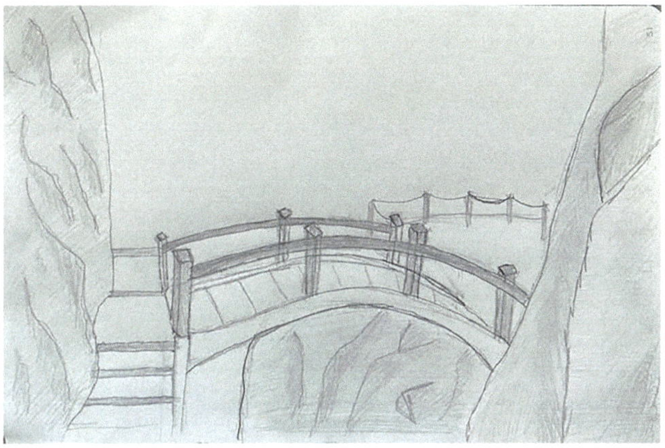

This bridge was selected by editor **Cathy Marcucci**. The wooden plank bridge is a short pedestrian span that connects an ascending pathway that hugs the face of the mountain and a small observation area. Mt. Huang, also referred to as Huangshan, literally means "Yellow Mountains." It is known as the "Magic Scenic Area" due to the foggy oceans of clouds surrounding the mountain peaks that can be glimpsed from the bridge and observation platform. It is located about 250 miles southwest of Shanghai in the south Anhui Province.

The editors of *Anesthesia Bridges* thank **Lisa Sandson**, who holds a BArch degree from the School of Architecture, Syracuse University and who formerly interned at The Architectural Team in Boston, MA, for her charming pencil drawing capturing the fairy-tale quality and romance of this tiny bridge.

Introduction

97

Catherine Marcucci

The focus of this section is on how we interact and communicate with our patients. You can be the best diagnostician and have excellent procedural skills, but if you can't communicate with your patients, you will just be another anonymous face that a patient runs into during their medical journey. Being a good communicator with patients involves aspects of empathy, humor, professionalism, and sharing yourself. You can distinguish yourself from others by how you listen to and develop a relationship with your patients.

In the operating rooms, we are at somewhat of a disadvantage. We have limited time with patients and families, before and after their procedures. We are meeting patients at times of extreme stress for many of them—even if the surgery is a life-saving event. But it is because of that stress that you can make an immediate impact on the patient.

In this section, we present a number of chapters about how to communicate with patients. Some of these chapters are stories of specific interactions and are very personal. We also get advice about communication in different sub-specialty settings—and this is important because different patient populations and settings may require a different touch to how you proceed. We hope that readers will find this information helpful and maybe help stimulate some thoughts about how to improve their relations with patients.

Author

Cathy Marcucci is a senior academic anesthesiologist and inveterate anesthesiology educator. She is also fellowship-trained in transfusion medicine. When not taking care of patients and/or putting the latest book together, she dedicates her time to mentoring junior colleagues, writing copy for animal rescues, and travel.

C. Marcucci (✉)
Department of Transfusion Medicine, Clinical Center, National Institutes of Health, Bethesda, MD, USA

S. Mohamed et al. (eds.), *Anesthesia Bridges*, https://doi.org/10.1007/978-3-032-08294-7_97

98 Why You Should Talk to Your Patients

Raymond G. Graber

Introduction

We work in an environment that increasingly values speed and efficiency. When you meet a patient for the first time, it is tempting and easy to just stick to acquiring the important data that is required for an adequate preoperative evaluation and then launch into your discussion of the planned anesthetic. However, it is important to realize that this short period of time can make a big difference with regard to your patient's perception of you, the care that you are giving, and even your institution.

Meeting, Greeting, and Getting the IV In

I had a mentor who used to say that part of his role in the operating room was to serve as a "greeter." Patients and families arrive at preoperative preparation areas, unsure of what to expect and are frequently filled with anxiety. Introducing yourself to the patient and family and giving them a warm greeting is a good way to start building a relationship.

Another thing to think about is the initial IV placement. There is a tendency for a junior member of the team to be responsible for IV placement, but they are also the person who is most likely to miss the IV or cause pain during placement. I never mind placing preoperative IVs—in fact I enjoy doing it. A smooth painless IV start with a decent amount of local anesthetic is a good way to start earning the trust of the patient. It can be a time of forming a bond with your patient. If you ever have a chance to look at patient surveys of their anesthetic care, *one of the things they will always comment on is a bad IV experience.*

When doing tasks like IVs, I have a habit of trying to engage patients in small talk. Questions like "What kind of work do you do?" or "How many kids do you have?" or "Where do your kids go to school?" are good questions that can lead to further conversation. Not infrequently, I find I have unexpected connections with patients, and when this happens, the patients are just a little less nervous and happier to be there sitting with you. The story that follows is a tale of one of those unexpected connections.

R. G. Graber (✉)
Department of Anesthesiology and Perioperative Medicine, University Hospitals Cleveland Medical Center, Cleveland, OH, USA
e-mail: raymond.graber@uhhospitals.org

S. Mohamed et al. (eds.), *Anesthesia Bridges*, https://doi.org/10.1007/978-3-032-08294-7_98

Second Patient of the Day

It was a Monday morning, and I was working with our joint replacement team, doing hips and knees. I went out to meet my second-round patient, whom we will call Jack. Jack was here for a total right knee replacement. He was in his 80 s, was reasonably healthy, and of sound mind. I introduced myself to him, reviewed his medical and surgical history, examined him, and discussed anesthetic options with him. I grabbed some equipment and proceeded to sit down in a chair next to him to place his IV.

As is my habit, while I was working on the IV, I asked Jack about his background. He told me about his career and the company he runs, and he mentioned that he learned his leadership skills in the Army. When I asked him where he had served, he told me he had fought in the Korean War. "My dad also fought in Korea," I told him. "He also was Army infantry and was wounded at the Battle of Pork Chop Hill, then evacuated to Japan." We chatted some more as I finished up with his IV, then I went to pick up some preoperative acetaminophen for him.

When I returned, Jack was looking at me with a gleam in his eyes. "Was your dad Jim Graber from Watervliet, New York?" "Yes!" I responded. "How did you know?" "Your Dad and I were buddies – we shipped over together on the troopship!" At this point, we were all astounded. My father had passed away about 10 years ago and had never really talked about his war experience. We chatted a little more, but soon it was time to go to his operating room. We agreed to talk more, after surgery. We went to the OR, where he had an uneventful spinal anesthetic and a nice nap.

Post-op Visit

The following morning, I went to visit Jack in his room. He was up and walking about, still reasonably comfortable with an adductor canal block that was still working. He was able to tell me more about his war time memories. He had met my father in basic training, during a leadership training class. They had shipped from the West Coast to Japan together and spent a lot of time together during that long cruise.

Eventually, when they reached Japan, they were separated. My father was transported to Korea, where he joined up with his group (seventh Infantry Division), and eventually went into battle. Jack had heard that my father had been severely wounded, and even that he might have lost an arm and a leg. He told me that he had always felt bad that he had not tried to track down my dad, to see what happened to him. He was glad to hear that my father had recovered from his injuries with all limbs intact! My father had been a platoon leader and apparently had suffered shrapnel injury while leading his platoon into battle. He had injuries to an arm and a leg and was eventually evacuated to Japan for further treatment. As previously stated, I never knew much about his injuries, because my dad never talked about the war. He did have some impressive scars, though.

So, how did we get from two Army buddies—one from Ohio, the other from New York—to the present time? Well, my father spent time working in the hospital lab while he was recuperating. He had been a chemical engineering student when he enlisted, but he returned to the states with a newfound interest in medicine. After graduating from college, he was accepted into medical school at the University of Buffalo. He developed an interest in anesthesiology and ended up staying in Buffalo to continue his training (Fig. 98.1). One of his co-residents and friends was John Lauria, who went on to become chairman of anesthesiology in Buffalo. My dad moved back home and became chief of anesthesiology at St. Peter's Hospital in Albany, NY.

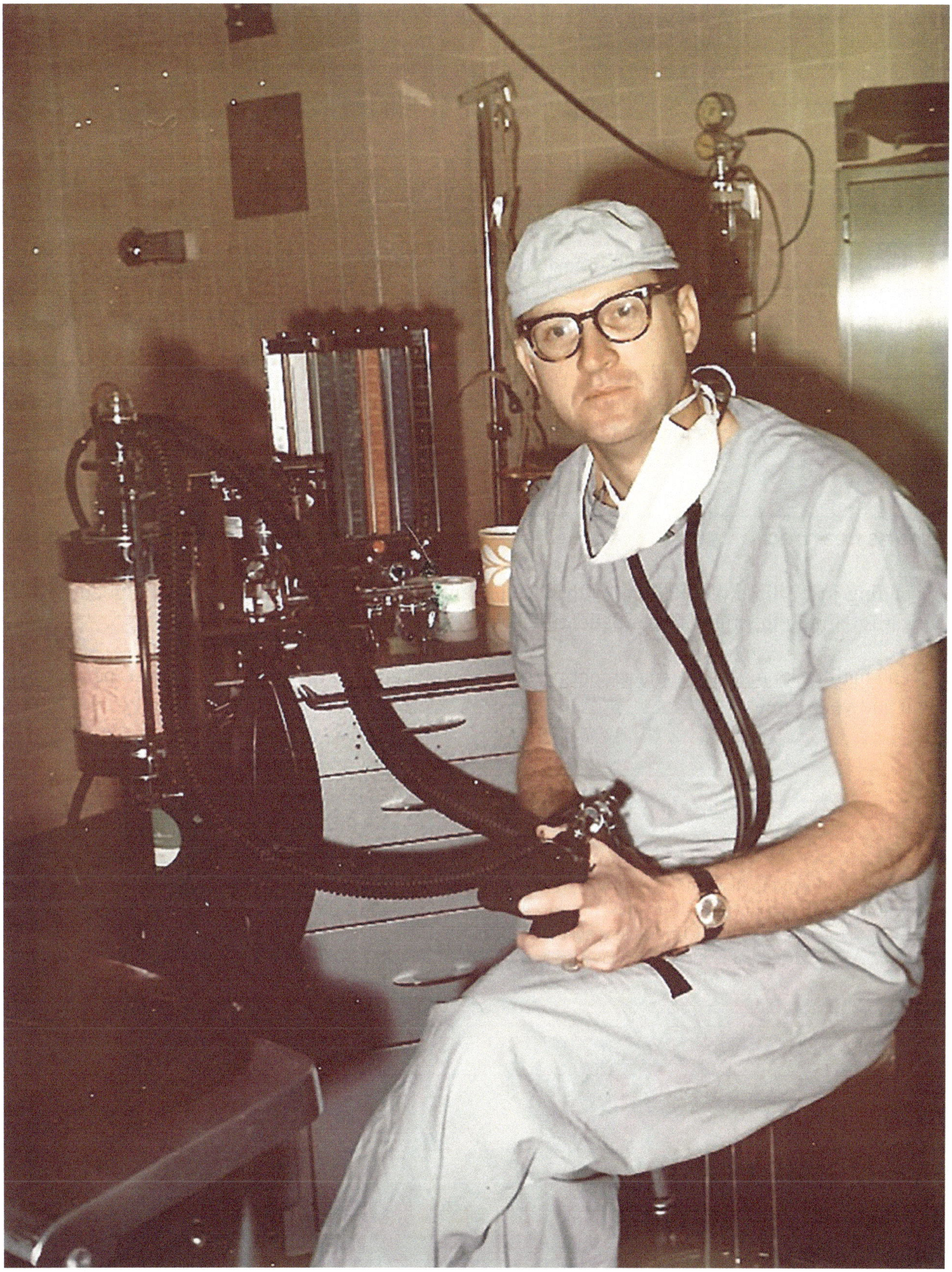

Fig. 98.1 Dr. James Graber circa 1965 while in anesthesia residency at the Meyer Memorial Hospital in Buffalo, NY. Photo: Collection of the Graber family

Along the way, he had six kids, and I (the oldest) got the medicine bug. I also wound up in Buffalo for medical school, where his old buddy, John Lauria, was an early mentor of mine. I went on to train and settle in Cleveland, and that is how, so many years later, I wound up taking care of this wonderful older gentleman who once went to war with my father.

Conclusion

The chain of events that led to me taking care of this gentleman was quite amazing. Jack had the satisfaction of hearing that my dad had recovered and flourished, and I got to fill in some missing history that I never knew about my dad.

So, in closing, I know that we all get rushed and pressed for time, and it is easy to just stick to medical facts. However, remember that getting to know your patients can lead to connections that patients really appreciate. And you never know what benefits it will bring you too.

Lessons Learned

- Spending just a little time talking with your patients can help ease anxiety and is a good first step towards earning the trust of your patient.
- Even small tasks like an IV placement performed well can lead to a patient's positive perception of you and your care.

Author

Ray Graber followed in his father's footsteps, from undergrad at RPI, to medical school at SUNY Buffalo, then into anesthesiology. He met his wife, Mary, just prior to finishing his training at University Hospitals of Cleveland. "Sorry Dad, I'm staying in Cleveland!" Jim Graber spent his career in private practice but took pride in teaching medical students from Albany Medical College. He was a past president of the New York State Society of Anesthesiologists.

Looking from the Outside In

99

Saundra E. Curry and Catherine Marcucci

The editors of *Anesthesia Bridges* are honored to posthumously publish the following essay by the late Dr. Curry, an esteemed author, teacher, mentor, and clinician.

Introduction from Dr. Curry

I became ill on March 12, 2020. It had nothing to do with COVID-19. I am on immunotherapy for cancer, and I was having a bad reaction to one of the medications. By the time it all resolved, it was 3 weeks later, and all hell had broken loose at my hospital.

Coronavirus Crisis and Conundrum

COVID-19 was all over the place. To nearly double hospital ICU capacity, most of our ORs were converted to ICUs (ORICU) with 4–6 patients apiece. As a result, we were performing only emergency surgery, so there was not much work for an OR anesthesiologist like myself to do. Our anesthesia staff were all converted to critical care physicians to staff the ORICUs. Residents, fellows, and faculty were playing a role. Yes, a few rotated through obstetrics and manned the emergency cases but most, along with surgeons, medical residents, and trained critical care doctors, took care of the impossibly sick patients in the now 80-patient ORICUs.

I was better now and under normal circumstances would be heading back to work. However, I had serious misgivings about this. I was in a very high-risk group, being over 60 years of age, with hypertension, and being treated for cancer. Did I have an obligation to go back to work in this situation, or should I be protecting myself? [1] Would I be doing anyone any good if I got sick and then my family and colleagues had to worry about me? If I did not go in, would I be considered shirking my duty as a physician and be thought less of by my colleagues? After all, one of the basic tenets of traditional medicine has always been going into the fray of war and disease, and this virus was both of those [2]. My primary desire was to help my colleagues during this crisis. I wanted to be useful.

S. E. Curry
Department of Anesthesiology, Columbia University, New York, NY, USA

C. Marcucci (✉)
Department of Transfusion Medicine, Clinical Center, National Institutes of Health, Bethesda, MD, USA

S. Mohamed et al. (eds.), *Anesthesia Bridges*, https://doi.org/10.1007/978-3-032-08294-7_99

Liaison

Then someone thought of something. The hospital closed to all visitors so the families of these ICU patients could not visit their loved ones. The ORICUs were not manned in the traditional ICU manner with occasional extra nurses, ward clerks, and even medical students. The clinical staff did not have the time to reach out as much as they would have liked to. Therefore, families had a hard time finding out what was happening to their loved ones. Sometimes, the first call they received was that their loved one had died. A network of volunteers was established to act as family liaisons to interact with the clinical staff and then connect with families. Best of all, it could be done by phone from home. I was not in the first group of volunteers, but as they opened more ORICUs, I found my place.

Some of the volunteers "attended" rounds via Zoom and participated in the care activities. I found this to be problematic. Though I had updated my computer and phone to be able to do this, often the connection was poor and my needing to reconnect was a distraction to rounds. Often, another patient was decompensating in the middle of rounds, so rounds stopped until things stabilized. This meant rounds could last for many hours and I thought my participation was more intrusive than helpful to the team. Others and I finally compromised and spoke to a senior member of the team after rounds. This meant my updates could be late in the day, but since my primary goal was to help my colleagues, that is what I did.

Many, though not all, of these volunteers were older members of the staff who had vast experience talking to patients and families, had solid medical backgrounds, and knew how to keep emotions in check while dealing with very emotional scenarios—including dying and death of patients. For example, one could be having a Zoom meeting with the family as they all watched as the patient took his last breath. As wrenching as these situations were, I personally felt it was worth it. Not only did my families get the information they needed, but I made phone friends.

***Note from the Editors:** A peaceful little bridge in a quiet wooded area (Fig. 99.1).

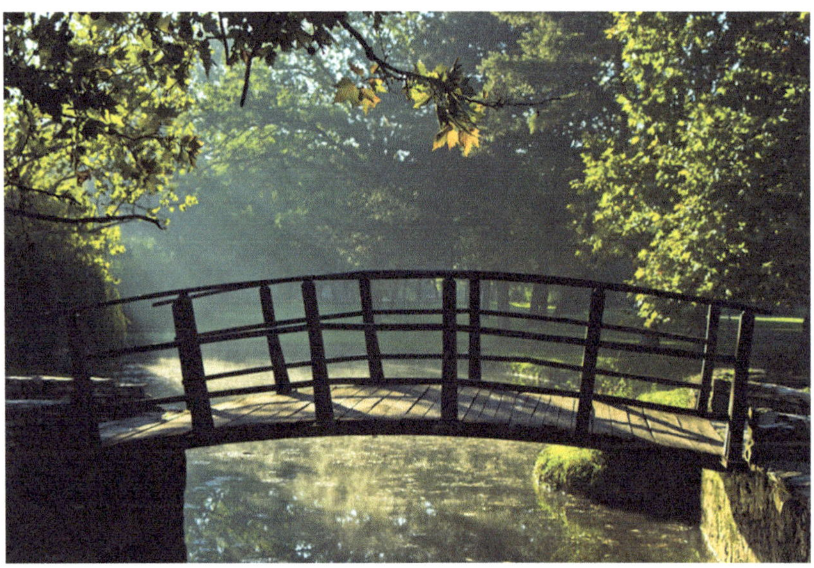

Fig. 99.1 A small rustic bridge in a peaceful forested location. Photo: Image used under standard license from stock.adobe.com

Different Conversations for Different Circumstances

My conversations were different with different people. While the patients were in the ORICU, the families were desperate for information. They hung on my every word and nuance, wanting to know why the patient needed a transfusion or why they were still on a ventilator and they would ever get better. A lot of patient families spoke only Spanish, and though my "anesthesia Spanish" is adequate, I did not think it was equal to discussing long-term goals and the fact that their loved one was dying. We have an excellent translator service which was quite helpful, but I still felt uncomfortable having difficult conversations through an interpreter. One of my colleagues is a native Spanish speaker, so we arranged for her to communicate with the Spanish-only patient families, and I would communicate with the English speakers.

Eventually, they began to close the ORICUs as the caseload decreased and the hospital began to restart elective surgery. This was a smooth process, but it meant that my patients were beginning to move out. The conversations with the families now were quite varied. I continued to follow my patients as they moved to another ICU. The patient's families could call the ICU and get information whenever they wanted, assuming someone picked up the phone. My conversations changed. They ranged from "I already talked to the ICU so unless you have something new, I don't need to talk to you," to "Yes, I talked to someone, but I'm only satisfied that I know everything once I've talked to you." I stopped calling the former and looked forward every day to talking with the latter.

One patient was extubated and moved directly to a floor bed. The conversation surrounding that event between the patient's husband and me was one of great rejoicing. The rest of my patients all received tracheostomies, so I had to explain that to families before the surgeons called for consent. After the trachs, the patients gradually moved out to trach units because they had stabilized enough.

One family had to go through the heart-wrenching decision to make their family member DNR. This was done with the great help of palliative care services. The patient was extremely ill, on dialysis, and had regular asystolic pauses. His condition precluded a pacemaker because of his infections. After the DNR order, the patient surprised everyone by starting to get better. His pauses stopped. His kidney function returned, so he no longer needed dialysis. His oxygenation improved with his trach. His sedation was decreased, and he became appropriately responsive. When he moved out to the trach unit, his wife and I had a joyful goodbye conversation. I told her I did not follow patients once they left our surgical-designated units. She was sad about that but happy for the reason.

I was very glad to get back to my usual anesthesia OR work once the pandemic was under better control. I derived a lot of satisfaction from being a family liaison for about two months and it seemed to help the families, too. Most importantly, I was able to relieve my colleagues of some added stress by carrying this burden for them. I felt useful.

Lessons Learned

- In times of crisis, normal processes can break down, and we as leaders may have to "think out of the box."
- Sometimes, there are other ways that we can contribute to patient care besides doing anesthesia.

References

1. Tsai C. Personal risk and societal obligation amidst COVID-19. JAMA. 2020;320(16):1555–6.
2. Koven S. They call us and we go. NEJM. 2020;382(21):1978–9.

Authors

Saundra Curry trained at Columbia and never left the mother ship. She was a clinician and spent her time teaching residents and medical students about anesthesia and medical professionalism. She was an active member of The Society for Education in Anesthesia (past president) and the ASA, serving on national committees and giving talks on education and professionalism nationally and internationally.

Cathy Marcucci is a senior academic anesthesiologist and inveterate anesthesiology educator. She spent several years of the pandemic training in transfusion medicine at the National Institutes of Health Clinical Center.

100 Adventures in London

James Berry

Introduction

During my fellowship year in 1989 in London, I was a "visiting registrar" at Guy's Hospital. The department was under the leadership of A.P. "Tony" Adams. He worked one afternoon a week doing pediatric dental cases. He actually only did one case most weeks, but he invited me along to watch and learn. The patient was a 3-year-old blonde girl, absolutely delightful and charming. The plan was an IV induction, as the Brits considered inhaled inductions in kids to be irresponsible.

Learning from the Best

Here's how it went: Patient on mother's lap, Prof telling her a story while patting her hand.

> This is the story of Tom Kitten. He was soft and lovely with black and white fur. He was usually well-behaved and kind, but occasionally he could be a bother. He could occasionally scratch or bite.
>
> And, the solution, should he scratch, is to say firmly to him, 'Stop that, Tom, you bad kitty.' Do you understand?

She nodded and the story went on in some detail. Quietly, the anesthesia assistant, known as an ODA, held her forearm a bit tighter as Prof slipped a butterfly needle into a hand vein.

"Stop that, Tom, you bad ki…" she said as the thiopental syringe was pushed. The Prof gathered her up in his arms, said goodbye to mum, and carried on with his intubation. It was the slickest pediatric induction I have ever seen and a great lesson in anesthesia.

J. Berry (✉)
Department of Anesthesiology and Pain Management, UT Southwestern Medical Center, Dallas, TX, USA
e-mail: James.Berry@UTSouthwestern.edu

S. Mohamed et al. (eds.), *Anesthesia Bridges*, https://doi.org/10.1007/978-3-032-08294-7_100

And Later...

As an aside, the Prof later that spring took me to the College of Anaesthetists dinner, where I was introduced to an elderly physician. He was small and soft-spoken, with wisps of grey hair and clear eyes. He seemed to be in his eighties, and I shook his hand as he quietly introduced himself, "Robert Macintosh, delighted to meet you." I didn't wash my hand for a week...

Sir Robert Macintosh died later that year at age 92.

We are all role models, whether we want to be or not... *James Berry, MD*

Lessons Learned

- It is instructive to watch experienced anesthesiologists at work. Many have developed stories or other strategies to distract patients during times of stress or pain.

Author

James Berry has spent his 34 years in academic medicine gaining perspective in four very different institutions: Univ Texas-Houston, Univ Mississippi, Vanderbilt, and now UT Southwestern. He also leads a busy non-academic life, with interests in aviation, radio/electronics, history, and home/auto repair. His life goal is to have some common ground with everyone he meets.

Putting Patients First

101

Neal Cohen

Introduction

When I began my career in medicine, the expectation was that when I assumed care of a patient, whether as a primary care provider, an anesthesiologist caring for the patient during the perioperative period, or in the intensive care unit, I "owned" the experience for the patient and had responsibility for managing the care. While the expectations may have been overblown, the concept was and remains critically important. Our patients expect us to guide their care, communicate the plan of care, get their input into decision making and implement strategies to ensure their health.

Evolution of Clinical Care Teams

Unlike what is illustrated in televisions and movies, the Marcus Welby, MD approach for those with long term memories of the television image of the perfect physician concept is naïve. In the current healthcare environment, particularly with respect to hospital-based care, clinical management is more commonly a team effort, including physicians, nurses, other health care providers, patients, and their families. No single provider is able to assume full responsibility for clinical management and decision making.

Anesthesia practice provides a vivid example of how health care delivery in general and the relationship with providers in particular has evolved. As an anesthesia resident, I recall meeting the majority of my patients the night before their operative procedure—even if that meant a Sunday night visit to perform the preoperative history and physical examination. On the day of surgery, I was not a stranger when I met the patient on arrival in the operating room, or may have personally transported the patient to the operating room (OR), obtained venous access, perhaps obtained blood samples for the blood bank or other lab studies, induced anesthesia, provided intraoperative care, and monitored the patient's course in the post-anesthesia care unit (PACU). The following day I make a postoperative visit to each patient to "check in "and determine if there are any anesthesia-related issues that needed to be addressed.

N. Cohen (✉)
Department of Anesthesiology, University of California, San Francisco School of Medicine, San Francisco, CA, USA
e-mail: CohenN@ucsf.edu

S. Mohamed et al. (eds.), *Anesthesia Bridges*, https://doi.org/10.1007/978-3-032-08294-7_101

Each patient, and most often their family members knew me by name and acknowledged my role in the care. We had established what I assumed was the normal patient-provider relationship, allowing me to fulfill my "contract" with the patient. Sound familiar? Unlikely. For many reasons, some related to improvements to optimize clinical care and make it more efficient and some related to changes in professional expectations, the course of perioperative care has changed dramatically.

Rarely does the anesthesia provider who will care for the patient during a procedure actually meet the patient until arrival in a preoperative holding area. Most often patients requiring anesthesia care no longer meet their anesthesia provider personally. Some are evaluated in a preoperative evaluation clinic, particularly if they have a complicated medical history or require more extensive preoperative management of underlying co-morbidities. Many others have telephone consultations with a nurse or anesthesia provider to review their history, medications, and other issues without undergoing any physical examination. The concept of a preoperative visit has become a preoperative assessment, often virtual and rarely involving the anesthesiologist responsible for intraoperative or postoperative care.

The perioperative course is now managed by a team of anesthesia providers, differentiating responsibilities for care in the operating room, PACU or ICU, and postoperative period. Anesthesia as a "team sport" undermines the ability to develop a meaningful relationship with the patient and to build a bond with the patient throughout the perioperative period. As a result, it is critically important to coordinate and communicate care among the diverse anesthesia care providers to ensure that the patient understands the role each plays; to optimize communication and facilitate safe transitions from the preoperative period throughout the perioperative course.

To do so, we must acknowledge how perioperative care is provided in our institutions and educate patients and their families about the collaborative relationships and commitment of all team members to their needs. Providing a single point of contact, either by providing a business card or single phone contact can ease patient and family concerns.

***Note from the Editors:** A charming bridge painting (Fig. 101.1).

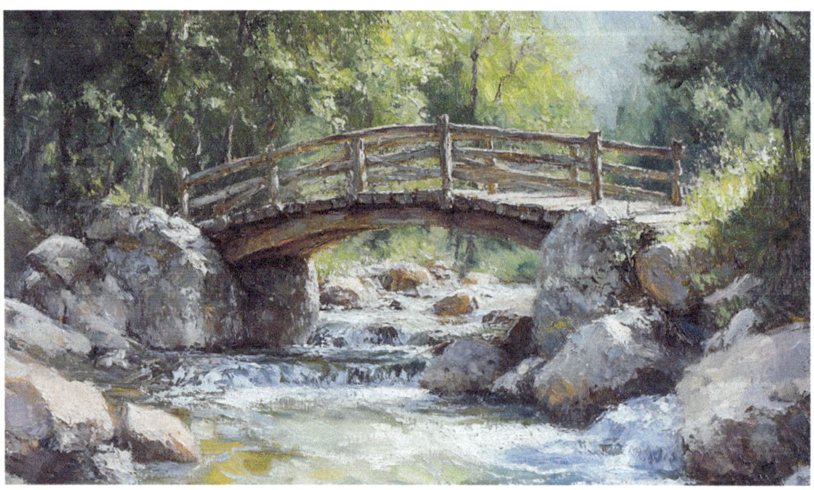

Fig. 101.1 Bridge painting by unknown artist. Perioperative care is now multi-layered with subtle overlaps, just like the artistic representation of this bridge. Photo: Image used under standard license from stock.adobe.com

Coordination of Care

When participating in any aspect of perioperative care, each provider should introduce her/himself to the patient (with mask removed, if clinically appropriate), define the role, and reinforce the fact that the team approach will not compromise care. In addition, it is important to explain to patients that care is coordinated, but that to ensure safety, repeated questioning about NPO status, medications, allergies, and site of surgery are not a reflection of lack of coordination but designed to ensure safe care.

In addition to the changes taking place in anesthesia care during the perioperative period, similar challenges exist in coordinating care with the other members of the team, including the surgeons. The surgical evaluation of a patient has become less rigorous, relying on the primary care provider and anesthesiologists to "clear" the patient for surgery.

At the same time, both the surgeon and anesthesiologist have responsibility for the perioperative care of the patient, particularly those undergoing complex surgical procedures and those with underlying medical conditions. To prevent misunderstandings and delays and minimize cancellations, there must be better communication between the anesthesia team and the surgical team throughout the perioperative course. Since direct communication is challenging, we have defined new ways to "communicate" and manage transitions of care.

Checklists, flow diagrams, and, in theory, the electronic medical record, can help with coordination of care across the continuum. In reality, while checklists and pre and postoperative huddles have improved communication and, in many cases reduced complications, they do not replace the need for both the anesthesia providers and surgical team to establish a relationship with each patient, to advocate on behalf of the patient, and support the patient's needs throughout the perioperative course. While "ownership" of the clinical experience is a different concept than it has been in the past, the need to ensure that each team defines a way to fulfill this responsibility is essential for patients, providers, and health care organizations.

Lessons Learned

- Medicine has moved from physician-centric care to team-based care. Consequently, it is harder for us as anesthesiologists to build a relationship with our patients.
- Good communication between surgical and anesthesia team members and with patients is essential to ensure great patient care.

Author

Neal Cohen has been a member of the faculty at the University of California San Francisco for the majority of his career. During his tenure, he has been fortunate to participate in the care of patients in the operating room and both pediatric and adult ICUs. In addition to his clinical opportunities, he has extensive experience in building relationships with other health systems and academic institutions internationally, primarily in the Pacific Rim. At the time Neal wrote this chapter for us, his academic role was vice dean for the school of medicine providing oversight of professional service relationships and affiliations as well as compliance, risk management, and regulatory affairs.

102 Communicating with Patients and Families

Neal Cohen

Introduction

Communicating with our patients and families is integral to the practice of medicine. For anesthesiologists, in addition to establishing a relationship with a patient, one of our primary responsibilities is to understand patient goals of care, to inform patients of our plans and associated risks, benefits and alternatives and to reassure each patient that we will provide the best care we can to ensure a good outcome. This communication takes many forms and has many implications.

Initial and Personal Experiences

Our initial interaction with a patient sets the stage for the rest of the relationship. Not only does it allow us to establish a therapeutic relationship, but we also use it to obtain "informed consent." The process for obtaining informed consent has changed over time, as patients request more information about the plans of care and its consequences. At the same time, the interaction with patients is short and often does not allow a lengthy discussion. In addition, patients are often frightened, perhaps intimidated and may not hear what they are told, may not understand what is said, and are often hesitant to ask questions.

I had a personal experience that reinforces the challenge associated with patient communication. My father had an appointment to meet with an oncologist to discuss management of his newly diagnosed leukemia. I happened to be visiting my parents at the time of the visit, so I joined them. Having cared for many patients with malignancies and seen them without hair, looking pale and gaunt, I was not fazed by what I saw. My parents, on the other hand, were overwhelmed.

When they subsequently met with the physician and a nurse practitioner, the physician provided as clear and thoughtful a discussion of the plan of care and its implications as I could have expected. He and my parents had a lengthy discussion, questions were asked and answered, and they were provided information to take home for their reference. I was impressed and pleased—until we walked out the door. As we

N. Cohen (✉)
Department of Anesthesiology, University of California, San Francisco School of Medicine, San Francisco, CA, USA
e-mail: CohenN@ucsf.edu

S. Mohamed et al. (eds.), *Anesthesia Bridges*, https://doi.org/10.1007/978-3-032-08294-7_102

left, I realized that although my parents interacted with the physician, they had no more idea about what to expect after the meeting than they did before they met him. Since I was witness to the discussion and plan, I was able to reinforce what had been told to them. Had I not participated in the interaction, my parents would have been lost.

ICU Experiences

This personal experience reinforced what I already experienced when meeting with patients and families when working in the ICU, though it never occurred to me that my experience would be the same. I learned early in my career to have the ICU social worker participate in discussions whenever possible. Her role was primarily to listen to the discussion, ask for clarification, if the message was not clear. After the discussion, I excuse myself and allow the patient and/or family to meet with the social worker alone. She is able to clarify what is "heard," not what is said—allowing us to address any misunderstandings and hopefully more effectively address questions and concerns.

The process used in the ICU has been very useful, not only for disseminating information, but also in clarifying goals. One more situation exemplifies the challenge. An ICU patient with a terminal illness was receiving full supportive care, despite his poor prognosis. In lengthy discussions with the patient and his family about goals of care, they were realistic, but "hoping for a miracle' 'and were insisting that full care be continued.

As we discussed options, we learned that the patient and his wife were recently married, and he had adopted her two children from a previous marriage. With help from the social worker, we also learned that he had a life insurance policy which he purchased just before his illness—and that it had a "waiting period" of another two weeks before being available to his family. If the policy was not available to his wife and children, they would have no resources and would lose their house.

Based on this information, we contacted the insurance company to request removal of the time restriction—and they agreed. The patient transitioned to comfort care and died in his wife's arms. Had we not "communicated" effectively with the patient and family, we would have been working at cross purposes and potentially created an antagonistic, rather than a therapeutic relationship.

Plan of Care

While the issues that arise when communicating with patients about to undergo a surgical procedure are more straightforward than the situations described, anesthesiologists must also be aware of the patient's goals of care and that each patient understands and consents to proceed with the plan of care. Since the preoperative interactions are short and often involve multiple different providers, this discussion can be challenging.

Some institutions are utilizing web-based tools that can be used by patients at home to educate them about their upcoming anesthetic and surgical procedure as a way to reinforce the message provided during the personal discussions with the providers. This web-based information also helps patients prepare questions for the provider to make the discussion more interactive and helpful. It does not minimize the need to review the plans and to discuss goals of care as part of the preoperative assessment.

Most importantly, whatever methods are used to obtain informed consent, we must understand the patient's goals of care. In order for us to make clinical management decisions, we need to confirm that the patient understands what has been discussed and has an opportunity to clarify any concerns and agrees to proceed. This discussion is a fundamental part of the patient-provider relationship. Your plan is **ALWAYS** based on your patient's plan (Fig. 102.1).

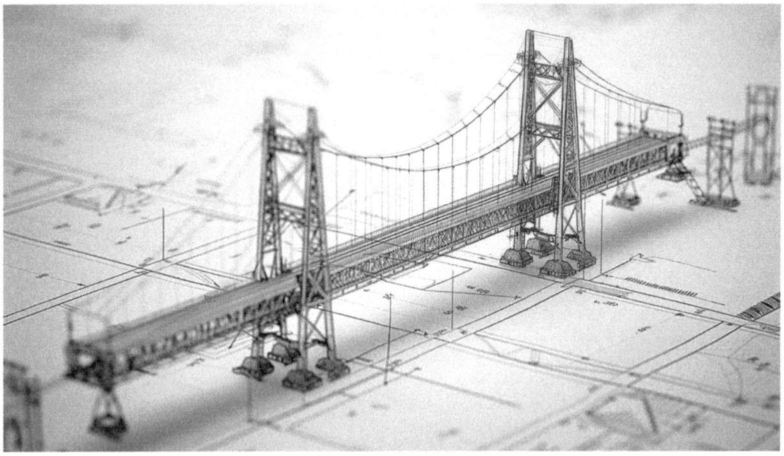

Fig. 102.1 Do not assume that the right thing or correct action is going to happen on its own. Think it through; *plan* it out! Photo: Image used under standard license from stock.adobe.com

Lessons Learned

- Our initial interaction with a patient sets the stage for the rest of the relationship.
- Anesthesiologists must be aware of the patient's goals of care and that each patient understands and consents to proceed with the plan of care.

Author

Neal Cohen has been a member of the faculty at the University of California San Francisco for the majority of his career. During his tenure, he has been fortunate to participate in the care of patients in the operating room and both pediatric and adult ICUs. In addition to his clinical opportunities, he has extensive experience in building relationships with other health systems and academic institutions internationally, primarily in the Pacific Rim. His current role is vice dean for the school of medicine providing oversight of professional service relationships and affiliations as well as compliance, risk management, and regulatory affairs.

A Case for Humanistic Traits as a Necessary Attribute for Physician Anesthesiologists

103

Mark E. Hudson

The practice of medicine is an art, not a trade; a calling, not a business; a calling in which your heart will be exercised equally with your head.—Dr. William Osler

I received a call recently from our preoperative holding area that a patient wanted to "change their anesthesiologist." In my discussion with the patient, he indicated that the physician was "in a rush" and "kept cutting him off" indicating that "he was too busy to answer my questions" and that "he barely looked at me." The patient's confidence in his prospective care was low, he felt unsafe, and was considering cancelling. After taking a few moments to understand his concerns and fears, and having reviewed his information and planned procedure, together we outlined a plan for his anesthetic, and I asked if he would allow me to care for him. He visibly relaxed and his procedure and anesthetic proceeded without incident. Later a glowing review was received by the hospital president regarding his overall patient care experience.

A Humanistic Approach

The anesthesiologist in question was one of our most knowledgeable and technically skilled physicians. However, his hurried interaction with this patient created a lack of confidence in the level of care he would provide in the operating room (OR), which created stress and fear for the patient.

Over the last decade, there has been an increasing incidence of patient dissatisfaction in our practice because physician anesthesiologists are not reflecting the humanistic qualities that patients expect. The preop evaluation has become just another task to complete, rather than serving as an essential tool in establishing a patient-physician relationship. This crucial interaction **should** allay stress and fear, act as a patient-centered anesthetic prescription, and set expectations for the patient. Unfortunately, it often does not.

While knowledge and technical skill are vital in what we do, our overarching role is shepherding patients safely through the perioperative period, while they are at their most vulnerable. With this in mind, a humanistic approach demonstrating empathy, compassion, and understanding specific-patient goals and fears contributes significantly to the quality of patient care we provide.

M. E. Hudson (✉)
Department of Anesthesiology and Perioperative Medicine, University of Pittsburgh School of Medicine, Pittsburgh, PA, USA
e-mail: HudsonME@anes.upmc.edu

S. Mohamed et al. (eds.), *Anesthesia Bridges*, https://doi.org/10.1007/978-3-032-08294-7_103

Managing Our Stress

Managing our own daily pressures and stressors is the first step in maintaining a humanistic outlook. Certainly, increasing production pressure demands, documentation burdens, and other non-clinical pressures related to our work has reduced the time available to interact with our patients. However, the degree of impact and the interference during our limited time to converse with patients can be moderated.

Often, the most difficult transition trainees have in becoming attending anesthesiologists is the requirement to manage multiple rooms at a time. In my experience, faculties who communicate well with their teams, are proactive in tasks associated with patient care, and develop routines and a set cadence in the management of their daily work are less stressed, and more able to have positive, valuable, interactions with their patients, with limited interference from other demands.

Then Manage the Patient's Stress

Approaching every patient engagement with an expected standard, with humility and empathy, in a patient focused way will enhance the value of your patient interactions, both in terms of developing the best anesthetic plan and in reducing anxiety and stress in the patient. The patient likely has an expectation for your behavior. Alignment with this expectation will confirm the trust the patient has in your care. Understand the honor associated with a patient's trust, in you, as their physician. Show humility; **"It will be my privilege to take care of you today."**

Treat patients as you would like to be treated. Seek a connection with the patient; ask them where they are from, what kind of work they do, what they do for fun. A patient's fear often extends beyond fear of their diagnosis or the procedure. They may be fearful of loss of autonomy or financial implications of the surgery and recovery. Self-reflection, understanding that **no matter how bad your day is going, the patient's day is most likely worse** can be a reminder of the need for patience, empathy, and compassion in your interactions, and decision making.

Likely, you already know much of the patient's history and medical condition from the medical record prior to meeting your patient. While confirming and expanding on those specifics will be necessary, time spent should have a specific goal to foster a connection, allaying fears, and instilling confidence, resulting in a reduction in stress and anxiety. Do not be hurried or gruff. If you are interrupted, politely disengage, and confirm you will return to talk more. Importantly, understand their specific concerns regarding care; **"What worries, or concerns do you have with your anesthesia care or surgery?"** Specifically addressing these concerns confirms your attention and focus on their care. Offer to answer any questions and disengage with a smile and an offer to be contacted if any questions or concerns arise.

This humanistic approach sets the stage for a patient centered approach, anchored by the establishment of a true doctor-patient relationship, with care grounded in empathy and compassion.

Healthcare has evolved dramatically over the last few decades and Physicians often lament the loss of the ideals that drew us to medicine. While our knowledge and technical skills have never been stronger as physician anesthesiologists, attention to essential humanistic habits have diminished. Develop and nourish your humanistic traits. These likely are the traits that attracted you to medicine. Approach each patient with humility, empathy, and compassion—the quality of the care you provide depends on it!

Lessons Learned

- Hurried and dismissive interactions with patients create a lack of confidence in care and contribute to the patient's stress and fear.
- Faculty who communicate well with their teams, are proactive in tasks associated with patient care, develop routines, and a set cadence in the management of their daily work are less stressed, and more able to have positive and valuable interactions with their patients.
- A humanistic approach demonstrating empathy, compassion, and understanding specific patient goals and fears, contributes significantly to the quality of patient care we provide.

Author

Mark Hudson is from a small Western Pennsylvania steel town. Owing to lessons in hard work and compassion, and with incredible sacrifices and support from amazing parents, he achieved his dream of becoming a physician. He has spent his entire 30-year career at the University of Pittsburgh, at all levels of leadership in the Department of Anesthesiology and Perioperative Medicine, buoyed by remarkable mentors and colleagues, and sustained by the incredible and unique opportunities presented to him.

Interacting with Patients: Small Gestures Can Be a Big Comfort

104

Zeyd Ebrahim

Introduction

One of the limitations of anesthesiology and acute care medicine is the amount of "face time" we spend with our patients. The preoperative period can be stressful and anxiety-provoking for the patient. It is extremely important that as anesthesiologists we work to create an environment of caring, respect, and stress reduction from the first time we meet our patients.

Small Gestures

I have always found that small things like getting them a warm blanket, conversations with them about medical concerns, and at times thoughtful humor or a funny comment will go a long way to reducing stress and creating a milieu of care. Fortunately, the morbidity and mortality associated with anesthesia is low, and outcomes are good. However, it seems that the patients we deal with are sicker and more complicated with an occasional adverse operative outcome. Thus, it is so important that the pre-induction conversations we have with our patients should be respectful, positive, and not taken for granted.

Lessons Learned

- Remember the small things—like getting a warm blanket, having thoughtful conversations, or sharing a moment of humor—to help reduce patient stress and bring them comfort.

Z. Ebrahim (✉)
Anesthesiology Institute, Cleveland Clinic, Cleveland, OH, USA
e-mail: EBRAHIZ@ccf.org

S. Mohamed et al. (eds.), *Anesthesia Bridges*, https://doi.org/10.1007/978-3-032-08294-7_104

Bonus Content!

We greatly appreciate Zeyd's advice and were motivated to take a peek into the literature to see what we could find as to why small acts have such a big impact. We were able to come up with a couple of simple concepts.

- **First**, we work at a unique position in the perioperative period, and we possess a specific agency—nobody else in the perioperative period does what we do.
- **Second**, we are positioned at the hub of activity—just think about us hustling around in the morning to get rooms started, right?
- **Third**, we work at the interface of communication with the patient—usually we are the first physicians to speak to the patient when they arrive at the door of the preop area, the last person to speak with them before the anesthesia starts and the first to speak with them when the surgical case and anesthetic is over.
- **Fourth**, we regulate access to the surgical care of the patient, to a large extent.
- An interesting aspect about the "small things" is that there are so many opportunities per day to do these things. These acts of kindness are accessible to both the giver and recipient and can often be done with little advance planning.
- The psychologists tell us that there are as many or more psychological, emotional, and even physical benefits for the giver as for the recipient. It is apparently a dopamine, serotonin, **and** oxytocin thing.
- There is quite a bit of hard science, if you want to delve deep into the psychology and the neurobiology of why small acts of kindness are so memorable [1, 2].
- For our patients, the perioperative period is one that is unfamiliar, such that all processing pathways—auditory, visual, and tactile—are activated.
- Many complex principles govern sensory perception, but to give a very simple overview, humans are very adept at multi-sensory processing, particularly of visual and tactile stimuli, which have similar neural processing pathways. There is also top-down processing of haptic stimuli, so a warm soft blanket will be processed both by the haptic sensory pathways and the early visual cortex (even in the absence of visual input), which may perhaps heighten the sensory experience and hence positive memories.
- Apart from the neuro-scientists, the social scientists have done quite a bit of work in the domains of kindness, gift giving, and service, particularly as society and the economy become more service based. You could write a PhD thesis on the subject (and many have), but small acts of service and kindness to our patients, while seeming to be marginalized and almost invisible, derive their importance from their highly symbolic nature.
- This involves something called the cultural technique of service. Superficially, we would seem to have all the knowledge and power over the patient. For instance, we are clothed, and they are not. We

are standing and they are in a dependent position. We understand the timeline of their planned care and the technology that is to be employed far more than they do.

- In actuality, the reverse is true—we exist in the milieu of the perioperative period to provide a medical service to the patient. We are actually there to do a good job for them, not the other way around. So, there is a dual reality in operation, which can create psychic tension. The social scientists tell us that small acts of kindness resonate so much with patients because on an emotional and psychological level, they lower the barriers between these realties and help the patient integrate the perioperative experience. To give a simple example—we can tell the patient that we are there to help them get through the perioperative period as comfortably and safely as possible but getting them a warm blanket **reinforces** that message by accessing visual and tactile sensory processing to present to them as well.

- You and your patient will benefit greatly from these gestures, but you have to do them. **As Oscar Wilde said, "The smallest gesture is worth more than the grandest intention."**

***Note from the Editors:** If you are going to build a small bridge in a landscape, why not give it maximum impact? This little bright blue bridge is a perfect illustration of this principle (Fig. 104.1).

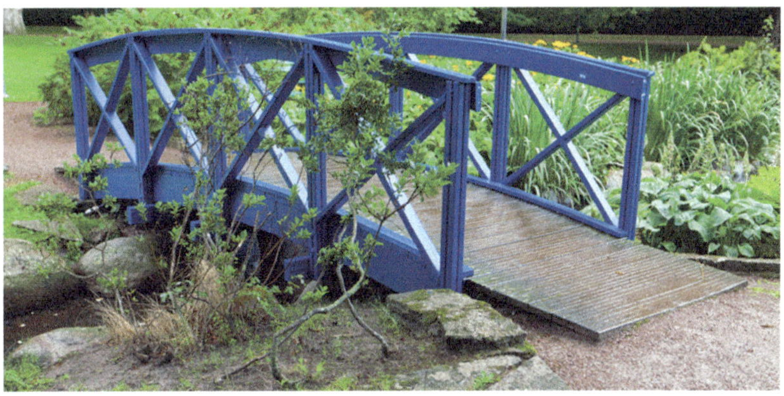

Fig. 104.1 A tiny blue bridge. Photo: voyagerix, image used under license from iStock.com

References

1. Krajewski M. The power of small gestures: on the cultural technique of service. Theory Culture Soc. 2013;30(6):epub. Accessed June 5, 2023
2. The science behind kindness and how it's good for your health. [Internet]. Ssmhealth.com. 2022 [cited 2025 Jul 27]. Available from: https://www.ssmhealth.com/blogs/ssm-health-matters/november-2022/

Author

Zeyd Ebrahim and his wife Lilian did their respective residencies at the Cleveland Clinic, and upon completing their training, joined the professional staff. Residents of Cleveland since 1977, they consider themselves fortunate to have had professionally satisfying careers at the Cleveland Clinic.

Connecting with Pediatric Patients and Their Parents

105

Nicholas V. Bishop and Kirk Lalwani

Introduction

Nicholas Bishop is a pediatric anesthesiology fellow at Oregon Health and Science University. He completed his residency training at the University of Washington and attended medical school at Thomas Jefferson University.

Kirk Lalwani is a professor of anesthesiology and pediatrics at Oregon Health and Science University. He completed his residency training and fellowship at King's College, the Royal London, and Great Ormond Street Hospital for Children in London, England, after attending medical school at St. John's National Academy of Medical Sciences in Bangalore, India. He has been an attending pediatric anesthesiologist for 24 years.

Below we give thoughts from Nick and Kirk on evolving your communication style to meet the needs of the pediatric anesthesia patient and, of course, the parents as well.

This Is a Learnable Skill!

Communicating and connecting with pediatric patients and their parents is based a bit on the inherent personality of the anesthesia provider but is also a learned skill and can be improved with careful observation and practice.

Familiarity with developmental stages of different age groups in children is helpful as you approach the preoperative interview. Remember you are privileged to be able to take care of this family's precious child, and you must earn their confidence that you will provide excellent family-centered care.

What does this mean? Establish rapport with the child based on their age and developmental stage. Conversations about favorite princesses works wonders for young girls, as do superheroes and video games for boys. Their favorite animated movie is another excellent topic, and all pediatric anesthesiolo-

N. V. Bishop · K. Lalwani (✉)
Department of Anesthesiology, Oregon Health & Science University, Portland, OR, USA
e-mail: lalwanik@ohsu.edu

S. Mohamed et al. (eds.), *Anesthesia Bridges*, https://doi.org/10.1007/978-3-032-08294-7_105

gists should be familiar with the current crop of popular children's movies and TV shows. Other popular topics are sports, hobbies, and cultural memes for older kids. We go into the practice of pediatric anesthesia because we are devoted to the care of children and it is helpful and great to show interest and develop an instant connection.

Sit down at the level of the child to converse if possible. Make the family comfortable by allowing them to express their apprehension and answer all their questions honestly. There is a lot of information on the internet about anesthesia for children and, in our experience, parents have often read it. **Make sure that you know more about whatever topic they might raise than they do**. The goal is to project a quiet, gentle knowledge and confidence about the topics and situations that might be causing anxiety to the parents, because the patient is certainly reading these signals from his family.

It is very helpful to get the parents' opinions about what approach would work best for their child, such as route of premedication, versus IV placement, distraction, child-life issues, and so forth. But it is also important to retain control of your clinical case. Here the trick is to maintain a respectful deference to the parents—do not **ever** argue or debate about a child with a parent or imply in the slightest way that they have provided substandard care for their child.

When interacting with the patient, a combination of approaches is often the best approach. Enter into conversation with your patient gently, perhaps by asking if she has a nickname that she wants the nurses to use. This acknowledges the patient's self and gives her a tiny bit of autonomy. It is also helpful to know and use the appropriate pronouns for transgender teenagers to make them comfortable.

Be wary of joking at the child's expense as this can easily backfire. Older children love "knock-knock" jokes or "Dad" jokes, but it is very child dependent. **IF** you use that technique, start by asking the (older) child what their favorite joke is. Lack of an enthusiastic response usually means the child is too nervous, or is not into jokes, in which case it is best to move on. If you get stuck on a communication point, a good segue is to make a neutral factual statement such as, "The nurse from the operating room who will be checking you in is named Patti. She has five kids (or a cute cat and a gigantic dog)."

To make things even more interesting, the practice of pediatric anesthesia has several special and delicate communication issues:

- **First**, the practice of pediatric anesthesia is one of the only clinical anesthesia situations that involves greeting and talking to the family as much, if not more, than the patient. Here is what we recommend and usually do: if the patient is less than two years old, greet the parents first and conduct the preoperative interview with the parents only. Interaction with the patient who is less than two years of age is only for rapport-building and playful, toy-related comments.

- We start talking to the patients at around age two years, with increasing detail as the age of the child increases, depending on maturity. At around age five years (approximately), we discuss consent to the process of undergoing anesthesia.

- Until around age 12, we greet the parents first and have the preoperative discussion with the parents, then speak with the patient. When the patient is an adolescent or teenager, we greet and speak with the patient first, then turn to the parents. In practice, parents will often involve their child in the conversation even when they are much younger or conversely try to answer for their teenager even when you address the patient! Follow their cues but always speak to older patients directly even if a parent is answering for them.

- **Second**, if your hospital culture allows parents to accompany a child to the operating room, communicate clearly about that. It is universally understood that the anesthesiologist makes the final decision as to the advisability of this and how to do it. If the parent would not be going to the OR with the child, briefly describe the induction of anesthesia in terms of the things the parent really wants to know. Will someone be holding the patient's hand? How long will the induction take? What will the child likely remember of being in the OR?

- Also, if the parents are staying in the waiting room, think about and develop something empathic and reassuring to say to the parents right as you transport the patient. For example, one of our colleagues who is also a pediatrician would mention that at the end of the preoperative conversation—quickly and just once. Or if you are a parent, you can mention that. This is just to find a kind way to help ease the difficult wait ahead for the parents.

- **Third**, communicate carefully about the immediate postoperative period. When will the parents be able to see their child? What are the after-effects of anesthesia? What should they expect? What is the plan to manage pain, delirium, and nausea? Families of adult patients expect that there will be something of an interminable wait and then the patient will have some amount of grogginess and pain when they can first visit their loved one in the postoperative period. Parents of children undergoing procedures know this on an intellectual level, but we have seen parents really get thrown for a loop when they experience it with their little one.

- **Fourth**, be extremely cautious about being cheery and humorous with children who have a serious diagnoses or chronic illness, or families with a new or recurrent grave diagnosis like cancer. Likewise, children with developmental issues often necessitate special consideration guided by the family's experiences and this is typically not a situation for humor.

- **Finally**, if you have the right patient and parents, you can use your experience and intuition to make it fun! The patient's Teddy Bear or Mr. Otter can definitely get a hat and a mask. Or explain to the child that they will get to choose a favorite scent for their space mask, decorate it with stickers, and then try to blow up a balloon with it, and if they pop it, they can have a popsicle for breakfast when they wake up and then go home!

***Note from the Editors:** Kirk Lalwani is a fan of mysteries and other crime and police shows. We are including the Oresund Bridge, connecting Sweden and Denmark, in his honor (Fig. 105.1) since the bridge and its environs are the setting of the Nordic *noir* television drama *The Bridge*.

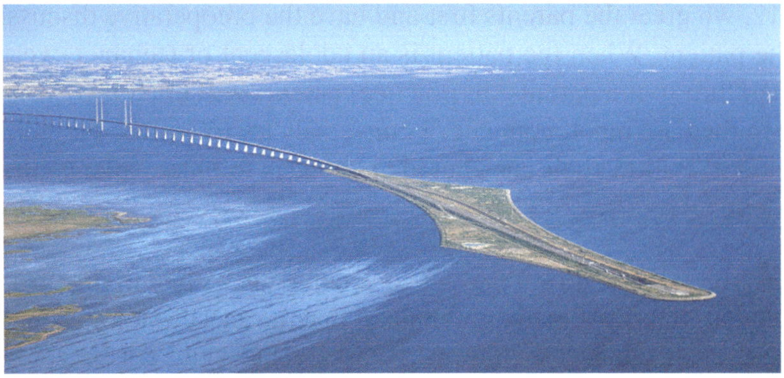

Fig. 105.1 The Oresund Bridge spans the Oresund Strait and connects Sweden and Denmark. It is a combined railway and motorway bridge. It is a most interesting bridge as one terminus is on a man-made island in the middle of the strait and the bridge then becomes the Drogden Tunnel that continues to Denmark. The justifications for the extra expense in digging the tunnel were to minimize interference with the nearby Copenhagen Airport, provide a clear shipping channel, and to minimize the effect of ice floes in winter. The submerged tunnel is now covered in marine organisms and has become an artificial reef. This is the view of the bridge when taking off from the Copenhagen airport. Photo: Image used under standard license from stock.adobe.com

Lessons Learned

- Adapt to the developmental stage of your patient with open body language and ageget and stay up to date on appropriate topics of interest which they are likely to be interested in order to establish rapport early on in the discussion.
- Involve the parents in the decision—making process; their invaluable knowledge of their child is a useful resource.
- Be cautious about being cheery and humorous, especially with children who have a serious diagnoses or chronic illness, or families with a new or recurrent grave diagnosis like cancer.
- Keep the atmosphere light when possible but always acknowledge any parental concerns by responding honestly and clearly.
- More than any other area of anesthetic practice, the goal when doing pediatric cases is to **communicate warm empathy and the utmost in calm competence.**
- These communication skills are something of a gift but can also be learned if you approach the issue with motivation and discipline and practice. Find senior practitioners who do this well and study them!

Authors

Nicholas Bishop was a pediatric anesthesiology fellow at Oregon Health and Science University in Portland, Oregon and then moved to Seattle for a job at Swedish First Hill Hospital. He enjoys music, travel, and the great outdoors. One of his dreams is to become a proficient sailor and to explore every last corner of Puget Sound in his native Washington state.

Kirk Lalwani is an attending pediatric anesthesiologist at Doernbecher Children's Hospital at Oregon Health and Science University in Portland, Oregon. He loves to travel, explore different musical genres, and is an avid SCUBA diver. He also considers himself a crime fiction and police procedural TV series aficionado. His dream is to live on every continent (only three to go!) and continue the agonizingly slow process of becoming a proficient pianist as an adult learner.

Connecting with Patients in the OB Suite

106

Brandon M. Togioka, Jennifer N. Tripi,
Christopher E. Swide, and Catherine Marcucci

Introduction

The authors have all practiced obstetrical anesthesiology for some or most of their careers. They all credit significant role models and mentors with providing instruction, guidance, and examples of masterful communication. We are delighted to include a photo of Brandon's favorite mentors—his parents, Bob and Patricia Togioka. They are superbly gifted teachers who have dedicated their lives to breaking down communication barriers (Fig. 106.1).

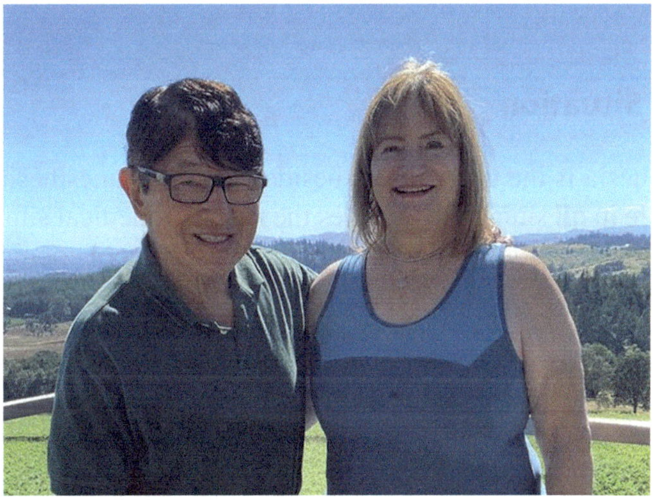

Fig. 106.1 Bob and Patricia Togioka—Brandon's parents, role models, and mentors. Aren't they great looking? At a young age, they dedicated themselves to Deaf education and attended Gallaudet University, the only university in the world where students learn through American Sign Language. After graduation they taught at the Oregon School for the Deaf for decades, where Patricia rose to the position of superintendent. Bob then refused to retire and worked for a number of years in a public school where he led the American Sign Language program. In Brandon's words, "They taught me to lead with humility and a serve-first mentality, without expectation for recognition, and to seek out the underserved." Photo: Collection of the Togioka family

B. M. Togioka · C. E. Swide
Department of Anesthesiology and Perioperative Medicine, Oregon Health & Science University, Portland, OR, USA

J. N. Tripi
Department of Anesthesiology, University of North Carolina at Chapel Hill, Chapel Hill, NC, USA

C. Marcucci (✉)
Department of Transfusion Medicine, Clinical Center, National Institutes of Health, Bethesda, MD, USA

S. Mohamed et al. (eds.), *Anesthesia Bridges*, https://doi.org/10.1007/978-3-032-08294-7_106

Basics: Meeting the Mom Where She's At

For most women, having a positive birth experience goes beyond remaining personally safe and delivering a healthy child. A positive birth experience is highly correlated with a feeling of personal achievement and involvement with medical decision-making. Anesthesia providers can promote this by offering true informed consent, timely supportive and empathetic words, and enabling patient autonomy, as much as is feasible.

We are all taught when we first rotate on the labor and delivery suite that the mother's health and well-being take priority over the baby's. However, as any person who has ever delivered a baby will tell you, that is not the mother's priority. The supreme concern of the parturient is that the baby does well and this anxiety can be paradoxically heightened after an uncomplicated pregnancy, as the mom-to-be is almost there in her prime and instinctual drive to deliver a healthy baby.

Though this is not formally taught and rarely discussed, parturients can also have a weird sense of aloneness, even while surrounded by medical staff, their partners, and other family members. It is a sense of being trapped in a process from which they cannot detach. More than one woman has been known to say, "You know what, I'm not doing this." It is a shock to look around and realize that there is only one person who has the job of delivering the baby and you are that person. What goes through your mind is, "Yeah, it's easy for you to tell me what to do, you don't have to do it."

Managing the Social Situation

The practice of OB anesthesia is the other place, besides pediatric anesthesia where you must remain calm, cool, and unflappable in **all** situations. Besides the range of medical situations and levels of medical, anesthesia, and obstetrical acuity, remember that you must be cool enough to deal with all kinds of "social" situations. We have seen:

- A 10-year-old parturient, crying hysterically, and calling for her own mother.
- A 60-year-old parturient (surrogate) delivering her own grandchild.
- A man on the L and D suite who was having babies with two different women at the same time. He kept going back and forth between the labor rooms.
- Enormous marital and relationship and family tension and drama. Once we saw a couple come in arguing about a marital infidelity. Actually, not arguing, screaming. They fought off and on throughout the whole labor period. At one point, the father was escorted out. The woman delivered the baby, asked to see the father, and when he leaned over to coo at the infant, she slapped him in the face.
- No matter what drama ensues, it is not our job or place to interact with it any more than is absolutely necessary. Our job is to focus on the vital signs and the fetal tracing and the airway, if necessary. You can even say that, if necessary, "My job is to make sure you stay safe from a medical standpoint and that we make the situation as safe as possible for the baby."

- Trauma-informed obstetric care has become a hot topic. Trauma-informed care requires that we first seek to understand a patient's trauma, then craft our anesthetic plan to meet their medical and psychosocial needs. This trauma can be related to a past birth or a non-medical experience. Perhaps the most common concern that we see pre-delivery is severe anxiety due to a past experience.

- As anesthesiologists we are especially prepared to deal with this situation. Listen, validate, and collaborate to create an anesthetic plan that meets the patient's needs. Ask, "I'm sorry for what you experienced, what can I do and avoid in order to help you have the best birth experience possible?" Also, do not be afraid to use anxiolytic medications and sedation, when appropriate. Benzodiazepines, dexmedetomidine, nitrous oxide, and opioids can be safely used in small quantities around the time of delivery.

- Another common source of stress on the labor floor is loss of control. Nowhere else in the hospital do patients come to the hospital with such detailed plans of care. Unfortunately, these plans are rarely followed, out of medical necessity. This can cause stress, anxiety, and sometime frustration. What can we do? First, we acknowledge their frustration and the fact that their birth plan was not followed. Something along the lines of, **"I am sorry that this birth has not gone according to your plan. We are here to make sure you are safe, and your baby is safe."** We explain what we are doing and why. Then, we try to empower the patient as much as possible—give them choices. Even small choice can be appreciated. For example, "what music would you like to listen to in the operating room?" "Do you want us to lower the drapes when the baby is delivered?" "Do you want your partner to cut the umbilical cord?"

Managing Medical Complications

When you first meet the parturient and her support people, perhaps you can acknowledge this—she's there to get a job done and you're there to do everything to support that! Also make it clear that you are available to discuss and answer questions regarding the impact of the anesthetic plan on the baby—this is the "true" informed consent mentioned above. The risks and benefits of analgesia for labor and anesthesia for cesarean delivery have evolved over the years. Do not practice in the OB suite if you do not know the current thinking backwards and forward. You will need to have a certain air of calm and quiet confidence because you will talk about some definite risks when the mother is at her most vulnerable.

Some patients arrive on the labor floor with a significantly elevated body mass index. This obviously makes neuraxial procedures and often intubation more difficult. Patients know this. Dwelling on the increased difficulty can impair the patient-physician relationship and decrease trust. Your job is to explain the risks and potential benefits of neuraxial anesthesia—these are pretty standard regardless of patient body mass index.

Another issue that can cause distress is gaps in continuity of care, which several of us can attest to, having delivered babies during change in shift. To reduce patient anxiety associated with necessary transfers of care, introduce the full anesthesia team, explain the transfer of care and sign out process, and clarify when staffing changes will occur.

***Note from the Editors:** Many locations where anesthesia is delivered now feature nature scenes and the benefits of this visual stimulation are well-known. We have seen meadows and flowers and forests put in the visual range of patients but not a lot of bridges, which is a shame, as bridges and their environs often make for lovely and relaxing pastoral scenes (Fig. 106.2).

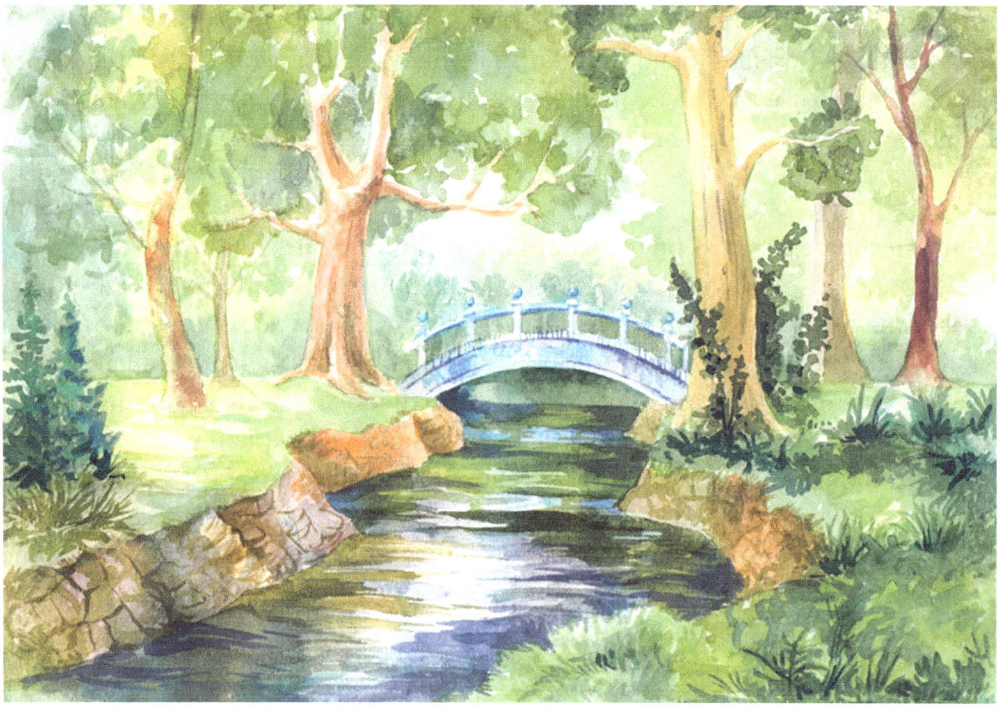

Fig. 106.2 A lovely painting of a stream and arched bridge. Photo: Image used under standard license from iStock.com

Epidural Issues

First, patients often have strong feelings about epidural analgesia. Some patients have strong desire to avoid it. This is fine. Do not be offended by a patient's desire to avoid epidural labor analgesia. It is their right and millions of women have delivered without the aid of an epidural.

However, we know that in certain scenarios an epidural can improve patient and fetal safety. These include preeclampsia with severe features and a non-reassuring fetal heart rate tracing, a trial of labor after cesarean delivery, and a twin gestation. In all these situations the need for urgent delivery or operating room treatment for hemorrhage can occur. Epidural analgesia provides a definite method of anesthesia that avoids maternal airway instrumentation, fetal exposure to systemic medications, and can facilitate faster operative delivery. In such situations we have found that a conversation with the mother that focuses on fetal wellbeing is helpful. We start by acknowledging the mother's desire to avoid neuraxial anesthesia and here is what we would say.

> We understand that your birth plan did not include epidural analgesia. We respect that and strongly desire to make your birth experience as pleasant as possible. Unfortunately, there are now reasons to think we may need to transition to the operating room quickly. If this is required, the safest plan is to have an epidural in place so that we

> can avoid general anesthesia. General anesthesia would expose your baby to multiple medications. In the same way that it will put you to sleep, it will sedate your baby. That may increase your baby's chance of needing to go to the NICU. Accordingly, we have talked with the OB team, and we all agree that it would be safer if you received an epidural now.

Conversely, some women will strongly desire epidural labor analgesia and will be unable to get it. Some examples include a tethered spinal cord, low platelet count, or treatment with anticoagulants. In these situations, we focus on the options the women do have:

> We understand you wanted an epidural. I am very sorry that we cannot provide this. While you cannot have an epidural because we are worried about your wellbeing, we can offer other medications such as nitrous oxide, nurse administered opioids, and an ultra-short acting opioid medication that you can self-administer with a button [remifentanil PCA].

Overall, the most common mistake we see junior obstetrical anesthesiologists make is to insufficiently describe the incidence of and risks associated with dural puncture. Especially if left untreated, post-dural puncture headaches can lead to chronic debilitating symptoms.

Hemorrhage

Also, remember that the average blood loss for uncomplicated vaginal delivery is 500 cc and it is up to a liter of blood for an uncomplicated operative delivery. Hemorrhage is common on obstetrics and compared to anesthesia in other parts of the hospital we are routinely underprepared. For example, is there any other surgery with an EBL of 1000 mL for which you would choose an anesthetic without a protected airway, no blood in the room, and a single intravenous line?

When hemorrhage occurs, patients realize something is wrong and moreover, their partners realize something is wrong. In a calm voice tell the partner, **"We are going to make sure your loved one is safe and comfortable, but we need you to leave the area now so we can focus on her."** Have a nurse escort the partner out of the room and assess how they are feeling. It is not uncommon for the partner to be more traumatized than the patient. After they have left tell the patient, "We have to put you to sleep, put in new lines, and likely give you blood. We have done this many times. We are working to keep you safe. Please take four big deep breaths."

Connecting with the Team

Once you have greeted the mother-to-be and her supporters, taken the history and physical, and obtained consent, do not make the mistake of thinking that "communicating and connecting" is done. You are just getting started. Your first task—get to know your charge nurses. They are often able to predict urgent patient needs. Take their calls promptly and respond to every question or issue they raise.

Next maintain the same professional demeanor and courtesy with the doula, if one is present. You should not be put in the position of having to justify your anesthesia assessments and plans to the doula, but you do want to maintain the utmost in professional courtesy. Having the doula on your side can be critical when patient acuity increases so do not let even the tiniest hit of tension creep into your attitude, affect, or interactions with or about her. Parturients often have a very strong, and long-established connection with their doula. Furthermore, payment for doula services often comes from the patient's pocket. The parturient has chosen this person as a highly valued and trustworthy member of their birth team.

In order to make the process of labor and delivery smooth and uncomplicated, it is of utmost importance that anesthesia and obstetrical physicians are on the same page. It goes without saying that complications test the anesthesia and obstetric provider relationship. Calm and effective communication can go a long way toward successfully navigating urgent and emergent patient needs.

Tragedy

Finally, the most difficult and devastating circumstance on the OB suite is when things do not go well, and the baby has not survived and will not be born alive. We have delivered care in this circumstance many times. Your job is to quietly express **sympathy** once, in as few quiet words as possible, such as, **"Ms. Johnson, I'm Dr. Smith, my deepest sympathies for your loss."** And to then be as invisible in your patient's care as possible.

Do not attempt to express **empathy** and do not, under any circumstances, share any personal details of any pregnancy losses you or your partner may have suffered, unless the patient directly asks you, which has happened to Cathy Marcucci twice (both times the patient was a physician). While well-meaning, these attempts to identify with the patient and empathize with her situation and grief are often not welcome. The experienced labor and delivery nurses will be the ones to watch and learn from in these tough cases.

Lessons Learned

- OB anesthesia is one of our specialty's most satisfying endeavors. Where else are you welcomed into a room and asked to utilize your skills to facilitate a safe and comfortable birth experience? And where else in our specialty do you get asked to take a photo with the patient, her family, and sign the baby book?! It really is the ultimate "connection" with your patient.

- As with a lot of the practice of anesthesia, learning how to communicate and connect in the OB suite is an art. Look around you to see who does it well and emulate them.

- When you walk into the patient's room, ensure you introduce yourself to the patient **and** all of her support people that are with her. This is critically important for building rapport and trust.

- If you can, sit down when talking to the patient. This will immediately place the mother and the entire room at ease.

- Do not dwell on the patient's weight. All pregnant women know how much weight they have gained; it is often more than they would have liked. Excessive mention will cause stress and tension.

- Make sure you are really up to date on anesthetic risks and benefits, especially labor epidurals. Those questions really have not gone away in the last decades.
- The mom-to-be deserves your utmost patience and kindness. It really is a life-altering experience.
- Project calmness and confidence in all situations, and sympathy in the situations when it is called for. But do not project yourself or your personal experiences where they would not be wanted or helpful.
- Know the names of the labor and delivery nurses and your obstetric colleagues. When you are in a patient's room and able to call your teammates by name, this shows the patient and her support people that you are a well-functioning team.

***Note from the Editors:** Here is another serene bridge that would be great for a labor deck (Fig. 106.3). What are childbirth and bridges both about but transition and renewal?

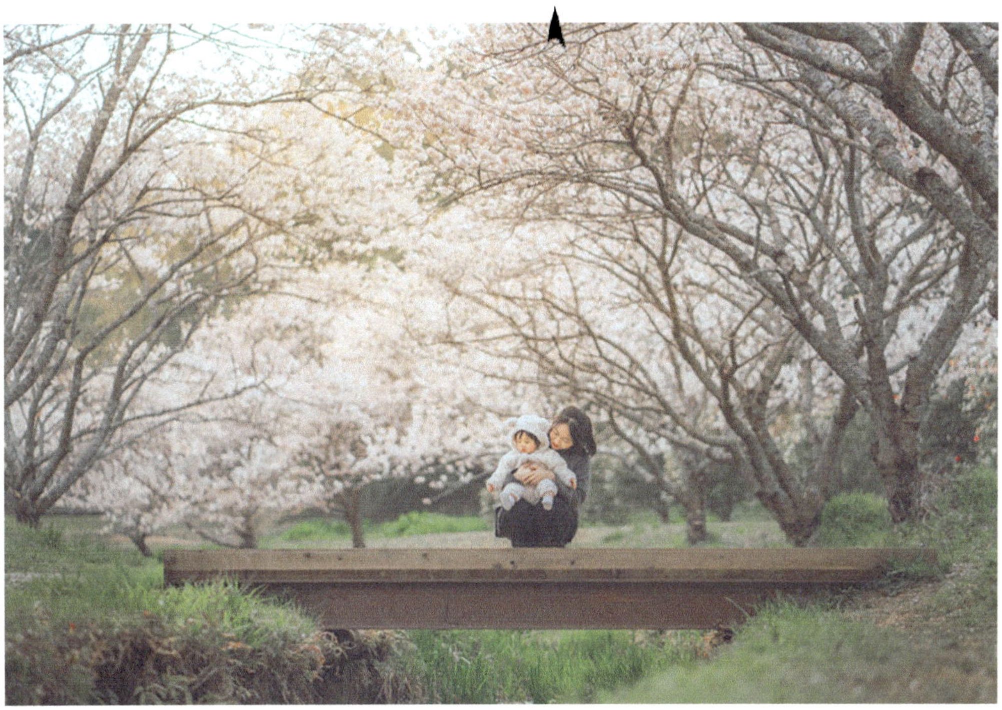

Fig. 106.3 A mother and child on a small footbridge bridge with cherry blossoms. Photo: Image used under standard license from iStock.com

Authors

Brandon Togioka is the vice chair of clinical research for Anesthesiology and Perioperative Medicine at Oregon Health and Science University, and the former director of obstetric anesthesia. He is married to Jennifer Togioka, a hospital accreditation director, with whom he has two daughters Ella and Brynn. When he is not working, Brandon enjoys jogging and watching his daughters participate in competitive swimming and ballet.

Jennifer Tripi was the chief resident of medical education of the anesthesiology residency at UNC-Chapel Hill. She then completed an obstetric anesthesiology fellowship and looks forward to her career ahead! When she is not working, she enjoys spending time with her husband, family, and friends, and travelling the world. She particularly loves hiking and exploring our beautiful national parks.

Christopher Swide is a professor of anesthesiology and perioperative medicine at Oregon Health and Science University. He is the associate dean for graduate medical education and served as the OHSU anesthesiology program director for 14 years. His specialty interests include obstetrical anesthesiology and regional anesthesiology. Chris lives in Portland with his wife. They have three adult children. He enjoys cooking, golf, running, bicycling, hiking, fishing, and reading. He is an avid Portland Trailblazer fan and longtime season ticket holder.

Cathy Marcucci was an obstetrical anesthesiologist early in her career, which she found very rewarding. She was fortunate enough to be able to attend the famous morning conferences of the late Dr. Robert A. Abraham, who was the chief of obstetrical anesthesia at Johns Hopkins for many years and an early leading advocate for regional anesthesia for parturients, as well as an expert in childbirth safety.

Connecting in the Intensive Care Unit: Building Trust

107

Jeremy C. Hoban

Introduction

Jeremy Hoban is double boarded in anesthesiology and critical care medicine. He completed residency and fellowship at the Cleveland Clinic and subsequently joined their staff. After several years he left academic medicine to lead a multi-disciplinary private practice group for 15 years. He has recently returned to academic medicine after assuming a position as division chief of critical care for the Department of Anesthesiology and Perioperative Medicine at University Hospitals Cleveland Medical Center and Case Western Reserve University. Jeremy shares his thoughts on communication issues in the ICU.

Trust

In my experience, what patients and families really want in a relationship with a healthcare provider is **trust**. Good communication is the foundation upon which trust can be built. The patient/family/physician (PFP) relationship is probably even more important in the ICU, in which patients can stay for an open-ended period of time than in an OR environment where interactions tend to be on a short-term basis. Patients often feel a loss of control and autonomy over their bodies and the situations they are placed in and can indeed be confronted with their own mortality. This obviously causes a significant amount of fear and anxiety for them and their families.

Creating a PFP relationship where trust exists that the physician will explain things honestly, help navigate difficult decisions related to treatment options and care goals, commit to providing the best possible pain/symptom relief, and allow the patient to retain as much autonomy as possible can go a long way in easing the previously mentioned fear and anxiety. Families usually have similar goals and needs as they struggle with feelings of helplessness as they watch their loved ones endure the diagnosis and subsequent treatments that necessitated their ICU stay.

J. C. Hoban (✉)
Department of Anesthesiology and Perioperative Medicine, University Hospitals Cleveland Medical Center, Cleveland, OH, USA
e-mail: Jeremy.Hoban@UHhospitals.org

S. Mohamed et al. (eds.), *Anesthesia Bridges*, https://doi.org/10.1007/978-3-032-08294-7_107

What was particularly disruptive during the Covid pandemic was the disruption of the normal communication channels employed for PFP interaction in the ICU. Speaking only for myself, I found it very difficult to obtain the same level of communication with families through something like a Zoom meeting that I had previously been able to achieve with a sit-down discussion. I have been told that patients found it difficult to hear and understand caregivers who were dressed in full protective gear.

Furthermore, all non-verbal clues that are usually subconsciously picked up during a normal conversation were essentially lost with the use of personal protective gear. I completely understand the need for the isolation and full protection needed to care for these patients, but I think going forward we will see higher levels of post-traumatic stress disorder (PTSD) in this cohort of ICU survivors.

I think the concept of rationing of care was something that had not been considered in ICU care in the United States prior to the pandemic. Certainly, the thought of not getting care was a significant source of anxiety for patients and their families. This was compounded by the disruption of the normal patterns of PFP communication. Luckily in our ICUs, while we made plans for rationing care under extreme circumstances, we never had to implement any limits on patient care.

Most physicians by their nature are confident people, unfortunately sometimes to an excess. What I think is more important than **projecting** confidence is **generating** confidence with patients and families. This is most easily done by being open and honest with them, including not knowing the answer to questions they may ask concerning the patient's condition and treatment. You do not have to be the most technically gifted surgeon or proceduralist or the physician who achieved a perfect score on a board examination.

What patients and families want to know is that you can be trusted. You can be trusted to help them navigate the complex decisions they are facing concerning their care, you can be trusted to advocate on their behalf in accordance with their wishes, and you can be trusted to make every effort to relieve the pain and anxiety associated with their diagnosis and subsequent treatment. Without this trust, patients and families will not have confidence in the diagnosis you make and the treatments you prescribe. The byproduct of being trusted is having the patient's and the family's confidence. Thus, communicate trust if you want to communicate confidence.

Lessons Learned

- What patients and families really want in a relationship with a healthcare provider is trust, and that is based on good communication.
- The byproduct of being trusted is having the patient's and family's confidence in the diagnosis you make and the treatments you prescribe. Without this trust, patients and families will not have confidence in you.
- Confidence is something you earn, not something you project!

***Note from the Editors:** The process of building strong trust is dynamic and complex. It involves flexibility but also consistency and congruity. You create it layer by layer; dishonesty and dissembling will wreck it in a moment. This bridge is a great metaphor (Fig. 107.1).

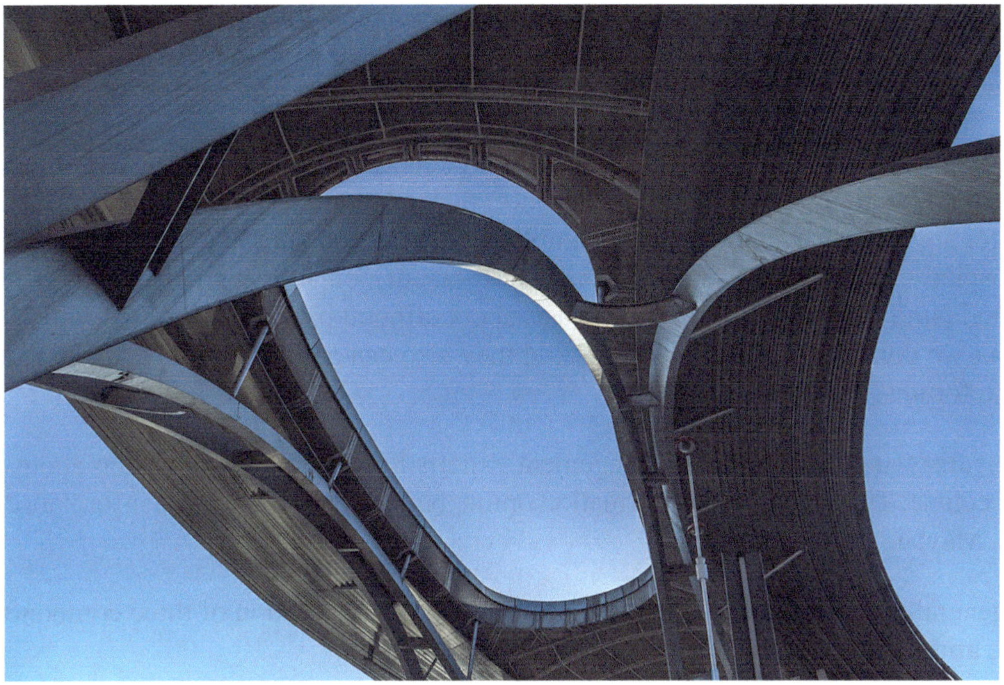

Fig. 107.1 A fascinating and complex bridge structure. Photo: hallojulie, image under standard license from stock.adobe.com

Bonus Content! A Primer on Trust

We think Jeremy Hoban has exactly captured the essence of how to communicate with those who find themselves journeying through the ICU, either in the bed or next to it. We wholeheartedly agree with his wisdom and advice that these patients and families want more than anything to know that **they can trust you**. But what is "trust" and how do you develop it? We searched online and spoke to several experts.

- Remember that "trust" is context specific. In medicine, it exists between parties with unequal knowledge and authority. This is very different than the trust that exists between parties on equal footing, sharing equal risk—think of interviews of former soldiers who found themselves in a foxhole under fire. They speak of trust as, "I had my buddy's back, and he had mine."
- A good definition for trust in medical situations is [1]:

> Willingness of a party to be vulnerable to the action of another party based on the expectation that the other will perform a particular action important to the trustor, irrespective of the ability to monitor or control that other party.

- Trust in the ICU is not equal between the parties because the patients have to trust us more than we trust them. We have the position and the authority—the power if you will—of knowledge that they do not have.
- But that does not mean that the relationship is completely unidirectional. We also have vulnerabilities relative to the patient and families. For instance, we must trust that they have been honest about the

patient's medical history—both remote and contemporaneous. Have they accurately reported preop medications, allergies, and functional and physical status? Is everybody who they say they are? Can we trust the families not to slip substances to the patients when we are not looking?

- Similarly, although we have the medical authority, patients and families have certain administrative remedies that we simply do not have. For instance, they can terminate the relationship if they are dissatisfied for any reason, even if they have simply decided they do not like us. They can also report us to the hospital executives or state medical board, but of course there is no method to report the patients and families. Somebody once said to us about difficult patients, "They can and do contact our bosses, but we don't contact their bosses." And they also can and do go to the lawyers, newspapers, and online forums.

- Social scientists and business and management experts have studied and written about trust extensively, of course. There are lots of information online but, unfortunately, little information in medical curricula. Maybe that should change.

- Trust is generally understood to consist of and exist at the intersection of three components: **ability, integrity, and benevolence** (Fig. 107.2) [1].

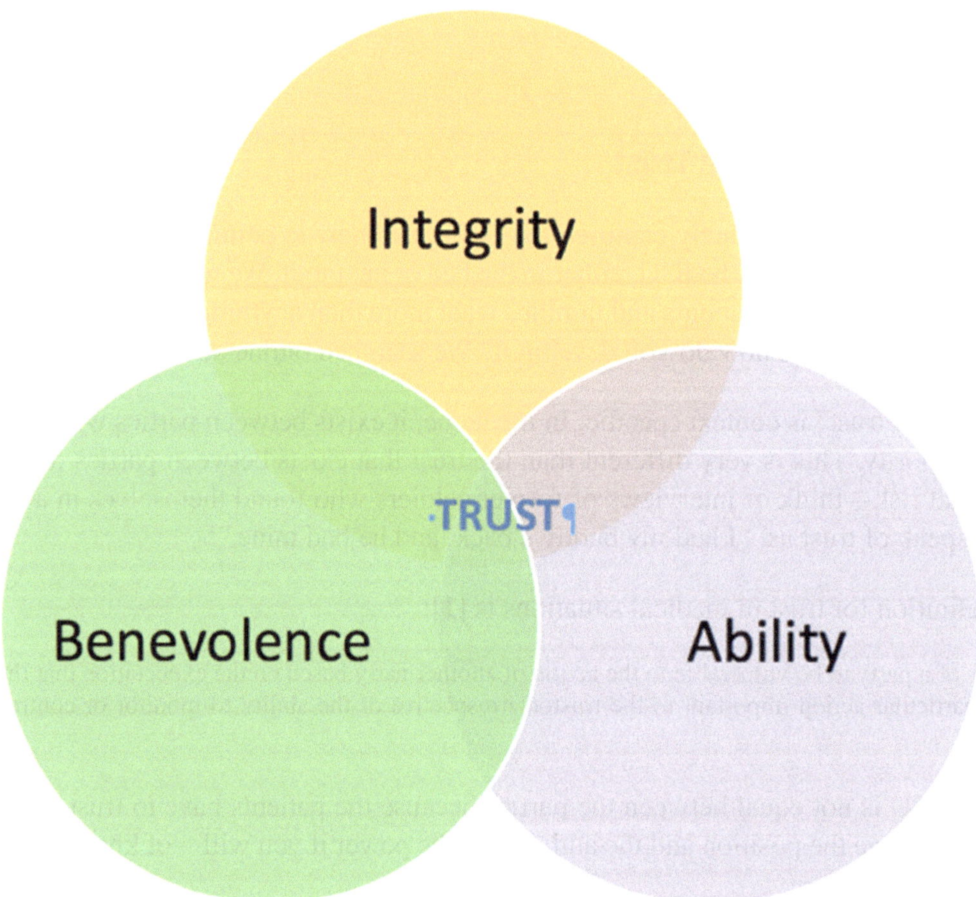

Fig. 107.2 A Venn diagram showing trust as the intersection of integrity, benevolence, and ability. The components are as important, if not more so, than the combined result, but you must have all three. Illustration: courtesy of Catherine Marcucci

- It also presupposes that an important relationship exists between the parties.
- Another formulation of trust is based on the development and deployment of four components—**consistency, compassion, communication, and competency**.
- Yet a third construct is that trust is comprised of **reliability, honesty, good will, competency, and openness**.
- Any of these formulations will work as long as you understand and use them. The point is not necessarily to accept one over the other. Rather, the point is to think and care about issue enough to be aware of which construct works for you. And then actively work on developing these aspects of your relationships with your patients and families.
- The trusted party might be the one that has the power and authority (and less perceived vulnerability) but keep in mind that the trusted party also has the greater burden in maintaining the trust relationship. All of the abovementioned components are required to establish and maintain trust, but a serious breach in any component will destroy trust, and quickly too.
- It has been our every day, common sense observation that the **quickest and easiest way to trash a trust relationship is to be dishonest**. All of the trust components are important, but we think that honesty is the most important. People just do not like to be lied to. They tend to take it very personally and do not forgive and forget very easily.
- The problem for us is that there is a difference between being wrong and being dishonest and it is sometimes hard for the patient to know the difference. We were taught that it is occasionally better to give the patients and families information that is incomplete rather than information that is specific but ultimately incorrect. It is a delicate line to walk.
- We have also found that patients and families have difficulties with the trust relationship when access to the medical providers (that is, the information source) is limited.
- One of the smartest and most effective patient relations strategies we ever saw was an ICU attending who had "office hours" every week in the ICU conference room for patients' families. He did not conduct it as a "seated" daily rounds on individual patients but rather made himself available to answer questions about general ICU care and just establish contact and rapport with families. If memory serves correct, it was usually two hours or so late on Friday afternoons or on Saturdays after morning rounds, so that he could meet with the families heading in for the weekend's vigil. He used the time to establish and deepen just about every component of the trust dynamic. As a result, the patients held him in the highest esteem, and it was very rare to have difficulties in the PFP relationships when he was on service. What prevents anger is access, availability, and answers.
- But not everybody is this skilled. And sometimes the trust quotient is established but then lost. So, how do you regain trust if it has been broken? This is a tricky matter indeed and we had to consult that ultimate and venerable source, *Psychology Today* magazine to get some answers [2].

- Here are the seven steps to regaining trust:
  1. Listen to the other person's anger and hurt feelings.
  2. Empathize with them.
  3. Ask what is needed to prevent a recurrence.
  4. Be conscientious to do all the things listed that show trustworthiness.
  5. Take full responsibility for your actions. Do not sidestep the issue or try to shift blame to the other person.
  6. Make a heartfelt apology expressing your regret.
  7. Continue to have open and honest communication.
- The overall seven tasks require considerable emotional and psychological energy and effort—they are just not that easy to do. It is much easier not to lose the trust relationship in the first place.
- Always, always guard the foundations of the trust you have in people and that they have in you with the utmost diligence and vigilance. Because the stresses of real life can erode them (Fig. 107.3). Which would be easier—doing routine maintenance on these bridge supports or trying to pick this pipeline up out of the sea?

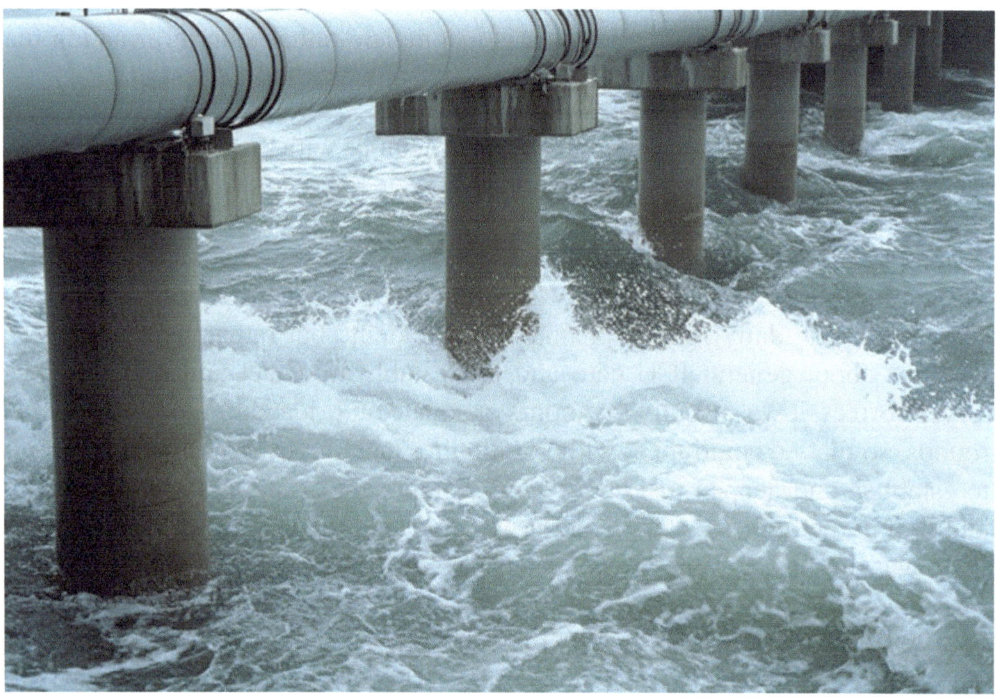

Fig. 107.3 Chemical and pipeline engineers are wary of this type of bridge most of all, for obvious reasons. Photo: Image used under standard license from stock.adobe.com

- If you wish to get deeper into this subject, read the work by Luke Chang, PhD. Dr. Chang runs the Computational Social and Affective Neuroscience Laboratory at Dartmouth.

- Dr. Chang studies and write on the science of trust. If you are interested in game theory and the application of economic games to the human condition, his work is a must read.

- Dr. Chang defines trust as "the psychological state of assuming mutual risk with a relational partner to gain an interdependent goal in the face of competing tensions." He also makes the crucial point that, "Trust is a dynamic state and evolves over the course of a relationship."

- Chang highlights the fact that trust is essentially a reinforcement phenomenon—it reflects the belief that a partner will take a specific action, especially in the context of a specific set of clues. The process of forming and updating these beliefs recruits the basic learning architecture of the brain.

- But trust is more than the partners assessing what has happened, it shapes the perception of future events, including losses and gains. Evidently, a loss in the face of pre-existing trust is perceived and adapted to differently from a loss that occurred without the context of trust. This makes sense—how many times have you heard someone say, "I *knew* I shouldn't trust him!" The process of forming and updating these beliefs recruits the basic learning architecture of the brain.

- The other fascinating subsection of the Chang paper discusses the fact that gossip can spread reputational information and hence impact trust. A common-sense take home message for us from this science—be careful what you and your staff say about each other to the patients and families! Words have a lot of power.

- In summary, trust is a complex yet fragile feature in the landscape of patient relationships. Trust issues are worthy of your closest attention. And most importantly, **trust yourself**!

***Note from the Editors:** Speaking of trusting yourself, would you cross this bridge (Fig. 107.4)? What's on the other side of the crumbling tower, maybe nothing? But what if you **had** to cross it? Who would you trust less, yourself or the bridge? The psychiatrists we know suggested that the only way to make this bridge less scary is to first imagine that you had to sprint across it naked emphasizing that trust (and fear) are context dependent.

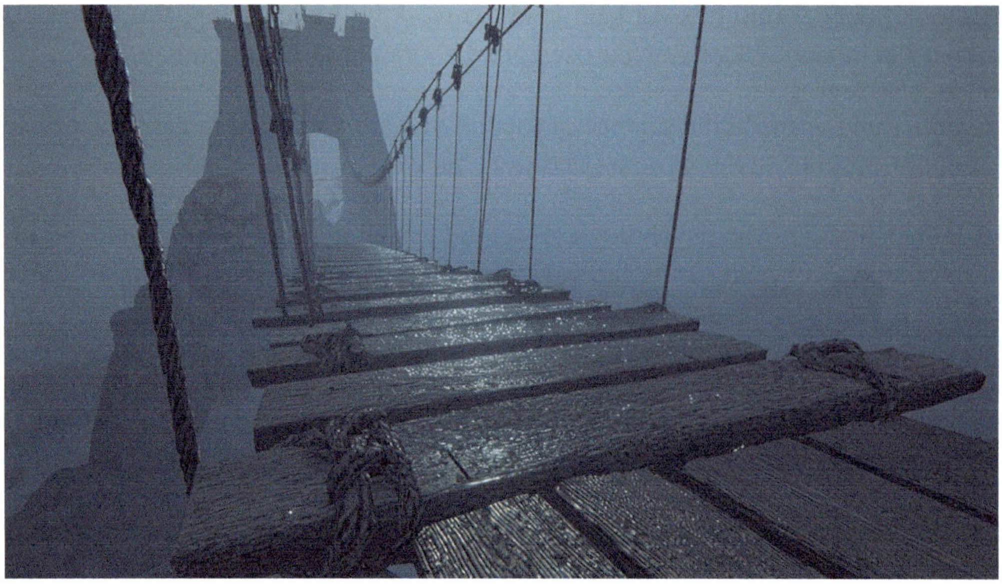

Fig. 107.4 A scary bridge image. Photo: Image used under standard license from stock.adobe.com

References

1. Gubbins C, MacCurtain S. Understanding the dynamics of collective learning: the role of trust and social capital. Adv Dev Hum Resour. 2008;10:578–99.
2. Lancer D. How to rebuild trust in 7 steps [Internet]. Psychol Today; 2012 [cited 2023 Apr 28]. Available from: https://www.psychologytoday.com/us/blog/toxic-relationships/202109/how-to-rebuild-trust-in-7-steps

Author

Jeremy Hoban is division chief of critical care for the Department of Anesthesiology and Perioperative Medicine at University Hospitals Cleveland Medical Center. When not at work, Jeremy enjoys spending time with his wife and their three children.

Connecting in the Intensive Care Unit: The Human Aspect

108

Jeremy C. Hoban

Introduction

In this chapter, **Jeremy Hoban** continues his discussion of important communication issues in the ICU.

Experience and Evolution

My communication style has definitely evolved as I have matured in my career. I have moved from more formal and technical patient/family/physician (PFP) discussions to a more patient/family-centric presentation style. Instead of hiding behind facts and figures, I make more of an effort to initially find out what the patient understands of his/her diagnosis, what it means to them at their particular stage in life, and what treatment options they are willing and able to pursue. The same diagnosis means different things to patients and families and thus, by default the treatment options they are willing to accept are often different. Given these differences, using the same presentation and presentation style to every patient/family you encounter throughout your career seems foolish. I try to tailor what I say and how I say it so that my interactions with patients and families is as beneficial as possible given their unique personality and make up. I also try to convey the human aspect of medicine.

In referring to the human aspect of medicine, I mean that medicine is not and never will be a hard science like chemistry. If you put two chemicals together, you are always going to get the same reaction. However, two patients with the same diagnosis will often have different outcomes. For instance, one of the most commonly asked questions post cardiac arrest concerns neurologic prognosis. I will often discuss with families what I am seeing on head CTs, on clinical examination, and what the current literature says about long term survival in these types of patients.

But I also tell them that the average outcome does not necessarily mean that their loved one will have the same outcome. I do not give them false hope, and I strive to be as honest about what I think the

J. C. Hoban (✉)
Department of Anesthesiology and Perioperative Medicine, University Hospitals Cleveland Medical Center, Cleveland, OH, USA
e-mail: Jeremy.Hoban@UHhospitals.org

S. Mohamed et al. (eds.), *Anesthesia Bridges*, https://doi.org/10.1007/978-3-032-08294-7_108

prognosis will be, but there is a human component that often plays a role in how a patient recovers. This human component is what separates their loved one from all of the other patients with the same diagnosis. This is the element which is also what separates medicine from chemistry. Only when you have seen enough patients do you realize that they all do not act the same way and are you comfortable in discussing this with patients and families.

Jokes?

The editors are split on the use of humor and jokes in the medical setting and specifically asked me to comment. I do not think I have ever told an actual joke to a patient/family, especially while delivering bad news. However, I do strive to be compassionate and not appear overly formal in patient/family interactions. As mentioned earlier, I try to tailor what I say and how I say it to the verbal and nonverbal clues that are present in every conversation I have ever had with a patient/family.

The goal is to provide as much information as possible on a level that can be easily comprehended (no overt use of medical jargon or acronyms) by patients/families to allow them to participate in the decisions that need to be made in the course of their care. If I ever had a patient who enjoyed humor and I thought this could be a way to further deepen the patient/physician relationship, I would not be opposed to incorporating some form of appropriate humor. The real problem would be that I can not remember any of the good jokes I have heard before!

***Note from the Editors:** Jeremy Hoban's favorite bridge is the Mackinac Bridge (Fig. 108.1). This is why:

> Probably my favorite bridge is the Mackinac bridge connecting the northern part of Michigan with the upper peninsula. I grew up in northern Michigan and have many fond memories of both crossing the bridge and sailing under it during family vacations

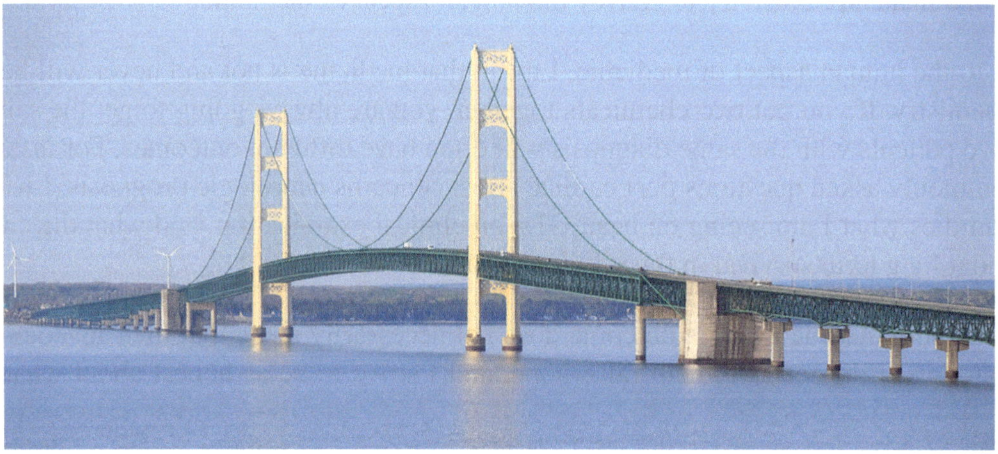

Fig. 108.1 The Mackinac Bridge is a beautiful suspension bridge that spans the Straits of Mackinac between the Upper and Lower Peninsulas of Michigan. It was opened in 1957 and is known as Big Mac or Mighty Mac. The original planning for the bridge started in the 1880s, inspired by the opening of the Brooklyn Bridge. Photo: Image used under standard license from iStock.com

Medical Patients and Families

Another interesting situation arises when caring for and communicating with patients and families who work in healthcare. I think communication with patients/families with medical backgrounds does change in some ways but remains the same in others. Individuals with medical backgrounds often have a more complete understanding of clinical diagnosis and a better understanding of the costs and benefits of various treatment options. Thus, there is less time involved in providing education that allows for informed decisions and autonomy when making important medical decisions.

On the other hand, I think the fundamental foundation of the PFP relationship remains the same. Patients/families still need to have trust in you, and the primary goal of any interactions should be to further enhance this trust and deepen the PFP relationship throughout the treatment process.

Organ Donation

Finally, there are the very important discussions with families about organ donation. These can be difficult and fraught with proverbial landmines that can destroy PFP relationships. Generally, I like the ICU team to lead these discussions personally as we often know the patient and their families better than others on the healthcare team. Hopefully we have also anticipated this clinical outcome and have spent a significant amount of time developing a trusting relationship with surviving families.

However, there are times when having a third party participate in the discussion can be of benefit, especially when the family is divided about the organ donation. In these scenarios, there can be a benefit in having families view the ICU team as having a primary interest in advocating for the patient rather than being seen as "speeding up the death just to harvest their organs." This accusation has been leveled at our ICU team in instances where the communication process with the family has broken down for various reasons. Having an independent third party outside of the broken PFP relationship can be beneficial, and can also be the source of the communication breakdown. My preferred goal would be to always lead the discussions around organ donation and never have a communication breakdown with families; however, in real world clinical practice, this is not always possible.

Lessons Learned

- As my career has progressed, my communication style has become less formal and more interactive. I listen as much as I talk!
- I find that I generally avoid jokes, jargon, and acronyms.
- My personal preference is to lead the discussions about organ donation, but at times having a third party is helpful and even necessary to foster a respectful and empathic discussion.

Author

Jeremy Hoban is division chief of critical care for the Department of Anesthesiology and Perioperative Medicine at University Hospitals Cleveland Medical Center. When not at work, Jeremy enjoys spending time with his wife and their three children.

Connecting in Interventional Pain Medicine: The Basics

109

Jeremy Jaffe

Introduction

Jeremy Jaffe Completed his residency at the Hospital of the University of Pennsylvania. After 1 year providing only general anesthesia services with the Allegheny health system, he joined the private practice at Abington Memorial Hospital, where he was also the departmental director of medical education, mentoring numerous medical students and residents. After 22 years, he transitioned from providing both anesthesia and pain management care to a practice devoted exclusively to outpatient chronic pain management. He is a founding member of SEPA Pain and Spine, an independent comprehensive interventional pain practice based in Horsham, PA. Jeremy is board-certified in both anesthesiology and pain medicine.

Jeremy sent us his thoughts and wisdom (in two parts) on transitioning from the general practice of anesthesia to a comprehensive pain management practice and the ensuing implications for physician-patient relationships and communication. Here are the basics. The following chapter has some advice on the nuances.

Basics

As anesthesiologists practicing in the OR, we are responsible for ensuring the safety and comfort of the patient and providing ideal operating conditions for the surgeon. Objective measures such as hemodynamic stability, degree of muscle relaxation, and adequacy of oxygenation and ventilation are routinely assessed with routine monitoring devices. Intraoperatively, we have the ability to accurately assess cardiac function. Though sometimes a source of skepticism, even absolute depth of anesthesia may be monitored.

Pain Management

But for many patients, what really distinguishes an anesthesiologist from other physicians is their ability to prevent or relieve pain. Unfortunately, our ability to objectively measure the complex constellation of physical and emotional distress that defines pain remains largely subjective—regardless of its source, whether it be classically nociceptive, inflammatory, neuropathic, functional, or emotional.

J. Jaffe (✉)
SEPA Pain and Spine, Horsham, PA, USA

S. Mohamed et al. (eds.), *Anesthesia Bridges*, https://doi.org/10.1007/978-3-032-08294-7_109

In the operating room, we often are alerted to the likelihood of inadequately controlled pain when our monitors indicate heart rate or blood pressure fluctuations or when we observe patient movement. However, multiple other explanations for these observations exist such as blood loss, medication effects, and disinhibition, and the absolute presence of pain may remain in doubt or be overestimated. Such is one of the more formidable challenges facing the anesthesiologist. Nonetheless, in the perioperative arena, however limited, at least we have a few objective tools for measuring our success or failure in controlling pain.

Throughout my training and in my early years as a practicing anesthesiologist, I became adept at using these objective tools and enjoyed observing patients smoothly emerge from their anesthetic and continue on in comfort to the post-anesthesia care unit (PACU). But I also struggled at times to explain why certain patients experienced a tumultuous emergence or why I was unable to control their postoperative pain.

In exploring subspecialty opportunities within anesthesiology, I considered the possibility that I could address some of these concerns by exploring pain management. My intuition was correct and my early experiences with pain management rotations allowed me to hone my skills in regional anesthetic techniques to better control intraoperative and postoperative pain. I also gained better insight into the rationale for a particular anesthetic plan and the pain medications I chose to utilize.

But the manner in which I explained my anesthetic choices and pain management strategies did not change very much: discussions with patients during typically brief visits before surgery were primarily focused on the acute challenge of how to safely shepherd that patient through their surgical procedure and deliver them to the post-anesthesia care unit (PACU) in stable condition and with good pain control. Patients rarely questioned why a certain anesthetic plan was offered and my role as an anesthesiologist was undeniably paternalistic and this dynamic suited the vast majority of patients (and their family members, when present) just fine.

When I elected to devote more of my clinical time toward chronic pain management, I was confident that I had attained expertise in assessing many forms of pain, conveying thoughtful, and hopefully empathetic, explanations of anesthetic care to my patients. I had familiarity with a potent arsenal of effective pharmacologic agents. I had acquired expertise in a variety of regional anesthetic techniques—first using only anatomic landmarks, and then techniques using nerve stimulation and ultrasound. Consequently, making the transition from an anesthesiologist to a pain management specialist seemed a very natural extension of my training and experience.

***Note from the Editors:** Jeremy Jaffe is from the Philadelphia, PA area and went to Temple University School of Medicine. In his honor of his hometown, we are featuring the lovely small bridge in the Japanese garden in Fairmount Park (Fig. 109.1).

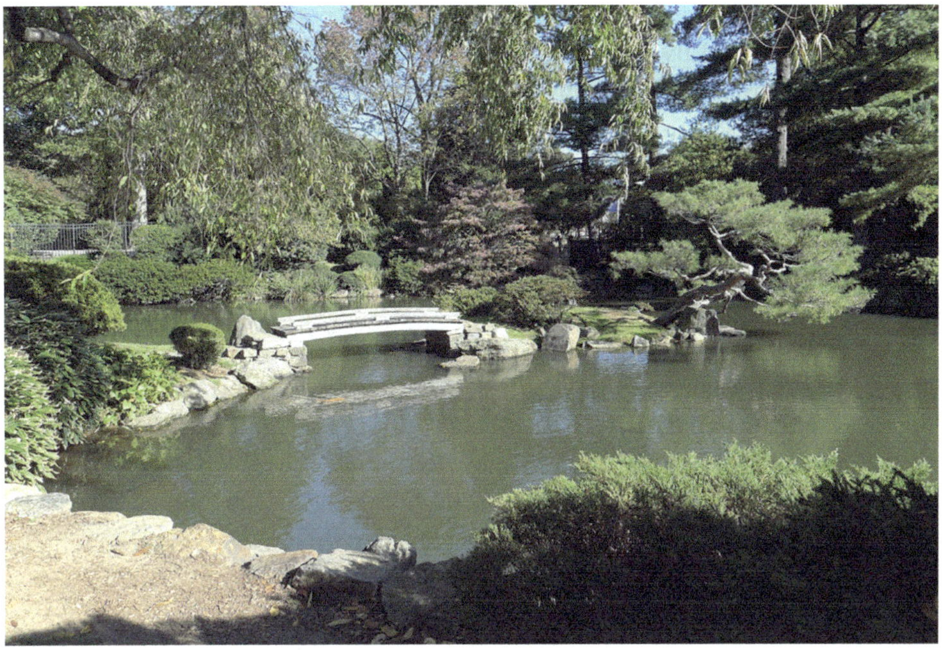

Fig. 109.1 The Japanese garden and bridge I Fairmount Park in Philadelphia, PA. It is part of the Japanese Cultural Center in the western part of the park. Fairmount Park is one of the most extensive, interesting, beautiful, and unusual municipal parks in the country. Philadelphia medical students are in it constantly. Photo: used under standard license from stock.adobe.com

Communications Skills Should Evolve as Practice Evolves

But there was an important and undeniable reality: as a pain management specialist, not only did I need to acquire a new set of procedural skills as part of an expanded armamentarium dedicated to chronic pain management, but perhaps most importantly, my success was dependent upon learning how to best relate and communicate with patients and their families. As an anesthesiologist who left the operating rooms for the pain management office and procedure rooms, some important differences in how I interact with patients have come sharply into focus. I have found certain strategies that allow me to better relate and most effectively communicate with pain patients, including:

1. **Listen and work hard to remain patient**

   Patients and their families have many questions, are often well-informed, may have already been treated by multiple other pain physicians, and **often already have an idea of the treatment they believe you should be offering**. I have found the paternalistic model of patient care less useful in the pain clinic. Many patients have strong opinions about medications, physical therapy, psychological support or interventional procedures that may be recommended. It is important to understand the value of "give and take" in earning the trust and confidence of a pain patient. By taking the time to listen to the patient and offer understandable treatment alternatives, from the simplest non-invasive to more complex invasive procedures, you will discover patients more quickly gain confidence in your treatment algorithms and skills.

Even in some cases where I have been unable to eliminate a patient's pain, I have been told that I was able to bring meaningful relief by merely taking time with them and listening. Chronic pain is rarely eliminated with a single treatment. Patients most often are seen over several visits, not infrequently over years, and functional improvement is often incremental. As an anesthesiologist I cared for a patient through a surgical procedure with minimal follow-up beyond the PACU or a brief post-op visit. As a pain physician, by listening and remaining patient, I develop lasting relationships with patients and their families.

2. **Remain empathetic and compassionate**

   Unlike the more concrete pharmacology and physiology that informs anesthesiologists and their treatment decisions and rationale, the subjective experience of pain is much more interpretive and multifactorial. I have found that pain patients need to know I am aware not only of their full medical history, but also how pain has affected their job, their families, and their ability to have a fulfilling life. Patients need to know I believe they are experiencing pain and the extent to which it is disrupting their lives.

   Furthermore, it can be challenging to convince patients you really do believe they are in pain. This point has been especially underscored as attention on a growing opioid epidemic has grown exponentially in the past decade. Patients often are defensive, even upon first meeting me, and I can sense they feel they must justify why they are taking opioids. They will relate stories of how other providers, pharmacists, friends, or family members have suggested they are drug seekers or "junkies." It is critical that as a pain physician I do my best to provide explanations that are evidence-based and avoid being judgmental, even in instances where I believe substance dependence or abuse needs to be considered.

   Sometimes it is just as important to provide these explanations to care givers or family members who accompany the patient. It is important to remind patients, their families and even myself, how subjective and unique the pain experience is for each patient. If I am unable to convey my belief and understanding, even when I believe the patient may be catastrophizing or irrationally fearful, I will be unable to gain the patient's trust and cooperation, and my treatment will be less effective.

   As an anesthesiologist explaining an anesthetic plan to a patient and their family, I always presented myself with calm and confidence, even when I had to be direct about significant anesthetic risks and how I would manage them. But beyond extending that same effort and demeanor toward pain patients, the critical importance of fully acknowledging, believing and in essence, legitimizing the patient's pain complaint is essential and largely unique to the practice of chronic pain management.

3. **Be clear about what treatments you can offer and when consultants are needed**

   Providing anesthetic care in the OR is typically the responsibility of a single anesthesiologist with or without assistance from a CRNA or AA. Providing chronic pain management often requires the expertise of several experts in adjuvant therapies such as physical therapy, acupuncture, massage therapy, psychological counseling, subspecialty consultations with orthopedic or neurosurgeons, addiction specialists, medical marijuana dispensaries, as well as with multiple medical subspecialties.

Clearly communicating the rationale for utilizing these experts improves patient cooperation, improves outcomes, and reinforces the pain physician's role as the expert coordinator managing a multimodal pain management approach. Ineffective communication will potentially give the patient the impression that they are being "pawned off on somebody else." Consequently, they will lose confidence in their pain doctor who "doesn't know what to do with me."

***Note from the Editors:** The "modern" theory of pain dates from the mid-1600s and began with Descartes' theory of pain specificity, which stipulated that nerves act as the bridges of pain transmission by propagating painful stimuli to the brain. To reflect the elucidation of the centuries-old and seminal physiological principle of pain management advance, we went looking for a bridge from the 1600s and found the Pennypack Creek bridge, right there in Abingdon, where Jeremy Jaffe practices (Fig. 109.2).

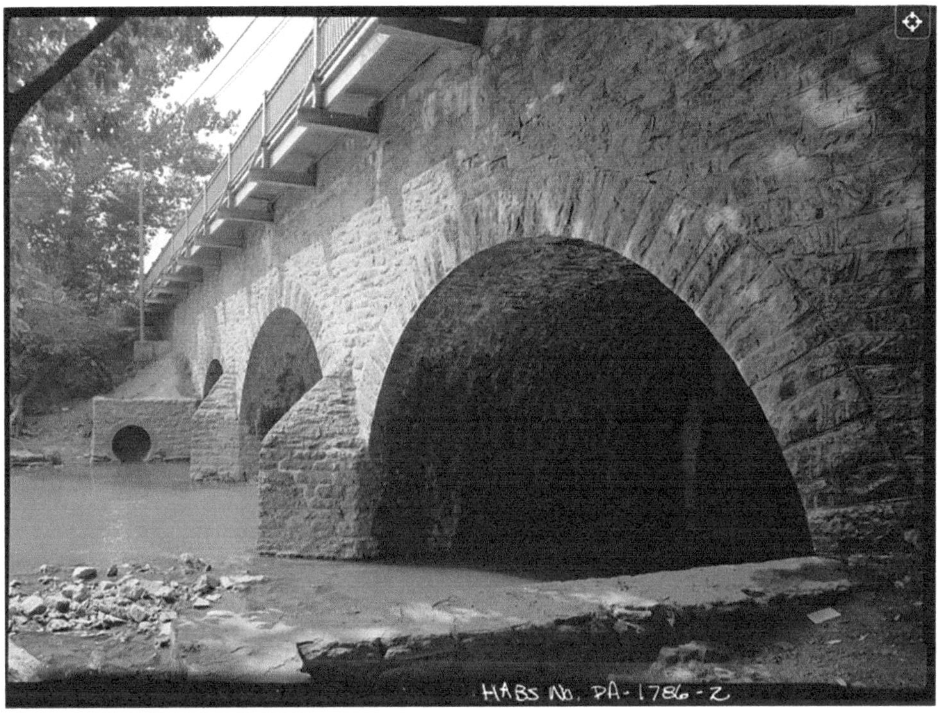

Fig. 109.2 The famous Pennypack Creek bridge, erected in 1697, is also known as the Frankford Avenue Bridge and the King's Highway Bridge. It is the oldest surviving roadway bridge in the US and was built at the request of William Penn to connect his mansion in present-day Bucks County to the new city of Philadelphia. The construction of the bridge was unusual in its time for the legislated width of 10 feet and the requirement of railings. Today, the bridge is recognized as both an historical and civil engineering landmark, as it did not require or receive significant rebuilding until 2018. Photo: Library of Congress, Historic American Buildings Survey

4. **Be prepared to explain medication choices and how and why you perform a certain procedure**

   Most patients heading to the operating room never asked me how a volatile anesthetic worked or the difference between techniques of central and peripheral neural blockade. In contrast, I have found that most pain patients want to understand a great deal about their pain management treatment plan. It is typical to be asked about my rationale for medication recommendations. Many pain patients have already had experience with a variety of over-the-counter medications or medications prescribed by their family doctor or another specialist.

Questions about the differences between muscle relaxants, neuropathic medications, and opioids are particularly common. The pain management physician must be prepared to address any concerns about pain medications and potential side effects. Having an app such as Epocrates® or an EMR equipped to readily review medication side effects or drug interactions is extremely helpful, especially when treating a patient population for whom polypharmacy is not unusual.

Beyond medications, many pain patients want to know how I perform a procedure and why I think it will benefit them. Being prepared with clear explanations, diagrams, models, radiographic studies, and outcome data not only allows the patient to make an informed decision, but also further demonstrates your expertise and confidence. When I provided anesthesia in the OR, the patient mostly had to assume I had the prerequisite experience that assured safe and competent care—after all, typically they did not have a choice. But as a pain management physician, **patients do have a choice**, and the better I am at explaining, answering questions and inspiring confidence, the more likely I will have the opportunity to provide effective treatment that most fully demonstrates my expertise and allows my practice to grow.

Lessons Learned

- A mentor once told me that "if you listen to a patient long enough, they will tell you what is wrong with them." While there is a limit to how much time you will have available for a patient, making the effort to be patient and actively listen gives you the best chance for successful treatment and a productive relationship with the patient. You will find that the initial evaluation is especially critical, as it is your best opportunity to get the full history and lays the foundation upon which all future treatment decisions are built.

- Empathy and compassion should be dispensed liberally. They are amongst the greatest tools a pain physician has to offer their patients and builds and maintains trusting relationships between physician and patient.

- Interventional therapies have become increasingly complex. Be prepared to fully review rationale, technique and sequela. Adequately detailed explanations, diagrams, models, and videos are indispensable.

- Maintain a good working knowledge of the medications you use most commonly. Apps such as Epocrates® and an EMR equipped with drug interaction checks are very helpful. Always be sure to query the Prescription Drug Monitoring System to know what controlled medications your patient has been receiving and from whom. Anticipate and plan for how you will manage refusal of recommended treatments or difficult conversations about non-compliance with medications. Have strategies to maintain a safe working environment for you, your staff, and the patient.

- Recognize that managing chronic pain requires you to consistently update any changes in history or exam and to vigilantly monitor patient response to treatment. Pain and co-morbid conditions often change over time. Be wary of "cutting and pasting" EMR templates with outdated or inaccurate information.

- We recommend that every physician who diagnoses or treats pain, **and who among us doesn't**, read the fascinating history of pain management in the US by Bernard et al. [1].

Reference

1. Bernard SA, Chelminski PR, Ives TJ, et al. Management of pain in the United States—a brief history and implications for the opioid epidemic. Health Serv Insights. 2018;11:1178632918819440.

Author

Jeremy Jaffe is currently a managing partner of SEPA Pain and Spine, with multiple offices and surgery centers surrounding the Philadelphia area. As a post-baccalaureate student, he was told he had to quit drumming in his rock-and-roll band if he ever hoped to make it to medical school, an admonition he ignored. In addition to his demanding clinical practice, Dr. Jaffe has continued to perform professionally and has opened for well-known acts while touring the East Coast.

110 Connecting in Interventional Pain Medicine: The Nuances

Jeremy Jaffe

Introduction

In this chapter, we hear more from **Jeremy Jaffe** as he discusses some of the nuances about his transition from the general practice of anesthesia to a comprehensive pain management practice.

What We Must Understand

Understand that the tenor and tone of communication in the pain clinic is different from the operating room. In the operating room (OR), no matter how relaxed I felt as a competent and confident anesthesiologist, there was always an appreciation, if not apprehension, that at any moment an otherwise routine case could evolve into a life and death situation. But with an anesthetized patient, I had no concern about how such apprehension might be conveyed toward (or need to be concealed from) that patient—they were asleep! There were certainly still the responsibility and challenge of relating and communicating with the surgeon and OR staff, especially when OR conditions were tense, but meeting that challenge is a topic beyond the scope of this discussion.

In the pain clinic, interactions may not deteriorate into a life and death situation, but tensions can become quite palpable, and escalations of emotions and even physical intimidation represent a challenge not found in the operating room. Patients, family or caregivers may have strong opinions about how a patient's pain is being managed.

To further complicate the situation, these opinions are often informed by a variety of factors: how established is the doctor-patient relationship? Does the patient have secondary gains? Do family members or caretakers have secondary gains? Has the patient had issues regarding compliance, poor experiences with other pain management doctors, or difficulties tolerating or getting insurance coverage for pain medications?

There are simultaneous complexities and subtleties amongst the many factors that impact the conversation and decisions made in the pain clinic. You must navigate these simultaneous challenges in real time, especially during heated discussion, when the focus and vigilance characteristic of the anesthesiologist in the OR becomes equally essential to effective patient care.

J. Jaffe (✉)
SEPA Pain and Spine, Horsham, PA, USA

S. Mohamed et al. (eds.), *Anesthesia Bridges*, https://doi.org/10.1007/978-3-032-08294-7_110

Although important, a calm reassuring demeanor will not suffice alone. In these situations, being well-informed and prepared to anticipate any issues specific to that patient is critical. Well-known strategies such as limiting number of persons in the exam room, positioning yourself closest to the door, maintaining a presence of support staff, verifying information such as reports of ER visits or claims of partial prescription fills ahead of time and even excusing oneself from the room, have all been employed. In relating and communicating with patients, these strategies further distinguish the pain physician from the anesthesiologist in the OR.

Understand that the chronicity of a patient's pain impacts the communication. An anesthesiologist generally compresses the majority of information that must be conveyed to a patient within a limited time span during the pre-operative visit. Postoperative communication is generally even more limited. In contrast, a pain physician treating chronic pain sees a patient over weeks, months, or years. It is important to foster understanding and manage expectations by communicating an anticipated treatment rationale during the initial consultation.

It is equally essential to recognize that as treatment progresses and pain and co-morbid conditions change, pain physicians must be certain to continue gathering feedback and adapt treatment accordingly. Not unlike the anesthesiologist in the OR monitoring an anesthetized patient, pain physicians are also monitoring their patients, but over a much longer time frame. They must be prepared to convey information, which may be technically complex. A patient may have more questions as their treatment progresses, and several discussions may be required before they are able to comfortably reach a treatment decision. The pain physician must allow for this extended time frame of care, allow themselves to revisit treatment decisions and allow the patient ample opportunity to contribute to these consequential discussions.

Lessons Learned

- Understand that chronic pain management most often involves a multimodal approach. Make sure the patient understands how co-morbidities impact care and why it is not unusual to coordinate care with other specialists such as physical therapy, psychiatry, physiatry, etc. Be clear that in managing the pain, you are coordinating the care and not simply passing the patient off to another provider.

- An anesthesiologist dedicates majority of his/her time monitoring cardiac, pulmonary, neurologic, and renal function to ensure a stable intraoperative course for the patient. Much of what we do in the OR is data driven and objective in nature. When you treat chronic pain patients, there will still be a need to understand the impact medications or other treatments have on critical organ systems. What distinguishes the pain physician from the anesthesiologist, however, is the additional focus that must monitor emotional, psychological, and behavioral changes impacted by chronic pain and its treatment. Accepting and embracing the responsibility of this much more subjective focus is perhaps the greatest challenge in transitioning from the operating room to the pain clinic.

Author

Jeremy Jaffe is currently a managing partner of SEPA Pain and Spine, with multiple offices and surgery centers surrounding the Philadelphia area. He is very active with charitable causes in his community and has helped raise hundreds of thousands of dollars for the Juvenile Diabetes Research Foundation (JDRF) as a co-chair for "Rockin' Docs for Diabetes Cure." He enjoys biking, tennis, and skiing and especially relaxing with his wife and two children while vacationing on Cape Cod or in Vermont.

Connecting with Cancer Patients

111

Valentina Baez Sosa, Richard W. Childs,
and Catherine Marcucci

What is your biggest fear?

Dying or having cancer?

–*Anonymous*

Introduction

The number of cancer survivors in the United States has significantly increased over time from approximately three million in the 1970s to over 18 million in 2022 [1, 2]. For some types of cancers, such as breast cancer, mortality rates have consistently declined primarily due to advances in early detection, surgery, radiation, and substantial progress in newly approved systemic therapies for patients with both early-stage and metastatic disease. At the same time, the worldwide incidence of cancer is increasing [3, 4]. Furthermore, the epidemiology is shifting for some cancers—such as the increased incidence in colon cancer in young adult patients. Most cancer patients that you will care for will undergo anesthesia and surgery as the first line of treatment, often for curative intent but sometimes for palliative treatment.

The Psychology of Cancer

Despite ongoing advances and new treatment options, most patients are terrified when they hear the word cancer for the first time. Even when you diagnose early-stage resectable disease, to the patient it is always a life-changing experience filled with uncertainty and fear. For them there is a sense of loss and grief after losing their pre-cancer identity and becoming a cancer survivor.

V. B. Sosa
National Heart Lung Blood Institute, Bethesda, MD, USA

Department of Transfusion Medicine, Clinical Center, National Institutes of Health, Bethesda, MD, USA

R. W. Childs
Rear Admiral, Commissioned Corps of the U.S. Public Health Service, Clinical Director, NHLBI, NIH, Laboratory of Transplantation Immunotherapy, National Heart Lung and Blood Institute (NHLBI), National Institutes of Health, Bethesda, MD, USA

C. Marcucci (✉)
Department of Transfusion Medicine, Clinical Center, National Institutes of Health, Bethesda, MD, USA

S. Mohamed et al. (eds.), *Anesthesia Bridges*, https://doi.org/10.1007/978-3-032-08294-7_111

In some cases, the patients want to "fight" cancer and they come to the clinic with their entire army of social support, tools, a new healthy diet, and a lot of information they "Googled" about how to beat this down. In other cases, there is a profuse sense of overwhelming fear, freezing their life. Whatever the scenario, one of the first things we can do as physicians are to assure them that they are not alone in this fight and that we, the ever-growing multidisciplinary oncologic care team, can be counted among their army of supporters. Our role is to not only to provide the patient with treatment options, but to arm them with encouragement and understanding so they can confidently navigate this long and at times tortuous path. It is very powerful to have this partnership shared decision-making ability throughout the entire cancer care plan.

Finally, when meeting with an oncologic patient, it is important to consider one of the most common cancer-related distress triggers: *fear of recurrence*. This applies to both patients and family caregivers and can happen anywhere along the treatment journey: in the days or weeks preceding routine visits, after laboratory testing, or after radiologic imaging, or before surgery. Some factors that can potentiate the fear of recurrence include age (younger patients, especially if diagnosed with cancer before 60 years old), more advanced cancer stage, a more recent diagnosis or prior recurrence, low level of education, and higher number of clinical visits, especially if more than five times a year, self-identification as a cancer patient, or the possibility of denial of the diagnosis [5].

The Perioperative Period

Fears of recurrence may loom very large in the perioperative period. What if the procedure that is intended to be curative somehow makes it worse? It is more than a fair question. It is well understood that tumor resection is a risk factor for metastasis. This can occur through hematological spread, lymphatic spread, localized spread into a body cavity, or occurrence of minimal residual disease even with apparent clear surgical margins. Because we do not control the surgical techniques, there is little that an anesthesiologist can do that will directly impact the occurrence of these untoward events. What then *can* we do and what can we tell the patients?

First, it is essential when caring for cancer patients that you show empathy and respect. Cancer patients want more than anything to know that they are doing everything they can do to be cured and get well. Do not trivialize or wave away their concerns or questions. You would have the exact same ones if you were the one with the cancer, we can pretty much guarantee it.

Second, you must know more about what they might have read than they know about what you have read. You should *assume* that they will have researched the concern (nervous belief?) that anesthetic drugs might affect the risk of cancer recurrence or metastatic spread of tumor cells during or after surgery. This material is readily available on the various websites.

Third, make sure that you yourself understand both the specific pathophysiology of the perioperative period and surgery as well as the overall clinical content. Here is a great summary [6].

- The surgical period creates a tumorigenic physiologic environment, with potential for both direct and indirect effects on tumor cell survival. Multiple perioperative factors combine to create a state of relative immunosuppression, including the surgical stress response, the inflammatory response to surgery, and direct effects of anesthetics, opioids, and other perioperative medications. Hypothermia and blood transfusion can also suppress immune function.

- The physiologic stress response to surgery causes relative immunosuppression through the release of hormonal mediators such as catecholamines, prostaglandins, and growth factors. Prostaglandins and catecholamines can cause activation of receptors that may increase the metastatic ability of cancer cells, for example beta-2-adrenergic, and cyclooxygenase-2 receptors.

- Inflammation associated with tissue trauma causes the release of cytokines, for example interleukin-6 and prostaglandins such as prostaglandin E2, that can cause inhibition of activity of natural killer (NK) cells. NK cells are essential in the perioperative phase as they are responsible for detecting and destroying circulating tumor cells.

Know the Literature!

Then, be prepared to discuss the literature as it is evolving. You can mention to your patients that the issue of whether anesthetic techniques and/or agents causing a worsening of cancer outcomes is complex, the answers to which are not fully known and may never be known. This is because it would be extremely difficult, and perhaps not even ethical, to design certain clinical trials to explore some questions, such as the effect pain medications have on recurrence. Of course, one should always tailor the discussion to the patient's knowledge and educational levels and try to focus on their specific concerns and questions.

There are a number of retrospective studies and a few recent randomized prospective studies, assessing the impact of various anesthetic techniques on outcome in a variety of cancer types. None demonstrate any significant overall difference in outcomes, including disease-free recurrence and overall survival. So, with our current state of knowledge, the data would suggest no need for a change in practice paradigms for cancer patients.

***Note from the Editors:** Drs. Baez Sosa, Childs, and Marcucci have all been on staff at the National Institutes of Health in Bethesda, MD. NIH post-baccalaureate intern Alex Pelayo sent us this wonderful picture of a nearby tiny bridge (Fig. 111.1). Alex, who is studying for an MBA and then med school and planning a career as an anesthesiologist, tells us:

> This is a small arched street culvert and creek bed located in Montgomery County, Maryland. The stream and bridge can be found alongside the Bethesda Trolley Trail, near the NIH campus. I didn't purposely try to photograph the rainbow, that was just a fortunate thing that happened!

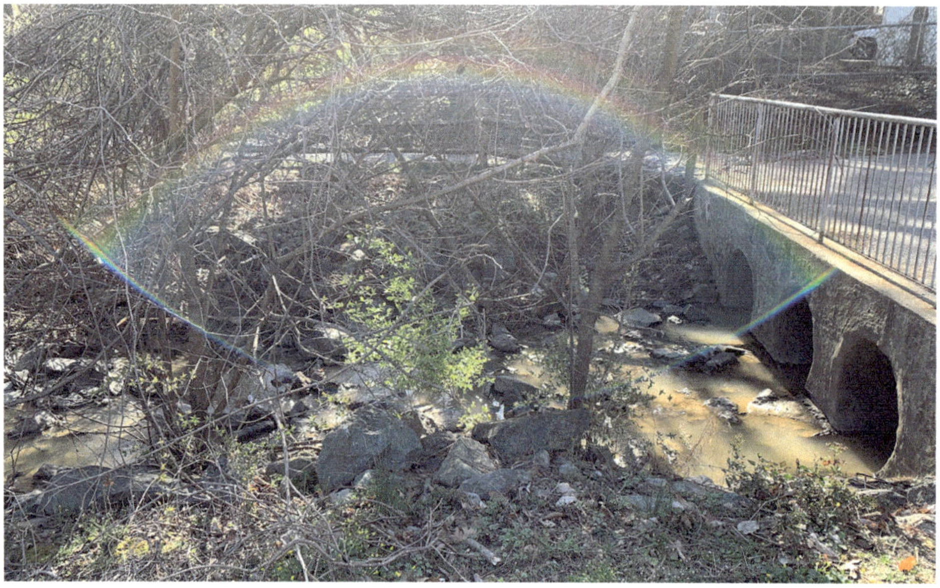

Fig. 111.1 Small stream and culvert adjacent to the Bethesda Trolley Trail in Bethesda, MD. Photo: Alex Pelayo

Large Retrospective Studies

As mentioned above, there are several large meta-analyses assessing outcome in thousands of patients. In general, these studies do not identify any significant difference in outcomes between different anesthetic techniques. The excellent review on Up to Date summarizes several key points the practitioner should be aware of:

(https://www.uptodate.com/contents/anesthesia-and-cancer-recurrence)

- A 2019 meta-analysis by Yap et al. of six retrospective studies looked at data from 7800 patients with breast, esophageal, or NSCL and found that TIVA had a small survival effect when compared with volatile anesthetics [7]. However, the conclusion was weakened by the heterogeneity of the patient cohort, including extent of surgery, types of cancers, and other patient characteristics.

- A subsequent retrospective Danish database analysis of over 8600 propensity matched patients undergoing surgery for colorectal cancer found an association between volatile anesthetic use and a small increase in cancer recurrence compared with TIVA with propofol (hazard ratio 1.12, 95% CI 1.02–1.13) [8]. However, there was no difference in overall survival.

- A 2022 study in *Anesthesiology* by Enlund et al. published overall survival data from a large cohort of 18,600 patients, derived from the Swedish Perioperative Registry and the National Quality Registry for Breast Cancer [9]. The median follow-up time was 33 months. They found that:

Among patients undergoing breast cancer surgery under general anesthesia, no association was observed between the choice of propofol or an inhaled volatile maintenance and overall survival.

Randomized Trials

Questions concerning general vs regional anesthesia and any potential differences among the general anesthetic agents are important to consider Regional anesthesia/analgesia could theoretically reduce cancer recurrence via several mechanisms: by reducing the stress response to surgery (via pain control or sympathetic block), by reducing the need for opioids or volatile agents, or via a direct effect of absorbed local anesthetics.

Again, there do not appear to be any high-evidence data showing a difference between local or general anesthesia and epidural-general vs general with postoperative opioid analgesia. Even though controversial concerns may exist about the proinflammatory effect of volatile agents such as isoflurane, sevoflurane, desflurane, and halothane, to date only pre-clinical models provide limited data suggesting a potential mechanism including upregulation of hypoxia-inducible factor 1-alpha (FIF1A) by isoflurane leading to an increase in angiogenesis and cell proliferation.

- The first large, randomized trial in this field compared two different anesthetic regimens for breast cancer surgery and was published in 2019 [10]. Approximately 2100 patients who underwent mastectomy or wide local excision with axillary dissection were randomly assigned to receive regional anesthesia/analgesia or general anesthesia. The regional technique was paravertebral block with propofol sedation; the general anesthesia technique was sevoflurane with opioid analgesia. Cancer recurrence was similar between patients who received regional anesthesia vs general anesthesia (hazard ratio 0.97, 95% CI 0.74–1.28), occurring in 10% of patients in each group over a median follow-up of 36 months. Whether these results can be applied to patients with other malignancies undergoing other cancer surgeries, particularly more extensive or painful procedures, is unclear.

- In a follow-up analysis of data from a trial including over 1700 patients who underwent major abdominal or thoracic surgery and who were randomly assigned to epidural-general anesthesia vs general anesthesia alone with postoperative opioid analgesia, overall and recurrence free survival were similar in the two groups at over 5-year follow-up [11].

- In a randomized trial including 400 patients who underwent video-assisted thoracoscopic surgery for lung cancer, recurrence free and overall survival were similar in patients who had general anesthesia with postoperative opioid analgesia, vs epidural-general anesthesia with postoperative epidural analgesia [12].

- A 2014 meta-analysis with data from over 3000 patients found no associated difference in cancer recurrence or survival in patients who received general-epidural anesthesia vs general anesthesia alone [13].

- Similarly, a 2017 meta-analysis of 28 studies (retrospective, observational, and randomized) including over 67,000 patients who underwent surgery for a variety of cancers found similar recurrence-free survival, overall survival, and biochemical recurrence-free survival in patients who had regional anesthesia with or without general anesthesia and those who had general anesthesia alone [14].

- A meta-analysis of 10 retrospective studies including approximately 13,760 patients who underwent radical prostatectomy for cancer found that regional anesthesia with or without general anesthesia was associated with improved overall survival, but similar cancer recurrence, compared with general anesthesia alone [15].
- A further meta-analysis has suggested that neuraxial anesthesia may be associated with improved overall survival, particularly in patients with colorectal cancer, as well as reduced risk of cancer recurrence [16].
- And serum from patients undergoing surgery for breast cancer using either propofol and paravertebral regional technique or opioid and volatile technique was examined in a number of studies to assess for a potential immunological effect. Those receiving a combined regional and intravenous agent technique demonstrated increased levels of immune cell infiltration into breast cancer tissue, increased levels of cancer cell apoptosis, and preserved NK cell cytotoxicity [17–19].

Volatile Agents

Here again, the data are not clear. Laboratory studies have shown that certain anesthetic agents may enhance metastatic potential and be cytoprotective for cancer cells, especially the volatile agents, which are known to be pro-inflammatory. However, there are also data that show that these effects might be cancer specific, as sevoflurane may actually *suppress* the proliferation of non-small cell lung cancer cells. Several studies have shown no appreciable difference:

- *Circulating tumor cells*—A randomized trial of 210 women who underwent breast cancer surgery reported similar circulating postoperative tumor cell counts in patients who received sevoflurane vs propofol anesthesia [20].
- *Immune cells*—In a randomized trial of 153 patients who underwent surgery for resection of colorectal cancer, the fractions of postoperative circulating natural killer cells, helper T cells, and cytotoxic T cells were similar in patients who had sevoflurane https://www.uptodate.com/contents/sevoflurane-drug-information?topicRef=117029&source=see_link vs propofol for anesthesia propofol or sevoflurane anesthesia [21].

There is little primary information on nitrous oxide. A secondary analysis of nitrous oxide vs nitrogen used with isoflurane/remifentanil anesthesia for colon resection for cancer showed no difference in recurrence or mortality outcomes in patients followed for 4–8 years.

Intravenous Agents

Propofol has been found in preclinical studies to have possible *antitumor* effects—which given its high use is a welcome finding that should be shared with patients to reassure them. There are a number of studies looking at different cancer cell lines, including gastric, breast, esophageal, endometrial, and lung cancer cell lines. In general, propofol seems to inhibit tumor cell proliferation and migration and reduce expression of genes associated with poorer outcomes. In a rat model of breast cancer, propofol did not suppress NK cell activity or increase metastasis. When tested in a murine allogeneic breast cancer model, propofol reduced lung metastasis compared with sevoflurane and similar to lidocaine.

Intravenous lidocaine is often given prior to induction and/or during multimodal anesthesia. Lidocaine is known to have anti-inflammatory properties, including reduction in inflammatory markers such as IL-1, IL-8, and tumor necrosis factor alpha. Lidocaine also blocks voltage-gated sodium channels on tumor cells. There is some suggestion that intravenous lidocaine administered during surgery may improve cancer surgery outcomes but unfortunately, the data are retrospective and lack adequate controls for key surgical variables [22, 23].

Ketamine and thiopental have known immunomodulating effects, and although rodent models and ex vivo data on cell lines suggest a potential deleterious effect, no high quality, human trial data currently exist to substantiate concerns with these agents, or available.

Opioids

The effect of opioids on the potential for increased metastasis and cancer recurrence is of obvious interest. Unfortunately, current data on the impact of opioid use are conflicting in outcome and mostly based on preclinical studies. For example, it is known that opioids can have effects that are immunosuppressive via both opioid and non-opioid receptors. They can also reduce NK cell cytotoxicity. Morphine has been shown to stimulate mast cell activation, which may increase concentrations of substance P and cytokines that have the potential to accelerate cancer progression.

Additionally, opioids may alter the profile of interleukins, such as IL-1, IL-4, IL-6, and tumor necrosis factor which can impact tumor growth. They also may interact with certain cancer-potentiating receptors that are over-expressed on certain cancer cell lines.

However, in some studies, the effects of opioids have been shown to be protective. For instance, morphine has been shown to have anti-tumor or antimetastatic effects in a breast cancer mouse model. Methadone has also been reported to have an anti-tumor effect in glioblastoma and leukemia models.

Adjunctive Agents

Non-steroidal analgesics are commonly administered intraoperatively or in the immediate postoperative period and there is increasing reliance on this class in ERAS protocols. It is known that long-term use of NSAIDS and aspirin is associated with improved survival from colorectal cancer. There is some suggestion that intraoperative NSAIDS may improve survival but the evidence to date is only via retrospective or very small prospective data [24–26]. However, NSAIDS may be associated with adverse events, such as bleeding and may not therefore be appropriate for all patients.

Supplemental oxygen is commonly used ubiquitously in the perioperative period. Surprisingly, we still do not precisely know how to optimally dose this agent nor do we fully understand the role that differing oxygen concentrations might play. It is known that tissue hypoxia plays a role in tumor angiogenesis and tumor progress. Conversely, tissue hyperoxia may have multiple deleterious effects as a consequence of oxygen free radical formation, as well as increased secretion and migration of tumor angiogenesis factors. Although few studies exist, physicians should be aware of the following [6]:

> The effect of FiO_2 on the risk of new or recurrent cancer was investigated in a post hoc analysis of the PROXI trial, in which patients who underwent abdominal surgery (approximately one-half for cancer) were randomly assigned to receive 30% or 80% oxygen during and for 2 hours after surgery [27]. The overall frequency of new cancers was similar between groups. However, the time to diagnosis of a new cancer and cancer-free survival were shorter in patients who received 80% oxygen.

Putting it All Together and Making a Plan

So, with current uncertainties over the effects of anesthetic agents and surgical techniques on cancer outcomes, what is the optimal way to communicate and connect with your cancer patients regarding these concerns? Currently, there is a shift in the practice of anesthesiology away from opioid-based anesthetics and towards regional anesthesia for intraoperative anesthesia and post-operative pain control. This practice shift already nudges the anesthetic plan ever so slightly in a direction that would be supported based on concerns emanating from current existing laboratory and clinical data regarding cancer outcomes.

Of course, as we all know, this recent shift in the clinical care paradigm has included a greater utilization of neuraxial anesthesia, peripheral nerve blocks, and perhaps propofol for sedation or light general anesthesia and non-opioid medications for pain control. This trend is fortuitous for the anesthesiologist who must reassure cancer patients. In our personal practice, we reassure patients that no clear data exist, but current anesthetic trends have moved in a direction that potentially would be of benefit to cancer patients. However, it is important to reassure patients that if a regional anesthetic approach is not feasible, there are no data that an alternative anesthetic plan would substantially worsen their outcome or negatively impact their survival.

***Note from the Editors:** Whatever you do, keep your patient and yourself focused on the big picture. Solid tumor cancers have to come out! But always remember, while you are considering the overall situation and trying to find a way through, that there is deep water on all sides for the patient (Fig. 111.2).

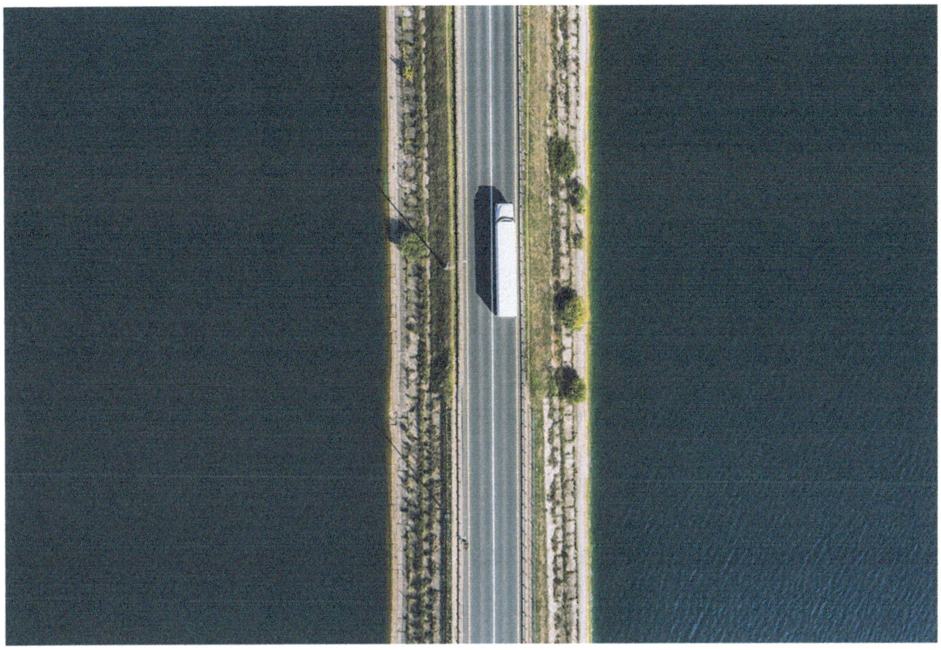

Fig. 111.2. A bridge across deep water. Photo: wmaster890, image used under standard license iStock.com

So, What Do You Do? Discussing and Deciding

Acknowledge that the perioperative period is associated with exposure to agents that potentially are pro-inflammatory, immunosuppressive, and may unfavorably influence tumor cell survival. The generalized stress response associated with the use of these agents may also be deleterious.

Laboratory and animal data may suggest an association between certain anesthetic techniques and tumor cell viability. However, clinical data are far less conclusive and do not mandate a practice change. Current existing studies are largely retrospective, are not sufficiently controlled for variables, and were not optimally designed to examine outcomes other than cancer recurrence.

Clinical studies comparing inhalational and intravenous anesthetics are mixed.

There is theoretical justification for regional anesthesia as it may block the stress response and /or reduce the need for volatile anesthetics and opioids. However, to date there are no clear clinical data showing a clear beneficial effect of this anesthetic approach on cancer outcome.

The strongest laboratory data in terms of specific agents pertain to intravascular lidocaine. Although in vitro data seem to indicate a protective effect on cancer recurrence, relevant clinical data to support these preclinical findings are limited.

Consider discussing the above points with your patient as appropriate, as well as a plan that incorporates what is currently known:

1. Minimize physiological and emotional stress and minimize the length of perioperative time interval and maximize pain control. It is already well-established that a competent, calm, and compassionate anesthesiology decreases anxiety and increases patient tolerance to and satisfaction with undergoing anesthesia.

2. Avoid or minimize the use of volatile anesthetic agents to the degree practical.

3. Consider the use of neuraxial anesthesia or regional blocks.

4. Utilize a propofol-based anesthetic plan, either for TIVA or as an adjunct for regional anesthesia.

5. Administer intravenous lidocaine if not contraindicated.

6. Administer NSAIDS if not contraindicated.

7. Avoid unnecessarily high inspired oxygen concentrations.

***Note from the Editors:** This drawing was inspired by the work of the great Dutch graphic artist M. C. Escher (Fig. 111.3). It simply yet dramatically captures the clinical complexities of the effect of surgery on cancer outcomes, as patients can feel they are traveling on a bridge to nowhere and that it is impossible to make their way through and out. The perioperative period may positively affect outcomes but how and to what degree does it introduce negative influences on outcomes and survival?

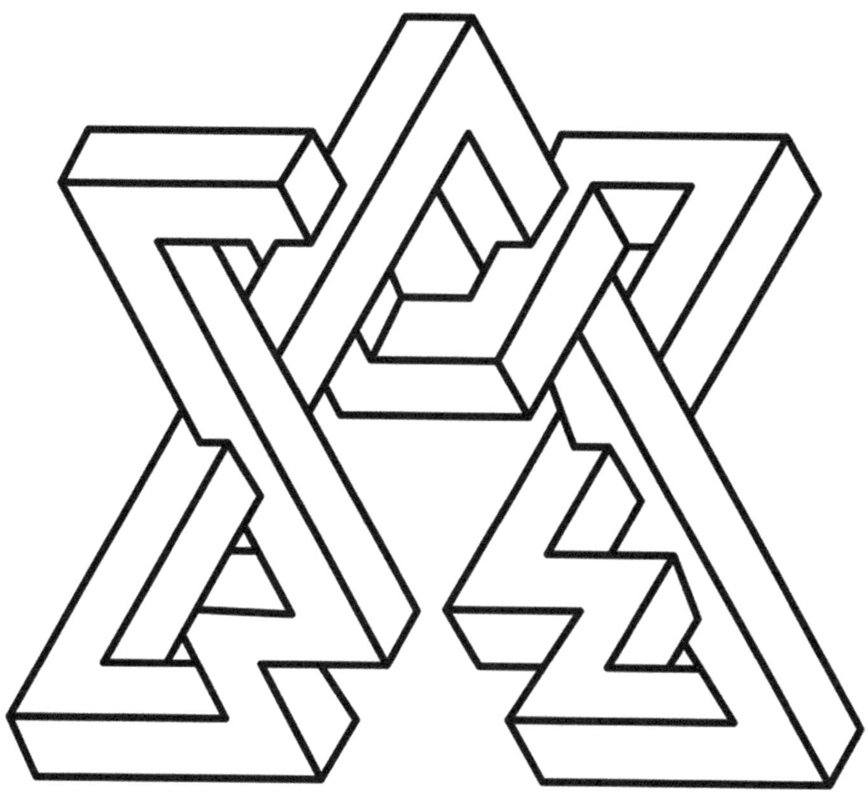

Fig. 111.3 Impossible geometric object inspired by MC Escher. Ilustration: Hanna Olekseichuk, image used under standard license stock.adobe.com

Lessons Learned

- The population of cancer survivors continues to grow due to advances in screening, diagnosis, and survival prolonging new therapeutics. Cancer diagnosis is a life-changing experience; every patient will cope differently.
- Some oncologic patients describe continuous hypervigilance, constant monitoring, and reporting of new and persistent symptoms. They have concerns about impact to family or significant others, as well as potential financial implications of treatment and recovery.
- Patients have difficulty managing stress from health needs, self-perceptions and body image changes, and increased awareness of vulnerability, even if it is shown or masked under different defense mechanisms. There is a special consideration for women, or any patient with children, regardless of age, as this can play an extra stressful factor.
- Oncologic care involves a multidisciplinary team and shared decision-making.
- Anesthesia and surgery are often the first lines of treatment for cancer patients, especially for curative intent. It is important to understand the most common triggers associated with cancer stress to provide care with empathy.
- Patients are likely to present for surgery with information and questions about the planned anesthetic technique, so be prepared to discuss these issues with knowledge and confidence. Never dismiss or wave away concerns related to anesthetic risks.
- There are laboratory and retrospective data that seem to indicate associations with anesthesia agents/techniques but no clear clinical data. Be prepared to discuss differences in these data with your patients.
- Our current understanding is that the effects of regional anesthesia or analgesia on cancer recurrence seem equivalent to general anesthesia. There is no high-quality evidence in humans that confirms a beneficial effect of regional anesthesia on cancer recurrence.
- Similarly, there are no conclusive data pertaining to specific analgesia or adjunctive agents that mandate a change in our current clinical practice paradigm. In the absence of contraindications, it might be prudent to utilize propofol, intravascular lidocaine, and NSAIDs when the clinically applicable.
- Providing cancer care is an honor and privilege that requires a wholehearted and dedicated team approach. We should take advantage of every opportunity to support the population of cancer survivors with love, kindness, and empathy and importantly, stay present for those who unfortunately fail therapy.

References

1. Miller KD, Nogueira L, Devasia T, et al. Cancer treatment and survivorship statistics, 2022. CA Cancer J Clin. 2022;72(5):409–36.
2. Siegel RL, Miller KD, Fuchs HE, Jemal A. Cancer statistics, 2022. CA Cancer J Clin. 2022;72(1):7–33.
3. Global Burden of Disease Cancer Collaboration, Fitzmaurice C, Akinyemiju TF, et al. Global, regional, and National Cancer Incidence, mortality, years of life lost, years lived with disability, and disability-adjusted life-years

for 29 cancer groups, 1990 to 2016: a systematic analysis for global burden of disease study. JAMA Oncologia. 2018;4:1553–68.
4. Ferlay J, Soerjomataram I, Dikshit R, et al. Cancer incidence and mortality worldwide: sources, methods and major patterns in GLOBOCAN 2012. Int J Cancer. 2015;136:E359–86.
5. Mehnert A, Koch U, Sundermann C, Dinkel A. Predictors of fear of recurrence in patients one year after cancer rehabilitation: a prospective study. Acta Oncol. 2013;52(6):1102–9.
6. UpToDate [Internet]. www.uptodate.com. Available from: https://www.uptodate.com/contents/anesthesia-and-cancer-recurrence.
7. Yap A, Lopez-Olivo MA, et al. Anesthetic technique and cancer outcomes: a meta-analysis of total intravenous versus volatile anesthesia. Can J Anaesth. 2019;66:546–61.
8. Hasselager RP, Hallas J, Gogenur I. Inhalation or total intravenous anaesthesia and recurrence after colorrectal cancer surgery: a propensity score matched Danish registry-based study. Br J Anaesth. 2021;126:921–30.
9. Enlund M, Berglund A, et al. Volatile versus propofol general anesthesia and long-term survival after breast cancer surgery: a National Registry Retrospective Cohort Study. Anesthesiology. 2022;137(3):315–26.
10. Sessler DI, Pei L, Huang Y, et al. Recurrence of breast cancer after regional or general anesthesia: a randomized controlled trial. Lancet. 2019;394:1807–15.
11. Du YT, Li YW, Zhao BJ, et al. Long-term survival after combined epidural-general anesthesia or general anesthesia alone: follow-up of a randomized trial. Anesthesiology. 2021;135:233–45.
12. Xu ZZ, Li HJ, Li MH, et al. Epidural anesthesia-analgesia and recurrence-free survival after lung cancer surgery: a randomized trial. Anesthesiology. 2021;135:419–32.
13. Pei L, Tan G, Wang L, et al. Comparison of combined general-epidural anesthesia with general anesthesia effects on survival and cancer recurrence: a meta-analysis of retrospective and prospective studies. PLoS One. 2014;9:e114667.
14. Grandhi RK, Lee S, Abd-Elsayed A. The relationship between regional anesthesia and cancer: a meta-analysis. Oshsner J. 2017;17:345–61.
15. Lee BM, Singh GV, Karam JA, et al. Regional anesthesia/analgesia and the risk of cancer recurrence and mortality after prostatectomy: a meta-analysis. Pain Manag. 2015;5:387–95.
16. Weng M, Chen W, Hou W, et al. The effect of neuraxial anesthesia on cancer recurrence and survival after cancer surgery: an updated meta-analysis. Oncotarget. 2016;7:15262–73.
17. Buckley A, McQuaid S, Johnson P, et al. Effect of anaesthetic technique on the natural killer cell anti-tumor activity of serum from women undergoing breast cancer surgery: a pilot study. Br J Anaesth. 2014;113(Suppl 1):i56–62.
18. Desmond F, McCormack J, Mulligan N, et al. Effect of anaesthetic technique on immune cell infiltration in breast cancer: a follow-up pilot analysis of a prospective, randomized, investigator-masked study. Anticancer Res. 2015;35(3):1311–9.
19. Ecimovic P, McHugh B, Murray D, et al. Effects of sevoflurane on breast cancer cell function in vitro. Anticancer Res. 2013;33:4255–60.
20. Hovaguimian F, Braun J, Z'graggen BR, et al. Anesthesia and circulating tumor cells in primary breast cancer patients: a randomized controlled trial. Anesthesiology. 2020;133:548–58.
21. Oh CS, Park HJ, Piao L, et al. Expression profiles of immune cells after propofol or sevoflurane anesthesia for colorectal cancer surgery: a prospective double-blind randomized trial. Anesthesiology. 2022;136:448–58.
22. Zhang H, Yang L, Zhu X, et al. Association between intraoperative intravenous lidocaine infusion and survival in patients undergoing pancreatectomy for pancreatic cancer: a retrospective study. Br J Anaesth. 2020;124:141–8. https://doi.org/10.1016/j.bja.2020.03.034. Epub 2020 May 28.
23. Cazenave L, Faucher M, Tourret M, et al. Intravenous lidocaine and cancer outcomes after radical cystectomy. Eur J Anaesthesiol. 2022;39:396–9.
24. Forget P, Bentin C, Machiels JP, et al. Intraoperative use of ketorolac or diclofenac is associated with improved disease-free survival and overall survival in conservative breast cancer surgery. Br J Anaesth. 2014;113(Suppl 1):i82–7. https://doi.org/10.1093/bja/aet464. Epub 2014 Jan 23.
25. Forget P, Vandenhende J, Berliere M, et al. Do intraoperative analgesics influence breast cancer recurrence after mastectomy? A retrospective analysis. Anesth Analg. 2010;110:1630–5.
26. Shasshua L, Shabat-Simon M, Haldar R, et al. Perioperative COX-2 and beta-adrenergic blockade improves metastatic biomarkers in breast cancer patients in a phase-II randomized trial. Clin Cancer Res. 2017;23:4651–61.
27. Meyhoff CS, Jorgensen LN, Wetterslev J, et al. Risk of new or recurrent cancer after a high perioperative inspiratory oxygen fraction during abdominal surgery. Br J Anaesth. 2014;113(Suppl 1):74.

Authors

Valentina Baez Sosa is an internist, hematologist, oncologist, transfusion medicine physician, certified bone marrow harvester by the National Marrow Donor Program (NMDP), and co-chair of the American Society of Hematology (ASH) Working Group on Well-Being and Resilience. She completed her transfusion medicine fellowship at the NIH Clinical Center. She is now the director of the Office of Translational Science in the Office of the Scientific Director of National Heart Lung and Blood Institute. In her spare time, she teaches gymnastics to Special Olympic athletes with intellectual disabilities such as Trisomy 21. She is a runner, yogi, and passionate salsa dancer.

Rick Childs is an internist and medical oncologist at the National Institutes of Health. He also serves as the NHLBI's Clinical Director and is a 2-star Rear Admiral in the Commissioned Corps of the United States Public Health Service where he serves as an Assistant United States Surgeon General. Besides being a devoted family man, Rick maintains an active interest in road biking, boating, fishing, sailing, and flying drones.

Cathy Marcucci is a senior anesthesiologist who has cared for thousands of cancer patients in her 30+ years of clinical practice. On behalf of the *Anesthesia Bridges* editors, she extends her thanks to Valentina Baez Sosa and Rick Childs for their assistance with this chapter.

112 Connecting with Palliative Medicine Patients

Amy J. Robbins

Introduction

Amy Robbins is or has been board certified in anesthesiology, pain medicine, and palliative medicine. She did her residency training at Johns Hopkins and was in general practice from 1995 to 2004. She began caring for palliative medicine patients in 2004. From 2004 to 2013, she practiced both general operating room anesthesia and palliative and pain medicine with full transition to palliative medicine in 2013 and continues to practice in that subspecialty today. Here are Amy's thoughts and advice on evolving your communication style to meet the needs of the palliative medicine patient:

Basics and Background

When meeting with palliative medicine patients, remember that it is almost always *the most* fragile and uncertain part of a patient's medical and life journey. Many physicians avoid having difficult conversations or discussing end of life issues with patients. The palliative provider is frequently viewed as an expert in these types of discussions, which tend to be more natural conversations than medical ones. Starting a difficult conversation can show the patient your interest and concern.

Make sure you have read the chart extensively before meeting with the patient or family, as palliative patients frequently have complex medical histories with multiple specialists involved in their care. Find a quiet space, one that is comfortable for patients and their family members. Set aside adequate time, an hour or more may be needed. Remember that advanced disease can have a great impact on a patient's ability to understand, respond, and communicate. Alzheimer's can impede communication skills, older individuals may have hearing deficits, pain medications can slow response time and alter mental status, fear and anxiety of one's medical condition and terminality may cause an inability to comprehend what is being said. Be prepared to repeat information as needed.

A. J. Robbins (✉)
Stanson Health, a Premier Inc. Company, Charlotte, NC, USA

Atrium Health, Carolinas Palliative Care and Hospice Group, Charlotte, NC, USA

S. Mohamed et al. (eds.), *Anesthesia Bridges*, https://doi.org/10.1007/978-3-032-08294-7_112

Do Not Burden the Patient

Many palliative patients do not want to hear a slew of details about their condition. Ask the patient what he knows and understands about his medical condition. A good opening line is “What have other doctors told you about your disease?” Inquire if he wants to know more details and only provide that information if he is agreeable to receiving it. “Would you like to know more about your condition?” It takes great patience to listen to the palliative patient, and you must provide adequate time to allow for the patient to express his concerns and feelings. If a patient is not able to communicate, if he is actively dying or on a ventilator, be ready to spend time in discussion with family members who know the patient and can speak on his behalf.

Talk about practical things at first. “Do you have a will, or living will?” Ask “Do you have any worries or concerns today?” If a patient says he is concerned about how his wife will cope with his death, move on to open-ended questions such as “Can you explain that a bit more to me?” Let the patient lead the way and summarize your understanding of what he expressed. Listen. Pause. Silence can be uncomfortable, and the pauses can be very difficult, but if you can pause for a significant amount of time, you may be surprised how much a patient will begin to speak and lead the conversation. Try counting to 20 slowly in your mind while waiting for the patient to speak.

Setting Goals

Finally, ask the patient what his goals are for this portion of his life. If a patient expresses fear of being in pain, reassure him of your full intent to allow him to be pain free. The treatment of cancer pain, pain of end-stage multiple sclerosis, contracture pain of end-stage Alzheimer’s, and shortness of breath and dyspneic chest pain in the end-stage ALS patient, are as urgent in the palliative medicine patient as they are in the surgical and ICU patient. If a desire to be at home at end-of-life is important, speak of your intent to make that happen. It is important to communicate your goal to care for the palliative patient with the utmost diligence, compassion, and care at this tender junction in his life journey.

Lessons Learned

- The entire communication paradigm for palliative medicine patients is based on a thorough chart review and adequate time. Do not skimp on this.
- The pace and amount of exchange of detailed medical information is dictated by the patient’s (or the surrogates’) needs and wishes. This is very different from what we are used to in the general practice of anesthesia.
- Start with simple focused questions and move to open-ended questions.

- The fear of pain is an overriding concern. This is what firmly ties the general practice of anesthesiology to palliative medicine practice. You must always be competent and ready to gently communicate a comprehensive pain treatment plan without overwhelming the patient.
- Care of palliative medicine patients is an honor for our specialty. Treat your responsibilities and your patients with the utmost dignity and respect.

Author

Amy Robbins lives in Charlotte and Boone, North Carolina. She and her husband Ray Koloski are the parents of five grown children and almost as many rescue animals. When they can get away from the demands of their busy lives, Amy and her family enjoy sports, cooking, traveling, collecting art, and hosting friends for skiing, mountain biking, and hiking in the beautiful Blue Ridge Mountains.

Connecting with Patients with Substance Abuse Disorders: Principles

113

Neil B. Sandson and Catherine Marcucci

Introduction

Drug and alcohol abuse and dependence are widely prevalent in the US, afflicting about 15% of the population and it is estimated that up to 70% of adults experiencing a substance abuse disorder suffered childhood abuse or neglect. No matter what branch of clinical medicine you practice, you will encounter patients who struggle with these issues, and accordingly it is important to develop skills and awareness around how to best communicate with this patient population. In tackling this, a good starting place is to examine some distinctive features of substance-abusing patients.

Basics

Perhaps the most fundamental distinction is that unlike many mental illnesses, *substance abuse and dependence are disorders of doing and not merely of being*. This is to say that substance users have engaged in conscious behaviors and choices that characterize their illnesses, as opposed to individuals with mood or psychotic disorders, in which the defining features of those illnesses are derangements in feeling states, perceptual experiences, thoughts content, and or thought processes, and the symptoms that follow from those derangements.

Depending on our individual philosophical/ideological learnings, we can conceive substance use disorders as dependent upon volition, or as representing a breakdown or overwhelming of volition, but in either case, these illnesses are intimately linked with the subjective sense of choice. As such, many of these patients experience powerful feelings of shame, emotional weakness, and inferiority. They are often very sensitive to any indication or suggestion by providers that their caregivers might share these feelings/opinions about them or similarly-situated patients.

N. B. Sandson
Department of Psychiatry, VA Maryland Health Care System, Baltimore, MD, USA

University of Maryland, Baltimore, MD, USA

C. Marcucci (✉)
Department of Transfusion Medicine, Clinical Center, National Institutes of Health, Bethesda, MD, USA

S. Mohamed et al. (eds.), *Anesthesia Bridges*, https://doi.org/10.1007/978-3-032-08294-7_113

Other frequent characteristics of substance abusing patients include a greater-than-typical intolerance of discomfort, and often frustration as well, though that is less specific to this patient population. They are often *somatically preoccupied and very focused on avoiding pain*. While no one is fond of pain or welcomes it as a possible result of a medical intervention, the substance-abusing patient will often make excessive demands to prospectively avoid or treat pain.

Lastly, many substance abusing patients have developed ways to escape detection for many years, and as such many of them are comfortable with being evasive and even frankly deceptive in providing information to medical providers.

***Note from the Editors:** A solitary figure on a bridge might be a slightly cliched metaphor for substance abuse disorders, but it is nonetheless apt. These diseases are often very isolating and these patients frequently live lonely and devastated lives (Fig. 113.1).

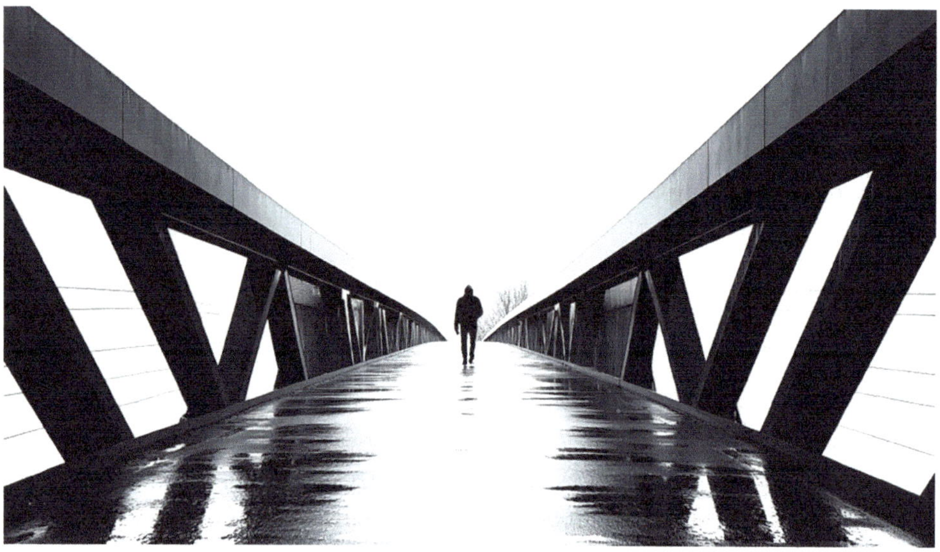

Fig. 113.1 Solitary figure on a lonely bridge. Remember, you do not know what difficulties and obstacles and trauma your patient has experienced. Do not judge. Photo: Image used under standard license from adobestock.com

Specifics

This brings us to specific advice on communication with this patient group:

- These patients are often fearful that providers will regard them as inferior, weak, selfish, shameful, or otherwise unworthy of quality care. It is critically important that *we treat them with the same caring, concern, and solicitude that we would mobilize for any other patient*, and that we hold them in similarly high regard.

- The reason to do so is because they are *not* inferior, weak, shameful, or otherwise unworthy of quality care, and they *do* deserve the same treatment that we would provide to anyone else. If you secretly harbor beliefs to the contrary, then please closely examine and hopefully change these beliefs, optimally with someone skilled and experienced in treating this patient population or absent yourself from clinical medicine.

- The formulation that substance abuse disorders are disorders of doing rather than being does not mean that the afflicted deserve our contempt, but rather our compassion. Whatever choices they have made that define the illness, *what none of them have ever chosen is to be afflicted with this illness in the first place*.

- While these disorders may not fit cleanly into a disease model *per se, they are unquestionably legitimate mental illnesses*, and neither contempt nor disdain should attach to the afflicted, any more than it should attach to other victims of disorders of doing, such as patients with eating disorders or trichotillomania. Accordingly, we should communicate with these patients in a respectful and concerned manner, without judgment or excessive detachment, just as we would for any other patient. They are afraid that we regard them as human garbage; the best way to communicate in ways that dissolve those fears is if we genuinely regard them as fellow human beings deserving of the best that we can provide.

- Uncertainty fuels anxiety, which will exacerbate intolerance to discomfort and frustration. To address this, communication of risks, benefits, and therapeutic options should be particularly clear and complete. Additionally, the more control one can provide to the patient, the better a medical encounter will go.

- It may seem paradoxical that a group of patients who have clearly lost control of their substance use might be particularly concerned with issues of therapeutic control. But even in the throes of addiction, when it could be said that the drug is in control and not the patient, it is nonetheless true that the patient is making the choices for themselves, albeit incredibly maladaptive ones, and they are very invested in preventing anyone else from having control over them.

- The 12 Steps of Alcoholics Anonymous/Narcotics Anonymous go right to the heart of issues of control, and patients who have worked that program are often less dominated by concerns of control, but many others are preoccupied with this concern. So, in communicating with these patients, it is also important to address issues explicitly and prospectively such as pain management and rehabilitative course, if appropriate. One might wish to adopt strategies that provide more control, such as a PCA pump, which meets both patient needs for control and clinician concerns about avoiding excessive dosing.

- Although many substance abusing patients are not completely honest with providers, it is not productive to engage in paradigm of trying to play detective or "catch" the patient in a falsehood. This leads very efficiently to an adversarial relationship in which provider and patient are at cross-purposes, and this of course will arouse patient concerns about being negatively judged.

- Rather, the best approach is to break down the paradigm of having conflicting agendas and demonstrate the ways in which you and the patient have common goals. The reason why this works so well is that it is not an exercise in rhetoric or sophistry, it is actually true. If one communicates to patients that in order to take the best possible care of them, to keep them comfortable without exposing them to danger, and to meet their shared objective of helping them, that you need to have the most accurate information available, then one is much more likely to get exactly that.

- Even in the not-so-hypothetical case of a patient who is malingering symptoms in order to obtain some secondary gain, Neil Sandson has had enormous success with stepping back and saying something like:

> My goal is to help you, not to deny or withhold care. Maybe the system hasn't always responded to you in helpful ways and hasn't provided what you've needed. But let's you and I come to an agreement between us right here and now. Please don't tell me what you think I need or want to hear that will steer me toward providing you with what you want. Please just tell me what you want or need, and in return I'll promise you that I'll do what I reasonably can to meet your needs.

He has had transformative results with this approach, not every time, but much more often than one might guess.

- *Nobody wants to become an addict.* This is no one's aspirational goal in life and it is a life of misery. If we approach our substance-abusing patients with the framework that in their own deeply dysfunctional ways, they are doing the best they can with the defenses and resources at their disposal, if we keep judgment at bay, then we create the space for honest interactions which allow us to provide they care that these patients need and deserve.

Lessons Learned

- Substance abuse disorders are disorders of commission. Nonetheless, *they are legitimate mental illnesses.*
- Nobody wants to become an addict.
- These patients often suffered significant childhood trauma. They also struggle with guilt, shame, anxiety, and bidirectional control issues.
- Do not play "gotcha" with your patient. It is disrespectful and very counterproductive to the physician-patient relationship.
- The best approach is one of common goals and a shared therapeutic plan.
- Effective communication with patients who are afflicted with substance abuse disorders is predicated on the ability to suspend judgment.

Authors

Neil Sandson is a psychiatrist who has cared for thousands of patients with substance abuse disorders. He would like to remind the readers that there is hardly a family in the country who has not been impacted in some way by this terrible constellation of diseases.

Cathy Marcucci went to Temple Med in North Philadelphia. She recalls that nearly every adult patient she saw on her rotations at Temple suffered from one or more substance abuse disorders. She also distinctly recalls that the faculty and house staff treated these ubiquitous and devastating comorbidities with competence and compassion.

Connecting with Patients with Substance Use Disorder—Practicalities

114

Catherine Marcucci and Neil B. Sandson

Introduction

In the previous chapter, **Neil Sandson** laid out a compassionate and commendable philosophical approach to the patient with substance abuse disorder. But what does this communication and connection actually look like in the preoperative clinic or the day of surgery?

From Cathy—Opening the Discussion

The first task is to find out what the patient has used and when. This applies to patients who are using illicit substances as well as patients who may be over-using legally prescribed substances. The best way to get this information is to say:

> We need to make sure that we give you enough pain medication during and after the surgery. The right amount can depend on what medications patients have taken in the last day, the last week, and the last month. We are not here to judge you. What's important is what you have used, how much, and when. I am also going to ask about cannabis because that can affect the profile of other drugs in the body. So, thank you in advance for working with us to take the best care of you that we can.

I also ask if they were nervous in the day before surgery and took any medications not prescribed to them but rather to somebody else at home. If you are matter of fact and non-judgmental, "just trying to make the anesthetic plan," patients will generally tell you.

Next is to find out if the patient has difficulty with tolerating any narcotic or sedating substances. This might seem a bit of a counterintuitive—I will admit that there can be a *tiny* tendency to think, "Jeez, this patient is injecting \$100 a day, every day, of street drugs, how can it be that oral oxycodone messes up their stomach?" Nonetheless, this is what you need to find out and then respect—just as you would for

C. Marcucci (✉)
Department of Transfusion Medicine, Clinical Center, National Institutes of Health, Bethesda, MD, USA

N. B. Sandson
Department of Psychiatry, VA Maryland Health Care System, Baltimore, MD, USA

University of Maryland, Baltimore, MD, USA

S. Mohamed et al. (eds.), *Anesthesia Bridges*, https://doi.org/10.1007/978-3-032-08294-7_114

any other patient who comes to the preop area and says they do not do well with a certain prescribed or over-the-counter medication and asks you not to give it.

Then, we advise that you discuss and agree on a plan for pain management with the patient. *Pain management starts with IV insertion*, remember that patients who abuse substances can develop hyperesthesia to certain skin stimuli, especially needles. Every anesthesiologist should have the narcotic equivalencies pretty much committed to memory, so that is an easy matter to discuss. I found early in my practice that intrathecal narcotics and other adjunctive medications had good efficacy. I could usually get a quick spinal in, using a small needle, without causing the patient significant discomfort. There is a school of thought that these patients should always have primary or at least adjunctive regional anesthesia, but I found that they often could not tolerate having the blocks done. Of course, a ketamine-based pain management plan is a good alternative strategy, but only for certain patients. I have had patients specifically request it and patients adamantly refuse it. Not to be flip about it, but it seems to depend on what all they use as part of their disorder.

I also developed a pre-induction technique of assessing what their baseline narcotic tolerances were using hydromorphone. After the monitors and oxygen were applied, I would titrate 0.2 mg every minute while talking to the patient until they yawned the first time, at which I would proceed with induction. I would often titrate as much as 2.0 mg before the patient got the slightest bit sleepy.

There are three special situations that deserve mention:

- **First**, is the patient on buprenorphine opioid replacement therapy? There are several buprenorphine formulations, the most common is Suboxone. It is a mixed agonist/antagonist with strong affinity for the *mu* receptor and antagonism at the *kappa* receptor. It is to be hoped that such a patient would not present to your preop area without previous consultation with their substance abuse clinicians and management of a suboxone wean. If a patient on active suboxone therapy comes to the OR or ICU on an emergent basis, then you must not rely on mu-agonist receptor pharmacology. In this case, the use of regional anesthesia and ketamine have a different risk-benefit ratio.

- **Second**, there is the situation of the patient who is in recovery from a substance abuse disorder. These patients are sometimes terrified of re-addiction and will request that they receive no narcotic medications at all. In fact, there is some literature that suggests that anesthesia is a risk factor for drug and alcohol craving and relapse in patients who are recovering from substance abuse [1]. So again, the best approach is one of respectful collaboration—do not try to argue them out of their position. Reassure them that you can create a plan that avoids narcotics, and they are free to change their mind at any time.

- **The third situation** that must be discussed with patients is their use of cannabis. Even a couple of days of smoked cannabis acts as a pan-inhibitor of CYP450 liver enzymes including CYP3A4 and CYP2D6. This may inhibit the metabolism and *raise the blood levels of benzodiazepines and local anesthetics*. It is also a P-glycoprotein transport inhibitor and may increase the levels and effectiveness of morphine.

Finally, remember that patients with substance use disorders also may have poor peripheral access. Ask them where the IV should go. If they give you a description of which veins to try and in what order, believe them.

Lessons Learned

- Do a calm, nonjudgmental survey of all substances used from all sources—prescription and illicit—in the last day, week, and month.
- Patients who have substance abuse disorders often have a lot of pain with needlesticks. Use your best techniques!
- Consider pre-induction titration of hydromorphone. Give some fractional doses until the patient yawns or slows down in conversation just a bit. Then use a "typical" amount of narcotic for the procedure.
- Ketamine is a great option for these patients. As is regional anesthesia—if you can get it done without the patient refusing.
- Patients who are recovering from substance use disorders have the right to refuse narcotics. And they often do. There is some rational behind this so you must honor the request.
- Smoked cannabis may have a clinically significant effect on benzodiazepines, local anesthetics, and morphine. It is important to elicit a history of chronic and recent use.
- Remember, it is very rare for a patient to use only one substance.

Reference

1. Sadgeghi P, Zacny JP. Anesthesia is a risk factor for drug and alcohol craving and relapse in ex-abusers. Med Hypotheses. 1999;53(6):490–6.

Authors

Cathy Marcucci has cared for this cohort of patients for her entire clinical career and has published a number of articles and book chapters on the clinical pharmacology of narcotics.

Neil Sandson is a psychiatrist who has a special interest in acute psychotic disorders and the CYP450 liver enzyme system. He estimates that about 75% of his clinical case load involves substance abuse work in some capacity.

Connecting with Patients with Special Needs, Including Disabilities

115

Carol F. Bodenheimer, Patricia M. Togioka,
Anthony A. Chico, and Catherine Marcucci

Introduction

It is imperative that every anesthesiologist, regardless of age, works to maintain elevated competency in caring for patients with special needs, including disabilities. Given the significant number of persons with disabilities in the United States, a doctor will be certain to work with special needs and disabled patients, families, and even colleagues. The Centers for Disease Control in Atlanta reports that 26% of adults in the US had or have a disability, with prevalence higher in the South and Southeast. The number of US children with a disability is 4.3%, with a greater proportion of disabilities experienced by children who live in poverty.

Basic Principles

The most important principle of communicating and connecting with patients with special needs disabilities is, of course, that *they are no different in their fundamental needs and rights than patients without disabilities*. They might also have an additional need or two or three, but they deserve the basic bedrocks of respect, consideration, and excellent medical care.

The other overarching principle is that patients with disabilities generally don't define themselves by their disabilities. Therefore, *always* assume that your patient with a disability or special need lives a full, complete, and independent life in their community and plan your care accordingly. For example, there is no change in recommendations for preoperative pregnancy testing for patients with a disability. Similarly, *do not* make assumptions about whether patients with disabilities do or do not have primary or life partners. Simply say to the patient, "May I ask who is accompanying you today?" if just as you would to a patient without a disability. The patient will readily enough say, "My spouse is with me today." It shows respect when you ask the patient directly and let that person tell you directly the information they want to divulge.

C. F. Bodenheimer
H. Ben Taub Department of Physical Medicine and Rehabilitation, Baylor College of Medicine, Spinal Cord Injury Care Line, Michael E. DeBakey VA Medical Center, Houston, TX, USA

P. M. Togioka (Retired) (✉)
Oregon School for the Deaf, Certified Interpreter for the Deaf and Hard of Hearing, Salem, OR, USA

A. A. Chico
Veterans Affairs Maryland Health Care System, Private Practice, Baltimore, VA, USA

C. Marcucci
Department of Transfusion Medicine, Clinical Center, National Institutes of Health, Bethesda, MD, USA

S. Mohamed et al. (eds.), *Anesthesia Bridges*, https://doi.org/10.1007/978-3-032-08294-7_115

***Note from the Editors:** This bridge and the beautiful reflection in the water are a great metaphor for always remembering that people with disabilities view themselves as whole and complete (Fig. 115.1). And they are looking for a smooth, strong journey through surgery and also through life—just like everybody else.

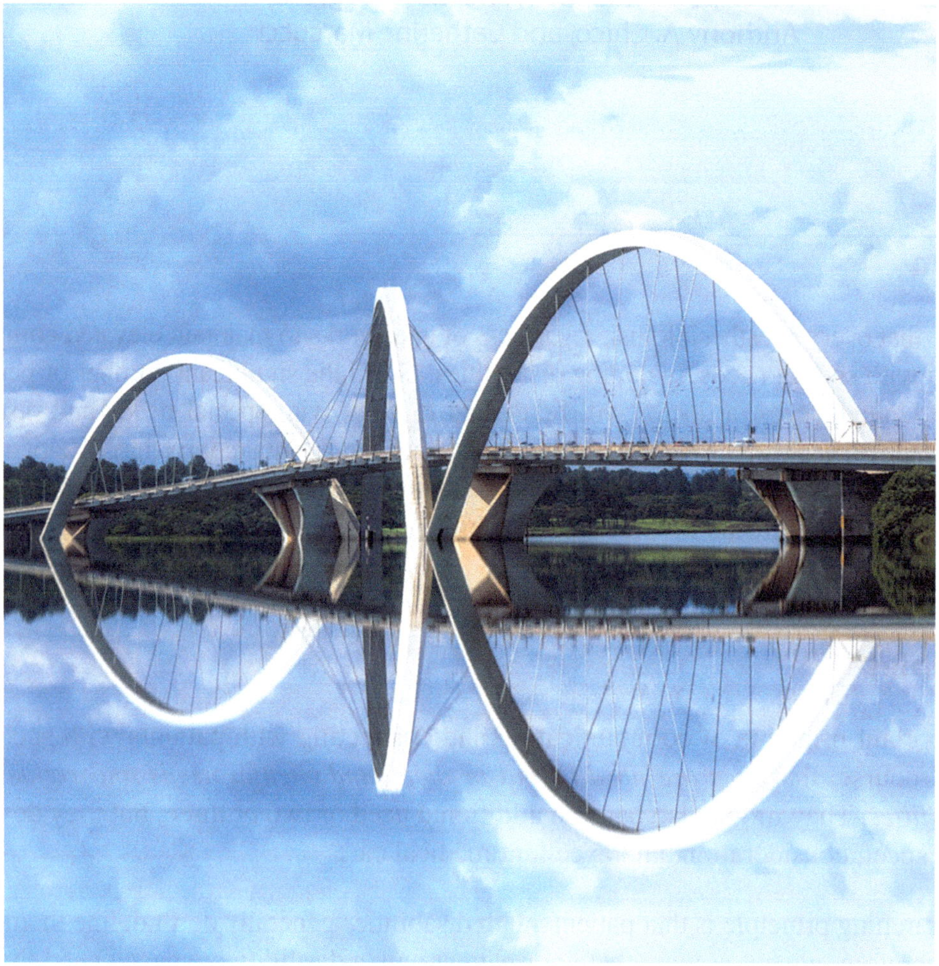

Fig. 115.1 JK Bridge in Brasilia, the capital of Brazil. Photo: R.M. Nunes, image used under license from iStock.com

Also, remember that there is no "disability day" on the OR schedule—you will care for disabled patients for procedures and treatments that are closely linked to their specific disabilities, but also care for patients with disabilities needing a new heart valve, an appendectomy, a labor epidural, or a broken bone pinned because they fell off their skateboard. In addition to the OR, you will also treat patients with disabilities in the pre-op and pain clinics, the ER, and the ICU. Patients with disabilities are every day, regular patients. It's such a mistake to think otherwise and can leave the patients with the opinion that you are looking down on, are afraid of, or worse, are feeling sorry for them.

The Importance of the Patient's History with the Medical System

Many individuals with disabilities unfortunately have had negative interactions with the medical system before meeting you. Keep this in mind and take the time to show your respect by looking at the patient directly, speaking to them and not others accompanying them, and using a normal tone of voice and language, unless the patient asks you to do otherwise. You will have done a good job caring for patients when you have done your usual excellent scope of anesthesia care, but have expanded your considerations and communications to cover the situations arising from their individual circumstances. It's what you *add to* communicating and connecting with patients with disabilities that renders your care excellent, not what you subtract.

It is a sad fact that individuals with disabilities also face significant barriers to health care access in the United States, so much so that at least a third will have an important medical condition that is undiagnosed, under-characterized, or undertreated. As you look at the entire patient situation, keep in mind that you may be providing anesthesia for a patient who unknowingly has diabetes, renal failure, hearing loss, or coronary artery disease.

General Communication Guidelines

The general approach to communicating with patients with disabilities is based on courtesy and common sense. It is important to use patient-centered language as completely as possible, keeping in mind that the preferred usages are somewhat fluid. However, if you approach patients respectfully and frame all discussions and questions from the viewpoint of a patient's free agency and *abilities*, the actual wording is less important.

Similarly, there is an excellent guide online that is a compilation of approximately 30 commonsense tips for anybody in any situation who is interacting with a person having a disability.** It is used by the court system in California and includes guidance on interacting with individuals who have physical, visual, or hearing disabilities. The authors recommend that all physicians review it for general applicability when caring for patients with disabilities.

**www.courts.ca.gov/partners/documents/5-Tips.pdf

Also, remember to use the same care in your notes. These days, most patients can read doctors' notes and documentation through their online chart access. It is unacceptable to use unnecessary subjective descriptors. It is fine to simply and factually describe both abilities and disabilities—"able to drive," "works part-time," or "uses a wheelchair."

Avoiding Anger and Anxiety

It is **Carol Bodenheimer's** experience that patients with disabilities are often most anxious that the acute care rendered in the perioperative setting will worsen their current baseline status or cause untoward setbacks to their medical or other treatments. Patients with disabilities often work hard in rehabilitative therapy on a continuing basis and are loath to sustain setbacks to that investment in their health and optimization of their status. A *patient with a disability usually has a valid reason for asking a physician not to take a specific action.* So, ask what they fear or have experienced during past medical treatments. Please accept their knowledge and experience and avoid doing what the patient has asked you not to do.

Similarly, what can cause a lot of anger for a patient is to be argued with about their disabilities or be put in the position of having to prove or defend their knowledge and expertise about their own disabilities. It is best to allow a patient with a disability to present their own story, as they see it, and your role is to respectfully listen.

However, the constraints of today's medical systems must be acknowledged—if time is growing short and the need for care is approaching, our suggested language is, "I hope there's time later to talk more, but right now I need certain specific information to make sure you get through this part safely." If you provide the context of why understanding specifics of their impairment is important to the medical care at hand, patients with disabilities will usually feel comfortable switching to just the relevant details that may impact the imminent treatment plan.

Do Not Assume That a Disability That You Cannot "See" Does Not Exist

Sometimes, it can be difficult to determine whether your patient has a hidden disability, such as if the chart mentions a diagnosis or disability that is not apparent on the first meeting. If you suspect this, initially greet the patient as you would for a patient having that procedure, then at the first opportunity, say, "As I go along, please let me know at any time what needs you have that I might not be anticipating or that might require more information or discussion." Pause to give the patient time to respond. As you continue your discussion, put any questions or discussions about the patient's disability in the context of why it is important to the delivery of anesthesia care.

Finally, one last general guideline is that short simple expressions of sympathy are appropriate, such as, "I am sorry you have a broken ankle." *But be very careful not to overdo expressions of sympathy and/or empathy to patients with disabilities*—you probably really don't know what it's like to be in their positions or to have experienced their acute and/or chronic medical issues. Also, physicians should be very cautious about sharing their personal medical information with patients. We now realize it does not have the effect that well-meaning physicians intend and can even worsen the connection to the patient.

***Note from the Editors:** First author Carol Bodenheimer is from Stamford, CT (Fig. 115.2). The city has a decently robust level of resources for people with different abilities and will provide communication aids such as qualified sign language interpreters and documents in Braille upon request and without extra charge.

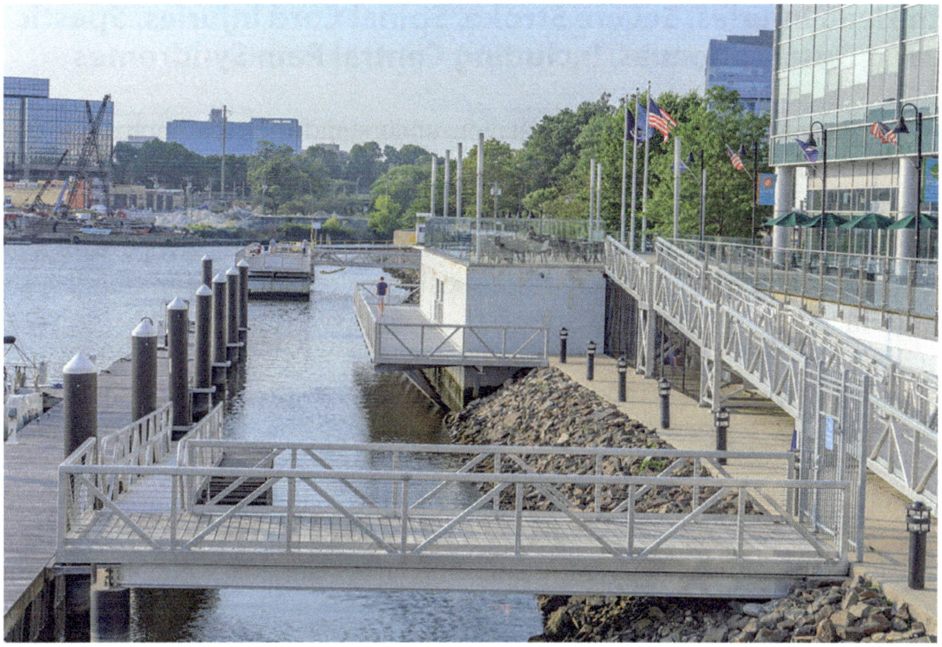

Fig. 115.2 This beautiful and affluent small city on Long Island Sound and the Nippowam River has a marina smack in the middle of the downtown area. The little bridge walkway looks pretty accessible, but what about getting into the boats? Rehab physicians and other rehab and disability professionals continually work toward a future when ADA resources are in place for residents regardless of locale or living situation. Photo: Image used under license from stock.adobe.com

Strategies for Specific Patient Cohorts

Of course, each patient with a disability deserves individualized and careful consideration before care is delivered. There are, however, several general guidelines that might apply to different patient cohorts as discussed below.

Patients with Amputations or Significant Peripheral Musculoskeletal Disabilities

Specific questions you might ask include:

- "Do you need any special support for positioning?"
- "Do you need any special skin care? How has your healing process been with previous procedures?"
- "Do you have any special concerns about pain that you want me to understand?"

Patients with Head Injuries, Severe Stroke, Spinal Cord Injuries, Spastic Conditions, and Dysautonomias, Including Central Pain Syndromes

It is often most important to these patients that you understand their pathophysiology as well as the untoward and even life-threatening risks that medications in the perioperative period may pose. Don't approach a patient without this knowledge. Also, *never* joke with a patient that their condition was a question on a recent exam you took. You can project an air of quiet competence with a brief discussion of how the anesthetic will be tailored to consider specific risks. With that in mind, specific additional questions could include:

- "Have you ever experienced any complications in surgery or after surgery such as hypertension or sympathetic overdrive?"
- "Do you have any information about your implantable device that you want to share with me?"
- "Do you have any information about your history of pain or pain management that you think I should know? How do you manage pain flares at home?"
- "What information can you share about placing IVs or other vascular access?"
- "What information can you share that will help us with comfortably and safely positioning you during the surgery?"

Patients with Intellectual Disabilities

This is a very nuanced topic. There are several key issues that must be resolved, and there is no way around them. First and foremost, does the patient have the capacity to consent? Remember, capacity to consent is not the same as competency! Competency is a legal designation that denotes the right to make one's own decisions. It is presumed unless established otherwise by the courts. Patients who have been deemed incompetent will generally have a court-appointed medical guardian. The medical guardian will provide the legal consent.

Capacity to consent involves the issues of whether the patient has sufficient understanding of the risks and benefits of a planned treatment and the capability to appropriately weigh those factors. It also involves the ability of patients to communicate their thoughts, questions, and concerns. Capacity to consent is situation-specific and can be fluid across time, such as in delirium.

Also, no specific cognitive level is, in and of itself, determinative for capacity to consent. For example, many patients with Trisomy 21 can give valid consents. If the patient does not have the capacity to consent, a substituted consent can be obtained. Most hospitals will have established practices and policies as to how this is done, usually on the order of the next of kin.

Once you have established that there is a valid consent, best practice mandates that the anesthesiologist stop and verify that the patient understood the questions asked or the information given about the procedure. For this reason, we believe that patients with cognitive disability might be the most difficult in terms of achieving a satisfactory level of communication and connection. You may need to allow extra time to interview these patients. Specific questions for these patients can include:

- "Is there anybody who helps you make medical decisions?"
- "Would it be helpful or make you more comfortable to have that person with you until we go into the OR?"

Nonverbal patients can be especially challenging, so you will have to work with family members on the best way to substitute a communication method:

- "Induction and emergence of anesthesia often involve verbal exchange between anesthesia staff and the patient. Can you advise us of any communication methods or strategies that we can substitute for your family member?"
- "What is the best way to reassure and comfort Ms. Johnson?"

Patients with Blindness or Low Vision

These patients generally do well and are very functional in their compensated environments, but the hospital setting is not a familiar (compensated) environment. In general, these patients will be very adept at telling you how to help them navigate the perioperative period. Again, provide the context as to why your queries are important to their anesthesia care. For example, you might ask:

> "There are things we routinely check and assess postoperatively. For example, we routinely ask patients if they are having eye pain to assess whether they have sustained a corneal laceration or abrasion, and we routinely ask the patients to open their eyes as they are emerging from anesthesia and even to wiggle sideways from the stretcher to the OR table and back. Are these questions going to be valid with your visual impairment?"

Patients Who Are Deaf or Hard of Hearing

First Things First: As when discussing other cultural communities, the terms Deaf, Blind, and DeafBlind are capitalized. This signifies a cultural as opposed to a disability identity.

A common story told in the Deaf community is this one. A Deaf person goes into a hotel that is having two conferences. The one to the left of the lobby is a series of seminars about the practicalities and psychology of coping with disabilities, and the one to the right is a conference with presentations about the effect of linguistics on cultural norms and identities. Where does the Deaf person go? To the right, of course!

Patients who are Deaf and Hard of Hearing who utilize a sign language or oral interpreter need face-to-face interpretation to ensure understandability. Never use a family member to interpret. There are numerous horror stories regarding this practice, and one should never assume a family member has any interpreting skills or even proficiency in a second language. Remember: you are one member of the communication partnership. An interpreter is needed equally for you as for the patient. If a patient says they don't need an interpreter and a family member can help or they "understand" well enough, you risk a situation where you are not receiving informed consent. Sometimes the interpreter will translate the written materials as well. Protect yourself and your hospital!

Patients using hearing aids to access communication need extra communication attention because there is usually so much background noise in hospital settings. It can also be difficult to establish privacy when using an interpreter or other in-person strategies, so do your utmost to find a quiet, private space. Make sure there is no direct sunlight behind you or the interpreter. Also, don't accept a "nod" as proof of understanding. Ask the person to summarize or explain back to you what their understanding is. Be careful about family members taking over the conversation. Talk to the patient, not an interpreter or family member. Don't say, "Tell him this." Speak to the patient directly and use second-person pronouns. Specific questions may include:

- "In this noisy environment, what's the easiest and most comfortable way for you to communicate what you need me to know?"
- "Is it helpful to have a pad and paper nearby and/or use more direct face-to-face communication to facilitate speechreading?"
- "Which arm is best for your IV so you can continue to communicate?"
- "Would you like the interpreter to remain with you until your anesthesia takes effect?"
- "We will have the interpreter waiting in the recovery room so that we can check in with you about how you are feeling."
- "We would like to take the time to work with you so that you can show us the signs that you might use in the OR to tell us that you are in pain or feel like you are having trouble breathing."

We recommend taking an induction mask and the other pre-op monitors to the pre-op area and having the interpreter help communicate the instructions that you would normally give to the patient in the preinduction period. Those of us who have been on OR tables can vouch that there is a bit of a helpless feeling in those moments before induction. You want to do everything possible not to compound those feelings for patients who need communication assistance.

Do not ask Deaf patients to move themselves from the stretcher and back before and after the case, as it will be difficult for you to communicate, "Just slide over about two more inches." Also, *do not forget* to include the fact that the patient is Deaf when you do a sign-out, even if it is just for you to leave the room on a break.

Finally, remember that *American Sign Language is a language*, just like Russian or French, or Hindi is a language. It is not just pantomime. Deaf patients in the perioperative period have the right to communicate with somebody who has fluency in their preferred language, just like every other patient.

***Note from the Editors:** The authors, like everybody else in the world, love Venice. We were delighted to hear that Venetian municipal authorities have announced plans for the construction of a number of wheelchair-accessible ramps and bridges (Fig. 115.3). The construction is also planned to accommodate visitors who are Blind and have Low Vision.

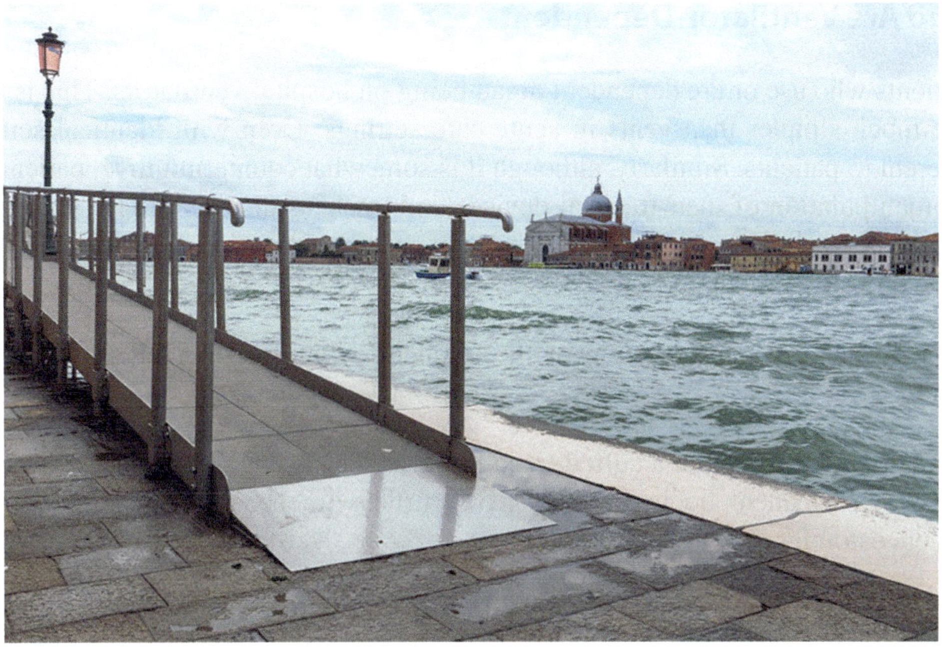

Fig. 115.3 A wheelchair ramp on a bridge adjacent to the Grand Canal in Venice. The new system of ramps and bridges is planned to allow wheelchair users and visitors with Low Vision to easily navigate a route from the city's main entrance at the Piazzale Roma to the iconic St. Mark's square. When completed, these public works will be the first time that Venice, since it was founded in 421 CE, will be widely accessible on land to people with disabilities. Photo: Arjan van deer Veer, image used under standard license from iStock.com

Patients Who Are DeafBlind

There is no one homogenized DeafBlind community. Some persons become blind early in life and lose their hearing as they age. Other people can be Deaf or Hard of Hearing and lose vision slowly, such as with Usher's syndrome, a rare genetic condition that leads to significant loss of hearing and vision but not a shortened lifespan. Other patients who are Deaf may also suddenly lose vision due to a variety of possible issues, including diabetes and trauma. A person who is DeafBlind may or may not know ASL or Braille. An individual might have no connection to others who have deafness and/or blindness.

When interacting with a patient who is DeafBlind, it is best to take their cue regarding communication. Often a family member or assistant may model effective strategies. Some people prefer an ASL interpreter, others may wish to touch your face to speech read, others may bring an enlarging device to read, while still others may depend on hearing aids. A specially qualified tactile interpreter may be required, so it is important that the perioperative team allows enough time for the patient's needs to be met. Whenever possible, let the patient handle the types of objects you will use when providing anesthesia prior to doing anything. As with all patients, clear explanations, a kind heart, and leaving adequate time for questions provide that all-important connection.

Patients Who Are Ventilator-Dependent

In general, patients who use or are dependent dread being on hospital ventilators. This is because home ventilators are much simpler than vents in acute care settings. Even with identical settings, hospital vents feel different to patients. Similarly, although it is somewhat counterintuitive, patients with tracheostomies find manipulation of their tracheal devices and tracheas distressing. Be sure to discuss why you are changing the tracheal device and when they can expect that it will be changed back to their usual device. Specific questions might be:

- "What can I do to make the insertion of the tracheal device for the OR more comfortable for you?"
- "How do you communicate with a cuffed trach in place?" This is particularly important since many individuals with permanent tracheostomies have cuffless tracheostomies or specialty fenestrated speaking tracheostomies.

Patients with Autism Spectrum Disorder—Anthony Chico, DO

Autism Spectrum Disorder (ASD), as the name suggests, is a condition that spans the spectrum of severity and involves a variable collection of symptoms that will sometimes necessitate a specialized plan based on the child's or adult's clinical needs. Remember always that the fact that ASD patients might have special needs in the perioperative period does not mean that they are being difficult. Although these can be happy and healthy patients who go to camp and play sports and do everything that everybody else does in both childhood and adulthood, this is not a fun diagnosis to have, and there is no longitudinal secondary gain for the patients or families.

Some key symptoms to factor into the treatment approach include:

- *Presence/severity of intellectual disability*
- *Presence/severity of communicative difficulties*
- *Ability/inability to engage in social reciprocity*
- *Ability/inability to self-soothe*
- *Common co-occurrence of anxiety and fear of new experiences, sensory stimuli, and/or items in the environment*

My general approach in the past in the emergency department would be to first meet with the parents and get a general sense of the patient's intellectual functioning and ability to communicate, and I strongly recommend this for anesthesiologists.

Here are some tips to provide the best possible care to this deserving patient cohort:

- **Comfortable Environment:** Create a calm and quiet environment in the preoperative area to reduce sensory overload. Minimize bright lights, loud noises, and overwhelming stimuli. Try to find the least noisy section of the pre-op area to minimize exposure to other patients and any crying or concerns they could overhear.
- **Sensory Accommodations:** Be aware of sensory sensitivities and provide accommodations as needed. For example, offering noise-canceling headphones or allowing patients to bring comfort items like a favorite toy or blanket can help. Be liberal about this, within the bounds of safety—use your discretion as the attending anesthesiologist to break a few rules, if necessary, about the number of teddy bears that can accompany the child back to the OR. Allowing the patient to keep a stuffed animal, special soothing item, or gaming device as long as possible can help aid in self-soothing and preparation to accept the next step in treatment.
- **Look for Signs of Discomfort:** Some patients are unable to interpret painful stimuli. Be aware that some children can have *decreased* sensory processing, especially to pain stimuli. The *Bridges* editors know of at least one case of a child, with age-typical communication skills, who walked around for a week with a broken arm.
- **Visual Aids and Social Stories:** Use visual aids, pictures, and social stories to explain the anesthesia process and what to expect during the procedure, which can help reduce anxiety and improve understanding. Be careful not to overdo this; however, as it may cause the patient to think of more anxiety-producing possibilities.
- **Clear and Simple Language:** When explaining medical procedures or asking questions, use clear, simple language. Avoid figurative language or idioms that may confuse individuals on the autism spectrum. Also, be very careful about jokes. Jokes only work if the joke is appropriate for the intellectual level, especially in terms of appreciating sarcasm, and play on words. Linguistic nuances may be misinterpreted or understood literally.
- **Empathetic Listening:** Be patient and attentive when listening to the patient and their caregivers. Acknowledge their feelings and concerns and validate their experiences. Model confidence in the patient's ability to manage the procedure.
- **Social Cues:** Recognize and respect the patient's unique social cues and communication style. Some individuals on the autism spectrum may have difficulty with eye contact or use alternative communication methods, such as gestures or AAC (Augmentative and Alternative Communication) devices.
- **Nonverbal Cues:** Pay attention to the patient's nonverbal cues to understand their comfort level and potential distress. Some people with ASD are very sensitive to physical touch, so be careful when offering touch-based signs of support.
- **Avoid Rushing:** Allow extra time for the patient to process information and make decisions. Rushing can increase anxiety and make communication more challenging.

- **Patient and Family Meetings:** Allow extra time for discussions with the patient and their family to address any concerns, answer questions, and build rapport.
- **Collaborate with Healthcare Providers:** Work closely with pediatricians, child psychologists, or other healthcare providers familiar with the patient's medical history and communication needs to develop a comprehensive care plan. Utilize the services of child-life consultants if available. If the procedure is one that is preplanned, consider making a phone call to the patient's occupational therapist, counselor, or special education teacher to explain the procedure so that this trusted person can prepare the patient in advance. A signed release from the parent may be needed. Alternatively, ask the parent about having the trusted professional do some prep work with the patient.
- **Medical Staff Training and Education:** Consider providing additional training for the medical staff regarding autism awareness and communication techniques. It is always very helpful to have a person with ASD who has experienced procedures speak to medical staff. This is always preferable when doing staff training about any disability or condition. You can often find speakers through a disability or medical disease support group.
- **Practice Patience and Flexibility:** Everyone on the autism spectrum is unique, so be prepared to adapt your communication approach based on the patient's needs and preferences.
- **Model Confidence in the Patient:** Assure the patient that you believe in them and have their best interests and needs in mind.
- **Courtesy and Respect Always:** Do <u>not</u> treat an adult patient with ASD like a child. Treat them like an adult who is dealing with a lifelong medical condition.

Here are just a few examples of specific language that you can practice and consider:

- "We always try to use the patient's/family's preferred language. When I do the sign-out to the PACU staff, what language should I use to describe your medical history?"
- "What has been particularly helpful or not helpful in the past?"
- "Do you like cherry popsicles or bubblegum? We can put a little of this on the breathing mask that will make it smell like cherries or bubblegum (and then show the patient both the mask and the syrup bottle). There won't be bubblegum on the mask; it will just smell like bubblegum. Do you want to ask your Teddy about this?"
- "If something is happening that you feel is too much for you to handle, how are you able to let me know that?"
- "You will wake up after surgery and be able to eat (or drink). I will see you, and your parents will be there. Your surgery will be all done, and you will be able to go home when you feel better."

  Patti Togioka tells about students with deafness who had never met an adult with the same disability. Some students mistakenly believed they would become hearing as adults. In the same way, some patients with ASD may believe they won't wake up after anesthesia or will lose a required body part.

Taking the time, in the beginning, to build rapport with the patient as well as listening to the caregiver's concerns and suggestions of engagement (behavioral, communication, and soothing techniques) will undoubtedly improve the care the anesthesiologist can provide as well as increase the likelihood the experience will be more positive and comfortable for the patients with autism spectrum disorder as well as the clinical staff caring for them. No matter how long the surgeons scrub their hands, anxiety and distress can quickly become infectious in the cold, sterile environment of the operating room without a proper plan to comfort this patient population.

***Note from the Editors:** This trail and bridge are in Sweden. In Scandinavia, people of all abilities are out in nature a lot even in winter, and the rope guide is as much an important bridge to the outdoors as the path (Fig. 115.4).

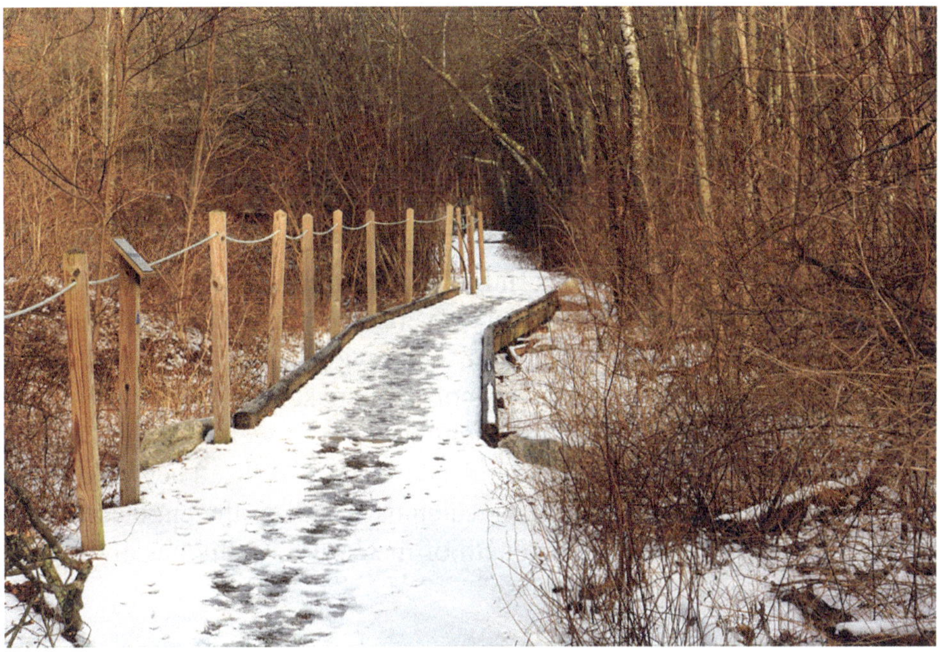

Fig. 115.4 Hikers or birders trace a rope with their right hand through the forest. The ropes on adaptive trails often have different textures that can warn them to watch their step or lead them to a QR code with an audio bird guide. This trail has signposts in Braille. Photo: Image used under standard license from stock.adobe.com

PACU and Postoperative Care

Finally, there are unique considerations for PACU and postoperative care for patients with disabilities. One of the most pressing issues is the lack of adequate pain control. Because patients may have limited ability to communicate their *symptoms* in the postoperative period, it is incumbent upon anesthesia staff to pay scrupulous attention to postoperative *signs*. Anesthesiologists covering the PACU must seek out and be vigilant for perturbations in airway reflexes and patency, respiratory pattern, skin tone and color, urine output and bladder distension, and mental status, including agitation. They may reveal to you what the patient cannot express.

Lessons Learned

- People with disabilities are the largest minority group in the United States—about 54 million people.

- It is also the most diverse minority group. People with disabilities constitute our nation's largest minority group, which is simultaneously the most diverse. Everyone is represented: all genders, all ages, all religions, all socioeconomic levels, and all ethnic backgrounds. *The disability community is the only minority group that anyone can join at any time* [1].

Remember, *"person first" language, always!* Patti Togioka referred us to the official policy of the State of Oregon for reference and examples. It can be found at ORS 410.710, "State Policy on Persons with Disabilities" [2]. The policy is a good summary of the requirements that were instituted when state business is conducted that concerns persons with disabilities. We recommend a quick look.

- The most important thing to remember is that patients with disabilities are not "less than" nondisabled patients. They see themselves and wish to be seen by their care providers as fully intact patients who have some additional features in their medical profiles. That is why the "person first" language was adopted.

- Once, several decades ago, Cathy Marcucci informally consulted Carol Bodenheimer about caring for an upcoming patient who was living with very severe cerebral palsy. The patient was 19 years old, and it was the third week of May. After Carol finished reviewing the general positioning issues, she remarked, "Remember, this patient is cognitively normal—make sure to ask her how college is going." So, at the end of the pre-op interview, Cathy inquired if finals were over and how they went. The patient was not able to walk or speak due to her disability, but she used her language device, and the answer came back quickly, "They sucked! Last calculus course in the engineering core curriculum. Next semester, engineering statistics and strength of materials." Cathy has always remembered this striking example of "person first, disability last."

- The information published by the California court system regarding interacting with persons with disabilities is a good general primer. It is recommended by Dr. Bodenheimer as a good basic introduction to respectful communication and interaction. Please, visit the link noted above!

- Accept that your patient with a disability likely has as much specific knowledge about their disability as you have general knowledge. In today's online world, it would be rare to have a patient who had not extensively researched their disability situation. The viewpoint of patients with disabilities is that the perioperative period is when two sets of experts get together to confer and collaborate before needed medical care is delivered. They are the experts in their disability, and we are the experts in the delivery of anesthesia.

- Patients with disabilities are often anxious when interfacing with the medical system for acute care, and rightfully so. They often have a long history of problems that have come up in previous medical situations. This is one reason it is so important to have persons with the disease process or disability be the expert speakers at medical staff trainings. There are lessons from "horror stories" that staff may never imagine that can be learned.

- At the time of this writing, the impact of COVID and long COVID disabilities on managing perioperative patients is unclear but is likely to be significant.

- A primary task when caring for patients with intellectual disabilities is to establish whether the patient has the capacity to consent. Remember that competency and capacity to consent are not the same thing. *Competency* is a legal concept, and all adults are presumed to have legal competency to make decisions unless a legal proceeding has resulted in a declaration of lack of competence. *Capacity* demonstrates the cognitive and emotional wherewithal to reasonably provide consent.

- *Do not* automatically rule out regional anesthesia for patients who are Deaf or Blind. Remember that even infants can safely receive regional anesthesia in the appropriate situations. We have seen ASL interpreters in scrubs in the OR with patients who are receiving regional anesthesia. Masks with clear front covers can aid in speechreading, if available.

- Flexibility and creativity in communicating with any patient with a disability can sometimes make a huge difference. Two examples regarding persons who knew sign language but were not deaf or hard of hearing made a real impact: one patient was working with staff and family to discuss the removal of a vent tube, which would result in death. The patient could not speak but knew ASL. Having an ASL interpreter provided the opportunity for the patient to explain his wishes. Another patient with ALS was a former sign language interpreter. When she could no longer speak, an interpreter was provided so that she could use signs she was still able to produce to communicate with staff, family, and caregivers.

- Probably the single biggest deficiency in perioperative care of patients with disabilities is lack of adequate pain control. In fact, while we were working on this chapter, Patti sent the following email to us:

  > I just read an article in the April 2023 *Anesthesia News* newspaper (Volume 49 #4) about a study of pediatric patients with Autism Spectrum Disorder getting less pain relief measures than non-ASD children. It is called 'Study Examines Peri-op experience of Children with Autism Spectrum Disorder'. It is written by Michael Vlessides and is on pages 18–19.

- ASD is a large umbrella group of conditions. Taking enough time to really listen to the patient and family is really the key to providing exemplary care.

- The parents/family members will guide you as to what is comforting and discomforting to their child or loved one. Truly, they are the expert as to what works, so don't waste your time trying to reinvent the wheel. Having someone with the patient in the OR, if possible, is a wonderful idea.

- Communicating and connecting with patients with ASD is all about appearing to go slowly and gently while actually swiftly and efficiently navigating the tasks that the patient might find difficult or unpleasant, such as putting the IV in or placing the monitors. Resolving this tension borrows heavily from the practice of anesthesia for neurotypical pediatric patients. It's really an art and a skill, and what expert anesthetic care is all about.

Avoiding Common Anesthesia Errors, 2nd Edition—also known as "*Green2*"—has several chapters with additional clinical advice for the care of patients with disabilities, both coauthored by Carol Bodenheimer, our respected physiatry collaborator and colleague. Please give them a look if you can.

The Green2 Chapter Titles on Patients with Disabilities Include

- Individuals with Cerebral Palsy and Other Spastic Disorders Need Your Best Positioning Prowess.
- Use Extra Care in Positioning Patients Who Have Had Amputations.

Reference

1. What is people first language. [Internet]. Thearc.org [cited 2025 Jun 20]. Available from: https://thearcoregon.org/wp-content/uploads/2018/10/9.2-People-First-Language.pdf.

Authors

Carol Bodenheimer is a physiatrist with appointments at several Texas academic institutions and the Department of Veterans Affairs. She has clinical expertise and research interests in multiple subspecialties of physical medicine and rehabilitation, including head injury, spinal cord injury, and gait and ambulation. She and her husband, Seth Alberts, live in Houston and have three young adult children. Her hobbies include cooking, traveling, and quilting.

Patti Togioka is an uber-experienced educator, administrator, linguist, and certified interpreter. She was first a teacher at and then the superintendent of the Oregon School for the Deaf in Salem, OR. She is fluent in American Sign Language. We are beyond impressed that she follows the anesthesia news and can cite it to us.

Tony Chico is board-certified in child, adolescent, and adult psychiatry. He is a staff and academic psychiatrist in the Maryland VA Health Care and University of Maryland systems, and also maintains a private practice in Towson. He and his wife Kim are the proud parents of two busy young men. Besides hanging out together at home, the Chico family enjoys traveling and sports.

Cathy Marcucci has been conferring with Anthony Chico for six months, Patti Togioka for nine months, and Carol Bodenheimer for 39 years. She has learned a great deal from all these professional collaborations and believes that seeking out colleagues from different medical specialties and professional communities makes for more well-rounded physicians.

Connecting with Patients Who Refuse Blood Due to Religious Concerns

116

Linda H. Song, Shelley Sahu Kalsi, Raymond G. Graber, and Catherine Marcucci

> Because the life of every creature is its blood. That is why, I have said to the Israelites, 'You must not eat the blood of any creature, because the life of every creature is its blood; anyone who eats it must be cut-off'.
>
> —New International Bible, Leviticus 17:14.

The very first fact on the American Red Cross's "Facts About Blood Needs" is: Every two seconds, someone in the US needs blood and or platelets [1].

As anesthesia providers, the concept of blood transfusion can seem so "normal." We are constantly ordering blood products: for the trauma patient, for the surgical oncology patient, for the patient with ongoing GI bleed and anemia in the ICU, or for the patient with severe cirrhosis and deranged INR. A 2017 study showed in a two-year review of all inpatient encounters that 12.5% of them involved a transfusion, with red blood cells being the most common product infused, followed by platelets and then plasma [2]. With just over one out of ten hospitalized patients getting blood transfusions as a national average, it's no wonder that we as clinicians are inured to the novelty of it.

Jehovah's Witnesses and Other Religious Communities

But for patients, the idea of receiving blood products can be entirely foreign or frightening, and for specific groups of patients, expressly forbidden. The Jehovah's Witness faith (JW) is famously one such group. The definition of who is counted as an active member of the JW faith is a bit complicated, but there are at least 1.2 million followers who have an active presence in most US counties. By some metrics, there may be as many as 8.5 million active practitioners. Most experts agree that the membership

L. H. Song · C. Marcucci (✉)
Department of Transfusion Medicine, Clinical Center, National Institutes of Health, Bethesda, MD, USA

S. S. Kalsi
Hematology Graduate Medical Education and Consult Service Section, Division of Intramural Research, National Heart, Lung, and Blood Institute National Institutes of Health, Bethesda, MD, USA

R. G. Graber
Department of Anesthesiology and Perioperative Medicine, University Hospitals Cleveland Medical Center, Cleveland, OH, USA

S. Mohamed et al. (eds.), *Anesthesia Bridges*, https://doi.org/10.1007/978-3-032-08294-7_116

is increasing—by as much as 20,000 followers since 2019. For comparison, there are about 7.6 million members of the core American Jewish community.

However, there are numerous other religious faiths that have proscriptions on accepting blood transfusions. For instance, the Muslim faith teaches that transfusion is a form of nourishment and, during Ramadan, may be considered to break the fast. There are also numerous cases in the medical literature and court system involving Christian Science practitioners who refused transfusions and blood therapies.

In 1996, Congress enacted the Child Abuse Prevention Act of 1996, which legislates that there was no federal requirement that a child must be provided "medical service or treatment against the religious beliefs of the parent or legal guardian." This provided a federal legal basis on which minority faiths were not required to provide medical treatment, including transfusion to their children.

Finally, there may be cultural and ethnic patient cohorts that refuse transfusion. Since the 1990s, the United States has served as a refuge to Hmong displaced from their native Cambodia. Some Hmong individuals eschew surgical interventions and employ shamans to effect cures for ailments, and this may extend to refusal of transfusion.

Diversity of Beliefs in the Jehovah's Witness Community

However, the religious objections that the authors have seen most frequently are those by the JW community. The Watchtower Society (WTS) is the official guiding organization for JWs. The WTS states that, according to the interpretation of specific passages within the Bible, JWs are to abstain from blood, and there is no special dispensation in emergency situations [3].

While this refusal of blood products can at times seem incompatible with medical care, JWs do seek out medical care and treatments. Additionally, JWs are not a monolith, and there can be considerable variation in interpretation regarding the use and consumption of blood products as well as procedures that involve the removal and return of blood from the body. The authors have personally cared for JW patients who died after refusing every blood product and therapy, but have also cared for JW patients who consented to a kidney transplant.

An additional point for us to remember is the necessity of medical confidentiality between the patient and their care team. A 2000 article in *The Journal of Medical Ethics* explores the hurdles and challenges a JW has to navigate when making blood acceptance decisions [4]. According to this article, WTS states that individual JWs are "free to choose" blood component therapies, but that freedom to choose also includes acceptance of the subsequent consequences of breaking with current guidance. Consequences can be as severe as "disfellowship," something akin to excommunication from the JW community, resulting in separation from family and friends. Unfortunately, family members and other JW hospital workers have been known to breach patient confidentiality and report patients who break from the blood policy to JW leadership [4, 5].

***Note from the Editors:** Since this chapter is about religious communities, we wanted to find a beautiful bridge associated with a place of worship and we definitely met our goal (Fig. 116.1).

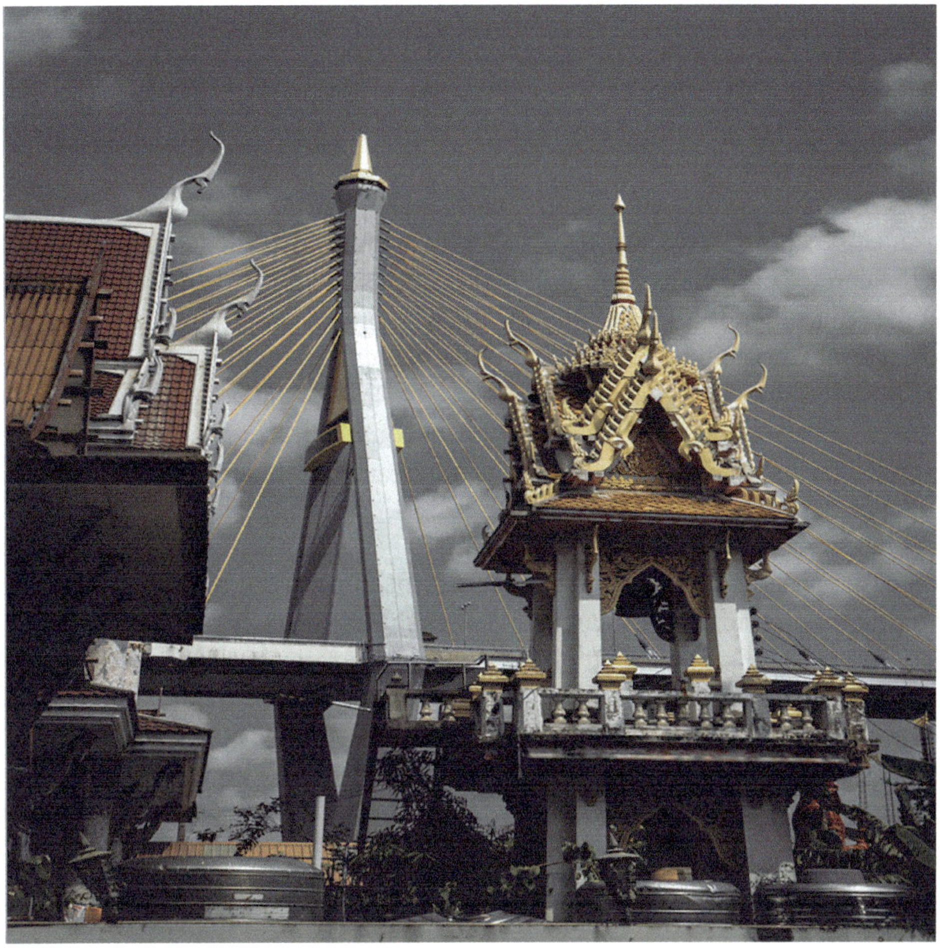

Fig. 116.1 Beautiful Buddhist temple with a modern suspension bridge in the background in Bangkok, Thailand. Photo: anutr tosirkul, image used under standard license from iStock.com

Caring for Jehovah's Witness Patients—Principles

So, how do we best take care of these patients within the constraints of the perioperative timeline? Hospital systems vary, of course, but we can share the approaches taken by our respective institutions.

First and Foremost Is Respect for the Patient's Beliefs: All patients have an absolute right to religious self-determination, of course. Nobody questions that. But the seeming lack of congruity in their specific decisions with respect to the individual blood components that they will and will not accept can be baffling. And lead to the urge to point out to them that their choices are not internally consistent. Once a resident said to us, "Gosh, when you read that quote from Leviticus, you'd think that JW patients would all be vegetarian instead of refusing blood for things like placental abruption." She wasn't being disrespectful; there's a valid point there.

But you must guard against these understandable feelings. Do not *ever* tell a JW that their individual or collective choices about individual blood components aren't logical or consistent. JW patients almost always have read and thought a lot about these issues. They generally already know what they believe and will consent to; occasionally, they will have questions about a component or technique they are not familiar with. Our job is to discuss and document those decisions and provide expertise on any remaining questions. Consenting a JW patient for "transfusion" is not one consent; it's a series of consents as you work through the discussion of the individual blood components and therapies. Show respect always and do not make any assumptions.

Second: You must be comfortable working within your hospital's medical, administrative, and legal framework for the care of patients with religious objections to blood. Sometimes the care of JWs and other patients takes place under a bloodless medicine umbrella, and the patients will have (we hope) undergone pre-op evaluation and optimization. But not every small hospital has such a program. Regardless, it's important that you give competent care to this patient cohort, and the patients are confident they are receiving the care they deserve. Make sure you understand the policies and procedures and that you are knowledgeable about the consent procedures and documents.

Third: The issues are considerably more complicated than the transfusion of the "main" blood products—red blood cells, plasma, and platelets. What also becomes very pertinent to anesthesia management is ensuring that the patient understands and verbalizes their consent/rejection of things such as cardiopulmonary bypass, cell salvage, and other extracorporeal circuits.

The current WTS guidance states that as long as a continuous circuit is maintained, external tubing for those above procedures can be considered an "extension of one's own circulatory system" [6]. But the ultimate decision to accept whether or not the continuous circuit is "self" is left up to the individual, and we have seen patients refuse intraoperative cell salvage techniques. However, we have also seen patients accept an epidural blood patch. Please note that there are several techniques in the literature describing how a blood patch can be done with continuous tubing and three-way stopcocks [7].

Fourth: Make sure that you are familiar with the major review articles on caring for patients who refuse transfusion and bloodless medicine. For example, Mason and Tran published a summary article pertaining to the JW parturient in 2015 [8]. There is also considerable information in the surgical and critical care literature on optimizing care throughout the perioperative period.

Case Western/University Hospitals

At Case Western/University Hospitals, the blood declination form has evolved over the years, as new product formulations and technologies have become available. Note that this is not labeled a "Jehovah's Witness form," because there are patients who refuse blood products for other reasons—such as fear of infection—which we cover in Chap. 117. This form serves as a concise checklist which guides the provider in his or her discussion with the patient and also allows the patient to specify what products or procedures they will accept. Our form has traditionally been paper, but future iterations will likely be integrated into the patient's electronic medical record.

In our checklist, we first discuss the products that most JWs will refuse—platelets, plasma, and packed red cells. We will then move on to talk about the protein derivatives such as albumin, cryoprecipitate, and fibrinogen concentrate—many of which are accepted. Then lastly, we discuss procedures like cell salvage and hemodialysis, if applicable to the surgical procedure. This form is filled out in the pre-op holding area, and then can be discussed as part of the huddle in the operating room.

We recommend that the patient not receive any sedatives prior to the huddle in the OR, so that the patient may participate in the huddle and make any last-minute changes or amendments to the form if they desire. The authors are aware of cases where last-minute changes were made in the transfusion plan/consent when patients were able to speak totally privately to the anesthesia and surgical care teams. The other advantage of having this form is that it is written documentation of what the patient wants—so that if there is a change in provider or the patient remains intubated and sedated post-op—the patient's desires are clearly delineated.

NIH—Alternate Transfusion Plan

At the Clinical Center at the National Institutes of Health (NIH), which admittedly is not subject to the same pressures as a busy private or academic medical center, coauthor Shelley Kalsi oversaw the development of the Alternate Transfusion Plan (ATP) that is used for JWs and other patients with objections to transfusion. The ATP covers the range of available transfusion-related therapies generally available at the NIH. This includes "medical" therapies like interleukins and interferons.

We think it's important that anesthesiologists have a good overview and reference point pertaining to the transfusion options that patients may read about in the JW literature and then ask about when they present for care. Knowledge of the expanded list of transfusion options is of value when caring for JW in the ICU and the extended care clinics. For instance, it's conceivable that fibrin sealant or dialysis would be considered for a critically ill surgical patient or an epidural blood patch for a parturient, and there may be value in having documentation on these options in the chart.

The following is a partial list to consider and discuss with JW and other patients who may consider refusing blood on religious grounds:

- **Whole Blood Components**
  - Red blood cells
  - White blood cells
  - Platelets
  - Plasma/cryoprecipitate
- **Plasma-Derived Components**
  - Albumin
  - Plasma protein fractions
  - Plasma-derived clotting factors

  - Immunoglobulins
  - Fibrin sealant
  - Fibrinogen
- **Medications to Promote the Production of RBCs (erythropoietin, etc.)**
  - Reconstituted with albumin
  - Reconstituted without albumin
- **Medications to Promote the Production of WBCs (filgrastim, etc.)**
  - Reconstituted with albumin
  - Reconstituted without albumin
- **WBC Derivatives**
  - Interferons
  - Interleukins
- **RBC Derivatives (Animal)**
  - Hemoglobin oxygen-carrying compounds
- **Medical Procedures and Techniques that Use Patient's Own Blood**
  - Apheresis
  - Auto-transfusion techniques—cell salvage, acute normovolemic hemodilution

When a JW patient is enrolled in an NIH clinical protocol and/or admitted to the Clinical Center, the study physicians and/or nurses order a consult with the Department of Transfusion Medicine (DTM). The patient is usually seen within 24 hours by a DTM fellow. It can take several visits to review the ATP document, answer questions about blood and blood-derived components, and techniques they may not be familiar with, and complete the patient's chosen transfusion plan.

The form is then signed and placed in the patient's chart, regardless of whether a blood transfusion is required or even anticipated at that time. Any transfusion refusal is also entered into the internal databases of the DTM as a second safeguard to the patient inadvertently receiving an unwanted transfusion. The ATP discussion is not a consent discussion *per se,* and a signed ATP is not a legal consent. The patient may change or amend the Alternate Transfusion Plan at any time for any reason.

However, when completed, the ATP serves as an *a priori* documentation of the patient's wishes. The transfusion plan is then available for use by any licensed independent provider, including the surgeons and anesthesiologists, when consenting the patients for transfusion. It is interesting to note that sometimes the nonanesthesia providers will refer questions about some of the techniques, such as cell saver and epidural blood patch, to the anesthesiologists and the anesthesiologists will refer certain questions about immunoglobulin therapy or interferons/interleukins to the internists and transfusion medicine physicians.

***Note from the Editors:** Several of the *Anesthesia Bridges* authors have lived or worked in Omaha, NE. Omaha is home to the unique and beautiful Abraham's Circle Bridge (Figs. 116.2 and 116.3). The Circle Bridge is part and parcel of the Tri-Faith Initiative, a consortium of three separate religious communities whose houses of worship are all located at points adjacent to the Bridge. Members of the three communities meet frequently to walk around the Bridge and discuss and debate the big issues.

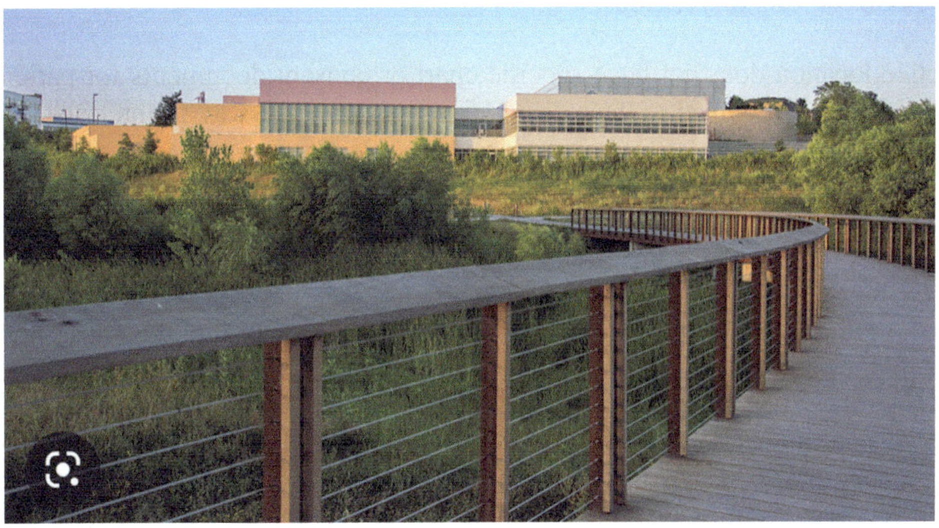

Fig. 116.2 The walkway of the Abraham's circle bridge in Omaha, NE. Photo: courtesy of Tri-Faith Initiative

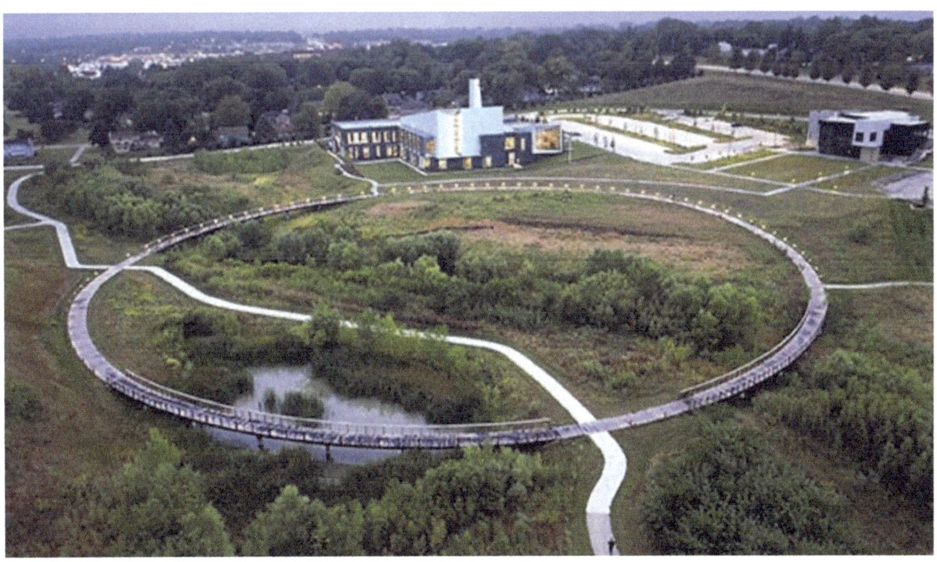

Fig. 116.3 An aerial view of the Abraham's circle bridge in Omaha, NE. Photo: courtesy of Tri-Faith Initiative

Lessons Learned

- Blood administration consents can seem mundane. But for many patients, and especially JWs, it can be riddled with challenges, misunderstandings, and hurdles. Thus, it is our duty to carefully address the issues, listen, educate, and above all, respect these patients throughout the blood product consent process.
- Keep in mind that patients may refuse blood for any of a number of reasons. There are many patient cohorts that may refuse blood for religious reasons, including JWs, Christian Scientists, Muslims at certain points in the religious calendar, minority sects, and some cultural/ethnic groups.
- Make sure you are very conversant and comfortable with your hospital's plan for caring for patients who refuse blood for religious reasons.
- If your practice location does not have specific chart or consent documents for patients who refuse blood, consider getting involved in their development. It's a great way to interface with the transfusion medicine service.
- The transfusion consent form used at Case Western/University Hospitals covers the major blood and blood components. It is efficient and easy to use.
- For reference, the form used at the NIH has a more complete list of blood components and products and blood techniques. It documents a transfusion plan, not a consent discussion.
- It is imperative that your consent to accept or refuse transfusion be done privately if the patient wishes. Remember that "consent" is the discussion, understanding, and agreement—not the piece of paper—but this is one situation when it's really best that they match. For that reason, Case Western/University Hospitals tend not to sedate patients until they can speak privately to their care team.

References

1. American Red Cross. Importance of the blood supply [Internet]. Redcrossblood.org. 2025. Available from: https://www.redcrossblood.org/donate-blood/how-to-donate/how-blood-donations-help/blood-needs-blood-supply.html.
2. Karafin MS. Demographic and epidemiologic characterization of transfusion recipients from four US regions: evidence from the REDS-III recipient database. Transfusion. 2017;57(12):2903–13.
3. Why Don't Jehovah's Witnesses Accept Blood Transfusions? [Internet]. JW.ORG. 2025 [cited 2025 Jul 27]. Available from: https://www.jw.org/en/jehovahs-witnesses/faq/jehovahs-witnesses-why-no-blood-transfusions.
4. Elder L. Why some Jehovah's Witnesses accept blood and conscientiously reject official Watchtower Society blood policy. J Med Ethics. 2022;26:375–80.
5. Muramoto O. Medical confidentiality and the protection of Jehovah's Witnesses' autonomous refusal of blood. J Med Ethics. 2000;26:381–6.
6. Waters JH, Potter PS. Cell salvage in the Jehovah's Witness patient. Anesth Anal. 2000;90(1):229–30.
7. De Andrade SL, de Carli D, et al. Epidural blood patch in Jehovah's Witness: two case reports. Rev Bras de Anestesiol. 2003;53(5):633–9.
8. Mason CL, Tran CK. Caring for the Jehovah's Witness parturient. Anesth Anal. 2015;121(6):1564–9.

Authors

Linda Song completed her pathology residency at the University of Maryland. She is board-certified in anatomic and clinical pathology. She completed a fellowship in transfusion medicine in the NIH Department of Transfusion Medicine and Center for Cellular Engineering and is now an assistant professor at MD Anderson in Houston, Texas. When she isn't at work, she and her partner are chasing or babywearing kids while booping two loving and dumb cats. When all that is said and done, she spends her free time eating and taking pictures of the local food scene or watching food documentaries.

Shelley Kalsi graduated from the Feinberg School of Medicine, Northwestern University, in Chicago, IL, and then completed residency training in internal medicine at the University of Maryland Medical Center in Baltimore, MD. After a hematology/oncology fellowship at the University of Pittsburgh Medical Center, she completed a fellowship in transfusion medicine/blood banking at the National Institutes of Health. She is currently deputy chief of the hematology consult service for the intramural program of the National Heart, Lung Blood Institute, in Bethesda, MD. Shelley lives in Maryland with her family and enjoys spending time outdoors.

Ray Graber is a senior anesthesiologist at Case Western and University Hospitals. He has had a career-long interest in transfusion-related issues and topics.

Cathy Marcucci is a senior anesthesiologist and is also fellowship-trained in transfusion medicine. She has cared for many patients who have refused blood on religious grounds in her 30+-year career.

117 Connecting with Patients Who Refuse Blood Due to Infectious Concerns

David Daniel, Kamille West-Mitchell, and Catherine Marcucci

Introduction

Over the past century, the practice of blood transfusion has doubtlessly saved millions of lives. However, the posttransfusion hepatitis crisis in the 1950s and the transfusion-transmitted HIV calamity in the 1980s have marred the image of a life-saving blood transfusion. This stigma associated with infected blood still exists today, with many patients unable to appreciate how far we have come in our ability to provide safe, quality blood products.

Questions and Concerns

Patients present with a wide range of concerns about infectious agents—those agents that are currently screened for, those that are not screened for, and new and emerging agents that may be in the news. Their concerns may range from hesitancy and questions before consenting to transfusion to an outright refusal. These should not be dismissed with vague and generalized reassurances, "the blood supply is really, really safe," as unfortunately, even in this day, bacteria, viruses, prions, and parasites can be transmitted in blood.

Weirdly, sometimes the opposite happens—the patient comes in assuming that the blood supply is guaranteed to be free of everything they've ever heard of and everything they haven't. And sometimes, the patient will have really unusual concerns—we know of patients who have refused blood, not due to concerns about infectious agents but concerns about the vaccine the donor might have received to prevent viremia associated with this particular agent. We have actually had patients who indicated that they would consent for blood only if they could be guaranteed that the donor had not received the SARS-CoV-2 and the annual influenza vaccines.

It's our job to sort through both underestimates and overestimates of the blood supply infectious risk competently and confidently. This chapter will outline what infectious diseases are currently screened for, what the actual current risks are to the patient as we currently understand them, and where to go for more help and information.

D. Daniel · K. West-Mitchell · C. Marcucci (✉)
Department of Transfusion Medicine, Clinical Center, National Institutes of Health, Bethesda, MD, USA

S. Mohamed et al. (eds.), *Anesthesia Bridges*, https://doi.org/10.1007/978-3-032-08294-7_117

Screening, Testing, and Treatment

There are several levels of safeguards that are required or permitted by the federal government to maximize the safety of the US blood supply. *The first level of screening is via the blood donor questionnaire at the time of donation.* This questionnaire has several dozen questions that a blood donor answers, and it is an epidemiology screen to safeguard the blood supply. Many questions are targeted toward the risk of unknowingly donating blood carrying an infectious disease. Donors are queried on place of residence, recent illnesses, travel to locations where there might be risk of acquiring infectious agents such as malaria, and certain activities such as use of intravenous drugs or recent tattoos. Potential donors will be deferred from donating blood for varying periods of time depending on their responses. The questions and deferral periods evolve over time, but are generally identical in every place in the country at a given point in time.

The second level of screening involves actual testing of donated blood for specific infectious agents. Again, this is required by federal law, and testing must be done using FDA-mandated assays. The current tests performed on donated blood are shown below (Table 117.1). We feel there is most likely a learning opportunity for anesthesiologists with this table. Most anesthesia practitioners know, for instance, that donated blood is tested for the hepatitis B virus (HBV), but how many are aware that three separate assays are performed? In actuality, "HBV testing" involves assays for HBV surface antigen, HBV anticore antibody, and nucleic acid amplification testing (NAT) for the virus.

Table 117.1 Federally mandated testing for pathogens in donated whole blood in the US. https://www.cdc.gov/bloodsafety/basics.html

Infectious disease pathogen	Laboratory tests used	Frequency of tests
Hepatitis B virus (HBV)	Hepatitis B surface antigen (HBsAg) detection Hepatitis B core antibody (anti-HBc) detection NAT for HBV	Every donation
Hepatitis C virus (HCV)	Hepatitis C virus antibody (anti-HCV) detection NAT for HCV	Every donation
Human immunodeficiency virus types 1 and 2 (HIV)	HIV-1 and HIV-2 antibody (anti-HIV-1 and anti-HIV-2) detection NAT for HIV-1 and HIV-2	Every donation
Human T-lymphotropic virus types I and II (HTLV)	HTLV-I and HTLV-II antibody (anti-HTLV-I and anti-HTLV-II) detection	Every donation
Treponema pallidum(syphilis)	Antitreponemal antibody detection	Every donation
West Nile virus (WNV)	NAT for WNV	Every donation
Bacterial Contamination	Bacterial culture	Every platelet donation unless PR is performed
Babesia	NAT and antibody for B. microti	Performed on donations in Babesia-endemic regions Not performed on PR platelets
Trypanosoma cruzi (Chagas disease)	*T. cruzi* antibody detection	All first-time donors tested
Cytomegalovirus (CMV)	CMV antibody detection	Performed on some donations for special needs recipients

NAT Nucleic acid amplification testing

Platelets

Platelet products have a unique risk of infectious transmission as they are usually stored at room temperature. In the United States, there are a few different ways to reduce this risk. The most common approach is to draw a small sample of the platelet product for bacterial cultures; some centers will also use a rapid bacterial detection test performed on the day of transfusion to extend the platelets' shelf-life.

The alternative method used to decrease the infectious risk of platelet transfusion is pathogen reduction (PR) or pathogen inactivation. Platelet pathogen reduction is done by using a chemical agent (amotosalen) that is activated by UV light to bind nucleic acids so that DNA cannot replicate and thus the cell cannot divide (Intercept method).

These approaches have decreased the incidence of septic platelet transfusions; however, the risk is still reported to be on the order of 1:50,000–80,000, with a few deaths reported each year. At present, pathogen reduction of platelets is licensed, but not universally performed or required. Some hospital settings transfuse only PR platelets, some have a partial inventory of PR platelets, and some have no PR platelets. If you are unaware of what is in the inventory of your hospital's blood bank, a simple phone call to the desk will get you the answer in ten seconds or less. There are also solvent/detergent treatment methods that are used for pathogen reduction for specialized plasma products—these are licensed but much less widely adopted.

The Big Three

The biggest players in transfusion-transmitted infections include HIV, and hepatitis B and C. For these pathogens, there exists ample evidence of the transmissibility via transfusion, as well as universal donor screening. In the 1980s, HIV contamination of up to 3.3% of the donor pool forever changed the practice of transfusion medicine. In response, practices have been implemented, such as deferral of "high-risk" donors and confidential exclusion of donated units, which have made the incoming donor pool safer. Enhanced laboratory testing, including fourth-generation HIV testing, has reduced the window period of detection to as low as 18 days. Currently, the estimated risk of a transfusion-transmitted HIV infection is modeled to be less than 1 in 2 million, although what is observed in clinical practice is thought to be less.

Besides HIV in the 1980s, hepatitis C contamination of the donor pool in the 1950s had the most lasting impact on the world of transfusion. Previously called non-A non-B Hepatitis, hepatitis C virus (HCV) was identified through the work of Dr. Harvey Alter at the National Institutes of Health (NIH). Patients were noted to have developed an unidentified hepatitis posttransfusion, later found to be hepatitis C. During this time, the use of paid donors for blood collection was standard, and in one study, 51% of those who received blood from a commercial donor developed posttransfusion hepatitis. The transition to using exclusively voluntary donors and the development of HCV nucleic acid testing have decreased the risk of acquisition of HCV from blood transfusion to 1 in 2.6 million. Fortunately, HCV infection is now considered to be a curable disease.

Syphilis was the first recognized transfusion transmitted infection. Documented in 1915, mandatory antibody testing of donors began in the 1950s. Continued testing has proven fruitful as well, with no new cases of transfusion-transmitted syphilis reported since the 1960s. There is an entire contingent of Transfusion Medicine professionals who feel that testing the donor blood supply for syphilis can safely be eliminated. However, bacterial contamination by organisms other than *T. pallidum* continues to be a concern in the contamination of blood products. This concern is especially important when considering platelet product transfusions, as they are stored at higher temperatures, 20–24 °C. These bacteria are most commonly gram-positive *Staphylococcus* species.

***Note from the Editors:** Coauthor Kamille West-Mitchell is from Jamaica, and in her honor, we are featuring the beautiful Iron Bridge in Spanish Town, Jamaica (Fig. 117.1). It is considered a national landmark and has been considered for inclusion as a UNESCO World Heritage Site.

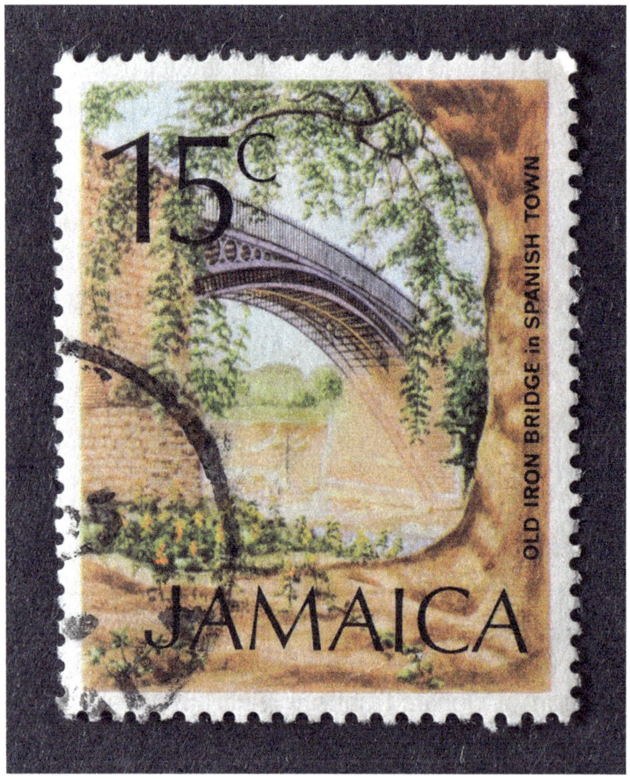

Fig. 117.1 A Jamaican postage stamp showing the historic Spanish Town cast-iron bridge. The bridge spans the Rio Cobre River and was built in 1801 after segments were cast in England and shipped to Jamaica. It is under extensive restoration, especially the stone abutments. Photo: Image used under standard license for editorial use nonfiction book from shutterstock.com

Rare Infectious Agents

There are a few rare and/or important infectious agents to consider. This includes entities such as cytomegalovirus and HTLV, which reside in white blood cells. Leukoreduction has proved to be valuable in keeping the blood products "CMV safe," and eligible for transfusion, even to a CMV-negative individual (all the red blood cell units at the NIH are leukoreduced).

Parasite species such as *Babesia, Plasmodium* (malaria), and *T. cruzi* (Chagas disease) are all rare, and are screened based on the donor questionnaire, and tested based on the incidence of the organism in the blood donor community.

No discussion of transfusion-transmitted infections would be complete without mentioning variant Creutzfeldt-Jakob disease. While only four total documented cases of transfusion transmission of this disease exist, and there is currently only a theoretical residual risk in the US population, previously there were strict and aggressive donor deferrals issued in response to concerns for this disease. However, most of these questions have been dropped as of May 2022. Similarly, although to a lesser extent, viruses such as Zika and Chikungunya have been a nidus for donor deferrals based on theoretical risk, without any documented cases of transfusion-related transmission in the US. However, cases of Zika virus transmission through platelet transfusions have been documented in Brazil.

It is important for anesthesiologists to be aware of the emerging and ultra-rare infectious agents that patients might ask about, especially the ones in the news. Based on the screening questionnaire, donors will be deferred for recent illness, but at this time, there are no serologic tests conducted for infectious agents such as *Ehrlichia* species, Eastern equine virus, Powassan virus, dengue fever, hepatitis A, or hepatitis E, all of which are associated with rare or theoretical risk of transmission via transfusion.

It's okay to tell your patients that the exact risks posed by these agents are still unknown and that they remain a concern. If possible, always mitigate these concerns with the current information on known and documented cases of transmission. For instance, despite the hundreds of millions of people who had documented COVID-19, at the time of this writing, there were no documented cases of transfusion-transmitted SARS-CoV-2 virus. Anesthesiologists should feel free to call the blood bank at any time for help with questions about the rare and new risks. Try not to have to deal with any "infectious" questions that you yourself have not already thought about and asked of the transfusion medicine staff at your hospital.

Risk-Benefit Ratio

The most important part of this discussion is not the risk part of the risk-benefit ratio; it's the potential life-saving aspect of transfusion. One strategy is to discuss the patient's preoperative hemoglobin and what value might trigger a transfusion. Concrete, but gently put, examples work: if a patient has lost approximately half of her blood volume (that is, if the hemoglobin has decreased from 15 to 7 gm/dL), and stroke, blindness, heart attack, or death are becoming concerns, the truly small risk of a transfusion-transmitted infection is more easily seen in perspective.

Don't bash the patient's psyche with fear tactics, but do make the points that are there to be made. Finally, most patients can be reassured and will then consent to a transfusion, but a patient has the absolute right to refuse any medical treatment or intervention at any time, as long as competency and capacity are intact. You can have the discussion, but you cannot make the final decision.

***Note from the Editors:** Coauthor David Daniel trained in Brooklyn. To honor that, we found a beautiful old bridge in Prospect Park. (Fig. 117.2).

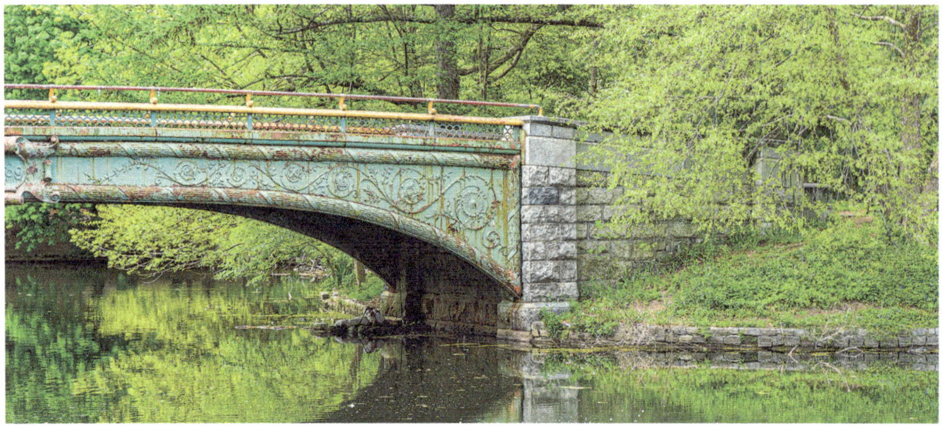

Fig. 117.2 The old iron bridge in Prospect Park, Brooklyn. Photo: Image used under standard license from stock.adobe.com

Lessons Learned

- The Food and Drug Administration is responsible for the regulation of the US blood supply. There is abundant information online, especially at the FDA and CDC websites and in the Transfusion Medicine literature [1].
- Donor blood is tested more than one way for the "big three" viruses—hepatitis B, hepatitis C, and HIV.
- Platelets carry the risk of bacterial contamination. There are several methods to reduce this risk, including bacterial cultures and pathogen reduction. If you are not sure about how your blood bank addresses these risks, a short phone call will provide the answer.
- While the history of blood transfusion has been implicated in the propagation of a few notable infectious diseases, overall, the risk of transfusion-transmitted infection is low. The risk of transfusion-transmitted disease is 1 in 2 million for HIV, 1 in 2.6 million for HCV, and 1 in 1.1–1.5 million for HBV. As far as we know, at this time, there are no documented cases of transfusion-associated COVID-19.
- Treat the patient's questions with respect, calmness, and confidence. Don't wave away or undersell the issues and concerns—they're legitimate—but don't overstate the risks, either.
- Seek help from your blood bank and the transfusion medicine physicians if questions arise about the rare and emerging infectious agents. Just pick up the phone and call the blood bank desk. Whoever answers the phone will direct you to someone who can help you with this reference work.
- In the future, emerging technologies, such as pathogen reduction, will surely further decrease the already low risk.
- Overwhelmingly, when transfusion is indicated, the benefits of transfusion greatly outweigh the risks, especially when taking into consideration the extensive donor screening and laboratory testing that is

currently available and standard of care. Our job is to present the facts, discuss the risk-benefit ratio, and document the patient's final decision. If the patient's final decision is to refuse blood, document appropriately, and let the surgical and Transfusion Medicine services know so that the appropriate record of the refusal can be entered into the overall hospital records and blood bank database.

Reference

1. Bloch EM. Transfusion-transmitted infections. Ann Blood [Online]. 2022;7.

Authors

David Daniel is board-certified in clinical and anatomic pathology and transfusion medicine. He did his clinical fellowship in transfusion medicine at the NIH Clinical Center and is now on faculty at Johns Hopkins. He and his wife, a transplant nephrologist, are both beyond proud and beyond busy to be the parents of twin boys.

Kamille West-Mitchell is board-certified in clinical and anatomic pathology as well as transfusion medicine. She is the director of the Blood Services Section of the Department of Transfusion Medicine at the Clinical Center, National Institutes of Health. When she is not busy in Bethesda overseeing the safety of the blood supply at the NIH, she can be found salsa dancing, at piano lessons, and enjoying nerdy discussions with her husband in her home island of Jamaica.

Cathy Marcucci is trained in both anesthesiology and transfusion medicine. She is always happy to build bridges between her two specialties.

Wisdom on Doctor-Patient Relations

118

Catherine Marcucci, Allan Gottschalk, Ronald S. Bank, Brian T. Gierl, Edward J. Damrose, and Amy J. Robbins

Contributors:

James Abernathy, MD (JA)

Michael D. Altose, MD (MDA)

Carol F. Bodenheimer, MD (CFB)

Catherine Cooper, MD (CC)

Steven M. Frank, MD (SMF)

Mark J. Lema, MD PhD (MJL)

Steven L. Orebaugh, MD (SLO)

Maria K. Orlic, MD (MKO)

Neil B. Sandson, MD (NBS)

C. Marcucci (✉)
Department of Transfusion Medicine, Clinical Center, National Institutes of Health, Bethesda, MD, USA

A. Gottschalk
Department of Anesthesiology and Critical Care Medicine and Neurosurgery, Johns Hopkins University, Baltimore, MD, USA

R. S. Bank
Department of Anesthesiology, INOVA Fairfax Hospital, UVA School of Medicine, INOVA Campus, Falls Church, VA, USA

B. T. Gierl
Department of Anesthesiology and Perioperative Medicine, University of Pittsburgh Medical Center Presbyterian, Pittsburgh, PA, USA

E. J. Damrose
Department of Otolaryngology—Head and Neck Surgery, Stanford University, Palo Alto, CA, USA

Department of Anesthesiology, Perioperative and Pain Medicine, Stanford University, Palo Alto, CA, USA

A. J. Robbins
Stanson Health, a Premier Inc. Company, Charlotte, NC, USA

Atrium Health, Carolinas Palliative Care and Hospice Group, Charlotte, NC, USA

S. Mohamed et al. (eds.), *Anesthesia Bridges*, https://doi.org/10.1007/978-3-032-08294-7_118

Introduction

To cap our section on doctor-patient relations, the editors have collected the following words of wisdom from our authors and contributors. Most of these thoughts are about how we connect with patients, but how we interact with family members is also important—these interactions make a big difference in how you and your hospital will be seen by your patients. Plus, kindness toward your patients and their families and loved ones is its own reward—it's just the right thing to do.

General Wisdom

Patients want state-of-the-art services, assured competency, altruistic intentions, integrity, accountability, honesty, objectivity, and compassion. In other words, treat them like you would want someone to treat your mother, grandmother, spouse, or children. We are the ultimate service profession.—**MJL**

- To distill Mark Lema's advice down to three words—what the patients and families need from you is calmness, courtesy, and common sense.—**AJR**

- And Mark Lema is also correct that you must never, ever express anger or frustration to a patient about any aspect of their behavior. The compassion part is so important. One of us once had a patient step into the bathroom of the pre-op area to inject IV drugs. The patient's explanation was, "I'm afraid you aren't going to give me enough stuff." What's the correct response to this type of event? It's not to judge, shame, or harangue the patient. It is simply to say that, "Okay, Mr. Smith, we understand. But can you tell us what you just injected, how much, and where is the needle?"—**Editors**

- *Patients have always spent more time with their disease than you have.*—**CFB**

- A corollary to this is that patients don't care about what happens to the medical population at large; they care about what happens to them (and their loved ones).—**Editors**

- Every single piece of this advice and wisdom applies to the families as well as the patient. And by "families," we also mean loved ones and support people.—**Editors**

- I think that the biggest need that the family has pertaining to the anesthesiologist is that they are confident and experienced and have done many such cases before.—**RSB**

- We are obligated to do the best we can, within reason, for our patients. Accordingly, it is important that we accept from the start that we will provide services, tolerate behaviors, support, and otherwise provide services for patients that we would otherwise seldom do in other roles in our lives, except parenthood.—**NBS**

- Of course, patients fear pain and death and a bad outcome. But they also fear humiliation. Shame is one of the strongest human emotions.—**NBS**

- Avoid complaining about *THE SYSTEM* in front of patients. It may be justified, but it's unprofessional, and it makes them question their care or our commitment to it. Things will always go wrong, given the complexity of the professional lives we lead, but it's best to keep the grousing in the locker room or the office. Patients just don't want to hear you talk about your problems; they would much rather talk about their own.—**SLO**

- People come to the OR embarrassed and worried about all kinds of things. For one, they are not in their underwear. And they are embarrassed about their teeth. Or they don't want to walk to the OR with just a pair of OR socks between them and the "dirty" floor. Once, we had a patient whose wife did not know that he had had a hair transplant, and he was extremely concerned about having his head shaved. A huge number of patients are worried about urinating or defecating under anesthesia, or vomiting on the staff, or that they might otherwise do something that is ridiculed. Be kind but don't be dismissive of their concerns. Rather, be a bit warmly indifferent, "It's okay, everybody worries about this. When I had surgery, I barfed on the anesthesiologist, and it was a friend of mine! But remember that we are doctors. And the nurses are nurses. Nothing about the human body is new to us or bothers us; there is literally nothing that we haven't seen. So, this doesn't bother us a bit. It's actually pretty common. We don't even think about it longer than it takes to fix it."—**Editors**

- A good pre-op includes finding something out about your patient. Where they're from. What they do. Even hobbies! Include the family members. Listen as much as you talk.—**SMF**

- Realize that many patients with expressive aphasia have no receptive deficits. Always speak to them in a manner consistent with their current mental status, age, and education level. "How's the food?" is often a good question for an inpatient with aphasia, as it is easy to express good or bad.—**BTG**

- Have empathy for your patients' requests to bring things into the OR, even if you have to say no. Remember it's sort of ironic: "You can trust us with your life, but not your glasses or your teeth."—**CC**

- Everybody has a different style, but we personally always try to say something positive and reaffirming to my patients both before and after anesthesia. Not too gushy, though. You can say something simple and neutral like, "Your family is nice." Or "It's good your kids could be with you today." Those statements will be burdensome to no one.—**Editors**

- We tend not to make any commiserating statements about wayward teenagers or husbands who doze off at inopportune times. Your patient doesn't need you to be an exasperated Mom or spouse. They need you to be an uber-competent professional who is hyper-focused only on them and their pressing need for a safe anesthetic, not your own frustrations.—**AJR**

- Also, don't make any remarks that highlight the distance between you, in your state of wellness, and the patient who is on the Island of Illness. If you ask the patient where they are from, don't mention that you were just there skiing. Because they probably weren't.—**Editors**

- Find something, anything, to say positive about the patient's clinical condition physiology in the preoperative period. This can range from being normotensive—"your blood pressure looks great, are you a swimmer?" to having a pulse ox reading of 98% or even "your skin looks healthy, so the IV should go in fine." Knock yourself out finding something positive about the patient's clinical status—"I see that your kidney function is perfect." The goal is to reflect to the patient as much as possible an image of vitality and health because that's what they will be clinging to. It's the empathic thing to do and means a lot to patients. I've been on that awful Island of Illness—now safely and thankfully back on the Mainland of Health—and I can tell you that it is emotionally devastating.—**CM**

- If you are stuck thinking of something reaffirming to the patient, some guerrilla tactics are in order. It doesn't matter if it's strictly true; what matters is what the patient hears in their time of need. When they are on the OR table and you are putting the monitors on, you can quietly say, "Gosh, Ms. Johnson, it's hard to believe you are X years old, you seem so young."—**Editors**

- Do not ever let the patient hear you mutter or swear under your breath if you miss something.—**Editors**

- Don't promise that you will get a procedure done, even the IV, in one try.—**Editors**

- Remember that while the patient is awake, everything you say to your trainee or the surgeons, you are also saying to the patient.—**Editors**

- There are different styles and time constraints, of course, but we were taught to always speak to the families of patients if they were transported to the ICU and/or remained intubated, even if there were no complications. Try to find something positive when you speak to the families, as it may be some time before the families can see their loved ones. We've had families tell us that the wait when their family member is out of the OR is as difficult as the wait while they are in the OR.—**Editors**

- So, the politics of the care teams being what they are, it's perfectly okay to let the patient know who the physician is heading the team and who the nurses are. We are not trying to stir up controversy but sometimes it's not made perfectly clear by every team member. We've talked to a lot of our own family and friends over the years about how "the anesthesia went," and often they are not really sure if the care providers they interacted with were physicians or nurses.—**CM**

- I have a chatty, informal style and usually don't introduce myself as Dr. Marcucci, even to the patients. I generally say, "Good morning, I'm Cathy Marcucci, I'm going to be your anesthesiologist today. I'm the physician who is leading the anesthesia team, and we will be with you until you get to the recovery area. I'm the same level as Dr. So-and-So (the surgeon), but on the anesthesia team. The nurse anesthetist who will also be taking care of you is Jane Doe."—**CM**

- A number of years ago, I was visiting Hopkins for the first time in quite a while, and I noticed something new (to me) at that time on the ID badges (Fig. 118.1) as the NIH does not have this type of ID badge. So, this is one way to do it! I have also seen scrub hats with "I am the doctor" embroidered across the forehead. But one way or another, find a low-key and courteous way to let the patients know That. You. Are. The. Physician.—**CM and JA**

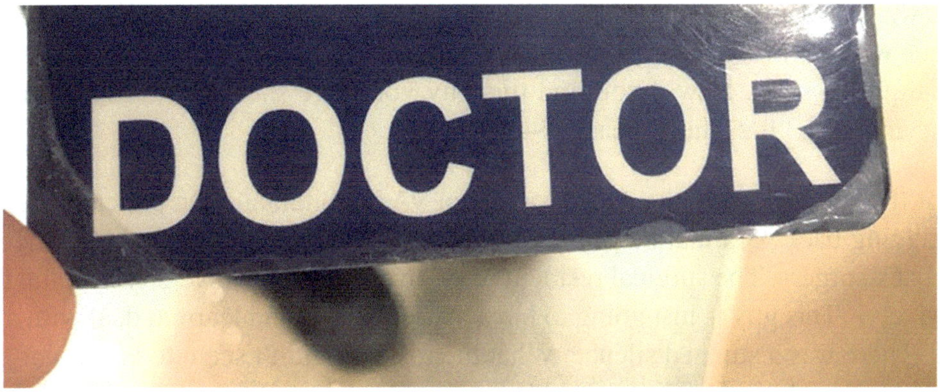

Fig. 118.1 It's okay to let everybody know exactly who you are and exactly what your job is! Photo: Cathy Marcucci

- Never editorialize in any way about a patient's weight, to the patient or in the chart. People are ultra-sensitive about it. Recently, I had outpatient surgery and was asked to step on a scale in the pre-op area, which was the first time I had seen that. I asked the pre-op nurse how they came to do that. He said that it just became too much of a problem with people falsifying their answers, and they just decided to go with hard data. So, if possible, just use a documented BMI and try to never use the words "obese" or "overweight."—**CM**

- The most interesting thing about doctor-patient relations is not to have patients of extraordinary fame and see if you can treat them like regular people, it is to have regular patients and find out what their extraordinary stories are.—**Editors**

- The salutation "thank you for your service" has become a bit trite and tiresome for some former and active-duty service members, or so I was told during the many years that I worked for the Department of Veterans Affairs. Try to think of something a bit more conversational and original. You can ask where they did their basic training and how difficult it was on a scale of 1/10. Or ask what their MOS (Military Occupational Specialty) was or where they were stationed—anything that indicates a bit of actual interest in their active service or tour of duty. If they went to a service academy, ask who their graduation speaker was—often it's a current or former President.—**Editors**

- There are some days when you hear the most amazing stories from the patients. We have had the wonderful opportunity to hear WW II stories, straight from the Greatest Generation. Because the 29th Division, which stormed Omaha beach at Normandy, was a Maryland division, Cathy Marcucci had the honor of caring for a number of D-day Veterans at the Baltimore VA many years later. She heard about what they had for breakfast on June 6, 1944, and how badly they needed a smoke on the way over. And she cared for many other WW II Vets, including a number of heavy bomber gunners—top turret and ball turret gunners and waist gunners. A former waist gunner told her that sometimes after a bombing run, they would be so immobilized from their heavy clothes, the extreme cold and fatigue, and empty shells up to their knees that ground crews would have to come into the fuselage of the planes to extract them from their battle stations and lift them out.—**Editors**

- And then there was the time I was in the pre-op clinic at the Philadelphia VA, talking to a Vet about the fact that he needed to postpone a dental implant surgery to go to a military reunion. He'd recently gotten back in touch with his WW II buddy after many years. They had had quite a time of it in the war. Shot down over France, escaped over the mountains into Spain, dragging and carrying another crew member with them. Evading the Germans and being hidden by the local population. I said, "Wow, that's quite a story. How'd you find this guy you were shot down with, after 65 years?" He looked at me and said, "It's Chuck Yeager."—**CM**

- Once, one of the editors was in the neuro room at a VA hospital, and the patient, a fine older gentleman with nagging back pain that he just couldn't seem to get the better of, was under general anesthesia for a back surgery. The surgical resident came over from the university hospital to scrub in and said dismissively, "This guy is just going to have to toughen up and learn to deal with a little pain and discomfort." There was a stunned silence. What the resident didn't seem to know was that "this guy" was a WW II Marine. As in Iwo Jima, 3rd Marines—on the island for all 36 days of that terrible, terrible battle. Everything stopped while calls went out in several directions and, it goes without saying, that the resident did not staff the case. Rumor has it that he was reprimanded for his idiotic and disrespectful remark by everybody from the anesthesia and surgical attendings up to the hospital director.—**Editors**

- One day in the PACU, I was talking to a WW II Navy Vet who had served in the Solomon Islands. I asked my patient if he had ever met John F. Kennedy. He said, "Yes, I sure did. Nice kid, skinny. He had a tiny sailboat with a red sail on his PT boat, and any chance he got, he'd sail around the lagoon. We used to see that little red sail early in the morning and say, oh, I guess the war is taking a break, Kennedy's out for a sail."—**CM**

- Sadly, these WW II soldiers and sailors and airmen are gone now. They were just regular guys—before, during, and after the war—but such tough old birds that it felt like they would never leave us. Each one that goes leaves a big space. It was such an honor to talk to them and take care of them. We advise that you talk to the Veterans of your generation, for your own sake as much as theirs.—**AJR**

- Consider using a generic picture when speaking with the family post-op or even pre-op to help them understand what their family member might look like in the ICU. You can take some op-sites to show the family and the patients at the pre-op visit. "Your Dad will have one of these on his neck." It helps decrease the family members' shock when they see their loved one.—**Editors**

- When doing the pre-op discussion, ask if there were any complications with previous anesthetics, of course. But also ask what they remember most about previous anesthetics—being afraid of going into the OR, the noise, feeling cold, having a sore throat. And then do your best to mitigate that. Ask them if they know their blood type and then inform them if they don't.—**Editors**

- I wouldn't use the phrase "vivid dreaming" when discussing the side effects of ketamine. That way understates the issue. It is downright hallucinogenic and therefore somewhat terrifying. After I myself had it (no benzodiazepine!), I switched to telling patients that it can be a bit "psychedelic" or "kaleidoscopic."—**CM**

- The term "twilight sleep" has been quite commonly used to describe sedation to patients and still has its proponents. I stopped using it after an annoyed patient said to me, "What does twilight sleep even mean? I've read up quite a bit on the anesthesia for this type of case. If I am going to be drowsy and sedated, why don't you just use those precise terms?" Fair question.—**CM**

- Tell your patients in the pre-op interview that you will be talking quietly to them when they are under anesthesia to let them know that they are okay and how the case is coming along. Ask if they would like any particular words of comfort or affirmation whispered to them during the case. And then, within reason, do what the patient asks you to do—for instance, say a prayer or read a passage or a message.—**Editors**

- Make sure to tell families that OR suites are staffed by anesthesia *teams*, and you may be seen in the hallway during the case. If a long case is planned, it is okay to let the family know that the anesthesia personnel do take breaks and how those breaks are covered. Reassure them that somebody will be with the patient every second.—**RSB and Editors**

- I make it a point to sit down, especially when getting to the anesthetic plan and risks part of the pre-op discussion. Sitting down seems so trivial, yet there is literature to show that patients and their families really appreciate this. They feel as though you are less rushed and really paying attention to them.—**RSB**

***Note from the Editors:** One of Ron Bank's favorite places on the planet isn't on land, it's the open sea (Figs. 118.2 and 118.3). Ron tells us about his fascinating travels below:

> There is an imaginary column of ocean water that extends from the deepest trenches of the ocean floor to the interface of the ocean and atmosphere. This is the zone of the oceans where animals can swim free in any direction without the constraints of continental topography, such as the continental shelf. Every night, a vast pelagic zone migration takes place as an immense array of deep-ocean animals travel through the layers of this vertical water bridge toward the surface to feed. There are a few dive shops that do open ocean night dives where divers can witness the incredible creatures that make this migration. These types of pelagic night dives are called blackwater dives. One of the very best is in Kona, HI—the Pelagic Magic dive. My kids and I have enjoyed it several times. It's an epic experience like no other.

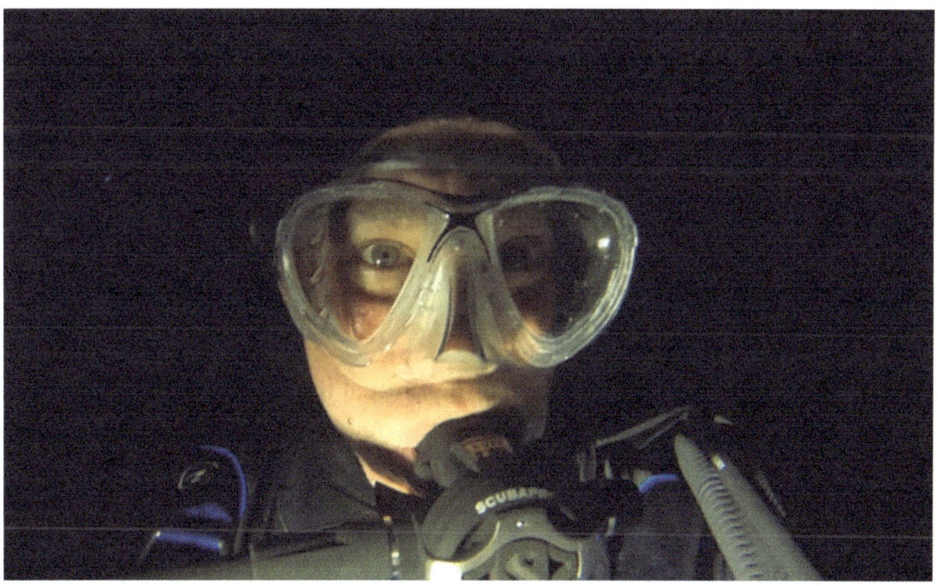

Fig. 118.2 Ron Bank, down in the black depths of the night ocean off Kona, HI, on a "Pelagic Magic" night dive. Rumor has it that he requests to be the first person off the boat and into the water. Ron is a truly expert diver and is certified as a Divemaster by the Professional Association of Diving Instructors. It still takes nerves of steel, even for an experienced diver. Would you do it? Photo: Ron Bank

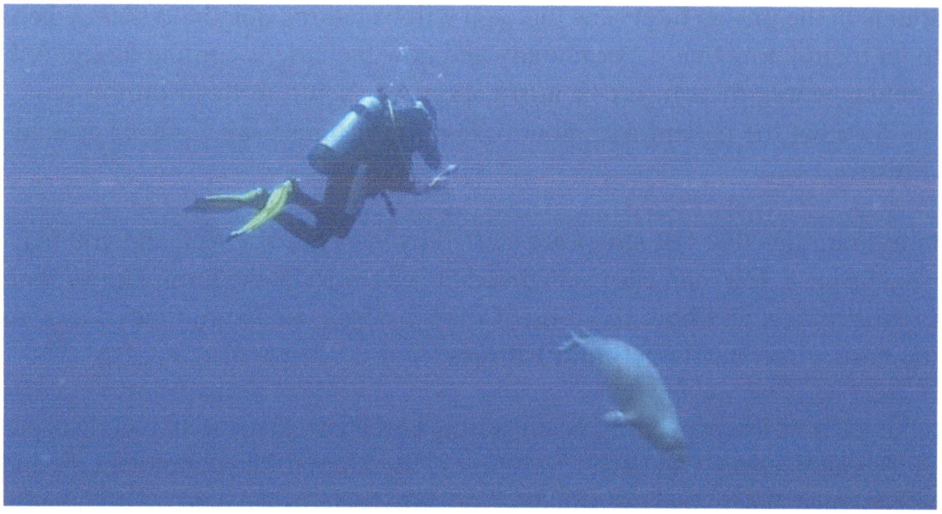

Fig. 118.3 Ron Bank partaking of the ocean's splendor on a "daylight" dive. He has been on countless dives in beautiful waters all over the world. Here he is diving in the remote waters off Niihau, HI. His dive buddy is a critically endangered Hawaiian monk seal. Photo: Ron Bank

- Don't tell a patient that they will have an awake intubation. Would that not cause tremendous anxiety? Even if you are only using analgesia without sedation, tell them that we will numb your mouth and your throat and place the endotracheal tube while you are still breathing. Assure them that if they are not comfortable, you will stop and make them comfortable. If you are using sedatives, tell them that they will be intubated while they are breathing on their own and stress again that you will stop and give them more sedation if they choose.—**BTG**

- Patients' families often ask how long the surgery should take. Do not give the surgeon a deadline. Explain that you can provide an anesthetic for 10 or 20 hours, or as long as it takes.—**BTG**

- It's not only what you say to patients, but also how you say it. It's also your appearance—always make sure there is not a spot on your clothes—not even a drop of blood on your OR clogs. Once, one of the editors was going for surgery and was greeted by a member of the anesthesia team who had blood on their scrubs, OR coat, *and* shoes.—**Editors**

- If you've reviewed the chart the night before or had a preoperative discussion with your team, it's fine to say that. "*We started getting ready for your case yesterday* and have a few questions for you" is not something that any patient minds hearing.—**Editors**

- Reassure patients with opiate use disorder that you will treat their pain appropriately. Titrating opiates in pre-op can help understand that you will appropriately treat them and their opiate receptor physiology.—**BTG**

- Regarding connecting with the families of cardiac surgery patients, I think that it's a delicate balance of truly preparing them for what they will see in the ICU (intubated, neck lines, and so forth) as well as a realistic assessment of the risks—which we're obligated to do—in the most reassuring manner possible. Of course, the risk and expectations will vary with the magnitude of the case and the patient's condition.—**RSB**

- I let them know that while this is a big surgery that we are an experienced cardiac anesthesia team and that our institution is one of the best and does many such procedures per year (assuming that it's not a rare procedure). I explain what to expect, and I then answer any questions. I also make it a point to speak in lay terms—"breathing tube in the windpipe"—and so forth. I think that this makes the patients and their families comfortable with the technical aspects of the case.—**RSB**

- We have said this in other places and other books, but don't joke and don't even be glib. Don't announce, "The guest of honor is here!" when you take the patient back to the OR. Maybe this is a party they don't want to be at. Just say to the nurses, "Please meet Mr. Johnson."—**Editors**

- Always remind the surgeons that the patient is *awake* if the patient isn't going to be under general anesthesia. And remind them that the patient could be *aware* if the patient is going to be under general anesthesia.—**Editors**

- Patients who are anxious and have had previous surgery often get to the OR and tell us that we're "doing it wrong, I was also asleep for this part the last time." It can be worthwhile to let patients know that they are usually awake in the OR and usually don't remember it afterwards.—**BTG**

- Insist on quiet and calm for the induction of anesthesia, even if the induction is the placement of neuraxial or regional anesthesia.—**Editors**

- Always ask the patient if there is anything you can do to make them more comfortable before induction.—**Editors**

- I swear to God, you feel like you are a frog on a lab table when you are flat on your back and the OR team is standing over you preinduction. Consider sitting down next to the patient, just for a second, to reassure them that you will be with them the whole time.—**CM**

- After reassuring the patients and optimizing their comfort, consider telling them you will be starting the anesthetic in 30 seconds, when you will be starting the anesthetic in 2 seconds. Why not give the retrograde amnesia a helping hand?—**Editors**

- Come up with something better than "a stick and a burn" when injecting subcutaneous local. That phrase is overused and needs to be retired.—**Editors**

- Never let a patient hear a saw or drill. For that reason, consider carefully before doing an amputation under spinal. If you do a spinal, consider also doing a green-mask general. One of us once (while in training) had a patient say, "Well, I guess they just fired up the saw to cut my leg off." We could hardly say, "No, that's not what's happening," could we? We grabbed the propofol, but about 20 seconds too late. And vowed to never let that happen again.—**Editors**

- Never, ever tell a patient, "Hang on, they're almost done." That is amateur anesthesia practice! Don't do it! You want the patient to open their eyes, warm and snug in the PACU, look around, and realize their case is over.—**Editors**

- A syringe of propofol at the ready helps avoid "hang on anesthesia."—**Editors**

- Remember that you can never tell a patient how they are feeling. And you can never, ever tell a patient that they are not in pain. "Pain" is the result of multiple complicated pathways, but it always involves the cortical processing of neurological signals. You can never tell a person what is going on in their cortex—what they are thinking—so by definition, you can never determine their pain level or pain quality.—**AJR**

- There are different styles and time constraints, of course, but we were taught to always speak to the families of patients if they were transported to the ICU or remained intubated, even if there were no complications. Try to find something positive (or at least neutral) and true when you speak to the families, as it may be some time before the patients themselves can tell their loved ones all about it.—**Editors**

- Be scrupulous and skilled and kind in what you say about the patients, not just what you say to them.—**Editors**

- Keep a file of wonderful notes that you get from patients. Read them when you're down on medicine.—**RSB**

- Don't accept any gifts of any material value from patients. Most hospitals have policies about this, but if your practice location doesn't, make it your personal policy. You can accept the kind wishes and thoughts, but not the item. But it's okay to accept token items that have no material value, such as a magazine or journal article that has been printed for you.—**Editors**

- It is now well understood that a strong and skilled anesthesia communicator who fosters good doctor-patient relations can decrease the risk of litigation, and poor doctor-patient relations can increase the risk. One really bad interaction is sometimes enough to make an unhappy patient decide to file a formal complaint or even sue.—**Editors**

- I have been told by risk management four times in my 30-year clinical career that a timely, thorough, and friendly visit to the patient and post-op to answer questions helped ward off litigation (for problems I didn't cause). I've done what, probably at least 10,000 post-op visits? At approximately 30 minutes to visit with the patient and family, answer questions, track down information for them, and write a note, that's 5000 hours or roughly two years of my career spent just in post-op visits. Is it worth that time to defuse four potentially litigious situations? I say it is. But that's not really why I did it. I did it because it was the right thing to do. Patients are often adrift in the modern medical landscape. They are just looking to connect and to know that someone cares enough to check to see that they are doing okay. I view post-op visits as the anesthesia equivalent of the house call.—**CM**

- One of our partners frequently said, "Remember, you're coming to work. Your patient is coming to a major life event."—**Editors**

- Conduct yourself so that your excellent communication skills and doctor-patient relations are mentioned in every reference that is given for you.—**AJR**

- Don't state or even admit that you are tired. We have heard from at least one patient who saw their anesthesiologist rubbing tired eyes and yawning as they came down the hall to do the preoperative interview. Splash water on your face or jog in place if you have to.—**Editors**

***Note from the Editors:** The Mt. Washington Arboretum is a small urban park in Mt. Washington Village, a historic section in northern Baltimore, MD. It is not a formal patient respite or recovery garden, but because it is located within five miles of six major hospitals, patients and families often find their way there. One of our favorite features in the arboretum is a small rain bridge from a rooftop green garden to a tiny reflecting pool (Fig. 118.4).

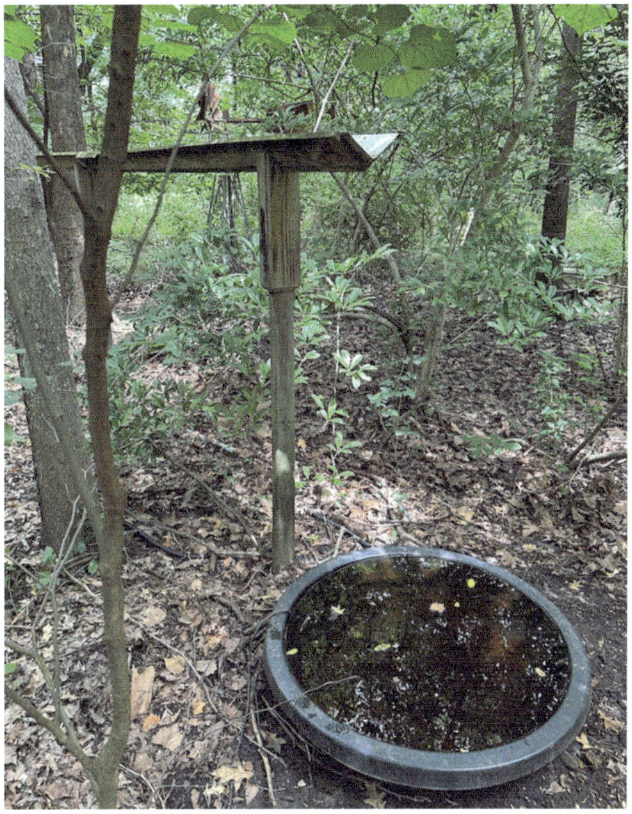

Fig. 118.4 The Rain Bridge in the Mt. Washington Arboretum in Baltimore, MD. Photo: Catherine Marcucci

- Don't allow yourself to become triangulated between the patient and family. The trick is to be clear, to everybody, what your role is—to be the caretaker for the patient, in conjunction with decisions made by the legally identified decision-maker, which is usually, but not always, the patient. You can provide information and answer questions, but do not referee arguments. And you can say that exact thing, "I am concerned that this conversation is heading off in an unproductive direction." Always make the point that arguments and disagreements among family members are not in the best interest of the patient.—**NBS and Editors**

- Along those lines, watch carefully how senior anesthesiologists establish and employ the lines of communication with the primary family contact.—**Editors**

- Whenever possible, err on the side of extra contact with the families. Just a few extra minutes of time can make so much difference to a family who is a bit adrift in the choppy waters of the perioperative period. We know of a situation (pertaining to a surgeon) that is still bothering the family ten years later. The surgery was successful, but in the hectic perioperative period, which included several days in the ICU, the family never saw the senior attending surgeon once. There had been an emergency in the preoperative period, and they hadn't met the surgeon then, either. If you ask this family, "What is Dr. So-and-so like?" they say, "Don't know, never even laid eyes on the guy." And they are not amused by this, either But they also don't want to see you in the cafeteria, either, so be sure to explain the anesthesia care team model and how the room will be staffed.—**Editors**

- *Patients who go to sleep crying, wake up crying.* Do your best to stabilize the patient's emotional state before starting the anesthetic. We've taken bank presidents and professional athletes to the OR with stuffed animals.—**Editor**

Neurosurgery Patients

- The one thing that comes to mind in neuro is about expectations. Part of that is making sure we know what kind of short- and long-term outcomes the surgeon is anticipating. Sometimes the outlook is bleak, but often it's not. In those cases, it's good to remind patients and families that they may be worse before they are better. Motor weakness, aphasia, and so forth can all be worse in the immediate post-op period due to swelling, but get better over time. Spine patients who are expected to regain function don't always regain it in the hours or days after surgery.—**MDA**

- I always remind patients and families that everything we intend to do to them—breathing tube, IVs, a-lines, central lines—all happen after they are asleep.—**MDA**

- Never, *EVER*, speak of "paralyzing" the patient. Especially a neurosurgical patient, who is already worried about waking up paralyzed—it is in the surgical consent. We don't use paralysis; we use muscle relaxation or "a relaxant." Everyone wants a relaxant.—**BTG**

- I tell spine patients:
  - Lying face down for several hours can make your face swollen, and it can also make your airway swollen, and sometimes that means it's not safe to take out the breathing tube until you've been sitting up for a little while. This is really uncommon, but I need to mention it, so that if you wake up in the ICU with a breathing tube, that doesn't necessarily mean that anything went wrong, we're just trying to be safe, and we'll keep you comfortable until it's safe to take it out. Believe me, I want that tube to come out at the end of the case as much as you do, and almost every time it does, but the main thing is to keep you safe.—**MDA**

- Modern surgical family lounges have tracking boards that display the time when the surgery starts. Families often don't realize that many steps that occur before the start of the case, for you to place an awake arterial line, preoxygenate, induce, intubate, and obtain additional vascular access, can be more than 30 minutes. A neurosurgical case may also include urethral catheterization, neurophysiological monitoring with or without baseline evaluation, pinning, shaving, positioning, image guidance system registration, and field preparation. Explaining this sequence beforehand and/or visiting the patient's family (with the consent of the patient) and explaining the perceived delay of an hour or two can ease their anxiety.—**BTG**

- When thinking about relationships with neurosurgical patients, much of what has already been said is valuable and will go far. It needs to be recognized that working on a patient's brain seems very personal to them and their families. When dealing with procedures of the spine and peripheral nervous system, pain is a major focus for many who have suffered terribly for years and worry, often with prior experience to back it up, that their surgical course will be even worse.—**AG**

- When seeing a patient preoperatively, I focus on telling them what I am going to do for them to make the experience better. If it is a craniotomy, I describe how I will perform a scalp block with a long-acting local anesthetic and that they will be awake immediately after the procedure. If it is an opioid-dependent patient presenting for a procedure of the spine, I describe the steps, beginning with preoperative medications, that I will take to get them comfortable. Then, I reinforce this discussion by titrating opioids, generally fentanyl, due to its rapid onset, until the patient is comfortable. Apart from getting patients to believe that their pain will be addressed effectively, this permits calibration of opioid dosing in the opioid-resistant patient.—**AG**

- As described above, one's conduct should clearly demonstrate that the focus is genuinely all about the patient. But we often do the opposite under the guise of medical or legal necessity. I continue to be impressed by how many anesthesiologists feel the need to list every possible major complication and then some while the patient is obviously melting down inside. I simply remind them that many things can happen under anesthesia and that I am happy to discuss any and all of them. Virtually nobody takes me up on this.—**AG**

- At the same time, if a patient has some comorbidity, I mention it as a concern and tell them what we will be doing about it. Most patients are already aware that their heart problems, for example, could be an issue during anesthesia and surgery. They want to know that you understand this and will be actively working to prevent complications. As for the medical-legal ramifications of this approach, in my many years serving as an expert witness, I have never seen where anyone has ever been protected by the reading of the riot act during the consent process. The goal is to exchange necessary information, education, and establish that you are both on the same team.—**AG**

- A patient-centered approach continues long after the consent is obtained. The anesthesia team should be talking to the patient, not about them. Conversations with another party about next weeks' vacation demonstrate to the patient that you are already on vacation. Be attentive to pain and disability when asking patients to move. Induce on the stretcher when necessary. When inducing on the stretcher, let patients remain where they are most comfortable—you can move them wherever you like once they are anesthetized.—**AG**

- Avoid placing additional lines while the patient is still conscious, just because it may be temporarily convenient. Also, how much do you really need a preinduction arterial line? Use your skills. The look of relief on the face of a patient who is always a difficult IV stick when you tell them that they can be anesthetized first is really worth it. I have never gotten in trouble performing an inhalational induction in such a patient.—**AG**

- Use your own experience to project empathy. When a patient tells me they are nervous, I tell them that I felt the same way as I waited for my hernia repair a few months back. When they mention their discomfort with the idea of placing a urinary drainage catheter, I simply tell them that I completely understand because all my friends were watching when that was done to me.—**AG**

- Don't forget to establish relationships with the family and friends that accompany a patient for their procedure. The confidence they feel will be projected to the patient. Having established a preoperative relationship with the support group, check in after emergence to let them know how things have gone. They may have already heard from the surgeon, or not, but this demonstrates concern. When there are potential issues at induction, such as awake intubation or anxiety, I will often find the family afterwards and let them know that this phase of the procedure was uneventful. For those concerned about protecting themselves from a medical-legal perspective, having the family on your side will go a long way.—**AG**

- All of the above set one up for success when performing one of the more esoteric neuro-anesthesia procedures, the awake craniotomy. When patients feel confident and in control, difficulties are rarely encountered. The issue of confidence also applies to the nurses and surgeons, who must not permit their anxieties and uncertainties to be projected to the patient. This is much less likely to happen if they believe that you've "got this."—**AG**

Thoughts from a Surgeon: Edward J. Damrose, MD

- Regarding the anesthesia team: Personally, I like going in to talk to the patient together—it creates a picture of solidarity and unity that is reassuring to the patient. Presenting your assembled team shows the patient how much thought and care have been put into their case and their special day.—**EJD**

- When bad things happen—and they will—there is the tradition of the surgeon speaking solely on behalf of the entire team as the proverbial "captain of the ship." I'm sure it has its roots in practicality—perhaps it allows a single individual to control the narrative. Perhaps it allows the family to focus their anger or other negative emotions on one individual—which perhaps allows the rest of the team to carry on and care for the patient. Or perhaps this was thought to have medicolegal benefits by somehow insulating team members. I don't know.—**EJD**

- I have seen this not work well—when surgery was canceled due to an anesthetic error, I have seen the surgeon contact the family first to state that the anesthesiologist "messed up" and the case had to be canceled. When the anesthesiologist went to speak to the family, the family was quite hostile and unreceptive.—**EJD**

- When bad things happen that involve anesthesia, it is best that the anesthesiologist and surgeon go together to explain to the family not only what happened, but what the plan is going forward to address the bad thing that happened. It is also important that the family hear from the team that they are indeed sorry for what has happened. I know that this advice is controversial and has changed over the years, but in my experience, families sue physicians they do not like, and one thing that they do not like is a lack of humility or empathy on the part of their doctor.—**EJD**

- I generally prefer to speak to the family alone when the adverse outcome was due solely to the surgery. I think this helps to insulate the team members from my actions and responsibilities.—**EJD**

- The situations I have found where anesthesia and I miscommunicated were usually in the setting of a complex patient needing a surgical procedure where we disagreed about the anesthetic risk or anesthetic plan. In one case I recall, a patient presented to the Emergency Department with an obstructing laryngeal tumor who was in significant respiratory distress. I had explained to the patient that this was an emergency, but the junior anesthesiologist wanted to wait several hours because the patient had eaten earlier in the day and was concerned about the aspiration risk. The patient was not doing well and had other factors which would have made front-of-neck access exceedingly challenging to obtain quickly. The anesthesiologist had made the decision without physically seeing and examining the patient. I requested a more senior colleague to intervene, and the patient was brought quickly to the OR, and we were able to secure the airway before the patient arrested.—**EJD**

- I also recall a very challenging awake tracheostomy on a very anxious patient who could only breathe comfortably sitting fully upright. Just as I reached the trachea, the tumor completely obstructed the airway, and the patient began to panic. He grabbed my arms, and I was simply unable to reach his trachea to complete my approach. His IV was in his left antecubital fossa, and when he pulled me toward himself, the IV was kinked, and we were simply unable to push the IV meds to relax him so I could finish. With the help of the OR team, we were able to pull his arm straight, infuse the medications, and relax him enough so that I could finish. We got our heads together about this afterward and decided we needed a safe word when it was OK to push meds in this situation.—**EJD**

- One of my general surgery instructors once told me: Not every patient needs to pass through the OR doors on their way to the morgue.—**EJD**

- BUT: Patients need hope. It is alright to share your hope and your belief that someone will be well, even when the odds and the data argue against that possibility. I have seen too many patients "beat the odds" to believe that death is certain, or even predictable. Patients need to believe that you believe they will be well—that your skill and talent are not a waste—that you wouldn't be wasting your time trying to help them if this wasn't the case.—**EJD**

- On the other hand, as surgeons and anesthesiologists, we always have something to offer patients—even when it isn't surgery or anesthesia. We can always offer compassion and empathy. We can listen. We can hold a hand. We can comfort. Sometimes we think that because a patient cannot benefit from surgery or anesthesia anymore, we have nothing to offer—this is untrue. Sometimes, patients just need us to be with them as they take their final steps in this world on their journey through life.—**EJD**

Cultural and Other Considerations

- It's really important to meet the patients where they are in their cultural landscape. It's not up to you to tell your patients anything about who they are and how they should live. Your job is to define your own practice boundaries and find a way to articulate them with the patients' needs. If you are asked to do something you do not think you can do, it is best to deal with this upfront, with as much calmness, collegiality, and courtesy as possible. Please see **Ken Abbey's** Chapter 284 in *Avoiding Common Anesthesia Errors, 2nd Edition* for a deeper discussion of the institutional, state, and federal polices and statutes that may apply to these difficult situations. Unfortunately, these are sometimes not just cultural, moral, or ethical situations. Sometimes they cross into legal liability issues.—**Editors**

- We have been asked whether we would be willing to do and/or not do all kinds of things—not to eat or touch meat on the day of surgery, to do an anesthetic for a patient in a full-body drape (eschewing certain standard monitors), not to discuss the details of a patient's medical situation with the patient or certain family members, and to restrict the actions of individual members of the anesthesia care team based on certain demographic factors. Some we could do, some we could not or would not. Each of these unusual and unique situations will have its own unique solution. Above all, do not (electively) do something you said you would not do.—**Editors**

- *Always* wait for the chaplain or other religious figure or person that is requested by the patient, unless the clinical situation does not permit. There is a great chapter (Chap. 269) in *Avoiding Common Anesthesia Errors, 2nd Edition* that covers a number of common faiths and the basic health beliefs, tenets, and premises that might apply in the perioperative period. This chapter alone makes getting the book worthwhile.—**Editors**

- Don't make a famous person be famous in the perioperative period. We took care of a lot of famous people at Hopkins when we were training and on the faculty there. The senior people had a variety of styles—sometimes we were even dealing with official security details. By and large, though, we saw the senior people pretend like they didn't even know who the patients were.—**AJR and RSB**

- Never, ever look at the chart of a famous person (who is not receiving your direct care) or any chart out of curiosity. You can get into so much trouble doing that, including being fired. It's amazing that this still happens, but it does.—**Editors**

- However, it is not true that you are going to treat a physician patient "just like anybody else." You are not, especially if the patient is another anesthesiologist. For one thing, you are going to show them the intraoperative anesthesia record, most likely, and alter your discussion of risks and consent. And they are going to be as concerned about doing a good for you as a patient as you are concerned about doing a good for them as a provider. We know this for a fact.—**Editors**

- In terms of "learning" pain medicine, the hardest thing for me has been learning to manage patient expectations for chronic pain relief and having the difficult discussions with patients who will likely never be pain-free. To complicate these discussions further, the availability of certain medications and procedures is heavily limited by insurance companies and affordability. My advice is that trainees need as much teaching on how to handle the cultural landscape of chronic pain as they do on the techniques and medications. No amount of teaching in this area would be too much.—**MKO and Editors**

More Wisdom from *Avoiding Common Anesthesia Errors, 2nd Edition*

There is a wealth of additional tips, teaching tidbits, and overall wisdom on doctor-patient relations in our previous book. Please check out this information and remember that every single penny of royalties goes to FAER in perpetuity!

Green2 Chapters with More Wisdom on Doctor-Patient Relations:

- Don't Underestimate the Role of Spirituality in Patients' Perceptions of Disease and Healing, and Remember to Uphold the Right to Self-Determination.
- What's In a Name?
- We Are Not the Only People Who Care About the Patients.
- The Physician as Patient—What I Learned During the Last Five Times I Went to the OR on the Stretcher Instead of Pushing It.
- Apologizing to Patients After an Adverse Event Is the Ethical Thing to Do and Just Might Keep You Out of Court.
- Refusal to Do a Case on Moral or Ethical Grounds: More Practical Navigation Through Choppy Waters.

Authors

Cathy Marcucci is a senior anesthesiologist who lives in the Baltimore area with her husband and *Anesthesia Bridges* author Neil Sandson, a psychiatrist. They often speak of the fact that her interactions with patients are usually never longer than ten minutes and Neil's are never shorter than one hour.

Allan Gottschalk is a senior neuro-anesthesiologist at Hopkins. He feels strongly that interacting with neurosurgical patients and their families requires a certain type of calm but gentle confidence. When not in the hospital, he spends as much time as possible with his family and on the beautiful Chesapeake Bay.

Ron Bank is a senior cardiac and trauma anesthesiologist at INOVA Fairfax Hospital in the northern Virginia suburbs of Washington, DC. He is widely known for his ability to establish rapport with his patients and earn their everlasting gratitude—they keep in touch with him for years—as featured in several *Bridges* chapters.

Brian Gierl is a senior neuro-anesthesiologist in the UPMC system in Pittsburgh, PA, and program director of the neuro-anesthesiology fellowship. He has a focused and ongoing commitment to overseas medical missions, including trips to Rwanda, Ghana, Uganda, Haiti, Guatemala, Vietnam, and Zambia. When not caring for his Pittsburgh or international patients, Brian is an avid outdoorsman.

Ed Damrose is a professor of otolaryngology—head and neck surgery and, by courtesy, of anesthesiology, perioperative and pain medicine at Stanford. He is also chief of the division of laryngology; director of the Stanford Voice & Swallowing Center and the fellowship program in laryngology; recent past chief of staff/Stanford Health Care; and medical director for professionalism/Stanford Health Care.

Amy Robbins is a health care executive whose work involves anticipating and resolving the issues that exist at the interface of patient care and the electronic health record. She has also remained a practicing hospice and palliative care physician and has thought deeply about optimizing doctor-patient relations for that most deserving cohort of patients. She lives in the Charlotte, NC, area with her husband, Ray Koloski.

GPSR Compliance

The European Union's (EU) General Product Safety Regulation (GPSR) is a set of rules that requires consumer products to be safe and our obligations to ensure this.

If you have any concerns about our products, you can contact us on ProductSafety@springernature.com

In case Publisher is established outside the EU, the EU authorized representative is:

Springer Nature Customer Service Center GmbH
Europaplatz 3
69115 Heidelberg, Germany

Batch number: 10622480

Printed by Printforce, the Netherlands

Anesthesia Bridges

Sharif Mohamed • Raymond Graber
Amr Abouleish • Edwin Avery IV
Jeffrey Kirsch • Catherine Marcucci
Editors

Anesthesia Bridges

Wisdom for Your Personal and Professional Journey

Volume II

Springer

Editors
Sharif Mohamed
Department of Anesthesiology
The University of Texas Medical Branch
Galveston, TX, USA

Amr Abouleish
Department of Anesthesiology
The University of Texas Medical Branch
Galveston, TX, USA

Jeffrey Kirsch
Department of Anesthesiology and Pain Medicine
University of Washington School of Medicine,
Seattle, WA, USA

Raymond Graber
Department of Anesthesiology and Perioperative Medicine
University Hospitals Cleveland Medical Center
Cleveland, OH, USA

Edwin Avery IV
Department of Anesthesiology and Perioperative Medicine
University Hospitals Cleveland Medical Center
Cleveland, OH, USA

Catherine Marcucci
Department of Transfusion Medicine,
Clinical Center
National Institutes of Health
Bethesda, MD, USA

ISBN 978-3-032-08293-0 ISBN 978-3-032-08294-7 (eBook)
https://doi.org/10.1007/978-3-032-08294-7

This Springer imprint is published by the registered company Springer Nature Switzerland AG
The registered company address is: Gewerbestrasse 11, 6330 Cham, Switzerland

Editors

Sharif Mohamed: To my parents Samy and Safy and to my wife Lobna. And also to my kids Lina, Amr, Ali, and Hamza—your support is my lifeline.

Ray Graber: To my wife, Mary, who lovingly keeps our household running. To our sons, Luke and Colin, who are both launched and finding success in their careers. To Bridget and Lauren—so great to have you with us in the family. And to Aubrie, who is growing into a lovely young woman and college student.

Amr Abouleish: To my most important mentors—my parents, Ezzat and Atiya Abouleish. I am who I am because of them.

Ed Avery: To my wife Lauren who is our family's always vigilant safety officer. To my daughter, Nicole, whom I am so proud of for her hard work at Northwestern University, and to my son, Edwin, who is a top student in his class.

Jeff Kirsch: To my granddaughters Noa, Romi, and Mika and to my grandson Dylan, who give me hope for a better tomorrow. And to my grandson, Daniel, whose tragic death indelibly revealed that medicine can and must do better. I love you all.

Cathy Marcucci: To Charlie and Lisa, as always! Being your Mom is the best thing that ever happened to me. And to Neil—many thanks for helping with yet another book.

Contributing Editors (Alphabetical)

Mike Axley: To my twin brother Chris, who is my personal hero. He is just a really thoughtful, caring person. I always try to live by his immortal words, "Could you, please, just attempt to be cool?"

Ron Bank: To my parents, Barron and Lois, whose support and encouragement carried me through to becoming a physician. To my family who support me and tolerate my long hours. To my patients, who entrust me with their lives—an honor greater than any other.

Andrew Barker: To my wife—I am forever grateful for your support and love. Your patience and belief in me are sustaining. To my wonderful children, whose curiosity and energy inspire me every day.

John Briggs: To KB, the real hero, love of my life, and forever partner. Thank you, JB and MB, for always leading by example and I am forever grateful. JB and WB—may the future be bright. I love you all.

Carol Bodenheimer: First, to my family who keep things busy and interesting, always! And to Temple University School of Medicine and Temple University Hospital staff, who taught me the importance of lifelong learning and professionalism.

Kirk Lalwani: To my wife Seema, who always puts family first and has cheerfully supported me through the years. To my kids Nikita and Rohan, as they forge their paths to adulthood and inspire me to be the best Dad I can.

Dan McCoy: To my mother, Peggy, who taught me, word by word, how to listen, how to think, and how to write. Your example of kindness and work ethic guides and inspires me to this day.

Raj Nathwani: To my wife Laura for keeping life together so that I can pursue medicine; to my children Ary, Zubin, and Kamy for keeping the sunshine flowing in; and to my parents for all their sacrifices.

Steve Orebaugh: To anesthesia trainees everywhere. We hope that this book can enhance your ability to care for perioperative patients and keep them safe!

Amy Robbins: To my parents, Gary and Marilyn Robbins, who instilled the pursuit of education and a long-lasting love of learning into me as a young child.

Neil Sandson: To my wife, Cathy Marcucci (you may have heard of her), and my children, Charlie and Lisa. Thank you for bringing purpose and richness to my otherwise bland life.

Jake Seagull: To Judy and my son Daniel, and our canine family member, Sasha, for their unfailing support, love, and tail wagging—although only one of them wags.

Brandon Togioka: To my father, a model of servant leadership and to my mother, who taught me how to write. To my wife Jennifer—my source of inspiration and support.

Jennifer Tripi: To my husband, for his unwavering love, patience, and support. To my sisters for their devoted friendship. And to my parents for their constant encouragement and guidance through life.

Brant Wagener: To my wife and kids whose love and support make my life possible.

David Zvara: To Bharathi—an amazing wife, mother, and companion; my driving inspiration.

We also thank Contributing Editors **Albert Liao** *and* **Kristin King Liao** *for their advice and assistance with the manuscript.*

In Memoriam

Saundra E. Curry, MD *1952–2024*

Richard A. Jaffe, MD PhD *1947–2023*

John S. Rogoski, DO *1961–2024*

Highland Park Bridge—Pittsburgh, PA

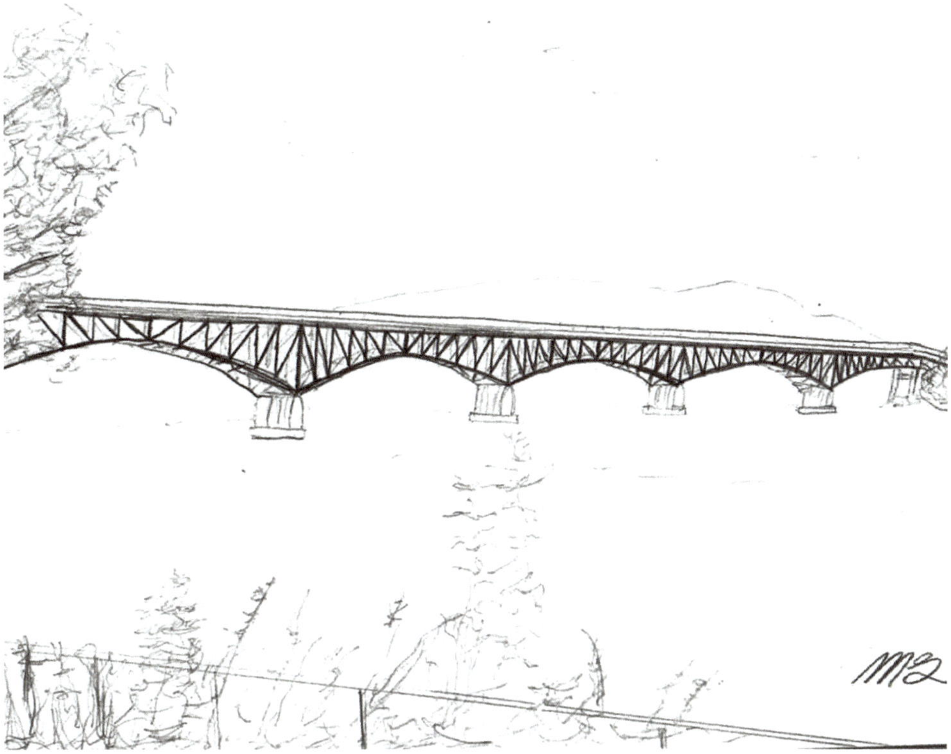

Author **Neil Sandson** chose the Highland Park Bridge in Pittsburgh as his favorite. He tells us that growing up in the Squirrel Hill section of the city but going to school in Fox Chapel meant that he crossed the bridge at least twice a day—thousands of times in total. The bridge was constructed between 1937 and 1939. It carries vehicular traffic across the Allegheny River between the Pittsburgh neighborhood of Highland Park and the suburb of Aspinwall northeast of the city.

Neil and the *Anesthesia Bridges* editors thank **Mitchell Godett** of The Architectural Team in Boston, MA, for his charming pencil drawing that perfectly captures the bridge in its riparian setting. We were delighted when Mitchell also sent us a detailed drawing of the bridge's trusses, below.

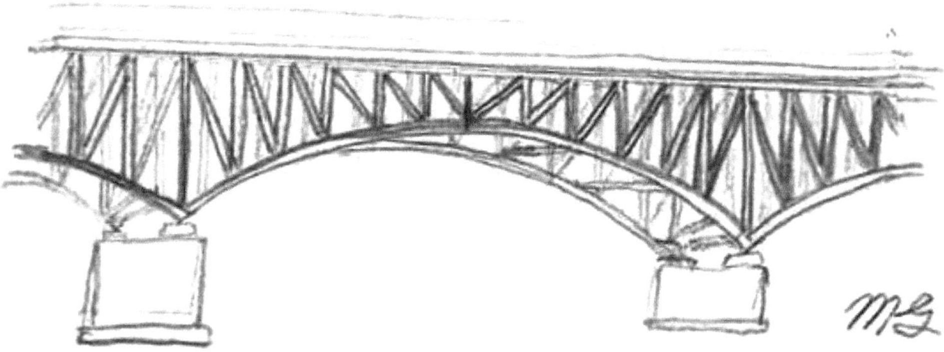

The steel truss design was created by the same engineer who was responsible for Pittsburgh's South Tenth Street and Homestead High Level Bridges. It replaced a much smaller streetcar bridge and was designed to handle "heavy commuter traffic." Construction costs were about $2.5 million (1930s dollars).

Foreword

I've always had a deep interest in thinking about how we can better support the professional development of anesthesiology trainees and those in practice with an eye toward understanding how we can more effectively guide individuals throughout their careers—no matter what trajectories, twists, or turns they might take. So when the editors of *Anesthesia Bridges* told me about their concept for a new book, I was immediately excited to learn more.

While I have been in continuous practice since finishing residency in 2008, I have also integrated a number of nontraditional activities into my professional portfolio. Since finishing training, I've served in combat deploying overseas as US Navy Commander, led the American Medical Association as its chair and president, developed novel artificial intelligence algorithms that have been deployed at scale across the globe, served on both for-profit and not-for-profit boards, overseen the launch of six tech-enabled healthcare companies, and currently direct a $560 million health philanthropy. Throughout my career, I've always yearned for a reference that could give me perspective on how to seek, prioritize, and best position myself for to look for and receive new opportunities. This book is that reference I have longed for.

On the surface, this book is a collection of 200+ essays spread out in ten sections: Communication, Professionalism, Leadership, Academic Promotion and Career Planning, Education and Training, Doctor-Patient Relations, Clinical Wisdom, More Wisdom on Clinical Anesthesia Practice, Personal Stories, and Life Stories. But the sum is very much greater and more powerful than the parts. Taken together, these stories, anecdotes, and pearls of wisdom provide the reader with an opportunity to reflect on how to bring their best self to the bedside, the profession, apply it, and look for the unexpected opportunities to impact the world around us.

While many of the authors are either known to me, or personal friends, I cannot remember a time when I so enjoyed reading the words of my colleagues because of the deeply personal nature of this work. I invite you to enjoy it, reflect on it, and let it guide you to the next chapter of your professional success.

Jesse Ehrenfeld, MD MPH
Professor of Anesthesiology
Senior Associate Dean
Medical College of Wisconsin
Milwaukee, WI, USA

Artists

Edwin Avery

Claiborne Pell Bridge

Ed is a professor of anesthesiology with a subspecialty in cardiothoracic anesthesiology. He immensely enjoys both detailing his sports car and traveling in his off time; a favorite getaway spot of his is the island of Providenciales in Turks and Caicos. He regularly gives lectures to his Turks and Caicos medical colleagues as well as sponsors free blood pressure clinics for the islanders when he visits.

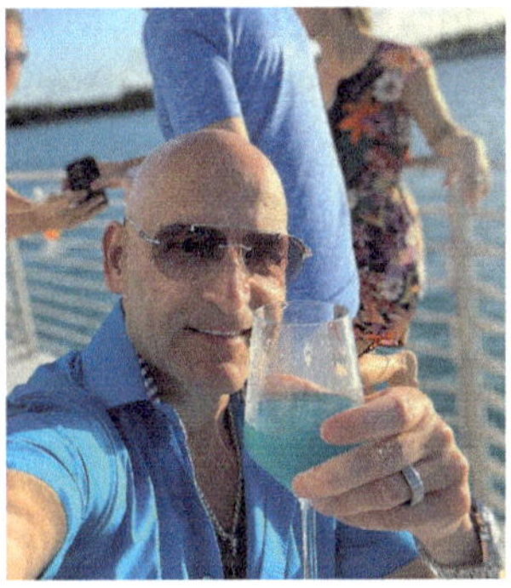

Nina Babbitt

Newport Bridge

Nina Babbitt holds a BS and a Master of Architecture degree from Wentworth Institute of Technology. She currently works at The Architectural Team in Boston. She enjoys working on a range of projects from historic rehabilitations to new builds. She especially likes to be involved in the schematic phase of the design process, studying how architecture can be woven into the fabric of a place. When she is not at work, she loves to travel, practice yoga, and spend time in the ocean.

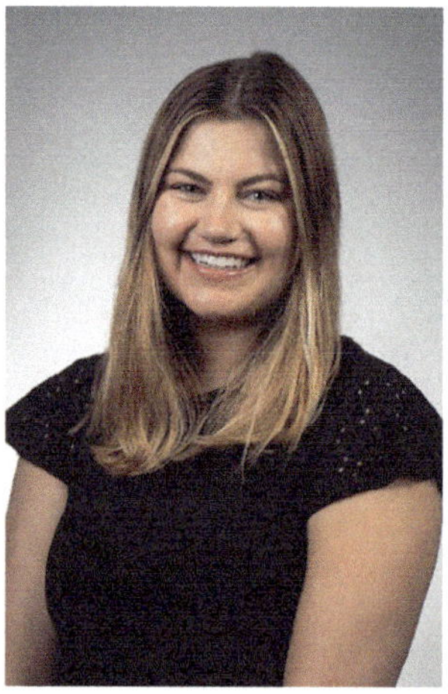

Niamh Curry

A Stone Bridge, Pennsylvania

Niamh Curry was born in Ireland and raised in Massachusetts. She has always been passionate about art and architecture, and is proud to work at The Architecture Team based out of Chelsea, MA. She graduated from the University of Massachusetts Amherst, in 2022 with a Bachelor of Science in Architecture. Her favorite projects to work on usually involve rehabilitations of old buildings.

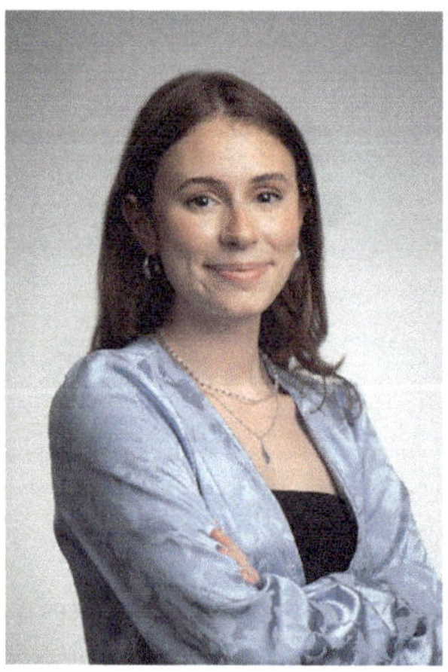

John Giacalone

Harrisburg Railroad Bridge

John Giacalone is an employee at The Architectural Team and former student of Roger Williams University. He is an enthusiast of modern architecture, and some of his favorite architects include Le Corbusier and Frank Lloyd Wright. Outside of architecture, his interests include staying active with things such as snowboarding and martial arts, as well as watching and performing stand-up comedy.

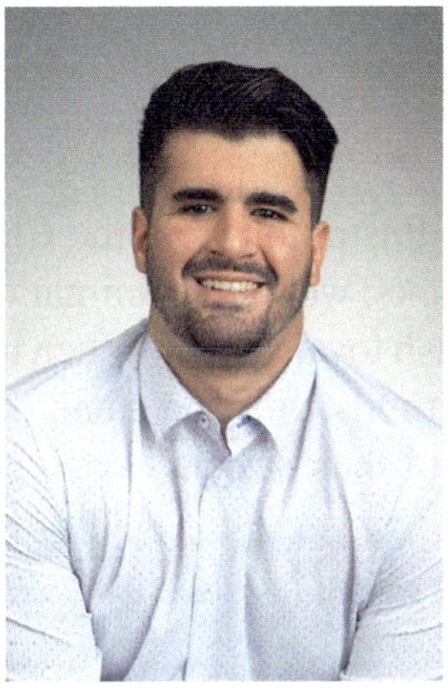

Mitchell Godett

Highland Park Bridge

Mitchell Godett was born and raised in New England. Since a young age, he has enjoyed spending time outdoors whether it be skiing in the mountains of New Hampshire or fishing Massachusetts's coastline. He has particular interest in the historic preservation of local architecture, and currently works as a project designer in Chelsea, Massachusetts, after receiving his master's degree from Northeastern University. He also brings the aspect of reusing something old to make something new into his passion for woodworking.

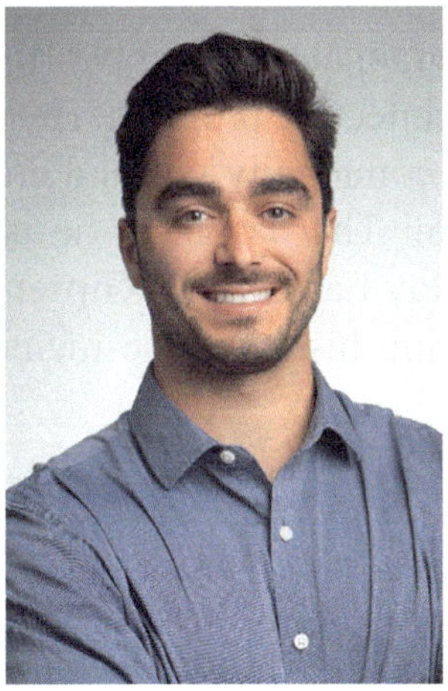

Luke Graber

Anatomic Drawings

Luke Graber has a BFA in illustration from the Cleveland Institute of Art. He has illustrated children's books, worked in animation, developed board games, and currently works as a plush toy designer. When he isn't doing creative work, he enjoys spending time with his wife and small dog at home and looking for new ways to create fun out of their simple lives together.

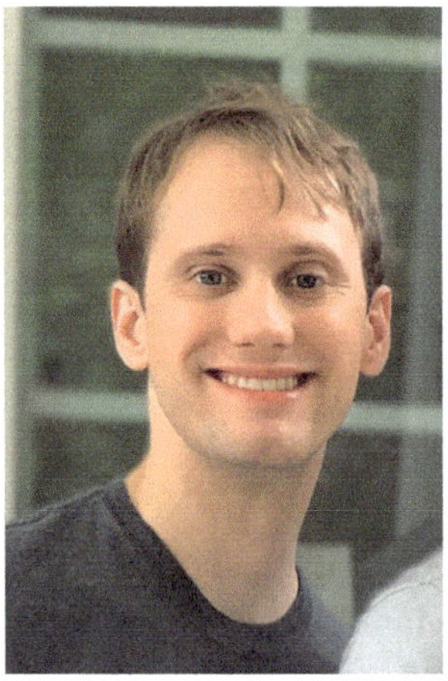

David Howe

Cooper River Bridge

David Howe is a recent graduate of Wentworth Institute of Technologies Bachelor and Master of Architecture program. He has a strong passion for creating designs that enhance community ties and create a more equitable environment through built form. The designers he is most inspired by include Renzo Piano, Charles and Ray Eames, Olaf Gipser to name a few. Some of the hobbies he partakes in during his free time include yoga, reading, furniture making, and antiquing.

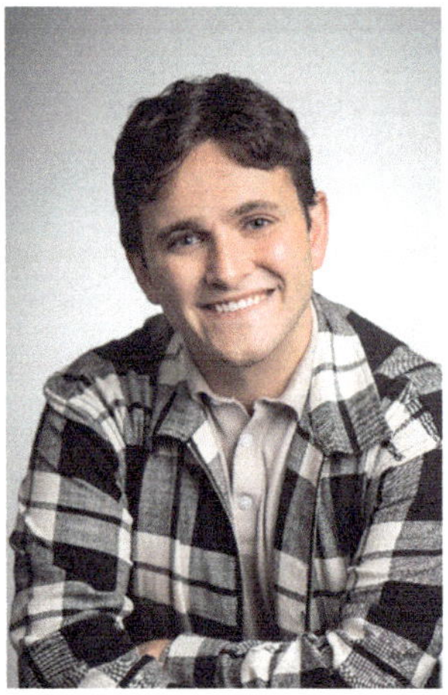

Mark Liu

Ambassador Bridge, Ankle Block

Mark is pursuing a fashion design program at Savannah College of Art and Design. His interests include photography and film. He is particularly interested in street fashion, a sensibility which is reflected not only in his admiration for avant garde designers such as Yohji Yamamoto but also in his extensive knowledge of underground hip hop and personal relationships he has developed with musical artists such as MF Grimm.

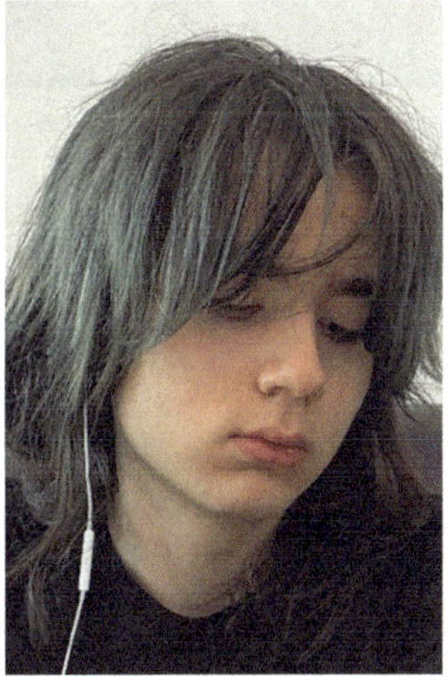

Michael Liu

Stari Most (Old Bridge)

Michael Liu is (emeritus) Senior Partner and Design Principal at The Architectural Team, Inc. where he has directed the design of numerous significant building and master plan commissions. He has been active in the recruitment and cultivation of staff and has been a regular guest design critic at the University of Notre Dame, Roger Williams and Northeastern schools of architecture. His design tastes are eclectic and include both contemporary and traditional architectural expressions. He particularly enjoys sketching buildings and urban venues in his overseas travels.

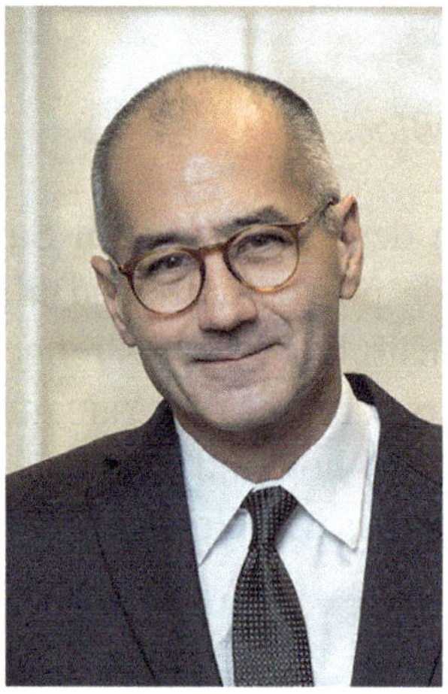

Daniel Nemec

Chesapeake Bay Bridge

Daniel Nemec is a designer and artist located in Boston, Massachusetts. Holding a master's degree in architecture from Northeastern University and a bachelor's degree from Roger Williams University, his work is focused around social-ecological design. Utilizing 2D and 3D mediums, the artwork explores their intersectionality through combining orthogonal and natural forms.

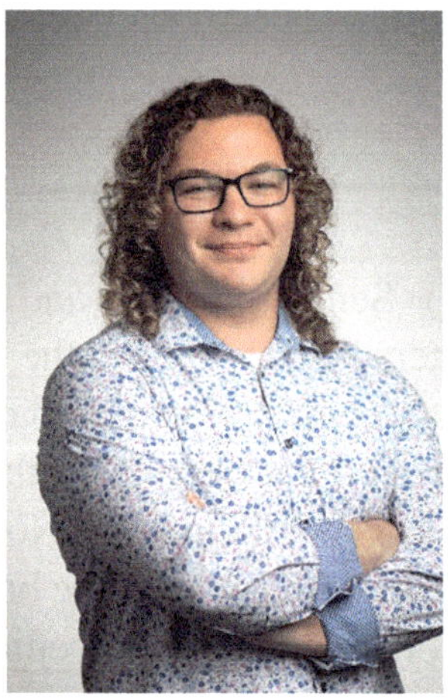

Kelsey O'Connor

Zakim Bunker Hill Memorial Bridge

Kelsey O'Connor, NCIDQ, is a designer located in Boston, Massachusetts. She earned a BFA in interior design from Suffolk University. She draws much of her inspiration from the built environment and the way that we experience space.

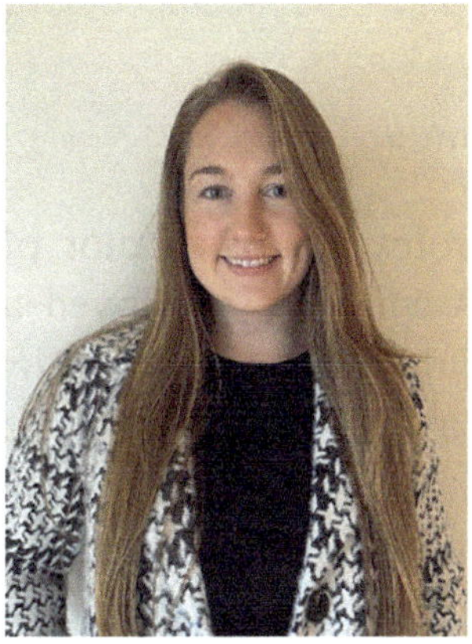

Craig Riley

Thurston Avenue Bridge

Craig Riley was drawn into the field of architecture at a young age due to his fascination of playing with Legos and Lincoln Logs. In order to pursue an education within architecture, he elected to attend the University of Massachusetts Amherst. There, he was able to harness his skills of elaborate designing and constant puzzle-solving.

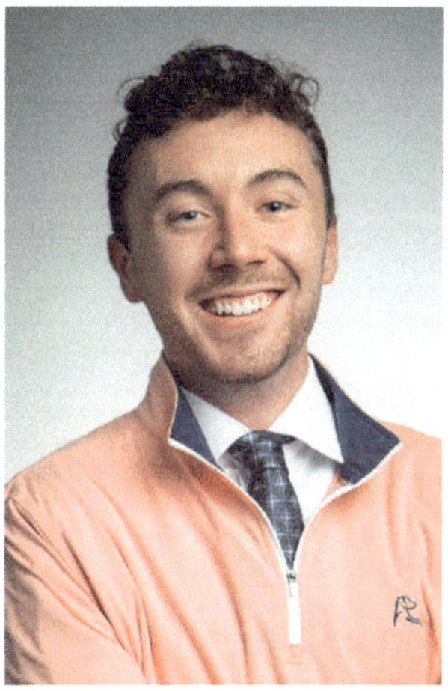

Lisa Sandson

Tiny Bridge on Yellow Mountain

Lisa Sandson holds the professional bachelor of architecture degree from Syracuse University and is currently employed at Cummings Properties in Boston, a unique design/build firm. She grew up loving the arts and has a background in realistic drawing and oil painting. She has always been interested in bridges, as they are the perfect example of a spatialized threshold. She has a black belt in martial arts and loves cooking, travel, and dogs.

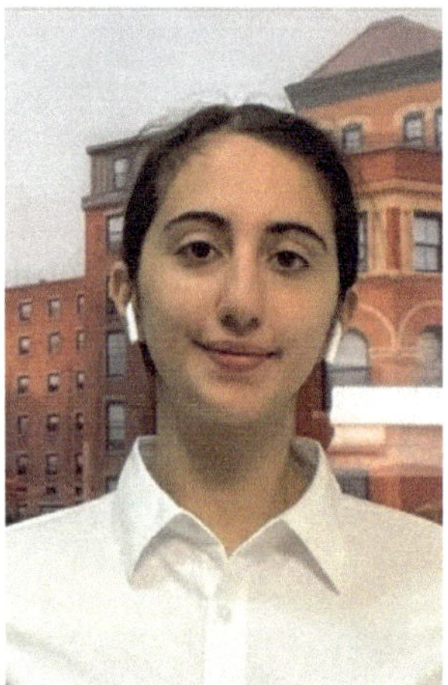

Photographers

Daniel Asher

Operating Room Panorama

Daniel is a cardiac anesthesiologist who actively seeks opportunities for creativity in his daily life. When he's not gardening or cooking, you will probably find him right next to his kids drawing sailboats in crayon or designing a new technological process for his hospital's actively evolving EMR.

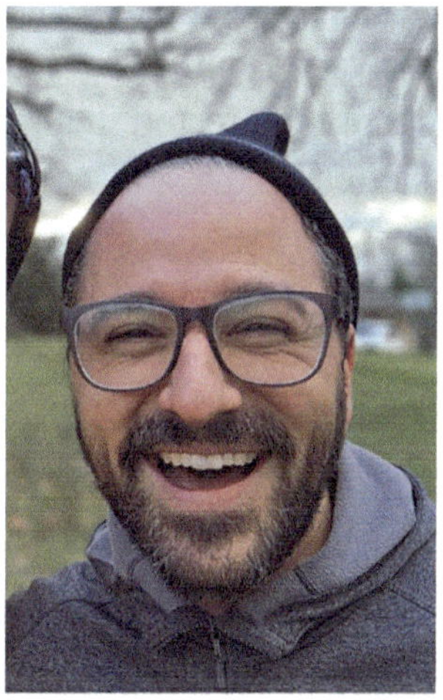

Michael Axley

Microscope, Gladstone Bag, Sellwood Bridge

Michael is an anesthesiologist in private practice with Oregon Anesthesiology Group. He lives in Portland, OR, with his wife, Kimberly Malek, and his three children. He has lived in Portland since he came out to go to school at Reed College and considers himself fortunate to make that wonderful city his home. His hobbies include general aviation, fishing, and the beach.

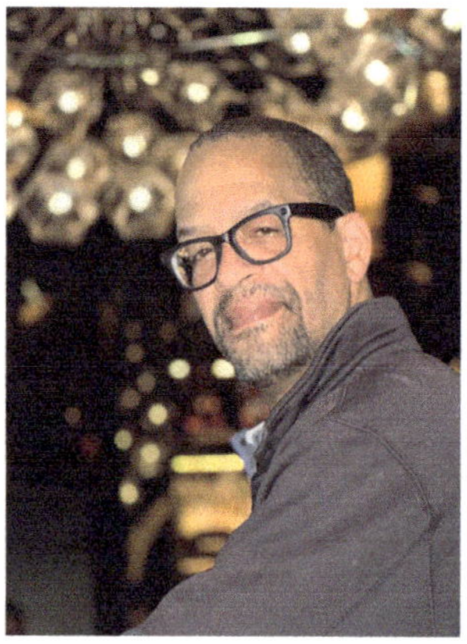

Jordan Bank

Memorial Bridge

Jordan is a student in the metropolitan Washington DC area with special interests in American, world, and aviation history. He is a very serious baseball player and participates in an intense showcase league. He is also a certified SCUBA diver, with multiple dive specialties in many different skill sets. In his remaining spare time, he is deeply interested in animal advocacy and writes for his local animal rescue newsletter.

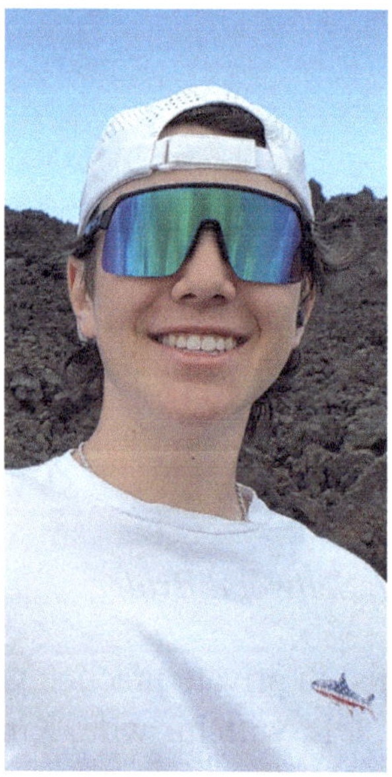

Emma Bailey

Benson Bridge

Emma Bailey is the creator of "Pines & Vines"—a Pacific Northwest travel blog with a focus on outdoor recreation. She is passionate about helping people connect with nature regardless of physical ability or previous experience. She enjoys hiking, photography, and nerding out about the local geology. She lives in Portland, OR.

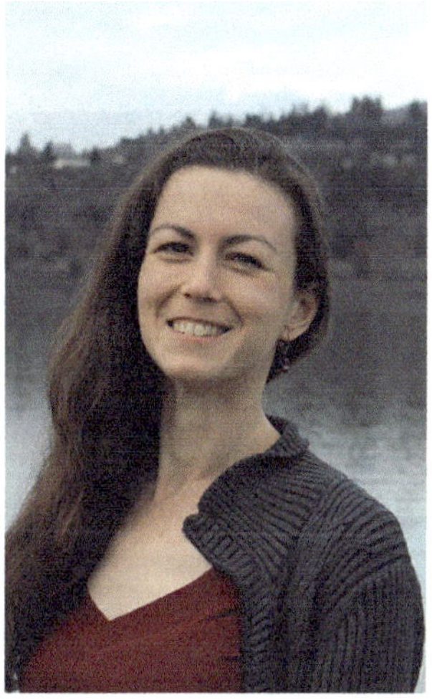

Marlee Chamberlain

The Tilikum Crossing

Marlee is a medical student at Oregon Health and Science University (OHSU). She obtained a BS in biology at Oregon State University, then went on to achieve an AS in paramedicine at OHSU and an MS in biomedical sciences at the University of Northern Colorado. She worked as a paramedic in Portland, and with a love of hiking and traveling, takes pictures where she travels or when she was stationed in an ambulance waiting for a call.

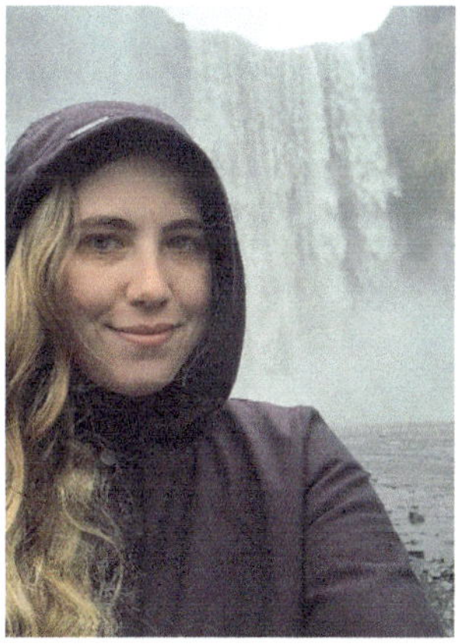

Harriet Chen

Jekyll Island Bridge, Porto Bridge, Boston Bridge

Formerly a NICU nurse and always a devoted mother of two, Harriet has been creating portraits for over 28 years. She absolutely loves connecting with people and allowing special and fun moments to happen naturally. Passionate about capturing light and reflecting the beauty in everyone, her images are original, organic, and have a bit of a documentary flair. She works both in the studio and on location. She currently lives in Alabama with her husband, five cats, and their dog.

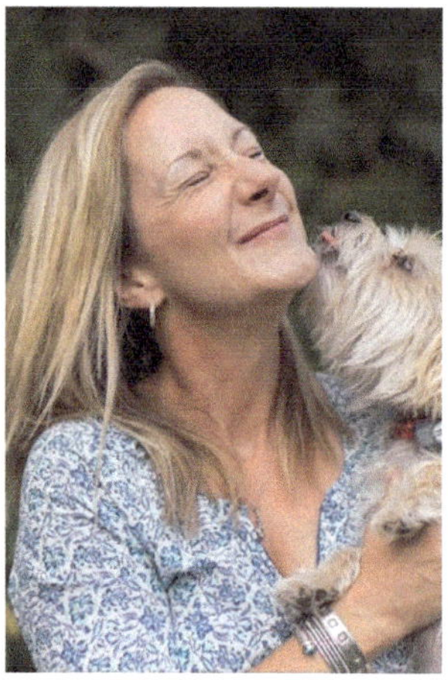

Laura Chess

St John's Bridge, Oregon

Laura is a double-boarded emergency and critical care physician in Portland, OR. She trained in Detroit but is grateful to now live so close to the ocean and mountains. When she is not spending time with her husband and three kids, she enjoys hiking, surfing, cooking, wine tasting, playing polo, and skiing.

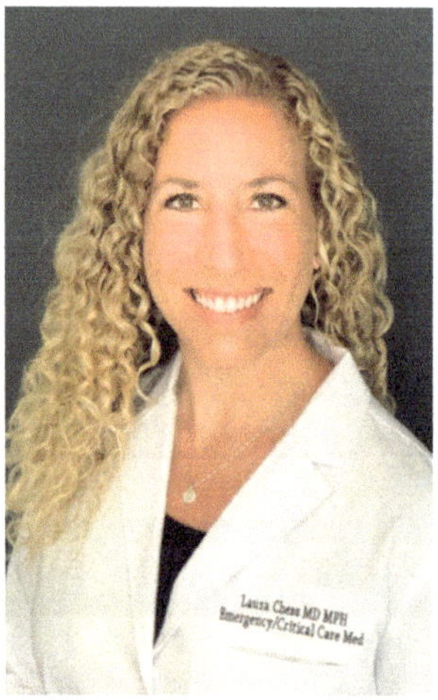

Benjamin Conner

Glen Canyon Navajo Bridge, Grand Canyon Silver Bridge

Ben is currently a physical medicine and rehabilitation resident at Spaulding Rehab Hospital in Boston, where he is already mentoring medical school students and applicants. When he is not spending time with his beloved wife and their animals, he enjoys a healthy balance of outdoor adventures and reclining seats at the movie theater.

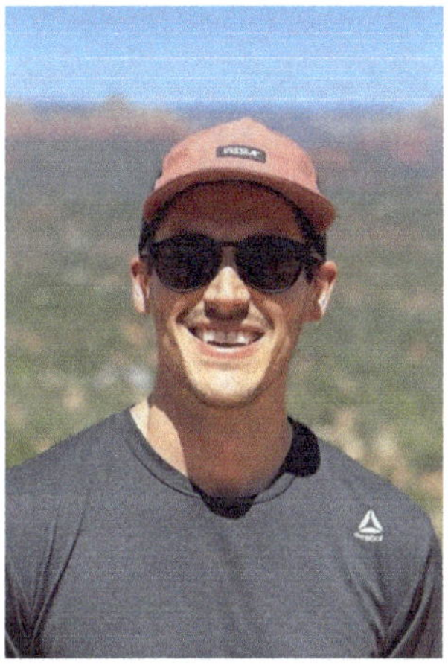

Lois Connolly

Earpiece

Lois is a professor of anesthesiology and medical director of the Master of Science in Anesthesia program at the Medical College of Wisconsin, Milwaukee. Additionally, in the ASA she serves as vice president for professional affairs. She deeply believes that the culture of our environment where we spend a great part of our day influences our health. Healthy clinician = healthy patients; meaning better patient outcomes. Lois and Patrick enjoy traveling the world experiencing cultures and history.

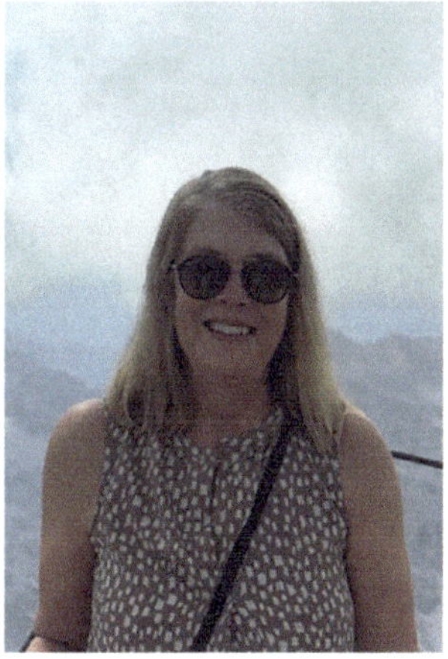

Abigail Crawford

Alaskan Bridge

Abigail is a graduate of the University of Alaska where she obtained a BS degree in natural sciences and a minor in psychology. She attends the University of Washington School of Medicine. Her hobbies include most things outdoors in the beautiful state of Alaska—she loves to hike, bike, kayak, camp, fish, play tennis, ski, and snow machine. She has also volunteered at Project Hope, which makes free naloxone kits for the state of Alaska.

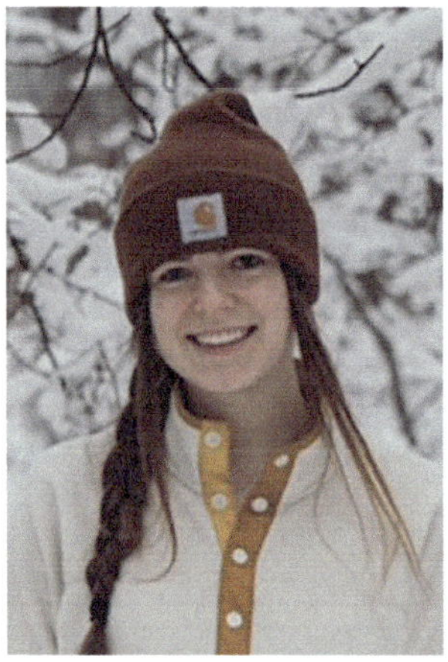

Isabella Giglio

Philadelphia Walkway Bridge

Isabella Giglio is a busy medical student at Sydney Kimmel Medical College pursuing her interest in surgery. She attended University of California Santa Barbara for her undergraduate degrees where she has dual degrees in Aquatic Biology and Sociology. She enjoys combining her passions of medicine and art through photography.

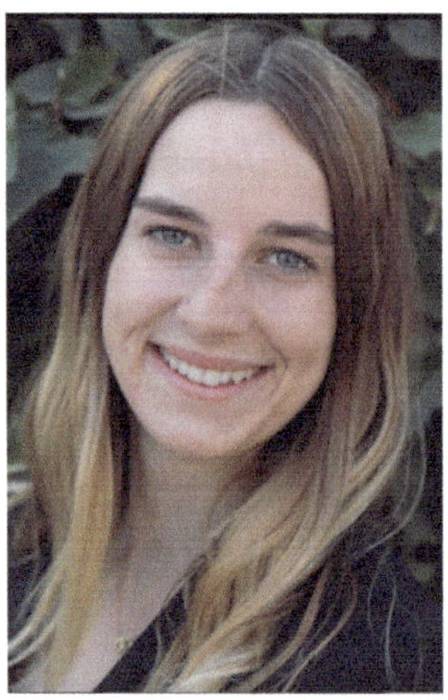

Aubrie Graber

Medical Text Books

Aubrie is a Cleveland native and cat aficionado who loves to chronicle life around her through photos and video. She is a former long time competitive cheer flyer and also varsity cheerleader. She developed a passion for doing sports photography at her high school, including for basketball, lacrosse, and wrestling. She is studying communications and media production at the University of Dayton.

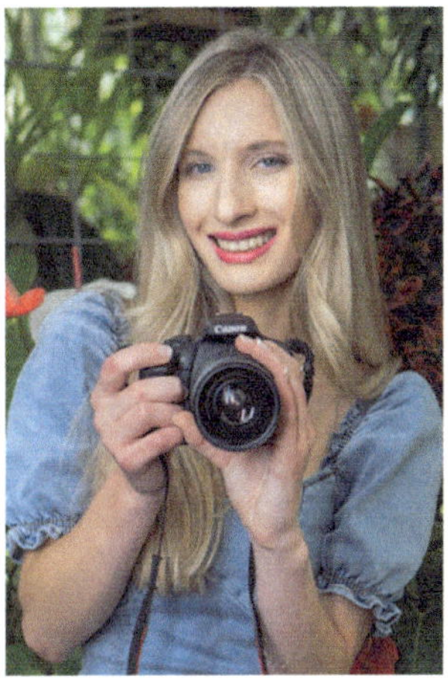

Mary Graber

London Tower Bridge

Mary graduated with a BA in interior design from Ashland University and formerly worked as a wallpaper designer. She is also the proud mother of three amazing children. In her spare time, she enjoys traveling, photography, decorating, gardening, biking, yoga, baking, and many other creative projects, but she especially treasures spending time with her family and three cats: Theodore, Tulip, and Angel.

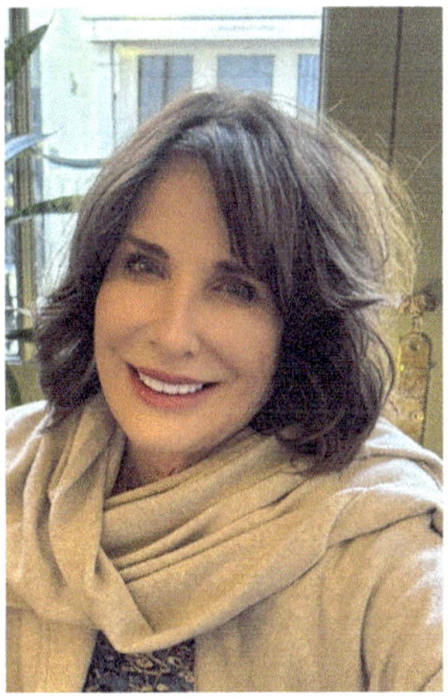

Gavin Hess

Bamboo Slide Rule

Gavin is a busy college student at Auburn University where he is majoring in business and finance and enjoying getting to know that part of the country. He enjoys traveling with his family, especially Hawaii and the beautiful South Carolina beaches. He is a sports and outdoors enthusiast and was a competitive wrestler throughout his school years.

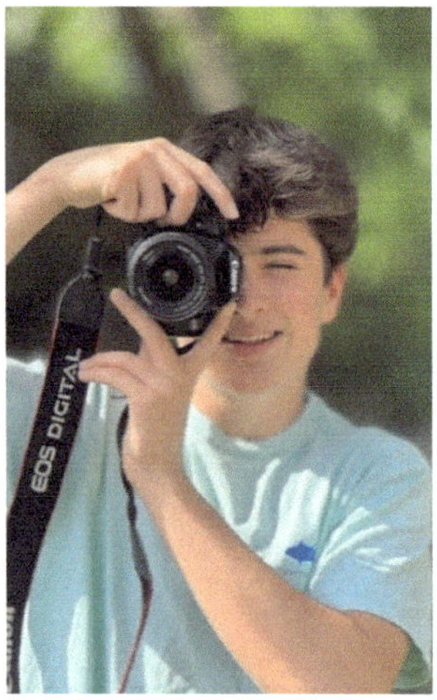

Harriet Hopf

Heaphy Track Pedestrian Bridge

Harriet is a professor of anesthesiology and biomedical engineering and president of the Academic Senate at the University of Utah. Her local and national leadership roles have positioned her for her current focus on nurturing career and leadership success in the next generation. Her husband Leo is an expert in strategy and decision-making and a peerless peer mentor. McKinley, their off spring, recently received a MA in history from the U of Utah and is busy reinventing the way history is told.

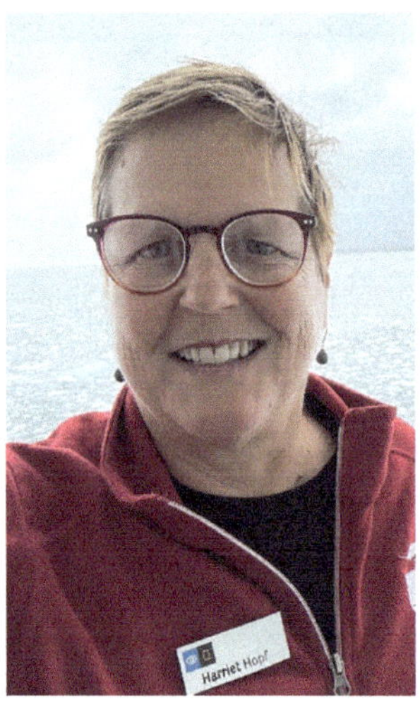

Scott Hull

Wheelhouse of the tugboat George L. Ostrander, Mackinac Bridge

Scott has been a chief engineer in the US Merchant Marine for the past 40 years, formerly on the Bering Sea and the Gulf of Alaska, but now sailing on commercial vessels in the Great Lakes. Home is a small lake in central Indiana, where he boats and rides his Indian motorcycle with wife and *Anesthesia Bridges* author Conni Walkup Hull. He also enjoys painting and photography in his shop while rocking out to Joan Jett and Blondie.

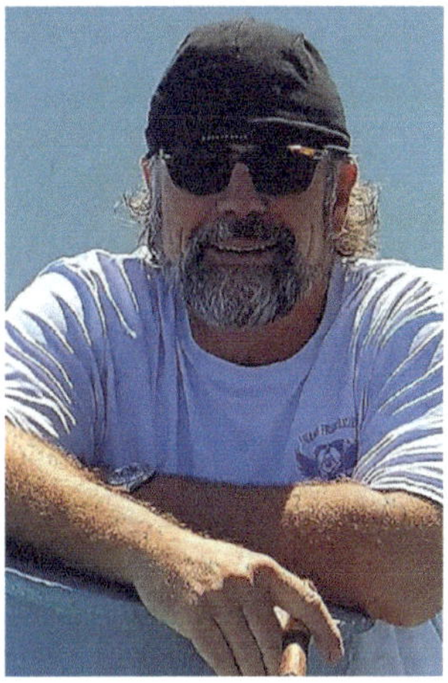

Hailey James

Sedona, Flying Dog Lennon

Hailey James is originally from Arizona. She still loves the Southwest but loves dogs more and relocated to East Texas several years ago to begin her career in dog rescue. She considers it the hardest but most worthwhile thing she has ever done. The 24/7 nature of dog rescue precludes a lot of free time, but she continues to enjoy doing photography when she can. Her photo of Lennon (below) won several contests and landed him a loving home in Canada.

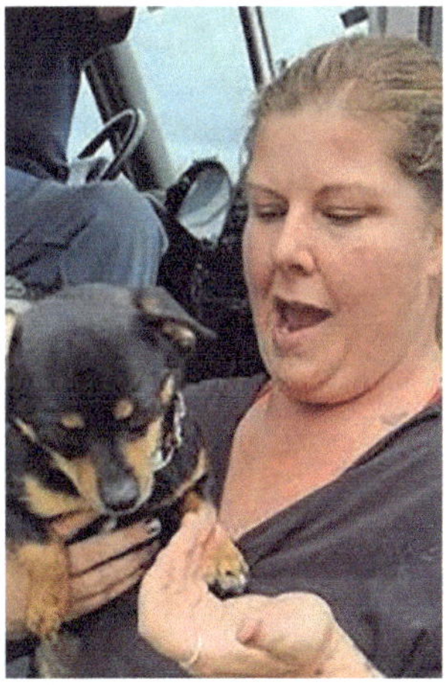

Randy Jensen

RJ Acres Farm Pictures

Randy Jensen lives and farms in Blair, NE, on a beautiful and historic 900-acre property. A devoted family man, he spends as much time as possible with his grown children and their spouses and his four beautiful grandchildren. He also enjoys volunteering at his church, traveling both in the US and internationally, and rooting for the Nebraska Cornhuskers.

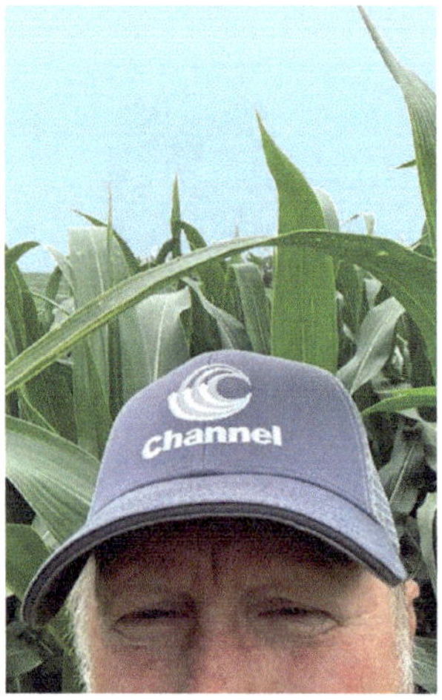

Ruth Jensen

RJ Acres Farm Pictures

Ruth's professional accomplishments include working for over four decades as a senior chemical engineer and engineering executive and holding an office in her family's farm corporations, all while never losing sight of her pre-eminent role as a mother and now grandmother. She is a dedicated churchwoman, expert cook, and world traveler. She also collects and has been asked to exhibit her beautiful antique jewelry.

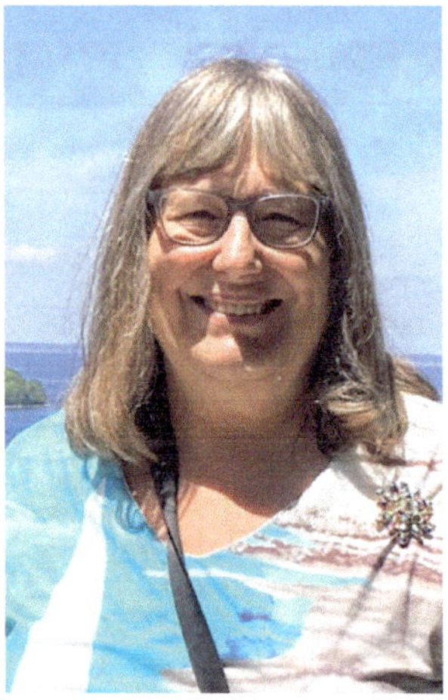

Bo Johns-Hennessy

C&O Canal Bridge, Arlington Memorial Bridge

Bo is a native Washingtonian and resides there with his husband and their Shih Tzu, Wally. He finds joy in exploring and photographing the wider DC area. He is a devoted volunteer, serving in leadership positions with GO BO GO Fund, the Foundation for Community Betterment, and Lehigh University. He was a consultant at McKinsey & Company before founding his own firm to collaborate with real estate and technology clients to shape the built environment.

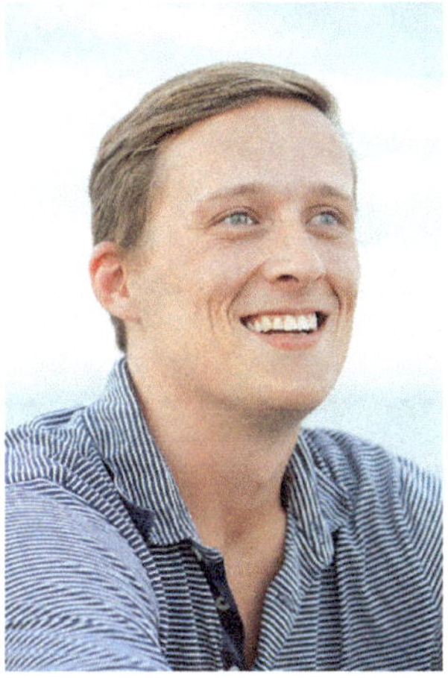

Caroline Koloski

Pullen Park Bridge

Caroline is from Charlotte, NC. She has a BA in psychology and is now a pre-med student. When she isn't hanging out with her cat Blackie, she can be found on the golf course or going to concerts with her friends. She also loves spending time with her large family. After finishing a study abroad semester in Florence, Italy, she is now an EMT and preparing for medical school.

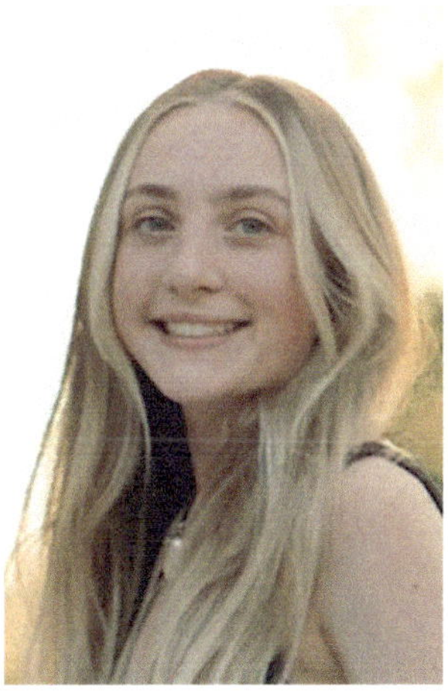

LouAnn Kopenhaver

Hanover Walkway

LouAnn is a retired reading specialist and literacy coach, having earned a BS in Education from Millersville University and an MEd in psychology of reading from Temple University. Since retiring, her favorite pastime is spending time with her grandkids, family, and friends, but she also enjoys golf, reading (of course), and traveling with her husband.

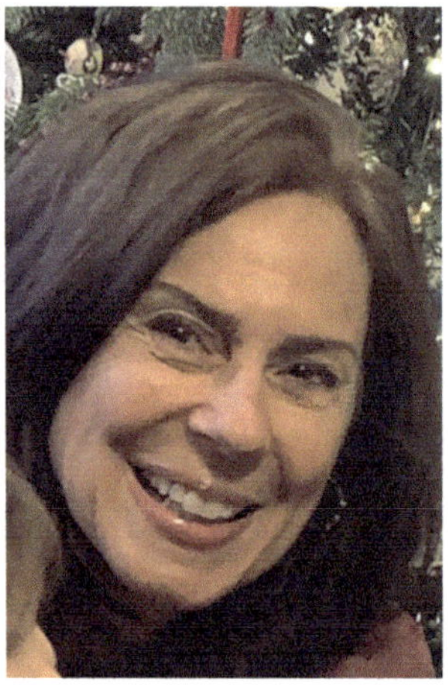

John Liao

Liao Gladstone Bag

John is an honors student, talented artist, musician, and aspiring pilot. He has studied violin for eleven years and has formally studied visual art for three years. He enjoys oil painting, sculpture, and drawing and is currently studying color theory. His many other interests include running cross country, engineering, space, film, science fiction, history, and anything to do with airplanes. He is the grandson of Dr. Schue-Yuan Liao.

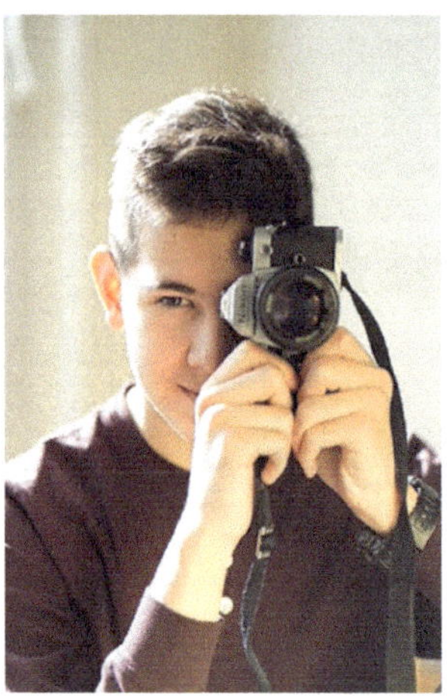

Catherine Marcucci

Rain Bridge in the Mt. Washington Arboretum, Brandywine River Bridge, Olentangy River Bridge

Cathy thinks of herself more as an editor than photographer, but she snaps a photo here and there. Her professional careers have been in engineering, anesthesiology, and transfusion medicine. Her abiding personal interest is her family and when she can find the time, she also enjoys traveling, swimming, minor league baseball, duplicate bridge, and helping out dog rescues.

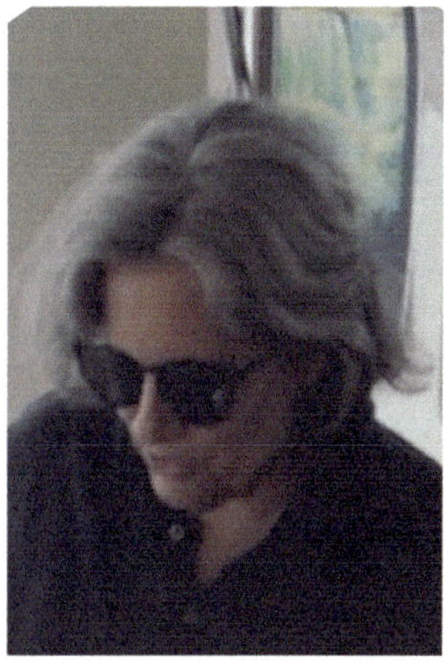

Elaine Matte Mut

St. Louis Arch

Elaine is a Houston-based amateur photographer who began her photography journey in earnest as a volunteer publicity photographer for three Houston public schools, as well as local community events. She has been fortunate to have her photography published in local papers and magazines and exhibited at several local galleries. Her main passion in retirement is traveling with family to areas with abundant wildlife and natural surroundings.

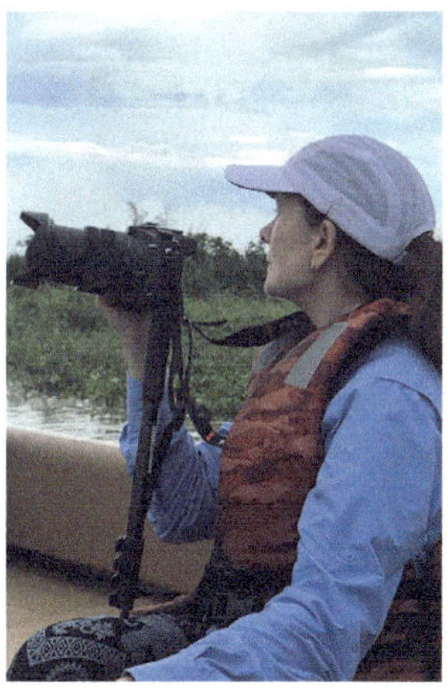

Kathleen Naughter

Washington Park Bridge

Kathleen received her BS in studio art from the College of St. Rose in Albany, New York, where she worked as an assistant in the photography lab back in the days of 35 millimeter film. She considers her greatest accomplishment to be raising her three wonderful sons, John, Patrick, and James. Her newest role is grandmother, and she is looking forward to spending time with Lucille, the most beautiful baby in the world.

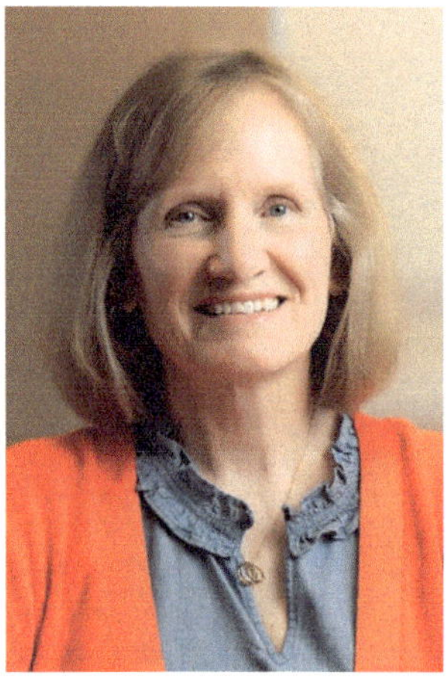

James Nguyen

Philadelphia Walkway Bridge

James is from Newport Beach, California, and is now a busy fourth year medical student at Thomas Jefferson University in Philadelphia who is in the residency interviewing process. In his free time, he enjoys exploring Chinatown and other Philadelphia neighborhoods as well as raising his kitten, Boh.

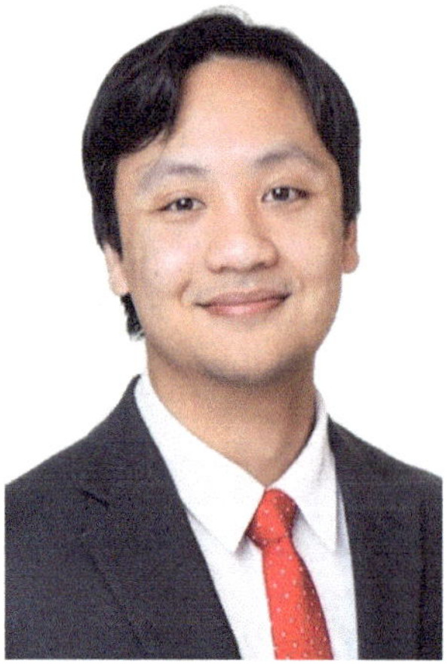

Anthony Passannante

UNC Skyway Bridge

Tony is a professor and executive vice-chair of anesthesiology at UNC Chapel Hill, and assistant dean for admissions for UNC SOM. His focus in anesthesiology practice has been vascular anesthesia and operating room management. His hobbies include hiking and traveling. His family continues to grow with two recent weddings and two grandchildren growing up at an astonishing pace.

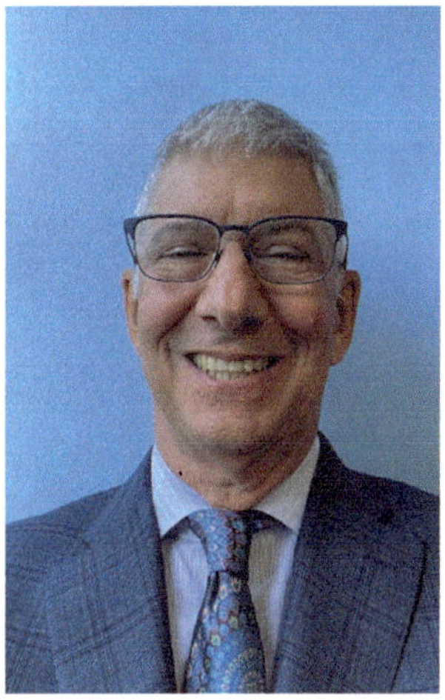

Alex Pelayo

Montgomery County Bridge

Alejandra is a San Francisco native who completed a research fellowship at the National Institutes of Health. She graduated from the University of Redlands with degrees in sociology and biology. She is passionate about diversifying medicine and science and has served on several boards. She is now an MBA student and is seriously considering medical school to follow.

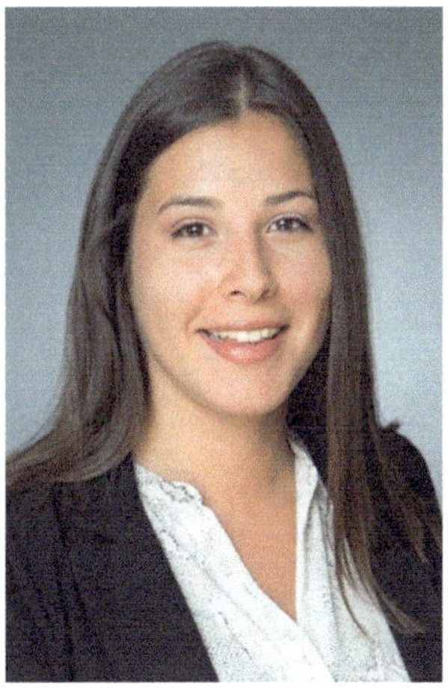

Amy Robbins

Aqueduct of Segovia

Amy is an anesthesiologist and medical executive who specializes in palliative medicine and cancer pain management. She remains deeply committed to both clinical work and the development of healthcare safety, quality, and clinical decision supports for best practices. She lives in NC with her husband, two dogs, and two cats. Her passions include her family, travel, animal rescue, and collecting art.

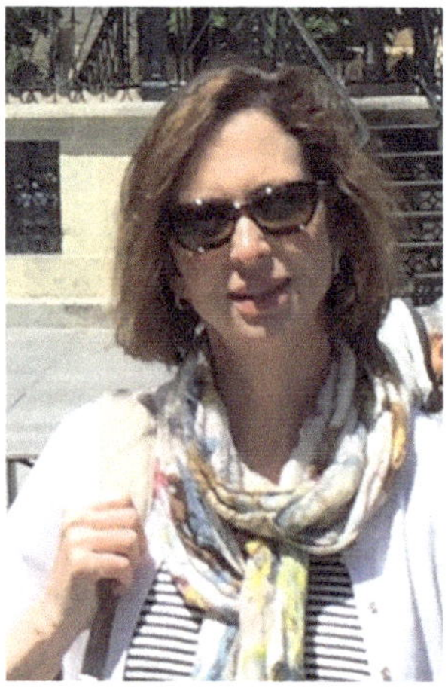

Neil Sandson

Stick Bridge

Neil Sandson is a psychiatrist, proud husband and father, and lifelong squash and duplicate bridge player, gamer, and science fiction buff. Fortunately, none of that distracted him from his newfound passion for the art and science of bridge building, edible or otherwise. He was especially honored to be asked to make a cheese bridge.

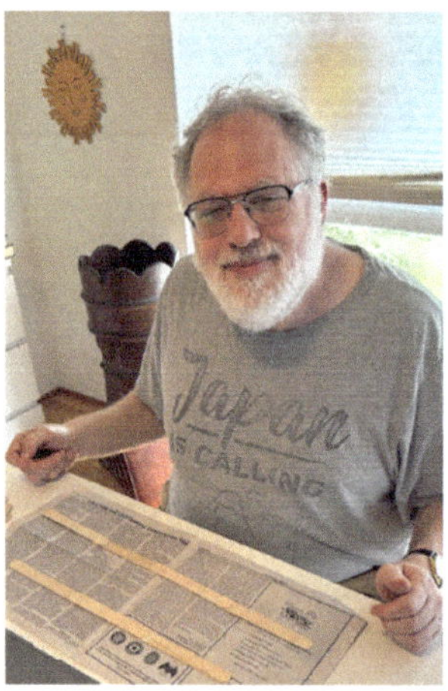

Daniel Sessler

Harbor Bridge, Sydney

Dan is a senior anesthesiologist who has authored more than 980 research papers. He has been a principal or co-investigator on grants totaling $100 million. He founded and directs the Outcomes Research Consortium—the world's largest anesthesia research group; it publishes a full paper every other day, for a total of more than 2000 papers. In his previous life, he was a photographer and still enjoys great images.

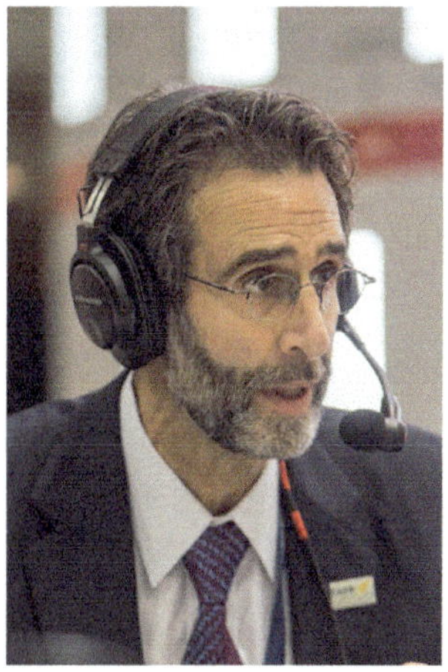

Richard Sheffield

Abril Bridge in Lisbon, Portugal

Richard is a retired technologist and is now fully occupied as a writer and author. After graduating from Georgia Tech, he learned that understanding the latest wave of high-tech gadgets and being able to write about them is a rare and valuable skill. He splits time between the heat of Atlanta and the more heat of Miami, where he loves spending time with his plastic surgeon girlfriend.

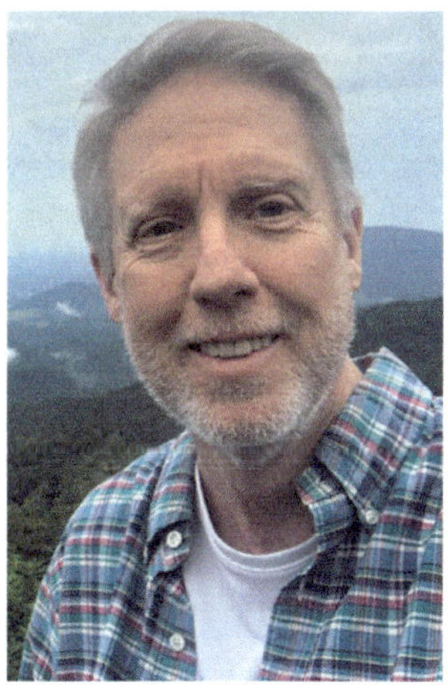

Dillon Shook

Gottschalk Bag

Dillon Shook is a software engineer working primarily on the web for the last decade. His other hobbies include photography and getting inspiration from other photographers like Albert Dros, Irene Rudnyk, and Markus Reugels, playing guitar and listening to lots of music, game development, cooking, gardening, and not having enough time in the day.

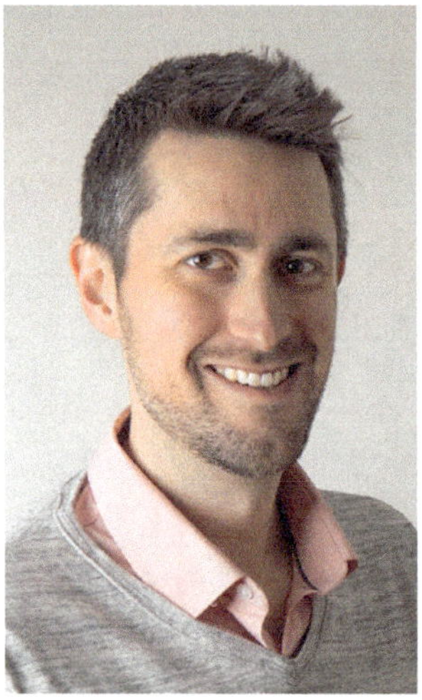

Joshua Stich

The High Line, New York City

Born in Atlanta, Georgia, Joshua grew up both there and on the Gold Coast, Australia. He attended New York University, where he majored in neural science and chemistry. He is now a medical student at Albert Einstein where he is naturally already interested in anesthesiology. In his spare time, he plays all the ice hockey he can, volunteers with a number of organizations, and travels.

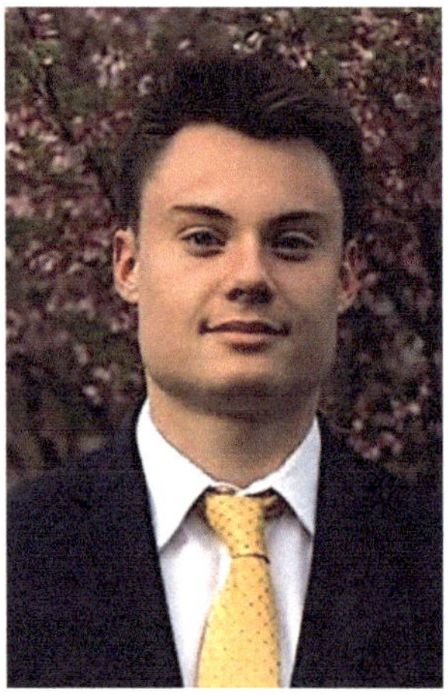

Jennifer Tripi

UNC Skyway Bridge

Jennifer (Jen) completed her obstetric anesthesia fellowship at UNC Hospitals at Chapel Hill this year and joined the Ohio State team as a general and obstetric anesthesiologist. When she isn't busy at the hospital, she enjoys spending time with her husband, family, and friends. She also loves exploring and hiking our country's beautiful national parks, traveling the world, playing board games, and interior designing.

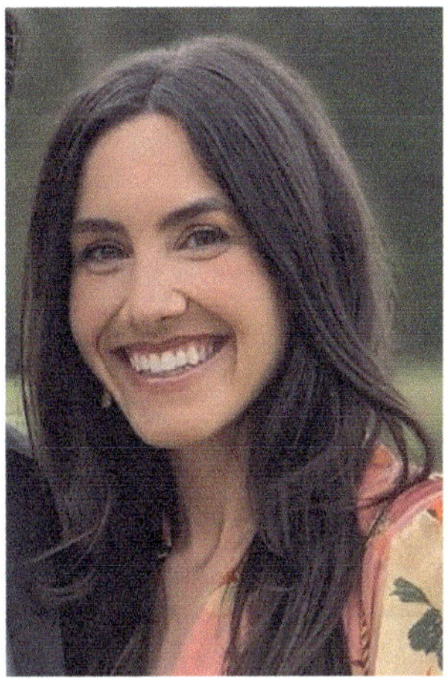

Chloe Wagener

The Natural Bridge

Chloe Landon Wagener loves to travel, reads voraciously, and writes short stories. When she has time away from her studies, she is working on the basics of a novel. She is endeared to all animals, especially dogs, and loves chocolate. She is a percussionist and pianist and wants to pursue a career in medicine or law.

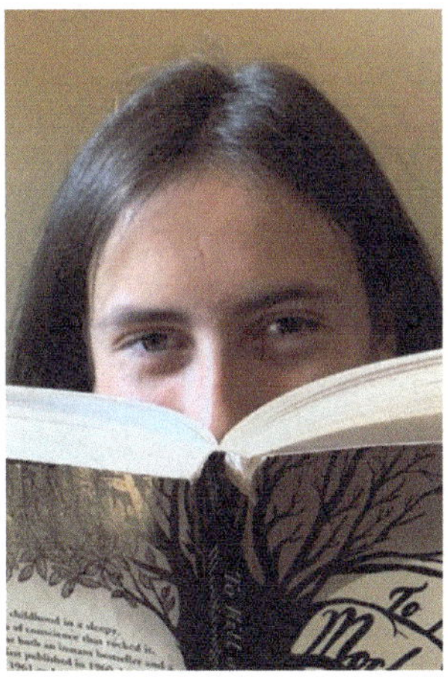

James Wyatt Wagener

Footbridge

James Wyatt is an energetic soul like his mother. He loves to try everything at least once like his dad. He loves to travel, wants to learn to cook, and dances like a fiend. He plays the violin and is learning the clarinet. He wants to learn the saxophone so he can play in the jazz band and is a member of the mountain biking team.

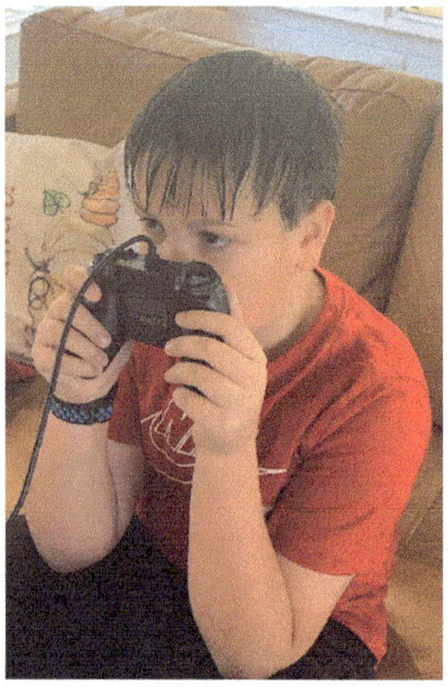

Nathaniel R. Wagener

National Bridge Park

Nathaniel Ryan is a boy's boy. His current love is soccer, and he idolizes Lionel Messi. He also loves to play games on his Nintendo Switch with his brother and is learning to play Pokémon with the help of his dad. He plays the piano when he has to and is a math wizard.

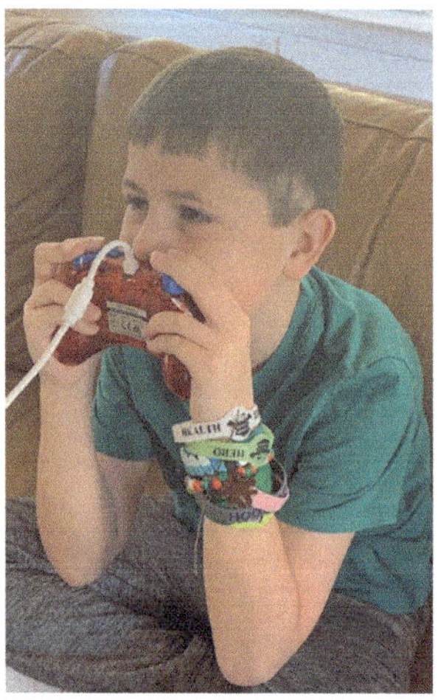

Daniel Walker

Alaskan Wooden Footbridge

Danny is a student in suburban Philadelphia, PA. He enjoys taking photos while working summers on his grandfather's commercial fishing boat in Southeast Alaska and already has a large collection of striking nature photos. Danny also enjoys sports, running cross country, traveling, soccer, and playing his cello.

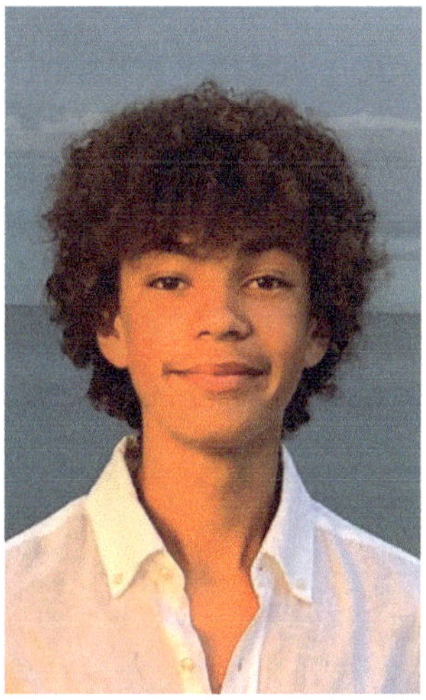

John Walker IV

Fairmont Park Bridge

John is a busy student at Drexel University. He is a premed major and is also taking extra coursework in psychology. He enjoys sports of all kinds, spending time with his family, exploring the most interesting places in Philadelphia, traveling, playing rugby for his school club team, distance running, and playing cello.

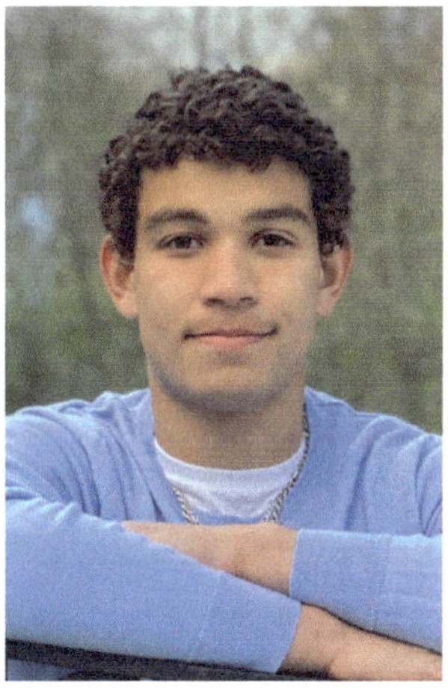

Marilyn Walker

Little Island at Pier 55

Marilyn was born and raised in Atlanta, Georgia. As someone with a strong passion for the sciences, she carried this interest into her undergraduate studies, where she pursued degrees in psychology and chemistry at New York University. As an intern at the Sigurdsson Neuroscience lab at NYU Langone, she hopes to continue to advance the field of medicine.

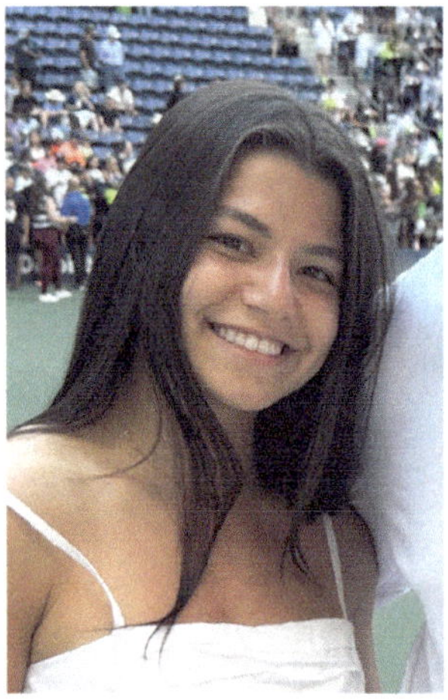

Christie Waters

Sandstone Natural Bridge, Jordan

Christie is a mostly retired chemical engineer and STEM educator who enjoys spending as much time outdoors as the upstate New York weather permits. In addition to taking too many photos of her grandkids, she tries to capture both the simple and the stunning beauties she encounters while traveling.

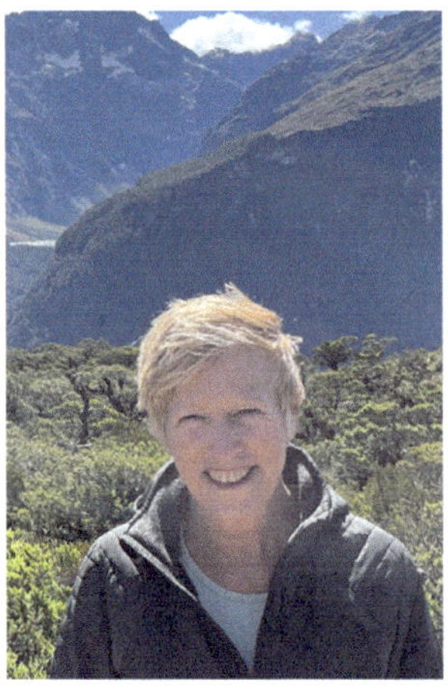

Toby Weingarten

Cold Creek Bridge

Toby Weingarten is a professor of anesthesiology at the Mayo Clinic and has been a member of their faculty since 2005. He has been very active in researching anesthetic outcomes with over 250 peer-reviewed publications, numerous abstracts, and book chapters. When he is not in the hospital, he is almost always outside, bird watching, fishing, gardening, tapping maple trees, or playing with his bees.

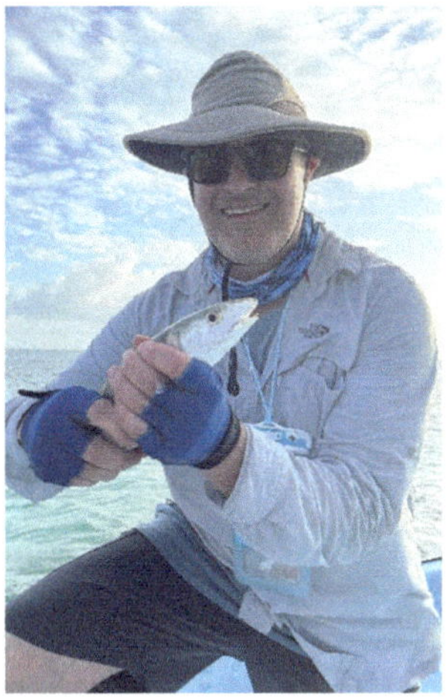

Brad Winters

BNSF Freight Train

Brad is a senior anesthesiologist and intensivist at Johns Hopkins. He is a devoted family person whose outside interests include hiking and mountain climbing, kayaking, ice climbing, mountain and road biking, movies, travel, collecting vintage slide rulers and antique microscopes, and of course trains.

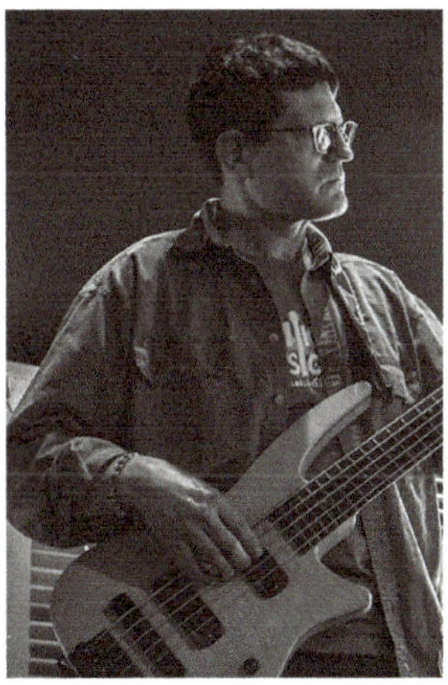

Eli Wright

Student Walkway at Towson U

Eli lives in the Baltimore area and is a busy executive and entrepreneur in the automotive industry, with expertise in the European luxury models. He followed the creation of this book from the start and finally agreed to join the project after several requests. In his very rare spare time, he enjoys music, sports, and photography.

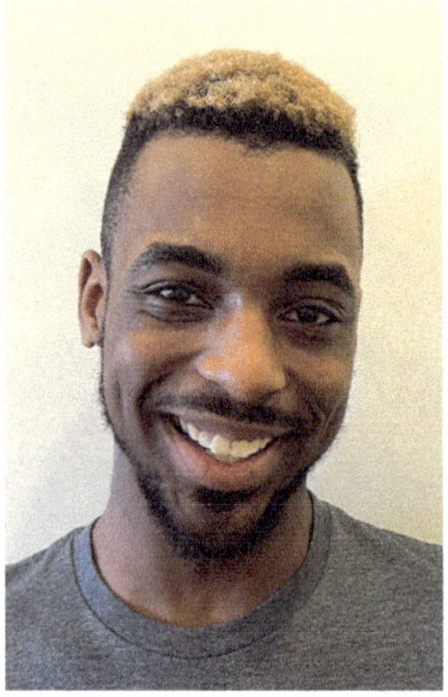

Charles Yeo

Philadelphia Main Line Bridges

Charlie Yeo is an internationally known pancreas surgeon and the eighth Samuel D. Gross Professor and chairman of the Department of Surgery at the Sidney Kimmel Medical College of Thomas Jefferson University. He is a sports fan, loves rock and roll music, and is an avid reader. He and his wife have a new puppy, Paxton—and many of their recent photos have been of him, of course.

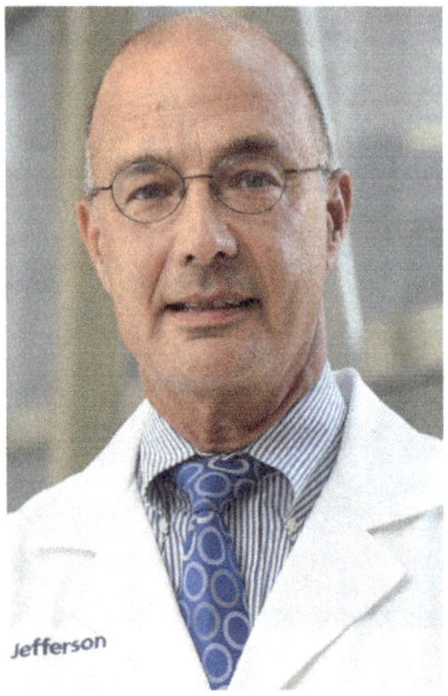

David Zvara

North Carolina Bridge

David is an avid iPhone photographer, capturing over 8664 images to include the grandkids' birthdays, grandkids' soccer, grandkids' first day of school, more grandkids with pets. In short, endless sources of creative inspiration! To date, the commercial translation of this work has fallen short of expectations, but opportunity abounds as the grandkids star in school plays nearly every weekend of the year.

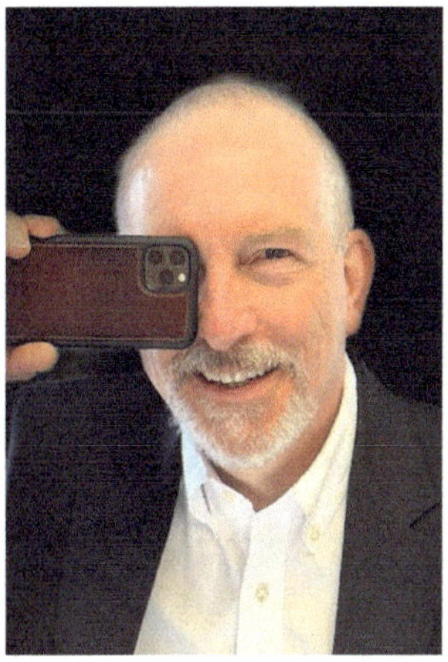

Jessica Zvara

Natural Log Bridge over Creek with Exuberant Dog

Jessica is a faculty anesthesiologist at the University of Virginia, where she specializes in cardiothoracic anesthesiology. Outside of the operating room, she loves romping around the woods with her two kids, her husband, and her dog Hobbes. A little late to the game, she is beginning to dabble in the art of baking and is currently loving homemade English muffins.

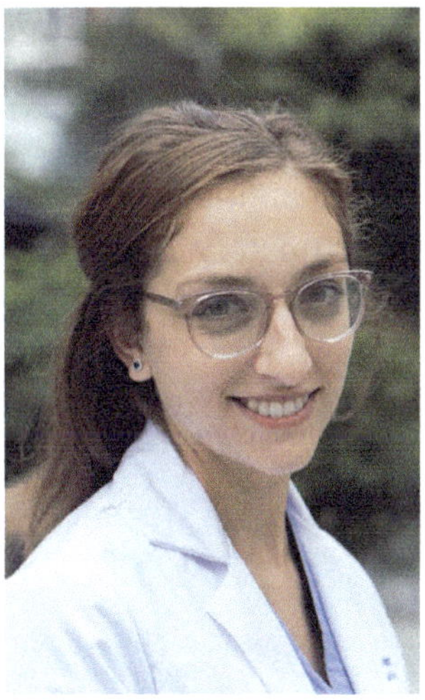

The editors also thank (in alphabetical order) the Abouleish family, the Altose family, the Auers-Jensen families, the Bank family, Barking Mad Animal Refuge, Inc, Amberly Hall Brown, Austin Brown, Hon. Christopher C. Conner, the Dalal-Taylor family, the DeCaria-Lupa family, Steven M. Frank MD, the Gottschalk family, the Graber family, the Harrison-Jordan-Marcucci family, Vincent L. Hoellerich MD, the Leffert family, the Lessinger-Wiener family, the Lien-Brinzac family, Sharon L. Milgram PhD, the Peterson family, the Prischak family, the family of Gary and Marilyn Robbins, the Robbins-McGahey family, Matthew Rorie, the Sandson family, F. Jacob Seagull PhD, the Togioka family, the Tung family, and the Zvara family for sending us photos and images from their personal files and collections.

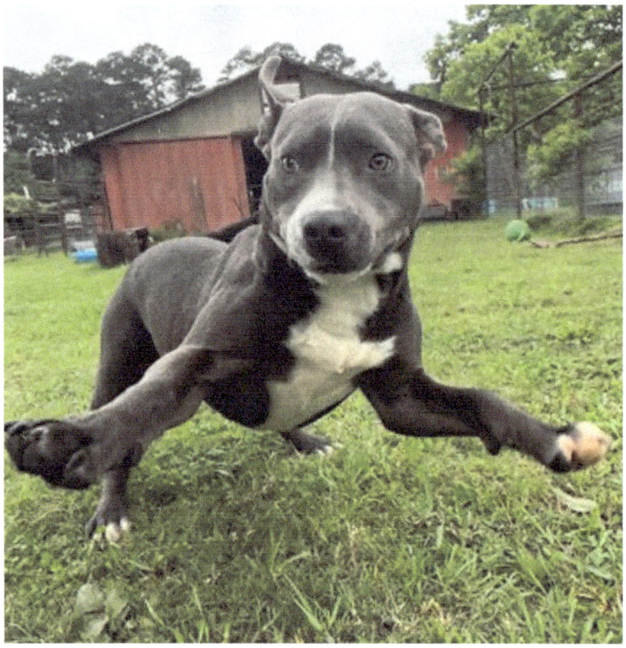

This is Lennon at **Barking Mad Animal Refuge** in Hemphill, Texas. He's such a handsome dog and a bit of a celebrity, having won several contests for best dog photo. Plus, he can fly! If you have room in your hearts and lives, please consider the millions of abandoned animals in rescues and sanctuaries who desperately need help. Fortunately for Lennon, a wonderful family saw this photo and offered him a loving home. **Photo: Hailey James**

BMAR *is online at barkingmadanimalrescue.com*

The Newport Town Bridge—Newport, Wales

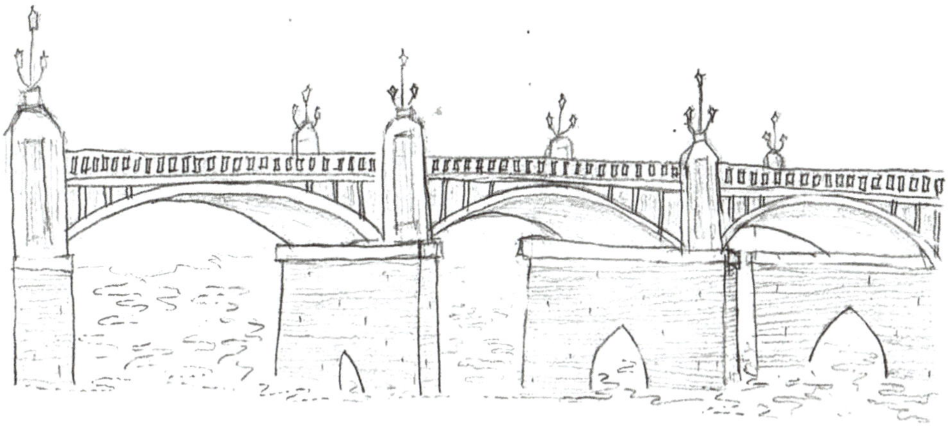

This charming little bridge in Wales is known to the locals as Town Bridge. It was selected as a favorite bridge by consensus of the editors. It opened in 1927 and spans the River Usk, connecting the High Street with Newport Castle. The five-span bridge replaces earlier wood and stone bridges.

The famous escape artist Harry Houdini jumped off the stone version in 1913 with his hands manacled and his feet shackled. He was arrested the next week for holding a public entertainment on the bridge and obstructing traffic. Four of the pillars of the current bridge are decorated with a painted stone cherub and shield design that has found its way onto British merchandise and even album covers.

The *Anesthesia Bridges* editors thank **Nina Babbitt** from The Architectural Team in Boston, MA, for her lovely original drawing that captures the romantic quality of the 1920s architecture.

Statement of Disclaimer

The views expressed herein are solely the authors' and contributors' own personal and professional opinions and experiences and should be used only to foster thought, reflection, and (we hope) lively discussion and further inquiry.

They do not represent superseding clinical mandates and should not be construed as the official statements, instructions, guidelines, recommendations, or positions of any employer, educational and/or academic institution, business, or professional clinical group including but not limited to the American Board of Anesthesiology, the American Society of Anesthesiologists, the Society for Pediatric Anesthesia, the American Society of Regional Anesthesia and Pain Medicine, the Society for Pediatric Anesthesia, the Anesthesia Quality Institute, the Closed Claims Program, the Anesthesia Patient Safety Foundation, and the Foundation for Anesthesia Education and Research.

The authors' opinions and advice also do not represent any official administrative, clinical, or academic position of any other company, institution, group, or practice, whether mentioned by name or not.

No aspect of this book represents the official positions of the National Institutes of Health, the US Food and Drug Administration, the Department of Health and Human Services, the Department of Veterans Affairs, the Department of Defense, or any other civilian or military entity or agency of the United States government.

Finally, the content and the proffered opinions in this book should not substitute for the appropriate legal, financial, or medical advice.

There is no disclaimer needed concerning the kindness, interest, and enthusiasm that the staff of Towson Hot Bagels in Timonium, Maryland, had for this project as they saw senior editor Cathy Marcucci every weekend for breakfast for **at least** three years (Fig. 1). As soon as she trudged up to the counter with her laptop the counter staff would automatically start her usual order—plain bagel toasted with a fried egg and sausage, no cheese. The staff even followed along closely enough to ask how specific chapters were coming along! Many thanks to the breakfast crew with the bagels!

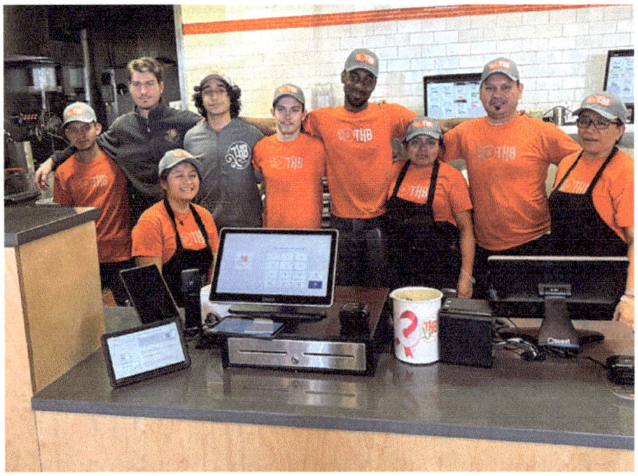

Fig. 1 The Saturday morning crew at Towson Hot Bagels in Timonium, MD

We once gave the THB crew a page of quotations planned for the book and asked them which were their favorites. They selected the important life wisdom below.

From Conni Walkup Hull: If you bleed in the water, sharks will come. It's the way of things. But it's a waste of time to blame the sharks - it's what they are. It's up to us not to look like a tasty snack.

From Neil Sandson and Coach Ed Serues: Never change a winning game, always change a losing game.

Acknowledgments

The practice of anesthesiology is more than a science, it is also an art. Several years ago, we realized that there was a generation of supremely wise and superbly competent anesthesiologists who were at or near retirement age. As these wonderful clinicians and mentors moved on to the next phases of their lives, we saw that an entire encyclopedia of knowledge, experience, wit, and wisdom would go with them. The science would still be found in the pages of the journals and the textbooks, but the art would be lost.

Our lead editor Sharif Mohamed had the great idea to develop a book project to build a wisdom bridge from that generation of practitioners to the junior people coming up behind us. But this bridge would not be made of concrete and steel, rather it would be constructed piece by piece with thoughts, advice, stories, and perhaps a gentle admonishment and warning or two. And so, the *Anesthesia Bridges: Wisdom for Your Personal and Professional Journey* project was created. Additional editors and a huge number of contributors were recruited and what followed were several years of emails, texts, and interviews as hundreds of the best physicians and clinicians (and nicest people!) in our specialty took the time the help us. As we began talking to and corresponding with the most senior and retiring anesthesiologists, we also spoke with many anesthesiologists who are still at the full pinnacle and prime of their careers and began to gather up and collate their wisdom and knowledge to pass on as well.

And so, this book became a heartfelt gift from the community of senior anesthesiologists to our junior physician colleagues.

The manuscript is organized into the topics that pertain to the life and careers of an anesthesiologist. Each section has essays ranging from short, pithy pieces of advice to longer contemplative pieces in a conversational style, as if you were chatting with the experts themselves. Each section ends with a collection of additional words of wisdom and short sayings. This book is not intended to be a clinical anesthesia handbook but of course some clinical topics found their way into the manuscript. They do not comprise comprehensive clinical coverage of any one topic but perhaps a clinical pearl or two will resonate and stay with the reader.

In every book project, there are always those individuals who go above and beyond. Co-editor Ray Graber has done a heroic amount of work on this book, especially in the middle third of the project, when he really kept the snowball rolling down (up?) the hill and the juggling pins in the air. Left to his own devices, he would eschew special mention, nonetheless the editorial group feels strongly that his absolutely critical contributions must be mentioned—there would be no book without him. We also thank senior editor Cathy Marcucci for devoting her time and focused effort to the project over many months and lending us her advice, expertise, and the benefit of her network. We appreciate having her wisdom in developing what we hope is a fun, easy-to-read book that is still packed with valuable content.

We would also like to give special mention to our colleagues who took on extra subjects and topics on short notice. These friends were hugely helpful in consulting on editorial decisions and even developing entire sections of the book by writing, editing, reviewing, and finding authors for us. Each of them fully deserves their positions as consulting and contributing associate editors. And so, we thank (in alphabetical order) Michael S. Axley MD, Ronald S. Bank MD, Andrew Barker MD, Carol F. Bodenheimer MD, John C. Briggs MD, Kirk Lalwani MD, Albert Liao LAc, Kristin King Liao LAc, Daniel J. McCoy MD '26, Rajen V. Nathwani MBBS BSc, Steven L. Orebaugh MD, Amy J. Robbins MD MBA, Neil B. Sandson MD, F. Jacob Seagull PhD, Jennifer N. Tripi MD, Brandon M. Togioka MD, Brant Wagener MD PhD, and David Zvara MD.

Neil Sandson, Carol Bodenheimer, and Jake Seagull are three of the best friends the anesthesiology community ever had. They all reviewed numerous chapters and provided expert addenda and comments. We couldn't imagine doing a book without them. The same is true of Kirk Lalwani, who has to be one of the best people in the entire country to do a large writing project with. David Zvara lent us his wisdom and advice at crucial points in the manuscript development and sent us his brilliant essay for beginning physicians.

Amy Robbins is a superb clinician who has boarded in anesthesiology and two anesthesiology subspecialties and who always replied within two minutes with suggestions, advice, and content. Brandon Togioka also was always immediately available and always correct and helped us immeasurably with his special expertise in obstetrical anesthesia. Steve Orebaugh was unfailingly generous with his expertise in two of major areas of the practice of anesthesiology—airway management and regional anesthesia. The University of Alabama at Birmingham associate editors—Andrew Barker, Brant Wagener, and John Briggs, were a rock-solid resource and sent us important content, great ideas and suggestions, and encouragement. Similarly, Al and Kristin Liao provided important editorial support on our acupuncture content.

Raj Nathwani popped onto our radar early in the project and provided us with such valuable content and advice that he was invited to join the editorial group on the spot. Mike Axley, who was a writer and journalist before going into medicine, was our go-to person for all questions and problems of that nature. A special acknowledgment and thanks goes out to Ron Bank, who wasn't involved in the earliest stages of the project but who instantly understood what we were trying to do and sent us pages and pages of ideas, suggestions, edits, clinical pearls, and words of wisdom, all while meeting the demands of a busy clinical practice. Finally, Jen Tripi had the firepower to undertake full editorial duties by recruiting contributors and developing content even while being a busy anesthesiology trainee.

Throughout this project, we were fortunate to draw on the knowledge and expertise of a number of guest authors, who are not part of the anesthesia community. We thank them for taking time from their studies and professional communities to contribute to ours. First, we thank Harvey Alter MD, who is the 2020 Nobel Laureate in Medicine or Physiology for the discovery of the Hepatitis C virus. There are many demands for Dr. Alter's attention, nonetheless he took the time to help develop a chapter on blood donation (and insisted that he appear only as a middle author) and write us a short essay on his life's priorities. We also thank James K. Gilman MD (Maj. Gen. ret.) who was the Director of the Clinical Center of the National Institutes of Health for sending us both clinical and life wisdom advice.

Other guest authors and contributors who assisted with content and from whom we learned much are (in alphabetical order):

Brian Adolph, Robert Adolph, Abdullah Alswied MD, Miya R. Asato MD, CJ Barilleaux-Badger, A.M. Coleman (Cole) Bank, Amberly Hall Brown, Austin Brown, Marina Bueno MLS (ASCP) SBB, Melissa Butynski MEM, Karen M. Byrne MDE MT (ASCP) SBB, Kathleen (Cathy) Conroy-Cantilena MD, Marlee Chamberlain MD '26, Richard W. Childs MD, Herbert Chen MD, Leonard N. Chen MD PhD, Xiaopo Cheng MS PhD, Anthony A. Chico III DO, Robert Christian MD, Ariana S. Cogan MT (ASCP)^{CM}, Benjamin C. Conner MD PhD, Hon. Christopher C. Conner, Emma R. Cooley BA, Abigail J. Crawford MD '28, Edward J. Damrose MD FACS, David Daniel MD, Willy A. Flegel MD, Deborah Gerson MS CCC-SLP, Chelsea L. Gottschalk MD, Laura M. Gottschalk MSW MPH, Michael D. Graham PhD, John Matthew Hess BS ME, Theodore C. Houk MD, Conni Walkup Hull JD, Jane B. Jacobs Esq, Randy G. Jensen BAnimSc, Ruth A. Jensen PE, Deb Waterman Johns BS, Shelley Sahu Kalsi MD, Oliver Karam MD PhD, Caroline C. Koloski BA, LouAnn Kopenhaver BS MEd, Stephen D. Lasday DPM FACFAS, Patricia Lee DO JD, Olivia Liao BA '28, Yafet T. Mamo MD, Daniel J. Marcucci PhD MLA AICP, Daniel J. McCoy MD '26, Carolyn B. Metzler PhD, Sharon L. Milgram PhD, Robert E. Minahan MD, Scott D. Mist PhD LAc, Logan Olson PharmD BCCCP,

Alejandra Pelayo, Marc P. Pelletier MD, Linda M. Peterson MD FAPM, Kailey L. Peterson, Kelsey Peterson Ostergren MPH CIC, Herleen Rai MD, Emily Rhinehart BS, Captain W. Mitchell Robbins BSAE MS, Matthew Rorie BS AgEcon, Charles H. Sandson BS IME, Joseph M. Schwartz MD, Richard Sheffield BS MA, Linda Song MD MPH, Valentina Baez Sosa MD, Joshua L. Stich MD '28, Grant Taylor MD, Nicholas B. Taylor MD, Zachary R. Taylor BS, Megan E. Terek MD, Patricia Togioka MA, Robert Togioka MA, Tsung-Lin Tsai MD PhD, Joanna L. Walker MD, John R. Walker IV, Marilyn X. Walker BS, Jenny Wang MD MBA, Kamille West-Mitchell MD, Hon. Jennifer P. Wilson, and Charles J. Yeo MD FACS.

We must also give a big shout-out to the artists and photographers who donated their original work to our project. There is a separate acknowledgment for each of these talented people in the pages that follow. Special thanks go to Michael E. Liu AIA NCARB, for arranging to have the talented young architectural designers at The Architectural Team do such beautiful drawings for us.

We also send our deep thanks to Jesse Ehrenfeld MD MPH for writing our Foreword.

Finally, we are extremely grateful for the superb skills and superb patience of everybody at Springer especially Sinchu Mohan, Nithiya Vadivazhagan, and Greg Sutorius. Thanks for hanging in there with us – the whole team was great to work with at all times!

As we developed the manuscript, each of the editors chose to acknowledge the special person or persons who built the bridges that we ourselves crossed in our personal and professional development. Sharif, of course, gets the lead-off acknowledgment. He is honoring his father, Dr. Samy Mohamed Rezk, a prominent OB-GYN in Saudi Arabia and Egypt (Fig. 2). Sharif credits his dad with being his first mentor and teacher and the most important life role model he has ever had.

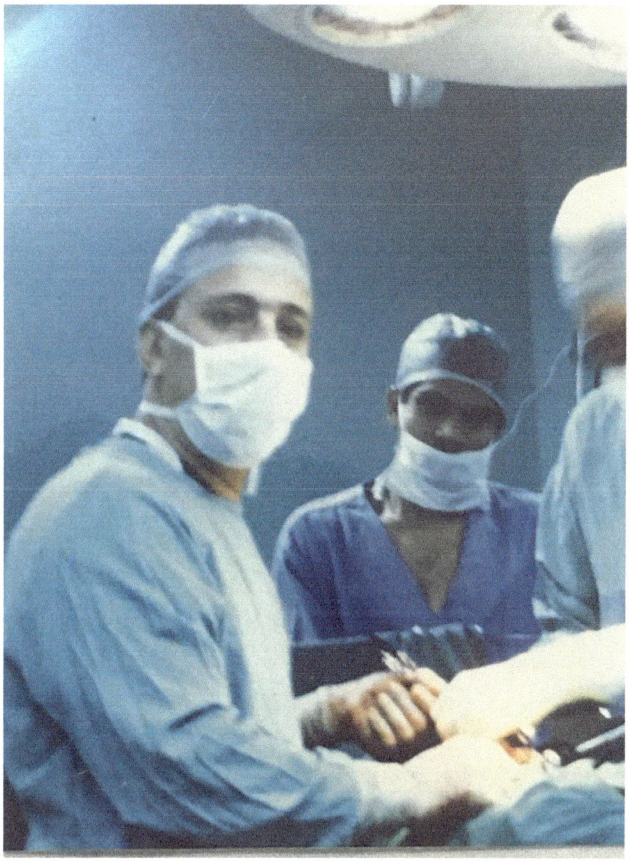

Fig. 2 Dr. Samy Mohamed Rezk operating on a large fibroid tumor in 1986 at Al Noor Specialist Hospital in Saudi Arabia. Dr. Rezk now lives in Dokki, Giza, Egypt, with his spouse (and Sharif's mom) Safy Ezzat. As we went to press, he was still in clinical practice! When not busy running his fertility clinic, he enjoys spending time with his 4 children, 12 grandchildren, fishing in the Nile, and leading the congregation at his local mosque

Finally, we thank our contributors and editors for their outstanding generosity to the Foundation for Anesthesia Education and Research—every person who contributed to this book instantly agreed that all royalties from this project be pledged in perpetuity to FAER. We are humbled and honored to be associated with and learn from this generous and caring group of professionals and providers.

Galveston, TX, USA Sharif Mohamed, MD
Cleveland, OH, USA Raymond G. Graber, MD
Galveston, TX, USA Amr E. Abouleish, MD
Cleveland, OH, USA Edwin G. Avery, MD
Seattle, WA, USA Jeffrey R. Kirsch, MD
Bethesda, MD, USA Catherine Marcucci, MD

Contents of Voume II

Part VII Clinical Wisdom

Contents of Voume I

Contributors

James H. Abernathy, MD MPH Department of Anesthesiology and Critical Care Medicine, Johns Hopkins School of Medicine, Baltimore, MD, USA

Amr E. Abouleish, MD MBA Department of Anesthesiology, John Sealy School of Medicine, The University of Texas Medical Branch, Galveston, TX, USA

Brian Adolph Adolph Citgo, Timonium, MD, USA

Robert Adolph Adolph Citgo, Timonium, MD, USA

Konstantinos Alfaras-Melainas, MD MSc Department of Anesthesiology and Perioperative Medicine, University of Pittsburgh School of Medicine, Pittsburgh, PA, USA

Abdullah Alswied, MD Center for Cellular Engineering, Department of Transfusion Medicine, Clinical Center, National Institutes of Health, Bethesda, MD, USA

Harvey J. Alter, MD Department of Transfusion Medicine, Clinical Center, National Institutes of Health, Bethesda, MD, USA

Michael D. Altose, MD PhD Department of Anesthesiology and Perioperative Medicine, University Hospitals Cleveland Medical Center, Case Western Reserve University School of Medicine, Cleveland, OH, USA

Gregory K. Applegate, DO Department of Anesthesiology and Perioperative Medicine, University Hospitals Cleveland Medical Center, Case Western Reserve University School of Medicine, Cleveland, OH, USA

Miya R. Asato, MD Departments of Neurology and Pediatrics, Johns Hopkins School of Medicine, Baltimore, MD, USA

Daniel I. Asher, MD Department of Anesthesiology and Perioperative Medicine, University Hospitals Cleveland Medical Center, Case Western Reserve University School of Medicine, Cleveland, OH, USA

Edwin G. Avery IV, MD Department of Anesthesiology and Perioperative Medicine, University Hospitals Cleveland Medical Center, Case Western Reserve University School of Medicine, Cleveland, OH, USA

Michael S. Axley, MD Oregon Anesthesiology Group, Portland, OR, USA

A. M. Coleman Bank, BS Medical Assistant, Pre-Medical Candidate, Fairfax, VA, USA

Ronald S. Bank, MD FASA Department of Anesthesiology, INOVA Fairfax Hospital, Falls Church, VA, USA
UVA School of Medicine INOVA Campus, Falls Church, VA, USA

David W. Barbar, MD BayCare Clinic, Green Bay, WI, USA

C. J. Barilleaux-Badger Barking Mad Animal Refuge, Hemphill, TX, USA

Andrew B. Barker, MD Department of Anesthesiology and Perioperative Medicine, Heersink School of Medicine, University of Alabama at Birmingham, Birmingham, AL, USA

Rodger E. Barnette, MD FCCM (Retired) AIC Kijabe Hospital, Kijabe, Kenya
Department of Anesthesiology, Lewis Katz School of Medicine, Temple University, Philadelphia, PA, USA

Brian P. Barrick, MD DDS Department of Anesthesiology, University of North Carolina at Chapel Hill School of Medicine, Chapel Hill, NC, USA

Mark J. Baskerville, MD JD MBA MA Department of Anesthesiology and Perioperative Medicine, School of Medicine, Oregon Health & Science University, Portland, OR, USA

James Berry, MD Department of Anesthesiology and Pain Management, UT Southwestern Medical Center, Dallas, TX, USA

Meena Bhatia, MD Department of Anesthesiology, University of North Carolina at Chapel Hill School of Medicine, Chapel Hill, NC, USA

Ali Bilal, MD Department of Internal Medicine, University of Texas Medical Branch, Galveston, TX, USA
John Sealy School of Medicine, University of Texas Medical Branch, Galveston, TX, USA

Nicholas V. Bishop, MD US Anesthesia Partners, Seattle, WA, USA
Department of Anesthesiology and Perioperative Medicine, School of Medicine, Health & Science University, Portland, OR, USA

Carol F. Bodenheimer, MD H. Ben Taub Department of Physical Medicine and Rehabilitation, Baylor College of Medicine, Houston, TX, USA
Spinal Cord Injury Care Line, Michael E. DeBakey VA Medical Center, Houston, TX, USA

Mark V. Boswell, MD PhD MBA Department of Anesthesiology, University of Toledo College of Medicine, Toledo, OH, USA

Denis L. Bourke, MD (Retired) Baltimore VA Medical Center, Baltimore, MD, USA
(Retired) Department of Anesthesiology, University of Maryland, Baltimore, MD, USA

John C. Briggs, MD MHSA Department of Anesthesiology and Perioperative Medicine, Heersink School of Medicine, University of Alabama at Birmingham, Birmingham, AL, USA

Amberly Hall Brown Austin Brown Music, Nashville, TN, USA

Austin Brown Austin Brown Music, Nashville, TN, USA

Marina Bueno, MLS (ASCP) SBB Department of Transfusion Medicine, Clinical Center, National Institutes of Health, Bethesda, MD, USA

Melissa Butynski, MEM PhD'28 Department of Biology, University of British Columbia, Kelowna, BC, Canada

Karen M. Byrne, MDE MT(ASCP)SBB (retired) Department of Transfusion Medicine, Clinical Center, National Institutes of Health, Bethesda, MD, USA

Michelle J. Capdeville, MD Department of Cardiothoracic Anesthesiology, Anesthesiology Institute, Cleveland Clinic, Cleveland Clinic Lerner College of Medicine, Case Western Reserve University, Cleveland, OH, USA

Christine Garcia Cattaneo, MD MBA Anne Arundel Medical Center, Annapolis, MD, USA
TeamHealth, Inc., Knoxville, TN, USA

Marlee Chamberlain, MD '26 School of Medicine, Oregon Health & Science University, Portland, OR, USA

Herbert Chen, MD Department of Surgery, O'Neal Comprehensive Cancer Center at UAB, Birmingham, AL, USA
Heersink School of Medicine, University of Alabama at Birmingham, Birmingham, AL, USA

Leonard N. Chen, MD PhD Department of Transfusion Medicine, Clinical Center, National Institutes of Health, Bethesda, MD, USA

Xiaopo Cheng, MS PhD Department of Chemical & Biologic Engineering, University of Wisconsin, Madison, WI, USA
Artificial Intelligence Technology, NVIDIA, Santa Clara, CA, USA

Anthony A. Chico III, DO FAPA Veterans Affairs Maryland Health Care System, Private Practice, Baltimore, VA, USA

Richard W. Childs, MD Commissioned Corps of the U.S. Public Health Service, Bethesda, MD, USA
Laboratory of Transplantation Immunotherapy, National Heart Lung and Blood Institute, National Institutes of Health, Bethesda, MD, USA

Katya H. Chiong, MD Department of Anesthesiology and Perioperative Medicine, University Hospitals Cleveland Medical Center, Case Western Reserve University School of Medicine, Cleveland, OH, USA

Robert J. Christian, MD Transfusion Medicine, Department of Pathology and Laboratory Medicine, School of Medicine, Oregon Health & Science University, Portland, OR, USA
Blood Baking/Transfusion Medicine, University of Washington/Bloodworks NW/ Seattle Children's Hospital, Seattle, WA, USA

Rose Christopherson, MD PhD Department of Anesthesiology, Portland VA Medical Center, Portland, OR, USA

Ariana S. Cogan, MT (ASCP)CM Department of Transfusion Medicine, Clinical Center, National Institutes of Health, Bethesda, MD, USA

Neal Cohen, MD MPH MS Anesthesia and Perioperative Medicine and Medicine, University of California, San Francisco School of Medicine, San Francisco, CA, USA

Norman A. Cohen, MD (Retired) Department of Anesthesiology and Perioperative Medicine, School of Medicine, Oregon Health & Science University, Portland, OR, USA
Committee on Late Career and Retired Members, American Society of Anesthesiologists, Portland, OR, USA

Daniel J. Cole, MD David Geffen School of Medicine at UCLA, Los Angeles, CA, USA
American Society of Anesthesiologists, Los Angeles, CA, USA

Christopher M. Conley, MD Boston University School of Medicine, Department of Anesthesiology, Boston Medical Center, Boston, MA, USA

Benjamin C. Conner, MD PhD Department of Physical Medicine and Rehabilitation, Spaulding Rehabilitation Hospital, Harvard Medical School, Boston, MA, USA

Hon. Christopher C. Conner Middle District of Pennsylvania, Harrisburg, PA, USA

Lois A. Connolly, MD Department of Anesthesiology, Medical College of Wisconsin/Froedtert Hospital, Milwaukee, WI, USA

Kathleen (Cathy) Conroy-Cantilena, MD Department of Transfusion Medicine, Clinical Center, National Institutes of Health, Bethesda, MD, USA
MedStar Washington Hospital Center, Washington, DC, USA
MTF Biologics, Edison, NJ, USA

Emma R. Cooley, BA Brand Experience Design Group, Charlotte, NC, USA

Catherine Cooper, MD Stony Point Endoscopy Center, Department of Anesthesiology, Virginia Commonwealth University School of Medicine, Richmond, VA, USA

Dane Coyne, MD Department of Anesthesiology and Perioperative Medicine, University Hospitals Cleveland Medical Center, Case Western Reserve University School of Medicine, Cleveland, OH, USA

Abigail J. Crawford, MD '28 School of Medicine, University of Washington, Seattle, WA, USA

Saundra E. Curry, MD Department of Anesthesiology, Columbia University Roy and Diana Vagelos College of Physicians and Surgeons, New York, NY, USA

Niloofer F. Dalal, MD Emory Clinic, School of Medicine Faculty, Emory Health Care, Atlanta, GA, USA

Edward J. Damrose, MD FACS Department of Otolaryngology - Head and Neck Surgery, Department of Anesthesiology, Perioperative and Pain Medicine, Stanford University School of Medicine, Stanford, CA, USA

David Daniel, MD Division of Transfusion Medicine, Department of Pathology, Johns Hopkins School of Medicine, Baltimore, MD, USA
Department of Transfusion Medicine, Clinical Center, National Institutes of Health, Bethesda, MD, USA

Beth Darnall, PhD Department of Anesthesiology, Perioperative and Pain Medicine, Stanford University School of Medicine School of Medicine, Stanford, CA, USA

Dawn Dillman, MD Department of Anesthesia, Carver College of Medicine, University of Iowa, Iowa City, IA, USA

David R. Dininny, MD Department of Anesthesiology and Perioperative Medicine, University Hospitals Cleveland Medical Center, Case Western Reserve University School of Medicine, Cleveland, OH, USA

Anis Dizdarevic, MD Department of Anesthesiology, Columbia University Roy and Diana Vagelos College of Physicians and Surgeons, New York, NY, USA

Sarah E. Dodd, MD Department of Anesthesiology and Perioperative Medicine, Mayo Clinic, Rochester, MN, USA

Karen B. Domino, MD MPH Department of Anesthesiology & Pain Medicine, University of Washington School of Medicine, Seattle, WA, USA

Susan D. Dumas, MD Obstetric Anesthesia Division, Department of Anesthesiology, Vanderbilt University Medical Center, Vanderbilt University, Nashville, TN, USA

Zeyd Ebrahim, MD Anesthesiology Institute, Cleveland Clinic, Cleveland Clinic Lerner College of Medicine, Case Western Reserve University, Cleveland, OH, USA

Charles W. Emala, Sr. MS MD Department of Anesthesiology, Columbia University Roy and Diana Vagelos College of Physicians and Surgeons, New York, NY, USA

Brenda G. Fahy, MD FCCP MCCM University of Florida College of Medicine, Gainesville, FL, USA

Joel M. Feinstein, MD University Hospitals, Heersink School of Medicine, University of Alabama at Birmingham, Birmingham, AL, USA

Brian C. Fitzsimons, MD Department of Anesthesiology and Perioperative Medicine, University Hospitals Cleveland Medical Center, Case Western Reserve University School of Medicine, Cleveland, OH, USA

Willy A. Flegel, MD Department of Transfusion Medicine Clinical Center, National Institutes of Health, Bethesda, MD, USA
Georgetown University Medical Center, Washington, DC, USA
Huazhong University of Science and Technology, Wuhan, Hubei, China

Lee A. Fleisher, MD Leonard Davis Institute for Health Economics, Department of Anesthesiology and Critical Care, Philadelphia, PA, USA
Department of Medicine, Perelman School of Medicine of the University of Pennsylvania, Philadelphia, PA, USA
Center for Clinical Standards and Quality, Center for Medicare and Medicaid Services, Baltimore, MD, USA

Patrick J. Forte, MD Department of Anesthesiology & Perioperative Medicine, University of Pittsburgh, Pittsburgh, PA, USA

Steven M. Frank, MD Johns Health System Blood Management Program, Center for Bloodless Medicine and Surgery, Department of Anesthesiology and Critical Care Medicine, Johns Hopkins School of Medicine, Baltimore, MD, USA

Sarah N. Fribance, MD Department of Anesthesiology and Perioperative Medicine, University of Pittsburgh School of Medicine, Pittsburgh, PA, USA

Daniel M. Frohwein, MD Interventional Pain Management, Orlando Orthopedic Center, Orlando, FL, USA

William R. Furman, MD MMHC (Retired) Department of Anesthesiology, Vanderbilt University Medical Center, Nashville, TN, USA
Physician Hospital Surveyor, The Joint Commission, Boston, MA, USA

Harley S. Geller, MD Senior Anesthesiologist, Charlotte, NC, USA

Deborah Gerson, MS CCC-SLP (Retired) Speech and Language Pathologist, Timonium, MD, USA

Brian T. Gierl, MD Neuroanesthesiology and Neuroanesthesiology QI, UPMC Presbyterian, Department of Anesthesiology & Perioperative Medicine, University of Pittsburgh School of Medicine, Pittsburgh, PA, USA

James K. Gilman, MD Office of the Director, Clinical Center, National Institutes of Health (Retired), Adjunct Professor of Medicine, Uniformed Services University of the Health Sciences, Bethesda, MD, USA

Allan Gottschalk, MD PhD Department of Anesthesiology and Critical Care Medicine, Department of Neurosurgery, Johns Hopkins School of Medicine, Baltimore, MD, USA

Chelsea L. Gottschalk, MD Lexington Eye Associates, Lexington, MA, USA

Laura M. Gottschalk, MSW MPH Health Promotions, American Lung Association, Chicago, IL, USA

Lindsey N. Gouker, MD Anesthesia Services Chatham Hospital, Department of Anesthesiology, The University of North Carolina at Chapel Hill School of Medicine, Chapel Hill, NC, USA

Raymond G. Graber, MD Department of Anesthesiology and Perioperative Medicine, University Hospitals Cleveland Medical Center, Case Western Reserve University School of Medicine, Cleveland, OH, USA

Michael D. Graham, PhD Department of Chemical and Biological Engineering, University of Wisconsin-Madison, Madison, WI, USA

Jeffrey A. Grass, MD MMM (retired) Department of Anesthesiology and Perioperative Medicine, University Hospitals Cleveland Medical Center, Case Western Reserve University School of Medicine, Cleveland, OH, USA

Ronald L. Harter, MD Department of Anesthesiology, Wexner Medical Center at The Ohio State University, American Society of Anesthesiologists, Columbus, OH, USA

Maya Jalbout Hastie, MD EdD Department of Anesthesiology, Columbia University Roy and Diana Vagelos College of Physicians and Surgeons, New York, NY, USA

Judith Hellman, MD Department of Anesthesia and Perioperative Care, University of California, San Francisco School of Medicine, San Francisco, CA, USA

Mada F. Helou, MD Department of Anesthesiology and Perioperative Medicine, University Hospitals Cleveland Medical Centerz, Cleveland, OH, USA

John Matthew Hess, BS Tessco Technologies, Inc., Hunt Valley, MD, USA

Jeremy C. Hoban, MD Department of Anesthesiology and Perioperative Medicine, University Hospitals Cleveland Medical Center, Case Western Reserve University School of Medicine, Cleveland, OH, USA

Vincent L. Hoellerich, MD Central Carolina Hospital, Sanford, NC, USA
Duke Health Community Division of Anesthesia, Raleigh, NC, USA

Jeffrey T. Hopcian, MD Department of Anesthesiology and Perioperative Medicine, University Hospitals Cleveland Medical Center, Case Western Reserve University School of Medicine, Cleveland, OH, USA

Harriet W. Hopf, MD Department of Anesthesiology, University of Utah, Salt Lake City, UT, USA
Member of the Board of Directors, Women in Anesthesiology, Salt Lake City, UT, USA

Theodore C. Houk, MD (Retired) St. Joseph's Hospital, University of Maryland Medical System, Towson, MD, USA

Mark E. Hudson, MD MBA Department of Anesthesiology and Perioperative Medicine, University of Pittsburgh School of Medicine, Pittsburgh, PA, USA

Conni Walkup Hull, JD Law Office of Conni L. Walkup, Columbia City, IN, USA

Michael P. Hutchens, MD MA Surgical Intensive Care Unit, Portland Veterans Administration Medical Center, Portland, OR, USA

Jane B. Jacobs, Esq Tarter Krinsky and Drogin LLP, New York, NY, USA

Jeremy Jaffe, MD SEPA Pain & Spine, Horsham, PA, USA

Richard A. Jaffe, MD PhD Department of Anesthesiology, Perioperative and Pain Medicine, Stanford University School of Medicine, Stanford, CA, USA

Randy G. Jensen, BS RJ Acres, Inc., Blair, NE, USA

Ruth A. Jensen, BS RJ Acres, Inc., Blair, NE, USA

Vesna Jevtovic-Todorovic, MD PhD MBA Department of Anesthesiology, School of Medicine, University of Colorado Anschutz Medical Campus, Aurora, CO, USA

Shawn Y. Jia, MD Department of Anesthesiology, The University of North Carolina at Chapel Hill School of Medicine, Chapel Hill, NC, USA

Deb Waterman Johns, BS Scout, Get Dressed, FIFI, Washington, DC, USA

Daniel M. Joseph, MD Emory Clinic, School of Medicine Faculty, Emory Health Care, Atlanta, GA, USA

Vilma A. Joseph, MD MPH FASA Department of Anesthesiology, The University Hospital of Albert Einstein College of Medicine, Montefiore Medical Center, New York, NY, USA

Tymoteusz J. Kajstura, MD PhD Cardiac Anesthesia Division, Department of Anesthesiology and Critical Care Medicine, Johns Hopkins School of Medicine, Baltimore, MD, USA

Shelley Sahu Kalsi, MD Hematology Graduate Medical Education and Consult Service Section, Division of Intramural Research, National Heart, Lung, and Blood Institute, National Institutes of Health, Bethesda, MD, USA

Inas Kamel, MD PhD Department of Anaesthesia and Intensive Care, Cairo University, Cairo, Egypt

Sharon T. Kapulek, MD Department of Anesthesiology, University of North Carolina at Chapel Hill School of Medicine, Chapel Hill, NC, USA

Patricia A. Kapur, MD Anesthesiology and Perioperative Medicine, David Geffen School of Medicine at UCLA, Los Angeles, CA, USA
Anesthesiology and Critical Care, Perelman School of Medicine, University of Pennsylvania, Philadelphia, PA, USA

Oliver Karam, MD PhD Department of Pediatrics, Yale School of Medicine – Yale University, New Haven, CT, USA
Pediatric Critical Care, Yale New Haven Children's Hospital, New Haven, CT, USA

Evan D. Kharasch, MD PhD Department of Anesthesiology, Duke University School of Medicine, Durham, NC, USA

Jeffrey R. Kirsch, MD FASA Department of Anesthesiology and Pain Medicine, University of Washington School of Medicine, Seattle, WA, USA
(Emeritus) Anesthesiology and Perioperative Medicine, School of Medicine, Oregon Health & Science University, Portland, OR, USA

Rachel Kirsch, MD Department of Anesthesia and Perioperative Care, University of California-San Francisco School of Medicine, San Francisco, CA, USA

Ziyad O. Knio, MD Division of Critical Care Medicine, Department of Anesthesiology, Columbia University Roy and Diana Vagelos College of Physicians and Surgeons, New York, NY, USA
Department of Anesthesiology, University of Virginia School of Medicine, Charlottesville, VA, USA

Lynn Knox, MD Department of Anesthesiology, John Sealy School of Medicine, The University of Texas Medical Branch, Galveston, TX, USA

Caroline C. Koloski, BA Velocity Clinical Research, Raleigh, NC, USA

LouAnn DePalma Kopenhaver, BS MEd (Retired) Capital Area Intermediate Unit, South Western School District, Hanover, PA, USA

Alexander S. Kuo, MD Department of Anesthesiology, Harvard Medical School, Massachusetts General Hospital, Boston, MA, USA

Julia K. Labovski, MD Department of Perioperative Medicine, Clinical Center, National Institutes of Health, Bethesda, MD, USA

Kirk Lalwani, MD FRCA MCR FASA Department of Anesthesiology and Perioperative Medicine, School of Medicine, Oregon Health & Science University, Portland, OR, USA

Meghan B. Lane-Fall, MD MSHP FCCM Department of Anesthesiology and Critical Care, Vagelos College of Physicians and Surgeons, Columbia University, New York, NY, USA

Stephen D. Lasday, DPM FACFAS Sarasota Memorial Hospital, Sarasota, FL, USA
West Coast Podiatry Center, Sarasota, FL, USA

Kathryn K. Lauer, MD Department of Anesthesiology, Medical College of Wisconsin/Froedtert Hospital, Milwaukee, WI, USA

Patricia Lee, DO JD Department of Transfusion Medicine, Clinical Center, National Institutes of Health, Bethesda, MD, USA

Sarah K. Lee, MD Department of Anesthesiology, Lewis Katz School of Medicine, Temple University, Philadelphia, PA, USA

Lisa Leffert, MD Department of Anesthesiology, Yale School of Medicine – Yale University, New Haven, CT, USA

Marc Leib, MD JD Healthcare Consultant, Phoenix, AZ, USA

Mark J. Lema, MD PhD Department of Anesthesiology, Roswell Park Comprehensive Cancer Center, SUNY Distinguished Service Professor and Chair, Jacobs School of Medicine & Biomedical Sciences, American Society of Regional Anesthesia, American Society of Anesthesiologists, Buffalo, NY, USA

Michael C. Lewis, MD FASA Department of Anesthesiology, Pain Management, & Perioperative Medicine, Henry Ford Hospital, Henry Ford Health System, Detroit, MI, USA

Albert Liao, LAc Liao Acupuncture, Towson, MD, USA

Kristin King Liao, LAc Liao Acupuncture, Towson, MD, USA

Olivia Liao, '28 Carnegie Mellon University, Pittsburgh, PA, USA

Cynthia A. Lien, MD Department of Anesthesiology, Medical College of Wisconsin/Froedtert Hospital, Milwaukee, WI, USA

Michael Lin, MD John Sealy School of Medicine, The University of Texas Medical Branch, Galveston, TX, USA

M. Concetta Lupa, MD Departments of Anesthesiology and Pediatrics, Department of Anesthesiology, The University of North Carolina at Chapel Hill School of Medicine, Chapel Hill, NC, USA

Yafet T. Mamo, MD Department of Transfusion Medicine, Clinical Center, National Institutes of Health, Bethesda, MD, USA

Andrew Mannes, MD ME MBA Department of Perioperative Medicine, Clinical Center, National Institutes of Health, Bethesda, MD, USA

Asad Mansoor, MD Department of Anesthesiology, University of Michigan Medical School, Ann Arbor, MI, USA

Catherine Marcucci, MD Department of Transfusion Medicine, Clinical Center, National Institutes of Health, Bethesda, MD, USA

Daniel J. Marcucci, PhD MLA AICP Center for Leadership in Global Sustainability, Virginia Polytechnic Institute and State University, Blacksburg, VA, USA

David P. Martin, MD PhD Department of Anesthesiology and Perioperative Medicine, Mayo Clinic, Rochester, MN, USA

David C. Mayer, MD Department of Anesthesiology, Department of Obstetrics and Gynecology, University of North Carolina at Chapel Hill School of Medicine, North Carolina Society of Anesthesiologists, Chapel Hill, NC, USA

Daniel J. McCoy, MD'26 The University of Arizona College of Medicine – Phoenix, Phoenix, AZ, USA

K. A. Kelly McQueen, MD MPH FASA Department of Anesthesiology, University of Wisconsin School of Medicine and Public Health, Madison, WI, USA

Rita B. Merman, MD Department of Anesthesiology and Perioperative Medicine, University Hospitals Cleveland Medical Center, Case Western Reserve University School of Medicine, Cleveland, OH, USA

Jay Mesrobian, MD MBA FASA TeamHealth Anesthesia, Milwaukee, WI, USA

Berend Mets, MB ChB PhD FRCA FFA(SA) Department of Anesthesiology and Perioperative Medicine, Penn State College of Medicine, Penn State Milton S. Hershey Medical Center, Hershey, PA, USA

Carolyn B. Metzler, PhD Senior Mathematician and Analyst, Gaithersburg, MD, USA

Lucas Meuchel, MD PhD Department of Anesthesiology and Perioperative Medicine, School of Medicine, Oregon Health & Science University, Portland, OR, USA

Frederick G. Mihm, MD Division of Critical Care Medicine, Department of Anesthesiology, Perioperative and Pain Medicine (Critical Care), Stanford University School of Medicine, Stanford, CA, USA

Sharon L. Milgram, PhD National Institutes of Health, Bethesda, MD, USA

Robert E. Minahan, MD Real Time Neuromonitoring Associates, Glen Burnie, MD, USA

Scott D. Mist, PhD LAc Department of Anesthesiology and Perioperative Medicine, School of Medicine, College of Nursing, Oregon Health & Science University, Portland, OR, USA

Sharif Mohamed, MD Department of Anesthesiology, John Sealy School of Medicine, The University of Texas Medical Branch, Galveston, TX, USA

Hanan Mohamed Mostafa, MD Anesthesia, Surgical Intensive Care, Pain Medicine, Kasr AlAiny School of Medicine, Cairo University, Cairo, Egypt

Ahmed Mukhtar, MD PhD Department of Anaesthesia and Intensive Care, Cairo University, Cairo, Egypt

Bryant A. Murphy, MD, MBAFASA Department of Anesthesiology, The University of North Carolina at Chapel Hill School of Medicine, Chapel Hill, NC, USA

Rajen V. Nathwani, MBBS BSc Department of Anesthesiology and Pain Medicine, University of Washington School of Medicine, Harborview Medical Center, Seattle, WA, USA

Mark Nelson, MD MEd Department of Anesthesiology, Virginia Commonwealth University School of Medicine, Richmond, VA, USA

David J. Ninan, DO FAOCA CPE Kansas College of Osteopathic Medicine, Wichita, KS, USA
Department of Anesthesiology, Riverside University Health System, Western University of Health Sciences, Pomona, CA, USA

Matthew P. Norcia, MD Department of Anesthesiology and Perioperative Medicine, University Hospitals Cleveland Medical Center, Case Western Reserve University School of Medicine, Cleveland, OH, USA

Mark C. Norris, MD Boston University School of Medicine, Boston Medical Center, Boston, MA, USA

Logan M. Olson, PharmD BCCCP PGY2 Critical Care, Nebraska Medical Center, Nebraska Medicine, Omaha, NE, USA

Steven L. Orebaugh, MD Department of Anesthesiology & Perioperative Medicine, University of Pittsburgh School of Medicine, Pittsburgh, PA, USA

Maria K. Orlic, MD Department of Anesthesiology and Perioperative Medicine, School of Medicine and Dentistry, University of Rochester Medicine, Rochester, NY, USA

Kelsey Peterson Ostergren, MPH CIC Health Policy Initiatives, Michigan Health & Hospital Association, Okemos, MI, USA

Anthony N. Passannante, MD Department of Anesthesiology, UNC School of Medicine, University of North Carolina at Chapel Hill School of Medicine, Chapel Hill, NC, USA

Alejandra Pelayo, BS National Institutes of Health, Bethesda, MD, USA

Marc P. Pelletier, MD Division Chief of Cardiac Surgery, Yale School of Medicine, New Haven, CT, USA

Nicholas L. Pesa, MD Department of Anesthesiology and Perioperative Medicine, University Hospitals Cleveland Medical Center, Case Western Reserve University School of Medicine, Cleveland, OH, USA

Linda M. Peterson, MD FAPM McLaren Greater Lansing Hospital, Lansing, MI, USA

Kailey L. Peterson Kohler Company, Kohler, WI, USA

William P. Peterson, MD Cardiac, Thoracic, and Vascular Anesthesia, University of Michigan Health, Sparrow Health System, Lansing, MI, USA

Emily T. Poynton, MD Department of Anesthesiology and Perioperative Medicine, University Hospitals Cleveland Medical Center, Case Western Reserve University School of Medicine, Cleveland, OH, USA

Donald S. Prough, MD Department of Anesthesiology, John Sealy School of Medicine, The University of Texas Medical Branch, Galveston, TX, USA

Marcelo J. Quezado, MD MedStar Medical Group Anesthesiology, Medstar Union Memorial Hospital, Baltimore, MD, USA

Herleen Rai, MD Division of Transfusion Medicine, Department of Pathology, Clinical Pathology Residency, The Johns Hopkins School of Medicine, Baltimore, MD, USA

Michael A. Ramsay, MD FRCA Department of Anesthesiology and Pain Management, Baylor University Medical Center, Dallas, TX, USA

Mojica Remskar, MD PhD MACM Department of Anesthesiology, University of Minnesota Medical School, Minneapolis, MN, USA

Emily C. Rhinehart, BS Pre-Medical Candidate, Fallston, MD, USA

LeeAnn Rhodes, MD Pain Medicine Interventionalist (Anesthesiology), Maryland Brain, Spine and Pain, Annapolis, MD, USA

Amy J. Robbins, MD MBA Stanson Health, a Premier Inc. Company, Atrium Health, Carolinas Palliative Care and Hospice Group, Charlotte, NC, USA
Atrium Health, Carolinas Palliative Care and Hospice Group, Charlotte, NC, USA

Wendye Robbins, MD Incendia Therapeutics, Boston, MA, USA
Blade Therapeutics, Inc., South San Francisco, CA, USA

W. Mitchell Robbins, BS MS Pilot and Airline Captain, Ponte Verda, FL, USA

John S. Rogoski, DO Department of Anesthesiology, College of Medicine, Wexner Medical Center, The Ohio State University, Columbus, OH, USA

Matthew L. Rorie, BS RJ Acres, Inc., Blair, NE, USA

Richard W. Rosenquist, MD Department of Pain Management, Anesthesiology Institute, Cleveland Clinic, Cleveland Clinic Lerner College of Medicine, Case Western Reserve University, Cleveland, OH, USA

Frank Rosinia, MD MHCM Department of Anesthesiology, Joe R. & Teresa Lozano Long School of Medicine, UT Health San Antonio, San Antonio, TX, USA

Charles H. Sandson, BS ZS Associates, Washington, DC, USA

Lisa L. Sandson, BArch Cummings Properties, LLC, Woburn, MA, USA

Neil B. Sandson, MD Department of Psychiatry, University of Maryland School of Medicine, Baltimore, MD, USA
VA Maryland Health Care System, Baltimore, MD, USA

H. David Sanusi, MD Physician Specialists in Anesthesia, PC, Atlanta, GA, USA

Joseph M. Schwartz, MD Senior Psychiatrist, Baltimore, MD, USA

F. Jacob Seagull, PhD Center for Bioethics and Social Science in Medicine, Michigan Medicine (University of Michigan Medical School), Ann Arbor, MI, USA

Troy G. Seelhammer, MD Department of Anesthesiology and Perioperative Medicine, Mayo Clinic, Rochester, MN, USA

Daniel I. Sessler, MD Department of Anesthesiology, Center of Outcomes Research, UTHealth, Houston, TX, USA

Ahmed Shash, MD Department of Anaesthesia and Intensive Care, Cairo University, Cairo, Egypt

Richard G. Sheffield, BS IM MA (Retired) Blog – Spend Your Retirement Money!, UPS.com, Atlanta, GA, USA

Kenneth T. Shelton, MD Division of Critical Care, Department of Anesthesia, Critical Care and Pain Medicine, Heart Center, ICU, Harvard Medical School, Massachusetts General Hosptial, Boston, MD, USA

Cobin Soelberg, MD JD Master of Bioethics Bend Anesthesiology Group, Bend, OR, USA

Linda H. Song, MD MPH MD Anderson Cancer Center, Houston, TX, USA
Department of Transfusion Medicine, Clinical Center, National Institutes of Health, Bethesda, MD, USA

Ziyan Song, MD Division of Cardiothoracic Anesthesiology, Division of Perioperative Medicine, Department of Anesthesiology, Adult Cardiothoracic Anesthesia, Heersink School of Medicine, University of Alabama – Birmingham, Birmingham, AL, USA

Valentina Baez Sosa, MD National Heart Lung Blood Institute, Bethesda, MD, USA
Department of Transfusion Medicine, Clinical Center, National Institutes of Health, Bethesda, MD, USA

Juraj Sprung, MD PhD Department of Anesthesiology and Perioperative Medicine, Mayo Clinic, Rochester, MN, USA

Joshua L. Stich, MD '28 Albert Einstein College of Medicine, New York, NY, USA

M. Christine Stock, MD FCCM FCCP Department of Anesthesiology, Northwestern University Feinberg School of Medicine, Chicago, IL, USA

Louise Y. Sun, MD Cardiac Anesthesiology, University Medical Line, Anesthesiology, Perioperative, and Pain Medicine, Stanford University School of Medicine, Stanford, CA, USA
Institute for Clinical Evaluative Sciences, Toronto, ON, Canada

Christopher E. Swide, MD Department of Anesthesiology and Perioperative Medicine, School of Medicine, Health & Science University, Portland, OR, USA

Edwin Tavarez, MD Department of Anesthesiology, Montefiore Medical Center, The University Hospital of Albert Einstein College of Medicine, New York, NY, USA

Grant Taylor, MD Wellstar Douglas Surgical Associates, Douglasville, GA, USA

Nicholas B. Taylor, MD General Surgery Residency Program, Jefferson Abingdon Hospital, Abingdon, PA, USA

Zachary R. Taylor, BS Chemist, Philadelphia, PA, USA

Megan E. Terek, MD Cardiac Intensive Care Unit, INOVA Fairfax Hospital, Falls Church, VA, USA

Michael M. Todd, MD Department of Anesthesiology, University of Minnesota School of Medicine, Minneapolis, MN, USA

Brandon M. Togioka, MD Department of Anesthesiology and Perioperative Medicine, School of Medicine, Oregon Health & Science University, Portland, OR, USA

Patricia M. Togioka, MA (Retired) Oregon School for the Deaf, Certified Interpreter for the Deaf and Hard of Hearing, Salem, OR, USA

Robert D. Togioka, MA (Retired) Oregon School for the Deaf, Certified Interpreter for the Deaf and Hard of Hearing, Salem, OR, USA
American Sign Language, Salem-Keizer School District, Keizer, OR, USA

Jennifer N. Tripi, MD Obstetric Anesthesiology, The University of North Carolina at Chapel Hill School of Medicine, Chapel Hill, NC, USA

Paul A. Tripi, MD Department of Anesthesiology and Perioperative Medicine, Division of Pediatric Anesthesiology, Rainbow Babies & Children's Hospital, Case Western Reserve University School of Medicine, University Hospitals Cleveland Medical Center, Case Western Reserve University, Cleveland, OH, USA

Christopher A. Troianos, MD FASE FASA Anesthesiology Institute, Cleveland Clinic, Cleveland Clinic Lerner College of Medicine, Case Western Reserve University, Cleveland, OH, USA

Tsung-Lin Tsai, MD PhD Bloodworks NW, Seattle, WA, USA
Department of Transfusion Medicine, Clinical Center, National Institutes of Health, Bethesda, MD, USA

Elizabeth A. Ungerman, MD MS Anesthesiology Residency Program, Department of Anesthesiology & Perioperative Medicine, University of Pittsburgh School of Medicine, Pittsburgh, PA, USA

Kamila Vagnerova, MD Department of Anesthesiology and Perioperative Medicine, School of Medicine, Oregon Health & Science University, Portland, OR, USA

Brant M. Wagener, MD PhD Division of Critical Care Medicine, Division of Molecular and Translational Biomedicine, Birmingham, AL, USA
Department of Anesthesiology and Perioperative Medicine, Heersink School of Medicine, The University of at Birmingham, Birmingham, AL, USA

Joanna L. Walker, MD Clinical Dermatology, Rare and Advanced Skin Cancer Clinic, Perelman School of Medicine, University of Pennsylvania, Philadelphia, PA, USA

John R. Walker IV Drexel University, Philadelphia, PA, USA

Marilyn X. Walker, BS Sigurdsson Laboratory, NYU Langone, New York, NY, USA

David A. Wallace, MD Department of Anesthesiology and Perioperative Medicine, University Hospitals Cleveland Medical Center, Case Western Reserve University School of Medicine, Cleveland, OH, USA

Jenny Wang, MD MBA VA Maryland Health Care System, Baltimore, MD, USA

Jonathan H. Waters, MD Department of Anesthesiology & Perioperative Medicine, University of Pittsburgh School of Medicine, Pittsburgh, PA, USA
Blood Management Program, University of Pittsburgh Medical Center (UPMC), Pittsburgh, PA, USA

Anesthesia Services, Magee Women's Hospital of UPMC, Pittsburgh, PA, USA
Department of Bioengineering, Swanson School of Engineering, University of Pittsburgh, Pittsburgh, PA, USA

Toby N. Weingarten, MD Department of Anesthesiology and Perioperative Medicine, Mayo Clinic, Rochester, MN, USA

Ronald H. Wender, MD Department of Anesthesiology, Cedars-Sinai Medical Center, Los Angeles, CA, USA

Kamille A. West-Mitchell, MD Blood Services Section, Department of Transfusion Medicine, Clinical Center,National Institutes of Health, Bethesda, MD, USA

Charles Whitten, MD Department of Anesthesiology and Pain Management, University of Texas Southwestern Medical Center, Dallas, TX, USA

Jeanine Wiener-Kronish, MD Harvard Medical School, Massachusetts General Hospital, Boston, MA, USA

Hon. Jennifer P. Wilson Middle District of Pennsylvania, Harrisburg, PA, USA

Bradford D. Winters, MD PhD FCCM Adult Critical Care Medicine, Department of Anesthesiology and Critical Care Medicine, Johns Hopkins Hospital Surgical ICUs, Bayview Medical Center Surgical and Burn ICUs, Baltimore, MD, USA
The Armstrong Institute for Patient Safety and Quality, Baltimore, MD, USA
RESQ Committee for Johns Hopkins Hospital, Baltimore, MD, USA
Johns Hopkins School of Medicine, Baltimore, MD, USA

Susan Wong, BS Office of Scientific Resources, Office of Research Services, National Institutes of Health, Bethesda, MD, USA
Friends of Rabbits, Columbia, MD, USA

Lee C. Woodson, MD PhD Department of Anesthesiology, John Sealy School of Medicine, University of Texas Medical Branch, Galveston, TX, USA

Charles J. Yeo, MD FACS Department of Surgery, Sidney Kimmel Medical College, Enterprise Surgery, Jefferson Health, Philadelphia, PA, USA
Pancreas, Biliary, and Related Cancer Center, Thomas Jefferson University, Philadelphia, PA, USA

David A. Young, MD MEd MBA FASA Department of Anesthesiology, Baylor College of Medicine, Texas Children's Hospital, Houston, TX, USA

Jordan S. Zunder, BSC MSC BMBS FRCPC University of Ottawa, Ottawa, ON, Canada
Department of Anesthesiology and Pain Medicine, The Ottawa Hospital, Ottawa, ON, Canada

Department of Anesthesiology and Pain Medicine, University of Washington School of Medicine, Harborview Medical Center, Seattle, WA, USA

David A. Zvara, MD FASA FAHA (Emeritus) Department of Anesthesiology, The University of North Carolina at Chapel Hill School of Medicine, Chapel Hill, NC, USA

Jessica Zvara, MD Vascular Anesthesia Division, Department of Anesthesiology, University of Virginia School of Medicine, Charlottesville, VA, USA

Part VII

Clinical Wisdom

The Iconic Pennsylvania Stone Arch Bridge

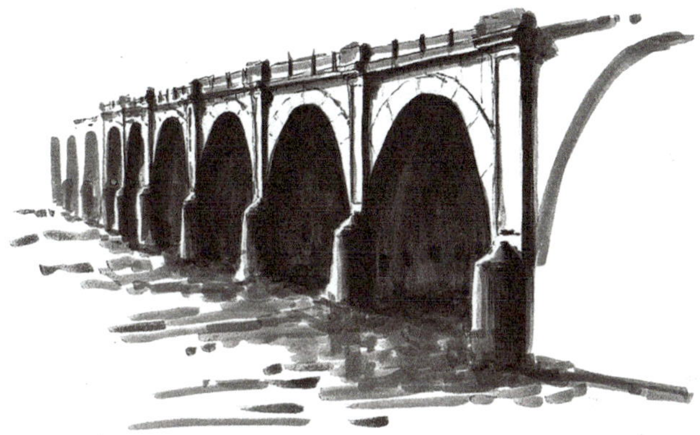

A huge number of the *Anesthesia Bridges* editors, authors, and contributors are from or have lived in Pennsylvania, so it is natural for us to want to introduce one of the most iconic Pennsylvania bridge forms to our readers. The earliest stone bridges date back to the Colonial era. They are all over the state—Johnstown has one, Lewistown has one, and Derry Township in Mifflin County has one. The highest concentration of stone arch bridges is in the southeastern part of the state. There were once 500 stone bridges in Pennsylvania; sadly, there are just over 300 remaining. They are being demolished due to the high cost of upkeep and also due to safety, as they are often only one lane wide.

The *Anesthesia Bridges* team thanks **Niamh Curry** of The Architectural Team, Boston, MA, for her magical drawing showing the muscular but beautiful quality of the Pennsylvania stone arch bridges.

119 Introduction

Raymond G. Graber

We all have stories to tell. On any given day, all kinds of interesting things happen during our daily work. These events get shared with colleagues in the hallways and in the break rooms. We learn from the things that happen to us and from the stories of others. Some stories get a life of their own and become local lore. Some events will permanently change how we as individuals practice medicine. Other incidents led to case reports and the development of national guidelines. Sometimes, experiences can be career-changing.

In this section, we present a mix of clinical stories and clinical strategies. The clinical stories reflect moments of profound impact on some of our authors. The clinical strategies are a synthesis of hard-earned lessons learned from the times when things did not go well. Anything that can go wrong will go wrong—and I can guarantee that you will see that happen during your careers. We hope that readers will find these stories interesting, and maybe help stimulate some ideas that can be adopted in their daily practices.

Author

Ray Graber serves as vice chair for quality in the anesthesiology department at University Hospitals Cleveland Medical. He has dual interests in cardiac and orthopedic anesthesia. During his 30+ year career, he has focused on process improvement, reduction of errors, and improving patient outcomes.

R. G. Graber (✉)
Department of Anesthesiology and Perioperative Medicine, University Hospitals Cleveland Medical Center, Cleveland, OH, USA
e-mail: raymond.graber@uhhospitals.org

S. Mohamed et al. (eds.), *Anesthesia Bridges*, https://doi.org/10.1007/978-3-032-08294-7_119

Think the Anesthesia Community Has Already "Borrowed" Everything It Can from the Airline Industry? Not Even Close!

120

W. Mitchell Robbins, Amy J. Robbins, Willy A. Flegel, Catherine Marcucci, and F. Jacob Seagull

Introduction

The practice of anesthesia has frequently been described as being similar to flying an airplane: Three minutes of intense activity at the beginning and end with intense boredom in between, with the possibility of being punctuated by moments of sheer terror in the middle. Of course, this annoying cliché is stupendously false in both cases. But what is true is that *both* aviation and anesthesia involve using advanced technology to achieve nearly magical results in a high-risk situation—suspending a person in a precarious situation that can easily result in death if managed improperly. And both are safer than ever.

Asking an Aviation Expert

Mitch Robbins is an aerospace engineer, former military pilot, and senior pilot for a major US airline. He recently took the time to have several long conversations with the authors about his background, training, and day-to-day life in the aviation industry. He answered some questions that we have been mulling over on the similarities and differences between our two industries, and still, there is a lot to be learned. He grew up in a military and flying family and is the older brother of **Amy Robbins,** who is the second author on this chapter (Fig. 120.1).

W. M. Robbins
Pilot and Airline Captain, Ponte Vedra, FL, USA

A. J. Robbins
Stanson Health, a Premier Inc. Company, Charlotte, NC, USA

Atrium Health, Carolinas Palliative Care and Hospice Group, Charlotte, NC, USA

W. A. Flegel
Department of Transfusion Medicine, Clinical Center, National Institutes of Health, Bethesda, MD, USA

Georgetown University Medical Center, Washington, DC, USA

Huazhong University of Science and Technology, Wuhan, Hubei, China

C. Marcucci (✉)
Department of Transfusion Medicine, Clinical Center, National Institutes of Health, Bethesda, MD, USA

F. J. Seagull
Center for Bioethics and Social Science in Medicine, Michigan Medicine (University of Michigan Medical School), Ann Arbor, MI, USA

S. Mohamed et al. (eds.), *Anesthesia Bridges*, https://doi.org/10.1007/978-3-032-08294-7_120

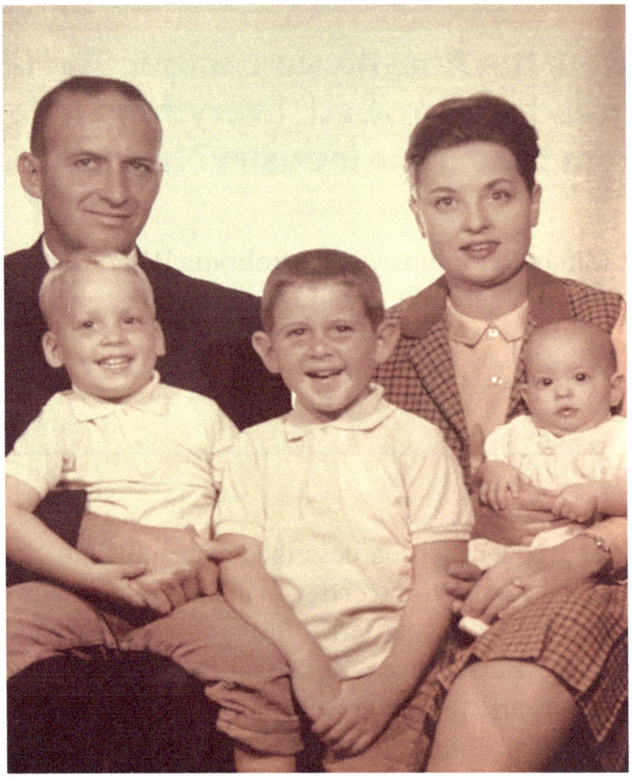

Fig. 120.1 The Robbins family, circa 1965. Mitch and Amy are on their parents' laps; late brother Martin is in the middle. Marilyn and the late Gary were cooler than the rest of us put together; there's no denying it. They were both pilots, highly educated, and successful professional people. Don't be fooled by that prim Peter Pan collar that Marilyn is wearing—she's always had the "right stuff"—then and now. When the family plane that her fighter pilot husband Gary was flying lost its engine and might have crashed with family fatalities, did she panic and become hysterical? Nope. Her only reaction was to decide, "Hey, I think it's time for me to get my own pilot's license in case I ever would have to do a dead stick landing." And she did. Amy and her brothers grew up being piloted around the country by both their father *and* their mother. Photo: Collection of the Robbins family

Evolution of Anesthesia Safety

The evolution of anesthesia safety that arose in the 1980s was a result of anesthesia adopting a systematic approach to reduce risk, through the CRICO insurance program to reduce medical malpractice, associated with Harvard hospitals, leading to the ASA standards for monitoring. The trend toward systematic safety continued in the 1990s, when the concept of "cockpit resource management" was borrowed from aviation and adapted into "crew/crisis resource management" for anesthesia and pioneered by people like Dave Gaba.

As a result, anesthesia safety has improved over tenfold since the 1980s and stands at around 4 deaths per million surgeries today. By comparison, there is one major crash per roughly seven million flights. From 2010 to 2020, there were 2 years with a single fatality in commercial aviation, and the other 9 years had zero fatalities, according to the National Transportation Safety Board.

We in Anesthesia Still Have a Lot to Learn

Pilots never study the performance and safety procedures of anesthesiologists. Neither the military nor the commercial flying communities pays any attention to the anesthesia community whatsoever. Rather, they see themselves as most closely aligned to the nuclear industry. Within medical specialties, the airline industry is perhaps most similar to the practice of transfusion medicine in its extremely high level of federal oversight and regulation.

Why would that be? Well, for starters, they take themselves, their training, and their culture of safety much more seriously.

Who Is a Good Pilot?

Because this book is being written for young anesthesiologists, we wanted to find out whether there was a single attribute that Mitch looked for when training young pilots—what predicts who is going to be a successful and excellent pilot. His immediate answer? "Willingness to undertake and maintain medical qualifications." The career-long medical and physical surveillance of pilots is a bit less than in previous years (for example, cholesterol meds are now allowed), but still prodigious and much more than physicians undergo. A working pilot submits health records and undergoes medical testing on an ongoing basis. This includes hearing and vision tests and even having yearly EKGs.

In terms of personality, there is no typical type of inherent character that makes an excellent pilot. Pilots are sometimes quiet and understated, but often very arrogant and type A. They are apparently often actually closer to surgeons in personality than anesthesiologists. But it's always true that people who wish to be professional pilots live a life of constant evaluation and proficiency testing. Airlines also know who they are *not* looking for, and the people who shouldn't be pilots tend to demonstrate that along the way. So, first, a good pilot must have the willingness and acceptance of the need to undergo constant training and surveillance. And second, the other important character trait is the ability to compartmentalize and focus on the job at hand.

There are more women commercial pilots now, of course, but the number is still very low. In the US, the proportion of women commercial pilots has hovered around 7% over the last decade (FAA statistics). Mitch estimates that he only flies with women on 5% of flights or less.

Training

Commercial pilots train constantly. And we mean constantly—way more than anesthesiologists train. Mitch described something called "chair training," which is a practice that young pilots do on a ubiquitous basis. This involves sitting in a chair before a poster of a cockpit, with all the switches, dials, and gauges, visualizing and pantomiming the actions involved in flying the plane. We asked him if he had ever done this, assuming that he was being facetious, and he said, "all the time!"

Another huge difference is the amount of simulation training professional pilots do. Each major commercial airline has its own simulation center(s). The simulation is so advanced and life-like that pilots sometimes can forget they are in the simulator. Mitch was really surprised to hear how little simulation training anesthesiologists do, even though we do it for much longer than 10 years ago. Pilots also do simulation training and undergo testing and certification on each *aspect* of flying.

Landing is a major area of pilot training and pilots will undergo courses of full-time training just on landing. They also do what's called "differences training"—intense simulator training and testing on systems and planes that are similar to each other but just different enough to have incremental margins of performance and hence safety. When Mitch was transitioning from flying the smaller A320 to the larger but essentially similar A330, he did several *months* of self-study, followed by about three weeks of full-time simulator work.

And a pilot who is going to transition from flying an Airbus A330 to an Airbus A350 would undergo at least a month of full-time simulator training and testing. This is for even the most senior and experienced pilots. The A350 is quite different for a pilot from the A330, although to an untrained eye they both look like huge and similar jet aircraft. The A350 is newer, larger, and more fuel-efficient. It has a mostly composite airframe and is very quiet in flight. Most importantly, there are additional active flight control systems to enhance the ride and efficiency. The avionics suite (pilots' office) is much more advanced with track balls, keyboards, six full-sized screens, and touch screens that can be electronically customized. It has more robust flight control systems to accommodate minor system failures automatically. It's also the first paperless cockpit. So, Mitch took himself off to the simulator center and did nothing else but train full-time on these differences for weeks. We had the first draft of the outline of this chapter ready for his review during this interval, but Amy said, "Hmmm, no, we really shouldn't interrupt a pilot who's in the middle of differences training."

Contrast this with the (relatively minimal) training that happens when new anesthesia equipment and systems are implemented. Perhaps we can compare the pilot's A320 to A330 to A350 plane transitions to the move from one hospital to the next hospital. The pilots find themselves with a new cockpit layout, with new computer systems, different checklists, and different crew management philosophies and routines. When moving to another hospital, there is little or no paid time for self-study for the anesthesiologist to acclimate to the new venue. We find ourselves in a new hospital, amidst a new OR layout, an unfamiliar OR crew, and with varying anesthetic machines, tools, and resources. As an anesthesiologist, has the quick transition in hospital settings ever compromised your confidence, or challenged your established routines?

And then there are the issues of training versus performance. Pilots would never dream of training during a commercial flight. The idea that we let anesthesiologists-in-training "practice" on real patients is somewhat horrifying to them. A pilot in training or pursuing certification does undergo in-flight training, but that happens only under the auspices of an accompanying instructor who is assigned to training duties and nothing else. Pilots don't fly empty planes in training—too costly—but if they are training on an actual flight, they have no responsibility for passenger safety. And the working pilots who are flying the plane have no responsibility for the trainee.

So, what this boils down to is that nobody flies a commercial flight without having already obtained full certification, and uncertified and unsupervised pilots never, ever fly a "live" plane. In contrast—how many anesthesiologists practice on a real patient before they have been certified on a simulator? How many times have you left a CA-1 resident alone in a room for an hour or more to attend to your other room?

Mission Briefings

In commercial aviation, a written flight plan is filed for every flight. The plan is comprehensive, including every waypoint, emergency diversion possibilities for weather, equipment degradations, and in-flight emergencies. Most contingencies are codified in a standard operating procedure.

In military aviation, before each unique combat mission, there is a briefing to review the plan, as well as a discussion of contingencies in case of adverse events. There may be simulations. Following every military combat mission, an extensive review of the action will take place to study what went right and what went wrong, to improve success and safety in subsequent missions.

In anesthesia, we aspire to state the plan during pre-op time out. But do we? A good time-out should include what we are concerned about, and major goals (waypoints). How often do we conduct a debrief? How often is it comprehensive? What do we do to learn from our operational flights and missions?

***Note from the Editors:** Mitch Robbins as a young military pilot (Fig. 120.2).

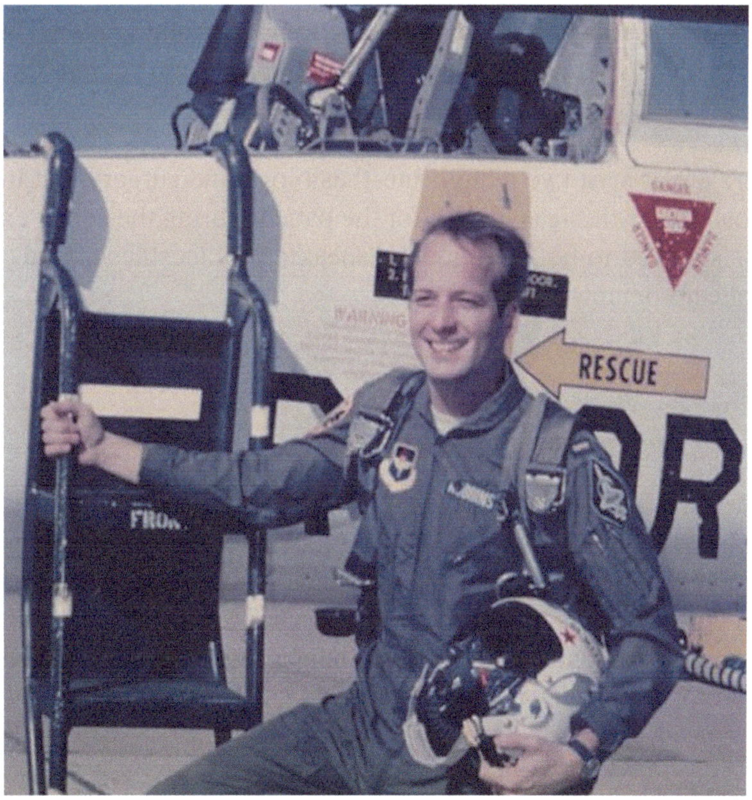

Fig. 120.2 Mitch Robbins in 1985, posing for his hero shot. The plane he is flying is the Northrup T-38 Talon supersonic jet trainer. Photo: Collection of Mitch Robbins

Preactivity Checks

In commercial aviation—every single flight—pilots review a preflight checklist. Out loud. As a team. It is never skipped for short flights. It is never completed for "once at the start of the day for all the flights that day."

In anesthesia, pre-op time-outs have been adopted as a policy, for example, by the Joint Commission or the WHO and its checklists. There are mixed data on how well the procedures are followed. It is sometimes challenging to ensure that anesthesia machines are fully checked out/calibrated before each procedure.

Teamwork

Pilots always work in teams. A long international flight for a major carrier will actually have four pilots in the (cockpit)—two teams of two pilots. It's rare to know the other members of the pilot team well, and there is not a lot of conversation between pilots on a flight—or as Mitch said, "We don't get on the plane to talk." Mitch's airline employs about 13,000 pilots, and there are about 500 pilots employed by his airline who fly the type of plane he flies. (Copilots are always copilots on every team). The team in a cockpit is concerned with one thing: flying the plane. They take off and land, and if they do that, the flight is a success. The goals of every member of the pilot team are absolutely identical.

Every pilot who is in a pilot seat is flying the airplane and doing nothing else. There is also no concept of a "mid-level pilot provider." There are no multiple training routes to get into the pilot's seat, and there is no consideration that there will be.

In anesthesiology, there are at least two teams: anesthesiology and surgery, but they don't always have identical goals. The goal of anesthesia is to care for the patient during the achievement of a second goal: surgery. Anesthesiologists need to be "bilingual"—speaking to anesthesia goals and surgical goals in every case. This complicates teamwork.

Sterile Cockpit

Whenever a plane is below 10,000 feet (including taxi, takeoff, and landing), there are no nonessential duties and activities. No conversation other than official aviation communications. No eating. No general interest announcements to the passengers. No chit-chat amongst the pilots themselves. Although, in aviation, talking about the weather is not considered chit-chat. We also asked Mitch if pilots listened to music at any time during flights, and his immediate answer was, "never." This is not just an informal pilot culture or custom; it's federal law (covered under 14 CFR Part 121.542).

During the critical portions of surgery (induction and emergence), do we ever talk about or do anything that is not an essential duty? Do the surgeons ever still have the music on during emergence and extubation?

- Interestingly, though, Mitch tells us that it is somewhat unclear where the origin of the common term "sterile" cockpit comes from. He suspects that this is one of the few things that was borrowed at some point from the medical industry. Flight decks are anything but sterile. Pilots reside there for about 50% of the lifecycle of the airframe—large airliners are airborne about half the time from delivery to retirement.

Culture of Talking About Errors

Pilots. Report. All. Errors If an adverse event occurs—including a near-miss where something bad almost happens—a pilot will almost certainly report the problem immediately. This is not because pilots are more conscientious than anesthesiologists. Rather, it is because aviation has adopted the culture of safety. Aviation is obsessed with failure and preventing failure. This is more than just an attitude by individual pilots. It is part of the structure of the entire industry and profession. The FAA has adopted an error reporting system called the Aviation Safety Reporting System/ASRS. The system rewards pilots, or anyone, for reporting a problem and punishes those who don't. If a pilot reports a problem, his or her report cannot be used in any way to prosecute the pilot; in fact, they gain immunity in all but criminal offenses. This seems very difficult to the practice of medicine with the wide discoverability that is permitted in civil medical malpractice and other tort cases.

Furthermore, the National Transportation Safety Board conducts an extensive review and creates a public record of any fatality that occurs in its industry. The public case files are astonishing in their complexity, depth, and detail for both civil and commercial aviation fatalities—they contain not just photographs, but drawings, maps, transcripts of the radio transmissions, in-depth analysis of equipment performance and failure, and even records of who was on duty at the control towers at the time of the fatality. They may take months to complete and compile. The Anesthesia Closed Claims Database, now maintained by the Anesthesia Quality Institute, is based on the same principles, of course. But there is an order of magnitude difference (or more!) in the scope of *post-hoc* review conducted in the case of an aviation death and an untoward anesthetic death—and of course, detailed investigations of iatrogenic deaths are not widely available in the public domain!

Authority/Canceling Flights/Primary Mission

A pilot does have the absolute authority to cancel or terminate a flight. But rather than cancel the flight, the pilot is more canceling the plane, as the passengers will be rerouted to other flights and most likely will continue to travel on the day of the canceled flight. In-flight emergencies do happen. If an airplane that is in the air needs to be landed, all the pilots will discuss and concur and make a unanimous decision. If a unanimous decision cannot be reached, certain calls, even by the "junior" cockpit members, have binding authority and cannot be questioned by the captain. The decisions by pilots to cancel flights are never questioned at the moment—can any anesthesiologist even imagine such a luxury? The aviation business is data-driven. Everything is thoroughly documented, reviewed, and analyzed at a later time, but there is no hassling of the pilot at the time of a cancelation. Pilots can also remove themselves from a flight with no penalty due to feeling sick or fatigued.

Job Satisfaction

Many, many pilots feel they have absolutely the best job in the world. They couldn't dream of doing anything else. They are human, of course, not infallible machines, and we mentioned to Mitch that we have read reports about burnout among pilots. This has not been his impression based on what he has observed amongst his colleagues. Pilots get flying assignments based on seniority and several types of bidding systems for dates, routes, and planes. So, as careers progress, pilots' day-to-day work life becomes increasingly optimized to their own preferences and needs. Pilots also almost always have aviation hobbies—whether they fly personal family planes or hobby planes. This is quite different from the practice of anesthesiology, which is not generally something that you think of having a lot of fun doing in your spare time.

***Note from the Editors:** While pilots are away doing the jobs they love, their families carry on at home, and this is true for both civilian and military pilots. This picture, taken around 1967, shows the pictures that Marilyn Robbins posted for her kids when their dad Gary was away on one of his two tours of duty in Vietnam (Fig. 120.3).

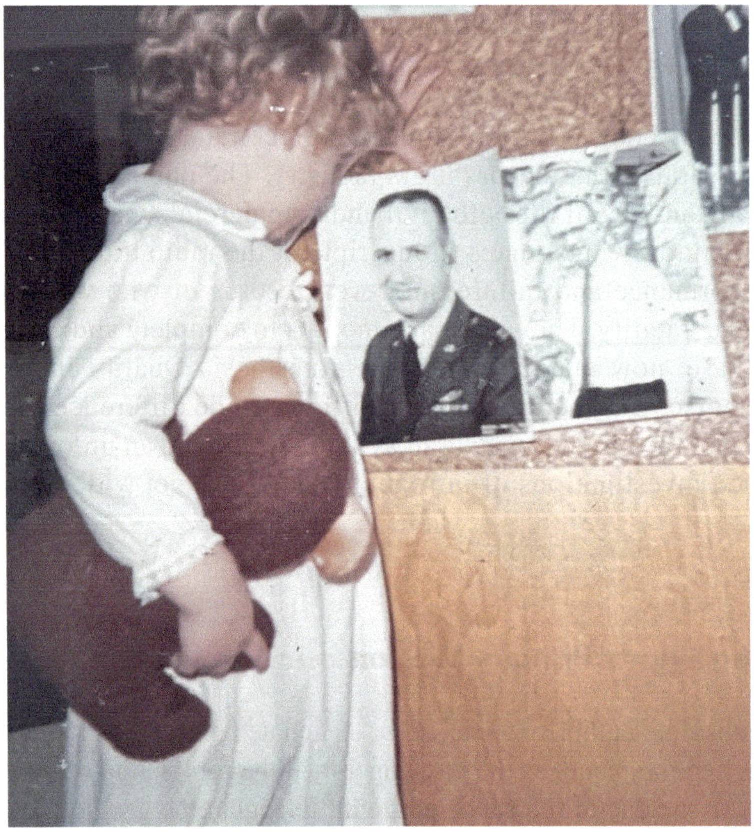

Fig. 120.3 That adorable tot with the light brown curls and her teddy bear is author Amy Robbins. She is looking at pictures of her father Gary Robbins that her mother posted for her so that she wouldn't forget him when he was away at war. In combat, Gary flew the F-100 Super Sabre, but he was also a West Point grad with a degree in aerospace engineering. As we can see in the photo on the right, he certainly looked like the typical mid-century engineer when he wasn't in uniform—crew cut, short-sleeved white shirt, skinny tie. Photo: Collection of the Robbins family

High Reliability: Do We Have It?

Are we obsessed with failure? Are we committed to being resilient in the face of a threat to safety? Do we refuse to simplify the interpretation of a procedure? These are some of the hallmarks of high-reliability operations. Being obsessed with failure would mean constantly thinking about what can go wrong. Commitment to resilience would involve having contingencies in place for every conceivable problem that might arise. Refusal to simplify would mean that we try and conceive those problems uniquely for each patient's condition individually.

Are We Going Where Aviation Is Going?

Aviation is moving toward the paradigm of "TEM"—threat error management. The emphasis of TEM is on defining time buckets. This involves deciding what pilots must do now and what isn't time critical, then team building to bring in all available resources to manage a nontime-critical event. Mitch tells us, "On the airplane, this is connecting with expertise on the ground via radio, datalink, and aircraft satellite phone. For example, if we have an in-flight passenger medical event, we need to decide if we need to divert immediately or can continue. This may be three hours from a place to land. We ask for onboard medical assistance but also connect to a contract medical provider on the ground to help make the decisions." This is really fascinating and something that isn't very common in the OR. Yes, you might call for help in an emergency—lost airway or arrest—but how often are we able to call for multiple resources in a nonemergent situation?

And Remember that the Pilot Flying the Plane Is Always First to Arrive at the Scene of an Aviation Accident

Safety is easier for pilots to embrace because they own the problem. Pilots think, "Hey, I have to keep myself safe for another day, so it's no extra chore to keep my passengers safe as well." Any problem with flight safety directly and immediately affects them, too.

Adage: There are bold pilots and there are old pilots, but no bold old pilots. *Even arrogant type A personalities cannot be bold if they want to grow old as pilots.* Many more pilots died in airplane crashes than passengers did in a century. Aviation is the industry with the most obvious track record of more casualties among its employees than customers.

Conclusions?

So, yeah. We're good. They're better. We could do more.

We are involved in safety. They are committed.

The difference between involved and committed can be illustrated by a breakfast of bacon and eggs. The chicken was involved. The pig was committed.

Lessons Learned

- The comparisons between aviation go so far and no farther. We've extensively studied their industry; they really never think about us.
- They train constantly and in a manner that is fundamentally different from the way we train. They certify on each aspect of piloting and flying skills before they fly passengers. This includes both simulator training and certification and examinations.
- Humility counts! Pilots must be humbly committed because they only survive if they maintain safety at all times and costs. We ought to be similarly humble whenever we address patient safety.
- The adage for the entire existence of human flight—there are old pilots and bold pilots, but no old, bold pilots have been said a million times. It's true for aviation, but not the practice of anesthesiology. Remember that if you ever feel like making a "bold" move in the OR or ICU, it's the patient who is carrying the risk of that boldness, not you, at least not immediately.
- They don't abbreviate or abridge their protocols and standard operating procedures. Ever.
- They always work in teams—a long flight will have four fully qualified pilots. Imagine having four board-certified anesthesiologists for every long OR case! Not possible due to costs, you are thinking? But remember, the commercial airline industry is for profit, and they find a way to make it happen.
- They are accountable to the federal government in ways that we are not.
- They are on the plane!

***Note from the Editors:** Speaking of being on the plane, here is Mitch Robbins on a vacation day in the cockpit of a large jet (Fig. 120.4).

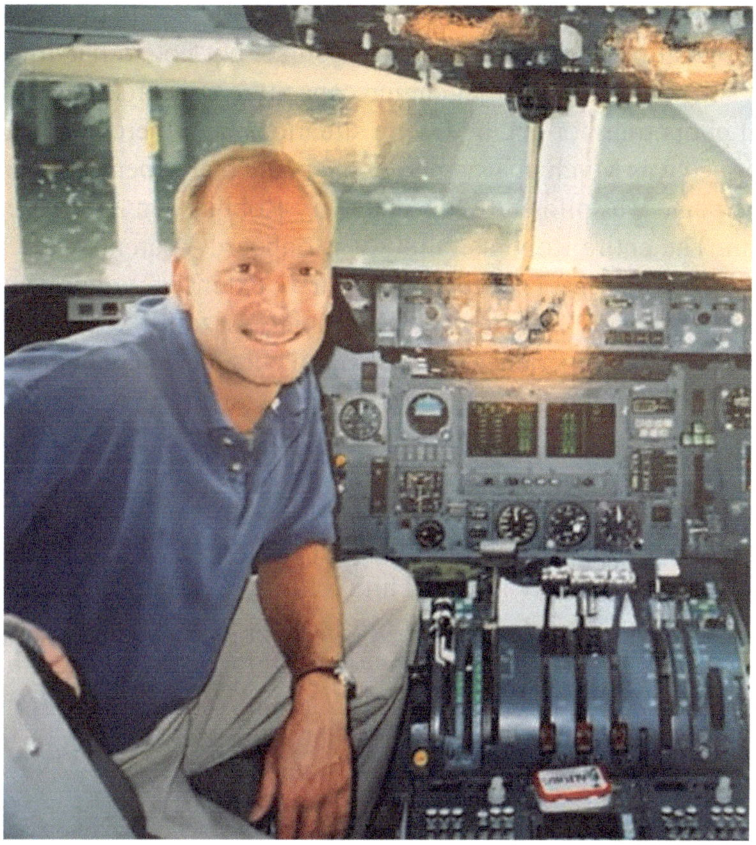

Fig. 120.4 Except when he is at home with his family or on his farm, this is Mitch Robbins' favorite place in the world. Photo: Collection of Mitch Robbins

Bonus Content!

Mitch was kind enough to take the time to extend the interview to answer some questions that we have always wondered about. Here are some additional fun facts about his life and world:

- It is true that pilots have sole control of the plane on take-offs and landings. However, it is not true that the rest of the time the plane flies itself, and the pilots wouldn't even need to be on it. It can take up to an hour to program in all the necessary information for a long flight. After take-off, the pilots spend a huge amount of time making sure the airplane is doing what it's supposed to do. Pilots are also in constant communication with air traffic control on a variety of subjects, including the weather—in fact, they are rarely not in communication with their control tower centers.

- On an international flight, all four pilots are qualified in both seats, and all four pilots are on the flight deck for take-off and landing. On the long flights, two pilots will be in front in the seats and two will be in the bunks, which are right behind and above the pilot seats.

- That pilot who is walking around outside the plane is not just there for his or her mere curiosity or to make a show for the people watching from the terminal. It is mandated before every flight that one pilot does a thorough visual inspection of the plane from the tarmac.

- Airplane engines do fail! Mitch has experienced five engine failures in his life, including his military time. These are notable situations for the pilots, of course, but not so much for the passengers on a commercial flight, as there is redundant jet engine capacity engineered into modern commercial airplanes. Commercial pilots train for engine failure situations, and there are a variety of plans that are implemented. Only once was Mitch in a single-engine plane that experienced engine failure—he was a young boy and the plane was piloted by his dad Gary Robbins, an Air Force fighter pilot who did two tours in Vietnam. The entire Robbins family was onboard—parents Gary and Marilyn and kids Martin, Mitch, and Amy (Fig. 120.1). Because of Gary's extensive training and experience, he was able to get the plane to ground in the desert of Kingman, Arizona, without injury to himself or his precious passengers. After this experience, Mitch's mom pursued and obtained her own private pilot's license! The family went on to travel the country in small planes, piloted by both Mom and Dad, and Mitch's love of flying blossomed.

- We asked Mitch if it's true that if you get on a flight and there is a pilot on the flight as a passenger that you can be assured that you are on a safer flight with a better pilot. His answer was no. Mitch has sometimes lived in locations that have required him to fly to where he was going to pick up his plane and then fly home as a passenger. He never gives a thought as to who might be flying the plane that he is catching a ride on. It is true that pilots often would prefer not to chat to other passengers, and for that reason, they often fly home in street clothes. They have had to put family and personal life thoughts and concerns aside while flying and are often trying to rest and get back into the mindset of their "civilian" lives.

- About the movies: Top Gun did actually have some degree of accuracy. Mitch admits there is a certain amount of hard-flying, hard-drinking fighter jock behavior that goes on, less now than in the past, but still not completely gone. The use of "call signs" that Top Gun made famous is a Navy thing, not so much with Air Force pilots. Mitch did not go by a fighter pilot nickname when he flew for the Air Force, although he has flown with "Bozo," the real-life pilot who was responsible for the aerial coordination and flying sequences in Top Gun. Bozo was also the pilot who flew the famous "buzzing the tower" scenes.

- Yes, Sully Sullenberger did a great job when he landed an Airbus A320, which Mitch flew for many years, on the Hudson River on January 15, 2009. But it wasn't an accident or really a miracle that he was in the position to do it. As Sullenberger said afterwards. "One way of looking at this might be that for 42 years, I've been making small, regular deposits in this bank of experience, education, and training. And on January 15, the balance was sufficient so that I could make a very large withdrawal."

Authors

Mitch Robbins is truly an expert on all aspects of piloting, aviation regulations, and safety. He has had a lifelong love of flying and grew up in the aviation industry. He obtained his private pilot's license at the age of 18. He graduated from the University of Michigan with a degree in aerospace engineering and then joined the Air Force. He attended US Air Force flight school in 1984–1985 at Reese Air Force Base, Texas. After completing several phases of pilot training, he eventually flew KC-135 refueling planes, also known as "heavies." He was stationed in South Dakota for 5 years—essentially because the northern tier bases were closer to the Cold War—although he flew all over the world. He also completed tours of duty as an instructor pilot and safety officer. He left the Air Force in 1992 with the rank of Captain and about 2500 flying hours.

After spending a year in engineering work, he joined the National Transportation Safety Board, where he continued to develop expertise in investigating aviation accidents. His first job at a commercial airline was as a flight safety manager, while he also flew part-time. He was in the air on the morning of 9/11, flying from Dallas to Detroit, and made his emergency landing in Indianapolis on that awful day. He has worked full-time as a line pilot for a major US carrier since 1997, first flying the Airbus A320, the Douglas DC-9, and then the Airbus A330. He is now a senior pilot, flying the Airbus A350, chiefly to Asia. He had "at least" 20,000 flying hours when he stopped counting closely years ago (his airline does maintain those records). Somewhere along the line in this busy career, he also completed a master's degree in systems engineering at USC.

Amy Robbins being the daughter of a career military pilot, grew up all over the United States. A few of her elementary school years were spent living in Papillion, Nebraska, when her father was stationed at Strategic Air Command headquartered at Offutt Air Force Base just south of Omaha. She was on that plane with the failed engine, along with her mother and two brothers, that her father brought down in the desert of Arizona. As she watched out the window, she vividly remembers seeing the desert sand and cactuses getting larger as they rapidly approached the ground. She recalls her father, while maneuvering a plane with no engine, saying, "I got you, you son of a bitch!" Meanwhile, her mother calmly told the children to put their heads down and hold onto each other. Amy and her brother Mitch have often wondered if the exemplary calm and cool nature of both parents during that traumatic event was instrumental in both children pursuing professions where one must remain calm and effective in emergencies—aviation and anesthesiology.

Bill Flegel was seriously considering a career as a pilot and even applied to the Lufthansa flight school, eventually realizing, however, that he was more interested in a career in medicine. After completing medical training, he pursued a private pilot's license in the EU and the US. Aviation safety has been a topic of great interest to him since his initial flight training in the mid-1980s, and he has published on its application to transfusion medicine. After 500 flying hours with "single-engine land" planes, he qualifies in the category of "old, not bold pilots."

Cathy Marcucci had a great time interviewing Mitch Robbins, as she loves nothing more than hearing about other people's lives and professional worlds. In the near future, she is hoping to travel to Asia on vacation with Amy Robbins' family—on a plane that Mitch is flying, of course. She has even been promised a preflight visit to the cabin.

Jake Seagull is a psychologist and human factors expert at the University of Michigan. His master's thesis topic was developing training methods for improving the performance of Apache attack helicopter pilots. He then did his PhD work at the University of Illinois Champaign-Urbana which has a famous aviation psychology program, and where his PhD advisor was Chris Wickens, a prominent expert in that field. Jake also has expertise and teaches CRM and simulation in the medical context. He is not a pilot but does enjoy jumping out of airplanes.

Learning from Medical Errors and Adverse Events

121

Karen B. Domino

Introduction

I trained as a resident at the Hospital of the University of Pennsylvania in the early 1980s, a time prior to today's monitoring standards, physiological monitors, video laryngoscopes, perioperative checklists, and faculty supervision for anesthesia care. During my training, several adverse patient events shaped my lifelong approach to clinical practice and served as the basis for my academic work in patient safety.

Adverse Events

During one of the early months of my residency, I found two nurses crying in the locker room near the OR. It turned out that two surgical patients were mixed up and underwent the wrong surgery. Both patients were middle-aged, overweight women. One circulating nurse took patient #1 to the OR for a parathyroid procedure, while patient #2 waited in the preoperative holding area. My fellow resident prepared patient #2 for an awake intubation prior to taking the patient to the OR for a cervical spine procedure, continually calling patient #2 by patient #1's name—the patient never corrected him. At patient #1's surgery, her parathyroid glands were normal, but a thyroid mass was found and removed. Patient #2 underwent a cervical laminectomy, but little pathology was found. After the procedures, the recovery nurses checked the patient's armbands and discovered that the patients had been mixed up and underwent the wrong procedures!

Obviously, patients #1 and #2 and their families were very unhappy. The "never event" resulted in financial and reputation losses for the hospital, resignation of the chief of the hospital's anesthesia department, a specialty change for one anesthesia attending, and loss of jobs for the two circulating RNs. After this transformative event, I've always checked patients' ID wrist badges myself when meeting a patient in the preoperative area.

There were many other adverse events during my residency that shaped my clinical practice. Some of the most memorable ones were unrecognized esophageal intubation resulting in patient death (mistak-

K. B. Domino (✉)
Department of Anesthesiology & Pain Medicine, University of Washington, Seattle, WA, USA
e-mail: kdomino@uw.edu

S. Mohamed et al. (eds.), *Anesthesia Bridges*, https://doi.org/10.1007/978-3-032-08294-7_121

enly attributed to capnograph malfunction with a reading of 0), florid postobstructive pulmonary edema after premature extubation, complicated by difficult reintubation, and cardiac arrest in a young healthy patient during spinal anesthesia.

Anesthesia Closed Claims Project

These adverse events inspired my interest in quality improvement and patient safety. The Anesthesia Closed Claims Project was started in the mid-1980s in response to high malpractice premiums for anesthesiologists, as improving patient safety would reduce malpractice premiums.

After moving across the US to the University of Washington, I joined the Closed Claims Project team and ultimately directed the project for over 25 years. My residency experiences taught me the critical importance of learning from adverse events in order to improve one's clinical care. Anesthesiologists worldwide have improved patient safety by learning from these tragic cases through the in-depth analysis of the types and sequences of adverse events and causes of clinician judgment problems. After all, pilots learn from near-misses and plane crashes by others, rather than having to experience them themselves!

Lessons Learned

The Closed Claims Project has also taught me a few other important lessons for clinical care:

- Humility: Medical errors and poor outcomes can happen to good anesthesiologists.
- Fight tendencies to become overconfident, cut corners, and lack vigilance over time in practice. Always keep your mind focused, prepared, and plan ahead for all contingencies.
- "To err is human" is one of the truest statements ever said or written. Systems changes are essential to improve patient safety.
- In today's complex medical world, communication skills, teamwork, and human factors are critical in preventing medical errors. Training in these "nonscientific" skills is essential to improve patient safety.

Bonus Content from the Editors

The Closed Claims file is now under the auspices of the Anesthesia Quality Institute. The entire anesthesiology community is indebted to Dr. Pierce, Dr. Ward, Dr. Domino, Dr. Lee, and their colleagues at the University of Washington for their brilliant work over many years on this landmark quality and safety initiative.

We want to highlight the text from the website of the Anesthesia Quality Institute, at https://www.aqihq.org/ACCMain.aspx:

> The Anesthesia Closed Claim Project's goal is to identify anesthesia-related major safety concerns, patterns of injury, and prevention strategies in areas where anesthesiologists provide care. To achieve this goal, ASA member anesthesiologists collect both quantitative and qualitative data to identify a sequence of events concluding in a narrative summary of care from malpractice insurance companies. The evaluated claims can be classified as rare and/or serious events. Analyzed data can be used in publications, presentations, and/or research studies.

Elsewhere in this book, we urge our readers to "review the Closed Claims file." But how do you actually do that?

***Note from the Editors:** The Anesthesia Quality Institute is located in Schaumburg, IL. Midwesterners love to be outside all seasons of the year, maybe it's because of the farming background and culture. This wonderful little footbridge is just outside of town (Fig. 121.1).

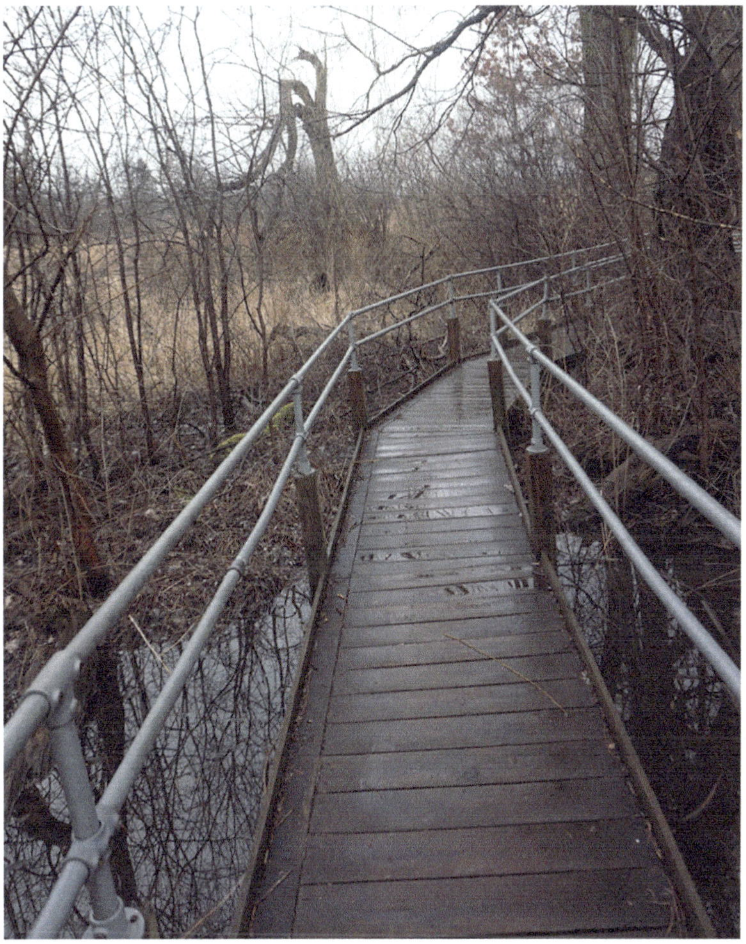

Fig. 121.1 A footbridge through a winter scene in Schaumburg, IL, the home of the AQI. Photo: Image used under standard license of stock.adobe.com

Open access to the Closed Claims file is not available, but applications can be made for limited analyses (Fig. 121.2). Short of that, we advise that you read through the data that have been mined from the project files. It is really the most valuable and clinically relevant data in the entire specialty of anesthesiology. The very first paper published with data from the Closed Claim file was a paper on unexpected arrest during spinal anesthesia [1]. Since that time, there have been a number of publications that have summarized data and outcomes from closed claims, and reading back through them is a great idea. A summary of some of our most important practice guidelines that are derived from closed claims data can be found at:

Application Process

- Application is completed by the ASA Member
- AQI reviews the application.
  Please note that you may be contacted for further clarifications on your request.
- An initial scientific review is performed by the Chair of the Closed Claims Committee.
- A second/final scientific review is performed by the Closed Claims Committee.
- Once the request is approved, a *Limited Data Use Agreement (DUA)* will be delivered to the investigator for review and signature.
- Upon the completion of the DUA, the investigator will receive analysis.

Please click link to the Data Request Application:
https://closedclaims.aqihq.org/CCReviewer/ReqIntro

Fig. 121.2 Application and review/ process for investigators accessing the anesthesia closed claim File, at https://www.aqihq.org/ACCDataUse.aspx

https://pubs.asahq.org/anesthesiology/article/113/4/957/10703/The-American-Society-of-Anesthesiologists-Closed

We also recommend reading two chapters in *Avoiding Common Anesthesia Errors, Second Edition*—"How Not to End Up in the Closed Claims File—Lessons Learned from the Anesthesia Closed Claims Project" (Chap. 278) by **Lorri Lee** and **Karen Domino** and "The Anesthesia Closed Claims Project—What's Trending Now" (Chap. 279) by **Cobin** Soelberg. These are great, quick-to-read reviews that touch on the highlights of *staying out of the file*. They discuss "what to do and what not to do" and include several hints as to what is trending in the database. Specifically, claims for MAC anesthesia cases, out-of-OR cases, and regional anesthesia and blocks are all on the increase. The chapters provide more detailed analysis and specific advice.

Reference

1. Caplan RA, Ward RJ, Posner K, Cheney FW. Unexpected cardiac arrest during spinal anesthesia: A closed claims analysis of predisposing factors. Anesthesiology. 1988;68:5–11.

Author

Karen Domino grew up in Michigan, but has spent most of her life in Seattle, where she lives on Puget Sound with her husband, dog, cat, and two reptiles. An East Coast colleague described Karen as a "true Seattle-lite" due to the "work hard-play hard" outdoors mentality of residents in the Pacific Northwest. Recently retired, Karen was always passionate about patient safety and learning from medical errors and devoted her research, teaching, and administrative career to improving patient care.

Additional Thoughts on (Clinical) Judgment

122

F. Jacob Seagull, Rodger E. Barnette, Ronald S. Bank, and Catherine Marcucci

Introduction

The "Part III Leadership" section of this book has two chapters on developing good judgment. We are grateful to our friends on the federal bench who found the time in their busy schedules to help us out with their ideas and advice. In the process of writing and revising those chapters, we circulated them amongst ourselves for discussion and comment. **Rodger Barnette** and **Ron Bank** wrote back with interesting additional thoughts on having and using judgment, particularly clinical judgment and decision-making. And Jake Seagull gives us a bit of expert insight to put everything in the correct context.

From Rodger Barnette

In the previous chapters on judgment, much weight is given to gathering facts and information and having the time to ponder the accumulated data. In medicine, you may have that luxury for some types of judgment calls—but not for all.

My definition of a difficult clinical decision is making a judgment call with an inadequate and incomplete database—and often doing so while under time pressure. And then you only know if you called it correctly when a time interval (minutes, hours, days) has passed. I think that is very different than what is discussed in the judgment chapters elsewhere in the book.

What I am describing is a subset of "judgment" that has time pressure as an integral part of the issue. Something I think most judges don't deal with on a frequent basis, but anesthesiologists deal with constantly. This is not meant to take anything away from the excellent and interesting advice from Judges Wilson and Conner, only to widen the discussion.

F. J. Seagull
Center for Bioethics and Social Science in Medicine, University of Michigan Medical School, Ann Arbor, MI, USA

R. E. Barnette (Retired)
AIC Kijabe Hospital, Kijabe, Kenya

Department of Anesthesiology (emeritus), Lewis Katz School of Medicine Temple University, Philadelphia, PA, USA

R. S. Bank
Department of Anesthesiology, INOVA Fairfax Hospital, UVA School of Medicine, INOVA Campus, Falls Church, VA, USA

C. Marcucci (✉)
Department of Transfusion Medicine, Clinical Center, National Institutes of Health, Bethesda, MD, USA

S. Mohamed et al. (eds.), *Anesthesia Bridges*, https://doi.org/10.1007/978-3-032-08294-7_122

Here is a brief example of clinical decision-making under pressure. Rather than being extremely remarkable, I am sharing this case because it is actually quite typical—the type of situation that we are consistently, if not constantly, faced with:

> A few years ago in Kenya, a patient presented who needed an urgent/emergent C-section. I was working with a Kenyan nurse anesthetist with 10 years of experience. I had worked with this particular nurse anesthetist many times and had huge respect for his skills.
>
> The patient had what appeared on our rapid exam to be a perfectly normal airway. However, after a rapid sequence induction, the nurse anesthetist attempting to intubate said, "I don't see anything I recognize, do you want to take over?" The SpO2 was already dropping, so I said no, grabbed a #4 LMA from the back table, and immediately inserted it.
>
> We could then ventilate easily, and the mother and baby did just fine. Yes, it was an unprotected airway. But, in retrospect, I believe attempting to intubate after the inability of a skilled practitioner to control the airway would have been a mistake and could have led to serious injury to the patients.

From Ron Bank

I absolutely agree with Rodger. He echoes points that I tell everyone, from high school students to fellows, about anesthesia, especially cardiac and critical care anesthesia, all the time.

I think that the judgment chapters coauthored by the federal judges are most relevant to more macroissues—such as making big decisions, giving advice, life in general. This is entirely distinct from the kind of judgment that is required in clinical anesthesia in general, and cardiac/critical care anesthesia in particular. In fact, I would add "seconds" to Rodger's "minutes, hours, days" timeline.

I've long said to all levels of trainees—as well as to colleagues from many areas of medicine—that you must know yourself. That while anything can be learned, you must know your personality—with regard to your ability to make literally life and death decisions sometimes in seconds, under stress, with incomplete information. This is entirely different from that with which a judge is faced, or an internist, family medicine, or many other doctors. In fact, you don't just have to have the ability to perform in that manner; you must thrive in doing so, or you'll never be happy in your field.

All anesthesiologists can be faced with sudden life and death decisions—for example, a can't intubate/can't ventilate airway or malignant hyperthermia. And anesthesiologists in some of the anesthesia subspecialties—such as cardiac anesthesia—are faced with particularly complex, critical decisions frequently. In doing so, they become more stress-inoculated and accordingly become better as they hone their skills.

We've all noticed that different fields are more compatible with different personalities. Different fields have different cognitive, temporal, psychological, and physical demands. Thus, similar people gravitate to a given field. I think that anyone who considers a career in anesthesia has to be able to consistently make good decisions—good calls—under pressure, and who enjoys the challenge of doing so. I think, for example, many family medicine doctors would just hate and be totally stressed out by cardiac anesthesia. Conversely, I think that most cardiac anesthesiologists would be bored and unsatisfied with the pace of family medicine.

I think that a lot of the ability to make such snap decisions well rests in a very solid understanding of the physiology, pharmacology, and the science that goes into our field. The larger the body of knowledge that one has to draw on, the better equipped one is to make what would appear to others to be snap decisions, while, to the anesthesiologist making them, they are fast but very well-informed decisions.

The other factor is clinical experience, which comes with time. While we cannot undo some of our incorrect decisions, we can avoid making some errors by relying on colleagues—especially senior ones—for advice in the moment if they're in the OR or just a phone call away.

I also think that, as I alluded to in some of my "words of wisdom" elsewhere in this book, a critical skill that evolves is the ability to prioritize what one is doing in a clinical situation so that catastrophic errors become less likely by being less distracted with less important things during critical times.

***Note from the Editors:** Speaking of judgment, the Hague in the Netherlands is the home of the International Court of Justice as well as several remarkable bridges, including this convex canal bridge (Fig. 122.1). We like it because it illustrates the old commonsense maxim that with a lot of things in life, what you put in is what you get out, and what goes around comes around.

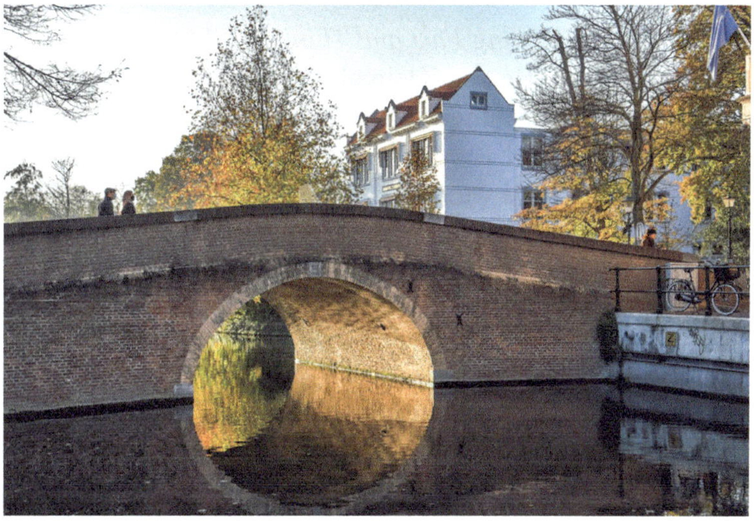

Fig. 122.1 The convex bridge of the Mauritskade at the Nassaulaan, The Hague, Netherlands, with a perfect reflection in the still waters of the canal. The bridge has been featured in many paintings and prints of the city. Photo: Image used under standard license from adobe.stock.com

From Cathy Marcucci and/or Jake Seagull

In reviewing the early versions of this essay, Jake noted that both Rodger and Ron went on to state their belief that there is an innate, DNA-derived ability or inborn "substrate" that must be present to exercise clinical judgment—that the ability to make appropriate or "correct" clinical decisions under intense time pressure is something you are born with.

Jake cautions us, however, that this has <u>not</u> been borne out by the science.

Clinical Decision-Making and Judgment, Like All Judgment, Is Learned

It is most definitely, in and of itself, not an inborn trait that rests in an anesthesiologist's DNA. People are born with differences in intelligence and personality traits and have different levels of discipline and motivation. And so, it is a combination of these circumstances that combine to make a superb clinical anesthesiologist, not an inborn ability to make clinical judgments.

Here Is a Summary of What Jake Wrote to Cathy on the Subject

- The concept of "innate ability to judge" is not correctly conceptualized.
- Gary Klein spent most of his life studying how the "innate expertise" and ability to make quick judgment is *NOT* innate but can be acquired. Throughout his work, Klein talks about "naturalistic decision-making" and "recognition-based priming" as decision-making that happens in context under time pressure. Naturalistic decision-making stands in contrast to the "classical decision-making" studies that involve weighing evidence and taking time to calculate probabilities.
- Daniel Kahneman's recent book *Thinking Fast and Thinking Slow* outlines and contrasts the two different types of decision-making [1]. He and Klein also wrote a seminal paper about the two different styles of "decision-making"/judgment under uncertainty. The paper's subtitle is "A failure to disagree" [2]. The Kahneman/Klein paper is very academic and a bit dry, but the book is not. It was on the New York Times bestseller list, and we recommend it as a really interesting read.

Put in the simplest terms, sure, there are personal cognitive styles, and there are people who are better at various tasks than others. True in every domain. But we should not over-generalize. It doesn't mean that situated cognition can't be learned or is an intangible, mysterious skill.

It is absolutely true that you can train to recognize contexts quickly. There are training principles for that type of skill. You can also learn strategies. For example, a chapter in *Avoiding Common Anesthesia Errors* is pertinent to the clinical vignette above—it reiterates the point about learning not to try and intubate over and over, but rather the "three strikes and you're out" rule.

We must keep in mind that those of us who are working in and writing for the anesthesia community have not invented the distinction between "thinking fast/thinking slow." These have been well-studied. The synopsis of the Kahneman paper cited above gives a tiny window into these basic principles [2].

- This article reports on an effort to explore the differences between two approaches to intuition and expertise that are often viewed as conflicting: heuristics and biases as opposed to naturalistic decision-making.
- Starting from the obvious fact that professional intuition is sometimes marvelous and sometimes flawed, the authors attempt to map the boundary conditions that separate true intuitive skill from overconfident and biased impressions.
- They conclude that evaluating the likely quality of an intuitive judgment requires an assessment of the predictability of the environment in which the judgment is made and of the individual's opportunity to learn the regularities of that environment. Subjective experience is not a reliable indicator of judgment accuracy.

Summary

Jake agrees with much of Rodger's and Ron's thoughts. The decisions we must make can be very different than those made in the courtroom. There *are* anesthesiologists who are better than others and even physicians who should not be anesthesiologists at all. But this is because they have decided, on some level, that they don't care to make the investment to be, not because they can't be in absolute terms. Anybody who wishes to improve their clinical judgment—even to a high level of performance—can do so with enough time, exposure to the clinical environment, interest, teaching or coaching, study, attention, dedication, and diligence.

Rodger Barnette knew what to do with the patient in the scenario above because he is smart, deeply interested in anesthesiology and his patients, and experienced. And because he cared enough at some point to do the work that allowed him to gain the expertise he would need to draw on, not because he was born instinctively knowing what to do. Keep in mind that Dr. Barnette is triple boarded—the care of critical patients has been his life's work. His clinical experience and excellence have become second nature to him—so much so that he feels like he was born with certain abilities (and we respect that), but he wasn't.

The same is true of Ron Bank, who is known as a superb clinician. Ron put the time and effort into becoming an expert as each new technique and piece of equipment became available, going back to his training days, and now, years later, his ability to make rapid decisions in clinically acute situations looks as if it "comes naturally" to him.

Lessons Learned

- What is meant by "good judgment" is very much situation-specific! In the courtroom, it involves evaluating all available evidence and taking the time to carefully conclude. In the practice of anesthesia, it almost always involves making sound clinical decisions under constant critical time pressures.
- When teaching, advising, and mentoring junior physicians, do not discount this aspect of our profession. Do the possible time pressures in clinical decision-making represent a fascinating challenge that you want to (possibly) do every day, or something to be dreaded and avoided?
- We believe that all great clinical anesthesiologists have a fundamental understanding of and affinity for physiology and pharmacology. We don't see how you can ever capably perform or enjoy the practice of anesthesiology without this.
- We urge all anesthesiologists who are interested in how we learn our specialty to spend a bit of time learning about the concepts of fast thinking and slow thinking.
- *Clinical judgment is learned.* It is a skill that is potentiated by interest, discipline, exposure, and practice. Isn't this the basis of simulator training?
- What we call *intuition, or a gut feeling, does exist*, but it is not innate or inborn; rather, these are learned skills.

- Rodger Barnette is correct when he writes, "Think back over your career and I'm sure you'll be able to remember very smart and very well-meaning colleagues who are not the right person(s) to be in charge of any emergency." But it is important to understand that this doesn't have much to do with a lack of an innate ability to make highly evolved clinical judgments. It's more the situation of that person not having *acquired* those skills, for whatever reason.

References

1. Kahneman D. Thinking, fast and slow. New York: Farrar, Straus and Giroux; 2011.
2. Kahneman D, Klein G. Conditions for intuitive expertise: a failure to disagree. Am Psychol. 2009;64(6):515–26.

Authors

Jake Seagull is a psychologist and human factors expert at the University of Michigan system. He is a great friend of and a frequent contributor to the anesthesia community. When not at home with his family, he is usually out traveling or fishing.

Rodger Barnette has had a fascinating career in clinical anesthesia both in the US and Kenya. He is triple boarded in anesthesiology, critical care medicine, and internal medicine and is chair emeritus at Temple University as well as a consultant in anesthesiology at Kijabe Hospital in Kijabe, Kenya. With his children now grown, Rodger and his wife enjoy living in both the US and Kenya and traveling constantly.

Ron Bank is in full-time practice in the INOVA health system in Northern Virginia, where approximately 50% of his clinical time is in a cardiac surgery room. He also holds a faculty appointment at the UVA School of Medicine and teaches students and trainees at all levels of medicine education.

Cathy Marcucci is a senior academic anesthesiologist and inveterate anesthesiology educator. She is also fellowship-trained in transfusion medicine. When not taking care of patients and/or putting the latest book together, she dedicates her time to mentoring junior colleagues, writing copy for animal rescues, and travel.

Every Label Deserves Your Utmost Attention

123

Raymond G. Graber and Daniel I. Asher

Introduction

If we could give our junior colleagues just one piece of "vigilance" advice (from our personal experience and learned the hard way), it would be that if there is a label, *any label*, give it your utmost attention. We will discuss medication vigilance and medication labels in the following chapter. But there are many other labels that MUST be reviewed and attended to correctly, or else there will be consequences to you and/or your patients. Here are some specific examples of problems that arise from failing to read the labels.

Patient ID

When meeting patients, get in the habit of checking their ID band with them. This not only verifies that you have the correct patient, but it also verifies that the patient indeed has an ID band. You don't want to transport a sedated and intubated patient to the OR and find on arrival that the ID band is missing, and thus there is no way to verify who the patient is during the pre-op huddle. And if you cut off an ID band during line placement, make sure a new one gets put back on! Sometimes, seeing the patient's birthday is a springboard to conversation—for example, we have shared the same birthday with patients.

Consent Forms

We have seen surgeons bring consent forms to bedside and put them in the wrong patient's chart. In addition, we can't tell you how many times we have seen patients go to the OR without a surgical consent form being filled out. You can stand there and witness the surgeon getting consent, but then, on review of the form, discover that he/she forgot to sign or neglected to have the patient sign. When a

R. G. Graber (✉) · D. I. Asher
Department of Anesthesiology and Perioperative Medicine, University Hospitals Cleveland Medical Center, Cleveland, OH, USA
e-mail: Raymond.graber@uhhospitals.or

S. Mohamed et al. (eds.), *Anesthesia Bridges*, https://doi.org/10.1007/978-3-032-08294-7_123

sedated patient goes to the OR without consent, we typically have to get hospital risk management involved; there's extra paperwork, *and no one is happy*. Take the time to verify that consents are complete and for the correct patient, prior to giving any sedation.

Patient Labels/Stickers

We draw blood samples, apply patient labels, and then send these tubes on their merry way to the labs or blood bank. Unfortunately, it's not an uncommon occurrence that patient labels found in the ORs are left over from prior cases. In addition, incorrect labels can find their way into a patient's chart. If you send a type and cross with a wrong name on it, you have caused a major problem. That is why many institutions will do a double check and require two separate samples to type and cross a patient. Always read the name on any label you attach to paperwork or a tube. If you find leftover labels after you are done with a case, make sure they are removed from the room and destroyed appropriately.

Blood Bags

Hemolytic transfusion reactions can occur when a patient is administered the wrong blood. That is why most institutions use two-person verification of patient ID and blood product information prior to administration. In addition, we have seen situations where the sticker on the blood product bag doesn't match the Red Cross label.

Lessons Learned

- *"Read the label" applies to patient ID bands, blood tubes, consent forms, and blood bags, and more—not just medication labels.*
- Read labels compulsively. Each label review takes only a few seconds. A good investment, considering the interminable time it takes to deal with problems, if something unthinkable happens.
- "Vigilance always" is not just a catchy phrase. Live it every day.

Authors

Ray Graber serves as anesthesia department vice chair for quality at University Hospitals Cleveland Medical. He has dual interests in cardiac and orthopedic anesthesia. During his 30+ year career, he has focused on process improvement, reduction of errors, and improving patient outcomes.

Dan Asher is a cardiac anesthesiologist at University Hospitals in Cleveland and is the medical director of the PACU, the system chief of the moderate sedation committee, co-chair of the perioperative quality council, and sits on numerous subcommittees that have a focus on improving the quality and efficiency of care that patients receive. His four kids, all school age keep him and his wife busy, but they make time to be active members of their local Jewish community.

124 Medication Errors

Raymond G. Graber and Daniel I. Asher

Introduction

Now, let's move on to the big stuff—the ways we can really hurt our patients. And, to compound the problems and peril, these errors are sometimes on us and us alone.

Let's Start Off with a True Story

A 21-year-old female underwent a cesarean section under epidural anesthesia around 1:00 AM. After delivery of the baby, cefazolin 1 gram was administered. The patient quickly complained of feeling short of breath, and this rapidly progressed to apnea. She was bag-mask ventilated, induced, and intubated. At the end of the case, she was reversed and extubated. It was discovered that the anesthesia resident had drawn up vecuronium rather than cefazolin. Both were in similar-looking vials with white caps—the resident had grabbed the wrong vial. Although the patient had no physical adverse effects, she did suffer from being awake and paralyzed.

Medication errors cause over 7000 patient deaths and cost our healthcare system over 40 billion dollars every year. They are a particularly big problem in the practice of anesthesia. It has been said that anesthesia is the only area where medications are typically prescribed, prepared, administered, and recorded by a single individual without any other health care professional to monitor the process.

There are many factors that predispose to medication errors. There can be look-alike packaging and labeling, with multiple drugs stored next to each other. Drug vials and infusions can be available in several different concentrations. Poor lighting can make it hard to identify meds. A noisy environment can impair communication. Practitioner fatigue can lead to a lack of attention when handling drugs and infusions, and failure to review patient allergies. The need for speed in emergency situations can lead to errors.

R. G. Graber (✉) · D. I. Asher
Department of Anesthesiology and Perioperative Medicine, University Hospitals Cleveland Medical Center, Cleveland, OH, USA
e-mail: Raymond.graber@uhhospitals.org

S. Mohamed et al. (eds.), *Anesthesia Bridges*, https://doi.org/10.1007/978-3-032-08294-7_124

In 1978, JB Cooper published a landmark paper that analyzed critical incidents that occurred during anesthesia. A critical incident was defined as an incident that led to an undesirable outcome or was a "near miss." Drug administration errors were one of the top three causes of all critical incidents and were responsible for 19% of incidents.

In addition, in a 1995 survey of anesthesiologists in New Zealand, 12.5% of responding anesthesiologists reported having harmed patients by a drug administration error. A review of the American Society of Anesthesiologists Closed Claims Database revealed that medication errors were involved in 4% of these cases. This all leads us to an equation for you to ponder:

Medication errors + patient harm = malpractice claims

Drug errors can occur in a variety of ways. The wrong drug can be administered due to incorrect labeling or grabbing the wrong syringe. There can be administration issues, where a medication is not completely flushed into the patient *or given at all*, given at the wrong time, or given via the wrong route, such as an epidural rather than intravenous. The correct drug can be administered in the wrong dose—commonly seen in pediatrics and also in infusion pump programming errors. An incorrect drug can be selected, such as when patients are given a drug they are allergic to or have a known intolerance to. The most common drug errors are preventable by just carefully reading the labels. Let's discuss these further.

Medication Vials We usually draw up our own meds, and this can lead to two kinds of errors—drawing up the intended drug but putting the wrong label on it, or drawing up the wrong drug and putting the intended label on it. The cefazolin/vecuronium swap described at the beginning of this chapter is an example of the latter. Either way, you now have a syringe of a drug with the wrong label on it.

This is called a *substitution error* and is the most common type of medication error. It's easy for "look-a-like" errors to happen—one drug vial may look like a different drug vial and can get misplaced into the wrong storage slot. So, don't just depend on the location of a vial; read the label. If you are scanning drugs when you remove them from a cart—read the scanning information as you do so—this acts as a double check.

Medication Syringes When selecting a drug for administration, we should always verify the label as we pick up the syringe. However, we sometimes also use secondary cues—like syringe location, size, and label color. As an example, we know of a situation where a patient under epidural anesthesia became hypotensive and was administered succinylcholine rather than ephedrine—because the person involved was rushing and relying on the secondary cues. People grab the wrong syringe all the time—but you protect yourself and your patient by compulsively reading the label as you pick up the syringe, and again as you are administering.

Medication Drips Many pharmacy-prepared bags have labels in small font—making them harder to read. Having multiple drip bags on multiple pumps can lead to problems if the wrong drug is plugged in or started.

***Note from the Editors:** Look closely at these bridges—parallel and very, very similar, but not the same! A metaphor for the problem of similar labels (Fig. 124.1).

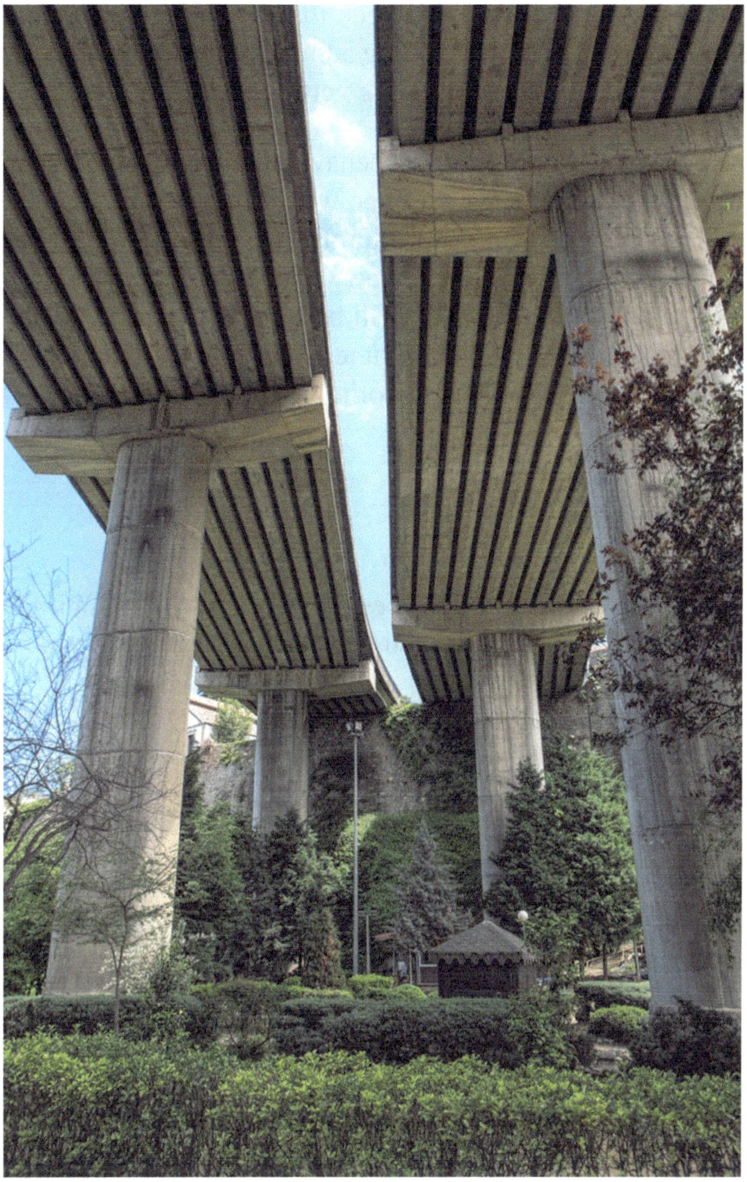

Fig. 124.1 Striking, and almost identical, highway bridges. Photo: Konoplytska, image used under license from iStock.com

What to Do

Besides reading the label, how else can we reduce medication errors? To start, make sure you know the patient's history and allergy list. Know the appropriate dose for all the drugs you administer, and if you are not sure—look it up! Know which drugs need to be given slowly, such as vancomycin and potassium. *All syringes must be labeled properly.*

For example, we have seen staff neglect to put labels on propofol syringes—but there are other drugs (clevidipine, lipid emulsion) that are also white. It is a Joint Commission mandate that all medications not immediately administered must be labeled. Check that you have the correct injection site and that the drug is fully flushed in. Develop compulsive drug administration practices—read the label when you pick up a syringe, and then one more time as you are getting ready to inject.

Fear often isn't a long-lasting motivator of human behavior. It's generally most effective for short-term behavioral change. But, in this instance, we do hope we have scared you, at least a little bit. Lack of attention to medication labels can cause all kinds of problems. During your training, and when you have that first job, you form the work habits that you'll carry with you for the rest of your career. Make compulsively reading labels one of those habits. You will be a better doctor with better outcomes and have fewer problems with your hospital risk management team because of it. And then at the end of the day, you'll be able to happily read the label on your favorite beverage and enjoy!

Lessons Learned

- Medication errors are common, and even the best physicians will commit them. When you have a quiet moment, ask the senior people around you what errors they have seen.
- Medication errors are particularly devastating because we have such autonomy with our medication management principles and practices.
- We all have moments of fatigue, or distraction, or trying to do too much. Forming good work habits early in your career (like compulsively reading labels) will help you reduce errors.
- There are other significant types of medication errors—such as administering drugs in the wrong order or failing to discontinue a medication—and some of these are covered in other sections of this book. Who among us has not forgotten to turn off the nitrous oxide at the end of the case or in other situations when 100% oxygen is called for? So every time you look at the label of a drug to give it, think about when you might or will need to discontinue it.
- Ask your senior colleagues what medication errors and near-misses they have seen or heard about in their careers. We all have seen them—all of us.

Further Readings

Cooper JB, Newbower RS, Long CD, et al. Preventable anesthesia mishaps: a study of human factors. Anesthesiology. 1978;49(6):399–406.

Webster CS, Merry AF, Larsson L, et al. The frequency and nature of drug administration error during anaesthesia. Anaesth Intensive Care. 2001;29:494–500.

Bowdle TA. Drug administration errors from the ASA closed claims project. ASA Newsl. 2003;67:11–3.

McCawley D, Cyna AM, Prineas S, et al. A survey of the sequelae of memorable anaesthetic drug errors from the anaesthetist's perspective. Anaesth Intensive Care. 2017;45(5):624–30.

Authors

Ray Graber has had a long-standing interest in medical error prevention as an aspect of departmental quality improvement work. He gives a talk about medication errors to each new class of anesthesia residents during orientation, with the hope that he can instill a little fear in them.

Dan Asher is a cardiac anesthesiologist at University Hospitals in Cleveland and is the medical director of the PACU, the system chief of the moderate sedation committee, cochair of the perioperative quality council, and sits on numerous subcommittees that have a focus on improving the quality and efficiency of care that patients receive. His four kids, ages nine years and under, keep him and his wife busy, but they make time to be active members of their local Jewish community.

Intravenous Fluids—A Practical Approach

125

Andrew B. Barker

Introduction

The *Anesthesia Bridges* editors think that **Andrew Barker** has put together just about the best summary of IV fluids ever. We recommend that our junior colleagues review this elegant summary of IV fluids frequently and adopt his philosophy and teaching tips that *IV fluids are medications*. We administer IV fluids constantly, yet often do not have a comprehensive understanding and/or of exactly what we are giving and why. Until now.

Basic Fluid Physiology

A. **Distribution of Total Body Water:** Water makes up around two-thirds of our total body mass. To be exact, men are 60% water, while women are slightly less at 55%. A 70 kg man will therefore contain about 42 liters, and a 70-kg woman will contain about 38 liters. The reason for this difference between the sexes is that women contain an extra 5% adipose tissue; the difference is only occasionally of clinical significance.

- 60% of total body weight in adult men
  - TBW = 0.6 × body weight (kg)
- 50% of total body weight in adult women
  - TBW = 0.5 × body weight (kg)
- Percentages decline with aging and increased body fat

A. B. Barker (✉)
Department of Anesthesiology and Perioperative Medicine, Heersink School of Medicine, University of Alabama at Birmingham, Birmingham, AL, USA
e-mail: abbarker@uabmc.edu

S. Mohamed et al. (eds.), *Anesthesia Bridges*, https://doi.org/10.1007/978-3-032-08294-7_125

B. **Volume of Distribution:** There are two compartments that water passes freely between in response to solute concentrations—this maintains osmotic equilibrium

- The Extracellular Compartment
  - Approximately 14 Liters
  - Further divided into the intravascular (plasma) compartment comprising 25% of volume and the extravascular (interstitial) compartments comprising 75% of volume
  - Composed of Na+ 140 mEq/L, 280 mOsm/kg
- The Intracellular Compartment
  - Approximately 28 Liters
  - Composed of K+ 140 mEq/L, 280 mOsm/kg

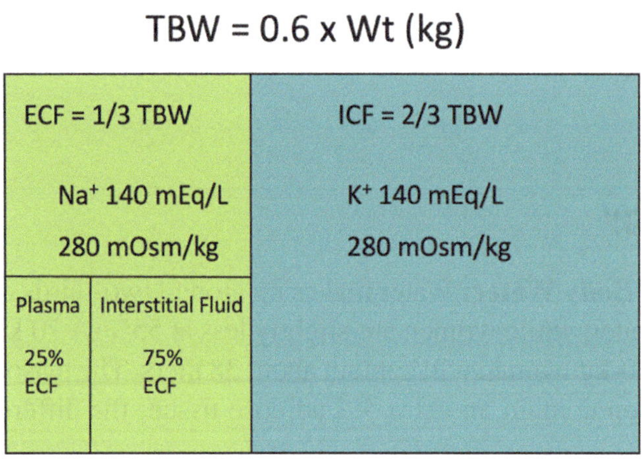

C. **Fluid Shifts:** Fluids can only be given into the intravascular space

- Fluid Loss
  - We lose fluid through our renal and gastrointestinal tracts, and this can be seen and measured.
  - The fluid we lose from our skin and respiratory tract cannot be measured with ease and makes up our insensible losses. These amount to 500 ml a day in health, on average, and increase in sickness, particularly when febrile.
  - In theory, it is possible to gain or lose pure water, but in most cases, fluid moves along with electrolytes, and the result is determined by the balance of water gains and losses, versus solute gains and losses.
- Fluid Gain
  - From iatrogenic IV fluid administration
  - From heart, liver, or kidney organ failure

Intravenous Fluids

A. **IV Fluids Should Be Viewed as a Medication:** the FDA defines a medication as follows:

- A substance recognized by an official pharmacopoeia or formulary.
- A substance intended for use in the diagnosis, cure, mitigation, treatment, or prevention of disease.
- A substance (other than food) intended to affect the structure or any function of the body.
- A substance intended for use as a component of a medicine but not a device or a component, part, or accessory of a device.

B. **Rationale for Fluids as Medication**

- Fluids are composed of a solvent and various solutes in different concentrations.
- Fluids are utilized to modify body composition in different settings.
- Type, amount, route, rate, and frequency of administration constitute a dose.
- Fluid administration has associated toxicity.
- Appropriate use of fluids requires consideration of context and knowledge of physiology.
- Dose-Effect Relationship
  - Fluids have a variety of types of fluids, a variable amount given, an administered route, an administered rate, and frequency.
  - Fluids affect volume status, hemodynamics, organ function, plasma composition, and compartment size.

C. **Indications for Fluids**

- <u>Maintenance:</u> For patients who cannot take oral or enteral fluids (preoperative NPO status, perioperative restriction, on ventilator) but will have ongoing routine requirements.
  - Requirements for adults can be broken into water and electrolyte requirements.
    - Approximately 2–3 Liters (25–35 ml/kg/day)
    - Adjust for insensible losses and other clinical conditions
    - Consider restricting fluid to 2–25 ml/kg/day in older patients, renal impairment, or cardiac failure
    - Use ideal body weight in obese patients
  - Daily water requirements—three approaches

    - 35 ml/kg/day
    - 4/2/1 rule (can be used for adults and children):
      - ml/kg/h for the first 10 kg (0–10 kg)
      - ml/kg/h for the next 10 kg (11–20 kg)
      - ml/kg/h for remaining weight (>21 kg)
    - Weight in kg (>60) + 40
  - Daily electrolyte requirements
    - Sodium and Chloride 1–2 mEq/kg
    - Potassium 0.5–1.0 mEq/kg
    - Calcium 0.2–0.3 mEq/kg
    - Magnesium 0.35–0.45 mEq/kg

- <u>Replacement:</u> Fluids in addition to routine maintenance to meet existing deficits or ongoing losses, such as insensible losses in fever, GI losses, and drain losses.
  - It is important to estimate fluid deficit (how much volume to give) and which fluid compartment is predominantly affected (which fluid to give).
  - Initial Therapy
    - Severe volume depletion required rapid administration of isotonic solutions or Lactated Ringers
    - Mild to Moderate hypovolemia
      - Choose a rate that is 50–100 ml/h greater than estimated fluid losses from urine output, insensible losses, GI loss, respiratory loss, or fever loss.
      - Choice of fluid is based on the type of fluid that has been lost and any coexisting electrolyte disorders.
- <u>Resuscitation:</u> Fluids may need to be given urgently as a bolus to correct symptomatic volume depletion and restore circulation. The following clinical parameters may indicate that urgent fluid resuscitation is required:
  - Systolic blood pressure less than 100 mmHg.
  - Heart rate greater than 90 beats per minute.

- Capillary refill time is more than 2 seconds, or the peripheries are cold to the touch.
- Respiratory rate is more than 20 breaths per minute.

***Note from the Editors:** Andrew Barker's favorite bridge is the Pont du Gard (Fig. 125.1). He tells us why:

> My favorite bridge is the Pont du Gard—a bridge but also a Roman aqueduct with significant history, amazing architecture, and political and economic importance! And since this chapter is all about fluids, I thought it would be fun to select a bridge that made its living down through the centuries by carrying fluids.

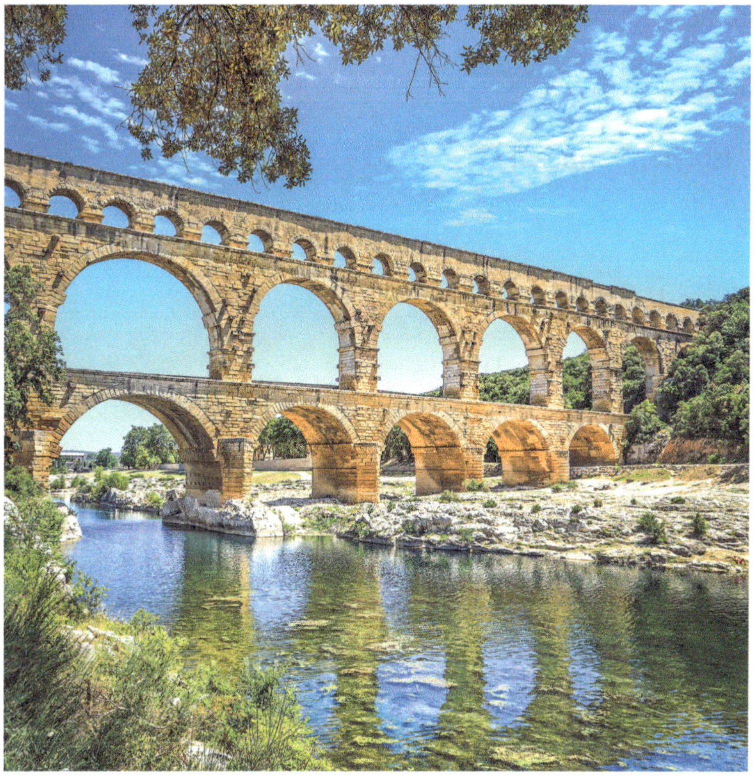

Fig. 125.1 The Pont du Gard is an ancient limestone aqueduct and toll bridge in Southern France, dating back to the Roman era. It was built in the first century AD as part of a 50 km aqueduct to carry water from natural springs near Uzes to a large basin near the Roman colony that preceded modern-day Nimes. It is estimated that it carried over 8,000,000 imperial gallons of water per day. It took only five years to build. The bridge was operational as an aqueduct for around 600 years and as an important tollway for several hundred years after that. It is considered to be one of the most stunning feats of engineering and architectural integrity in all of history. Photo: Image used under standard license from adobestock.com

D. **Types of IV Fluids:** It is important to know your IV fluid formulary and the components in each type of fluid.

- Fluid Types
  - Crystalloid
  - Dextrose in water: D5W, D10W, D50W

- Saline
- Isotonic (0.9%)
- Hypotonic (0.45%, 0.25%)
- Hypertonic (1.5%, 3%): Used in patients with symptomatic hyponatremia, such as in seizure, coma, or cerebral edema
- Combination of D5 and saline
- Balanced (isotonic)
    - Ringer's Lactate
    - Plasmalyte, Isolyte, Normosol
    - Bicarbonate
        - 50, 75 mEq in 1L 0.45% saline
        - 50, 75, 100, 150 mEq in 1L D5W
- Colloid
    - Albumin (5% or 25%)
    - Hetastarch
    - Dextrans

- <u>Fluid Contents</u>
    - Each type of fluid has different components of electrolytes, pH, and Osmolality. These are always listed on the IV fluid bag.
    - Influences the effect on the fluid compartments and the acid-base, electrolyte, and nutritional homeostasis.
    - Careful attention to the contents and clinical context is imperative to mitigate side effects.
- <u>Fluids Effects and Clinical Use</u>
    - Crystalloid
        - Isotonic (0.9% NS and balanced solutions)
            - Osmolality matches inside the cells, therefore no net change in osmolality, no net movement of water into the cells, and fluid remains in the extracellular space.

    - Expands the extracellular space by 1/3 the volume administered.
    - Used for resuscitation, maintenance, and replacement
  - Dextrose in water
  - 5% dextrose infused into the intravascular compartment will redistribute throughout the whole-body water space, both extracellular and intracellular.
  - Used for dehydration and hypernatremia treatment, not for resuscitation.
  - Hypertonic—shifts fluid from intracellular to interstitial and intravascular space.
- Colloid
  - Remains only in the plasma portion of the extracellular space.
  - Does not redistribute from the plasma space quickly.
  - Most colloids are hypertonic.
  - Used for plasma expansion during resuscitation.

Lessons Learned—A Practical Approach

- *Treat IV fluids as medications!*
- Know your formulary
- Understand where fluids go in the body
- Understand how fluids affect organ systems in the context of coexisting disease and modify your prescription accordingly
- Identify your clinical goal for fluid therapy—*maintenance, replacement, or resuscitation?*
- Choose the fluid type to administer. Identify electrolyte abnormalities that may influence your choice of fluid.
- Choose the rate of fluid administration based on weight and minimum daily requirements.
- Always reassess for therapeutic endpoints, side effects, and continued indication for fluids.

Author

Andrew Barker is an associate professor in the Department of Anesthesiology and Perioperative Medicine at the University of Alabama at Birmingham, Heersink College of Medicine. He is also the critical care medicine fellowship program director and co-medical director of the surgical intensive care unit. His research interests are in postoperative cognitive dysfunction, ICU delirium, patient safety, and coagulopathy. He is grateful for his very supportive wife and three beautiful children. He enjoys playing guitar and fly-fishing when he has time.

Help the Blood Bank Help Us

126

Willy A. Flegel, Ariana S. Cogan, and Catherine Marcucci

Contributors:

Karen Byrne MDE, MT (ASCP) SBB
Marino Bueno MLS (ASCP) SBB

Marina Bueno is the reference technical specialist for the DTM Immunohematology Reference Laboratory, where her expertise is constantly relied on by even the most senior TM staff and physicians. She is originally from the beautiful Tucuman Province in the northwestern region of Argentina. She loves hiking, being in nature, and learning about other cultures.

Karen Byrne was an education coordinator for 25+ years and believes that lifelong learning and professional relationships help keep patients safe and the work environment healthy.

Introduction

It is the editors' conviction that every anesthesiologist, junior and senior, should know a bit more about transfusion medicine than they do. There's an entire department down there, and their sole job is to help us get the right blood and blood products safely and appropriately into patients. A lot of anesthesiologists do not take the time to get to know those colleagues and do not spend much time thinking about how we can best help them help us. This is a mistake.

From Cathy Marcucci

And it's one I made myself, back in my salad days. I blush now to think of the clueless and anxious calls I made to the blood bank when I was a resident first doing big cases, which certainly did not impart any efficiency to the proceedings. I also remember once standing at the blood bank window waiting for

W. A. Flegel · A. S. Cogan · C. Marcucci (✉)
Department of Transfusion Medicine, Clinical Center, National Institutes of Health, Bethesda, MD, USA

S. Mohamed et al. (eds.), *Anesthesia Bridges*, https://doi.org/10.1007/978-3-032-08294-7_126

blood and realizing that I had no idea how many units of blood Hopkins even had at any one time. I asked the tech, "If you gathered up every single unit of packed red blood cells in the hospital tonight, how many units would be in the pile?" And she said, "About six hundred." (Hopkins was a smaller hospital back then than it is today). Made sense, but I could not have come up with that number on my own for anything.

So, we thought it would be fun to get the input of the staff in the Department of Transfusion Medicine (DTM) at the NIH Clinical Center of the National Institutes of Health on how anesthesiologists can do better by the blood bank. As a quick aside, the term Transfusion Medicine ("Transfusionsmedizin") was first used in Germany around 1970 and eventually adopted by blood bankers in the US who quite rightly wanted a term that noted the expanded role of blood banks in blood donation, component preparation, immunohematology, apheresis, therapeutic phlebotomy, and stem cell medicine. Anesthesiologists still tend to refer to "the blood bank," and the terms can generally be used interchangeably without huge harm.

At any rate, DTM at the NIH is the department where **Dr. Harvey J. Alter** did the historical work that led to the discovery of hepatitis B and hepatitis C—the latter of which earned him the 2020 Nobel Prize in Medicine or Physiology. DTM remains a top academic department as well as critically supporting a lot of the NIH's leading stem cell research. **Dr. Willy (Bill) Flegel** is the current medical director of the Transfusion Services Laboratory section of DTM and also has a distinguished national and international position in the TM community with wide-ranging research interests and an astonishing CV. I asked him and several members of the technical staff for their philosophical and common-sense advice for the anesthesia community. They were kind enough to share their thoughts in conversation and correspondence, as summarized below.

Principles of Professionalism

- First and foremost, blood is the most potent therapeutic agent in medicine. Treat it with the utmost respect.

- Second and also foremost, transfusion medicine (TM) physicians and technicians are as much a part of the perioperative care team as we are. Or as **Dr. Flegel** wrote to me, "Transfusion medicine specialists work with you, like you work with them. Treat your colleagues in transfusion medicine like you want to be treated by your colleagues from surgery."

- Never, ever display an impatient or peremptory attitude toward blood bank staff. Ever. The efficient management of personnel resources in a blood bank is key, more so in critical situations. While you may be supporting one patient only, transfusion medicine must remember the needs of many patients in the hospital.

- While we are on the subject of staff, transfusion medicine technologists all have college degrees and are board-certified. Many staff also have a Specialist in Blood Banking (SBB) qualification as well. This involves a year or more of clinical and didactic training at the master's degree level and a separate and rigorous exam. Do not make the mistake of thinking that you know more about the clinical or laboratory medicine aspects of blood banking than the techs do. You don't.

- Blood group matching is a high-risk activity with an impeccable safety record achieved by thorough quality assurance and meticulous documentation. When perplexed about some attitudes in that special field, consider why they foster such mindsets. The blood group laboratories ought to be managed like the cockpit of a plane. Their checklists are called "standard operating procedures" or "SOPs" and were among the first introduced to the hospital setting.

- As a corollary, do not even *THINK* about asking a TM staff member to go against an SOP. Especially when it comes to patient identification or blood component labeling. You can have emergency release blood type O blood if the rollout of the new EMR has gone haywire and you can't scan the patient's ID bracelet, but the blood bank cannot and will not release type-specific blood to a patient who has not been properly identified. Don't even ask.

- Transfusion medicine departments tend to be close-knit working groups. The physician staff will be readily available to consult and collaborate with the technical staff, if necessary. In turn, TM physician staff will work closely with and consult their quality assurance officers. This is necessary and arises from the highly regulated nature of blood banking.

- Like us, transfusion medicine staff must be eternally vigilant and strive to have a perfect safety record, for example, in ensuring that transfusion of wrong ABO-type blood cannot and does not occur. Transfusion medicine and blood bank directors also bear a lot of personal, professional, and even legal liability. It is not unheard of for a TM conference discussion to conclude with, "Well, we are just not doing that, because I'm not going to jail on this issue." This is only half a joke.

Day-to-Day Operations

- Take every opportunity to interact with your transfusion medicine department. Feel free to call or even go there to discuss inventory, schedules, and special issues such as the presence of antibodies. Unless there is an emergency, your attempts to collaborate will be most welcome, and you will only be helping yourself. For example, Cathy Marcucci once asked how long it would take to get additional cross-matched blood and was told, "three days." Unbeknownst to her, the patient had a rare antibody situation, and the two units of fully compatible blood that were available had required involvement of the American Rare Donor Program in Philadelphia. She discussed this with the surgeons, and modifications were made to both the surgical and anesthetic plans.

- The most important thing we can do for our transfusion medicine colleagues is to give them sufficient time. It seems simple, but the earlier we enter our blood orders, the better. Transfusion medicine hates the "night before/morning of" rush to get a patient ready for the OR as much as we do. So, please, do not make blood bank staff chase you down to find out if you want blood.

- And remember, it can take up to three days even to do the type and screen if an antibody workup is required, much less to procure needed units. It is best to try to get a sample to the blood bank at least a week before the anticipated need, even if the sample has to be repeated in the immediate preoperative period.

- Know your institution's parameters for type and screen samples, and keep in mind that there is some variability in this. For instance, at the NIH, a type and screen is valid for three days for both medical and surgical patients. The day the sample is drawn is day 0. The sample expires at midnight on the third day. So, a sample drawn on Tuesday at 10 AM will expire on Friday night at midnight.

- At other institutions, the day the sample is drawn is considered to be day 1. Some institutions will also have a longer interval for a valid type and screen if the patient has not been pregnant or transfused within the last 90 days. This is a simple thing to find out. If you don't know, just place a quick call to the blood bank desk and they will be able to tell you immediately. But regardless of the type and screen policy, if you receive a message to draw a sample or a new sample for type and screen, even if it's in the middle of a trauma case, please comply as promptly as possible.

- Transfusion medicine staff—physicians, supervisors, and techs—spend a lot of time getting to know patients well and closely following their clinical course. Medical charts and records, what's going on in the ICU, and the upcoming OR schedules are reviewed on a constant basis. It is not unusual for a critically ill patient who requires ongoing transfusion to have TM departmental review twice a day.

- Leave decisions on all blood group and HLA questions to the experts in transfusion medicine; they do it all the time and usually know best. That said, if you don't understand why O-positive blood has appeared in a trauma case or why a patient who is A-negative is now receiving A-positive blood, or if you think the wrong component has been sent up to the OR, do not hesitate to immediately call the issue desk or designated call phone to double-check. They will explain it as fully as they can within the time constraints, and you won't get yelled at. Really, do not hesitate to call. Even the blood bank might have made a mistake.

- Remember, platelets do carry ABO blood group antigens but do not express the Rh antigen. A platelet product that is labeled B-positive means that it was collected from a B-positive donor and that trace amounts of red blood cells in the product will be B-positive, not that the platelets themselves are carrying antigens from the Rh blood group. In a perfect world, every hospital would be able to uphold a strict policy of providing exclusively ABO-compatible and Rh-compatible platelet transfusions, but even this is not always possible. Again, if you are concerned about this, ask, but don't argue.

- Don't panic! When you panic, you tend to over-order. This rarely helps the patient and never helps the blood bank. If you are new to a hospital or new to doing big cases, take the time to review the hospital's massive transfusion protocol (MTP). These have usually been created with a lot of time and thought. There will be a designated contact person in the blood bank for the OR staff to work with during MTPs. The most common mistake for anesthesiologists to make is to bombard a variety of TM staff, techs, and physicians with verbal orders for products. The requests for blood components should all be directed through the MTP contact person.

- The problem of over-ordering cannot be completely eliminated, but can be mitigated if you make every effort to keep blood and blood components within the temperature range for that product. If appropriate temperatures are maintained, they can be returned to inventory. Do not, for instance, put an unused platelet product into a cooler for return to the blood bank. And do not pull units out of coolers until they are ready to be checked in and transfused, and never prop the lid of a cooler open. Red blood cell units that are sent to the OR and returned within temperature can be put back into inventory until the original expiration date. However, fresh frozen plasma that is thawed, sent to the OR, and returned can only be in inventory for five days, even if it stays within temperature.

- Generally, it's best not to put a component of any type in the trash. Every blood product in the hospital, no matter how or where it ends up, must be tracked and accounted for. Even if a product is obviously out of temperature or damaged, bag it, and return it to the blood bank, so it can be wasted there.

- Anesthesia staff often use the terms "red" and "yellow" to mean packed red blood cells and plasma. Transfusion medicine staff never use these terms because other components besides plasma are yellow—think platelets and cryoprecipitate. So, say precisely what you need, not the color of what you need.

***Note from the Editors:** Speaking of red and yellow, here are our two favorite bridges that would be right at home in a box of Crayola crayons (Figs. 126.1 and 126.2).

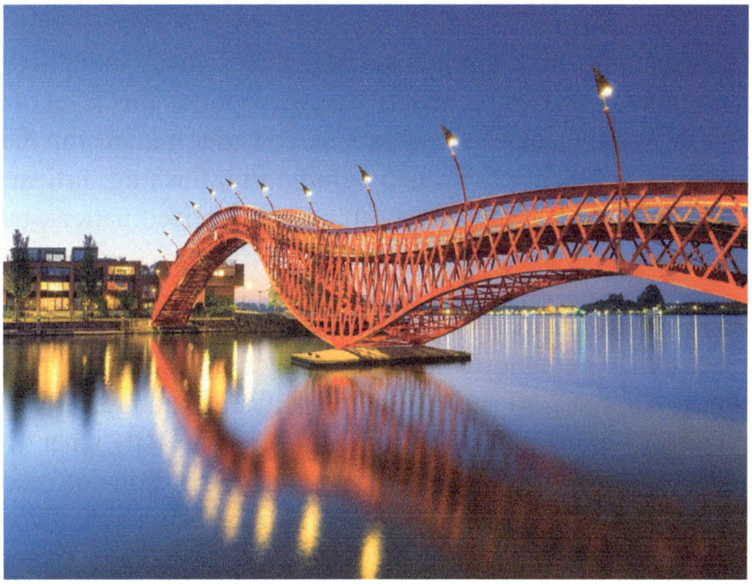

Fig. 126.1 The Python Bridge in Amsterdam. Photo: Image used under standard license from shutterstock.com

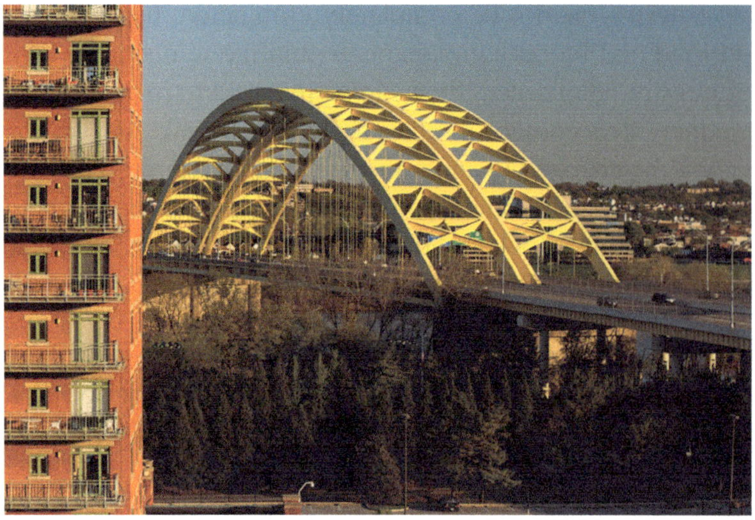

Fig. 126.2 The Daniel Carter Beard Bridge in Cincinnati, OH. Photo: Image used under standard license from adobestock.com

- If you have an evolving or tricky clinical situation, consider calling the blood bank to discuss what your needs are. For example, it may be helpful to ask what product they would recommend or what they can do to help if hyperkalemia is becoming a problem.

- Keep a watchful eye for intraoperative transfusion reactions. They are way under-recognized and underreported. Transfusion reactions ranging from mild to severe are thought to occur in about 1% of all transfusions. It's our thought that you probably haven't reported this level of transfusion complication in your practice to date. In an anesthetized patient, consider transfusion reaction if you are faced with unexplained hypotension, tachycardia, hemoglobinuria, flushing, urticaria, and microvascular bleeding. This last finding might be hard to spot in an anesthetized patient, but pay attention to the patient's eyes and oral mucosa.

- If you suspect that you are dealing with a transfusion reaction, stop the transfusion and call the blood bank immediately for help. Do not ignore the signs and symptoms and try to push through a transfusion reaction using fluids and standard anesthesia drugs. Transfusion reactions can be fatal, although this is fortunately quite rare. The blood bank staff will tell you exactly what to do and what blood to draw to help them rule out clerical errors, hemolytic and allergic transfusion reactions, and the always-serious transfusion-associated lung injury (TRALI) and transfusion-associated circulatory overload (TACO). The sooner you get this done, the sooner you can get the okay to continue transfusing the patient, if possible.

- Consider becoming proficient in thromboelastogram (TEG) and related technologies. There is a learning curve, to be sure, but it can help with solid point-of-care information. Remember, a TEG is really just a pictorial representation of the lifetime of a clot. There's a cute graphic online that represents coagulopathic states as different sizes and types of wine glasses that can help you get started [1].

- If you happen to "mis-spike" a unit and poke through the wall of the component bag, it must be discarded. Do not try to re-spike it.

- **O-negative blood is for O-negative patients!** There are occasional situations where emergency blood is truly needed, but these situations should really be rare. Unfortunately, O-negative blood is sometimes transfused when there has been a failure to plan and/or coordinate. Do not do this.

Final Thoughts from Dr. Flegel

As I have worked as a physician for more than 30 years in transfusion medicine, the practice has changed in many ways and much improved. The blood supply has become safer, and was nevertheless not considered unsafe at the time 30 years ago. The progress in blood product quality will continue unabated and quite possibly accelerate. Transfusion medicine will hence be needed in another 30 years for tasks barely imagined today. Treat our discipline nicely, otherwise we will not be able to maintain and less to recruit the qualified personnel needed for transfusion medicine specialization.

Lessons Learned

- The editors strongly concur with all points above!
- About half the blood that is transfused in the US is administered by anesthesia personnel. What we know about blood and blood components is not always matched by how much we give.
- We would also like to suggest that you consider joining your institution's transfusion committee. It's sometimes hard to get anesthesiologists to sit on this committee, and the transfusion medicine folks don't quite understand why.

Reference

1. FOAMcast. Thromboelastography (TEG) guided resuscitation [Internet]. FOAMcast; 2019 Jul 31 [cited 2025 Jun 13]. Available from: https://foamcast.org/2019/07/31/thromboelastography-teg-guided-resuscitation/

Authors

Bill Flegel started in bone marrow transplantation and infectious disease before completing a transfusion Medicine residency, possibly at the time in West Germany. Although TM physicians do not physically see as many patients as usual in other disciplines, he has nonetheless made decisions based on laboratory samples and tests for hundreds of thousands of patients and millions of blood donors in settings designed for safety and high throughput.

Ariana Cogan trained in a Level 1 trauma center before relocating to the NIH. She is known to be calm and effective in massive transfusion protocols, even when the OR is not. She and her husband and a very cute American Staffie mix live in the Northern Virginia suburbs and enjoy hiking and sightseeing.

Cathy Marcucci has enjoyed doing big cases since her residency days. She is fellowship-trained in vascular, thoracic, and transplant anesthesia (and transfusion medicine) and once gave 1000 units of blood products over the course of just one week in the OR.

What Could Possibly Go Wrong? Why We Huddle

127

Charles H. Sandson, F. Jacob Seagull, Catherine Marcucci, and Raymond G. Graber

Introduction

An operating room suite can be a complex beast. We want our ORs to be efficient and crank out cases, but on the other hand, we need to do this in a safe manner with excellent outcomes. It is easy to see how these goals can conflict. Rushing to get cases started can lead to a range of errors that result in anywhere from minimal to catastrophic harm. Many times, a change in individual patient results may not be obvious, but population outcome studies tell a different story.

You might say, "Wait a minute, we are all highly trained and skilled professionals, compulsive at our jobs, and would never make a serious mistake!" Well, guess what, we all make mistakes. We all have periods of inattention, or times when we might miss something important in a patient's history, or trust that someone else has completed a task. When multiple different personnel miss something, all the holes have lined up in the Swiss cheese model of medical error causation.

So, what are some examples of errors that can occur in the process of trying to get surgical cases going?

Patient Identification

We have all heard horror stories of patients who were not identified properly and have been taken to the OR and had someone else's surgery. And we strongly urge you to read Karen Domino's chapter "Learning from Medical Errors and Adverse Events" elsewhere in this book. Patients should always be identified by at least two identifiers (name and date of birth), and wrist ID bands should be checked on meeting a patient or transporting a patient to the OR. Any ID stickers placed on paperwork or blood tubes should also be verified—we know of cases where blood has been sent for type and cross with the wrong patient label affixed.

C. H. Sandson
ZS Associates, Washington, DC, USA

F. J. Seagull
Center for Bioethics and Social Science in Medicine, University of Michigan Medical School, Ann Arbor, MI, USA

C. Marcucci
Department of Transfusion Medicine, Clinical Center, National Institutes of Health, Bethesda, MD, USA

R. G. Graber (✉)
Department of Anesthesiology and Perioperative Medicine, University Hospitals Cleveland Medical Center, Cleveland, OH, USA
e-mail: raymond.graber@uhhospitals.org

S. Mohamed et al. (eds.), *Anesthesia Bridges*, https://doi.org/10.1007/978-3-032-08294-7_127

Surgical Site Identification

We also know about patients who were identified correctly, but the wrong side was operated on. For example, cases like knee scopes and burr holes are being carried out on the wrong side. In addition, we have seen nerve blocks performed on the wrong (non-operative) arm or leg. That is why surgical sites should always be marked by the surgeon prior to going to the OR.

Antibiotic Prophylaxis

The data are clear that timing has an effect on the ability of antibiotic prophylaxis to be effective. Most antibiotics are best given in the one-hour window prior to incision. In addition, antibiotic choice matters, too. You need to know about significant antibiotic allergies. Methicillin-resistant *Staphylococcus* (MRSA) screening is done prior to some types of surgeries, and a positive result will change your antibiotic strategy. Getting the antibiotic type or timing wrong will lead to an increased risk of infection.

Thromboprophylaxis

Perioperative deep vein thrombosis and pulmonary embolism are complication of many types of surgery. Appropriate use of preoperative subcutaneous heparin, compression stockings, and intraoperative sequential compression devices can help reduce these risks. Failure to address this issue can lead to significant morbidity and even mortality. It is our experience that this particular perioperative complication is especially devastating for patients and families—they may understand intellectually that it's a risk, but the occurrence of a blood clot is often anatomically distant from the surgical site and therefore takes on an especially "unnecessary and untoward" aspect. A patient once told us, "They were operating on my gallbladder and that went okay but I guess no one was paying attention to my leg."

The Preoperative Huddle

To try to deal with issues such as these, the Joint Commission inserted the practice of preoperative time-outs into its hospital accreditation standards in 2003, and this was expanded into pre-op "huddles" by the World Health Organization in 2009. These two measures, consciously or unconsciously, saw the incorporation of industrial engineering techniques into the pre-op process.

Since communication failures are major contributors to over 70% of sentinel events, it makes sense to take steps to improve communication within the perioperative team. Huddles foster communication. Huddles are intended to break down communication barriers, as well as build up a shared understanding of the perioperative plan.

For the uninitiated, the pre-op huddle is a conference between the various teams taking part in an operation, at a minimum nursing, surgery, and anesthesia. The huddle covers a variety of topics, including patient identification, planned surgical procedure, equipment, allergies, antibiotic and DVT prophylaxis, blood availability, and anesthetic technique. It is basically a checklist, where the whole perioperative team can make sure that all necessary protocols are being followed.

For Charlie Sandson, naturally, the newfound standardization these measures have brought is an industrial engineer's dream, especially when you consider what was commonplace before the implementation of the huddle. Surely many nurses and physicians can recall trying to figure things out on the fly when actual case planning information was not readily available or discussed ahead of time. However, Jake Seagull's thinking, with his human factors expertise and extensive experience pertaining to medical mistakes, is that it is not as much about standardizing practice as standardizing the creation of a plan and then communicating it. This should include creating contingencies for unanticipated events—turning them into anticipated events and then making sure the whole team knows what's going on.

***Note from the Editors:** Charlie Sandson attended Rensselaer Polytechnic Institute, where he majored in industrial and management engineering and was a keeper for their NCAA DIII soccer team. This bridge is instantly recognizable to anybody on the RPI campus (Fig. 127.1). Go Engineers!

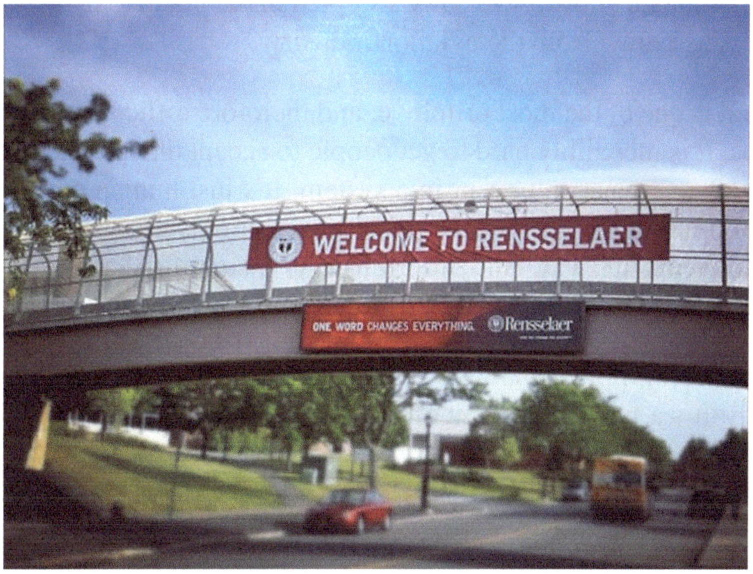

Fig. 127.1 This pedestrian bridge spans 15th Street on the campus of Rensselaer Polytechnic Institute in Troy, NY. Photograph: Courtesy of the Sandson family

The implementation of the huddle helped replace this often-chaotic scramble with a steady structure, the ability to stop and take stock of the situation, ensuring that all stakeholders are working with the same information once surgery commences. This is especially important at teaching hospitals, where the surgeon or anesthesiologist might have a team of junior residents and students. The result is one more layer in the Swiss cheese model, and a reduction of perioperative errors.

In spite of the advances in patient safety that have resulted from huddles, there is still the psychological instinct to resist them. At a certain profound level, the innate human tendency is to think, "This is stupid. Why do we need to waste time going through this formality? We know what we are doing and taking time to stop my prep will delay everything. Plus, it's stupid." Resistance can come from time and production pressures ("we are already running late"), to non-participation by surgeons or thoughts that, "This surgery doesn't need a huddle! We do 15 quick surgeries in a row... we aren't going to stop before each one....".

But if you do a huddle well, it takes less than two minutes, it can prevent errors from happening, and if an error happens, it can make recovery from the error easier. Huddles ideally should shift a group of individuals working separately to do their job toward a team of people working together. So, resist the urge to resist them.

Lessons Learned

- The anesthesia community has always been fairly accepting of and successful at identifying safety needs and implementing strategies to improve care. Be part of keeping that momentum going!
- The concepts of preoperative time-outs and preoperative huddles are based on human factors and industrial engineering principles. These were further developed and expanded by national and international health entities and are now universally accepted in the practice of anesthesia. As discussed in another chapter, they also draw from the aviation industry.
- But remember, denial is one of the most primitive, and therefore difficult to extinguish, psychological defense mechanisms. It is incredibly hard to get people to accept that they themselves are or might be the weak link or the dangerous component in a system. It's just human nature to have the view that surveillance is appropriate for others, while greater autonomy is appropriate for self. The problems arise when everybody feels this way. And unfortunately, unstructured and unsupervised systems will inevitably trend toward decreased levels of performance and safety.
- *This is a fertile area for future research.* Do not think that everything that would benefit from being "huddled" already is. It's a fascinating area of anesthesia practice, and there is still a lot of room for improvement.

Bonus Content!

We advise our readers to try to be thoroughly conversant on the most important and latest quality assurance, quality management, and safety concepts. Flipping the saying, it's important to be able to competently talk the talk, not just walk the walk. So, what is the "Swiss cheese model" referred to above, anyway? It's become one of the dominant paradigms of safety. We all *think* we know precisely what the exact model is and what it means, but do we?

In 2005, Thomas Perneger published an interesting paper titled "Swiss cheese model of safety incidents—are there holes in the metaphor?" [1] He summarized the model, first published in 2000:

> James Reason proposed the image of "Swiss cheese" to explain the occurrence of system failures, such as medical mishaps. According to this metaphor, in a complex system, hazards are prevented from causing human losses by a series of barriers. Each barrier has unintended weaknesses, or holes—hence the similarity with Swiss cheese. These weaknesses are inconstant—i.e., the holes open and close at random.

When by chance all holes are aligned, the hazard reaches the patient and causes harm (Fig. 127.2). This model draws attention to the health care system, as opposed to the individual, and to randomness, as opposed to deliberate action, in the occurrence of medical errors.

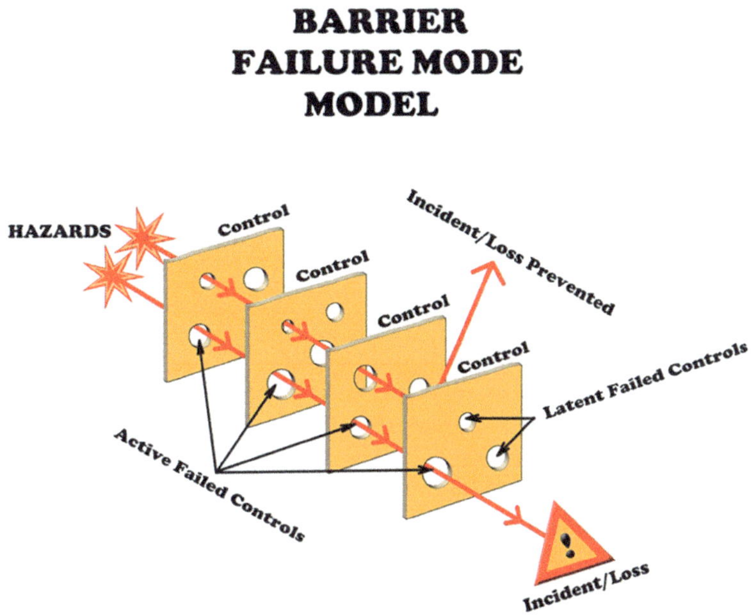

Fig. 127.2 Representation of the Swiss cheese model, first published by James Reason in 2000. Photograph: Image used under standard license from shutterstock.com

He also quotes safety expert Ronald Westrum, who gave the following testimony in testimony to a US Advisory on Blood Safety and Availability, in April 2000:

> Reason's model has become the common language through which complex accidents can be understood. I remember being at one conference where six speakers in a row got up and showed Swiss cheese diagrams as a kind of academic overkill.

Perneger used the figure (Fig. 127.2), without labels or comments, to survey 85 safety and quality improvement professionals, doctors, nurses, and pharmacists at a major safety conference and online. All respondents said they were familiar or very familiar with the model. The survey asked the following questions: What does the slice of cheese represent? What does each hole represent? How or where is an active error represented on this figure? How could we make the healthcare system safer, using the Swiss cheese model? The author supplied five possibilities and asked each respondent to select all that applied. For example, for "What does each hole represent?" the choices were:

- A latent error
- A loss in terms of health or money due to an error
- An opportunity for error
- A weakness in defenses against error
- An unsafe act

The results were fascinating. And all over the place. Perneger summarized them as follows:

- Most respondents correctly identified the slice of cheese as a barrier that protects patients from harm and hence a defense that prevents the occurrence of an error. However, only a few recognized that procedures that alleviate the consequences of an error may also appear as barriers.
- Only a few respondents understood that a hole is either a latent error or an unsafe act.
- The most obvious interpretation of the arrow (path from hazard to harm) was chosen by only half of the respondents. The majority choice (series of events leading to an error) is not entirely correct, as it is patient harm, not an error, that is represented by Reason at the tip of the arrow (however, the error may be equivalent to patient harm, as in wrong-site surgery).
- Only three out of ten respondents correctly identified an active error as one of the holes. Making the system safer by plugging a hole was correctly selected by most respondents, but the solution of adding a barrier (a slice of cheese) was not.

The author's discussion and concluding statements neatly sum up the problem:

> **This survey shows that among quality improvement professionals, the meaning of the Swiss cheese model of medical error is far from univocal.** On average, respondents gave answers that were compatible with the model to about two-thirds of the proposed statements. This is better than half—the proportion that would be expected by chance—but far from a general consensus. This suggests that invoking the Swiss cheese model will not necessarily lead to effective communication, even among quality and safety professionals.
>
> There was substantial variability among respondents as to what the various features of the model represent. The murkiest notion appeared to be the representation of the medical error itself. Few of the respondents recognized that an active error is a type of weakness in defenses against patient harm within the health care system, represented by a hole in the Swiss cheese model (a "hole" is either an active or a latent error). The model is almost too successful in placing emphasis on systemic causes of patient harm, as opposed to an individual's failure.

Since we are in the safety business, it is incumbent on us to make sure we understand the ubiquitous models, catchphrases, and even buzzwords as we use them in our daily conversations and considerations. Also, please don't assume that your listener has the knowledge that you (and they) think they do—we know from the Perneger paper that even the safety "experts" often do not.

Reference

1. Perneger TV. The Swiss cheese model of safety incidents: are there holes in the metaphor? BMC Health Serv Res. 2005;5:71.

Authors

Charlie Sandson is a management consultant in Washington, DC, with a lifelong interest in the principles of safely managing human capital and other resources in interconnected systems. He holds a degree in industrial and management engineering from RPI. He is an expert outdoorsman and also enjoys sports of all kinds, skiing, and traveling when he can get away.

Jake Seagull has spent his professional life swimming with the sharks in the safety pond. He has manifest respect for those among us who can resist thoughts of "no need to check—it'll be alright."

Cathy Marcucci first developed her unending interest in safety as a chemical engineer working in hazardous chemical and natural gas production facilities. She remembers chipping in for personalized safety gear—hard hats and steel-toed boots—when engineering colleagues got promoted.

Ray Graber has been a practicing anesthesiologist in Cleveland since 1988. Early in his career, he developed an interest in process improvement, reduction of errors, and improving patient outcomes. Checklists, protocols, and guidelines are the way to go—especially for the more complex cases!

I've Never Seen It Done This Way

128

Michelle Capdeville

Introduction

Like a number of my contemporaries, my career in anesthesia came as an afterthought. I had matched in a categorical general surgery program at the University of Michigan in 1989, well before a 2-week anesthesiology rotation in my fourth year of medical school in California. After two years of residency, my interests shifted toward anesthesiology and ultimately a cardiothoracic sub-specialty. This was more than 25 years ago, and I still have vivid memories of my beginnings as an attending anesthesiologist at a premier tertiary center renowned for its cardiovascular care. Mind you, this was a time when cardiothoracic surgeons were a bit gruff—yes, this is a polite understatement—and there were very few women cardiac anesthesiologists. I happened to be one of two working full-time in my department.

One Fine Saturday, Early in July…

I have learned time and again over the years never to be complacent, because just when you think you've seen it all, there will always be something lurking out there that tests your ability to fly by the seat of your pants. For instance, I believe I may be one of the only (if not only) cardiac anesthesiologists to start a pump case without an endotracheal tube. More than 25 years later, I still have vivid memories of that experience, and much to my amazement, this story has continued to be passed along like some sort of urban legend—only it really happened!

I was a new staff member, having finished my cardiothoracic anesthesia fellowship just two weeks prior, and was taking call for the very first time—alone. It was a Saturday, so as one can imagine, I was "*it*" for the next 24 hours. The on-call fellow (keep in mind, this was July) and I had gone to pick up an 82-year-old patient in the coronary care unit who was on an intra-aortic balloon pump for emergent coronary revascularization.

Nothing about this cardiac case seemed out of the ordinary from an anesthesia standpoint, other than perhaps the patient's advanced age. I had done plenty of these types of generic cardiac cases as a fellow

M. Capdeville (✉)
Department of Cardiothoracic Anesthesiology, Anesthesiology Institute, Cleveland Clinic, Cleveland, OH, USA
e-mail: capdevm@ccf.org

S. Mohamed et al. (eds.), *Anesthesia Bridges*, https://doi.org/10.1007/978-3-032-08294-7_128

and was in a good comfort zone for my first solo flight. Transport had been uneventful, and after my fellow smoothly inserted an arterial line and PA catheter, I gathered up my syringes for anesthetic induction.

As I looked up at the monitor during pre-oxygenation, hoping it was just a loose EKG lead, I realized that the patient was in ventricular fibrillation. I swore under my breath, promptly gave resuscitation drugs, and instructed the fellow to intubate immediately—no point in hitting the code light since nobody was around. Almost simultaneously, the surgeon, known for his intimidating personality, raged that I had "messed up" the patient (he actually used a more graphic term).

No Endotracheal Tube? No Problem

Naturally, the whole room was flustered, akin to a grizzly bear at a picnic. I myself had two main goals: *first*, take immediate care of the patient; and *second*, give an outward appearance of cool and calm, as I didn't want to come across as a meek member of the female species who couldn't take the heat. As fate would have it, just when things couldn't get worse, my fellow stated he couldn't see anything at laryngoscopy. I stepped in, literally stuffed an oral airway into the patient, and easily mask ventilated him with the intention of reconsidering our approach at securing the airway.

Despite the patient being out of v-fib and relatively stable, after a rapid Betadine prep, the surgeon proceeded to open the chest. With Betadine up my left arm and a sternal saw heading in my direction, I pulled back the mask and reached for the heparin syringe. Before I knew it, we were cannulated, and the surgeon was asking with a hint of sarcasm if I had given him heparin. Inside of me, I wanted to scream, "Did you ask for it?!" but decided this was probably a bad idea.

On Pump

Once we were on the pump at full flow, I stated that the lungs were "down" and tossed the circuit and mask aside. As my fellow and I stood at the head of the OR table staring at our non-intubated patient, I can vividly remember him saying, "I've never seen it done this way." It wasn't until after the aortic cross-clamp was on that we pulled in the difficult airway cart and intubated the patient with laryngoscopy-assisted fiberoptic bronchoscopy under the surgical drapes. By that point, the atmosphere was as though nothing unusual had transpired. Fortunately, the patient had a favorable outcome, and I managed to conceal my own catecholamine surge. By Monday, when I returned to work, this story had made the rounds, with one of my more senior colleagues stating simply, "better you than me."

***Note from the Editors:** Not every bridge has to be hundreds of feet in the air. Sometimes you just need something so that you get across the creek without getting your feet wet (Fig. 128.1). We think this picture is a great metaphor for how Michelle Capdeville made her way through the cases she describes in this chapter—working her way from one little safe spot to the next as the events of the day flowed past her.

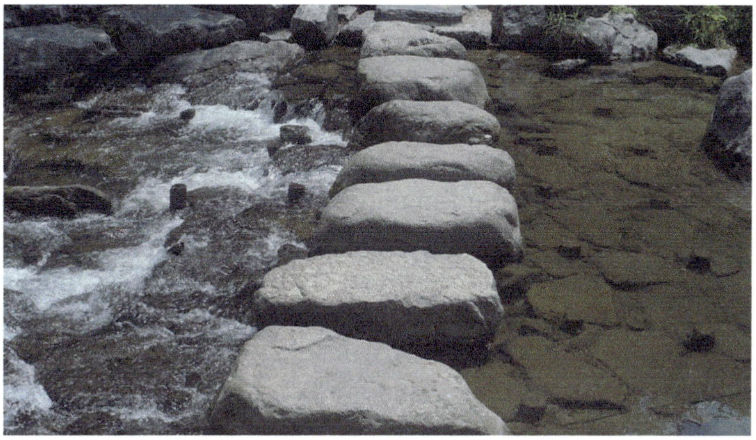

Fig. 128.1 Stepping stones form a small but sturdy bridge and spillway six inches above a creek. Photograph: Image used under standard license from shutterstock.com

Another Saturday, Another Crazy Case

Needless to say, the rest of my calls were a walk in the park. This even includes the time when I was called in to do a lung transplant with a fairly high-strung surgeon who was covering the transplant service (by default, not by choice) after the main transplant surgeon had left the institution. Naturally, this was on a Saturday, and as a new attending, I had never staffed these types of cases before. I kept that little tidbit of information under my hat to minimize any additional stress in the OR.

As luck would have it, about a third of the way through the case, the big OR monitor had frozen up completely, but the display of vital signs and hemodynamics just happened to be picture perfect. Every time the surgeon looked up to glance at the monitor, he was pleased to see that all was well. In the meantime, I had hooked up a small portable transport monitor under the drapes that gave me basic heart rate with audible beeps, blood pressure, and oxygen saturation information, but no end-tidal or other useful display. I kept the blood gas lab busy that day!

When I quietly called the clinical engineer on-call to ask him what to do, he gave me two options: Reboot the monitor and hope for the best or stay the course. I chose option B, because the surgeon would have gone mad if he were to look up at the monitor only to see a blank screen. I chose wisely, because as it turned out, there was a major problem with the monitoring equipment's electronics - I believe the term "fried" was used - and by Monday, a new monitor had replaced the now-defunct piece of equipment. To this day, the surgeon never learned what actually happened - all he knew was that everything was "picture perfect."

Keep Calm and Ride Out the Crisis

These and numerous other experiences have taught me the value of remaining calm in a crisis and to never take anything for granted. Even the simplest of cases or routine procedures can take a turn for the worse, a notion I try to keep in mind every time I enter the operating room. To this day, as one of the more senior members of my department, I am regularly challenged, as our patient population has become older and sicker. I make a point of conveying the importance of taking charge of unstable situations to our trainees.

In a crisis, taking the lead with a calm but firm demeanor can make a chaotic situation more controllable, focus all efforts on the problem at hand, and minimize confusion and panic. Fortunately, the days of adversarial behavior in the operating room are, generally speaking, long gone, but the need to convey a sense of calm authority when the unexpected occurs or a patient is in a life-threatening situation cannot be overstated. And of course, knowing when to call for additional assistance is more of a badge of honor than a perceived weakness.

Lessons Learned

- Always be prepared for the unexpected—it will find you sooner or later.
- Be calm in a crisis. The OR team takes direction better when cooler heads prevail.
- When circumstances allow, call for an extra pair of experienced hands to assist—you will never regret doing so.

Author

Michelle Capdeville has been a cardiothoracic anesthesiologist for over 30+ years. She served as the adult cardiothoracic anesthesia fellowship program director at the Cleveland Clinic from 2008–2017, has been a member of the editorial board for the *Journal of Cardiothoracic and Vascular Anesthesia* since 2005, and a section editor for the journal since 2014.

Protecting the Patient: Points of Pressure

129

Daniel I. Asher and Raymond G. Graber

Introduction

One of the first things we are taught as physicians is *primum non nocere*—first do no harm. Harm can be caused by action, like giving the wrong medication, or by inaction, by not protecting a patient from harm. Let's discuss how we protect our patients on a daily basis in the operating room—specifically things that can get injured by contact such as the skin, nerves, and eyes.

Protecting the Skin

Many of our patients are at increased risk of perioperative pressure injuries. Elderly patients with poor mobility, poor nutritional status, increased or severely decreased BMI, peripheral vascular disease, and thinner subcutaneous tissue are at the highest risk, but any combination of those risk factors in younger patients can also put your patients at risk. Exposing them to a long and complex procedure further complicates matters. Pressure ulcers tend to develop at points of bony prominences, such as the elbow, sacrum, scapulae, coccyx, and heels, and are exacerbated by shear forces exerted when applying angular pressure, such as when shifting a patient without lifting them up off the bed.

Pressure points will vary with the type of positioning—we have seen forehead and chest ulcerations from prone positioning for spine surgery. Many operating rooms use a variety of gel padding, memory foam, and egg crate type foam padding in efforts to protect pressure points. Multilayer foam dressings can be applied prophylactically over pressure points (like the sacrum) to disperse the pressure and minimize the shear forces, and they have also been shown to reduce pressure ulceration risk. Also, be aware of the risk of skin injury during repositioning to and from prone or lateral positions. We have seen skin tears in patients with tissue paper-like skin as a result of these movements.

D. I. Asher (✉) · R. G. Graber
Department of Anesthesiology and Perioperative Medicine, University Hospitals Cleveland Medical Center, Cleveland, OH, USA
e-mail: Daniel.Asher@uhhospitals.org

S. Mohamed et al. (eds.), *Anesthesia Bridges*, https://doi.org/10.1007/978-3-032-08294-7_129

Protecting the Nerves

Unfortunately, peripheral nerve injuries (PNIs) can occur as a consequence of poor protection of our patients during anesthesia and surgery. Nerve injuries can be a complication of an injection of local anesthetic or the surgical procedure but also may occur as a preventable complication of patient positioning—where either excessive stretch or compression is usually the culprit. Awake patients can feel the effects of nerve ischemia and will adjust body position to avert injury; however, the anesthetized patient is unable to do so. *In a study of the American Society of Anesthesiologists Closed Claim Database, nerve injury accounted for 16% of legal claims.*

Some patients have pre-existing conditions that may predispose them to PNIs—specifically issues that affect the microvasculature of nerves, such as hypertension, diabetes mellitus, and smoking. Pre-existing peripheral neuropathies may predispose to PNI. Anatomic variations can also contribute to a given patient. For example, patients with thoracic outlet narrowing may be predisposed to brachial plexus injuries. Men have a 2:1 greater incidence of ulnar neuropathy than women, and this is thought to be due to the larger coronoid process and less adipose tissue over the medial aspect of the elbow. Patients with extremes of body fat, both low and high, may also be predisposed to PNIs.

Surgical Factors

Many PNIs are out of the anesthesia team's control and occur as a consequence of the surgical procedure. Where nerves are adjacent to bone, repairs of fractures of those bones can lead to injury. The radial nerve wraps around the humerus and is at risk in a mid-shaft humerus fracture repair. The brachial plexus lies under the clavicle and can be injured during fixation of a clavicle fracture. Common peroneal nerve injury can be seen after total knee arthroplasty—possibly related to the stretch of the nerve that occurs during correction of excessive valgus deformity or flexion contractures. Sciatic nerve injury has occurred with hip arthroscopy, total hip replacement, and as a result of an acetabular fracture or surgical repair. Excessive tourniquet pressure or time can lead to perioperative nerve injury.

In cardiac surgery, sternal retraction can compress and stretch the brachial plexus. Many nerves travel with vascular structures, and these can get injured when these vessels are dissected, accessed, or harvested. The saphenous nerve can be injured during saphenous vein harvesting. The radial nerve can be injured during radial artery harvesting. Brachial plexus can be injured as a result of axillary artery cannulation. Phrenic nerve injury can occur as a result of internal mammary artery dissection.

Know the Risk Factors and the Safeguards to Take!

Where we can have an impact is in the prevention of PNIs related to positioning. It is important to know the nerves at risk for each type of surgical positioning. In general, the ulnar, radial, and common peroneal nerves, along with the brachial plexus, are anatomically most vulnerable to injury due to intraoperative positioning. These nerves need to be protected with adequate padding and the avoidance of excessive stretch during positioning.

In addition, key sites should be periodically monitored to check that the patient hasn't shifted position during surgery from changes in table position or retractor use. For example, if a head falls off to the side of a foam ring, it may place additional stretch on the brachial plexus. Make sure limbs are secured in place. Arms can fall off arm boards, and similarly, legs can fall off tables. Nerve injuries still occur despite adequate positioning and padding—most likely due to exacerbation of pre-existing neuropathy.

Let's talk about some general strategies for protecting our patients' nerves:

Brachial Plexus: Limit arm abduction in a supine patient to 90°. Keep the head and neck neutral to the rest of the spine to avoid extra stretch on the plexus. In the lateral position, use a roll under the chest to reduce compression of the plexus—and make sure the roll itself isn't compressing the axilla. Avoid the use of shoulder braces in a steep head-down position—this practice can lead to stretch of the brachial plexus.

Ulnar Nerve: When supine with arm on an arm board or tucked at side, position the arm so as to decrease pressure on the ulnar groove of the humerus—this means the forearm is typically neutral ("thumbs up" or mildly supinated). Arms can be wrapped with blankets or protected with foam cushioning. In the prone position, make sure the ulnar groove area is adequately cushioned.

Radial Nerve: Watch out for pressure on the radial nerve as it wraps around the humerus. We have seen a radial nerve injury due to pressure against the nerve from a beanbag being used for lateral positioning.

Peroneal Nerve: Padding should be used to prevent pressure of any hard surface against the peroneal nerve at the fibular head. Although commonly associated with the lithotomy position, peroneal nerve injury has also been seen after lateral positioning.

One last thing to consider—nerve injuries can also occur postoperatively. Splints, casts, and braces can cause compression to nerves. A rare (but additional) cause of perioperative nerve injury is post-surgical inflammatory neuropathy (PSIN). In this condition, surgical trauma results in immune stimulation, and is primarily expressed as inflammation of neural tissue—with resultant nerve dysfunction. This may occur in the region of the surgery but can occur at a completely remote site elsewhere in the body.

***Note from the Editors:** The key to preventing nerve injuries is to keep the 3D spatial orientation of the nerve, bony, and soft tissues in mind. We thought the Nanpu Bridge in Shanghai, China, would be a good metaphor for the complexity of the anatomic geometry (Figs. 129.1 and 129.2).

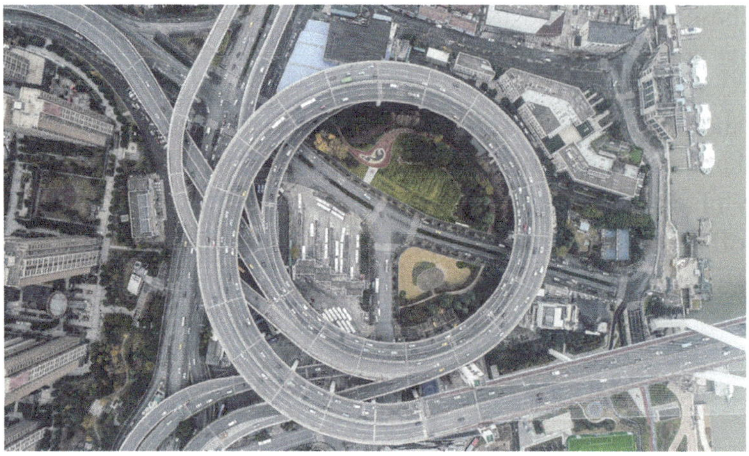

Fig. 129.1 Aerial view of the approach to the Nanpu Bridge in Shanghai, China. Photograph: Image used under standard license from stock.adobe.com

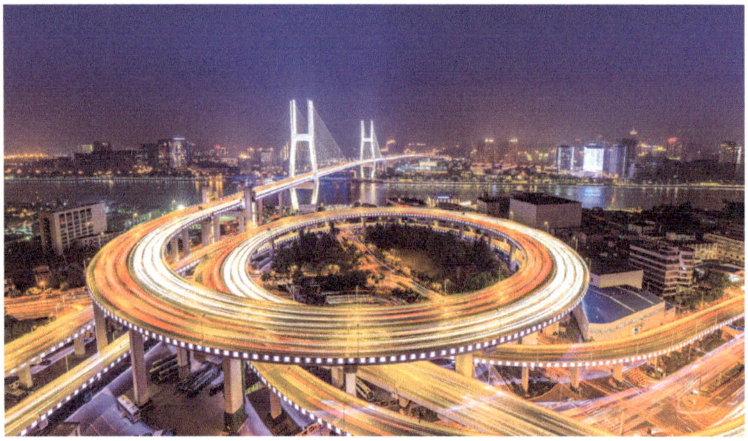

Fig. 129.2 Nanpu Bridge at night. The highway access to the bridge is even more spectacular than the actual span. Photograph: Image under standard license from iStock.com

Protecting the Eyes

In this section, we will talk specifically about corneas. The corneal epithelium can be injured via a variety of methods—including trauma, exposure, and chemical irritation. The result is a defect in the corneal epithelium. There is a tendency to group all these mechanisms together and use the generic term "corneal abrasion" for any of these causes of epithelial defect. However, this is misleading because the most common cause of perioperative corneal epithelial defects is probably not trauma, but rather exposure and drying.

While under general anesthesia, basal tear production is about 25% of normal, lack of complete eye closure (lagophthalmos) occurs in 59% of patients, and blinking does not occur. In addition, patients are frequently exposed to high flows of oxygen by face mask in the recovery period or while under sedation in the operating room. The incidence of corneal injury depends on patient and procedure risk factors and the type of preventive care used. *Overall, if no preventive care is used, such as lubrication and taping, the incidence is 10–30%.* With lubrication and eye taping, the incidence drops to 0.05–0.15%.

Patient risk factors include age greater than 50 years, Sjogren's syndrome, protrusion of the eyeball (proptosis or exophthalmos secondary to hyperthyroid disease), facial palsies with incomplete eye closure, and a history of recurrent erosions from contact lens use.

Certain surgical procedures have a higher incidence of corneal injury. Procedures involving the head and neck seem to have an increased risk of corneal injury, either due to antiseptic chemical irritation or direct trauma. Another risk factor appears to be the development of conjunctival edema (chemosis). This bulging of the conjunctiva may cause loosening of the eye tape and lead to conjunctival exposure.

Significant conjunctival edema can be seen in multiple scenarios, such as when patients have received a lot of IV fluid, in prone cases, in the dependent eye in lateral position cases, and in the Trendelenburg position. For example, it has been reported that long laparoscopic or robotic prostatectomies, which are typically performed in a steep Trendelenburg position, have a higher incidence of associated corneal injury. There appears to be a higher risk of corneal injury in general when cases exceed 90 minutes.

The key to the prevention of corneal injury is maintenance of complete lid closure. Tape or transparent IV dressings are generally used to seal the eyes shut. Ophthalmic ointments or gels also provide protective benefit, especially if you have a patient or procedure that falls in one of the risk groups described above. Most corneal epithelial defects will heal rapidly in a few days, but in the meantime, they are extremely uncomfortable for the patient.

Conclusions

While under anesthesia, patients lose some of the protective responses and reflexes that keep their bodies safe and functioning while in an awake state. It is our job to take over these protective functions while a patient is in our care, and also to limit the complications that occur as a result of our care.

Lessons Learned

- Skin injuries are more common than you think—learn the pressure points and make sure your operating room staff are protecting them appropriately.
- Nerve injuries are devastating. Know the common mechanisms of nerve injury for each position.
- Most corneal injuries are due to drying of the epithelium. Keep them lubricated and sealed shut.
- Make the prevention of nerve injuries part of every teaching case and every sign-out.

- *Advice from the editors*: If we could add one piece of caution to this excellent summary, it would be to redouble efforts to prevent nerve injuries in parturients. We've seen some significant and long-lasting deficits in these patients. It seems as if everybody is focused on getting the baby safely delivered and the fact that the patient is undergoing a major medical and/or surgical intervention gets lost in all the excitement.

Further Readings

American Society of Anesthesiologists Task Force on Prevention of Perioperative Peripheral Neuropathies. Practice advisory for the prevention of perioperative peripheral neuropathies 2018: an updated report. Anesthesiology. 2018;128:11–26.

Cheney FW, Domino KB, Caplan RA, et al. Nerve injury associated with anesthesia: a closed claims analysis. Anesthesiology 1999;90:1062–9.

Martin DP, Weingarten TN, Gunn PW, et al. Performance improvement system and postoperative corneal injuries: incidence and risk factors. Anesthesiology. 2009;111:320–6.

Spruce L. Back to basics: preventing perioperative pressure injuries. AORN J. 2017;105(1):92–9.

Authors

Dan Asher is a cardiac anesthesiologist at University Hospitals in Cleveland and is the medical director of the PACU, the system chief of the moderate sedation committee, co-chair of the perioperative quality council, and sits on numerous subcommittees that have a focus on improving the quality and efficiency of care that patients receive. His four kids, ages nine years and under, keep him and his wife busy, but they make time to be active members of their local Jewish community.

Ray Graber serves as anesthesia department vice chair for quality at University Hospitals Cleveland Medical. He has dual interests in cardiac and orthopedic anesthesia. During his 30+ year career, he has focused on process improvement, reduction of errors, and improving patient outcomes.

Protecting the Patient: The Airway

130

Emily T. Poynton and Raymond G. Graber

Introduction

Let's continue our discussion about protecting the patient. Airway management is one of the cornerstones of anesthetic care. Let's talk about how we protect the teeth, larynx, and lungs during intubation and ventilation.

Protecting the Teeth

A patient's smile is part of how they greet the world—and part of having a great smile is having great teeth. Unfortunately, these teeth are at risk every time the airway gets instrumented. The incidence of dental injury during anesthesia probably depends on how closely one looks—and has been reported to be in the range of 1:1000 to 1:4500 in retrospective studies, but as high as 25% in a prospective study. Injuries can range from loosening or dislodging teeth to damaging the surface of enamel or veneers. *The maxillary incisors have the highest risk of getting injured.*

Prevention of injury starts with a good preoperative history and examination of the teeth. You need to find out where the at-risk areas are. Teeth that are already significantly loose from periodontal disease are at risk for further loosening during airway management. Patients should be cautioned that these teeth are at risk for dislodgement. The presence of crowns and veneers, and bridges should be noted. If general anesthesia is planned, dentures are removed prior to going to the operating room.

A number of methods have been advocated to try to protect the teeth. A strip of microfoam surgical tape can be wrapped around a laryngoscope blade to give a slight cushion to the surface. Custom or off-the-shelf dental guards can be used to protect the teeth. The downside to these is that they do take up at least some space and may make visualization more difficult in the scenario of limited mouth opening. They can also fall out and drop into the pharynx. Video laryngoscopy has also been shown to produce less pressure on teeth than traditional laryngoscopy blades.

E. T. Poynton (✉) · R. G. Graber
Department of Anesthesiology and Perioperative Medicine, University Hospitals Cleveland Medical Center, Cleveland, OH, USA
e-mail: emily.poynton@uhhospitals.org; raymond.graber@uhhospitals.org

S. Mohamed et al. (eds.), *Anesthesia Bridges*, https://doi.org/10.1007/978-3-032-08294-7_130

Teeth injury can also occur during emergence. Patients can bite down on endotracheal tubes, suction devices, or oral airways. Rolled cotton gauze bite blocks can be used to prevent patients from biting on their tubes. These are best positioned laterally in the mouth between the molars. Molars anatomically handle compression forces well, while front incisor teeth are not meant for that purpose and can be levered out.

***Note from the Editors:** We try to include the number system for the dentition in every book we do (Fig. 130.1). We think it's helpful as well as best practice to include the correct name and number of any problem teeth in the preop assessment and/or postop notes.

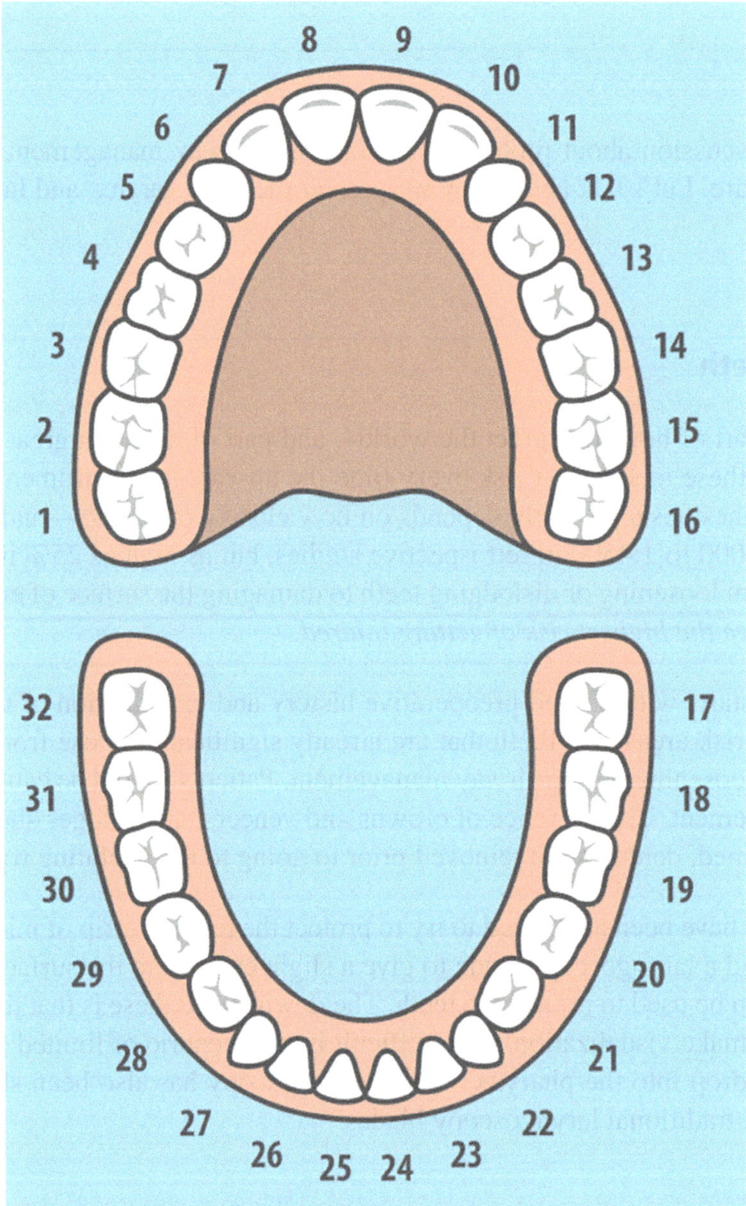

Fig. 130.1 We are airway professionals, and the dentition is the part of the airway that we see the most, so try to use the precise name and number of the tooth if there is a dental issue with a patient, either preop or postop. Remember that the teeth that are numbered 1, 16, 17, and 32 are wisdom teeth—not always present in children and often extracted in adults. (Photograph: Image used under standard license from shutterstock.com)

Protecting the Vocal Cords

We depend on our voices to function in our daily worlds. Some of our patients may be singers, actors, clergy members, lawyers, or other professionals who get up before people and are dependent on having a good "voice." Unfortunately, there are a number of potential vocal cord injuries that occur as a result of intubation.

A large percentage of patients will have sore throat and hoarseness (up to 70%) after short-term (2–3 hours) intubation, with the vast majority resolving in 3–4 days. Hoarseness is typically due to edema or swelling of the vocal cords. However, studies in patients who have been intubated in an ICU setting for even relatively short periods show an additional finding—vocal cord ulcers and granuloma formation at the point of contact with the endotracheal tube.

A prospective study of 3093 adult patients examined the time course of hoarseness after intubation. Hoarseness was observed in 49% of patients on the day of surgery and in 29%, 11%, and 0.8% on 1, 3, and 7 postoperative days, respectively. In the 25 patients who were still hoarse at 7 days, ENT evaluation revealed arytenoid cartilage dislocation in 3 patients (0.097%) and vocal cord paralysis in 4 patients (0.13%).

Patients with unilateral vocal cord paralysis clinically present with changes in voice quality, intensity, and vocal fatigue. These patients aren't able to cough as well, either. The mechanism of this injury is thought to be due to high-endotracheal tube cuff pressures causing injury to the recurrent laryngeal nerve. Remember that the anterior branch of the recurrent laryngeal nerve can be compressed between the endotracheal tube's cuff and the lamina of the thyroid cartilage.

One anatomic study showed that the nerve was at risk of compression when the cuff was just below the cords—and recommended that the upper end of the cuff should be at least 1.5 cm below the cords. The risk of vocal cord paralysis appears to be increased in patients who have risk factors for poor tissue perfusion—age greater than 50, history of diabetes or hypertension, ICU patients who are unstable and are on vasopressors. Duration of intubation and high-endotracheal tube cuff pressures also increase the risk. Recurrent laryngeal nerve injury can also occur as a consequence of surgical injury during thyroid, carotid, and anterior cervical spine surgeries.

So, what strategies can we use to try to protect the vocal cords of our opera singing patient? Well, to start with, if the surgical procedure is amenable, use a regional anesthesia technique and avoid instrumenting the airway. When appropriate, laryngeal mask airways have less effect on vocal cord function than endotracheal tubes. However, a sore throat still occurs, and rare events like arytenoid dislocation are still possible. Preoperative dexamethasone has been advocated to reduce inflammation of vocal cords, and preoperative proton pump inhibitor has been recommended to reduce the risk of acid reflux irritation of cords.

When intubation is planned, the patient should be adequately relaxed prior to intubation attempts. If you don't get a good view with direct laryngoscopy, switch to video laryngoscopy, so that you are not blindly poking at the vocal cords. Using a smaller tube size (6.0–7.0) has resulted in decreased incidence of sore throat and hoarseness.

Make sure the cuff is adequately past the vocal cords and that cuff pressure is in a good range. Ideally, measure cuff pressure and maintain it in the range of 20–30 cm H2O. Keeping the pressure above 20 cm H2O helps prevent aspiration, and keeping it below 30 cm H2O reduces the risk of recurrent laryngeal nerve injury.

Be aware that the volume of air to achieve that pressure range will depend on tube and patient size, but ranges from 3–5 ml in adults. Beware helpful assistants who inflate the cuff for you—there is a tendency to want to inflate with a full syringe volume. Remember that nitrous oxide will diffuse into a cuff and elevate cuff pressure over time. In an intensive care setting, the shorter the duration of intubation, the better. Make sure the cuff is completely deflated prior to extubation. Try to minimize coughing with extubation—via either deep extubation, if not contraindicated, or pharmacologic methods such as intravenous lidocaine or IV dexmedetomidine.

***Note from the Editors:** Emily Poynton went to college at Notre Dame University. We selected the LaSalle Street Bridge in her honor (Fig. 130.2).

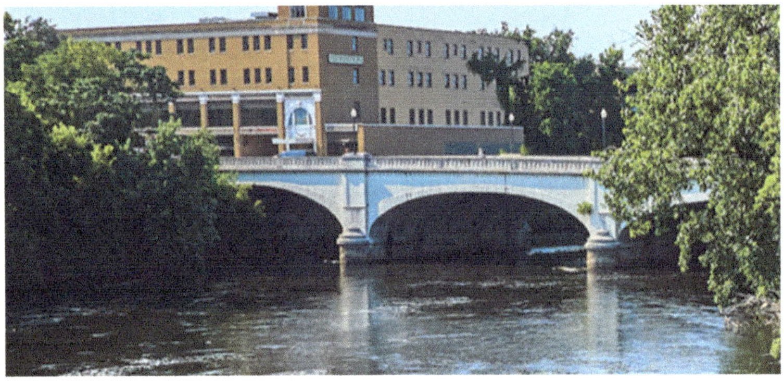

Fig. 130.2 LaSalle Street Bridge in South Bend, IN. It was built in 1907 and spans the St. Joseph River. It is listed on the National Register of Historic Places. Photograph: Image used under standard license from stock.adobe.com

Protecting the Lungs

There are a couple of key concepts to consider when talking about protecting the lungs. The first is protecting from aspiration, and the second is protecting from ventilator-induced lung injury.

Maybe one of the first things we think about when preparing to induce a patient is whether the patient is at risk for aspiration. If the patient is low risk for aspiration, we do a "standard" induction. It is our practice to always induce with the patient at least mildly head up, because it is easier to ventilate if the abdomen is "downhill." The bigger the stomach, the more head-up we will go. This positioning is also associated with less reduction in functional residual capacity.

We also believe in early use of nasopharyngeal or oral airways and jaw thrust assist as needed. These maneuvers all allow for easier ventilation and also decrease the amount of air you may inadvertently ventilate into the stomach. On the other hand, if the aspiration risk is high, then you will have to decide between a rapid sequence induction/intubation versus an awake intubation and think about whether you want to use any of the pharmacologic strategies to reduce stomach acid.

After the airway is secured, it is now time to choose ventilator settings. Many of us older faculty will remember the days when tidal volumes (TVs) were routinely set to 10–15 ml/kg, using actual body weight. The current standard of care is to use what has been termed protective lung ventilation. Protective lung ventilation has been shown to improve outcomes in ventilated patients with acute respiratory distress syndrome (ARDS) and is a reasonable default ventilation strategy in all mechanically ventilated patients. The basic concept is to use lower tidal volumes and reduced airway pressures to decrease the risk of volutrauma and barotrauma to the lungs. This strategy may also decrease the release of inflammatory mediators.

TVs should be based on predicted body weight in kg, which is 50+ 0.91 (height cm −152.4) in men and 45+ 0.91 (height cm −152.4) in women. TV is set to 6 to 8 mL/kg and is adjusted to keep ventilator plateau pressures less than 30 cm H_2O. In cases where one lung ventilation is being used, TV is set to 4 to 6 mL/kg, and is again adjusted to keep ventilator plateau pressures less than 30 cm H2O. In patients with ARDS, TV is typically set to 4–6 ml/kg.

Respiratory rate is titrated to achieve the desired minute ventilation and end tidal CO_2. Use of the lowest acceptable FiO_2 is recommended, titrating for adequate SpO_2 and PaO_2. Positive end expiratory pressure (PEEP) should be used in most patients, with a starting setting of 5 cm H_2O (and titrated up as needed), because it reduces atelectasis and promotes alveolar ventilation. In laparoscopy surgery, the patient may benefit from PEEP of 8–10 cm H_2O.

Conclusions

Airway management is a key focus of anesthetic management. Understand the potential complications and work to avoid them.

Lessons Learned

- Prevention of teeth injury starts with a good preoperative history and examination of the teeth. Find out where the at-risk areas are. Use the correct number if a specific tooth has to be noted in the chart.
- In general, the maxillary incisors are at risk.
- Use smaller endotracheal tubes and appropriate cuff volumes to reduce hoarseness and the risk of vocal cord injury.
- It's been suggested to have the cuff placed at least a centimeter below the vocal cords.
- Incorporate protective lung ventilation into your routine anesthetic management.

Further Readings

Mourão J, Neto J, Luís C, et al. Dental injury after conventional direct laryngoscopy: a prospective observational study. Anaesthesia. 2013;68(10):1059–65.

Warner ME, Benenfeld SM, Warner MA, et al. Perianesthetic dental injuries: frequency, outcomes, and risk factors. Anesthesiology. 1999;90(5):1302–5.

Yamanaka H, Hayashi Y, Watanabe Y, et al. Prolonged hoarseness and arytenoid cartilage dislocation after tracheal intubation. Br J Anaesth. 2009;103:452–5.

Young CC, Harris EM, Vacchiano C, et al. Lung-protective ventilation for the surgical patient: international expert panel-based consensus recommendations. Br J Anaesth. 2019;123(6):898–913.

Authors

Emily Poynton is a native of Cleveland, Ohio, and a graduate of the University of Notre Dame. She completed residency in anesthesiology and fellowship in critical care at University Hospitals Cleveland Medical Center, where she stayed on as faculty after graduation. Her academic interests include critical care medicine, transplant anesthesia, and critical care quality improvement, for which she is the resident rotation director. Outside of work, she can be found spending time with family and watching Notre Dame and Cleveland sports.

Ray Graber serves as anesthesia department vice chair for quality at University Hospitals Cleveland Medical. He has dual interests in cardiac and orthopedic anesthesia. During his 30+ year career, he has focused on process improvement, reduction of errors, and improving patient outcomes.

Protecting the Patient: Unintended Consequences

131

Dane A. Coyne and Raymond G. Graber

Contributor:

Lisa L. Sandson, BArch

Introduction

In this last chapter about protecting the patient, let us talk about some unintended consequences of anesthetic administration and what we can do to reduce these risks.

Preventing Hypothermia

Intraoperative hypothermia is a common occurrence, due to anesthetic-induced vasodilatation, cold operating rooms, open body cavities, and lack of shivering. It has potentially deleterious effects on a patient's immune function and coagulation system and can even cause antibody-mediated red blood cell hemolysis in susceptible patients.

When recovering in the postanesthesia care unit, a hypothermic patient will experience prolonged shivering, which is an obvious discomfort. However, in addition, there is an associated increase in catecholamine levels, resulting in increased cardiac output, heart rate, and arterial pressure, along with an increase in oxygen consumption and carbon dioxide production. Thus, there is physiological stress associated with recovering from hypothermia, and numerous studies have shown poorer outcomes in most, if not the majority of, survival metrics.

Perioperative hypothermia is also associated with psychological stress in a wide range of patients. This is also fairly common in military veterans, many of whom have unpleasant memories or even low levels of post-traumatic stress disorder due to being exposed to extreme cold for prolonged periods.

D. A. Coyne (✉) · R. G. Graber
Department of Anesthesiology and Perioperative Medicine, University Hospitals Cleveland Medical Center, Cleveland, OH, USA
e-mail: Dane.coyne@uhhospitals.org; raymond.graber@uhhospitals.org

S. Mohamed et al. (eds.), *Anesthesia Bridges*, https://doi.org/10.1007/978-3-032-08294-7_131

The best treatment is prevention. Always monitor core body temperature closely even if you do not expect the case to be lengthy. Use underbody and over-the-body warming devices, such as forced warm air convective blankets, hydrogel energy conduction pads, and circulating underbody warm water gel pads. Wrap arms to help insulate them. Warm any intravenous (IV) lines with significant fluid volume or blood products being administered through them (platelets do not need to be warmed). Use a heated humidified circuit in cases with a higher risk of hypothermia or to help recover from hypothermia if it occurs.

***Note from the Editors:** Winter activities and sports can be wonderful to experience but only if you can get warm at will (Fig. 131.1).

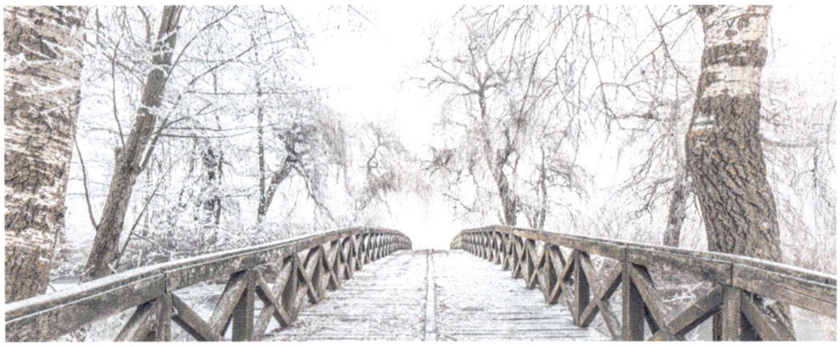

Fig. 131.1 A snowy bridge in a lovely but cold landscape. Photo: Image used under license from shutterstock.com

Protecting from Infection

Perioperative infections can be a devastating and costly process for patients. There are multiple things we can do to help prevent infections. First and foremost is timely administration of prophylactic antibiotics. In general, antibiotic prophylaxis works best when administered in the hour prior to incision. Ideally, your institution should have guidelines for which antibiotics to use for specific surgery types as well as alternatives for patients with significant beta lactam allergy or who are colonized with, or who have risk factors for, methicillin-resistant *Staphylococcus aureus* (MRSA). If not, work with your pharmacists and infectious disease doctors to develop them.

Remember though, it is not just about the antibiotics. Are you a potential cause of infection? Are you washing your hands? Are you wearing gloves and frequently changing them? Are you keeping your anesthetic workstation clean? (It is so easy to contaminate this site with patient secretions.) Are you using maximal barrier precautions and chlorhexidine prep when placing central lines? Are you wiping IV ports with alcohol prior to injecting medications or hooking up infusions?

Protecting from Awareness

Awareness is a fairly uncommon occurrence: 0.1–0.4% of general anesthetics. However, when it occurs, it can impose severe long-term psychological consequences on patients who experience it. Intraoperative awareness occurs when a patient becomes conscious during a procedure performed under general anesthesia and subsequently has recall of these events. It does not include the time before general anesthesia is induced, during emergence, or when under sedation for cases performed under local or regional anesthesia. The American Society of Anesthesiologists (ASA) has developed practice advisories to reduce the incidence of intraoperative awareness [1].

Preoperative assessment should include identifying patients at a high risk of awareness before the anesthetic is started. Patients with a personal history of awareness should be interviewed with regard to their previous experiences. Some procedures are known to have a higher incidence of awareness, typically because the patients are potentially unstable, and we are limiting our anesthetic doses; examples would include cardiac surgery, trauma, potentially difficult airways, or those patients with ASA IV or V classification. Patients with rapid sequence induction and intubation have an increased risk of awareness, and this group includes women who are being induced for cesarean delivery. Patients who are chronically dependent on opioids, alcohol, or other central nervous system (CNS) depressants may have higher anesthetic requirements and thus may also be at risk.

Prevention of awareness begins in the preinduction phase. Room setup should verify that the anesthetic infusion pumps are working and that the vaporizers are adequately full. Benzodiazepine premedication should be considered in most patients who have an increased risk of awareness. There is controversy regarding using benzodiazepines in C-section patients in the preinduction period because of fear of fetal depression. Many obstetric anesthesiologists prefer to administer midazolam after the umbilical cord is clamped. The downside to benzodiazepine use is delayed emergence in some patients.

During the intraoperative phase, patients are monitored for somatic signs of inadequate anesthesia. This can include patient hypertension, tachycardia, hyperventilation, diaphoresis, tearing, and nonpurposeful movement. If the patient is "light," we can make them "deeper." End-tidal agent monitoring can be performed to tailor a volatile anesthetic to the desired alveolar concentration level appropriate for the specific agent, considering the patient's age. Brain electrical activity monitoring is another option. Most of these devices use proprietary algorithms to convert electroencephalogram (EEG) data into an "index" score from 0 to 100. These devices may be helpful when utilizing a total intravenous anesthesia (TIVA) technique or in patients with a known history of awareness.

If awareness is suspected intraoperatively, make sure you are actually delivering the planned anesthetic. Does the vaporizer have an adequate level, and what is the end-tidal agent level? Are your intravenous drugs being properly infused into a functional IV? Increase your depth of anesthetic and consider adding additional benzodiazepine. Your goal is to ensure amnesia going forward (antegrade). Unfortunately, you are unlikely to be able to accomplish retrograde amnesia of any prior awareness.

A patient who may have experienced unintended intraoperative awareness may be identified during PACU care or during routine postoperative physician or nursing care. Once such a patient is identified, the anesthesiologist who was responsible for the patient's care, or a qualified designee, should interview the patient and document the details of the patient's experience.

If the anesthesiologist determines that unintended intraoperative awareness has occurred, the following steps should be taken:

- Assure the patient of the credibility of his or her account and sympathize with their experience. *Do not attempt to tell the patients they aren't remembering what they believe they are remembering!*
- Explain what happened and why if a reason can be given; for example, the necessity to administer light anesthesia in the presence of significant cardiovascular instability. We know of a patient who was aware at the end of a lung volume reduction while spontaneous ventilation was reestablished. She had a thoracic epidural in place and was not in any pain or paralyzed. We asked her to describe her experience, and she said, "It wasn't bad at all. I just remember thinking, hmm, I wonder if this means the surgery is almost over."
- Offer the patient support, including referral of the patient for counseling if appropriate.
- Document any referrals or treatment provided to the patient.
- Notify the patient's surgeon.
- *Notify your hospital's risk management department.*

***Note from the Editors:** Speaking of protection, one of our favorite bridges is the Széchenyi Chain Bridge in Budapest, Hungary (Fig. 131.2). It is one of many beautiful bridges that mounts its own guard.

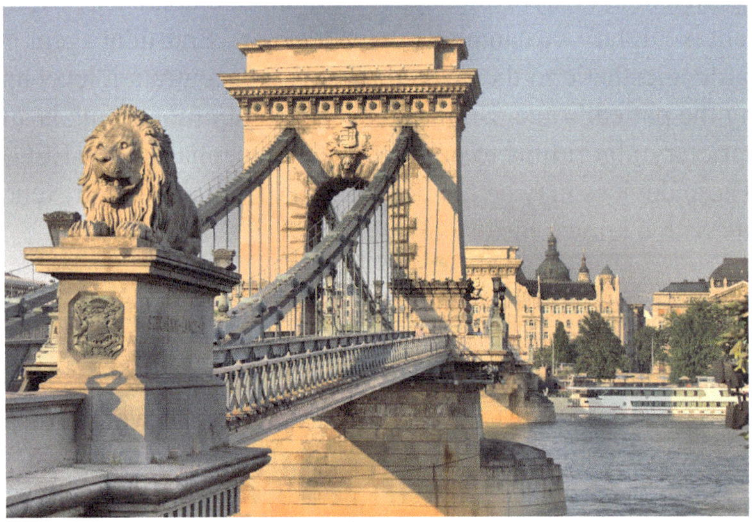

Fig. 131.2 The Széchenyi Chain Bridge in Budapest, Hungary, protected by majestic stone lions. It was designed by the British engineer William Tierney Clark and opened in 1849. It spans the Danube. Photo: Image used under standard license from stock.adobe.com

Protecting from Airway Obstruction

Neuromuscular blocking drugs are effective weapons in our anesthetic arsenal, but incomplete reversal at the end of cases can lead to aspiration, airway obstruction, or hypoventilation. So, to start, use "train-of-4" (TOF) twitch monitoring to guide redosing of muscle relaxants. Try to avoid total twitch suppression during a case; this will make it easier to reverse at the end.

As a quick review, when we do TOF monitoring, we deliver four supramaximal stimuli (at intervals of 0.5 seconds) with a peripheral nerve stimulator and measure or observe the response. This test is based on the concept that acetylcholine is depleted by successive stimulations. Quantitative devices analyze evoked muscle contractions or the muscle action potentials that result. Qualitative assessment is our best guess assessment of what we observe by "eyeball." First, we observe the number of twitches after the four stimuli. We call this a twitch count. If four twitches are present, the fourth twitch response is compared with the first twitch response and a ratio of 0–1 is calculated. This is known as the TOF ratio (Fig. 131.3).

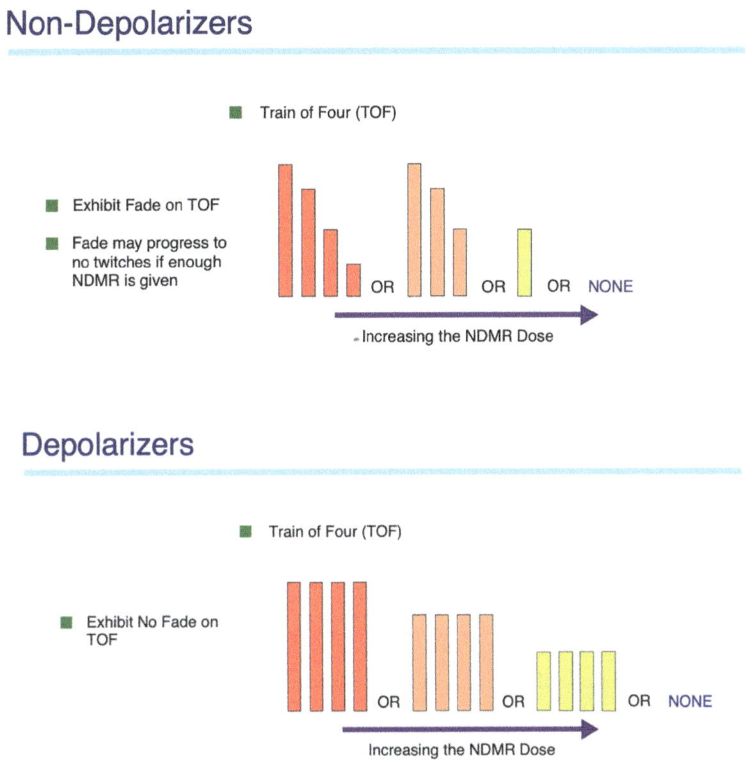

Fig. 131.3 Train-of-four monitoring for non-depolarizing vs. depolarizing neuromuscular blockade. Illustration: Lisa Sandson

Use a muscle relaxant reversal strategy that is tied to the current TOF twitch count. For example, when the TOF count is 0 or 1, use sugammadex to reverse. Neostigmine will not reverse this depth of block. If the TOF count is 2, you can use either neostigmine or sugammadex, realizing that sugammadex will reverse in 2–3 minutes, while neostigmine may take >30 minutes. If the TOF count is 3 or 4, either neostigmine or sugammadex can be reasonably used.

Even if you have apparent full recovery of all four twitches by "eyeball," you should still administer a reversal drug. Remember, the human eye is not capable of distinguishing whether the TOF ratio is between 0.4 and 0.9, which would indicate clinically significant weakness, or > 0.9, which would indicate full recovery. Use TOF assessment after reversal to assess the adequacy of reversal. You can use clinical tests in conjunction, but do not depend on them. Keep an eye out for new technology in quantitative analysis of neuromuscular blockade.

Lessons Learned

- Hypothermia prevention starts at the beginning of a case [2].
- We can all do better when it comes to hand washing and cleaning injection ports [3].
- Awareness under anesthesia can have devastating mental consequences to a patient. How the anesthesiologist handles a report of intraoperative awareness can make all the difference to the patient's satisfaction and the anesthesiologist's legal exposure [4, 5].
- Use TOF monitoring to rationally choose a neuromuscular blockade reversal strategy [5]. The human *eye does not* have the capability to distinguish between clinically significant weakness and full recovery. Extubating a weak patient is a distressingly common error and leads to hypoventilation, inadequate cough, hypoxemia, and reintubation. We believe it's one of the most common causes of "failed extubation."
- Minimizing unintended consequences of anesthesia requires the vigilance and compulsive care that the practice of anesthesia is known for.

References

1. Practice Advisory for Intraoperative Awareness and Brain Function Monitoring. Anesthesiology. 2006 Apr;104(4):847–64.
2. Sessler DI. Perioperative thermoregulation and heat balance. Lancet. 2016;387:2655–64.
3. Loftus RW, Koff MD, Birnbach DJ. The dynamics and implications of bacterial transmission events arising from the anesthesia work area. Anesth Analg. 2015;120(4):853–60.
4. Brull SJ, Kopman AF. Current status of neuromuscular reversal and monitoring: challenges and opportunities. Anesthesiology. 2017;126(1):173–90.
5. American Society of Anesthesiologists Task Force on Intraoperative awareness. Practice advisory for intraoperative awareness and brain function monitoring: a report by the American Society of Anesthesiologists task force on intraoperative awareness. Anesthesiology. 2006;104(4):847–64.

Authors

Dane Coyne arrived in Cleveland to pursue residency training, successfully graduating from University Hospitals as both an anesthesiologist and a critical care physician. He serves as the chair for resident competence and is the section chief/residency rotation director for thoracic anesthesia. Clinically, he is interested in developing strategies for crisis management and advanced airway techniques. In terms of hobbies, he is an avid reader, mixologist, chef, and fairly newly established father.

Ray Graber serves as anesthesia department vice chair for quality at University Hospitals Cleveland Medical. He has dual interests in cardiac and orthopedic anesthesia. During his 30+ year career, he has focused on process improvement, reduction of errors, and improving patient outcomes.

132 Does Labor Epidural Analgesia Increase Cesarean Delivery Rate? A Simple Question with a Complicated Answer

Brandon M. Togioka and Catherine Marcucci

Introduction

The following internal dialogue is common amongst parturients on the labor floor, "I'd like to decrease the pain and suffering that I am feeling right now, but I am very worried about how an epidural may affect my baby." You will be asked about the link between epidural labor analgesia and birth outcomes, including the rate of cesarean delivery. *Unfortunately, this is a simple question without a simple answer*.

The Stats

In the United States, one in three babies is born by cesarean delivery, an unprecedented rate. Cesarean delivery rates vary significantly by hospital, in an astounding range of 7–70%, and by state, in a range of 23% (Alaska) to 38% (Mississippi) [1, 2]. It has been argued that differences in acuity account for a significant proportion of this variation; however, the rate of cesarean delivery amongst parturients deemed at a lowest risk also varies significantly across hospitals: in a range of 2–36%. Indeed, obstetric (OB) provider preferences, institutional staffing models, and patient preferences have all been shown to impact cesarean delivery rate. Given that cesarean delivery is associated with a higher rate of maternal mortality, severe maternal morbidity, future placenta accreta spectrum disorder, neonatal injury, and neonatal respiratory complications, the maternal desire to avoid cesarean delivery is well-founded [3].

Although cesarean delivery can be life-saving for both mother and baby, oftentimes the indication for it is less clear. The most common indication for a primary cesarean delivery is dystocia. Dystocia, or "difficult birth," is defined as prolonged labor. Labor is the process by which regular contractions of the uterus push the fetus down the birth canal, eventually resulting in its expulsion. The "normal" rate of cervical dilation was originally defined by Friedman. You may have heard of the Friedman curve, which plotted cervical dilation on the y-axis and time on the x-axis. Freidman separated slowly progressing labor (latent phase labor) from more rapid cervical dilation (active phase labor).

B. M. Togioka
Department of Anesthesiology and Perioperative Medicine, School of Medicine, Oregon Health & Science University, Portland, OR, USA

C. Marcucci (✉)
Department of Transfusion Medicine, Clinical Center, National Institutes of Health, Bethesda, MD, USA

S. Mohamed et al. (eds.), *Anesthesia Bridges*, https://doi.org/10.1007/978-3-032-08294-7_132

Based upon this curve, practitioners could call a cesarean delivery if latent labor lasted for longer than 20 hours in a nulliparous woman or 14 hours in a multiparous woman. Similarly, a cesarean delivery could be called if the active phase of labor was abnormally slow (protracted labor) or if cervical dilation paused (arrest of labor). Arrest of labor was defined as lack of cervical dilation for >2 hours in a woman at ≥4 cm cervical dilation.

The problem is we now know that few women transition from latent to active labor at 4 cm (6 cm is the threshold for most women) and that cervical dilation in the active phase of labor occurs more slowly than originally believed. Thus, the most common indication for primary cesarean delivery, dystocia, is wrought with misinterpretation. As a consequence, it is very difficult to determine to what extent epidural labor analgesia may contribute to the decision to call a cesarean delivery.

The effect of epidural analgesia on the duration of labor has been extensively investigated. The observation is consistent: epidural analgesia is associated with an increased incidence of oxytocin administration, an increased incidence of operative vaginal delivery (use of forceps or vacuum), and a prolonged second stage of labor, defined as the time between full cervical dilation and fetal expulsion [4, 5].

The effect of epidural analgesia on the first stage of labor is less clear. The first stage of labor begins when regular, painful, productive (meaning they lead to cervical dilation) contractions commence and ends when the cervix is fully dilated (10 cm). It is important to note that it is impossible for a woman, or a researcher, to know exactly when the first stage of labor has begun because no one knows when cervical dilation begins. We can say, however, that strong evidence that epidural analgesia increases the duration of the first stage of labor is lacking. Additionally, the intravenous fluid bolus that is coadministered with neuraxial placement is associated with reduced endogenous oxytocin release from the posterior pituitary, where the antidiuretic hormone is stored, which would be expected to slow labor.

The preceding explanation would clearly be confusing to a new mother in extremis from labor pain. How then, may we answer the question?

Association Is Not Causality

First, multiple observational studies have found an association between the provision of epidural labor analgesia and cesarean delivery; however, severe pain during labor is associated with dystocia and a higher rate of cesarean delivery. In other words, association does not equal causality.

Second, epidural analgesia is associated with factors such as oxytocin administration and protracted labor, which are associated with cesarean delivery. These data come mostly from older studies, which assessed epidural solutions that contained a high-concentration local anesthetic; modern epidural solutions contain a lower concentration of a local anesthetic, are associated with less motor block, and cause a smaller decrement in perineal tone and expulsive force.

Third, before-and-after studies assessing the introduction of anesthesia service with an associated rapid increase in the rate of epidural labor analgesia found no increase in the rate of cesarean delivery [6, 7].

Fourth, meta-analyses of randomized controlled trials are the gold standard for evaluating the impact of interventions. They have found no correlation between epidural analgesia and the rate of cesarean delivery [4, 5].

Fifth, there are many other reasons to support the provision of epidural labor analgesia. Labor is extremely painful, and high-dose opioids induce neonatal depression and alter the fetal heart rate pattern. Also, the presence of an epidural decreases the requirement for intubation and general anesthesia, and epidural analgesia facilitates active maternal involvement in the birth process. Perhaps, most importantly from a maternal perspective, epidural analgesia is associated with improved patient experience [4].

Lessons Learned

- The likelihood of cesarean delivery is greatly impacted by the obstetric provider who makes care decisions and the institution where the woman delivers.
- Dystocia, or "difficult birth," is commonly misdiagnosed and accounts for the majority of primary cesarean deliveries in the United States.
- Epidural labor analgesia is associated with factors such as oxytocin administration and protracted labor, which are associated with cesarean delivery.
- Before-and-after studies as well as meta-analyses have not found an association between epidural labor analgesia and a higher incidence of cesarean delivery.
- Epidural labor analgesia has many benefits including improved maternal satisfaction with the birth process and reduced requirement for intubation and general anesthesia.
- If you provide anesthesia for OB patients, think about your answers to these questions before you are asked. It's okay to start discussing the issue with the exact statement in the title of this chapter.

You might be asked if you or your partner had or would have an epidural, and we think this is one of the few instances where it is okay to share your personal experiences and medical information. A patient once asked one of our authors Cathy Marcucci if she had ever considered natural childbirth. Her Cathy's answer was the truth, "Not even for one second!" We don't actually know of any anesthesiologists who have chosen to have their babies without an epidural (if not contra-indicated). Do you?

References

1. Kozhimannil KB, Law MR, Virnig BA. Cesarean delivery rates vary tenfold among US hospitals; reducing variation may address quality and cost issues. Health Aff (Millwood). 2013;32(3):527–35.
2. Centers for Disease Control and Prevention. Cesarean delivery rate by state [internet]. CDC; 2020 [cited 2022 Jun 22]. Available from: https://www.cdc.gov/nchs/pressroom/sosmap/cesarean_births/cesareans.htm
3. Liu S, Liston RM, Joseph KS, et al. Maternal mortality and severe morbidity associated with low-risk planned cesarean delivery versus planned vaginal delivery at term. CMAJ. 2007;176(4):455–60.
4. Halpern SH, Leighton BL, Ohlsson A, et al. Effect of epidural vs parenteral opioid analgesia on the progress of labor: a meta-analysis. JAMA. 1998;280(24):2105–10.
5. Sharma SK, McIntire DD, Wiley J, et al. Labor analgesia and cesarean delivery: an individual patient meta-analysis of nulliparous women. Anesthesiology 2004;100(1):142–148; discussion 146A.
6. Gribble RK, Meier PR. Effect of epidural analgesia on the primary cesarean rate. Obstet Gynecol. 1991;78(2):231–4.
7. Yancey MK, Pierce B, Schweitzer D, et al. Observations on labor epidural analgesia and operative delivery rates. Am J Obstet Gynecol. 1999;180(2 Pt 1):353–9.

Author

Brandon Togioka is the vice chair of clinical research for anesthesiology and perioperative medicine at Oregon Health and Science University and the former director of obstetric anesthesia. He is married to Jennifer Togioka, a hospital accreditation director, with whom he has two daughters, Ella and Brynn. When he is not working, Brandon enjoys jogging and watching his daughters participate in competitive swimming and ballet.

Cathy Marcucci did a lot of OB anesthesia in her residency and very early in her career and has retained an interest in this challenging and rewarding subspecialty. She distinctly recalls the placenta accreta question she was asked during her oral boards. She was so nervous that she attempted to pantomime the clinical situation, wiggling her fingers to try to make air drawings to convey placental invaginations, as if she was in a high-stakes game of charades, which she sort of was actually. Fortunately, the examiners took pity and passed her.

Do We Have to Go Over Drug–Drug Interactions Again? Yes, We Really Do

133

Catherine Marcucci and Neil B. Sandson

Introduction

Are we going to have a drug–drug interaction (DDI) section in every single book we do, and do we really need to do that? Yes, we are, and, yes, we do. There are two main reasons:

> **First**, DDIs are common and costly. Even in developed countries or in tertiary care facilities in developing countries, it is estimated that as many as 15–40% of significant DDIs may go unrecognized, including in intensive care units. DDI software and the availability of dedicated pharmacy staff help but do not solve the problem. We feel that "DDI protection" is ultimately the responsibility of the prescriber.
>
> **Second**, unfortunately, we are still not seeing that DDIs have become a routine topic in anesthesia resident lectures and rarely see a discussion of DDI issues in papers concerning anesthesia pharmacology or medication mishaps. The refresher information below is a condensation of our previously published DDI educational material.

Remember, it is impossible to memorize every significant DDI that you might be faced with, and the electronic chart "DDI programs," while better than even 10 years ago, are unwieldy to the point of being unusable.

Instead, we recommend that anesthesiologists continue to work on mastering the basic principles of drug metabolism, understand the six types of DDIs, have a passing familiarity with the P-glycoprotein transport system, and then concentrate on the drugs most relevant to your particular anesthetic practice. We don't generally advocate for the rote memorization of huge tables of DDIs.

C. Marcucci (✉)
Department of Transfusion Medicine, Clinical Center, National Institutes of Health, Bethesda, MD, USA

N. B. Sandson
Department of Psychiatry, VA Maryland Health Care System, Baltimore, MD, USA

University of Maryland, Baltimore, MD, USA

S. Mohamed et al. (eds.), *Anesthesia Bridges*, https://doi.org/10.1007/978-3-032-08294-7_133

So Here Goes...

- Remember that in general, pharmacodynamics is what drugs do to the body and pharmacokinetics is what the body does to drugs. Every molecule that enters the body must have a final disposition and humans have evolved a variety of mechanisms to accomplish this.
- Pharmacokinetic drug handling occurs in four main ways: *absorption, metabolism, distribution, and excretion.*
- Metabolism occurs via phase I (oxidation) reactions and/or phase II (conjugative) reactions.
- There are two parts of the DDI universe: pharmacodynamic DDIs and pharmacokinetic DDIs.
- DDIs are distributed across the pharmacokinetic domains. For instance, DDIs involving the P450 system (much more below!) are interactions that affect metabolism. DDIs involving the P-glycoprotein transport system involve absorption, distribution, and excretion (more in Chap. 135).
- One very important galaxy in this whole big pharmacology universe are those DDIs that are mediated by cytochrome (CYP) P450 enzymes. These enzymes effect phase I metabolism and are found chiefly, but not exclusively, in hepatocytes.
- The most important of the CYP450 enzymes are **CYP3A4, CYP2B6, CYP2E1, CYP1A2, CYP2D6, CYP2C9,** and **CYP2C19.**
- Each enzyme has substrates, inducers, and inhibitors (except for **CYP2D6**, which has no known inducers).
- There is also considerable variation in the genetic expression of individual enzymes.
- Activity of the enzymes can vary in disease states.
- We briefly review the highlights of each enzyme below.
- A significant amount of the original landmark CYP450 DDI work pertaining to anesthesia drugs was done by Evan Kharasch, MD PhD*, who is also a contributor to this book. We have all his papers on file and review them frequently.

***Note from the Editors:** *Anesthesia Bridges* editor Cathy Marcucci and author Evan Kharasch are both big minor league baseball (MiLB) fans, although they have never attended a game together. While searching for the best MiLB parks and the best bridges in America—for the bucket lists, of course—the editors found Modern Woodmen Park, the home field of the Quad City River Bandits (Fig. 133.1).

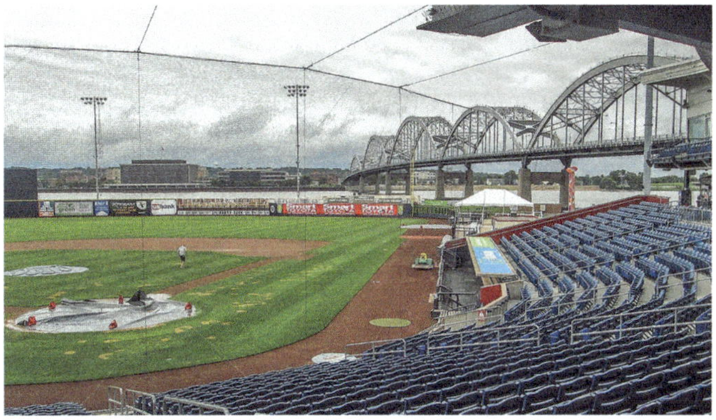

Fig. 133.1 Modern Woodmen Park, formerly known as John O'Donnell Stadium, with a stunning view of the Centennial Bridge and the Mississippi River over the outfield fence. The bridge connects Rock Island, IL, with Davenport, IA. Photo: Image used courtesy of ballparkbrothers.com

CYP3A4

- **Cytochrome P450 3A4**: A "must-know" for perioperative providers, this enzyme is the "workhorse" of the CYP450 system. It catalyzes the majority of phase I biotransformations of both endogenous biochemicals and xenobiotics and has a meaningful role in metabolizing from 50%–70% of the currently administered supplements and medications.
- **CYP3A4** functions as a sort of "backup" enzyme if its enzymatic action at other P450 "locations" is strongly inhibited or lacking due to genetic variability.
- There are no **3A4** poor metabolizers (inconsistent with life), and there is very little **3A4** genetic polymorphism; however, there is a 10- to 30-fold variability of metabolic efficiency based on ethnic, cultural, age, gender, dietary factors, and the presence of liver and intestinal disease.
- There are many substrates, inducers, and inhibitors of **CYP3A4**. Many commonly used analgesic and sedatives drugs are **CYP3A4** substrates. These include midazolam, ketamine, fentanyl, alfentanil, sufentanil, methadone, buprenorphine, and most local anesthetics. Other **3A4** substrates include calcium channel blockers, many statins, steroids, tricyclic antidepressants, antipsychotics, macrolide antibiotics, and carbamazepine.
- **CYP3A4** inducers include ritonavir, many anticonvulsants, rifampin, and St. John's wort.
- **CYP3A4** inhibitors include "azole" antifungals such as ketoconazole and itraconazole, some selective serotonin reuptake inhibitors (SSRIs), and some quinolone antibiotics. Grapefruit juice is such a potent inhibitor of intestinal **CYP3A4** that it is not allowed on some hospitals' dietary menus.

CYP2B6

- **Cytochrome P450 2B6**: The importance of this enzyme is only just being fully understood. It comprises about 2%–10% of the CYP450 system found in the liver, lung, kidney, and intestine.

- Expression and inducibility of **CYP2B6** are highly variable based on age and ethnicity.

- **CYP2B6** has an emerging profound role in anesthesia since it is considered the chief metabolic enzyme involved in clearance of propofol. It also metabolizes ketamine when it is given at subanesthetic dosages. **CYP2B6** is a main mediator of the metabolism of methadone. This is a CYP enzyme to watch as new studies appear in the literature.

CYP2E1

- **Cytochrome P450 2E1**: This enzyme is found in hepatocytes and is important for detoxification. It performs partial metabolism of ethanol, isoflurane, sevoflurane, desflurane, enflurane, and halothane.

- There is considerable genetic variability of **CYP2E1**, which has emerging importance with regard to ethanol-mediated liver damage and changes in the metabolism of other drugs.

- Inducers of **2E1** are ethanol, tobacco smoke, and isoniazid.

CYP1A2

- **Cytochrome P450 1A2**: This enzyme is found exclusively in the liver and accounts for about 10%–15% of the metabolism accomplished by the major CYP450 enzymes. It is a highly polymorphic enzyme with at least 15 alleles identified to date, and single point mutations can cause variability in enzyme expression. Clinically significant DDIs may be difficult to predict as enzyme expression can vary up to 40-fold from individual to individual, based on ethnic factors as well as enzyme induction or inhibition by foods, tobacco smoke, and medications.

- This is the enzyme that is significantly affected by foods: **1A2** is induced by brassica vegetables (kale, cauliflower, broccoli, greens, brussels sprouts, cabbage), charred meats, and grape juice. This enzyme is inhibited by apiaceous vegetables (carrots, celery, parsley), caffeine, and grapefruit juice.

- **CYP1A2** is strongly and rapidly induced by smoked tobacco.

CYP2D6

- **Cytochrome P450 2D6**: This enzyme constitutes about 2–5% of the body's CYP450 enzymes but metabolizes about 25% of the current drugs. There is great phenotypic variation due to genetic polymorphisms; patients can be:
  - Poor metabolizers (no **CYP2D6** function).
  - Intermediate metabolizers, extensive metabolizers (normal 2D6 function).
  - Ultrarapid metabolizers (increased **2D6** function).
- Ethnicity is a factor in **2D6** variability. Caucasians (5%–10%) and 2% of Chinese patients are poor metabolizers. Reduced metabolism may be as high as 50% in some Asian populations. Populations that may exhibit ultrarapid metabolism are persons of Mediterranean/North African descent (up to 30% of those populations) and Caucasians (up to 1%–2% of that population). The Roche Amplichip analyzes polymorphisms for **2D6** and **2C19.**
- There are no known inducers of **2D6**.
- Common perioperative drugs metabolized by **2D6** are opioids (tramadol, hydrocodone, codeine), although it bears mentioning that these are all prodrugs with regard to this enzyme. The parent drugs are only modestly effective analgesics and require metabolic conversion to significantly more analgesically effective metabolites.
- Other perioperative drugs that are **2D6** substrates include beta-blockers, some antiarrhythmics, tricyclic antidepressants, and several antipsychotics. Inhibitors of **2D6** include several SSRIs, ritonavir, bupropion, quinidine, and goldenseal.

CYP2C9

- **CYP2C9**: This enzyme metabolizes a number of anesthesia medications including propofol (30–50% of total metabolism), ketamine (30–40%), diazepam (5%–10%), and halothane (10–20%).
- **CYP2C9** metabolizes pain medications including celecoxib, hydromorphone, and several nonsteroidal anti-inflammatory drugs (NSAIDs) including ibuprofen, indomethacin, naproxen, and diclofenac. It also metabolizes a number of important perioperative drugs such as barbiturates (which also induce the enzyme), warfarin, clopidogrel, carvedilol, glyburide, glipizide, angiotensin receptor II antagonists, and sertraline.
- Inducers of **2C9** include the pan-inducers phenytoin and carbamazepine.
- **CYP2C9** inhibitors include amiodarone, fluconazole, and sulfamethoxazole.
- There can be a ten-fold difference in **CYP2C9** activity between individuals; this is one of the enzymes that is sometimes genotyped to determine dosage parameters.

CYP2C19

- **CYP2C19**: This is another CYP enzyme that is characterized by genetic polymorphism, resulting in poor and extensive metabolizers. About 5% of Caucasians, 5% of Africans, and 20% of people with Asian ethnicity are thought to have deficient 2C19 activity. It is not noted for metabolism of anesthetic agents but metabolizes other important perioperative medications such as clopidogrel, proton pump inhibitors, and several antidepressants and anticonvulsants.

- Inhibitors of **2C19** include omeprazole, cimetidine, ritonavir, fluoxetine, fluvoxamine, and isoniazid.

- Inducers of **2C19** include phenytoin, carbamazepine, and rifampin.

***Note from the Editors:** *Anesthesia Bridges* editor and author Neil Sandson is very interested in Japanese art and culture. We are including this unusual Impressionist painting of a beautiful Japanese landscape print to acknowledge the contributions Neil has made to the anesthesiology community over the years (Fig. 133.2).

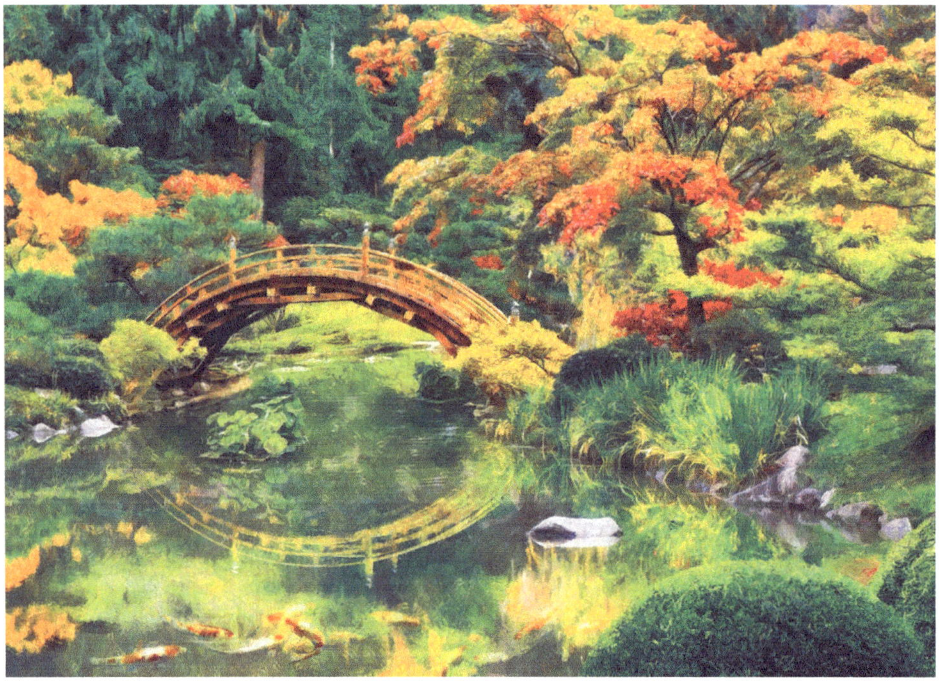

Fig. 133.2 Many artists have collected and admired Japanese paintings and prints and rendered them in the Impressionist style. This landscape painting is striking for its beautiful fall colors. Photo: Image by V. Lukas, used under standard license from adobe.stock.com

CYP450 Metabolism of the Most Common Operating Room Drugs

- **Inhalational anesthetics**: Metabolized by **CYP2E1** in the liver.
- **Propofol**: Metabolized by **CYP2B6** in the liver and also at extrahepatic sites, and about 30–50% of the metabolism is by **CYP2C9**.
- **Ketamine**: Metabolized by **CYP3A4** at anesthetic doses with some metabolism also by **CYP2B6** at subanesthetic doses.
- **Midazolam**: Metabolized by **CYP3A4**; lack of sedative efficacy can be seen when coadministered with 3A4 inducers such as carbamazepine and phenytoin. Increased sedation may be seen when coadministered with **3A4** inhibitors such as diltiazem, itraconazole, and goldenseal.
- **Fentanyl**: Metabolized by **3A4**.
- **Codeine**: As a prodrug, it requires metabolism by **2D6** to morphine for analgesic efficacy.
- **Methadone**: Metabolized mostly by **CYP3A4** but also by **2B6** and **2D6.**
- **Local anesthetics**: Ropivacaine, lidocaine, and mepivacaine are metabolized by **1A2** and **3A4**. Bupivacaine is metabolized by **3A4**, **2D6**, and **2C19**.
- **Vecuronium**: Multifactorial metabolism by CYP liver enzymes and also metabolized in the kidney. Metabolism is enhanced when coadministered with the CYP pan-inducer phenytoin.
- **Rocuronium**: Multifactorial metabolism by CYP liver enzymes and also exhibits enhanced metabolism when coadministered with the pan-inducers phenytoin and carbamazepine.
- **Notes**: Morphine and hydromorphone are chiefly metabolized by **UGT2B7.** The UGT enzymes are "first cousins" to the cytochrome P450 system and are involved in phase 2 conjugative metabolism. Morphine is also eliminated by the P-glycoprotein transport system.

Lessons Learned

- One of the most important ways you can start to master perioperative DDIs is to master the basic CYP450 enzymes that are relevant to the drugs we use most.
- **CYP3A4** is the workhorse of the cytochrome P450 system. It metabolizes midazolam, ketamine, fentanyl, alfentanil, sufentanil, methadone, and most local anesthetics including ropivacaine, lidocaine, mepivacaine, and bupivacaine.
- **CYP2B6** metabolizes propofol, most probably in the liver, but also at extrahepatic sites.
- **CYP2E1** metabolizes the inhalational anesthetics.

- **CYP1A2** metabolizes lidocaine, ropivacaine, and mepivacaine. This is one of the enzymes that is significantly affected by diet—both in terms of induction and inhibition. Smoked tobacco is a strong 1A2 inducer.

- **CYP2D6** metabolizes some of the opioids, such as tramadol, codeine, and hydrocodone, as well as bupivacaine. It has abundant genetic polymorphisms, and patients can range from poor metabolizers to ultrarapid metabolizers. There are no known inducers.

- **CYP2C9** is also partially responsible for the metabolism of many perioperative anesthesia drugs including propofol, ketamine, diazepam, and halothane. It is one of the enzymes for which genotyping is done to establish dosage parameters.

- In 2016, we put together a compendium of clinical case scenarios with this publisher (we love Springer!) that reviews this material in greater depth and breadth (Fig. 133.3). *The royalties are pledged in perpetuity to the Foundation for Anesthesia Education and Research (FAER)*, so we feel free to promote the book a bit. We are delighted that it received favorable reviews.

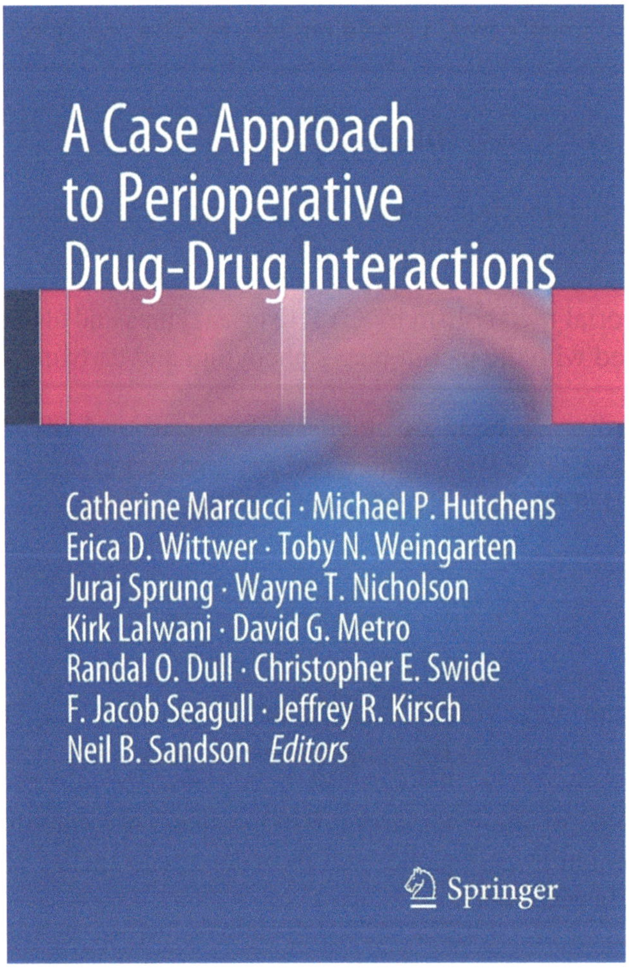

Fig. 133.3 Our DDI book, published in 2016, aka "the Blue Book." Photo: Courtesy of Catherine Marcucci

- If we may be so bold as to quote the concluding paragraph of the review by Ken B. Johnson, MD, that appeared in the July 2016 issue of *Anesthesiology*, as below ☺.

In the realm of perioperative clinical pharmacology textbooks, *A Case Approach to Perioperative Drug-Drug Interactions* stands alone as a comprehensive compilation of hundreds of clinically relevant DDIs presented in an organized and easily accessible format. It is a timely piece that integrates the basic science behind DDIs with case reports describing the clinical presentation of DDIs. It introduces clinicians to important concepts in pharmacogenomics, an advance in personalized medicine that will likely have a significant impact in perioperative care. This book embodies the future of what should be expected of perioperative clinicians with regard to their awareness and understanding of DDIs.

Final Thoughts from the Editors

- Do not stress about this material; just pick up your fork and start eating this elephant one bite at a time. In addition, do not fret because help from AI applications is out there in the not-too-distant future.

- May all your interactions be benign….

Suggested Readings

1. Kharasch ED, Thummel KE. Identification of cytochrome P450 2E1 as the predominant enzyme catalyzing human liver microsomal defluorination of sevoflurane, isoflurane, and methoxyflurane. Anesthesiology. 1993;79(4):795–807.
2. Kharasch ED, Thummel KE. Human alfentanil metabolism by cytochrome P450 3A3/4: an explanation for the interindividual variability in alfentanil clearance? Anesth Anal. 1993;76(5):1033–9.
3. Rao LK, Flaker AM, Friedel CC, et al. Role of cytochrome P4502B6 polymorphisms in ketamine metabolism and clearance. Anesthesiology. 2016;125(6):1103–12.
4. Crews KR, Gaedigk A, Dunnenberger HM, et al. Clinical Pharmacogenetics Implementation Consortium. Clinical Pharmacogenetics Implementation Consortium guidelines for cytochrome P450 2D6 genotype and codeine therapy: 2014 update. Clin Pharm Therap. 2014;95(4):376–82.
5. Blake CM, Kharasch ED, Schwab M, et al. A meta-analysis of CYP2D6 metabolizer phenotype and metoprolol pharmacokinetics. Clin Pharm Therap. 2013;94(3):394–9.
6. Dresser GK, Spence JD, Bailey DG. Pharmacokinetic-pharmacodynamic consequences and clinical relevance of cytochrome P450 3A4 inhibition. Clin Pharmacokinet. 2000;38(1):41–57.
7. Labroo RB, Paine MF, Thummel KE, et al. Fentanyl metabolism by human hepatic and intestinal cytochrome P450 3A4: implications for interindividual variability in disposition, efficacy, and drug interactions. Drug Metab Dispos. 1997;25(9):1072–80.
8. Paine MF, Khalighi M, Fisher JM, et al. Characterization of interintestinal and intraintestinal variations in human CYP3A-dependent metabolism. J Pharmacol Exp Ther. 1997;283(3):1552–62.
9. Wang B, Wang J, Huang SQ, et al. Genetic polymorphism of the human cytochrome P450 2C9 gene and its clinical significance. Curr Drug Metab. 2009;10(7):781–834.
10. Wang B, Zhou SF. Synthetic and natural compounds that interact with human cytochrome P450 1A2 and implications in drug development. Curr Med Chem. 2009;16(31):4066–218.
11. Wang B, Yang LP, Zhang XZ, et al. New insights into the structural characteristics and functional relevance of the human cytochrome P450 2D6 enzyme. Drug Metab Rev. 2009;41(4):573–643.
12. Court MH, Duan SX, Hesse LM, et al. Cytochrome P-450 2B6 is responsible for interindividual variability of propofol hydroxylation by human liver microsomes. Anesthesiology. 2001;94(1):110–9.

13. Sandson NB. Drug-Drug Interaction Primer: A Compendium of Case Vignettes for the Practicing Clinician. Arlington: American Psychiatric Publishing, Inc., 2007.
14. Marcucci C, Hutchens MP, Wittwer ED, Weingarten TN, Sprung J, Nicholson WT, Lalwani K, Metro DG, Dull RO, Swide CE, Seagull FJ, Kirsch JR, Sandson NB, editors. A Case Approach to Perioperative Drug-Drug Interactions. New York: Springer Science & Business Media; 2007.

Authors

Cathy Marcucci spent eight years of her life putting together *A Case Approach to Perioperative Drug-Drug Interactions* as the lead editor and considers it to be her *magnum opus*. She is very happy to be pen pals with Dr. Kharasch, whose brilliant original work deeply informed the educational outreach of the Blue Book on the deeply fascinating subjects of DDIs and minor league baseball.

Neil Sandson recalls first hearing about DDIs in medical school in the late 1980s and distinctly remembers the professor (a hepatologist) going on at some length about "debrisoquine!" His curiosity was further piqued by two lectures on DDIs that he heard at his 1996 national meeting. Besides his crucial participation in the Blue Book, he has written two other DDI textbooks, published numerous articles and book chapters, and lectured extensively on the subject.

The Six Types of Pharmacokinetic Drug–Drug Interactions

134

Catherine Marcucci and Neil B. Sandson

Introduction

There are many types of drug–drug interactions (DDIs), both pharmacodynamic and pharmacokinetic. An important subset of pharmacokinetic perioperative DDIs are those mediated by the cytochrome P450 enzymes found chiefly in the liver microsomes. These enzymes are chiefly responsible for the phase I metabolism of drugs. It is important to learn the CYP450 enzymes and what drugs serve as substrate, inducers, and inhibitors for those CYP450 enzymes when the drugs are administered concurrently. But sequence also matters! The chronologic patterns in which substrates, inhibitors, and inducers are combined has significant implications for detection of potential DDIs and thus clinical consequences. There are six basic chronologic patterns of DDIs.

Pattern 1: An Inhibitor Is Added to a Substrate

This pattern generally results in increases in substrate levels. This is one of the easiest DDI patterns to detect. If the substrate has a low therapeutic index, toxicity may result unless care is exercised, such as closely checking blood levels or lowering substrate dosages in anticipation of the interaction.

<u>**Example:**</u> Trimethoprim–sulfamethoxazole (TMP/SMX) is added to warfarin.

Warfarin is a **CYP2C9** substrate, and TMP/SMX (Bactrim®) is a **2C9** inhibitor. The addition of TMP/SMX impairs the ability of **2C9** to metabolize warfarin, leading to an increase in the international normalized ratio (INR). This particular interaction might be encountered by clinicians in the preoperative evaluation center.

C. Marcucci (✉)
Department of Transfusion Medicine, Clinical Center, National Institutes of Health, Bethesda, MD, USA

N. B. Sandson
Department of Psychiatry, VA Maryland Health Care System, Baltimore, MD, USA

University of Maryland, Baltimore, MD, USA

S. Mohamed et al. (eds.), *Anesthesia Bridges*, https://doi.org/10.1007/978-3-032-08294-7_134

For example, consider the situation in which you have a 65-year-old lady who is on warfarin for a history of leg deep vein thrombosis and has been experiencing recurrent urinary tract infections. Another example of a potential inhibitor-added-to-a-substrate DDI might occur when amiodarone (also a **CYP2C9** inhibitor) is added to the medication regimen of a patient on warfarin, perhaps in an ICU setting.

Pattern 2: A Substrate Is Added to an Inhibitor

This pattern may cause difficulties if the substrate has a low therapeutic index and is titrated according to preset guidelines that do not take into account the presence of an inhibitor. If the substrate is titrated to specific blood levels or to a therapeutic effect or with an appreciation that an inhibitor is present, then toxicity and/or excessive drug effects are less likely to arise.

Example: Midazolam is added to diltiazem.

This is a possible scenario in the OR. Midazolam is a **CYP3A4** substrate and one of our most commonly used drugs, both in the oral and intravenous forms. Diltiazem is a frequently used antihypertensive medication, and it happens to be an inhibitor of **3A4.** The use of midazolam in standard dosages when coadministered with diltiazem has been reported to increase midazolam levels and thus prolong sedation and delay the time until extubation can be safely accomplished.

Pattern 3: An Inducer Is Added to a Substrate

This pattern generally results in decreases in substrate levels. This is also a fairly easy pattern to detect. A decrease in levels of the substrate may result in a loss of efficacy of the substrate, unless blood levels are followed and/or the substrate dosages are increased in anticipation of the interaction.

Example: St. John's wort (SJW) is added to ethinylestradiol oral contraceptives.

This scenario might occur in the pain clinic. St. John's wort (SJW) is an herbal supplement that is most commonly taken for its supposed antidepressant effects. Commercially available extracts of St. John's wort contain varying amounts of several compounds including hyperforin. Hyperforin is an inducer of **CYP3A4** and **CYP2C9.** Many oral contraceptives contain ethinylestradiol and a progesterone component, both of which are primarily metabolized by **3A4.**

St. John's wort extracts with hyperforin contents of <1% are not likely to result in an unintended pregnancy. However, a number of commercial SJW products contain up to 5% hyperforin and may pose a risk for patients and caregivers who are not aware of the potential DDI. Another example of an inducer added to a substrate involves the addition of a pan-inducer, such as rifampin, to methadone.

***Note from the Editors:** This is one of most architecturally interesting bridges we have come across (Fig. 134.1). It is both energizing and calming. We thought this somewhat headachy chapter would be a perfect place for it, since both are needed to master DDIs.

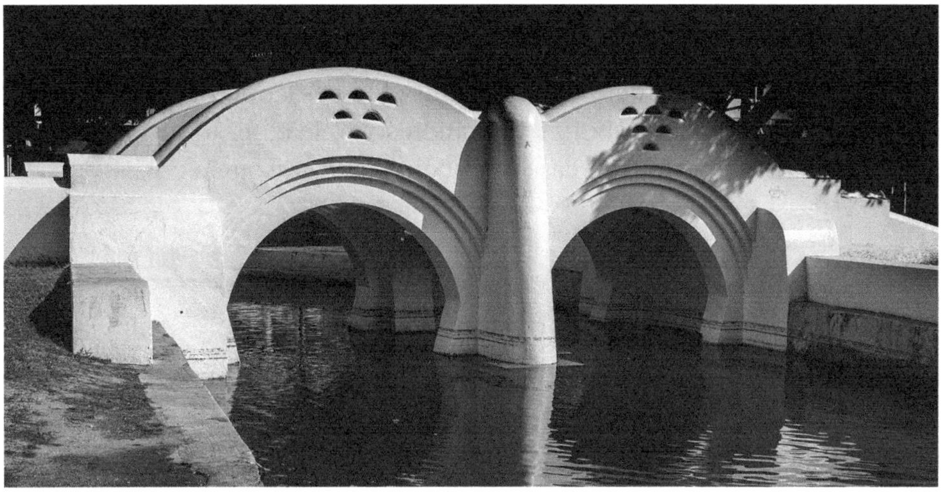

Fig. 134.1 An unusual and striking bridge in Hawaii. Photo: Image used under standard license from shutterstock.com

Pattern 4: A Substrate Is Added to an Inducer

This pattern may lead to a decreased drug effect of the substrate if the DDI is not taken into account. It may also lead to ineffective dosing of substrates if preset dosing guidelines are followed that do not take into account the presence of an inducer. If the substrate is titrated to specific blood levels or to a clinical effect, or with an appreciation that an inducer is present, then dosing is more likely to be effective.

Example: Vecuronium is added to phenytoin.

This is a possible scenario in the OR. Metabolism of vecuronium occurs primarily in the liver by liver microsomes to 3-desacetyl vecuronium. Only about 25% of the metabolism of vecuronium occurs in the kidney. Induction of the **CYP450** system by phenytoin and many other antiepileptics has been well-described. Phenytoin is a pan-inducer of multiple hepatic microsomal enzymes when administered on a chronic basis. Thus, the effect of vecuronium given to a long-term phenytoin patient is to exhibit increased clearance of non-depolarizing neuromuscular blocking agents, probably through substrate–inducer interaction at multiple enzymes.

Pattern 5: Reversal of Inhibition

After a substrate and an inhibitor are coadministered and equilibria is achieved, the inhibitor is discontinued. This leads to a resumption of normal enzyme activity and generally results in decreases in levels of the substrate and increased metabolite formation. This may result in loss of efficacy of the substrate unless blood levels are followed and/or substrate dosages are increased in anticipation of the reversal of inhibition.

Example: Fluconazole is discontinued in the presence of prednisone.

This is a possible ICU situation. Fluconazole, a **3A4** inhibitor, and prednisone, a **3A4** substrate, can be stably coadministered at appropriate dosages, yielding appropriate prednisone blood levels and clinical efficacy. The fluconazole is then discontinued, resulting in a cessation of **3A4** inhibition. **3A4** is then more available to more efficiently metabolize the prednisone, leading to a significant decrease in the prednisone blood level, and, in one known case, producing an Addisonian crisis.

Pattern 6: Reversal of Induction

After a substrate and an inducer are coadministered and equilibria is achieved, the inducer is discontinued. This results in decreased amounts of the available enzyme, leading to increased levels of the substrate and decreased metabolite formation. This may result in substrate toxicity if the substrate has a low therapeutic index, unless blood levels are followed and/or substrate dosages are decreased in anticipation of the reversal of induction. Reversal of induction is generally a gradual process that takes 1–3 weeks, but, when the inducer is smoked tobacco, this can occur more quickly, often within 1 week.

Example: Smoked tobacco is discontinued in the presence of clozapine.

Smoked tobacco is a **CYP1A2** inducer. Clozapine (Clozaril®) is an important medication for patients with treatment-resistant schizophrenia. It is principally a **1A2** substrate. Unfortunately, smoking is highly prevalent in the schizophrenic population.

Consider the situation of a schizophrenic patient who is a heavy smoker, has been stably maintained on clozapine, and whose dosage has been titrated to clinical efficacy with serial blood levels. If this patient is then admitted to a surgical or trauma service with sudden, enforced cessation of smoked tobacco, he will experience a sudden cessation of **1A2** induction. This will result in decreased metabolism of clozapine and a resulting increase in clozapine blood levels, possibly to a degree of toxicity that includes seizures.

Remember That These Clinical Effects Are Reversed if the Substrate Is a Prodrug!

Prodrugs require metabolism from an inactive parent compound to an active metabolite for clinical efficacy. When prodrugs, such as hydrocodone, tramadol, and cyclophosphamide, are the substrates in question, the clinical concerns of the above drug–drug interaction patterns are reversed.

Let us look at this a bit more closely. In the **pattern 1** example above (an inhibitor is added to a substrate), warfarin is the substrate and Bactrim® is the inhibitor. When Bactrim® is added to the medication panel of a patient on warfarin, the metabolism of warfarin is impaired, leading to excessive and unintended anticoagulation. In other words, the clinical concern is "toxicity."

However, if the substrate is an analgesic such as hydrocodone, it requires metabolism by **CYP2D6** to its active form, which is hydromorphone. If the patient on hydrocodone is then placed on a **2D6** inhibitor such as ritonavir or quinidine, the parent drug will not be metabolized to its active form and the clinical result is loss of efficacy and not toxicity. Similarly, the **pattern 3** concern would be toxicity and not loss of efficacy and so forth..

Lessons Learned

- The sequence in which interacting drugs are added to a regimen affects the likelihood of detecting a DDI.
- The six patterns are:
  - **1:** Inhibitor added to substrate
  - **2:** Substrate added to inhibitor
  - **3:** Inducer added to substrate
  - **4:** Substrate added to inducer
  - **5:** Reversal of inhibition
  - **6:** Reversal of induction.
- Patterns 1 and 3 are the easiest to detect, patterns 2 and 4 are somewhat more difficult, and patterns 5 and 6 are the most difficult to detect.
- For patterns 5 and 6 (reversals of inhibition and induction, respectively), detection of these DDIs is unlikely to be aided by DDI software or electronic medical record programs. Only an integrated understanding of this paradigm will provide reliable protection from falling victim to these patterns!
- If the substrate in question is a prodrug (requires metabolism to convert into a pharmacologically active form), then the clinical effects of the DDI are reversed.

Authors

Cathy Marcucci is a senior anesthesiologist in Maryland. Although she would never claim to be a true expert in DDIs, she does consider herself a somewhat experienced DDI educator. She remains a fan of the groundbreaking research and publications of Evan Kharasch, MD, PhD.

Neil Sandson is a senior psychiatrist in Baltimore, Maryland. He has published numerous peer-reviewed articles and four books on DDIs and given hundreds of lectures and presentations on all aspects of pharmacokinetic and pharmacodynamic DDIs. He has recently authored a comprehensive review and summary of DDIs with clinical relevance to the psychiatry community and remarked that he found himself frequently citing Dr. Kharasch's work.

Don't Forget About the P-Glycoprotein Pump

135

Catherine Marcucci and Neil B. Sandson

Introduction

As anesthesiologists, we must be prepared to function as specialists in perioperative medicine. This includes a thorough understanding of the drugs commonly given in the OR *and* the perioperative period. This "understanding" doesn't just mean drug dosages and effects; it also means routes of administration, pharmacodynamics, and pharmacokinetics including the specifics of elimination. Although pharmacokinetics usually focuses on metabolism and excretion, the emerging importance of the P-glycoprotein (P-gp) transporter also highlights the relevance of absorption and distribution.

Physiology of the P-Glycoprotein Transporter

The P-glycoprotein (P-gp) transporter is an adenosine triphosphate (ATP)-dependent pump that lines the lumen of the small intestine and extrudes various compounds or substrates. When a P-glycoprotein substrate is absorbed across the concentration gradient into the cytosol of an enterocyte, the transporter acts to extrude that drug or compound back into the gut lumen. P-glycoprotein also lines the blood–brain barrier, acting as one of the mechanisms that minimizes access of xenobiotic substances to the central nervous system. The pump will move substrates that have diffused from the blood into the cytosol of blood–brain capillary endothelial cells back into the vasculature.

Substrates of the P-Glycoprotein Pump

P-gp shares many substrates with cytochrome *P450 3A4*. These include morphine, ondansetron, tacrolimus, carbamazepine, corticosteroids, cyclosporine, dexamethasone, digoxin, quinidine, diltiazem, phenytoin, risperidone, and tricyclic antidepressants. Before a drug gets final Food and Drug

C. Marcucci (✉)
Department of Transfusion Medicine, Clinical Center, National Institutes of Health, Bethesda, MD, USA

N. B. Sandson
Department of Psychiatry, VA Maryland Health Care System, Baltimore, MD, USA

University of Maryland, Baltimore, MD, USA

S. Mohamed et al. (eds.), *Anesthesia Bridges*, https://doi.org/10.1007/978-3-032-08294-7_135

Administration (FDA) approval, dose-finding studies are done to determine the effective doses of these and other P-gp substrates that have already incorporated the effect of P-gp.

Inhibitors of the P-Glycoprotein Pump

P-gp inhibitors decrease the efflux of P-gp substrates from the enterocytes into the gut lumen. The net effect of a P-gp inhibitor is greater systemic absorption of substrates at a given dose. Similarly, at a given intravascular concentration of a P-glycoprotein substrate, the coadministration of a P-gp inhibitor will result in more influx past the blood–brain barrier and into the central nervous system. In this situation, drug toxicity may be a concern.

Significant P-glycoprotein pump inhibitors include midazolam, lidocaine, omeprazole, atorvastatin, erythromycin, fluoxetine, lovastatin, propranolol, simvastatin, and verapamil. Several common fruit juices are known to inhibit P-glycoprotein, including grapefruit juice, apple juice, and orange juice.

Inducers of the P-Glycoprotein Pump

Inducers of P-gp will act to increase transport of a substrate back into the blood. The net effect is to decrease the amount of drug that will cross the blood–brain barrier, for instance. In the case of induction of the P-gp transporter, there may be loss of efficacy. Significant P-glycoprotein inducers include aspirin, rifampin, St. John's wort, and trazodone.

Lessons Learned

- The P-glycoprotein transporter is an ATP-dependent pump that is relevant to the absorption and distribution of a number of important drugs in the perioperative period.
- *Substrates* of the P-gp pump that are especially relevant to us are morphine, digoxin, and ondansetron.
- The most relevant *inducers* are aspirin and St. John's wort. The most relevant *inhibitors* are midazolam and fruit juices.
- This is just a partial list of substrates, inhibitors, and inducers. Don't give or prescribe a drug that is new to you without knowing if it has significant P-gp pump effects. A more complete list is readily accessible on the UpToDate website.
- *Be especially careful when the patient is on drugs with a narrow therapeutic index, such as digoxin or tacrolimus.* In these cases, it is prudent to attend closely to the coadministration, addition, or deletion of P-glycoprotein inhibitors or inducers from the patient's regimen.
- Consider developing a checklist for your pre-op clinicians of the most relevant substrates, inhibitors, and inducers.

Authors

Cathy Marcucci and **Neil B. Sandson** have been interested and involved in drug–drug interaction education for anesthesiologists and psychiatrists for many years. They have collectively given hundreds of talks and published numerous articles and three books on the subject. Rumor has it that the government of New South Wales (Australia) even loaded the entirety of one of their books on a public health website somewhere, but that may just be a rumor.

136 Vigilance Always Is Not Just for the Operating Room

LeeAnn Rhodes

Introduction

Vigilance: that is the word that has echoed in my mind for several decades. It is the mantra anesthesiologists live by. I have been in the practice of pain management since completing my fellowship, and both my basic anesthesia training and advanced training have left me with invaluable lessons. As anesthesiologists, we are often in the position where we must conduct a rapid multisystem assessment of American Society of Anesthesiologists (ASA) 3 and 4 patients, forming differential diagnosis that may have gone unnoticed. This vigilance has informed my pain practice repeatedly through the years and allowed me to give better and more complete care to my patients.

Every Case Is an Opportunity

A number of cases stand out in my mind. For instance, I once was consulted on a gentleman who had several months of crushing chest pain. He had been seen at four prominent hospitals throughout our country and came back with a negative cardiac workup. He realized something was amiss, yet he felt as though he had been passed from one specialist to another, while continuing to deteriorate through lack of energy and loss of appetite. On exam, I noticed that he had a sensory change at his left T4 dermatome. I then ordered a thoracic MRI, which unfortunately revealed a metastasis at T4, which later turned out to be multiple myeloma. If I had not been trained to look at each system, I too probably would have missed this finding.

Over the years, I have seen plenty of cases canceled due to something being amiss. I tend to think of these "missed" opportunities as an opportunity to help patients, and the healthcare teams, by furthering everybody's knowledge of the patients' healthcare status. Typically, in these events, fear fills the patients. However, I do my best to reframe the situation. Often in the patients I see, it is the result of uncontrolled diabetes. A short conversation may reveal poor food choices, and, most commonly, sodas and other sugar drinks are the culprit. A brief educational intervention can go a long way.

L. Rhodes (✉)
Maryland Brain, Spine, and Pain, Annapolis, MD, USA

S. Mohamed et al. (eds.), *Anesthesia Bridges*, https://doi.org/10.1007/978-3-032-08294-7_136

Staying Steady During the Pandemic

The year 2020 rocked our world in a way that it never had previously in our lifetime. Our skills were summoned to the ICUs across the nation. In my world of pain management, I often was the only clinician who had recently seen the patient in person. For over a year, most of their ongoing care had been via televisits. Again, because of the training I received, I was able to diagnose several cases of atrial fibrillation, neoplasms, cardiac ischemia, and femoral stenosis, all of which enabled these patients to get the care for symptoms that were pushed aside, often due to their fear of entering into a healthcare system that had been consumed with COVID-19. Anesthesiologists are trained to be the calming force, and this has come into play at such a crucial time!

Lessons Learned

- In anesthesia training, we learn early how to evaluate complex patients for care in the OR.
- Carry this training forward into all aspects of your career, including the anesthesia subspecialties. In looking at and evaluating the overall health status of my pain patients, I have been able to diagnose and further their care of medical issues that are not strictly pain-related.
- A canceled case is an opportunity to further learn about and manage a patient's healthcare status.

Author

LeeAnn Rhodes has been a lifelong Marylander. After taking pain management as an elective during her residency, she found this to be her true passion. For 25 years, she worked in a teaching healthcare system and loved hearing the different perspectives from students' life experiences. Now, in her 26th year of practice, she has entered the private practice arena. When not working, she enjoys reading, traveling, boating, and spending time with her children and family! She attributes her accomplishments directly to the amazing mentoring she received during her medical training.

Reducing Noise

137

Raymond G. Graber

Introduction

You are probably thinking that this chapter will be a rant about surgeons and nurses who are having loud discussions as you are getting ready to induce your patient. Alternatively, it could be about music blasting in your room during key parts of cases, rendering communication difficult. Well, sorry to disappoint you, those topics will have to wait for another time. This chapter is about noise in another sense—the statistical sense. Noise refers to unexplained variation or randomness that is found within a given data sample. Specifically, we are going to talk about how we have tried to improve medical care by reducing variations ("noise") in care.

A Primer on Noise

If you want to read a good book on this subject, pick up *Noise—A Flaw in Human Judgment,* by Kahneman, Sibonyn, and Sunstein [1]. This book explores the topic of why people make bad judgments, and how to reduce variation and biases in decision-making. They include a chapter on decision-making in medicine and include examples of how different physicians can see the same patient or same data and come up with different conclusions and prescribe different treatments.

The medical profession has tried to address this issue through improved training and continuing education, and in the future, we will see more and more use of artificial intelligence applications to assist physicians. But maybe the most successful strategy has been by the development of guidelines of care. The book uses the Apgar score, developed by anesthesiologist Virginia Apgar, as an example of a guideline that works well and has improved quality of care.

R. G. Graber (✉)
Department of Anesthesiology and Perioperative Medicine, University Hospitals Cleveland Medical Center, Cleveland, OH, USA
e-mail: raymond.graber@uhhospitals.org

S. Mohamed et al. (eds.), *Anesthesia Bridges*, https://doi.org/10.1007/978-3-032-08294-7_137

Standards and Guidelines

When you think about it, standards and guidelines are attempts to improve outcomes by reducing variability, or "noise," in care. Typically, a group of experts is convened, they review the literature and discuss their personal experiences, and then a consensus document is written. Many of these are written in response to a perceived problem.

For example, in the early 1980s, anesthesia malpractice costs were soaring in response to lawsuits brought after cases of hypoxic brain injury due to undiscovered esophageal intubations or ventilator disconnects. The leadership of the American Society of Anesthesiologists (ASA) assessed current practice and decided that part of the problem was variability in how patients were monitored during the course of an anesthetic.

In response, the first ASA standard, the Standards for Basic Anesthetic Monitoring, was produced in 1986. Note that this was written as a *standard*, not a *guideline*. Standards are meant to be strictly followed—they are requirements—and there are medical liability ramifications if you don't follow them and there is a bad outcome. Standards can evolve over time.

For example, mandatory use of pulse oximetry and capnography was added in as these technologies became reliable and widely available. This standard was extremely successful, as evidenced by a drop in hypoxic brain injury cases, and a significant drop in malpractice insurance costs. Best practices were identified and implemented, variability was reduced, and outcomes improved. At present, the ASA has three published standards: "Basic Standards for Preanesthesia Care," "Standards for Basic Anesthetic Monitoring," and "Standards for Post-anesthesia Care."

Standards vs Guidelines

How do guidelines differ from standards? Whereas standards are typically meant to be mandatory, a guideline is typically a list of strongly recommended practices. A guideline allows for deviations based on clinical judgment for specific patients or situations. Thus, there may be less legal risk if one deviates from a guideline of care. Here is a direct quote from the 2022 ASA "Practice Guidelines for Management of the Difficult Airway." [2]

- Practice guidelines are systematically developed recommendations that assist the practitioner and patient in making decisions about health care. These recommendations may be adopted, modified, or rejected according to clinical needs and constraints and are not intended to replace local institutional policies.

- In addition, practice guidelines developed by the American Society of Anesthesiologists (ASA) are not intended as standards or absolute requirements, and their use cannot guarantee any specific outcome. Practice guidelines are subject to revision as warranted by the evolution of medical knowledge, technology, and practice. They provide basic recommendations that are supported by a synthesis and analysis of the current literature, expert and practitioner opinion, open forum commentary, and clinical feasibility data.

It is worth reading and understanding guidelines because they generally are the current best practices and will likely improve the quality of care you deliver. The ASA has produced multiple guidelines, most of which are published in *Anesthesiology*, then posted on the ASA website. In my practice, I have frequently referred to the ASA "Practice Guidelines for Management of the Difficult Airway" and "Practice Guidelines for Moderate Procedural Sedation and Analgesia" (I have rewritten our hospital sedation policy multiple times!).

Our subspecialty societies are also in the guideline business. A guideline that has been very helpful to me personally is the American Society of Regional Anesthesia (ASRA) produced "Regional Anesthesia in the Patient Receiving Antithrombotic or Thrombolytic Therapy." [3] This is available on their website and in App form for your phone. ASRA leadership realized in the late 1990s that there was an increasing potential to have neurologic complications as neuraxial techniques became more popular, and at the same time, more and more patients were receiving anticoagulant or antiplatelet therapy. This document has been updated multiple times as the pharmaceutical industry keeps pumping out new coagulation poisons.

***Note from the Editors:** Ray Graber is from Albany and went to Rensselaer Polytech in Troy, NY. We are including the Thaddeus Kosciusko Bridge in his honor (Fig. 137.1).

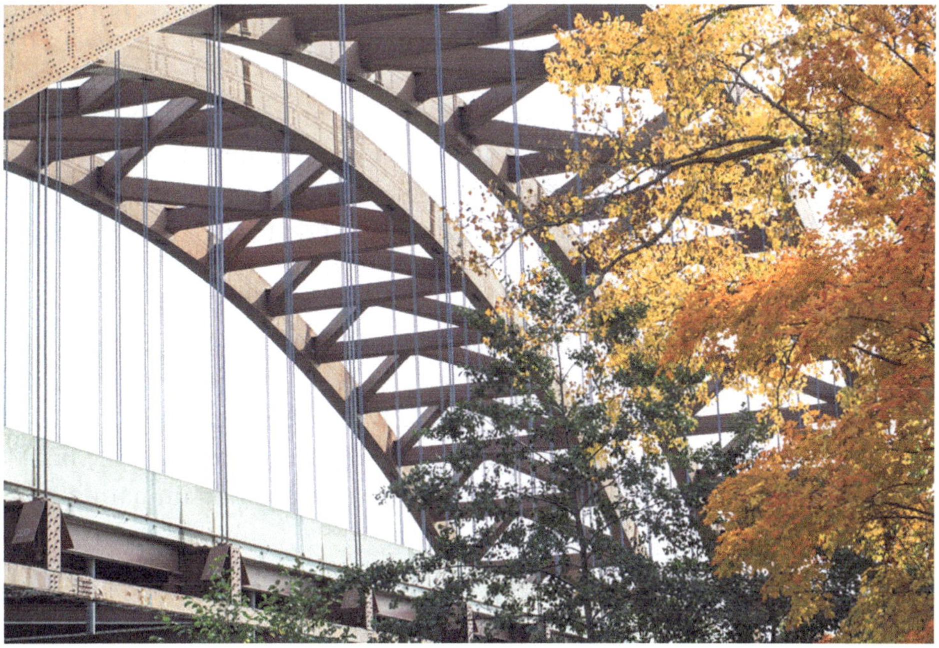

Fig. 137.1 The Thaddeus Kosciusko Bridge spans the Mohawk River in the greater Albany area. It opened in 1959 and carries three lanes of Interstate 87 highway traffic on each span. It is named after a notable Polish leader and soldier who contributed greatly to the Colonists' victory in the Revolutionary War. Photo: Image used under standard license from stock.adobe.com

Echocardiography

Let's switch gears and talk about echocardiography. I would guess that all of us who practice anesthesia will have requested or reviewed echo reports on our patients. We use this information to understand the cardiac physiology of our patients, and also to help risk stratify. Those of us who are cardiac anesthesiologists are in the business of performing transesophageal echos (TEEs) and writing reports. We trust that the information we get from these studies is reliable, repeatable, and accurate.

However, when I started doing TEEs in the 1990s, this was probably not the case. We learned how to perform TEEs on the job, went to national meetings, read multiple textbooks, and had mentors we worked with. However, at the time, there were no national consensus guidelines on how measurements were made, and how to use these measurements for grading valve disease or chamber size. The end result was potential for lots of variation in measurements and in interpretation.

The American Society of Echocardiography (ASE) has worked to reduce this noise in the system by writing recommendations that specify exactly how measurements are to be made, and how chamber size and valve disease should be quantified. The ASE and Society of Cardiovascular Anesthesiologists (SCA) jointly developed a certification process for perioperative echocardiography and created review courses to teach TEE principles to prepare practitioners for this exam. If you are performing echocardiography, you should be using the ASE guidelines so that your data and interpretations are reliable and accurate. In effect, you are working to reduce your personal noise.

As a last example, let's think about this topic as it applies at your local hospital and department level. There may be certain treatment protocols you don't want variability in. An example is perioperative antibiotics—we want specific drugs for specific cases given at specific times. This can be written into a hospital protocol. Many of us have worked to create ERAS protocols to support specific surgery types.

For example, in many centers, there is a move to send patients who are having hip and knee replacements home on the same day. This can only be successful if the joint replacement teams work together to standardize treatments to achieve this goal. We have switched to shorter acting spinals, such as mepivacaine or lower dose bupivacaine, to facilitate early discharge, but if you have an attending that uses longer acting spinals, the end goal is sabotaged. Eliminating noise in our local processes improves care.

About the Music Blaring in the OR…

In my opening paragraph I stated that this chapter was not going to be about loud conversations or music. Instead, I have tried to demonstrate the value of standards, guidelines, and protocols. They generally represent attempts to formulate best practices and reduce variability, both at the national level and within our own departments. But what about conversations and music in the operating room? I will conclude with the following thought: It's okay to have some favorite tunes playing in your operating rooms but try to keep the *noise* down!

Lessons Learned

- Standards and guidelines that have been written by our national organizations have the goal of improving care on a national level.
- You can improve care at your local level by participating in writing guidelines and protocols for your individual departments.
- Department protocols and guidelines should be well communicated and posted where members have easy access to refer to.
- All guidelines and protocols need to be periodically reviewed and revised as new technology, medications, and treatment goals are developed.

References

1. Kahneman D, Sibony O, Sunstein CR. Noise: a flaw in human judgment. 1st ed. New York: Little, Brown Spark; 2021.
2. Apfelbaum JL, Hagberg CA, Connis RT, et al. 2022 American Society of Anesthesiologists practice guidelines for management of the difficult airway. Anesthesiology. 2022;136:31–81.
3. Horlocker TT, Vandermeulen E, Kopp SL, et al. Regional anesthesia in the patient receiving antithrombotic or thrombolytic therapy: American Society of Regional Anesthesia and Pain Medicine evidence-based guidelines (fourth edition). Reg Anesth Pain Med. 2018;43(3):263–309.

Author

Ray Graber has been a practicing anesthesiologist in Cleveland since 1988. Early in his career, he developed an interest in process improvement, reduction of errors, and improving patient outcomes. Checklists, protocols, and guidelines are the way to go—especially for the more complex cases!

138 Resourcefulness

Lee C. Woodson

Introduction

During a career, anesthesiologists will be confronted with clinical dilemmas without an available conventional solution. You should be prepared to go outside of your usual bag of tricks.

Solutions

With regulations as they are today you probably will not use your own blood to resuscitate a baby as might have occurred before my time. But you might need to do an exchange transfusion to correct severe anemia when a bleeding infant is volume resuscitated before PRBCs are available.

Or you might cut an ETT short and extend the stylet out the end when a bougie is not available, or have a colleague illuminate the larynx with a laryngoscope when the light for the fiberoptic scope dies in a remote location or give volume through an arterial catheter. Everyone has their stories.

There is almost always a solution if you take a breath and consider what resources are available. But don't be too proud of yourself after a success, as another humbling experience is just around the corner.

L. C. Woodson (✉)
Department of Anesthesiology, University of Texas Medical Branch, Galveston, TX, USA

S. Mohamed et al. (eds.), *Anesthesia Bridges*, https://doi.org/10.1007/978-3-032-08294-7_138

Lessons Learned

- As you listen to war stories told by colleagues, keep in mind that their innovative solutions to problems may someday help you out when you most need it.
- But don't be proud, no need to brag or boast, the next problem situation is coming down the pike.

Bonus Content!

As with other topics in this book, we went to the literature to see if resourcefulness can be learned. And the answer is, of course it can!

- What's a good general definition of resourcefulness? It's not just surviving a lousy situation or coping with deprivation—that is more stoicism than anything. Resourcefulness is generally agreed to be the ability to use optimism, confidence, and creativity to find efficient and innovative ways to overcome challenges. These skills also involve optimizing resources to make something—a product, a process, or a system, new or better.
- Here's another way to look at it: **resourcefulness is knowing who/what to look for and what to ask to solve a problem**. *Sometimes the answer could be just one question away.*
- Two mottoes—*"redefine the possible" and "resourcefulness is innovation turned inward."*
- Being resourceful doesn't only involve creative and even outside-the-box solutions to problems in the moment. It also involves being resolutely proactive. Meaning you are full of resources—books, courses, online content, knowledge and, very importantly, your network.
- *Resourcefulness should be thought of as a skill.* It is very responsive to practice. It can be logged and tracked as well—most business and psychology websites on resourcefulness suggest that you keep notes on problems you have solved, problems you are working through, and problems you are likely to face. The very definition of resourcefulness is using what you have, to get to where you want to go, even in the face of obstacles. Being mindful of past problems and their solutions—what worked and what didn't—is very valuable. Experience is a fantastic resource, and you should use it.
- *Resourcefulness is also a mindset.* More than intelligence or stubbornness, it is based on *curiosity.* Other attributes of resourcefulness are adaptability, coordination/communication, creativity, patience, and persistence.

***Note from the Editors:** The Frederick Douglass Memorial Bridge spans the Anacostia River (Fig. 138.1). Frederick Douglass was enslaved in his youth and had no schooling or real education of any kind, as it was illegal to teach those children how to read. So, he secretly taught himself to read by studying the letters and words on packing crates on the Baltimore dockside and by carefully watching white and free children of color at their lessons. He is widely considered to be one of the most brilliant figures in American history.

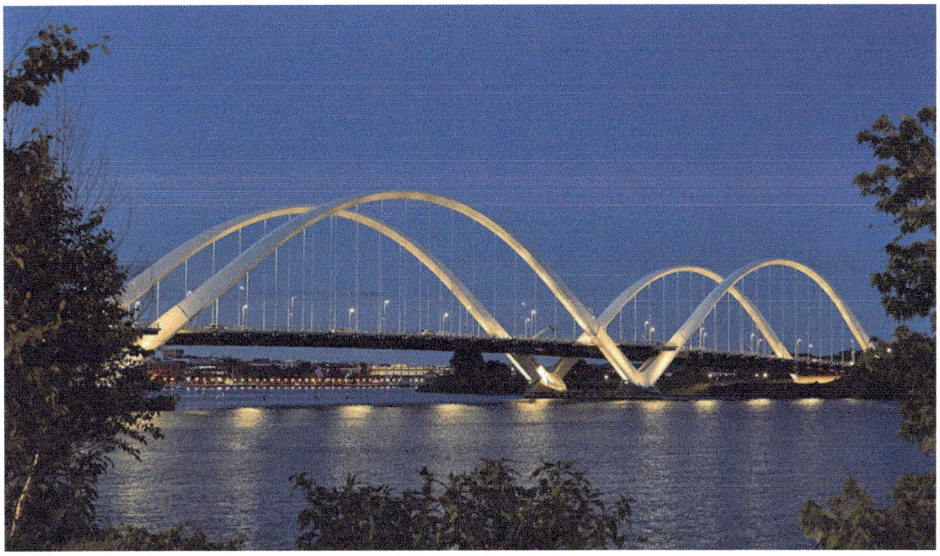

Fig. 138.1 The beautiful Frederick Douglass Memorial Bridge in the Anacostia section of Washington, DC. It was completed in 2021 and replaced an older swing bridge known as the South Capitol Street Bridge. Photo: Image used under standard license from shutterstock.com

How do you practice getting better at resourcefulness?

- Be receptive—don't automatically think "No, I can't do that." Instead, think, "I wonder how that would work."
- Learn from others—no need to reinvent the wheel. You can watch and learn *and/or* ask and learn. A simple query will do, such as, "What do you think are the two resources that are most valuable to a cardiac anesthesiologist?" Then, no matter the answer, set about looking into and/or acquiring these for yourself. Also ask about subsets of these questions—what are the best interpersonal resources, online resources, and free resources?
- Be willing to learn new skills, including research skills.
- Accept feedback and criticism.
- Be willing to share your resources with colleagues.
- From blogger Dan Lucas [1]:

> By far, my favorite example of being resourceful is the genius device that saved the Apollo 13 crew from dying in their emergency return to Earth, as photographed during that trip using one of their Hasselblad cameras.
>
> After Mission Control decided to cancel Apollo 13's moon landing following an explosion of an oxygen tank in the Service Module, the astronauts moved to the Lunar Module in order to save power that was going to be needed later for re-entry. The only problem with this plan was that the Lunar Module was designed for only two people for a 36-hour period, not three astronauts for 96 hours. They quickly discovered that carbon dioxide was building up fast, putting their lives in extreme danger. They had to change the circular CO_2 scrubbers in the Lunar Module for clean ones, but they only had spare square CO_2 scrubbers from the Command Module.
>
> In record time, the Crew Systems Division put together an improvised adapter using all sorts of weird and random parts, like a flight manual cover, suit pants, and socks. CAPCOM (Capsule Communicator) transmitted the

instructions to the astronauts in order to assemble this "mailbox" rig—as they called it—working against the clock and trying to survive the effects of the poisonous gas, which was quickly asphyxiating their brains. Talk about being under pressure! Wow!

Other inspiring and historical examples of resourcefulness can be found online [2].

- Susan B. Anthony was an early women's rights activist. The early suffragists used every available legal resource to win the right to vote for women. This included state and federal legislative campaigning, registering to vote and casting ballots, proposing a Constitutional Amendment, and litigating under the 14th Amendment to test the limits of women's rights.

- Jesse Owens was a track star and Olympic gold medalist. Owens was a fascinating and complex man, and he drew on his astonishing athletic prowess to make his way in the world. He insisted on competing in the 1936 Olympics as he viewed them as an opportunity to make his mark in the world and begin to make the impact that he wished to make.

- Ernest Shackleton and the crew of the Endurance survived in the Antarctic after their ship sank. Shackleton was another intriguing leader. He was cautious by nature, intuitive, inspirational, and innovative. Sir Raymond Priestley, the acclaimed scientist who served on Antarctic expeditions with both Scott and Shackleton, once wrote: "For scientific leadership, give me Scott. For swift and efficient travel, Amundsen. But when you are in a hopeless situation, when there seems no way out, get on your knees and pray for Shackleton." Shackleton used his available resources, first and foremost, for safety and survival. He once turned back just short of an expeditionary goal when he realized that his food was running out. He later remarked to his wife, "I thought you would prefer a live donkey to a dead lion."

- Jacqueline Cochran and the WASPs (Women's Airforce Service Pilots) played a crucial role in WW2. Cochran was highly intelligent and highly ambitious. She used her early childhood poverty and good looks to fuel her drive to achieve in the beauty business and then in the early days of civilian and military aviation. She also used the blank slate of the future as a resource —always looking for the next opportunity as she invented and reinvented herself as she went along.

Our final thoughts:

- Resourcefulness and resiliency are closely related, although resiliency is more an internal state, and one fosters the other.

- Great resourcefulness is a *sine qua non* of great leadership.

References

1. Credo Finance. Great leaders are uniquely resourceful—Week 12 [Internet]. Credo Finance; 2022 Apr 6 [cited 2025 Jun 13]. Available from: https://credofinance.com/great-leaders-uniquely-resourceful-week-12/
2. WorldStrides. Resourcefulness: history & social-emotional learning [Internet]. WorldStrides; 2020 Jun [cited 2025 Jun 13]. Available from: https://resources.worldstrides.com/wp-content/uploads/2020/06/Resourcefulness-History-SEL.pdf

Author

Lee Woodson has been retired for several years, after 30 years on the anesthesiology faculty at the University of Texas Medical Branch in Galveston. The last 20 years focused on the care of burn patients, especially pediatric patients at the Galveston Shriners Burn Center. Now his time is spent with his wife, Anne, and hobbies: fishing, traveling, cooking, gardening, and grandchildren. Also, he has learned that a professor emeritus has much in common with being a grandparent. You can show up from time to time and offer unsolicited advice but not stick around for the consequences.

Be Ready for Anything!

139

Berend Mets

Be Ready for Anything

– *Roger Eltringham*

Early Days

This sound advice, I heard first from Dr. Roger Eltringham. I had traveled from South Africa to England to start anesthesia training, and the good doctor was my faculty tutor. I was a serious young man at the time; a bit too intense and humorless for my own good ☹.

He had offered me a senior house officer job in anesthesia at the Gloucestershire Royal Hospital, sight unseen, taking a chance on the young Hollander who had received medical training at the University of Stellenbosch—he liked foreigners in his department. In fact, so much so that the Anesthesia Department that he directed had representation from four continents: Americans, Asians, Africans, Australians—a few Englishmen and Scots were also in evidence.

A more international department was not to be found anywhere.

This proved useful because Roger was very well connected with the World Federation Societies of Anaesthesiologists and had set out to create educational opportunities for many young anesthetists from around the world. He included me in his fold. Here he set about preparing us for the fellowship examinations of the Royal College of Anaesthetists. An examination at which he considered himself an expert: he told me that he had failed it three times ☺.

***Note from the Editors:** Dr. Mets' parents were Dutch, and this is the Veluwemeer Aqueduct, the coolest bridge in the Netherlands (Fig. 139.1). Both the engineering and architecture are stunning. The water depth on the bridge is 3 meters so small boats and other shallow-water craft can cross.

B. Mets (✉)
Department of Anesthesiology and Perioperative Medicine, Penn State College of Medicine, Penn State Milton S. Hershey Medical Center, Hershey, PA, USA
e-mail: bmets@pennstatehealth.psu.edu

S. Mohamed et al. (eds.), *Anesthesia Bridges*, https://doi.org/10.1007/978-3-032-08294-7_139

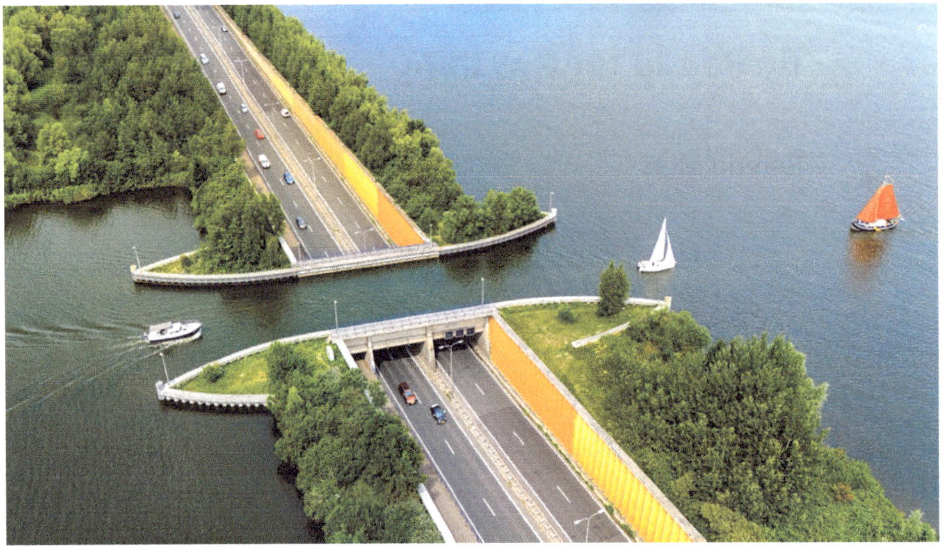

Fig. 139.1 The Veluwemeer Aqueduct connects two sections of a lake. *The water is the bridge.* The road, named the N302, connects mainland Netherlands to Flevoland, a large man-made island. Photo: Image used under standard license from shutterstock.com

International Experiences

None of this was in evidence however when I worked with Dr. Eltringham in the operating room and the intensive therapy unit in Gloucester, or when providing lectures in countries such as Vietnam and China where I traveled with Roger to educate via WFSA refresher courses around the world.

Roger would start off by advising me to always: *Be ready for anything.*

In theatre, that was crucial advice. To this day when I am in the OR, I project out in my imagination what is the worst thing that can happen now, and then plan how I will respond to that emergency in my mind: pick up this syringe—inject there; adjust ventilation—here; call for help—on that phone, etc.

In international health education and care even more so.

I remember one incident in New Zealand when I was giving a very complicated lecture. To do this well you need absolute concentration from the start of the presentation and need to know your opening lines perfectly to gain both your own, and the audience's confidence in your oration.

Well, the slides were up, and I gave my first introductory remarks. And then all the lights in the auditorium went off. And then magically on. I started again. A little non-plussed. They went off. And then on. And then all off! I started again for the third time—we worked out what it was. Somebody was standing at the back of the auditorium toggling the light switch—on and off—as he scratched his itching back against its lever.

I remember another incident in Ethiopia, under halothane anesthesia, with a double lumen tube for lung resection. I had positioned the double lumen tube the way I had learnt to do that at the University of

Cape Town, at a time when fiberoptic scopes were not yet in usual practice. And then heard the Bosun whistle going off: the alarm shrilly sounding the failure of the anesthesia machine's oxygen supply ☹.

A ready explanation only affording itself when I turned around in fright to see what the problem was—to conserve oxygen supplies to their last, the single freestanding oxygen cylinder feeding the anesthesia machine was being switched out by a nurse with a spanner after everyone was doubly sure that the tank was completely empty. During the tank swap—there existed no emergency cylinders nor central oxygen supply to provide continuous oxygen while in flight during this complicated case.

Room air was required for a short period of time—*be ready for anything*—and treat it all with good humor ☺.

Lessons Learned

- When doing medical mission work, be aware that equipment and supplies and practices will be different than in your home country. Prepare for the unexpected!

Author

Berend Mets was born in Indonesia of Dutch parents and lived on three continents before settling in South Africa where he studied medicine and anesthesia. He served as the anesthesia residency director at Columbia University in the 1990s before becoming Chairman of anesthesiology and perioperative medicine at Penn State University.

How to Be Ready for Anything: A Supplement to the Wise Words from Dr. Mets

140

F. Jacob Seagull, Charles H. Sandson, and Catherine Marcucci

Introduction

Be Ready for Anything is indeed good advice for anyone. But the question remains: how? What does it really mean to be prepared? How do we prepare ourselves for anything? How do we prepare our systems for anything?

Murphy's Law

It is a sentiment closely related to the widely misunderstood *Murphy's Law* that states, "Anything that can go wrong will go wrong." Surprisingly, Edward A. Murphy, Jr. was not a pessimist; he was a West Point grad, WWII veteran, and aerospace engineer who worked on safety-critical systems. The Law came into being in the late 1940s when he was conducting high-speed rocket sled experiments at Wright-Patterson Air Force Base.

In actuality, it arose from years of observing systems strive for protection and inevitably fall short. Far from being a fatalistic statement on the sad state of the world and resigning yourself to a poor outcome, his 'law' was a warning, with an implied conclusion of, "…so be sure to be ready for it." The path to safety leads through forethought and preparation. The point of Murphy's Law is not to merely accept the inevitable failures, rather to avoid that fate with action and actualization. In other words, to create systems so robust that no matter what does go wrong, the core objectives of the system can be achieved by competent professionals.

Experts have failed more times than beginners have tried. You can argue, and we do, that trying and failing is the activity that turns a beginner into an expert. What's more, it's not just failing at the same thing

F. J. Seagull
Center for Bioethics and Social Science in Medicine, University of Michigan Medical School, Ann Arbor, MI, USA

C. H. Sandson
ZS Associates, Washington, DC, USA

C. Marcucci (✉)
Department of Transfusion Medicine, Clinical Center, National Institutes of Health, Bethesda, MD, USA

S. Mohamed et al. (eds.), *Anesthesia Bridges*, https://doi.org/10.1007/978-3-032-08294-7_140

over and over that makes an expert. One key to becoming an expert is to try, and fail, in all sorts of different situations. True experts have a vast array of experiences to draw upon, usually including different scenarios, with unique technical constraints, or varying amounts of time pressure, and ever-changing margins of error. Experts use these different experiences to understand the options available in all the variations that occur. They are ready for anything. If something can go wrong, it will, and experts will be ready for it.

That's why none of Dr. Roger Eltringham's failures were in evidence when Dr. Mets worked with him.

He was being prepared by:

- *Planning for contingencies*
- *Being vigilant to threats to safety*
- *Being obsessed with failure*

This strategy of "imagining the worst" is sound advice, proven by studies of high-risk industries that boast impressive safety records. One of the hallmarks of an organization in a high-risk industry that has an exceptional safety record (High Reliability Organizations), is that the people in the organization are obsessed with failure, and the various ways things could go wrong. They think about failure because they are committed to resilience—being able to withstand adverse conditions without compromising safety. They plan for it. They adapt themselves to compensate for it. They are ready for it.

***Note from the Editors:** Speaking of being ready for anything, this is Cathy Marcucci's late father, Nicholas J. Marcucci, who served in the 81st Division and the 1629 Engineer Battalion in the Pacific Theater in WW2 and the Occupation of Japan (Fig. 140.1). Technical Corporal Marcucci once related that he had carried "field weight," including his pack, steel helmet, and rifle, of at least 70 pounds. And, besides all his regular gear and rations, he also carried engineering and construction gear. Apparently, this included surveying equipment and a pup tent if the engineers were out in front of the regular troops and had to carry everything they would need with them. However, his slide rule was made of bamboo and extremely lightweight so it would float in water (Fig. 140.2).

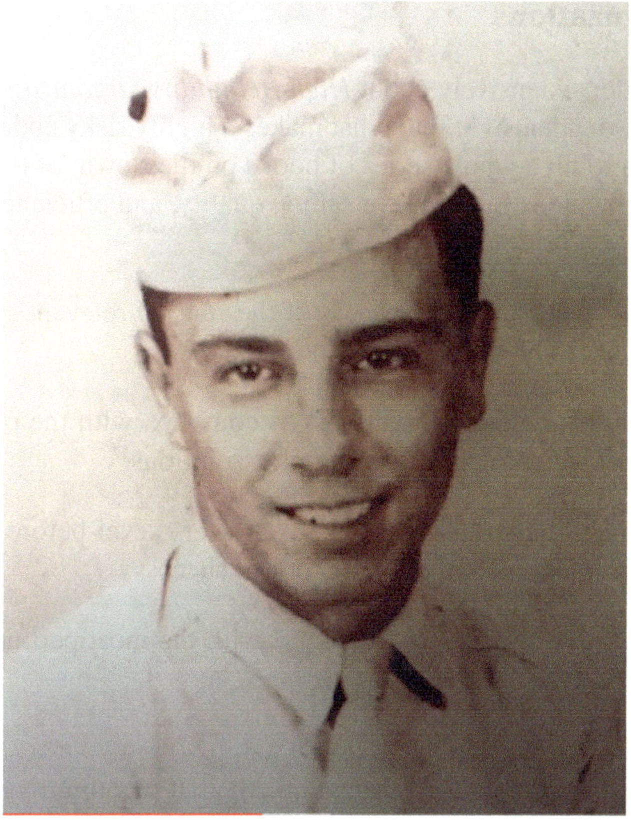

Fig. 140.1 The Defense Technical Information Center states that the 1629th, along with several other Engineer battalions "was organized for the purpose of furnishing support to combat operations in all theaters of the war. In the zone of communications, temporary landing strips for bombers, warehouses for medical, quartermaster, and ordnance supplies, and many roads and docks had to be built to keep the materiel moving to the front." Basically, the WW2 Engineers had the incredibly difficult job of insuring preparedness and combat readiness for the troops. Cathy's Dad once described that the landing strips were made of giant sheets of corrugated metal. Photo: Collection of the Marcucci family

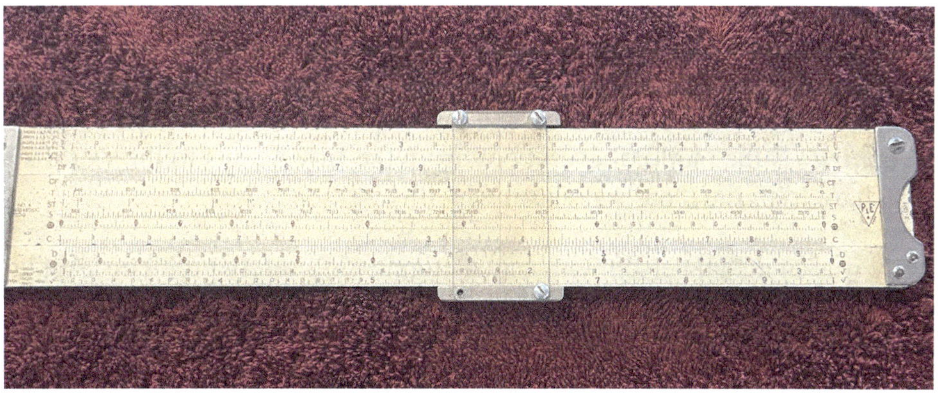

Fig. 140.2 This is Nicholas Marcucci's bamboo slide rule, used to help engineer American victory in WW2. Can you imagine designing laying out and building an airfield with this as your "computer"? Photo: Gavin Hess

High Reliability Organizations

Kathleen Sutcliffe has written extensively about *High Reliability Organizations* (HROs), and her work provides fascinating and in-depth insight into what makes a highly risky endeavor a highly reliable one. These concepts are enough to fill a whole series of books on their own, of course. But in general, High Reliability HROs are organizations that achieve safety, quality, and efficiency goals by employing five basic principles [1]:

- *Sensitivity to operations*—heightened awareness of the state of relevant systems and processes, and listening to the people who know the situation first-hand.
- *Reluctance to simplify*—the acceptance that work is complex, with the potential to fail in new and unexpected ways; complex situations require complex solutions.
- *Preoccupation with failure*—fix potential problems at every level before they occur and view near misses as opportunities to improve, rather than proof of success.
- *Deference to expertise*—to value insights from staff with the most pertinent safety knowledge over those with greater seniority.
- *Practicing resilience*—make sure a problem doesn't stop you in your tracks—always create contingencies; prioritize emergency training for many unlikely, but possible, system failures.

As we have discussed elsewhere, the aviation and nuclear industries were in the forefront with these principles. There still is ample work to be done implementing them in the medical universe, and they lend themselves perfectly to the practice of anesthesiology. Great area for research, don't you think?

Lessons Learned

- Be ready for anything really means be ready for failure.
- There is no big secret to readiness and success. It just requires consistent and proactive thought about failure. "*Be prepared*" is the motto of everybody from the Boy Scouts to the world's most advanced militaries—you have to figure there's a reason why this is.
- Edward Murphy was an actual person with actual engineering safety problems. Apparently, he hated the corruption of his life's work into a sort of resigned, fatalistic "shit happens" cliché.
- Experts are essentially master pattern-recognizers, using their plethora of experiences to understand all the options available at every decision point within a situation, especially a crisis.
- There is a lot of pop psychology that urges people not to even let the idea of failure cross your mind for one second. We think this is so wrong. *People succeed by steeping themselves in the possibility of failure.* You win by making sure there is always a path leading away from failure. "Failure is not an option" only works if you have spent the time and gained the expertise to minutely examine how failure might happen and how it can be avoided. There is also a maxim in popular psychology that it

takes 10,000 hours or 10,000 attempts to master a subject or technique. This might be true, depending on how that time is spent.

- We must think of failure constantly and look at our process of delivering anesthesia care. How can we break down our normal operating procedure into its component parts. What can go wrong at every step? What will we do if it does? What will the system around us do? Answer these questions, and we will be well on our way to disaster-avoidance expertise. And remember, planning for and dealing with failure depends more on what you do than on what you don't do.
- *The time spent on learning about High Reliability Organizations is well worth it! Start with the work of Kathleen Sullivan or try "High Reliability Organization Research: A Literature Review for Health Care" by Tolk et al. [2] This is an interesting article because it's in the engineering literature—the Engineering Management Journal. There is little doubt about it—anesthesiologists may be in the forefront among the medical specialties but medicine in general has not been at the cutting edge of this work.

Bonus Content!

As the authors were writing this chapter, an interesting discussion developed on the nature of errors in anesthesia practice and the commonly misunderstood principles. It became apparent that although she has published several previous books on "anesthesia errors," these really are handbooks and manuals of teaching points as opposed to scholarly treatises on error reduction [3]. Cathy was therefore not too proud to admit that she needed a refresher on several basic principles. Jake and Charlie corresponded back and forth, and Jake was kind enough to summarize several key points for her, as below.

First, don't fall into the trap of thinking that the best defense against Murphy is expertise. That would be the exact *opposite* of the best defense against Murphy. The actual best defense against Murphy is to design *SYSTEMS* (not people) that are fault tolerant/fail-safe. The last ten to twenty years in healthcare have seen an effort to move away from the idea of "being good enough to not make mistakes." This evolution in thinking is progress. We don't want to get involved in promoting messages that can be interpreted as going against this progress.

Second, we need to disabuse ourselves of the idea that, "Anesthesia is a field with zero margin for error." This is both false and dangerous. It is a dangerous way of thinking because "be safe" or "try not to make mistakes" is a recipe for disaster. And it is a recipe that is used by a lot of "old school" doctors. "I don't need all this 'team building' kumbaya safety mumbo jumbo. My patient safety is just being excellent!"

Anesthesiology *of course* has a margin of error. There are anesthetic errors all the time. All. The. Time. And this is not even getting into the most rigorous use of the term "error"— because that's a whole other thing. But the essential task for anesthesiologists is to design a system with lots of margin for error. Error and recovery.

Third, expertise is good and necessary. It is good to practice for contingencies. We need to make sure that the message of Murphy's law **isn't** "so be sure not to make mistakes."

More Bonus Content

In the ongoing friendly discussion and debate, Charlie also gave us a bit of insight into his industry. The details are different from our industry, but it seems like there might be some interesting analogies.

From Charlie Sandson

- I work for an industrial and management engineering consulting firm specializing in the healthcare and pharmaceutical industries. We serve a wide variety of clients, whose products do billions in revenue annually.

- Consulting is an expertise-based profession. Firms are hired to provide expert knowledge in a targeted area, be it strategic and focused expertise around C-suite business planning, or projects as tactical as salesforce deployment. Their whole value proposition is that consulting firms know what you don't, and any question you may have, they have thought about and know the answer to. *These firms don't sell perfection, they sell preparation.*

- As such, a consultant's greatest failure is to not know, to be confronted with an unexpected question that sends the whole team scrambling. This is embarrassing for the project team, weakens the client's confidence, and hurts the ability of the firm to deliver strong results and grow relationships (read: revenue) with the client team. As such, I never show anything to the client without having supporting data less than two clicks of a mouse away. For every slide in a PowerPoint the client team sees, there are three more sitting ready to deep-dive and pounce on any question the client team may pose. These are our redundancy systems.

- Usually, no one will see these appendix slides. A lot of cost and time goes into producing them only to have them never see the light of day. We plan to never have something come up that we haven't already asked ourselves and plotted a response for. Well, that's the goal anyway. Of course, things go wrong occasionally, as no one is immune from Murphy's reach entirely, but by preparing contingencies in advance, my job is to help my team be able to weather the occasional hiccup and consistently deliver valuable input to my client teams.

Much like the client never sees most of Charlie's appendix slides, our patients usually never "see" our redundancy systems. They will not know the time and cost it takes us to align our nurses, surgeons, and hospital staff on what the answer is, not if but when, something starts to turn into disaster. Mostly, these procedures will sit unused, and we may even get pushback about whether they're truly necessary. Rest assured, however, they are. One day Edward Aloysius Murphy, Jr. will call everybody's name. When the steely light of disaster shines upon us, only expertise, practice, and a strong system will provide our bulwark.

References

1. Veazie S, Peterson K, Bourne D. Evidence brief: implementation of high reliability organization principles. Washington (DC): Department of Veterans Affairs (US); 2019 May. Available from: https://www.ncbi.nlm.nih.gov/books/NBK542883/
2. Tolk JN, Cantu J, Beruvides MG. High reliability organization research: a literature review for health care. EMJ. 2015;27(4):218–37.
3. Marcucci C, Gierl, Kirsch JR. Avoiding common anesthesia error. Lippincott Williams & Wilkins—Wolters Kluwer; 2019.

Authors

Jake Seagull is a human factors expert at the University of Michigan. He'd be thrilled if the readers remembered forever that Murphy's Law is about how to succeed, not conceding to inevitable failure.

Charlie Sandson lives and works in Washington DC. In his free time, he enjoys sports of all kinds, travel to national and international spots, and spending time with friends. He is an Eagle Scout so he is more than familiar with "Be Prepared."

Cathy Marcucci is a senior anesthesiologist and less senior transfusion medicine physician who lives in suburban Baltimore. Speaking of failure, she just ripped out her entire garden for the fourth time after once again underestimating and failing to outwit the deer. However, she now knows for sure that they will climb up the stone steps to get to the specimen plants in the planters on the porch and she will not be making that mistake again. She remains grateful to Jake Seagull for his outstanding knowledge and patience in continually straightening her out on the most important key concepts.

141 Our Practices Are Shaped by Our Worst Experiences: Lessons from the Burn Unit

Lee C. Woodson

Introduction

Despite a career teaching residents at a university hospital, it is with a little reluctance that I set down words of advice to younger clinicians. Formal lectures are a conventional means of disseminating information. Guiding a resident while caring for a patient is more like collaboration where we both exchange experiences. Writing chapters is summarizing others' original work, with a little analysis. But using one's own experience as a model for others and writing in the first person seems a little pompous and unnatural.

Live and Learn

Still, much of the knowledge most useful to my practice came from well-intended misadventures, and sharing some of these lessons may provide information without the stressful experience, just as morbidity and mortality conferences help reduce the chance of the same mistakes being repeated. One piece of advice I shared with residents was my belief that *our practices are shaped by our worst experiences*. A rare complication is no longer rare when it enters your experience. Whether a stressful event was of our own making or not, we can identify situations where we can say, "I'll never do that again!"

Lessons Learned from Pediatric Burn Patients

Even if your hospital does not have a burn unit, acute burn patients may present through the ED. During the initial resuscitation, anesthesiologists' skills and experience match the needs of burn patients very well. When you take care of burn patients, you have ample opportunity to learn from "worst experiences." Here are some of the things I have learned from working for 30 years at a pediatric burn hospital.

L. C. Woodson (✉)
Department of Anesthesiology, University of Texas Medical Branch, Galveston, TX, USA

S. Mohamed et al. (eds.), *Anesthesia Bridges*, https://doi.org/10.1007/978-3-032-08294-7_141

Burns to the face and upper airway can be life-threatening, and intubation can be life-saving for some. At the same time, during the last 20 years of my career, our hospital saw at least seven deaths and numerous other severe morbidities in patients transported while intubated. The etiology of these injuries included a variety of mechanisms including accidental extubation, unrecognized circuit disconnection, mucous plug, or mechanical failure of the ventilator device. Neither I nor my colleagues can recall a serious complication from lack of an endotracheal tube (ETT). Securing an endotracheal tube (ETT) in the presence of facial burns and sedating intubated acute burn patients is difficult. Not all patients with inhalation injury require intubation. Intubation prior to transport to a burn unit should have clear indications and be coordinated with the receiving burn unit.

Fiberoptic Intubation (FOI)

Flexible fiberoptic intubation (FOI) is the most versatile technique for intubation. In the presence of respiratory distress, FOI allows intubation during spontaneous breathing and diagnosis of inhalation injury. Securing an oral ETT in the presence of facial burns is very difficult since tape will not stick and the head is swelling or shrinking for several days. A nasal ETT can be secured with great confidence with a septal bridle. Commercial devices are available, or red rubber catheters and 1/8-inch umbilical tape can be used.

If oral intubation cannot be avoided, the ETT can be most effectively secured by passing a red rubber tube (or a feeding tube) through a nostril and out the mouth. When this is tied to form a loop, the ETT can be fastened to it. One important point is not my bias but general consensus. If pediatric burn patients require intubation, a cuffed ETT should be used. If pulmonary compliance later decreases, necessitating positive end-expiratory pressure (PEEP) and higher peak pressures, it can be very difficult and dangerous to change from an uncuffed to a cuffed ETT.

Arterial Lines

Radial arterial catheters are difficult to maintain in burn patients, and these sites are often unavailable due to burn wounds. Femoral arterial catheters can be maintained for prolonged periods and have been found to be relatively safe in pediatric burn patients, but, because complications can be serious, clear indications are needed. For acute burn surgery, there are three main indications for an arterial catheter: if the blood pressure is expected to change more quickly than the interval between noninvasive cuff measurements, if vasoactive infusions are required (excluding dobutamine), or if arterial blood gases are required to manage mechanical ventilation. Otherwise, pulse oximetry along with FiO_2 can be used to monitor oxygenation.

Venous Access and Fluids

Peripheral venous catheters cannot be maintained for prolonged periods or allow blood sampling in patients with extensive burns. Central venous catheters sutured in place provide secure vascular access as well as a means for blood sampling. In adults, the intravenous (IV) is small relative to the patient and it is easier to get behind, which can be poorly tolerated depending on the coexisting disease. In infants, the IV is large relative to the patient and it is easier to overload and cause injury. Following the central venous pressure (CVP) during rapid blood loss and fluid resuscitation helps avoid overload in small children.

Having a central venous catheter in place allows us to not only monitor preload but also to easily get venous blood samples to monitor metabolic status and hematocrit. As a result, many large burn wound excisions can be managed without an arterial catheter. This is especially relevant during the early course for infants when patients are hypovolemic and vasoconstricted. Cannulation of the femoral artery at this time is difficult, and attempts can cause injury. A day or two later when systemic resistance is low and cardiac output is high, it becomes much easier and safer.

It is crucial to coordinate intraoperative care of burn patients with ICU course and goals. One issue is fluid management. Studies in burn patients show decreased volume required when colloid solutions are used rather than crystalloid. It is inappropriate to load a patient with liters of crystalloid after a week of fluid restriction and diuresis in the ICU.

Phenylephrine

One of my soap box topics is the inappropriate use of phenylephrine to treat hypotension. My persistent comments about this during our M&M conferences were probably a source of some annoyance. Phenylephrine is the drug of choice for hypotension in a number of circumstances, including Tet spells, hypertrophic obstructive cardiomyopathy, and hypotension during C-sections. In the absence of hypovolemia, phenylephrine is well-tolerated, but it is inappropriate to use during hypotension due to hypovolemia. Flow requires pressure, but we cannot easily measure flow. We measure blood pressure as a surrogate monitor of perfusion. However, by increasing afterload, phenylephrine decreases left ventricular ejection, cardiac output, and, thus, perfusion. Cerebral and coronary circulations are less sensitive to phenylephrine, but all other tissues suffer.

Phenylephrine infusion during burn wound excision can provide railroad track blood pressure recordings accompanied by progressive metabolic acidosis. It is more than a little perverse that we should intervene in a way to support a surrogate monitor at the expense of actual perfusion we are trying to support. Compared to phenylephrine, equipressor doses of norepinephrine increase contractility and maintain left ventricular ejection volume as well as after load so that cardiac output and tissue perfusion are maintained.

Lessons Learned

- We carry forward the lessons we learn when things go bad.
- If you can identify the cause of a problem or incident, then you can start thinking about how to prevent it from happening the next time.
- From the editors: Do *not* use phenylephrine to treat hypotension that is due to hypovolemia. You will "fix" the patient's blood pressure readings but progressively "unfix" the patient's overall physiological status.

Author

Lee Woodson has been retired for several years, after 30 years on the anesthesiology faculty at the University of Texas Medical Branch in Galveston. In the last 20 years, he focused on care of burn patients, especially pediatric patients at the Galveston Shriners Burn Center. He now spends his time with his wife, Anne, and hobbies: fishing, traveling, cooking, gardening, and grandchildren. Also, he has learned that a professor emeritus has much in common with being a grandparent. You can show up from time to time and offer unsolicited advice but not stick around for the consequences.

Digging Out of a Hole

142

Raymond G. Graber

Introduction

Does this scenario sound familiar? You take over a case from a trusted partner, and it's a well-managed disaster of a case, but still a disaster by all standards—and now it's your turn. The patient is not oxygenating well and is hypotensive, acidotic, and bleeding. You are wondering what you've got yourself into! How do you attempt to dig yourself out of this hole? Trust your training, and consider the following strategies:

The Handoff

Of course, it's important to get a good handoff when taking over a big case. This should include the following key elements—we can worry about the small stuff later: patient medical history, especially details about impairment in any of the major organ systems—respiratory dysfunction, cardiovascular dysfunction or arrhythmias, renal and/or hepatic insufficiency—and what the planned surgical procedure is, what the airway was like, allergies, antibiotics, lines/access, intraoperative problems specific to the case, preexisting clotting issues, blood loss, blood products available, and any periods of pulseless electrical activity (PEA) arrest. Also, as with any handoff, do let the surgical team know that you are taking over the case and that there has been a "change of the guard." Always get their perspective on what they are struggling with, as it helps us prepare for instability if we know what their challenges are.

When and if you have time, do a quick chart review to check for any missed details. Even the most diligent colleague can forget about an important fact in the stress of the moment, especially after hours of vigilant care. For example, has the patient recently been given any blood thinners or antiplatelet drugs? Is there a recent echo or cardiac imaging study, which shows evidence of and significant cardiac dysfunction or valvular issues that may be impacting hemodynamic stability?

R. G. Graber (✉)
Department of Anesthesiology and Perioperative Medicine, University Hospitals Cleveland Medical Center, Cleveland, OH, USA
e-mail: Raymond.graber@uhhospitals.org

S. Mohamed et al. (eds.), *Anesthesia Bridges*, https://doi.org/10.1007/978-3-032-08294-7_142

Survey the Scene

Take a look at the setup you are inheriting. What are the current vital signs? How are your intravenous (IV) lines organized, and which ones are large bore and good for volume transfusion? Do you need a rapid infusion/warming device? Are transducers in the proper position and providing accurate data?

What infusions are running, and is everything connected? How are medications organized? Are blood products and factor concentrate products immediately available in the room? What is actively being done to maintain normothermia? What are the surgeons working on at present, and what's left to do? If you are working with a resident or anesthetist, how experienced are they and did they start the case or have they also been handed off the case? Take the time to talk with your resident or anesthetist to get their perspective on the case and also to lay out your plan for how you want to tackle the ongoing issues. Knowing how deep you are buried will go a long way toward helping you dig yourself out.

Get Baseline Data

Although the case has been underway, it is new to you, so get some fresh data. What is the current blood loss total? How is the urine output? Get a blood gas to check hemoglobin, electrolytes, acid/base, lactate level, and ventilation issues. Do you need to send labs to check clotting status?

Temperature Management

We know that when patients get cold, it can affect the coagulation system. Remember that the ability of the coagulation system to function optimally rests on normothermia and optimal acid–base balance. If the core temperature is 33° Celsius, one can expect coagulopathic bleeding. Hypothermia also appears to increase the risk of surgical wound infections. So, when you take over a case, see what the patient's temperature is and also what is being done to keep the patient warm. Are volume lines being warmed? Is a rapid IV infusion-warming device in use? Is there a forced warm air convective warming blanket over or under the body or a continuous warm water flow mattress warming device in use? If the patient is cold, adding a heated humidifying device to the breathing circuit can help maintain and raise body temperature.

Do You Need Extra Help?

There are cases that are the anesthetic equivalent of going into battle. You may need more help to perform tasks such as drawing labs, checking and administering blood products, and checking on IV drips to make sure you are not running out of hemodynamic support drugs. Don't forget to use the other resources available to you—extra anesthesia staff who are not currently deployed. Nurses, surgical assistants, or cardiovascular perfusionists can help obtain/run equipment and check blood products.

***Note from the Editors:** We think that an overview of the types of bridge structures is fitting for Ray Graber's great overview of the "structure" of an OR case (Fig. 142.1).

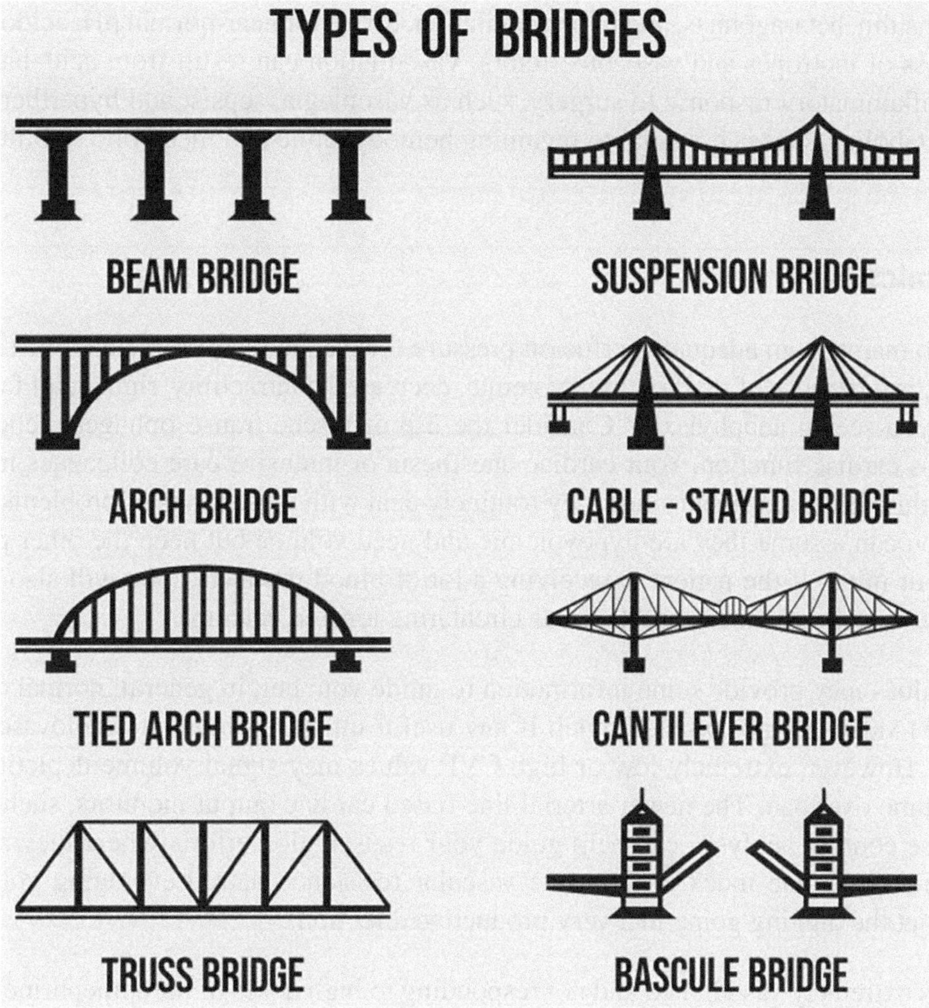

Fig. 142.1 A graphic representation of the basic types of bridges. There is no "safest" type of bridge, just as there is no safest type of anesthetic. In both, the bridge engineering and medical worlds, safety and performance depend on careful analysis, thoughtful planning, and skilled execution by motivated practitioners. Illustration: Image used under standard license from shutterstock.com

Intravenous and Arterial Access

Do you have adequate IV access? It can be difficult to place a central line under the drapes, but it is possible if the patient is not lateral or prone. Do you have trustworthy working arterial access? I once took over an ascending aortic dissection case with arms tucked and no art line because the patient crashed on induction and the surgeon decided to crack the chest. I scrubbed, gowned and gloved, and placed a femoral arterial line with ultrasound during the pump run. We do what it takes to get the job done, even in the most compromised circumstances.

Metabolic Issues

Sometimes you are running your own mini-ICU. In the OR! Keep the glucose <180 mg/dl. Maintain your potassium in the 4–5.5 mmol/l range. And always be aware of the things that will drive your potassium lower—insulin, beta-agonists, and hyperventilation. Strive for near-normal pH; acidosis can reduce the effectiveness of inotropes and vasoconstrictors. Vasodilation can result from acid–base imbalance, an abnormal inflammatory response to surgery, such as vasoplegia, sepsis, and hyperthermia. Tackling all of these metabolic issues is essential to regaining hemodynamic and metabolic stability.

Hemodynamics

Are you able to maintain an adequate perfusion pressure for the kidneys, brain, and heart? If the patient is hypotensive, is it because of rhythm, hypovolemia, decreased contractility, right heart failure, or vasodilation? Are you seeing anaphylaxis? Consider the use of rescue transesophageal echocardiography (TEE) to assess cardiac function. Your cardiac anesthesia or intensive care colleagues may be able to help you with this TEE assessment since they routinely deal with these kinds of problems. If the patient is bleeding, you can assume they are hypovolemic and need volume but keep the other possibilities in the back of your mind. If the patient is receiving a lot of blood products, they will also need frequent calcium supplementation because citrate binds circulating ionized calcium.

Central line values may provide some information to guide you, but, in general, normal central venous pressure (CVP) values do not provide much if any useful information about cardiovascular hemodynamics/filling. However, extremely low or high CVP values may signal volume depletion, right heart failure, or volume overload. The newer arterial line-based cardiac output monitors, such as those used in arterial pulse contour analysis, can help guide your resuscitation efforts where they are needed the most by providing cardiac index or systemic vascular resistance data. Leveraging your physiologic monitors can get the digging going in a very productive direction.

If the patient is extremely vasodilated and not responding to high doses of norepinephrine and vasopressin, consider adding either intravenous methylene blue, cyanocobalamin, or, in the most extreme cases, angiotensin, as these agents can be effective in helping restore arterial tone. Although controversial, hydrocortisone may also have benefits in some patients.

Respiratory

If the patient is not oxygenating appropriately in response to the fraction of inspired oxygen (FiO_2) you are delivering, think about some of the following. Has your endotracheal tube migrated down so that you are ventilating just one lung? Do you need to add more positive end expiratory pressure (PEEP) to combat pressure on the lungs from high intraabdominal pressures from positioning or insufflations? Are there secretions that need to be suctioned out?

Is the patient in pulmonary edema—and requiring diuresis and additional PEEP? Pulmonary edema can result from volume overload, acute hypertension, acute congestive heart failure, transfusion-related lung injury, air embolism or preeclampsia. Is there pulmonary embolism? Is there a pneumothorax? If you are developing severe hypoxia that is unresponsive to measures, my go-to diagnostic aids are bronchoscopy to check tube position and suction out mucus plugs and TEE to check for signs of pulmonary embolism or right-to-left shunt across a patent foramen ovale.

If a patient is deteriorating and not responding to other therapies, an option may be to consider the use of mechanical circulatory and respiratory support through the use of either veno-venous or veno-arterial extracorporeal membrane oxygenation (ECMO). ECMO support is reserved for the most acute situations, and, in many centers, a potential ECMO candidate will have to be evaluated by a shock team before proceeding with initiation of this therapy.

***Note from the Editors:** Every *Anesthesia Bridges* editor loves visiting the United Kingdom, so this photo is in everybody's honor. There is nothing like a British bridge (Fig. 142.2).

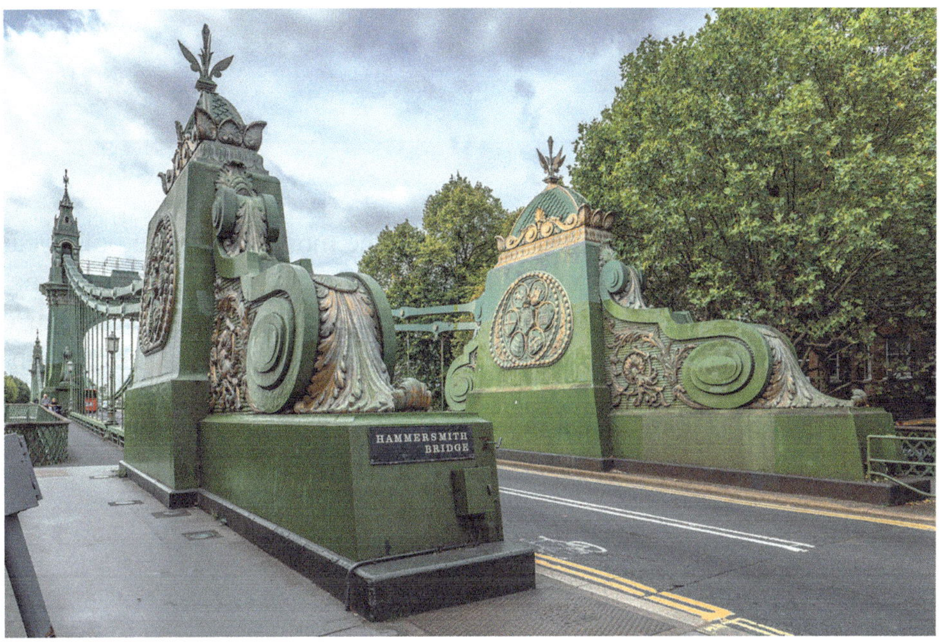

Fig. 142.2 The beautiful Hammersmith Bridge, spanning the Thames River in West London. The bridge was so important to Great Britain that it had its own act of Parliament—the Hammersmith Bridge Act of 1827. It has been repaired and renovated several times but still rests on the original foundations. It was closed indefinitely to vehicle traffic in 2019 but remains open to pedestrians and cyclists. Photo: Apostolos Giontzis, image used under license from iStock.com

Coagulation

If you are involved in a large blood loss situation, start thinking early about supplementing with allogeneic blood products, such as fresh frozen plasma, platelets, and cryoprecipitate. If you are using cell salvage, remember that these devices wash out most platelets and clotting factors. Activate your hospital's massive transfusion protocol (MTP) or order products separately. There are excellent trauma data to support administering packed cells–plasma–platelets–cryoprecipitate in a 1:1:1:1 ratio.

Remember the things that will deleteriously affect clotting—acidosis/alkalosis, hypocalcemia, and hypothermia—and focus on correcting those issues. Keep a regular check on the patient's clotting status, by checking hemoglobin concentration, platelet count, fibrinogen, and prothrombin time (PT)/partial thromboplastin time (PTT)/international normalized ratio (INR). Even better, use a point-of-care monitor of viscoelastic clot strength like such as thromboelastography (TEG) or rotational thromboelastometry (ROTEM)—the results come back much quicker and are well-proven to reduce the use of allogeneic blood product transfusion. Consider the use of tranexamic acid (TXA) or aminocaproic acid (ACA), which, by their antifibrinolytic effects, can be extremely helpful in reducing intraoperative blood loss.

Endgame

If the patient is unstable and likely to remain so, start talking early to your surgical and ICU colleagues and get a bed set aside for your patient. Make sure you give them a comprehensive report, specifically focusing on what the ongoing issues are.

Conclusions

We value and trust the colleagues we work with, but even the most experienced of us can be subjected to fatigue and confirmation bias and miss alternative diagnoses. So, when you take over a highly complex case going poorly, you have the opportunity to look at the case with a fresh pair of eyes. If one focuses on the details mentioned above, you can possibly make incremental changes that can redirect the patient's course and give the patient a fighting chance of a more positive outcome. With effort and perseverance, you can begin to drag your patient out of the proverbial hole!

Lessons Learned

- When taking over a complex case that may be going poorly, take the time to get a comprehensive report, and make sure you understand the current challenges of the case. Get fresh lab and hemodynamic data so you know where you are starting from.
- Once you figure out what the issues are, take the necessary steps to work toward fixing them.
- We shouldn't feel alone when in the middle of a complex case—so don't hesitate to call for backup!

Author

Ray Graber is a member of the cardiac anesthesia team at a busy tertiary care and trauma center. He is lucky to have excellent co-workers when it is time to go into anesthesia battle! Thanks go out to Ed Avery for his suggestions and comments regarding this piece.

Traumatic Events, Difficult Outcomes, and the Second Victim Process

143

Christopher M. Conley and Mark C. Norris

Introduction

During the daily navigation through the high-stakes realm of airway management and resuscitation, the specter of patient injury or catastrophe looms for every anesthesiologist. When bad stuff happens, one of your first thoughts may be "how am I going to deal with the patient's potentially distraught family?" What you may not initially think about is the emotional consequences that <u>you</u> may have after being involved in a catastrophic event. There are things that immediately need to be done and things that need to be dealt with in the long term. In this chapter, we will attempt to discuss our thoughts and experience with these issues.

The Family

If and when a sudden unexpected complication occurs, and once the situation (and hopefully the patient) is stabilized and you can be safely relieved from clinical duty, you need to prioritize speaking with the patient's family or loved ones. This task is often very difficult. Take a moment to gather yourself, clean yourself up, and change scrubs if they are soiled. The conversation that follows will be etched into the minds of that family for a long time.

Activate your hospital's patient relations team early. They are immensely helpful during these difficult moments—aiding in finding an appropriate, quiet conference room to talk as well as providing resources, both big and small, for families. You should notify someone in your department leadership—you want your leaders to hear about the existence of an event from you and not someone else. Bring a senior, more experienced colleague if you can. They can help field the more difficult questions and assist you if you stumble or are overwhelmed during the conversation.

Facts, not guesses, are very important here. You may describe the circumstances of the event and your best assessment of the patient's status, but accuracy and honesty are paramount. "We don't yet know" is

C. M. Conley (✉) · M. C. Norris
Department of Anesthesiology, Boston Medical Center, Boston, MA, USA
e-mail: Christopher.Conley@bmc.org

S. Mohamed et al. (eds.), *Anesthesia Bridges*, https://doi.org/10.1007/978-3-032-08294-7_143

a powerful, valid statement in the immediate aftermath of an emergency. Families latch onto hope. Be tempered in your optimism.

Share the plan moving forward. Reassure the family that the team continues to provide vigilant, compassionate care to the patient, enabling you to step away from the bedside to keep them informed. Answer, to the best of your ability, any questions they have in the moment, and, then, describe the next steps in the process of care. This plan should include when they might expect the next contact from the team regarding progress and when the family can go see and touch the patient. Again, patient relations can be a huge help with the continuity planning here.

Expressing sorrow for what happened is not an admission of guilt. It's okay to care and to cry with your patients and their families. But remember that in this moment, the family's experience, and not our own, needs to be center stage.

***Note from the Editors:** We think that this chapter is an appropriate place for this serene and snowy bridge (Fig. 143.1).

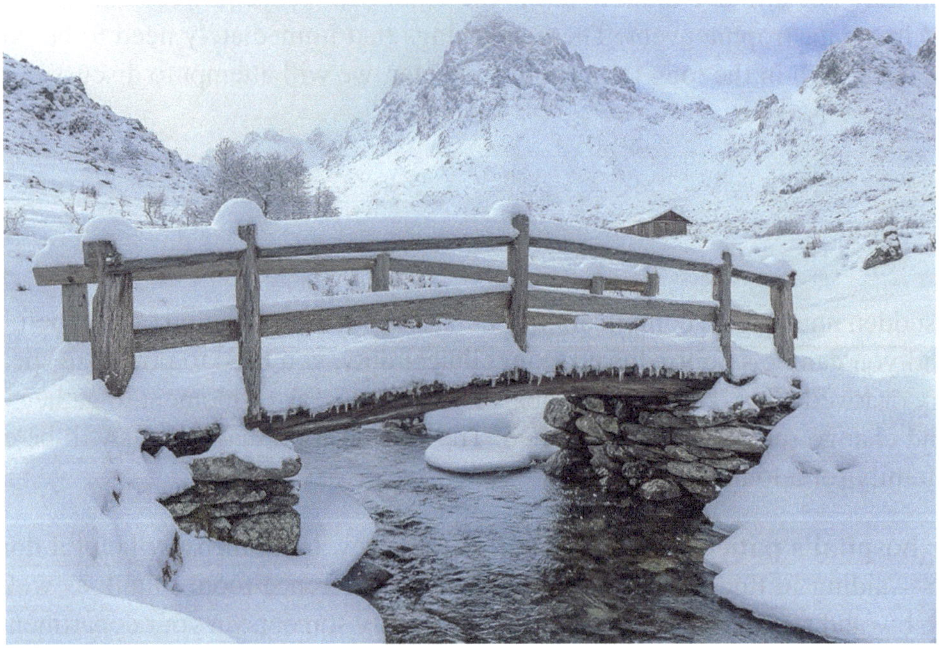

Fig. 143.1 Which is more peaceful—the mountains, the bridge, the snow, or the stream? Answer all of them. Photo: Image used under standard license from adobestock.com

You, Immediately After

Immediately following a traumatic event, the last thing you're going to want to do is to journal about it. But for better or for worse, this note could be one of the most important things you write in your professional lifetime. As soon as you are done informing the family and the "need to know" group we just described, your biggest priority must be to document the event as completely and accurately as possible.

- Ensure that your record is accurate and complete, including medications, airway documentation, and communications, including calls for help and ***stat*** calls. In these instances, often, multiple teams (physician and nursing) will be documenting the same incident, including code records. Whenever possible, confirm that timelines and interventions are in agreement.

- Character limits of the electronic anesthesia record may make it difficult to fit your full description of the event. We recommend writing a separate narrative of the incident in the form of an event note in your hospital's electronic medical record (EMR). EMRs track and archive changes, and you may be called away while writing the note, so it helps to draft it on a separate sheet of paper or in a word document before saving it in the chart.

- Running your note by a senior colleague or risk management professional can help you recall critical steps you took but forgot to write down. When you are writing your description of the event, state the facts. You may describe your thought process and why you chose your specific course of action, but never guess and do **NOT** editorialize. While it may be tempting to distance yourself from fault and to shift blame, families, and their lawyers, pick up on this disunity within the team. The chart is not a chat room. It is a legal document.

In these moments, departments need to circle the wagons and support their faculty. As soon as they can safely transition away from the bedside, the providers involved in the event should be excused from clinical assignment. Cases that were to follow should be postponed or assumed by a separate team.

You, in the Long Term

As soon as you're done writing about an event, you will begin to really start to feel the aftereffects of it. In the hours, days, weeks, and months that follow a traumatic case, anesthesiologists may experience what Susan Scott describes as "intrusive reflections," including anxiety, flashbacks, nightmares, insomnia, a deep depression, and a crisis of confidence as a physician. This mindset changes the lens through which you experience being a physician and saps the joy from your work. Breathing tightens while driving into the hospital parking lot. Every patient is another potential disaster.

Dr. Albert Wu first described this phenomenon of "the second victim" in 2000 [1]. The constellation of shame, self-doubt, and guilt can be devastating and debilitating to healthcare professionals. If left unchecked, it can lead to depression and even suicide. Susan Scott's pioneering work describes the second victim phenomenon as having six stages [2]. The process begins with the experience of a devastating outcome and ends when we move forward and move on. Scott suggests that the second victim syndrome concludes in one of three distinct trajectories: "dropping out, surviving or thriving." Each of us, to some degree, ponders each path, before choosing our final trajectory.

- **Dropping out** may manifest in a number of ways. It may mean leaving medicine as a profession. At its worst, it may mean succumbing to depression, suicide, or falling into the trap of self-medication with alcohol and substance dependence.

- **Surviving** is the middle pathway. In this state of mind, anesthesiologists shift from enjoying their work to dreading it. Every patient is a potential plaintiff, a bad outcome, or both. We get through the day, rinse and repeat. Many of us have walked this path, at least temporarily, in the wake of a catastrophic outcome. This "survival" approach and mindset is a loss for both physicians and our patients. When we're in the "surviving mode," we're not far from veering off into the "dropping out" group.

- **Thriving** involves a path that takes time and effort. We have to actively ***choose*** this path each day or it won't happen. When we commit to thriving, we enjoy our work and are humbled at the faith that our patients and our colleagues place in us each day as anesthesiologists. Use every modality that works for you to thrive (Fig. 143.2).

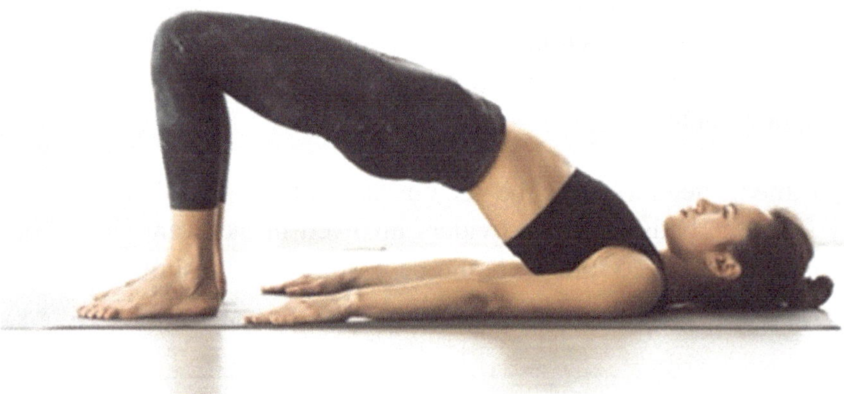

Fig. 143.2 Remember this type of bridge if you are trying to recover from a traumatic event at work or at home. Complementary modalities work! Photo: Image used under standard license from shutterstock.com

Which trajectory we ultimately take hinges upon the penultimate of Scott's six steps, which she dubs "emotional first aid." Emotional first aid encompasses all the systems and supports needed to navigate the aftermath of a catastrophic patient care event. It includes having strong support at home. Your whole family, spouse, kids, and others will go through this hurting and healing process with you. So, choose your family wisely! Support from colleagues, including condolences, a squeeze of the shoulder, and reassurances in their faith in us as people and as physicians may also be immensely helpful.

As important, however, is getting connected with a professional counselor. Having a seasoned expert to help navigate through the emotions of a tragic case (or the litigation that sometimes follows) can provide the tools needed to rebuild a physician's confidence and rediscover one's love for this specialty.

Lessons Learned

- After a traumatic event, you need to remember to take care of the patient, their family, and yourself.
- Meet with the family and give them an update as soon as you can safely do so. Involve the patient relations team and consider bringing a more experienced colleague with you.

- Time spent writing a detailed, accurate event note can be invaluable in the long term.
- Anesthesiologists are vulnerable to becoming “second victims“in the wake of tragic outcomes and tough cases. Recognize the symptoms and seek support early!

References

1. Wu AW. Medical error: the second victim. The doctor who makes the mistake needs help too. BMJ. 2000;320(7237):726–7.
2. Scott SD, Hirschinger LE, Cox KR, et al. The natural history of recovery for the healthcare provider “second victim” after adverse patient events. BMJ Qual Saf. 2009;18:325–30.

Authors

Chris Conley is a New England lifer. He completed his anesthesia residency at BWH, followed by a fellowship at Boston Children’s. His work passions include feedback systems in graduate medical education, physician wellness, and perioperative optimization in children. He married the love of his life, Anne, and they are the proud parents of Ben and Charlie.

Mark Norris has been practicing anesthesia, in both academic and private settings, for over 40 years. His interests include obstetric anesthesia, resident education, and expanding the diversity of the medical workforce. Outside of the hospital, he enjoys his family, cycling, and cooking.

Question Established Dogma

144

Michael A. Ramsay

Introduction

In early 1970, I was a resident in the intensive care unit (ICU) at The London Hospital. We always had a number of patients that had acute respiratory distress syndrome (ARDS) and were intubated and being mechanically ventilated. It appeared to be the standard of care that all patients on ventilators would be in a drug-induced coma. Many of these patients with ARDS did not survive, but, occasionally, we would get a patient whose pulmonary function would improve, and the order would be given to wake the patient up and wean them off the ventilator.

Outcomes

However, this would take days and sometimes weeks to occur, and the weaning process was slow to get to extubation. The patient would then spend days in the ICU before being sent to the ward. When I tracked these "successes," I found that they were very deconditioned and spent many more weeks in the hospital and then off to a rehabilitation facility. I called some patients that had been discharged home to see how they were doing. The spouse would answer the telephone and would say that the patient was doing well, not back at work, but was looking at the television. When I asked what show they were watching, I received the reply that they were not actually watching a program—they were just looking at the television set!

A New Sedation Scale

This was a success?! Somewhere in the process of treating these patients the brain function had become impaired. It could have been caused by many factors: hypoxia, hypotension, sepsis, etc., but I wondered if prolonged drug-induced coma could cause this. At this time, a new sedative drug had been released in Europe called Althesin (alphadolone–alfaxalone), which could be given intravenously and had a very short half-life. It was marketed as a total intravenous anesthetic. I wondered if it could be used in the

M. A. Ramsay (✉)
Department of Anesthesiology and Pain Management, Baylor University Medical Center, Dallas, TX, USA
e-mail: michael.ramsay@bswhealth.org

S. Mohamed et al. (eds.), *Anesthesia Bridges*, https://doi.org/10.1007/978-3-032-08294-7_144

ICU to control sedation. Instead of having patients in a coma, could we have them in a comfort state? To be able to achieve this, the drug would have to be prescribed to a sedation level rather than a dose. We put together a clinical trial to test this and came up with a controlled sedation scale.

At this time, there were no sedation scales published, not even the Glasgow Coma Scale. So, with the help of the ICU nurses and my colleagues, we developed a simple controlled sedation scale that could be used in the ICU to direct the administration of the new sedation drug Althesin. We published the results of our clinical trial in the *British Medical Journal* in 1974 [1]. So, for the first time, patients did not have to be in a drug-induced coma when being mechanically ventilated. Unfortunately, there were too many hypersensitivity reactions to the drug, and it was withdrawn from the market.

(Slow) Emergence of a New ICU Paradigm

However, a few years later, propofol was introduced, another intravenous medication that could be used for controlled sedation. Similar clinical trials were performed with propofol, and the controlled sedation scale that we developed was used in these trials but was renamed the Ramsay Sedation Scale.

This opened many doors for me personally, in speaking engagements and publishing. However, ICUs continued to have patients on mechanical ventilators in drug-induced coma, and the concept of controlled sedation was slow to gain acceptance. Unfortunately, it took another 30 years before the "animated ICU" became accepted with patients awake on ventilators, even walking the halls while being ventilated. The results were less time on the ventilator, less time in the ICU, and less delirium. New sedation scales came along and addressed agitation more thoroughly and are now the standard of practice not only in ICUs but across healthcare.

Lessons Learned

- Always keep thinking "outside the box" when assessing current practice.
- Be innovative, but change must be evidence-based.

Reference

1. Ramsay MA, Savage TM, Simpson BRJ, et al. Controlled sedation with alphaxalone-alphadalone. Br Med J. 1974;2:656–9.

Author

Mike Ramsay was born in Dublin, went to medical school in London, and after two years on the faculty of the London Hospital, he moved to the Baylor University Medical Center in Dallas. He says: "This was a strong decision of my wife Zoe, and the best decision in my career. I am not sure where my accent has landed. In London they are critical and call it Yankee and in Texas most say I am Australian!? The move has allowed us both to travel together around the globe on lecture tours. This has resulted in many international friends as well as local friends and also great memories. Along the way we have managed a few influences on medicine and providers as well. What an exhilarating and fun career!"

145 Don't Be Shy About Discussing Anatomy and Block Techniques with the Surgeons: It Builds Rapport and Everybody Wins

Jeffrey T. Hopcian, Stephen D. Lasday, and Catherine Marcucci

Introduction

We've got to admit it: we have always really liked to be posted in the podiatry rooms, especially on Fridays! At the VA hospitals, there can even be a bit of jockeying to get those rooms as they are often a little oasis of Zen in a busy operating room theater. The podiatric surgeons she knew at the Baltimore and Philadelphia VAs were smart, funny, low-key, and supremely good at what they did.

Ankle Blocks Are Accessible!

Of course, podiatry cases at the VA often included lower extremity blocks, which the anesthesia team were not only always happy to perform but also more than happy to teach. In fact, they were sometimes a bit bemused that so many anesthesiologists are happy to hand over these blocks. Their point was that these are low-risk blocks of superficial nerves and can easily be redone during surgery if necessary. Their working assumption was that the necessity for five injections required for a complete block of the foot was somewhat off-putting.

The anatomy notwithstanding, a podiatrist once said to us, "This block is well, well, well within the skill set of the anesthesia practitioner and trainee. The key is to do it without too much windup and not to give up doing the block if you fail to anesthetize one or more of the nerves for your first couple of times." The podiatrists also feel that more anesthesiologists would be eager to do ankle blocks if they stayed just a bit more comfortable and conversant on the innervation of the foot (Fig. 145.1).

J. T. Hopcian (✉)
Department of Anesthesiology and Perioperative Medicine, University Hospitals Cleveland Medical Center, Cleveland, OH, USA

S. D. Lasday
West Coast Podiatry Center, Sarasota, FL, USA

C. Marcucci (✉)
Department of Transfusion Medicine, Clinical Center, National Institutes of Health, Bethesda, MD, USA

S. Mohamed et al. (eds.), *Anesthesia Bridges*, https://doi.org/10.1007/978-3-032-08294-7_145

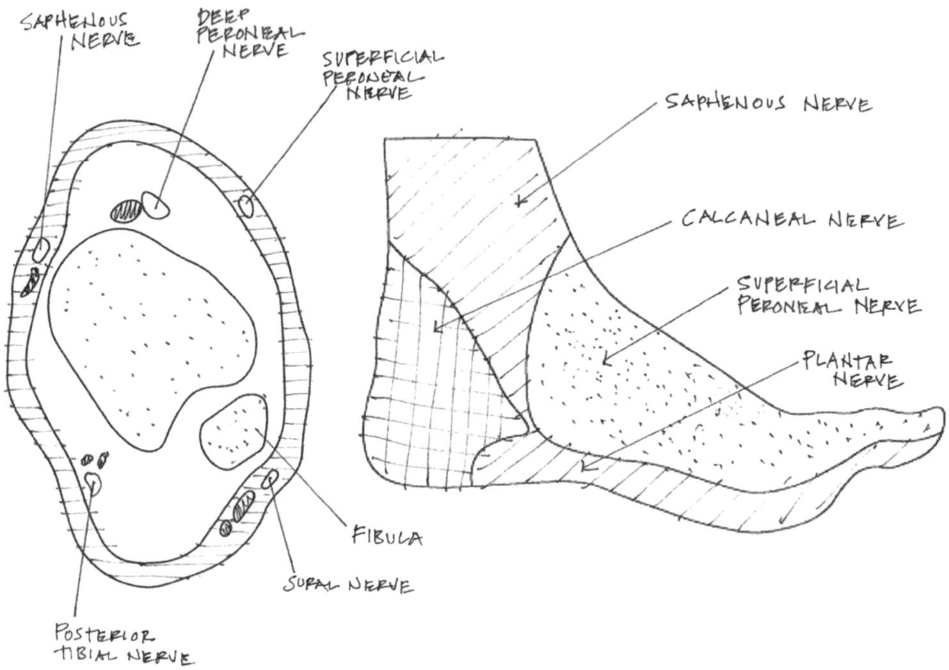

Fig. 145.1 Innervation and sensory dermatomes of the foot and ankle. Note that the calcaneal branches of the tibial nerve innervate the superficial tissues of the heel. Illustration: Mark Liu

Podiatry Pointers

Steve Lasday, who was formerly the chief of Foot and Ankle Surgery of Sarasota Memorial Hospital and is now the principal owner of the West Coast Podiatric Center, was kind enough to send us some notes on how he does his ankle blocks for maximum efficiency and smoothness.

He generally uses about 20 ml of a 50–50 mix of 2% lidocaine and 0.5% bupivacaine. It is important to note that the posterior tibial (PT) and deep peroneal nerves are deep to the fascia and innervate the deep structures (bone and muscle) in addition to their skin areas of coverage. The other three nerves are all superficial to fascial planes and provide innervation to the skin. He usually blocks the nerves as follows:

- Perform the posterior tibial block with the leg externally rotated. For most people, just the relaxed, externally rotated leg is sufficient, and, using the medial border of the Achilles tendon as a landmark, feel the PT pulse and aim posterior, aspirating before injecting.

Additional note from Steve: I learned this using methylene blue on cadavers and the first few times I provided a great flexor hallucis longus block or I would have if the patient had been alive. I use 5 mL of a local anesthetic direct to this nerve and divide the rest of the local anesthetic equally among the remaining nerves.

- Although we probably won't learn this technique on cadavers as Steve did, we can do this block a few times with ultrasound to learn the anatomy.

- Do the deep peroneal block next. At the level of the malleoli, make a skin wheal lateral to the extensor hallucis tendon (identify by having the patient extend the big toe). Advance the needle down to bone, pull back a millimeter, then aspirate and inject.

- From the entry point for the deep peroneal block, infiltrate laterally toward the medial malleolus to get the saphenous nerve and then laterally toward the lateral malleolus to get the superficial peroneal branch. Thus, you can infiltrate three nerves from the same site.

- Lastly, infiltrate subcutaneously from behind the lateral malleolus to the Achilles tendon to get the sural nerve.

Some podiatrists will basically do a ring block after the posterior tibial and deep peroneal nerve blocks. They generally do not use ultrasound for ankle blocks and rarely have to repaint the fence after the case is started. If they miss a nerve and have to redo a nerve, it's generally apparent before the case has started.

Request Other Refreshers!

Obviously, this is not a regional anesthesia textbook, so why are we talking about ankle blocks? First of all, they have become somewhat of a forgotten block in our repertoire, with the emphasis nowadays being placed on doing more proximal blocks in fascial compartments with the help of ultrasound. But even more importantly, this chapter should also serve as a reminder that we learn things not just from our anesthesia colleagues but also from our very skilled surgical friends.

There are many learning opportunities that can present while working in the operating room. Our hand surgeons are very adept at doing blocks at the wrist and digit level. Our orthopedic colleagues can be frequently found dissecting out nerves during fracture or tumor surgery. Ask if they can go over the living anatomy with you. Similarly, for the oral-maxillo-facial and ENT folks with head and neck and airway blocks, just ask for a brief professional-level refresher on the real live nerves. You might encounter the occasional grump who doesn't have the patience, but, by far, most of our surgical colleagues are happy to show us the relevant anatomy of the patient they are working on. Take advantage of any chance to learn from any of our surgical colleagues.

Lessons Learned

- Podiatrists generally will do this block for the anesthesia team, but we can do it, too!

- The trick is to stay current on the innervation of the foot and anatomical approach to the nerves, not just for the in-service and board exams.

- Podiatrists do the ankle block quickly and without a great deal of fuss, generally after the patient is already sedated.

- Even they will occasionally miss a nerve and then perform a redo. This is accepted as a matter of course for the podiatrists.

- Take every opportunity to review anatomy and learn blocks. Remember, the surgeons are our allies!

Authors

Jeff Hopcian moved to Cleveland 10+ years ago following his medical training in Ann Arbor and Chicago, to begin his anesthesiology career at University Hospitals in Cleveland, Ohio. He works as an interventional pain physician as well as an OR anesthesiologist and has a particular interest in regional anesthesia. In fair weather, he can be found outdoors running, cycling, and sailing. In foul weather, he tinkers away at the piano and ukulele.

Steve Lasday is originally from Pittsburgh but has lived in Sarasota, FL, for the last 25+ years. Together with his partner and associates, he has steadily been growing the West Coast Podiatry Center into the “go-to” practice for foot and ankle care. His greatest success in life was persuading his wife, Renae, to marry him. His passions are his two sons, Spencer and Max, and collecting and trading luxury timepieces.

Cathy Marcucci was in full-time clinical practice in the VA Health Care System from 2000 to 2019, where she was fortunate to work with a number of fun and smart podiatrists who patiently reviewed the ankle block whenever she needed. She recalls that she was asked to discuss and describe the innervation of the foot and ankle and how to do an ankle block as part of a “short question” during her oral boards. Fortunately, she had looked at this at 10 p.m. the night before the exam.

ERAS: Is This Just the Flavor of the Month?

146

Edwin G. Avery IV and Raymond G. Graber

Introduction

In this chapter, we interview **Ed Avery,** who was an early adopter and champion of enhanced recovery after surgery (ERAS) at his previous institution.

What Is This ERAS Stuff I Keep Hearing About? Is This Just the Flavor of the Month?

Ed Avery: Thanks for reaching out to me for an overview on the enhanced recovery after surgery (ERAS) topic. ERAS is one of those things that is new to many perioperative clinicians but has been studied intensely over the past decade and continues to be a very hot topic of investigation. If we consider ERAS from a 30,000-foot view, we know (based on the massive amount of international current peer-reviewed published literature—5192 PubMed references as of the date of this writing) that select interventions in the perioperative period can really make a big difference in improving clinical outcomes in a very meaningful way.

Let Us Talk About ERAS Interventions!

Ed: In general, ERAS interventions are broken up into things that can be done preoperatively, intraoperatively, and postoperatively to optimize one's readiness for surgery. For example, take a nutritional supplement (arginine-rich) with meals for the 5 days just prior to your surgery as this will help your wound healing after surgery and reduce the incidence of infection.

Another common ERAS principle focuses on improving preoperative hydration. The American Society of Anesthesiology first published nil per os (NPO) guidelines in 1999 and has always rec-

E. G. Avery IV (✉) · R. G. Graber
Department of Anesthesiology and Perioperative Medicine, University Hospitals Cleveland Medical Center, Cleveland, OH, USA
e-mail: edwin.avery@uhhospitals.org

S. Mohamed et al. (eds.), *Anesthesia Bridges*, https://doi.org/10.1007/978-3-032-08294-7_146

ommended a two hours fasting interval for clear liquids (excluding alcohol). It is also a good idea to avoid caffeine-containing beverages in the time immediately before your surgery as they will dehydrate you.

With ERAS protocols, the shift in focus is to actually encourage hydration in that period up to two hours prior to surgery. This practice allows patients to stay hydrated and take in calories in the form of carbohydrates, which subjectively makes them feel much better and stronger before their surgery. Imagine you are having surgery at noon tomorrow and are told no solid foods for at least 8 hours before your surgery and also not to have a high-fat meal when you do eat your last meal before surgery. You are going to be very hungry/hangry by noon the next day and will feel a bit lethargic if you go 12–16 hours without calories.

By taking clear liquids containing carbohydrates, such as sports drinks like Gatorade or Powerade, or even plain old apple juice, cranberry juice, or cranapple juice if you like, you get calories and hydration. This makes a big difference in how you feel going into surgery, for example, no headache from dehydration and not starved for calories.

An example of an intraoperative intervention that has repeatedly been proven to be helpful, especially in bigger, open surgeries, is the use goal-directed fluid therapy (aka GDFT). The goal is to optimize body fluid balance so that patients are not dehydrated during or after their surgical procedure, which can lead to acute kidney injury or perioperative hypotension. GDFT also avoids the opposite situation where they are "flooded," which can lead to prolonged mechanical ventilation and possibly ventilator-associated pneumonia.

There are several commercially available invasive and noninvasive devices available to help precisely titrate intravenous fluid administration both intra- and postoperatively. Furthermore, pulmonary artery catheters are being used less frequently in many surgeries as the newer GDFT technologies are less invasive and yield similarly accurate hemodynamic information. Put simply, it is safe to say that the days of anesthesia teaching regarding the 4-2-1 rule for intravenous fluid administration are long gone, like the caveman/stone age.

Postoperative ERAS interventions focus on getting patients up, moving, and engaging in their recovery while effectively managing postoperative pain using a multimodal analgesia approach. Multimodal analgesia strategies employ lower doses or complete elimination of narcotics. The strategies also use non-narcotic analgesics such as acetaminophen, nonsteroidal anti-inflammatory drugs, gabapentinoids, and nerve blocks, with or without indwelling catheters, to better extend the duration of analgesia.

***Note from the Editors:** Ed Avery is interested in architecture as well as driving, so we thought this would be the perfect bridge for this chapter (Fig. 146.1).

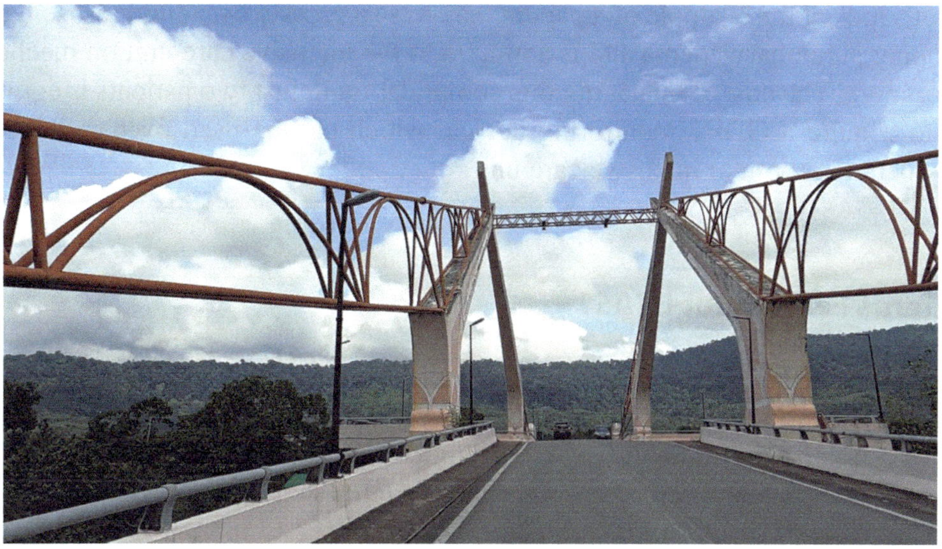

Fig. 146.1 A highway bridge with an unusual and visually striking canopy. Photo: Alla; image used under license from iStock.com

Do Surgeons Support These ERAS Efforts?

Ed: The few examples of ERAS techniques that are noted above just scratch the surface of this vast topic, and it should be recognized that different surgical subspecialties are finding ways to customize their developing ERAS protocols to improve outcomes. Indeed, our surgical colleagues are fast becoming familiar with and embracing ERAS interventions and protocols, are utilizing more minimally invasive approaches, and are comfortable with supplementing their procedures with local anesthetic injections. For a real impact, we need all of the perioperative clinicians to help go that extra mile and develop and follow ERAS protocols.

Do Hospitals Support This Effort?

Ed: The use of ERAS techniques has been repeatedly proven to improve clinical outcomes in multiple types of surgeries. The most notable clinical outcomes are a highly significant reduction in hospital length of stay as well as a reduced incidence of postoperative complications. Both of these outcomes contribute to decreased costs of care, and this will make your hospital and surgeons very happy.

Any Downsides to This Approach?

Ed: Using the ERAS interventions may take time and effort on our part, but, when done correctly, they are clearly effective. There can be financial costs secondary to new monitoring equipment, pharmacy expenditures, minimally invasive surgical equipment costs, slower surgical times, etc. But this is balanced by shorter hospital stays and improved outcomes.

For example, let's look at the example of a patient that gets so grossly over-fluid resuscitated that he/she ends up developing pulmonary edema and is admitted to the intensive care unit on mechanical ventilation for a day or more. The cost of managing this complication in just two patients is equivalent to what it would cost to acquire a GDFT monitoring device, which can be used over and over on different patients in the operating room or intensive care unit.

How Do Patients Feel About ERAS?

Ed: It's our job to educate our patients on how these ERAS techniques are changing our practice and how it will help them have an easier time with their recovery from surgery. We can expect that many of our patients will not know much about ERAS techniques. However, most patients will be extremely happy to have less thirst and hunger before surgery, less pain, a shorter length of stay, and fewer perioperative complications!

Lessons Learned

- Because ERAS principles contribute to improved patient outcomes, they are here to stay.
- ERAS techniques are best implemented in a multidisciplinary manner. Get your surgeons and partners involved!
- This is a rapidly evolving area. Keep an eye on the literature for new developments.

Authors

Ed Avery is a New Englander who trained and worked at the MGH for over a decade before moving to Cleveland. He is a cardiac anesthesiologist with multiple areas of interest, including blood pressure control, the coagulation system, and improving patient outcomes, and has participated in numerous clinical trials. In his spare time, he enjoys a good glass of wine and working on his cars, usually not at the same time!

Ray Graber is a senior anesthesiologist at Case Western. He has multiple areas of clinical expertise and is highly interested in quality and safety issues and initiatives.

147 Managing Surgical Patients Who Are Breastfeeding: And Finding an Area of Clinical Expertise

Sarah E. Dodd and Toby N. Weingarten

Introduction

In her first year on the faculty of the Mayo Clinic, **Sarah Dodd** cared for a lactating patient who was frustrated and tearful that she had received multiple sets of conflicting instructions that had left her unsure of what to do to have her surgery and safely continue breastfeeding her infant. This started a now years-long interest in educating and supporting providers and giving patients consistent and accurate information. It also is a great example of keeping your eyes and ears open for perioperative clinical issues that you can look into and help resolve.

Background

It is recommended to provide infants human milk exclusively until 6 months of age and as an adjunct to solid food until two years of age. While not every parent chooses to breastfeed, those that do may present for elective or urgent surgery. Historically the recommendation was to express milk for a period and discard it so as not to expose the infant to medications administered in the perioperative period in the milk.

More recently, the clinical recommendation is that patients are provided a lactation-compatible anesthetic and may resume feeding or pumping milk with intent to use as soon as they are awake and alert after anesthesia recovery. This recommendation recognizes that a period of milk expression and discarding is often unnecessary and may create a negative experience or outcome for the patient or infant. The anesthesiologist is well-positioned to create an anesthetic plan using lactation-compatible medications, and to assist with planning perioperative, and rarely intraoperative, breast-emptying to prevent mastitis or decrease in future supply.

Initiation of milk production in the breast occurs after infant and placental delivery; however, milk supply is maintained by demand created by frequency and volume of emptying. Patients should empty the

S. E. Dodd (✉) · T. N. Weingarten
Department of Anesthesiology and Perioperative Medicine, Mayo Clinic, Rochester, MN, USA
e-mail: Dodd.sarah@mayo.edu

S. Mohamed et al. (eds.), *Anesthesia Bridges*, https://doi.org/10.1007/978-3-032-08294-7_147

breasts preoperatively, as close to the start of the operation as possible, either by feeding or expression. An accurate separation time should be estimated, and additional intraoperative or postoperative emptying should be planned.

At our institution, intraoperative milk expression is offered to patients undergoing extended length surgeries and a protocol is available to guide the multidisciplinary anesthetic and surgical team. Depending on postoperative disposition, arrangements may need to be made for infant visitation or presence on a non-obstetric unit.

Clinical Care

Choosing medications for anesthesia and postoperative care need not be complicated (Table 147.1). Many medications do cross into breastmilk, but then cross back into the plasma as levels fall and the concentration gradients are reversed. The recommendation that patients may breastfeed once awake and alert after anesthesia is based on a low plasma level of sedating medications that correlates with only trace levels of medications in milk.

Ideal lactation-compatible medications are large molecules, hydrophobic, protein bound, short-acting, and with poor oral bioavailability. Most frequently used anesthetic medications exhibit these qualities and are compatible with breastfeeding.

There are multiple reliable sources for investigating whether a medication is compatible with uninterrupted breastfeeding after anesthesia, including LactMed and Infant Risk [1, 2]. If infants are preterm or have health concerns, involvement of their pediatrician is prudent to determine whether medication recommendations for healthy, term infants should be modified. Consider regional techniques, multimodal analgesia, and prevention of postoperative nausea and vomiting. If a planned medication is found not to be compatible with lactation, the anesthesiologist should identify an alternative when possible.

Lessons Learned

- Meet with the patient preoperatively to talk about lactation, paying close attention to their goals, concerns, and usual schedule.
- Advocate for lactating patients. They may need time and/or space to express milk or feed infants, education, and a comprehensive perioperative plan.
- Choose lactation compatible medications whenever possible (and it is almost always possible!) and pay attention to intervals between breast emptying.

Editor's Note: As a result of Sarah's interest in this aspect of perioperative care, she has developed an area of clinical expertise. She found a mentor in Toby Weingarten and went on to write the protocols at Mayo that have been successfully used on multiple patients with success. She has also been able to publish on this topic. Please see "More Wisdom on Career Development" (Chap. 81) for Toby's thoughts on mentoring Sarah and others.

Table 147.1 Lactation-compatible anesthetic medications by class

Class	Compatible
Anesthetics	propofol, midazolam, dexmedetomidine, lidocaine, bupivacaine, etomidate, volatile agents, nitrous oxide
Pain medications	acetaminophen, fentanyl, NSAIDs (PO), morphine, oxycodone (</=30 mg/24 h), ketorolac (IV), neuraxial opioids, remifentanil, low-dose ketamine
Antiemetics	ondansetron, dexamethasone, metoclopramide, haloperidol
Other	succinylcholine, NDMRs, neostigmine, glycopyrrolate, sugammadex, gadolinium and iodinated contrast

This is a summary for quick reference, but details may be found in the resources referenced below. Intravenous administration in standard doses unless specified

References

1. Montgomery A, Hale TW. ABM clinical protocol #15: analgesia and anesthesia for the breastfeeding mother, revised 2012. Breastfeed Med. 2012;7(6):547–53.
2. Mitchell J, Jones W, Winkley E, et al. Guideline on anaesthesia and sedation in breastfeeding women: guideline from the Association of Anaesthetists. Anaesthesia. 2020;

Authors

Sarah Dodd is an anesthesiologist at the Mayo Clinic in Rochester MN. Professionally, she is dedicated to women's health and specifically to the safe and coordinated care of patients who are lactating who require medical or surgical care. She is a Colorado native who loves the outdoors. Her husband and children are her greatest gifts in this life and her core values are showing **LOVE** to others and lifelong curiosity.

Toby Weingarten is a senior anesthesiologist at the Mayo Clinic. He has collaborated with numerous colleagues and is always happy to mentor motivated and energetic junior colleagues.

148 Strengthen and Safeguard Your Hands Throughout Your Career

Carol F. Bodenheimer, Albert Liao, and Catherine Marcucci

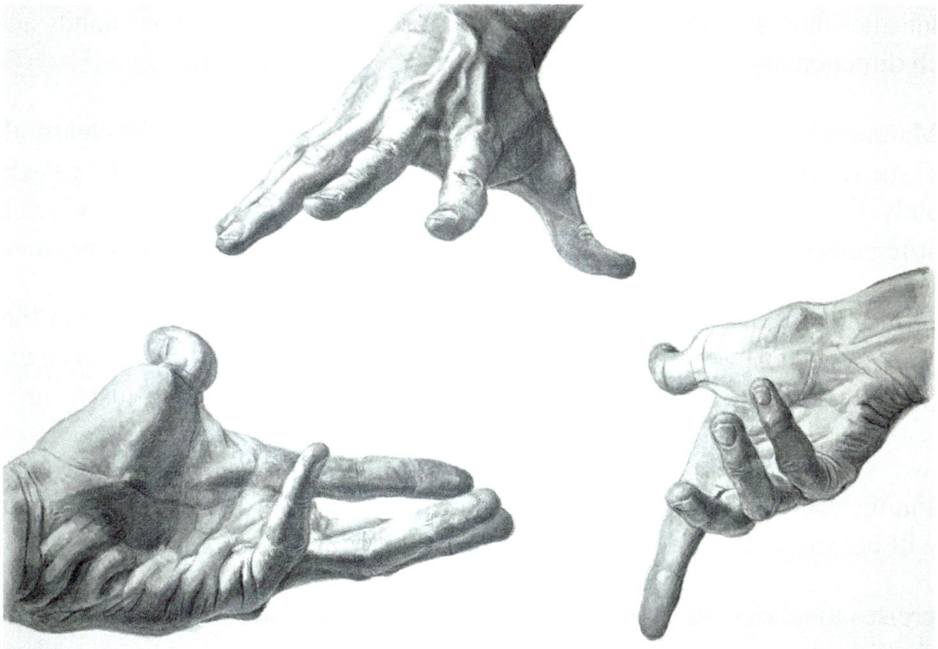

Fig. 148.1 Every technique and procedure in the entire field of anesthesiology starts with the correct placement of your hands. They are the most important pieces of anesthesia equipment and machinery we possess. These beautiful drawings illustrate their complexity, flexibility, and adaptability. Illustration: Luke Graber

C. F. Bodenheimer
H. Ben Taub Department of Physical Medicine and Rehabilitation, Baylor College of Medicine, Spinal Cord Injury Care Line, Michael E. DeBakey VA Medical Center, Houston, TX, USA

A. Liao
Liao Acupuncture, Towson, MD, USA

C. Marcucci (✉)
Department of Transfusion Medicine, Clinical Center, National Institutes of Health, Bethesda, MD, USA

S. Mohamed et al. (eds.), *Anesthesia Bridges*, https://doi.org/10.1007/978-3-032-08294-7_148

Introduction

Your fingers, hands, and wrists have 27 joints, 34 muscles, and 100+ tendons. The median, radial, and ulnar nerves each provide both sensory and motor function to the hands and there are 17,000 touch receptors in the palm alone. Our hands are considered one of the most exceptional developments in all of human evolution both in their ability to move and rotate in multiple planes (Fig. 148.1).

Hands are also acute sensory organs—the human hand can feel uneven surfaces that the human eye cannot see. It is critically important that anesthesiologists maintain all this wonderful anatomy, not just day-to-day, but over the course of a long career. Remember that if you start your anesthesia training in your mid-twenties and retire in your mid-sixties you will likely have a minimum of 9000 days of anesthesia "handiwork" to accomplish.

Advice from Our Colleagues and Friends

Maintaining your hands—strength, flexibility, and dexterity—is first and foremost accepting that you must do it and then devoting yourself to do it. Other hand professionals (musicians, painters, and jewelers) routinely do hand exercises, especially warmup exercises before practicing or performing. We haven't seen anesthesiologists routinely do this beyond perhaps wringing your hands and fingers once or twice in each direction and/or cracking the knuckles of each hand—ugh!

When Cathy Marcucci went on maternity leave back in the 1990s, she was unpleasantly surprised at how "unhandy" she felt on her first couple of days back. Even a simple peripheral IV gave her a moment's pause. Fortunately, Carol Bodenheimer was able to give her the following advice, which has carried her through her entire career. We are passing along Carol's professional advice and wisdom:

- At the barest minimum, daily hand exercises should include warmup exercises in the morning and relaxation exercises in the evening. Strengthening, stretching, and joint maintenance exercises should be done twice a week. Make sure you include your shoulders and arms, not just your hands.

- The easiest way to warm up your hands is to literally warm them—make sure you wear gloves on cold days and running your hands under warm (not hot) water—even for two minutes will help. Then, hand yoga will help as well, especially a routine that includes a variety of postures.

- Evening exercises to relax your hands can be based on tendon glides. There are lots of short routines for this on YouTube [1].

- If you will be off duty for maternity leave or even a two-week vacation, do your daily hand exercises but also hand strengthening. There are all kinds of inexpensive devices available. Cathy got some hand putty off the internet for just a couple of dollars.

- Also, if you are going to be off duty for a period of time, you can maintain hand dexterity with needle-crafts or coloring.

- Invest in regular hand and arm massages—30 minutes every two weeks would not be excessive. A great health habit to get into if you have the budget.

- The same with acupuncture—there are lots of specific meridian points that are beneficial for a hand professional, which we detail below. There is also an acupuncture approach for Raynaud's syndrome, which is a somewhat complicated condition. When used as a complementary adjunct, acupuncture may have efficacy in a multi-modal treatment plan.

- If you don't have the budget for professional massage or acupuncture, try qi gong routines for arms and hands. They are very low impact, take only 20 minutes or so, and really get your hands energized and soothed at the same time. Again, these are very easy to find on the internet [2].

- Of course, trouble with your hands can be a sign of trouble in your neck or shoulders or elbows. Practice good posture and body positioning habits and avoid repetitive-motion stress from tennis, softball, etc.

- It is not known what causes carpal tunnel syndrome, but it is known that poor ergonomics and repetitive motion worsen carpal tunnel symptoms. Make whatever adjustments are necessary to your desk and computer setups. If you find you are getting into a hand compartment syndrome, don't ignore it and hope it will go away. There are non-surgical options. We know of at least one plastic surgeon who recommends a course of Feldenkrais Method therapy before she will operate on the carpal tunnel.

- Swimming and/or water aerobics is one of the best cardiovascular exercises for the hands—all that low impact water resistance is great for strengthening.

- An anti-inflammatory diet will help keep your hand anatomy in smooth working order. Cathy swears by three cups of decaffeinated green tea to keep her hands loose and limber.

- It is incredibly important to prevent untoward hand injuries. Don't put your hands into blind spots. Don't even put them under the top of an old table at a flea market—too likely to have nails sticking out where you can't see them. Always keep your dog in front of you where you can see him so you

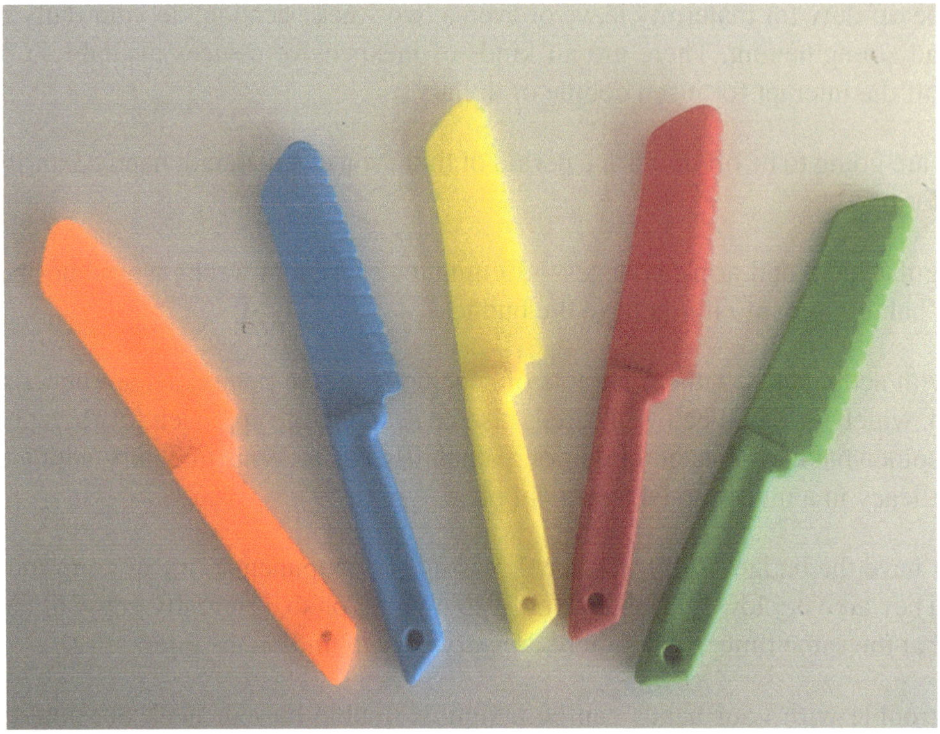

Fig. 148.2 The children's safety knives that the Sandson kids grew up with, widely available online and at discount stores. They slice fruit, vegetables, and bread just fine! Photo: Cathy Marcucci

don't go down on your hands and wrists. And use caution with manicures—they have been known to lead to finger and nailbed infections and abscesses.

- Similarly, think **VERY** carefully before you take up woodworking or use a lot of power tools.

- Rethink your knife inventory. Carol and Cathy have at least four friends between them who have sustained serious tendon injuries when a wet chef's knife slipped out of someone's hand and cut a phalangeal soft tissue structure. Therefore, these are the children's knives (and the only knives) that populate Cathy's kitchen to this day, with the exception of one small metal paring knife (Fig. 148.2). The Marcucci-Sandson group isn't fileting any sea bass or deboning any chickens with this knife set, that's for sure. So be it—that's what Wegman's is for.

- Consider a silicone wedding ring. They are safer in terms of avulsion injuries (which can be very, very serious) as the silicone band will break before your finger sustains enough force to cause grievous injuries. They also do not conduct electricity.

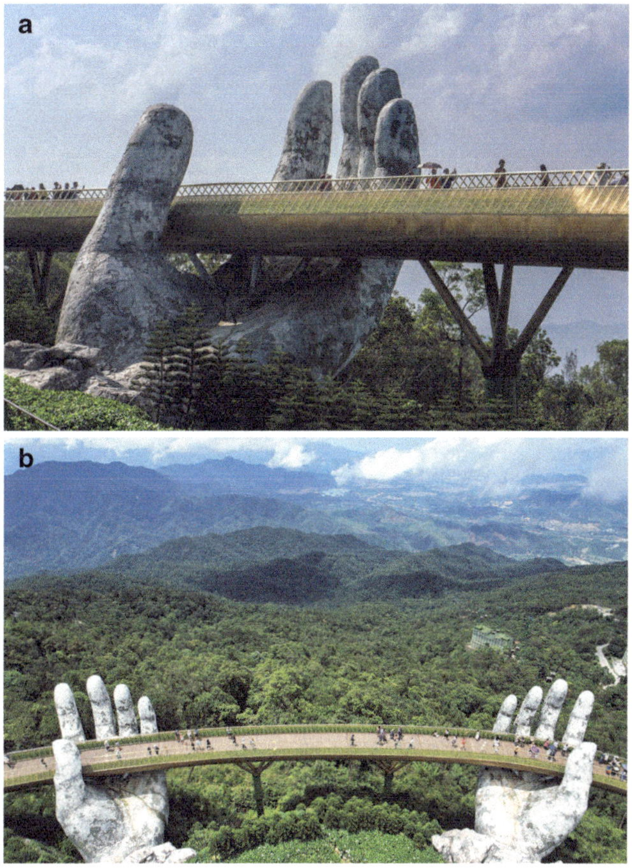

Fig. 148.3 (**a**) A stunning sculptural feature of the Golden Bridge. Photo: Image used under standard license from iStock.com. (**b**) An aerial view of the Golden Bridge, overlooking the coast city of Da Nang. The pedestrian walkway in the Ba Na Hills amusement park became an international sensation immediately after opening in 2018 and has been named as a "New Wonder of the World." The hands are made of wire mesh and fiberglass and provide only minimum support for the walkway. Photo: Image used under standard license from stock.adobe.com

- Sunscreen your hands every day. An extensive MOHS surgery for a wide squamous cell carcinoma would require significant recovery.

- If you do have hand surgery or sustain a serious hand injury, you may be looking at surgeries, pins, and an extended hand rehab period with a certified hand rehab professional. A friend who recently cut a tendon with a knife has had a three-month ordeal with her injured hand. This is one situation where the best hand surgeon in your region of the country would be worth it, even if you must travel.

***Note from the Editors:** No mystery as to why the Golden Bridge in Da Nang Vietnam was selected for this chapter (Fig. 148.3a and b).

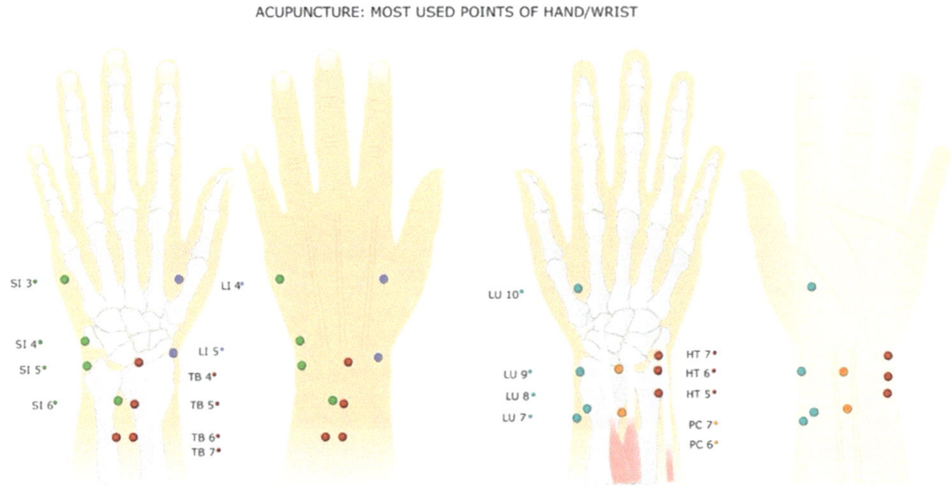

Fig. 148.4 Meridians are comprised of chains of specific acupuncture points. A number of specific points are shown above including those for Small Intestine, Lung, Heart, and Pericardium. Illustration: Image used under standard license from stock.adobe.com

Bonus Content! Acupuncture for the Hands—A Primer

Brush up on the information below before your first appointment to interview acupuncturists.

- There are 14 regular meridians on the body including Du and Ren meridians that run on the midline back and front, respectively.
- And there are 12 other meridians that represent the zang/fu organs of the body. There are six yang meridians and six yin meridians. These are further differentiated as six meridians of the foot (three yin, three yang) and six hand meridians (also three yin and three yang).

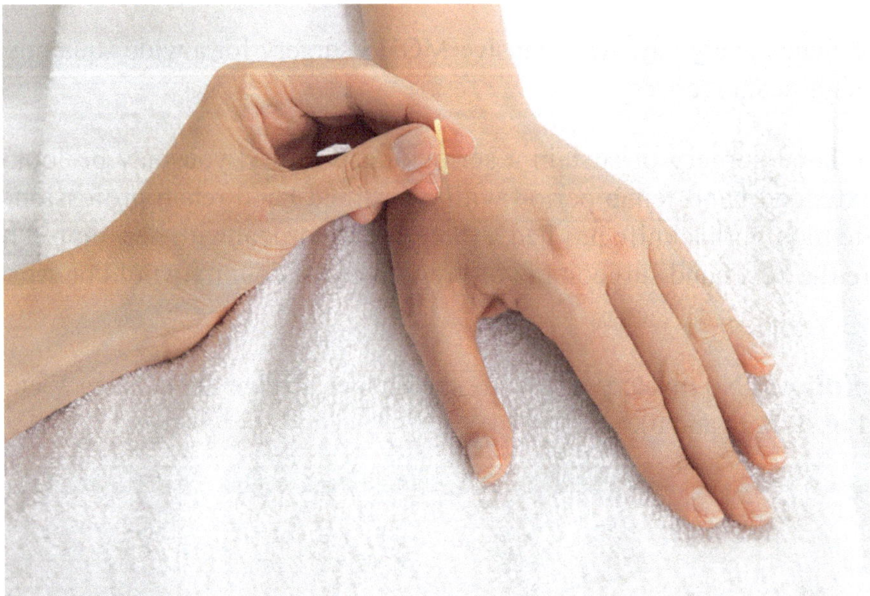

Fig. 148.5 The HeGu acupuncture point. Photo: Image used under standard license from stock.adobe.com

- The three yang hand meridians which run on the lateral part of the arm, are Large Intestine, Sanjiao, and Small Intestine (anterior to posterior), and the 3 yin meridians are Lung, Pericardium, and Heart (anterior to posterior), which run on the medial part of the arm. Several points on the Lung meridian on the hand are shown in Fig. 148.4.
- These 12 meridians run parallel to the extremities (arm or leg).
- For local pain on the extremities, we usually select points nearest the painful joint or area. Because the meridian runs parallel to the arm points, any of the arm meridians can be selected to treat a corresponding area on the shoulder, elbow, wrist, or joints of the hand and fingers. For lateral wrist or fingers pain, we choose yang meridian points, and for medial wrist or hand pain, we choose points on the yin meridians.
- The point Large Intestine 4, or HeGu, is on the hand between the thumb and first finger's proximal metacarpal bone (Fig. 148.5). It is a famous point for many ailments but is also the 'master of the hand.' Other most commonly useful points for the hand are Sanjiao 5, Waiguan, and Small Intestine 3, Houxi.

Lessons Learned

- Plan to keep your hands in the best possible shape—you more than likely will need them for high level performance for 40+ years!

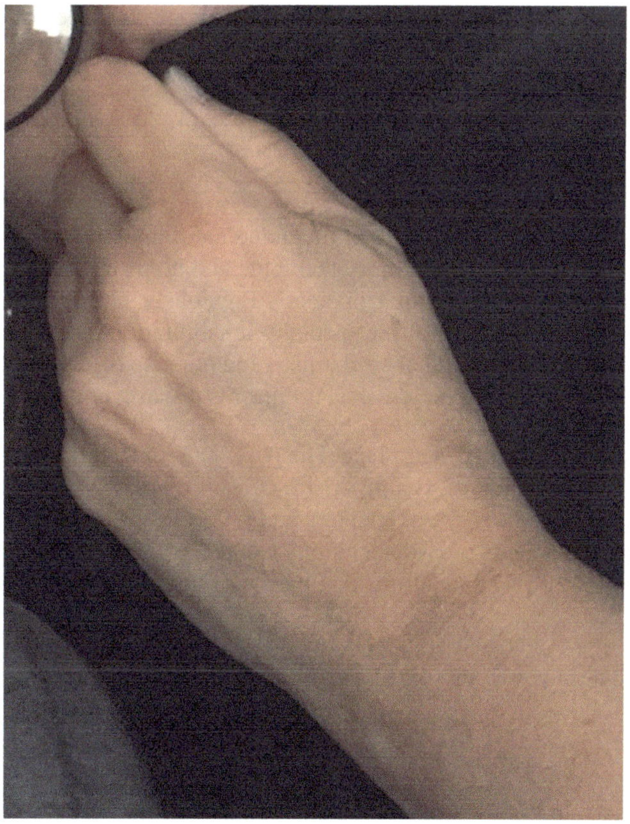

Fig. 148.6 "Senior" anesthesia hands after 35+ years of clinical practice. Photo: Courtesy of Catherine Marcucci

- A hand program should involve day-to-day warmup and relaxation and week-to-week stretching and strengthening.
- Hand gadgets don't have to be a bit expensive—a couple of dollars of putty will do the trick.
- Get professional help if you can afford it—massage and/or acupuncture. But, if not, the hand yoga and qi gong routines on the internet are free, short, and easy to do.
- Also, always guard against hand injury—power tools, rusty nails, and kitchen knives are some of the biggest culprits for hand injuries.
- Your hands are probably one of the most sun-exposed parts of your body—use sunscreen daily!
- Cathy Marcucci was really taken aback when she went back to work after a 4-month maternity leave. She has practiced the above advice from Carol Bodenheimer since 1998 more or less faithfully. Here are her hands today (Fig. 148.6). Not too bad for a senior anesthesiologist after 35+ years of clinical practice.

References

1. Southlake Health. Tendon gliding—Southlake hand therapy [video]. Youtbe; 2015 [cited 2025 Jun 19]. Available from: https://www.youtube.com/watch?v=dUhjUBAQv30
2. Qigong Meditation. 10 Minute MASSAGE HANDS | Simple Way to Relax and Heal Hands | Qigong For Beginners [video]. Youtbe; 2022 [cited 2025 Jun 15]. Available from: https://www.youtube.com/watch?v=D2-E4iIf4H4

Authors

Carol Bodenheimer is board-certified in both physical medicine and rehabilitation and electrodiagnostic medicine. She has a subspecialty certification in spinal cord injury medicine and holds a faculty appointment in the Department of Physical Medicine and Rehabilitation at Baylor University. Previously, she was president of the medical staff at Memorial Hermann/TIRR and medical director of the specialty rehabilitation unit. Carol has a wide range of clinical and research interests, including brain injury, spinal cord injury, and other spasticity syndromes as well as neurological and neuromuscular disorders, such as multiple sclerosis, Parkinson's disease, and post-polio syndrome.

Al Liao is a licensed acupuncturist in Towson, Maryland. His wife, Kristin King Liao, is also a licensed acupuncturist, and they practice jointly at Liao Acupuncture. Al and Kristin consult regularly with Cathy Marcucci on clinical acupuncture questions and have contributed to several chapters and publications including *Avoiding Common Anesthesia Errors, 2nd Ed.* They are the proud parents of two accomplished and young adult children. In his previous career, Al was a photojournalist based in Hong Kong and admits that his love of the "film arts" still burns brightly.

Cathy Marcucci is very grateful for her ongoing professional collaborations with Carol Bodenheimer and Al Liao. She thanks her coauthors for their ongoing interest in and contributions to the national anesthesia community.

Three Pieces of Advice

149

Ahmed Mukhtar and Hanan Mohamed Mostafa

Introduction

For this chapter, Ahmed Mukhtar was interviewed by Hanan Mohamed Mostafa.

Basics

In the early years of my training and career as an intensivist and anesthesiologist, I developed interests in clinical nutrition, ventilatory support, and antimicrobial therapy for critically ill patients. All these services are provided by other specialties—for example, dietitians, respiratory therapists, and infectious disease specialists. However, this multidisciplinary approach is helpful and serves the patients' best interests.

My First Piece of Advice: The intensivist must have minimum knowledge of all these disciplines. In fact, I believe it would be detrimental to intensivists if they do not. The intensivist must be able to make decisions on what is optimum for patients and be able to get all these multidisciplinary teams to work in harmony.

Here Is My Second Piece of Advice: As technologies advance—for example, the development of portable ultrasound—the diagnosis and management of patients has improved. However, I feel that we need to balance teaching such technologies and skills to our residents with teaching basic bedside clinical skills. Educating about new technologies should be in parallel to classic teaching so that residents will have the clinical depth needed in case of technological failure.

My Last Piece of Advice Is This: All young physicians are keen to learn and adopt new clinical guidelines, which is great. However, we need to remember that all guidelines are dynamic and evolving. Being a young physician, you need to focus on developing your clinical skills, while continuing to read and learn about new evidence as it gets published.

A. Mukhtar
Department of Anaesthesia and Intensive Care, Cairo University, Cairo, Egypt

H. M. Mostafa (✉)
Anesthesia, Surgical Intensive Care, Pain Medicine, Cairo University, Cairo, Egypt
e-mail: Hanan.mostafa@kasralainy.edu.eg

S. Mohamed et al. (eds.), *Anesthesia Bridges*, https://doi.org/10.1007/978-3-032-08294-7_149

Lessons Learned

- A good intensivist must have a broad range of knowledge, including understanding of ventilator support, nutrition, and infectious diseases.
- Using technology is fun and helpful, but do not forget to learn basic bedside diagnostic skills.
- It is good to learn about clinical guidelines, but be aware that they are not fixed in stone; they will evolve.

Authors

Ahmed Mukhtar is a professor of anesthesia and surgical intensive care at Cairo University. He earned his medical degree from Cairo University. He is passionate about the quality and safety of intensive care patients. Dr. Mukhtar is the director of the surgical and trauma intensive care unit at Cairo University Hospitals. He is board-certified in transesophageal echocardiography. He has special interest in critical care ultrasound. He is also the director of the critical care services of the liver transplant program at the Air Force Specialized Hospital. He is also a regional representative of the Liver Intensive Care and Anesthesia Group of Europe (LICAGE) in Egypt. He has more than 50 published studies in leading anesthesia and intensive care journals.

Hanan Mohamed Mostafa is an anesthesiologist and intensivist at Cairo University. She also has additional qualifications in healthcare management and spent time at Cincinnati Children's and Shriners to build her skills in PICU and burn critical care. She and her husband (an interventional radiologist) are the busy parents of two adolescent boys. In her spare time, she learned to play the flute and is a proud bookworm in all topics.

150 Truth

Raymond G. Graber

Introduction

This is a true story, from the author's personal files.

Tragedy

The sad part of the story starts in October of 1989, when a preteen girl was kidnapped from a shopping center in a nearby community. The kidnapper had apparently tricked her into thinking he was a friend of the family. The following February, the girl's body was found in a field, about an hour's drive away. She had died from multiple stab wounds and blunt trauma to the head.

The local police and FBI conducted an extensive investigation into her disappearance and murder. The case generated thousands of leads. Dozens of suspects were identified and questioned. In 1990, an FBI investigator came to the local VA Medical Center to interview a psychiatric patient who had made some suspicious remarks. After an initial interview, he thought he may have found the killer. The investigator left a message for the chief of anesthesia at that VA, requesting a call back.

Enter Me

That's where I enter this story. I had finished my training program in 1988, and I took my first job at this VA hospital. After a year, the current chief retired, and I was given the job. So, here I was, a little over a year out of training, and I had no clue as to what the FBI would want with me. With a little trepidation, I made the return call. The FBI agent proceeded to explain the situation and then made a request. He wanted to know if I would participate in a "barbiturate interview"—in effect, administering "truth

R. G. Graber (✉)
Department of Anesthesiology and Perioperative Medicine, University Hospitals Cleveland Medical Center, Cleveland, OH, USA
e-mail: raymond.graber@uhhospitals.org

S. Mohamed et al. (eds.), *Anesthesia Bridges*, https://doi.org/10.1007/978-3-032-08294-7_150

serum" to the suspect patient to facilitate questioning. My training had never prepared me for such a thing, and I wasn't sure how to respond. I told him I would get back to him.

There were so many questions that came to my mind. Is this a valid technique? Is it ethical? How is it done? How could I even research these questions? Remember, back in 1990, the Internet was just being conceived. Google was not established until 1998. If you needed to look something up, you went to the library. Alternatively, you talked to the smartest and wisest person you knew. So, in my case, I called my department chairman, Dr. Helmut Cascorbi.

Before we go any further with this story, let's learn more about this concept of truth serum.

History of Truth Serum

"Truth serum" is a term that has been popularized to describe a range of psychoactive drugs used in an effort to obtain information from subjects who are unable or unwilling to provide it otherwise. Alcohol could be considered to be one of the first agents used for this purpose. Many know the Latin phrase "In vino veritas," which translates to "In wine there is truth."

In the early 1900s, scopolamine, in combination with morphine, was administered to women in labor to ease their pain. An obstetrician, Robert Ernest House, noted that women who were given scopolamine during childbirth could answer questions accurately even while in a state of twilight sleep and were often times "exceedingly candid" in their remarks. In 1922, he promoted the idea that it could be administered to those accused of crimes so that the truth would come out during questioning. He believed this would help prevent false convictions.

House arranged to administer scopolamine to two prisoners in Dallas County jail. Both men were believed to be guilty, both denied guilt under scopolamine, and both were eventually acquitted. Enthusiastic at this success, House concluded that a patient under the influence of scopolamine "cannot create a lie ... and there is no power to think or reason." Thus, the concept of truth serum was born.

The next drug in our story is amobarbital (also known as sodium amytal). It is a barbiturate derivative, with sedative and hypnotic properties, and was first synthesized in Germany in 1923. It was noted that while under the influence, a person sometimes would divulge information that under normal circumstances they would block.

The drug was first employed clinically by Dr. William Bleckwenn at the University of Wisconsin to circumvent inhibitions in psychiatric patients. In the 1920s, Bleckwenn began studies on the use of barbiturates to treat catatonic mutism, a form of schizophrenia. He found that intravenous (IV) amobarbital was effective in producing a "lucid interval" wherein catatonic patients could converse normally, respond to questions appropriately, and provide information about their thought processes and backgrounds that would otherwise have been impossible to obtain. This beneficial effect was given the name "narcoanalysis."

In 1931, Bleckwenn injected a suspected murderer, John Whalen, with amobarbital. Whalen's testimony while under the drug led to his release from custody. Bleckwenn and his partner Lorenz administered the drug to several more criminal suspects over succeeding years. They decided that the test had limited applicability and was not infallible: "Up to present, we would conclude that the method is satisfactory and successful in the case of innocent people charged with crime. In the case of guilty persons, we have not always been successful in obtaining a confession."

Probably, the drug most commonly associated with "truth serum" is sodium thiopental or "Pentothal." This barbiturate entered clinical use in the mid-1930s. It was once the most common drug used to induce general anesthesia, and it was the drug I trained with during my residency. Besides being used for anesthetic induction, it was also used for several other medical indications: to induce burst suppression/ pentothal coma and to treat status epilepticus. Pentothal was eventually supplanted by propofol, which was approved in 1989. During WWII, both amobarbital and Pentothal were used as treatments for "shell shock," now known as post-traumatic stress disorder. It was also used on prisoners of war to enhance interrogation. Incidentally, Pentothal is no longer available in the United States. Manufacturers stopped producing it because of fear of the legal consequences of its use in lethal injection cocktails, along with pancuronium and potassium.

Does Truth Serum Work?

The US Office of Strategic Services (OSS) experimented with the use of mescaline, scopolamine, and marijuana as possible truth drugs during WWII. They concluded that the effects were not much different from those of alcohol: subjects became more talkative, but that did not mean they were more truthful. In the 1950s and 1960s, the CIA also studied various agents as possible truth serums, including LSD. A CIA report from 1961, released in 1993, concludes:

> No such magic brew as the popular notion of truth serum exists. The barbiturates, by disrupting defensive patterns, may sometimes be helpful in interrogation, but even under the best conditions they will elicit an output contaminated by deception, fantasy, garbled speech, etc.

In summary, it takes concentration to make up a lie and concentration is impaired while under the influence. It's likely more difficult for one to lie than tell the truth. However, these drugs do not completely inhibit a subject's ability to lie. These drugs lower inhibitions and make people more cooperative. Unfortunately, they also put people in an extreme state of suggestibility. Memories may be subject to reconstruction and fabrication. Subjects can be coerced into having a "false memory" of an event.

***Note from the Editors:** Speaking of truth, if you ever see a sign like this, *believe it*! (Fig. 150.1)

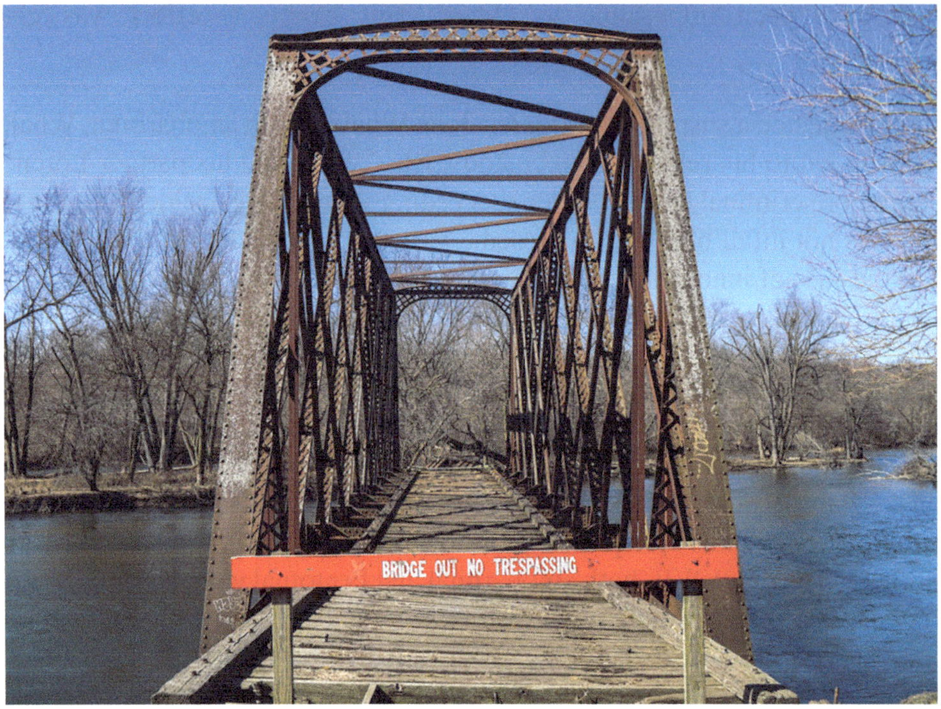

Fig. 150.1 A dilapidated wooden bridge with cautionary signage. Photo: Image used under license from stock.adobe.com

Ethical and Legal Issues

In 1963, the US Supreme Court ruled that confessions produced as a result of ingestion of truth serum were "unconstitutionally coerced" and therefore inadmissible. These were seen as a potential violation of the Fifth Amendment of the US Constitution—the right to remain silent. Ethical concerns have also been raised internationally in the European Court of Human Rights. It was argued that use of a truth serum could be considered a violation of the human right to be free from degrading treatment and could be considered a form of torture.

Back to Our Story

Let's return to 1990. I called my old chairman, Dr. Cascorbi, and informed him of what was being requested of me. Much to my surprise, he told me that he himself had participated in similar requests in his past. He told me that it was basically a way to loosen inhibitions. He felt that it was ethical as long as the patient was willing to consent to the process. He described his past experience and how to do it. So, I called the FBI agent back and agreed to participate.

Before the interview, I went to meet the patient. Given what he was suspected of, I was somewhat apprehensive to meet him. I did a routine preoperative evaluation. I described the procedure and got written consent. He was actually enthusiastic about the process. Meanwhile, a conference room was set up for the interview. Video cameras were brought in to record the interview. I had standard American Society of Anesthesiologists (ASA) monitors set up and airway equipment ready to go.

The appointed time came. The patient was brought in. After monitors were set up, I titrated small increments of Pentothal. The idea was to have the patient relaxed, mildly sedated, but awake enough to be able to listen to and respond to questions. The interview commenced. The FBI agent asked the patient a series of baseline questions with known answers. It came out during questioning that he actually did have some personal knowledge of the victim—he had worked at a stable where the victim had ridden horses. Then, the hard questions were asked. He denied any involvement in the crime. No new information came out of the interview. There was no evidence to incriminate him.

Conclusions

Although the administration of truth serum exists in movies and fiction, this does not appear to be a reliable technique. However, this has not stopped interrogators from continuing to consider using it. For example, the CIA considered the use of various pharmaceuticals like midazolam to facilitate questioning of prisoners after the events of 9/11. Ethical issues were raised by the CIA medical staff. The CIA ultimately decided against asking the Justice Department to approve drug-assisted interrogations.

Could a similar scenario play out in this day or age at your local hospital? I discussed this with one of my hospital's legal counsels. She told me that at minimum she would want to see a court order and an extensive discussion and documentation of the medical and legal risks and benefits. There would also have to be an anesthesia practitioner freely willing to participate. Pentothal is no longer available, but other sedative/hypnotics could be substituted. A suitable out-of-OR location could be found—even a postanesthesia care unit (PACU) slot. It is not clear what the point would be, if the results are unreliable and inadmissible in court. I don't know if current law enforcement personnel believe there is any validity to this process, but I would hope not.

When these events originally unfolded, I was naïve and was willing to go along for the ride with my friendly FBI agent. After all, it was for a good cause and the patient was a willing participant. Now, I'm a little wiser—I hope! I know more about the history of this process and the ethical and legal issues involved. Would I do it again? Maybe. A key thing to remember is that the patient involved wanted to do it. He believed that it would help clear his name. And maybe it did.

One thing I would do the same is talk it over with my chairperson first. This applies to any number of unexpected situations that might arise that you have not dealt with before or heard discussions about. It might be an unusual medical issue, or it could be a behavioral or social issue that you have witnessed. Some of these may make for great storytelling someday, but, in the meantime, you need advice on how to deal with the situation. Go to your chairperson first, and, then, keep him or her informed at every step of the way.

So, what was the outcome of this case? As I write this, it is now 30 years later. Suspects and leads are still being tracked down, and I still see stories about this case in the news. Unfortunately, the case was never solved. We never got to the truth.

Lessons Learned

- You will run into novel and unforeseen circumstances during the course of your career. Don't hesitate to discuss these situations with your mentors or chief. It's good for you to get advice. It is good for the chief to know what is going on.

Author

Ray Graber has fond memories of his mentors from his days training and working in the VA system and is glad to have had the chance to take care of our veterans. After two years, he returned to the mothership at University Hospitals Cleveland Medical Center, where further adventures awaited!

Twenty-Five Memorable Cases

151

Ronald S. Bank, Amy J. Robbins, and Catherine Marcucci

Contributors:

Andrew B. Barker, MD

Rodger E. Barnette, MD

Meena Bhatia, MD

Denis L. Bourke, MD

Norman A. Cohen, MD*

Dawn Dillman, MD

David R. Dininny, MD

Joel M. Feinstein, MD

Brian T. Gierl, MD

Raymond G. Graber, MD*

Jeremy Jaffe, MD

Daniel Joseph, MD

Kirk Lalwani, MD

R. S. Bank
Department of Anesthesiology, INOVA Fairfax Hospital, UVA School of Medicine, INOVA Campus, Falls Church, VA, USA

A. J. Robbins
Stanson Health, a Premier Inc. Company, Charlotte, NC, USA

Atrium Health, Carolinas Palliative Care and Hospice Group, Charlotte, NC, USA

C. Marcucci (✉)
Department of Transfusion Medicine, Clinical Center, National Institutes of Health, Bethesda, MD, USA

S. Mohamed et al. (eds.), *Anesthesia Bridges*, https://doi.org/10.1007/978-3-032-08294-7_151

David Sanusi, MD

Brandon M. Togioka, MD

Christopher A. Troianos, MD*

Toby N. Weingarten, MD

David A. Zvara, MD

Introduction

In every career, there are the cases that stay with you—the cases that made you the physician that you are. Even decades later, you can remember who you were working with and what room you were in. We asked our senior colleagues if they could share the details of those cases that remain in their hearts and minds. These are their stories.

A Box of Chocolates?—Kirk Lalwani, MD

When I was a resident in London, I had anesthetized a 75-year-old gentleman for a suprapubic catheter placement. He had an uneventful induction and a laryngeal mask airway. The procedure began and the surgeon inserted the trocar towards the distended bladder. When he pulled out the obturator, blood shot up and splashed off the ceiling back on to the field. The trocar was in an undiagnosed abdominal aortic aneurysm. We moved from an LMA to intubation, lines, and an emergent AAA repair. Fortunately, all went well, and the patient survived to leave the hospital with no ill effects.

Lessons: The motto of the story is **Be Prepared!** Anesthesia is like a box of chocolates…you never know what you're gonna get.

Super Bowl Sunday—David Sanusi, MD

It was Superbowl XXV Sunday, the NY Giants were to play the Buffalo Bills in Tampa Stadium. I was the chief anesthesia resident on call at Tampa General Hospital—a busy 1000 bed Level 1 trauma center. There were three other (junior) residents on call with me. We had finished most of the semi-elective/urgent cases by mid-afternoon and we were all excited to be able to watch the big game despite the in-house call. My attending decided to assign the next case to me because I was more senior and would require less monitoring on his part while they watched the Super Bowl. Arggh! I was not very happy because I had to work while my junior residents were sitting on their butts.

Anyway, the case was a cardiac transplant on a 19-year-old male named Ryan who needed this surgery due to viral cardiomyopathy. When I went to the floor to do his preoperative assessment, it was obvious that Ryan had been there for months. He had posters and photos on the wall of girls, water skiers, and motocross bikes. He had made his hospital room his home for months. Ryan was a young, buff, great-looking college kid with four beautiful sorority girls in his room. I was able to meet his family and his friends, and they were all so excited that there was finally a compatible match for his failing heart. When he saw me enter the room, he smiled ear to ear and said "DOC, let's get this show on the road! I'm sooo excited, I've been waiting a long time for this!"

I felt like such an idiot. My attitude before I entered the room was not exemplary. I had put a football game's importance in front of a human's life. I had forgotten why we train so hard and so long to do what we do. I didn't even remember who won that game, nor did I care. And when others tried to give me a break during Ryan's case, I refused and wanted to do his case personally.

Lessons: To this day, I still think of Ryan when I have the dreads of doing a case and I try to put myself in the patient's shoes. Thank you, Ryan, for such a valuable lesson!

Give Me a Light!—Christopher A. Troianos, MD*

I was a relatively junior cardiac anesthesiology staff providing anesthesia care to a 66-year-old man undergoing coronary artery revascularization and possible aortic valve replacement on a hot summer day in Pittsburgh. The outside temperature was 90° Fahrenheit with 85% relative humidity and air-conditioners were working at full capacity.

Six minutes after the aorta was cross-clamped and cardioplegia was administered, a power outage affected the entire hospital and operating rooms, during vein graft anastomosis to an open distal coronary artery.

The cardiopulmonary bypass (CPB) machine did not have a built-in battery back-up, and so the roller head supporting the patient's circulation was manually cranked to maintain a venous saturation of greater than 70% according to a battery-powered saturation monitor. This required a significant amount of work and energy expenditure and was continued until an alternative power source could be established. The operating suite lacked any type of overhead lighting in operating rooms, hallways, anesthesia workroom, and post-anesthesia care unit.

Surgeons could not visualize the operative field, except by relying on flashlights and laryngoscope blades found within the anesthesia machines. Personnel collided with one another in the hallways in their attempts to help caregivers in supporting vital patient needs. Cell phones were not available at that time, as everyone relied upon an intercom system to communicate, which of course was not functioning without electricity. Oxygen powered suction devices were secured from paramedics in the emergency department. All patients in the intensive care units who were on a ventilator, relied upon hand bagging to maintain oxygenation and ventilation, while communication with concerned family members was undertaken to calm their fears.

A decision was made to remove the aortic cross-clamp for my patient once the distal anastomosis was completed, in order to allow the heart to recover function and separate from CPB until power was restored to the hospital. This was not easily accomplished as the patient was hypothermic and the CPB heater was not operable. A dopamine infusion allowed sufficient return of spontaneous circulation to enable separation from CPB until power was restored. Cardiopulmonary bypass was reinstituted 85 minutes after the first loss of power, and the operation proceeded uneventfully with no further loss of power episodes. The patient awoke, neurologically intact the following morning and was discharged from the hospital 8 days after surgery. A complete description of this case along with our management of cardiac surgical patients during a power outage can be found in *Anesthesiology*: Volume 82, pages 298–302, 1995.

Lessons: Don't take anything for granted (even electrical power to a hospital), and as we are taught during our training, always prepare for the worst-case scenario, as you hope for the best!

***Note from the Editors:** Chris Troianos lives and practices in Cleveland, Ohio as do *Anesthesia Bridges* editors Ray Graber and Ed Avery and several other authors and contributors. We asked them what the most notable bridge in that metropolitan area is and they all said the Hope Memorial Bridge with its beautiful and slightly eerie Guardians of Traffic (Fig. 151.1).

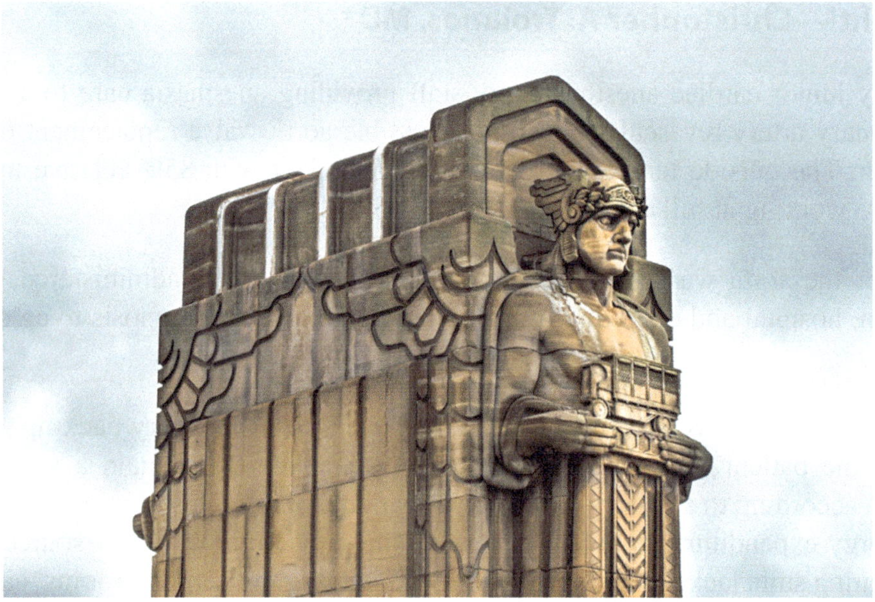

Fig. 151.1 A Guardian of Traffic figure on the Hope Memorial Bridge in Cleveland, Ohio. The statues were designed by sculptor Henry Hering and architect Frank Walker. There are four pairs of Guardians—each holds a different vehicle, including a stagecoach, a covered wagon, a hay wagon, a 1930s automobile, and four types of motorized trucks used in the construction of the bridge. The bridge crosses the Cuyahoga River and connects Lorain Avenue and Carnegie Avenue. The Art Deco truss-style bridge was completed in 1932. Photo: Image used under standard license from stock.adobe.co

On the Beach—Ronald S. Bank, MD

In 2013, while vacationing at Ocean City, we were at the beach on a cold and windy day for the time of the year. I wanted to head back to the hotel, but my kids convinced me to stay on the beach. Because of the wind, the waves were higher than usual.

My oldest son came running over to me and said that one of the girls, Samantha as we later found out, that had been in the water with a group of friends right next to us was lying face down in the water and that it looked like she couldn't move. I ran over and could see exactly that. Someone else was running toward her. I yelled to him to please not touch her as I had figured out that she had a C-spine fracture. I stabilized her head and neck to her body and turned her in the water with the help of a couple of others and the life-guards. One of the guys was going to pick her up and run her back to shore. I told him not to do that and that I'd have to stabilize her neck while she was carried back.

In the meantime, I had sent one of my kids back to my car to get my kit that I always had due to my work in tactical medicine with area law enforcement. The kit is complete with intubation equipment.

Her fracture was not high enough that she needed ventilatory support—we later found it was a C6 fracture. I held her in neutral C-Spine alignment on the beach and reassured her until the medics arrived.

One of the medics told me to release her neck so that she could put a collar on her. I reminded her that it was sand and that I could hold the C spine while she dug away a couple of handfuls of sand to place the bottom of the collar, which she did. For some reason they wanted to take her to a smaller regional hospital. I suggested Shock Trauma. They obliged. She was flown there by MD State Police.

She underwent anterior and posterior spine surgery throughout the night only to be told that she would be a quadriplegic. I ran the case by many of our spine surgeons who thought the same. She had an incredibly strong spirit. I stayed in touch with the family. I was able to assist them in having her transferred to Hopkins for rehab. They did an amazing job. Weeks or months (can't remember) after her initial surgery her family invited my wife and me to come to Kennedy Krieger to see her. When Samantha came out with one of the physical therapists walking with a quad cane with assistance my wife broke down in tears.

A year or so later Samantha's mom asked if they could visit us. We kept asking how Samantha was doing. She just said that we would see for ourselves. When they arrived Samantha walked up our driveway totally unassisted and gave my wife a hug. It was a very special moment given that she had been told by so many that she'd be permanently paralyzed in all four extremities.

Samantha went on to a full recovery. We have kept in touch with her family to this day and The Baltimore Sun even did a story on these events. What a great profession we have—to have training which enables us to have such a profound impact on peoples' lives.

Lessons: While she didn't need intubation, I was very glad to have my kit in my car. I suggest that physicians with substantial emergency skills such as anesthesiology or emergency medicine carry a kit in their vehicles. It would be a shame to have the knowledge and skill to help a critically injured person but not the equipment.

On the Plane—Ronald S. Bank, MD

In the early 2000s, my wife and I were flying home from a trip. During the first flight, the plane had to abort its climb and put down emergently due to a serious mechanical issue. The second flight took off well after midnight. I was sleeping when my wife and a flight attendant grabbed my arm and asked for help. My wife had heard the call for medical help and raised her hand.

Toward the back of the plane was an elderly woman, unconscious, lying across her husband. She was not moving, had a large amount of vomit in her mouth and was extremely pale. I could not feel any carotid pulse. The flight attendant brought me the medical kit. It had one dose of each of the ACLS meds of the time plus a few other meds, an IV bag, suction device, and other items. There was no AED as this was many years ago before they were widely available.

I asked the flight attendant to help with the suction device so that I could clear the vomit from her mouth. The device totally sucked in that it wouldn't really suck. So, I used the green plastic laryngoscope to intubate somewhat blindly. There was no pulse ox nor colorimetric capnometer. I thought that I was in the trachea based on chest rise. I couldn't hear much with the cheap stethoscope.

I gave her a milligram of epinephrine via her external jugular and did a few chest compressions while the flight attendant used the AMBU bag to ventilate her via the ETT. I was able to quickly get return of spontaneous circulation. I gave her a sedative (can't remember what they had) so that she would not try to self-extubate and I placed an nitroglycerin tablet under her tongue. I was able to start an IV. There was nowhere to hang the fluid bag. So, I put some tape through the hole in the bag, tied the ends to form a loop with a knot, and closed the luggage compartment door on it to hold it above the pt. There was also no oxygen. So, I was just delivering an FiO2 of 0.21. They said that they don't keep pressurized O2 on the plane due to its combustion hazard.

The pilot came back and asked if we had to do an emergency landing, which I found out later is extremely expensive for the airline. I said that she had arrested and that we did. So, she put the plane down emergently. As soon as we landed, the paramedics took over. They took my contact info. I later found out that the patient had a full recovery. I was never contacted by her family. I did receive a nice letter from the medical director of the airline and two free tickets for a future trip. Once the paramedics took her off most of the cabin broke out in applause. When we landed at our intended destination a lot of folks said thanks.

This event gave me a lot of respect for the conditions that first responders have when they do intubations in far less ideal conditions than we do. Also, before they'll give you a medical kit they ask for your medical license. So, carry your pocket card with you.

I later found out at an ASA talk about medical care during commercial flights that the kits are totally not standardized so one never knows what they will or won't have.

Lessons: One of the takeaways for me was to think about how you'd respond to a medical crisis in such an out of hospital environment. Overall, it was a memorable experience.

On the Train —Catherine Marcucci, MD

I know the exact date—December 18, 2009. It was a Friday night, one week before Christmas Day. I was in a very busy stage of my life and career and had scheduled ten days off over Christmas and Christmas week. I was sitting in 30th Street Station in Philadelphia, waiting for my train home (at that time, I commuted daily from Baltimore to the Philadelphia to do my cases at the Philadelphia VA) when I heard the loudspeaker—"Is there a physician in the station? Please report to Stairway 5!" I glanced around and saw that no one was paying the slightest attention to the announcement. Dang it! I took a deep breath and stood up. The lady next to me said, "Oh, you're a doctor! Good luck! Should I hold your handbag for you?"

As I hurried over, the Amtrak people were motioning down to the train platform. A second physician—a cardiology fellow from Jefferson—appeared and introduced himself as "Tom." To this day, I don't know

Tom's last name. We ran down the stairs, expecting to see someone lying on the pavement, only to be told, "On the train, on the train!" The only "train" seemed to be a one completely dark passenger car on an otherwise deserted platform.

There we found a youngish male slumped down in one of the seats. He still had a (very) weak, thready pulse but he wasn't breathing. When I told the Amtrak staff that the patient was in respiratory arrest one of them said to me, "We don't mean to be disrespectful, but do you have the training to know that for sure?" "It just so happens that I do," I said. Apparently, he had type 1 diabetes and had been talking to his wife when he became confused, started slurring his words, and eventually stopped responding to her. While she frantically tried to contact Amtrak to report her husband was likely in hypoglycemic shock, the train pulled into the station, and all the other passengers had exited, assuming that our patient was merely asleep.

No equipment or meds of any kind were available, except a cup of orange juice that was already at the scene. Emergency responders had been called but were 20 minutes away. "Can someone turn on the lights?" we asked. Not possible we were told; all power to the car had been cut. This was before the days of cellphones with flashlights were in every pocket, so Tom and I looked at each other and said, "Okay, I guess we're doing this in the dark."

He looked for the insulin pump, which he found and pulled out of the patient's thigh. I got in the seat behind the patient and gave him a brisk jaw thrust with both hands. The patient took one gasping breath. We asked the staff to run up to one of the coffee stands in the station and get some sugar packets, call the paramedics back to report a true arrest situation, and find a flashlight. Tom sloshed small amounts of orange juice and poured sugar in the patient's oral gutters to get some mucosal glucose absorption while I did jaw thrusts to keep the patient breathing—as I recall, it took about 25 or so before the patient resumed spontaneous respirations.

Removing the insulin pump and the sugar loading had a fairly rapid effect. By the time the paramedics got there about 20 minutes later, the patient was much more responsive although not completely alert. He was confused and wasn't sure where he was but was able to state his name. Supported by the paramedics, he walked out of the train car to the gurney (it's hard to get a stretcher into and down the aisle of a passenger train car) and was taken to a nearby hospital where he was evaluated and released several hours later. Tom and I quickly gave our names to the Amtrak authorities, shook hands, and headed in our separate directions. We never received any thanks or acknowledgement from the patient or his family at all. They contacted Amtrak to retrieve a briefcase left behind and were told that the patient had stopped breathing and two physicians had responded but didn't seem to have any interest in who we were or any of the details.

Ten days later, on my first day back to work after vacation, I was in the same station heading home at the same time. As I started to go down the stairs to the trains, there was a little commotion and a small crowd of Amtrak management people surrounded me, including the train master, the station master, and the Amtrak police supervisor. The train departure was put on hold for twenty minutes. The executives had heard about the incident and wanted to offer me compensation in the way of a free train tickets or passes. Since I was a regular commuter, the executives had come to the top of the stairway for several evenings in a row until I resumed my regular schedule after the holidays and the boarding attendants could point me out to them.

I must say that they were very appreciative and grateful for our willingness to help their passenger. Apparently, it is a *gigantic event* when a patient dies on a train, in addition to the tragedy itself, of course. I ended up declining the free tickets.

Instead, they agreed to give my kids (who were 8 and 11 at the time) an insider's behind-the-scenes tour of the whole train station, including the trains, dispatch rooms, and the big dispatch board. We couldn't tour the switching yards due to insurance purposes, but the train master hosted us for lunch before the tour and helped my son Charlie with his Boy Scout Railroading merit badge. Amtrak also wrote me a nice letter and wrote a separate letter of commendation to my hospital director as well.

I wish I could say that we performed heroic and advanced life-saving techniques for this passenger, but we didn't. With no equipment, no meds, and no light, we just went back to Medical Training 101—remove the inciting agent, treat to the extent possible, and support respirations and circulation as best you can. All those years of anesthesia training and practice and I resuscitated somebody with jaw thrusts, for Pete's sakes. Really, I could have saved the guy after one week of residency. It seems so ironic. The other thing that has stayed with me is the fantastic coincidental nature of it all. He would have died, probably, if he hadn't pulled into a station where someone with airway skills was sitting but, fortunately for him, he did.

I occasionally think about this gentleman and wonder how he is doing. I know his name and where he lives. I could look him up on the internet, but I never have. Honestly, it feels a bit strange to me that nobody in that family ever thought to thank us or even had the slightest curiosity about who had come forward. If a physician in a train station saved my family member, I'd send them flowers or a letter, wouldn't you? But they didn't, and so my first lesson learned is that using our medical expertise to assist or even save the lives of strangers on the street is its own reward. And second, the people that you *really* want acknowledgement from already know. When I finally rolled through the front door late in the evening I said to my husband, "Well, I ran into a train car tonight in the dark and saved a guy." And he said, "Of course you did."

Lessons: You will save somebody on the street at some point in your career and you will have the quiet satisfaction of knowing that you could do it and did do it.

***Note from the Editors:** Cathy Marcucci rode across this Amtrak train bridge across the Susquehanna River on her way home the evening of the escapade in the dark train car (Fig. 151.2). It's not a beautiful bridge or a scenic view and is often in fog as in the photo, but it got her where she wanted to go—home—on that eventful evening.

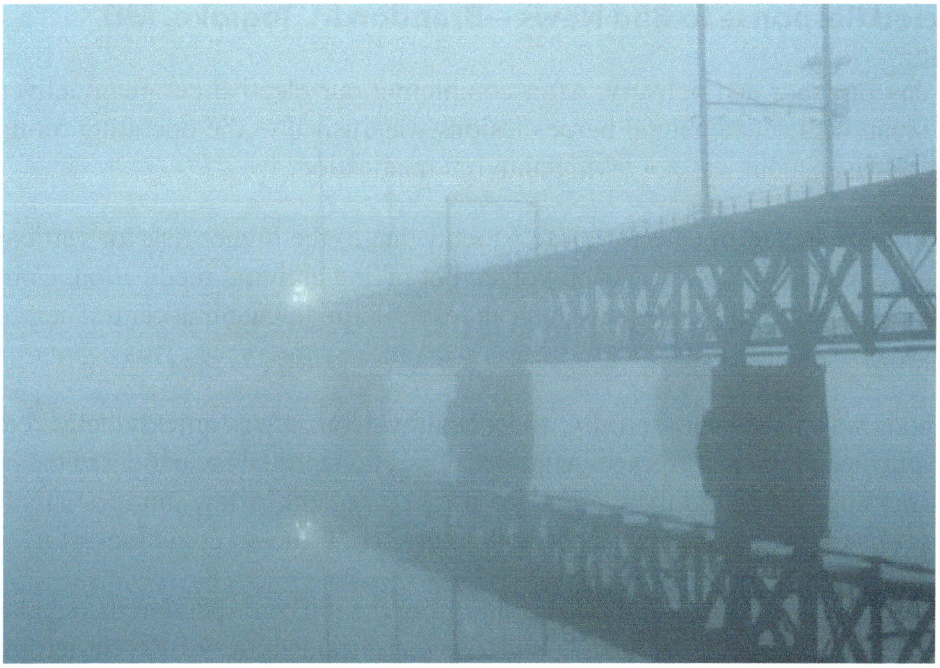

Fig. 151.2 The Amtrak train bridge across the Susquehanna River between Havre de Grace and Perryville—two Maryland Chesapeake Bay towns. Photo: Image used under standard license from stock.adobe.com

Always Remember the Goal Is for the Patient to Forget—Catherine Marcucci, MD

There is a memorable case in my head for the very reason of how routine and unremarkable it was. I was still fairly new in training and had done a general anesthetic for a routine GI case—removal of a pretty big tumor that was pressing on the inferior vena cava, but the pathology was fortunately benign. I had done the usual standard case—careful preoperative interview, general anesthetic, spinal morphine for pain control for the overnight postop stay in the ICU. The usual, standard case. I went to see the patient just after he arrived on the floor for the postop note. I was talking and asking some questions, when the patient politely interrupted me. "Excuse me," he said. "Have we met?" He just had no idea who I was.

I asked him the last thing he remembered before induction of anesthesia. "Nothing," was the reply. I asked the first thing he remembered when the case was over, "Again, nothing." He said to me, "I know I had a big surgery and I guess I had anesthesia, but really, it's like it never happened. The day is just gone. My gut feels different though."

Later my attending said to me, "Did you happen to get the postop done on that guy from the other day?" When I related the story, he said, "Okay, you probably won't remember the patient's name. But always remember what he said to you. This type of case is as important as any of the big or complicated or 'heroic' cases we do. Right here, this is what the practice of anesthesia is all about."

Lessons: Our job is to make it so that patient practically forgets they even had anesthesia and surgery. Couldn't have learned a better lesson than this case.

An Unexpected Response to Bad News—Brandon M. Togioka, MD

It was a busy day on labor and delivery. After completing our elective cesarean delivery schedule, a multiparous woman with active genital herpes lesions was rushed to the operating room for an urgent cesarean delivery. The patient was not taking antiviral medication.

Cesarean delivery is standard of care for these patients due to the higher risk for vertical transmission with vaginal delivery. This risk is greater in women not taking antiviral medication. Congenital herpes simplex disease manifests with skin lesions and can result in life threatening central nervous system and disseminated disease.

A spinal anesthetic was placed uneventfully, and a healthy neonate was quickly delivered. Uterine tone was adequate, and blood loss was average. After delivery, I transported the patient to the post-anesthesia care unit, gave nursing report, and then left to see my next patient. A few minutes later a frantic nurse ran toward me, "Dr. Togioka the baby has a lesion on its face! Can you come look at it?"

I am still uncertain why the nurse asked me this question; the job of inspecting the neonate is primarily the responsibility of the pediatrician and secondarily the responsibility of the obstetrician. Perhaps it was the combination of the nurse's shock and my proximity, which led the nurse to ask me. It may have been that the other clinicians had left the immediate area to see other patients and the nurse, knowing that the new mother might be questioning and upset, approached the physician she could find.

At any rate, I try to never disregard nurses, ever, if they have a clinical concern. If a nurse runs to find a doctor and you are that person, you don't tell them it's not your problem and to go find somebody else. So, I walked back and looked at the baby. I was horrified at what I saw. The baby had a significant burn on its cheek, likely from the electrocautery used during the cesarean delivery. I felt absolutely horrible telling this new mother that her beautiful baby girl had been scarred by our team. Her response was quite surprising, "I am *SO GLAD*. I thought she had gotten herpes from me!"

Normally, delivering news of an iatrogenic injury to a neonate's face would be met with anger and sadness. This mother's response was quite the opposite—gratitude and happiness. I was not considering the patient's diagnosis of herpes simplex when I delivered the news.

Lessons: Always consider the context when you are delivering news and patient expectations and concerns have a significant effect upon how medical information is received.

Don't Underestimate the Power of a Few Milligrams of Local—Joel M. Feinstein, MD

Practicing anesthesiologists sometimes get into the habit of putting everyone to 'sleep' and forget about the powerful effects of a few milligrams of local anesthetics placed in the exact right location. Being part of the regional anesthesia team, we are often contacted as a last option for critically ill patients that need surgery. Regional can be particularly helpful when an extremity surgery is necessary and no one thinks it is safe for the patient to undergo general anesthesia. It is not uncommon for us to do surgical blocks for upper and lower extremity amputations and even an occasional mastectomy, but every once in a while, we get some unusual requests for surgical blocks.

As a young attending, we had a patient present with a non-healing wound after femoral artery access by vascular surgery. Plastic surgery was planning for a rotational rectus femoris flap to cover the defect. The patient was dependent on supplemental O2 with severe COPD. The consensus was that if she required general anesthesia with intubation, she would likely not tolerate extubation and become ventilator dependent.

Unfortunately, her coagulation status prevented consideration of a neuraxial, so the regional service was consulted. The groin and medial upper thigh innervation are a complex web of nerves that are not traditionally amenable to surgical blockage. After discussing with the patient and surgery team, we offered a surgical TAP and low volume femoral and obturator blocks. The surgery was successfully completed with minimal sedation, and the patient was ultimately discharged home without significant complications.

Lessons: A good understanding of anatomy and knowledge of various regional anesthesia techniques can save the patient and the perioperative team from embarking on avoidable misadventures in the operating room.

What It Means to Be a Physician—David A. Zvara, MD

At the start of my career, I was called for a "red trauma" for a hunter accidentally shot by his partner in the field. The wound was terrible, and the weapon was a high velocity deer rifle. As I came to the bedside, this young man looked at me with pleading, fading eyes and asked, "Will I be ok?" I remember thinking in the split second of that moment that the nature of the wound was not survivable. Everything was happening fast. This young man was on the verge of consciousness, intubation, and rush to the OR. There was noise, shouting, and confusion in the ED bay as we prepared for lines, airway management, and transport.

And in that moment, as if all action about us were suspended, and the only communication was between the two of us, I looked him square in the eye and lied. "Yes," I said. "You will be ok. We're going to get you through this." I spoke these words with total confidence. There was a shocking calm and ease of pace in my voice. I had no idea where this came from within me. I will never forget that last look he gave me. One of trust. Hope. Comfort.

These were his last words. He died a short time later. I was the last person to whom he spoke. Somehow, I knew in the moment that our skills would not be enough, but that what he needed most in his time of terrifying realization, was comfort.

I was moved by that encounter and remember it some 30 years later. Sometimes the best we can do is provide comfort. A glimmer of hope. To lie to a patient is unethical. Still, to this day, I stand by my lie.

In anesthesiology, especially cardiac anesthesiology, we know that our words may be the last a person hears. Our conversation may be their last.

Lessons: In that golden moment of trust, be there, in whole, for the patient. Listen, comfort, care.

Two Days in the OR—Amy J. Robbins, MD

As a very young anesthesiology physician several decades ago, I was on call one night when we became aware of an emergency situation involving a young person who had been in an accident on a rural farm. I was there when the patient arrived on a stretcher and was rolled off the helicopter. After the patient rolled by, two men in scrubs followed quickly behind with the patient's detached arm in a bucket. Literally, we saw an arm sticking out of a bucket of ice. This arm had been completely severed from the patient in a farming machinery accident.

The patient was brought into immediate emergency surgery in an attempt to reattach the arm. Reattachment was not a common procedure at the time, and we were a mid-sized regional hospital, not a major academic or research center. Surgery lasted over 24 hours, and I was lead anesthesiologist for about 20 of those hours.

We challenged the blood bank supplies on this single case. Through all my years at Hopkins, I transfused more blood products to this patient than I ever had done in a single case, and this includes lengthy liver transplants and extensive vascular cases back in the day. We could barely keep up with the patient's needs. I have a vivid image in my mind of seeing the blood oozing and dripping off the draped arm, onto the laps of the two surgeons who were bent over the patient's draped arm, and pooling on the floor below. Altogether, the surgery and anesthesiology teams persevered for upwards of 36 to 48 hours with a successful result. It was exhausting for all. It challenged the team physically, mentally, and emotionally.

Thankfully, the young patient was healthy and survived the lengthy surgical process and I do know to this day he has use of that arm! It was one of the handful of cases that I've done that has gone into a second day with the patient still on the table. The visuals remain with me today—I saw an arm in a bucket of ice walk by, and 2 days later, it was again part of the patient.

Lessons: What I learned is that well-trained, disciplined medical teams can achieve great results against the odds.

Fly-By—Amy J. Robbins, MD*

I was on call one afternoon when we got word that there was an emergency landing at our local metropolitan airport. The level one trauma center downtown that typically received trauma and emergency patients was on bypass, and with few emergency and trauma resources nearby, our small hospital was selected to receive and care for this patient in critical condition with a life threatening ruptured aortic aneurysm.

We received the patient from the airline. He was unconscious, his blood pressure was in the 50 mmHg range on entry into the OR where resuscitation and surgery began. The hospital did not have a cardiac program, and the typical procedures at this hospital were routinely bread and butter cases for the most part. The anesthesiology, surgical, and nursing teams worked together in concert. Some of the team had not done arterial and central lines in years! This patient was in great hands! All involved drew on our collective experiences working with patients in larger systems and especially in our training years and were able to provide the patient with a level of care commensurate with what would have been received in a larger and more sophisticated setting. The OR team can be a well-oiled machine working together in the most stressful circumstances. We used the knowledge we gained in our training and we succeeded.

Lessons: What I learned is that I left Hopkins, but Hopkins didn't leave me.

***Note from the Editors:** Contributing editor Amy Robbins has always had a love of railroad bridges. One of Amy's favorite train bridges is the Poughkeepsie Railroad Bridge (Fig. 151.3).

She shared the following with us:

> My maternal grandfather, Coy William Foster, was a lifelong train dispatcher for the Illinois Central Railroad. I also grew up on trains and our family would walk the tracks and the train bridges and he would impart his knowledge. Tons of history in those train rides and walks!!

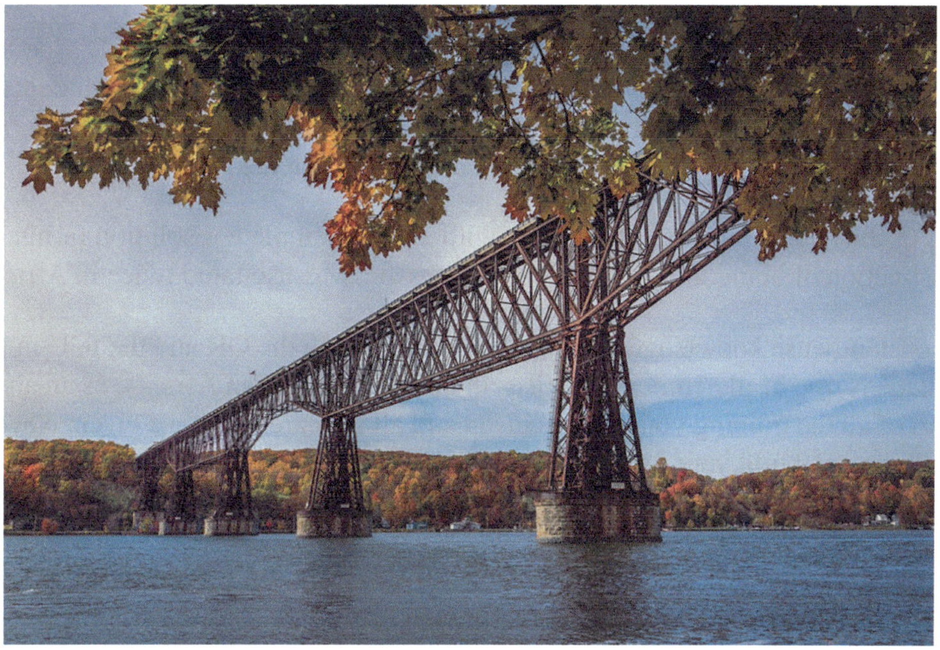

Fig. 151.3 The beautiful Poughkeepsie Railroad Bridge, also known as the Walkway Over the Hudson. It is a steel cantilever bridge that spans the Hudson River, connecting Poughkeepsie, NY on the east with Highland, NY on the west. It was originally a double-track train bridge that was part of the line of the New Haven Railroad. It was completed in 1889 and remained in service until 1974. It is now the second-longest pedestrian bridge at 1.28 miles and is part of the Walkway Over the Hudson New York State Historical Park. It is also designated as a National Civil Engineering Landmark. Photo: Image used under standard license from stock.adobe.com

A Case from East Africa—Rodger E. Barnette, MD

You must understand we were structured like a small ICU. I was the only consultant (attending in our system) with nine anesthetic locations. This, of course, is not the typical ratio in the US, but of necessity, it's what we had in a setting of limited resources, which includes limited trained personnel. The KRNAs (Kenyan Registered Nurse Anesthetist) were to notify me of difficult patients, and I would periodically "round" through theatre.

I was called into an OR because the KRNA could not intubate. The patient had a large hemangioma involving the lips and tongue. And I had not been informed because neither the surgeon nor the KRNA anticipated a problem. The KRNA in several attempts to intubate had caused bleeding and an increase in size of the lesion.

Within a very short time of my arrival, I realized we were in a cannot intubate, cannot ventilate situation. I was told of the nature of the lesion by the surgeon, so I took a 7 ETT and placed it via the left nares to a depth of about 17 cm. I then compressed both nares with one hand (which also kept the ETT from moving), compressed the mouth closed with the other hand, and asked the KRNA to connect the circuit to the ETT and hand ventilate.

We were able to ventilate easily, and I then requested a tracheostomy by the surgeon.

In adult men, an ETT introduced in this way to a depth of 17–19 cm places the tip of the tube just above the glottic opening. The technique is useful only if you know the ETT will bypass the obstruction.

Interestingly, when this patient returned later in the week he arrested in the OR, due to the surgeon injecting a large amount of absolute alcohol into the lesion. Since alcohol in high concentrations is a myocardial depressant, I was able to obtain return of spontaneous circulation with 3 mg of epinephrine. I then placed him on an epinephrine drip and weaned him over the next 24 hours.

He walked out of the hospital about a week later with almost complete resolution of his lesion. He has the dubious distinction of being the only patient I successfully resuscitated twice in Africa.

Lessons: I constantly use knowledge and experience from both the OR and the ICU in the care of my patients. The same is true of my clinical practices in both the US and in Africa—as an anesthesiologist, you are the sum of all the training you have received and all the care you have given. Never overlook an opportunity to learn and build your experience base.

Triple Check—Denis L. Bourke, MD

When I began my anesthesiology residency in the early 1970s, we started most IVs with a straight needle. Butterflies were a luxury, and Medicuts, awful as they were, were reserved for only the biggest cases. I was taught to never the trust an IV if you didn't start it yourself and, if at all possible, to use the back of the hand to insert an IV. Those guidelines served me well for a number of years, but times change.

By the 1990s, nurses usually started the IVs in the preoperative area. At our VA, the preop nurses started the IVs and, for obvious reasons, the policy was to connect the IV to an infusion pump. In one instance, nobody in the preop area was able to start an IV in an obese patient. They called upon a recovery room nurse to have a try. She was successful in starting an IV in the antecubital space. When the patient came to the operating room, I wasn't particularly happy with the infusion ports in the pump IV line and decided to switch to one of our standard infusion sets with a stopcock. When I disconnected the IV line, bright red blood came pumping out of the IV catheter. The line was obviously in an artery. We removed the catheter and applied pressure while looking for another site to start an IV.

After obtaining a satisfactory IV, the case proceeded with no further complications. There are numerous case reports of everything from minor problems to major disasters resulting from inadvertent intra-arterial injections.

Lessons: Triple check any IV not started by yourself before using it.

Peripheral Venous Pressure and Becoming an Academic Anesthesiologist—Toby N. Weingarten, MD

In medical school I connected with a great anesthesiologist, Jim Munis, whose enthusiasm for our specialty and physiology sealed my determination to become an anesthesiologist. A couple of years later, much to my surprise he had moved to Mayo and was now my attending as a CA-1 resident. During a morning presentation, he lectured about peripheral venous pressure. The idea of this concept is that measurement of pressure at a peripheral vein would give a more accurate understanding of volume status than either arterial or central venous pressure. The reason being is that it would not be influenced by arterial constriction or dilation or performance of the heart.

The next day I was assigned to a case of a resection of a large and very active pheochromocytoma tumor. I decided to monitor it and see what happened. I attached pressure transducers to my arterial, central, and peripheral lines. It was a wild case with big fluctuations in hemodynamics despite only minimal fluid administration and loss. Fortunately, the patient did well and the outcome excellent.

That night, I meticulously copied each value and time of these pressure measurements into Excel and calculated correlation constants between the three vessel pressures. My hypothesis was that because the peripheral venous pressure was isolated, it would not correlate with the other two systems. I was very wrong: correlations were strong! This was a refute to the hypothesis that peripheral venous pressure would be devoid of influence other than volume status; at least in the setting of huge swings of catecholamine levels during surgical manipulation of a massive pheochromocytoma. I wrote it up and got it published in Anesthesia and Analgesia as a case report.[1]

This hooked me on academics, a journey that started with case reports then case series and eventually turned into sophisticated studies of large patient cohorts.

Lessons: My work over the past two decades has taught me two very important lessons. First, the cliché "medicine is always changing" is true, and as a clinician it is incumbent to stay abreast of the literature. What was thought to be true yesterday changes as more and more studies validate or invalidate practices. What is your practice? Examine your protocols every few years. Does current evidence still support the inclusion of this particular drug in your ERAS protocols? Maybe something safer or better or more economical can now be used?

Second, the value of continuously auditing ones' practice. In the era of electronic medical record systems, the barrier for examining outcomes has gone down, you no longer have to work at the big academic center to do this. Always ask yourself, "How are we doing with PONV, sedation scores, pain levels?" Then "do we have a problem with a particular outcome or is there something we can be doing better?" Then circle back to the current literature and revise your protocols. Never stop doing this, your patients will thank you for it.

The Case Is Cancelled—Brian T. Gierl, MD

Our patient was a 63-year-old woman without relevant past medical history who presented for C3-C5 ACDF six weeks after a motor vehicle collision. She went to an outside hospital Level 2 trauma center after the MVC where her C-spine CT showed moderate-severe central canal stenosis at C3–4 and C4–5. Her symptoms were pain in the area with numbness to the associated dermatomes bilaterally. Those symptoms were exacerbated by cervical extension and led to nausea and presyncope. We recognized that she did not have a study of her neck vasculature and that her nausea and presyncope with cervical extension could be related to a cerebrovascular injury. A subsequent study showed a vertebral artery dissection with occlusion and the case was canceled.

Lessons: Sometimes, your best case is the one that you don't take to the OR.

Lessons Learned—Norman A. Cohen, MD

I had one very impactful case my first year of residency. It was an on-call urgent case on a Saturday at the VA. An elderly man, with aortic stenosis, presented with hydrops of the gallbladder for an open cholecystectomy—this was before laparoscopic cholecystectomy was an option. As was the custom at my institution, I handed my induction drugs to my attending. She proceeded to give around 200 mcg of sufentanil and around 8 or 10 mg of midazolam during the induction very quickly and in sequence. She told me after the fact what she gave and never asked my thoughts on dosing. No surprise that the blood pressure tanked and did not respond to phenylephrine, epi, etc. Patient coded, CPR didn't help, and the patient died. I subsequently had to present this case to M&M rounds and was raked over the coals. My attending took no ownership at all of her decision-making in giving essentially all the drugs I handed her to the patient.

(Big) Lessons: I learned from that was that I wasn't handing off my drugs to anyone if I was going to be the one held accountable and that I had to develop a much better understanding of the pathophysiology of cardiac valve diseases. It also changed the way I operated as a leader of an anesthesia care team with both residents and CRNAs throughout my career.

***Note from the Editors:** Norm Cohen is a big fan of suspension bridges and remembers reading books about the Golden Gate Bridge as a kid. He has a short list of other favorite suspension bridges, including the Bosphorus Bridge in Istanbul, which connects Europe to Asia (Fig. 151.4). We think it may have been the first intercontinental bridge. Norm had the opportunity to cross it on a visit to Turkey in 2009. He found it to be impressive and inspiring, both scenically and due to its engineering.

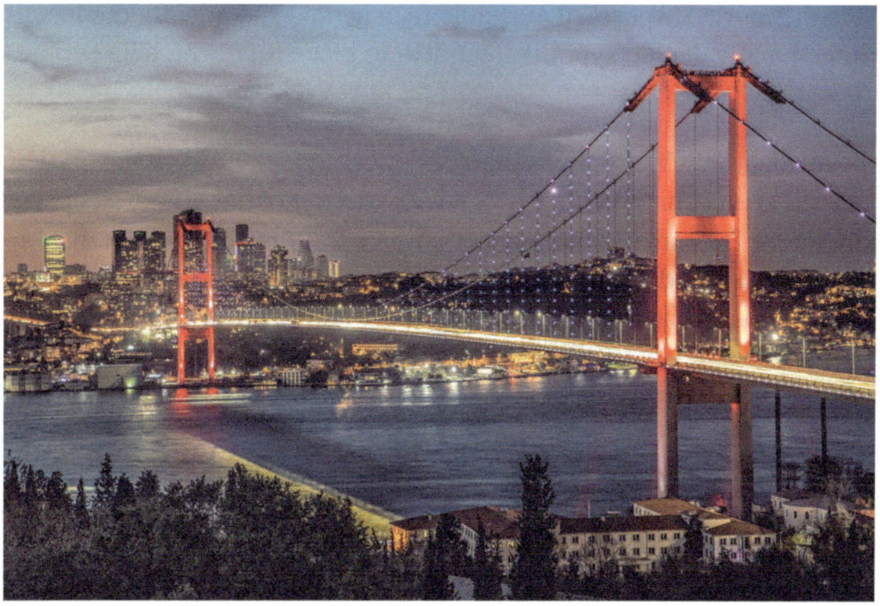

Fig. 151.4 The Bosphorus Bridge, known officially as the 15 July Martyrs Bridge and also known informally as the First Bridge, spans the Bosphorus Strait. It is one of three bridges to span the strait and the southernmost bridge. It is a gravity-anchored suspension bridge with steel towers that was completed in 1973. It is known that that at least one pontoon bridge across the strait existed in antiquity; Leonardo da Vinci was the first to suggest that a suspension bridge could be built. Photo: Image used under license from stock.adobe.com

Context and Culture—Dawn Dillman, MD

When I was a CA2 resident on overnight call, a roughly 20-year-old patient was rushed to the OR for an exploratory laparotomy for a gunshot wound to the abdomen. For context, this was around 2000, at the Johns Hopkins Hospital. Hopkins is located in Baltimore, MD, which had the highest rate of murder in the country at that time. That is to say, it was relatively common to be receiving trauma victims in the OR to perform life-saving surgery. Frequently, the patients would say as they were rolling in "Don't give me the bag, doc!" It was a common result of this type of injury and surgery to end up with a colostomy bag, which was then seen as a social stigma.

In this case, however, the patient said, "I don't want you to put me to sleep." This seemed targeted specifically to me, and I remember being confused and asking the patient why not as we moved him over to the other table and started putting on monitors. He responded, "Because you are going to give me AIDS." That puzzled me more, and I said I promised I wouldn't give him AIDS, and the attending, senior resident, and I got him off to sleep.

What I was too young and naïve to know at the time was the context of that comment. The patient was a black man from a neighborhood in Baltimore, and I was a white woman from a Midwest town. I knew no one personally who had AIDS, and as I understood it, it was very clear that HIV was transmitted by blood or body fluids. While antiviral treatment was available, we were still close to the time when AIDS was a death sentence, and it was very much in the Baltimore community. As I later learned, one of the theories that circulated amongst the black community was that HIV and AIDS were specifically designed and given to black persons by white persons, as a way of keeping the black population in control. This was believable given the myriad aspects of systemic racism, and specifically the insults of the Tuskegee experiments that intentionally denied syphilis treatment to black men which had come to light in a similar timeframe as the advent of AIDS.

I still reflect on this incident in which I, my senior resident, and attending were all white. We did something that a person asked us specifically not to do, which was to not put him to sleep, because in our view it was the safer thing to do. I wonder about what emotional trauma he felt from that on top of the physical trauma of the gunshot wound. Indeed, the patient did make it through the surgery and ended up surviving the injury and hospitalization without acquiring HIV. However, I wonder about what I might have said that would have acknowledged his fear and let him know I understood so that I could reassure him that he was safer proceeding with me. I also wonder if he would have had the same fear and request if his anesthesiologist was black, or his surgeon or any other person in the operating room would have been black.

Lessons: We work in context of our culture, and it is on us to understand the implications of our privilege to be able to provide care that is sensitive to the needs of others. It is also imperative to work towards training a diverse workforce that reflects our community.

A Near-Miracle Is Not Always Enough—Andrew B. Barker, MD

I had a Jehovah's Witness patient that underwent a nephrectomy and IVC reconstruction. He came and refused all blood products and was not optimized by alternative methods prior to surgery. He came to the ICU postop with a hemoglobin of 4.5 g/dL. We drew labs twice a day only using an ABG syringe, gave IV iron, erythropoietin, and albumin. He recovered well after about 10 days and went to a floor bed for further recovery. As he resumed a regular diet, he choked while eating a turkey sandwich and ultimately died after that event.

Lessons: What I learned is that we can work near medical miracles, but we can't stop death when someone's time comes.

***Note from the Editors:** There are many spooky and abandoned bridges in the US that carry legends of ghosts and haunting (Figs. 151.5 and 151.6).

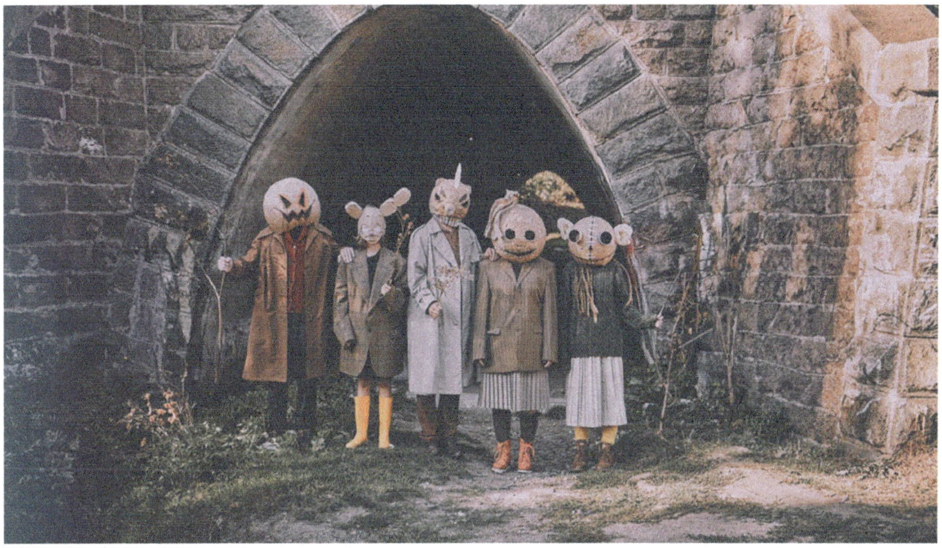

Fig. 151.5 What better place for goblins to gather than under a spooky old bridge? Photo: Image used under license from stock.adobe.com

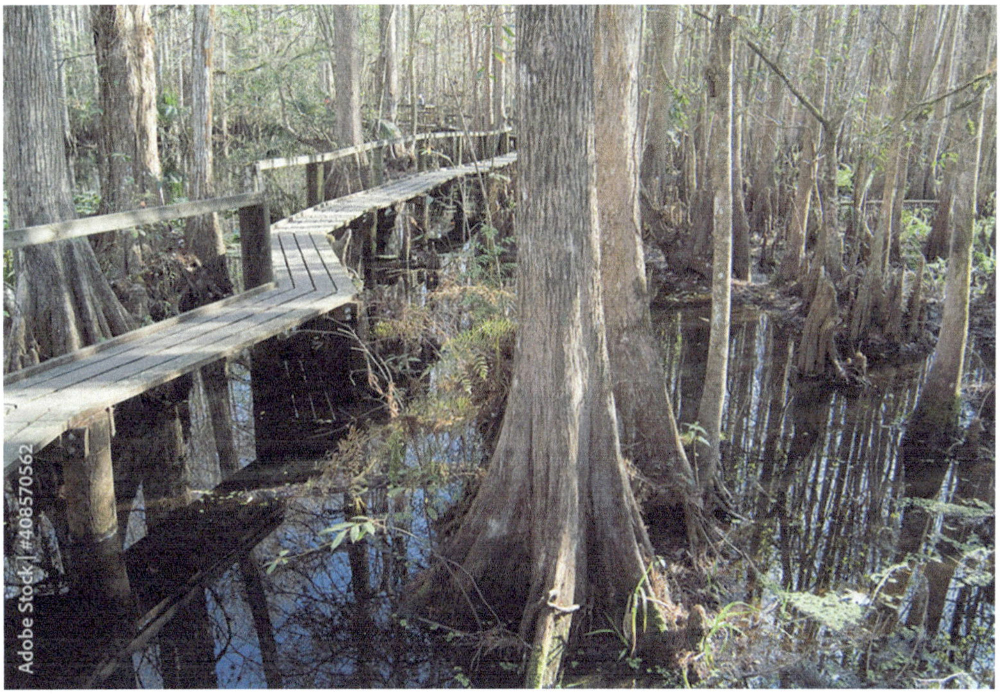

Fig. 151.6 The bridge through the cypress swamp, Highland Hammock State Park, Florida. Scary bridges aren't always broken-down structures that look ghostly at night. Notice that there is a railing only on **one** side of that footbridge. It doesn't look like it would be too difficult to find yourself in that water—in other words, in a swamp of dark water. In Florida. Need we say more? Photo: Image used under standard license from stock.adobe.com

One Snowy Night—Raymond G. Graber, MD

It was a December night in Cleveland in the early 1990s, and the lake effect snow was coming down hard. I was on cardiac call, and I was paged to come in for a heart transplant. The drive in was marred by poor visibility, but at least it was late, so the traffic was minimal. We had a relatively new transplant program at our institution, but we had hired a very experienced and internationally known surgeon to head it up. This would be the first heart transplant where I was the lead anesthesia attending—in the early days of our program we frequently paired off with another attending so we could all learn from each other.

After the organ was formally accepted by the organ retrieval team, we induced and lined up our patient. This process was uneventful, and soon we were prepped, draped, the chest was opened—and we sat waiting for the retrieval team to return with the heart. There was a problem, however.

The organ was coming in from out of town on a small private jet. Our organ harvest team typically landed at a small airport on the shore of Lake Erie, which is relatively close to our hospital. The blowing and drifting snow shut this airport down. The plane detoured to Cleveland's main international airport, but the pilot was forced to circle because conditions were not suitable for landing.

We sat in the OR waiting, wondering what the delay was. Remember, cell phones were a novelty back then, and there was certainly no texting. We finally got word that the organ was on the ground, on the way. But there had been a complication.

The retrieval team had been circling for a while and finally had to make a decision. Do they detour to another city and abort the transplant, or do they take the risk and try to land? The pilot agreed to go for it. The pilot successfully got the jet down on the runway but was not able to stop the jet on the snow-and-ice covered surface. The jet went off the runway, down an embankment, and took out a radar tower. Thankfully, no one was injured, and the team climbed out of the plane, carried the organ up the snow-covered hill, climbed into the waiting ambulance, and were then driven to the hospital.

We greeted our intrepid colleagues as they finally arrived with the organ. We heard about the story in bits and pieces as they set to work. The organ was successfully implanted, and the patient was weaned off pump with dobutamine and amrinone, which was the phosphodiesterase inhibitor in use at the time. The patient was taken to our SICU for recovery.

This story made our local news—it was a great human-interest story of courage and perseverance. Unfortunately, it did not have a happy ending. A couple days postop, the patient had been extubated and seemed to be doing OK, but the right heart began to fail. The patient had significant pulmonary hypertension, and the new right heart was not tolerating the load. These were the days prior to milrinone, nitric oxide, ECMO, or ventricular assist devices. The patient deteriorated over the course of several days, and none of our pharmacologic therapies were able to turn things around. He soon expired.

This case was filled with emotional highs and lows. It is always a "high" to see a transplanted heart start beating, especially when you are relatively new to this game. But to see that patient start out so well, and then rapidly deteriorate, was heartbreaking for the whole team. We did our best work, but the treatment options that were available to us at that time were not up to the task. Success in high-risk surgeries such as this is not measured by just getting out of the operating room, but by seeing the patient walk out of the hospital.

Lessons: This case impressed on me a career long mindfulness of the risks of pulmonary hypertension and right heart failure. In our preop evaluation of patients, we tend to focus on left heart issues—coronary artery disease, left ventricular ejection fraction, aortic and mitral valve disease, and so forth. Right heart issues can just as easily kill a patient, too.

It's a Go!—Meena Bhatia, MD

"It's a go!" I could only imagine the power those words had on my patient who was named "Robert." That night, Robert, a 47-year-old man struck down by a sudden and debilitating cardiomyopathy heard the heart was a match. The transplant was on. I imagined him with his wife and two children in the pre-operative waiting area. I'm sure they were excited, beyond all words, at the new life before them. And terrified of the unknown. Opposite emotions, side-by-side, interpreted privately by each in the family. I can imagine my patient sharing a kiss and a squeeze of the hand as he rolled alone with the surgical team to the operating room. I know the pre-induction banter.

I was not part of the surgical team. I was the ICU attending that night. I was alerted to the transplant and readied the team for the anticipated arrival. One delay followed another. Finally, the patient arrived in my ICU. Report given: the transplanted heart never gained recovery. There was a profound rhythm and mechanical failure post reperfusion. My patient arrived on venoarterial ECMO in a raging coagulopathy and with a prayer for either cardiac recovery or a plan for emergency re-listing and re-transplant. My job was to keep him alive long enough to give him this long shot chance.

We worked the rest of night balancing vasopressors and mechanical support. The bleeding never let up. One massive transfusion protocol followed another. My arms tired from pumping blood. The surgeons were ever present and the blood flowing, flowing. We were losing. The heart never recovered.

"Can you speak with the family?"

"Sure," I said. This was one of many conversations with Robert's wife. Each time, I shared our hope for his turning this around. "He's a fighter," I said. Hope was palpable in the ICU waiting room.

Many hours into this ICU admission, I received a call from our blood bank. "We're 100 units into this resuscitation. Is it time to stop?"

I know the chief of the blood bank was doing her job. As the administrative, legal, and medical steward of this resource, and concerned about all our patients, not just this one, she posed a legitimate question. Our data, recently reviewed, demonstrated the near complete futility of heroic efforts such as this despite the rare anecdotal save. She was asking me, "Is it time to stop?"

"No," I said without hesitation. 'We go on. There is still hope." And we did. Long into the night, and through the couple of days, we did all we knew how to do in his ICU course.

The heart never recovered. The bleeding subsided, but, ultimately, Robert was declared unsuitable to re-list given the multi-system organ failure. He died soon thereafter, wife and children beside him. I wrote the final note in his chart.

I will never forget this case. *I know resources are limited.* The blood bank was doing their job and following protocol when they inquired about terminating the transfusion protocol. As a physician responsible for the allocation of precious healthcare resources, I must weigh the needs of my patient against the needs of all our patients. I know all these things, and in the moment, the decisions are clouded by the reality of this patient's life. This patient's family. I wish I could say we saved Robert. But in spite of the massive resources we used and despite all our efforts, we failed. I think about this case, and I have no regrets. Should we have stopped our efforts sooner? Was the blood bank chief, one step removed from the patient and their family, right? Did we expend precious resources in a doomed effort? My answer is an emphatic "*No.*"

Lessons: At the end of the day, after all the hope washed away from their faces and only sadness left, I looked the family in their eyes and said that we did absolutely everything in our power to save a life, a husband, a father. Perhaps that provided a measure of comfort for them. For a while, we flew on hope. Sometimes, that is all we have as caregivers. We fought to the last and I will do it again if needed.

Note*: the editors thank David Zvara, MD for his mentorship of the author and assistance with this essay.*

Saturday Call—Daniel Joseph, MD

I was on call for the weekend at the orthopedic and spine hospital doing solo MD anesthesia. I went in on Saturday AM expecting to do an "old lady hip fracture" case and on arrival found out she was bumped for an urgent posterior cervical spine decompression/fusion case which was a revision after recurrence of cervical spine osteosarcoma. The case was challenging and took about 6 hours but went well.

I thought we were going to follow that with the hip fracture case but then found out there was an add-on for urgent decompression/fusion of the thoracolumbar spine. Also, another six-hour case!

The patient was a 46-year-old male who was discharged from the VA Hospital two days earlier with a diagnosis of spinal plasmacytoma associated with myeloma. There was a concern about possible coagulopathy as well as impending paralysis due to cord compression. Apparently, he was married with children.

Now I'm really feeling sorry for myself, another complicated six-hour case with invasive lines, positioning, and transfusion of blood products and no help in sight. And I'm thinking, they knew about this when he was at the VA two days ago, why didn't they just do it there?

Well, I did my normal preop evaluation and we were starting to head back to the operating room in the mid-afternoon, and the patient says, "Doc, wait a minute!" And I start thinking "what now, come on, we want to get this case started already." But, of course, I stop and say "Sure, what's on your mind?" And the patient then pauses for just a couple of seconds, looks at me, and says "Doc, do you think I will ever walk again?"

Well, that made me take a real deep breath and realize why we went into medicine in the first place.

Lessons: This certainly put into perspective that we are generally very fortunate to be the ones responsible for taking great care of patients and not be the person lying on that stretcher—who is sometimes, and often rightfully, scared out of their mind! A moment I will always remember!

***Note from the Editors:** This is the Island in the Mur (Fig. 151.7). This iconic structure, in the middle of the Mur River in Graz, Austria has always fostered discussion—is it an island or a bridge? The

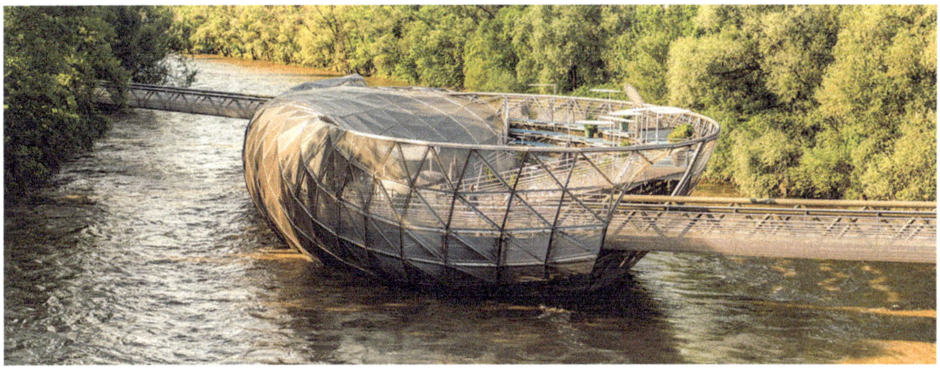

Fig. 151.7 The island in/bridge across the Mur in Graz, Austria. It was intended to be a temporary installation but was so popular that residents chose to make it part of their cityscape. The structure houses a café, playground, and performance space. Photo: Image used under standard license from stock.adobe.com

answer, of course is that it is both. We think this is a good metaphor for these memorable cases—do they define the pinnacle of the careers of these anesthesiologists or are they just an expected part of the ongoing training of an anesthesiologist? The answer, of course, is that this type of case is both.

Multiple Lessons Learned—Jeremy Jaffe, MD

Here's one I've never forgotten:

Very early in my career as an anesthesiologist doing pain medicine, I had an occasion to treat patient Jane Doe ("JD") with occipital neuralgia. I had performed Ms. Doe's initial occipital nerve block without complication, and they got good relief. She returned three months later for a repeat injection. The injection was performed routinely, but within seconds of completing the procedure, the patient complained of severe lightheadedness and then fainted. It became clear to me that some of the local anesthetic must have crossed the occipital bone. I later learned that JD had neglected to report who a past history of a partial craniotomy, a contraindication to occipital blocks.

After summoning help immediately, I made a point of telling the patient, who was entirely unresponsive, that I knew what had happened and that hopefully she could hear me. I advised her that we were starting an IV to administer medicines to stabilize her blood pressure and that she would be intubated and then transferred to the emergency room. I cancelled my remaining cases, and I met the ambulance at the emergency room. Within two hours of arriving in the emergency room JD was extubated.

While in the hospital in the emergency room, it was noted that the patient's blood pressure was very low. A decision was made by the admitting service to keep the patient in house. There was much speculation that the injection had caused some kind of prolonged sympathetic block. I advised the treating physicians that I did not think an extended sympathetic blockade adequately explained the patient's low blood pressure, which persisted for several days.

Ultimately, a cardiology consult was requested and upon further investigation, the cardiologist discovered that my initial history and physical had noted that the patient had a history of Graves' disease for which the patient had not yet followed up for treatment. JD was subsequently diagnosed by further work up with a cardiomyopathy associated with Graves' disease. She was treated and recovered. Upon discharge, the patient thanked me for my attentiveness to her case. Ms. Doe advised me that, in fact, she had heard me speaking to her during her resuscitation and was relieved that I continued to speak with them throughout this critical event up until she was transferred into the ambulance. She also acknowledged that I had previously recommended that she seek out care for their Graves' disease and admitted that although she had intended to follow up, she had not.

This case becomes even more interesting a year later. At that time, the patient requested that I personally administer their anesthetic for an upcoming surgery. I consented to take care of Ms. Doe. Several days before the procedure I received a message on my voicemail at my anesthesia office. The message was from the patient's spouse. The basic gist of this message was an acknowledgement that I was scheduled to take care of Ms. Doe on a certain date. However, while stating happiness that I was going to care of JD, the spouse also stated that they "knew I would do a good job because they owned a gun and knew how to use it."

Although I initially thought this comment was made in jest, I found it quite unsettling. I immediately advised my chairman that I had received this message. My chairman immediately notified the local police and arranged to have the patient's spouse join a conference call with the police, myself, and my chairman. During this conversation my chairman expressed that it is never acceptable to threaten a healthcare provider, even if intended to be a joke. The police concurred, corroborated my report of the incident, and then further admonished the patient's spouse for leaving a threatening message.

My chairman then advised the couple that he would not permit me to take care of the patient because of that message. Furthermore, he advised them that he would not allow <u>any</u> of his anesthesiology staff to take care of the patient. Therefore, the patient had to seek care at another institution. The patient was very upset with the spouse indeed. I had no further communication with either the patient or the spouse.

<u>Lessons:</u> This episode early in my career taught me several important things.

- Regarding the occipital injection: We can only know a patient's history if they provide it or by reviewing available records. Exam clues can also help. But this incident demonstrates that perhaps by more carefully probing and confirming the medical history, this complication may have been avoided.

- My training in anesthesia served me well in calling for immediate help, understanding the problem, and being able to execute the airway and resuscitative efforts that saved this patient's life.

- The less well-taught lesson was my continued communication with the patient, despite the fact that she was unresponsive. This turned out to be very important to her throughout this critical incident. She later expressed to me that although she was very frightened, she was confident that I had matters in hand and that ultimately, she would be OK. No doubt, this communication also played a role in her desire to have me provide anesthesia care in the OR later that year.

- Persistent follow-up of a critical case and maintenance of communication with the hospital teams proved to be essential to this patient's ultimate diagnosis and recovery. While I had not been given the history of a prior craniotomy, I had elicited the history of untreated Graves' disease and to this day, I emphasize to all students how critical an accurate and detailed initial history and physical can be. During my early training as an intern, I personally made it my mission to uncover at least one important aspect of the patient's medical, surgical, social, or family history that had not yet been documented by other providers. It was my way to make sure I was being as thorough as the patient deserved.

- Medicine places physicians at risk. In addition to infectious diseases, burn out, and on the job injuries, direct threats from patient's and/or their families can occur and must be taken seriously—anesthesia and pain management can be stressful enough!

The Rookie—Jeremy Jaffe, MD

Here is a brief story my first year as attending when an obese bring-back uvulopalatopharyngoplasty (UPP) for bleeding came to the OR in the middle of the night. The patient appeared to have a thick neck, Mallampati 3 airway, and large tongue—the makings of a difficult airway. I expressed concern to the ENT who responded that post-UPP there would be no issue. He also assured me he could help if any problems. So I did a rapid sequence intubation and couldn't intubate. Moderate trouble ventilating. The ENT couldn't intubate either. Fortunately, I grabbed an LMA, was able to ventilate better through it and the patient was allowed to awaken in stable condition. He was rescheduled for that morning and had fiber optic intubation.

Lessons:

- Rookies make rookie mistakes.
- Never trust a surgeon when it comes to the airway—we anesthesiologists are the experts.
- Overnight emergencies are sometimes less emergent than advertised.
- Thank goodness for good training!

The Case I Will Never Forget—David R. Dininny, MD

It was the end of my eleventh month of my critical care fellowship. I thought that I knew a lot. She was 19 years old and pregnant. The fetus looked good, ultrasound consistent with a normally developing infant on the small side and almost twenty weeks gestation. She was intubated and from another hospital. Her head CT looked bad, very big intracranial bleed, not survivable. Her mother and the father of the unborn child were devastated. They wanted to know if we could save the baby.

I was clueless. A quick literature search found several case reports of prolonging the life of a brain-dead pregnant woman with successful delivery of a viable fetus, the longest being 108 days. Theoretically, what they asked was possible. What was the right thing to do? After several meetings with the hospital ethics committee, ob-gyn, neurosurgery, and the ICU team, it was concluded that attempting to prolong the life of the body was reasonable.

As a fellow, I had spent the last 11 months trying to keep people alive. I managed their pressors and inotropes, their ventilators, their renal replacement, their nutrition until they recovered and left the ICU, or I was not successful, and they expired. This was a little different. She was already dead, but her unborn fetus was not.

We got lucky. She got a corner room in the ICU. Every day we rounded on her. Nothing changed. Her lungs worked. Her kidneys worked. Her heart worked. Her GI tract worked. Her placenta worked and the baby slowly grew. No one in the media found out so there was nothing in the news.

Each week ob-gyn checked the placenta and the fetus by ultrasound. I became an attending. Now my fellow took care of her, and I supervised. As the fetus gradually grew, the placenta began to show signs of deterioration. How long could we go before we had to deliver the baby? As the baby approached 30-weeks' gestation, ob-gyn felt the placenta was at its end.

It was time. Before she went to the OR, with the family's consent, Lifebanc was contacted. The organs looked good and the process of placing the heart, liver, kidneys, and pancreas was started. After successful placement, she was taken to the OR for an operative delivery. A viable female baby was delivered and whisked away by the neonatologists. The uterine and lower abdominal incisions were closed. The transplant teams prepped and draped. Her organs were procured. The heart, one kidney, and the pancreas left for other hospitals. The liver and one of the kidneys were transplanted in our institution.

I felt weird. As the ICU attending, I was not involved in any of the OR cases, but I watched. It seemed surreal that the baby and the organs were gone, and her brain-dead body was all that was left. In those days, each patient had plastic card like a credit card that we used to stamp all their paperwork with their info. I took her card and put it in my desk drawer. Whenever I opened the drawer, I saw the card and thought of her.

After a year had passed, I was curious about the outcomes. One of the ICU nurses had stayed in contact with the family and was able to tell me that the little girl was developing normally. A conversation and explanation of my position with the people at Lifebanc got me the information that all of the transplanted organs were functioning well and the recipients were all doing well. A tragedy for one person had become a miracle for five others.

Lessons: I am now a much older (and I feel wiser) anesthesiologist. I am also much humbler. I no longer practice critical care medicine, choosing years ago to only work in the OR. I now believe that all we can do is temporize the insults our patients undergo. We do not make them live or die. At best, we give them the opportunity to fix themselves. I did not make the brain-dead mother survive. I helped to give her body what it needed, and it survived on its own. The things a human body can survive continues to amaze me.

I still think of her often. I recently cleaned out my desk and finally discarded her plastic card, but I will never forget her name. The honor of taking care of her body, organs, and unborn child left a mark on me that will never disappear.

Authors and Contributors

Ron Bank originally trained at Hopkins and is a general and cardiac anesthesiologist in the INOVA health care system. He maintains a busy full-time clinical practice and has certainly done his share of fascinating and challenging cases!

Meena Bhatia currently practices critical care medicine and cardiothoracic anesthesia at the University of North Carolina at Chapel Hill. Meena and her husband, Justin, live in Chapel Hill with their three little Tar Heels: Niam, Nora, and Bodhi. She enjoys traveling, crafting with the kids, and hiking around the state. Her favorite family activity is cheering on UNC's basketball, football, and soccer teams.

Norman Cohen retired from clinical practice at Oregon Health and Science University as a Professor Emeritus at the end of 2019—just in time to miss the ravages of COVID. He continues to live in Portland, Oregon with his wife Anna, two cats, Vern and Luigi, and a Labrador puppy arriving in early 2023. Norm has spent his retirement improving his golf game, which desperately needed attention, and, after the lifting of travel restrictions, SCUBA diving and visiting family in the United Kingdom.

Dave Dininny trained at CWRU and spent his professional career at University Hospitals-Cleveland Medical Center. His practice has focused on anesthesia for complex vascular and hepatobiliary surgery. When not at work, he is most likely on his boat or on the beach.

Jeremy Jaffe completed his anesthesiology residency at the Hospital of the University of Pennsylvania. He spent 23 years providing anesthesia and pain management services at Abington—Jefferson Hospital outside Philadelphia. He then transitioned to 100% private practice, exclusively providing comprehensive interventional pain management as a founding partner of SEPA Pain and Spine. His outside interests include drumming, biking, tennis, and traveling.

Kirk Lalwani trained in anesthesia and pediatric anesthesia in Norwich and London in the U.K. and arrived at Seattle Children's as a "Rent-a-Brit" following which he has spent the bulk of his career as a pediatric anesthesiologist at Oregon Health and Science University. When he is not traveling or scuba diving, he enjoys hiking, biking, skiing, police procedurals, and crime shows.

Amy Robbins also trained at Hopkins and is board-certified in general anesthesiology, pain medicine, and palliative medicine. She continues to maintain a part-time clinical practice in the Charlotte, North Carolina metro area. She and her husband Ray Koloski are the proud parents of five young adult children.

Toby Weingarten lives in southeastern Minnesota where he is a busy dad to Chloe, Ben, and Elise; dogs Macaroni and Ziti; and his betta fish Dominic. When he is not writing papers or running kids around including to the airport at 3:30 AM to get back to college, he is outside gardening, tapping maple trees, tending beehives, and enjoying fly fishing on the many fine trout streams of the Driftless area of Minnesota.

***Note from the Editors:** This isn't Toby Weingarten's fish but we're sure his looks just like this (Fig. 151.8). Who amongst hasn't spent a few minutes looking at the fish bowl before heading to bed the night before (or after) a big case.

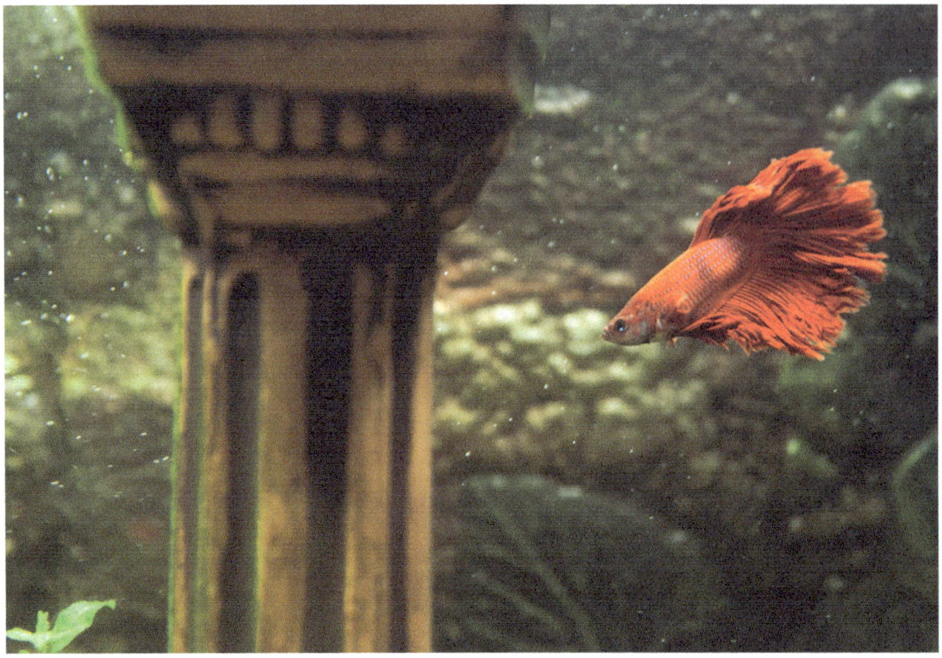

Fig. 151.8 A red betta fish swims underneath the classical Greek bridge in its fish bowl. Photo: Mariana Mikhailova, image used under standard license from iStock.com

Part VIII

More Wisdom on Clinical Anesthesia Practice

Philadelphia and Reading Railroad Bridge—Harrisburg, PA

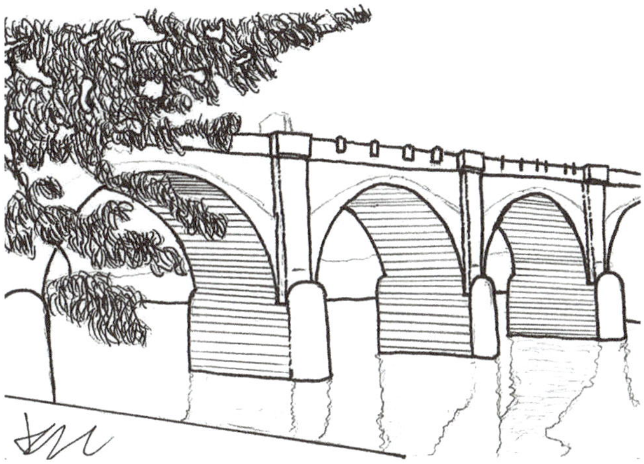

This is just one of the many bridges spanning the Susquehanna River in Harrisburg, PA, that are imprinted in the memories and minds of *Anesthesia Bridges*, contributor Dan Marcucci, authors Steve Orebaugh, Kit Conner, and Jen Wilson. and photographer LouAnn Kopenhaver. In fact, US District Judges Wilson and Conner could see this bridge from certain locations in the old Ronald Reagan Federal Building and Courthouse in downtown Harrisburg.

The bridge carries freight rail traffic of the Norfolk Southern line between Harrisburg and Cumberland County on the West Shore of the river to its further destination in Hagerstown, MD. The bridge has a complicated history as its 51 concrete arches were rebuilt and extended over the stone arch base of an earlier truss bridge. The rebuild was started in 1924 and not completed until the 1940s. The bridge also has a 7% grade from west to east, which reduces the height of the tracks above normal water level from 24 to 17 meters. The bridge has been in the rail system of multiple railroads including the historic Pennsylvania Railroad. It was designed to withstand the transit of up to 75 trains per day.

The editors of *Anesthesia Bridges* thank **John Giacalone** of The Architectural Team in Boston, MA, for his fantastic ink drawing of this treasured Harrisburg landmark.

152 Introduction to Clinical Wisdom Section

Raymond G. Graber

Medical decision-making is a challenging task that requires clinical wisdom. Clinical wisdom comes from having a good knowledge base, from books, journals, and a plethora of online sources. It is also tempered by individual experience and what we have learned from our mentors. It has been said that we learn from our mistakes—these can be painful experiences but valuable sources of wisdom. If we do not reflect on our experiences, then we ae doomed to repeat our mistakes.

One of our favorite quotes is from Lauris Kaldjian, as below [1].

> Physicians and other health professionals need practical wisdom because they strive to identify the best means to ends that are good and worthwhile as they care for patients as persons. They do this by making an astounding array of decisions that are individualized, evidence-based, ethically justified, goal oriented and context-sensitive under conditions that are often complex, uncertain or challenged by multiple perspectives or competing priorities. The connection between practical wisdom and medicine is so direct that it encourages the conclusion that clinical judgement is inseparable or indistinguishable from practical wisdom in medicine.

In the following section, we have invited authors from across the country to give us a peek into their areas of expertise. We hope that their hard-won clinical wisdom will benefit the reader's clinical practice.

Reference

1. Kaldjian LC, Yoon J, Ark TK, et al. Practical wisdom in medicine through the eyes of medical students and physicians. Med Educ. 2023;57(12):1219–29.

Author

Ray Graber serves as vice chair for quality in the anesthesiology department at University Hospitals Cleveland Medical. He has dual interests in cardiac and orthopedic anesthesia. During his 30+ year career, he has focused on process improvement, reduction of errors, and improving patient outcomes.

R. G. Graber (✉)
Department of Anesthesiology and Perioperative Medicine, University Hospitals Cleveland Medical Center, Cleveland, OH, USA
e-mail: raymond.graber@uhhospitals.org

S. Mohamed et al. (eds.), *Anesthesia Bridges*, https://doi.org/10.1007/978-3-032-08294-7_152

Physiology Wisdom

153

Elizabeth A. Ungerman, Daniel I. Asher,
Rajen V. Nathwani, and Catherine Marcucci

Contributors:

Ronald S. Bank, MD (RSB)

Brian Barrick, MD (BB)

John C. Briggs, MD (JCB)

Carol F. Bodenheimer, MD (CFB)

Brian T. Gierl, MD (BTG)

James K. Gilman, MD (JKG)

Raymond G. Graber, MD (RGG)

Michael D. Graham, PhD (MDG)

Michael P. Hutchens, MD (MPH)

Kirk Lalwani, MD (KL)

Logan Olson, PharmD BCCCP (LO)

E. A. Ungerman (✉)
Department of Anesthesiology and Perioperative Medicine, University of Pittsburgh, Pittsburgh, PA, USA
e-mail: ungermanea@upmc.edu

D. I. Asher
Department of Anesthesiology and Perioperative Medicine, University Hospitals Cleveland Medical Center, Cleveland, OH, USA

R. V. Nathwani
Department of Anesthesiology and Pain Medicine, University of Washington School of Medicine, Harborview Medical Center, Seattle, WA, USA

C. Marcucci
Department of Transfusion Medicine, Clinical Center, National Institutes of Health, Bethesda, MD, USA

S. Mohamed et al. (eds.), *Anesthesia Bridges*, https://doi.org/10.1007/978-3-032-08294-7_153

Rajen V. Nathwani, MD (RVN)

Anthony N. Passannante, MD (ANP)

Amy J. Robbins, MD (AJR)

Neil B. Sandson, MD (NBS)

Introduction

Physiology is the foundation of everything we do as anesthesiologists. Understanding it on a deep level is a sine qua non for being an anesthesiologist. It's a subject that is always worthy of review, no matter how well you think you know it. We could have provided hundreds of pages of physiology wisdom but had to limit ourselves to the basics plus a few additional thoughts.

Basics

- Physiology is about biological processes moving with or against the gradient. That's all it is. Energy expenditure lets a process move against the gradient; gravity and entropy move it down the gradient.—**Editors**
- Never hesitate to ask for help from anyone, especially if you don't understand why something is happening. No one wants a patient to do badly.—**EAU and Editors**
- It's difficult to provide a solution if you don't understand the problem.—**LO**
- Think about *why* something has happened—do not jump to conclusions! For example, high lactate *does not* automatically equal give more fluid, low blood pressure does not automatically mean give more pressor, acute kidney insufficiency does not automatically equal give more fluid.—**RVN**
- But just don't think about it, teach it! Don't tell you trainees what to do or not to do, make sure they understand the physiology of why or why not.—**Editors**
- And don't only think about what is going on in that instant. Every single time you interface with a patient, think to yourself, "*What might happen next?*"—**CM**
- Every consideration of the of a clinical problem should include consideration of the associated anatomy and pharmacology. The point is that things don't just happen in the human body. There is always a reason. Even "idiopathic" events are caused by something, we just don't fully understand the etiology yet.—**Editors**

- With this in mind, you will find that clinical management in a MICU is quite different than management in an anesthesiologist-run SICU. In the MICU, the focus tends to be on management of the disease symptoms. In an anesthesia intensive unit, it is almost always on management of the physiology of the disease. There is a subtle but significant difference in these two clinical approaches. And of course, the airway and access management will be much, much different in an anesthesia unit. It's always good to foster professional collegiality but generally not efficient or helpful to try to convert MICU docs to our way of thinking on clinical management.—**Editors**

- Don't every assume that any bad physiologic data are artifacts. Be certain that they're not before believing that they are.—**RSB**

- Sit down every once in a while, and fish out your basic study materials—the ones you used to study for the boards. Review the classics—the Starling curve, gas exchange in the lungs, cerebral autoregulation, the autonomic nervous system, and so forth. This is especially helpful before you give a talk to non-anesthesiologists. It's surprising how many questions after your talk will be about basic physiology.—**Editors**

- You don't really and fully understand the cardio-pulmonary circuit until you have to get your patient through several days of ECMO.—**Editors**

- We think so much about the "mechanical" physiology—the heart as a pump, the vasculature as the plumbing, and so forth. But we should also never lose track of the "metabolic" physiology. For example, every consideration of pathophysiology should include the acid-base state of the body. Always think back to med school and the basics! Such as vomiting = metabolic alkalosis from acid loss. And diarrhea = metabolic acidosis from base loss. Basics are basic.—**EAU and editors**

- My personal opinion is that Stewart acid base physiologic understanding is important but difficult to grasp at a deep level. Superficially, the body cares far more about transmembrane potential than it does pH. As evidenced by what patients will tolerate from electrolyte disturbances compared to pH derangements. It's easier to move stuff intracellularly than it is to diuresis excession.—**JCB**

- Pulse does not necessarily equal flow!—**CM**

- Malpractice attorneys like to ask defendants about the physiology basics. There is much accepted factual information, and expert witnesses will often advise the plaintiff to attack a defendant on a physiology issue.—**Anonymous**

- Remember, all we can really do is observe the physiology and make limited short-term interventions. What we can see and do pales in comparison to the homeostatic mechanisms of the human body (Fig. 153.1).—**Editors**

***Note from the Editors:** We love the photo of our working environment (Fig. 153.1). It symbolizes how far the practice of anesthesiology has come. It also serves as a reminder that what we do pales in comparison to what the human body does on its own.

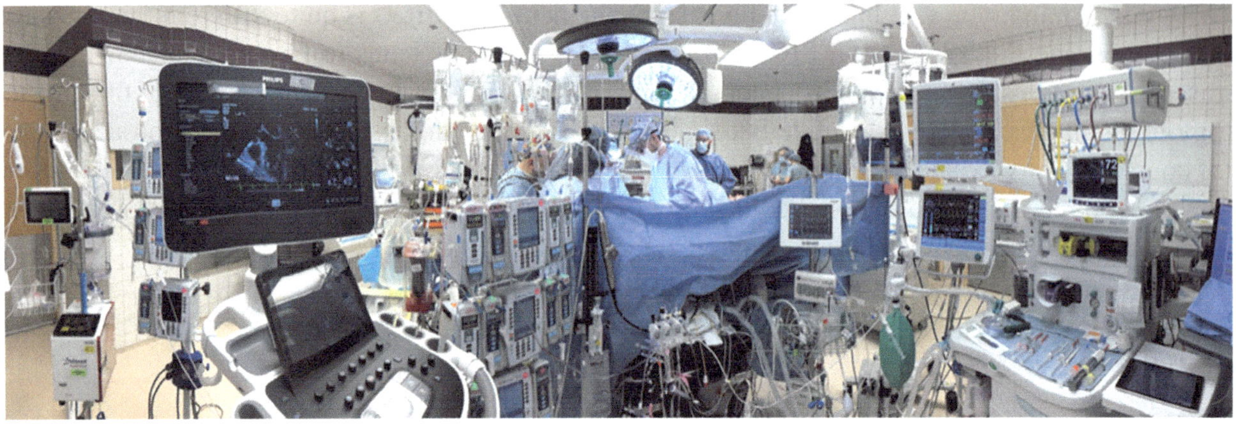

Fig. 153.1 A busy operating room at University Hospitals. This scene could also be titled "what we do to keep the patient stable so that the surgeons can operate on 25 square inches of the body." Photo: Dan Asher

Vital Signs

- You can learn a lot about patients by taking two sets of vitals—one before "the doctors" meet them and one after.—**EAU**

- Rather than just considering systemic mean arterial pressure, consider organ perfusion pressure.—**RVN**

- We agree with Raj Nathwani. You might talk about managing the vital signs, but you must keep in mind that you are really managing the physiology and pathophysiology of each organ system.—**AJR and EAU**

- Sinus bradycardia scares me way more than sinus tachycardia unless the patient is a trained athlete. In that case, the heart rate has gone where it needs to go for homeostasis. And in athletes the HR can be very, very low—easily in the range of 50–60 bpm. So don't mess with it.—**CM**

- But if the patient isn't a trained athlete, sinus bradycardia is scary because it's that much closer to zero! Bradycardic reflexes can occur as a parasympathetic response to intracranial hypertension or emotional distress. They also happen in an instant due to specific triggers such as cold-water immersion (polar bear plunges are nuts if you ask us), pressure points, or oculo-cardiac reflexes. Always keep the possibility of these reflexes in the back of your mind.—**Editors**

- I have had two patients who had an asystolic arrest due to reflex bradycardia in my career. The first was as a resident when the OLHN team was prepping the neck for resection of a laryngeal cancer and put heavy pressure on the carotid sinus which caused progressive bradycardia. The patient then went into sinus arrest over about fifteen seconds. We gave both an anti-cholinergic and a small dose of epinephrine and had to do chest compressions for a minute or so to circulate the medications. We had resumption of NSR and went on and did the case as the cancer had to come out. The patient had complete post-op cardiac studies that were negative.—**CM**

- The second patient had sudden and complete asystole in an eye room when the resident tugged on something in the orbit. In this case, all three anesthesia personnel who happened to be in the room said simultaneously, "*Let go of the eye*!" Fortunately, there was immediate spontaneous resumption of normal sinus rhythm, and the patient was under general anesthesia for some reason. The lesson I learned with that one is to always ask the eye surgeons to let you know when they are going to manipulate the eye and *focus* on the field and the monitor—no talking, no charting during that short interval. If you are going to be in your other room(s) when the surgeons get started, remind your trainee to pay attention to what the surgeons are doing!—**CM**

- Oculo-cardiac reflex bradycardia is something to ask the more senior anesthesiologists about. It's not just something you read about that really never happens. We've all had it happen at least once.—**Editors**

- I've actually never seen a case, but trigemino-cardiac reflex has been described due to both mechanical and thermal stimulation to the trigeminal nerve. The reflex results in both bradycardia, hypotension, and gastric hypermotility.—**CM**

- If we could have only three modalities on a desert island and had to manage a critically ill patient or one that was bleeding profusely, we would pick an echocardiogram (to see what is going on in the central circulation and by inference the pulmonary system), an arterial line—to also evaluate the pulmonary circuit and oxygen delivery in the periphery, and a temperature monitor.—**Editors**

- We are taught that when a patient complains of being in pain, that they will be tachycardic and hypertensive. This may be true in the patient who has acute pain, it may be true for the patient in the OR under an anesthetic and we use respiratory rate and blood pressure to guide our administration of opioids and inhalation agents. Be careful, though, about translating this learning point to the patient in chronic pain. One with chronic pain may be hypertensive, or tachycardia, or with increased respiratory rate as we see in the acute pain patient.—**AJR**

- But unfortunately, many chronic pain patients are misunderstood, misbelieved, and not treated appropriately for their pain because their heart rate and blood pressures are normal and within range. Don't fall into this misconception and remember a chronic pain patient frequently has normal vital signs. If you don't remember this, you will no doubt under treat the patient with long standing pain whose body and physiology have accommodated.—**AJR**

- There are two categories of vital signs in palliative care patients. There is the group of patients who have life threatening illnesses, are seeking aggressive and/or curative care, and many of whom do conquer the disease and live with remission and continued quality of life. These are the patients whose vital signs we watch, we care if they are hypertensive, or hypotensive, or with decreased respiratory rates. All of these signs can indicate adequate or inadequate symptom management and pain control, as well as indicate the management if other co morbid conditions such as diabetes, hypertension, and heart disease are in good control.—**AJR**

- The second category is the palliative patient at the end of life. Vital signs are frequently not monitored at this time. We can look at respiratory rate and blood pressure as an indication of imminent dying, but much of the time we do not measure or monitor the vitals. We focus on the patient, what is their color—is it pink or dusky? Are they responsive or unresponsive? Do they have skin mottling as a sign of organ shut down? Are they breathing deeply, or shallowly, or not at all as opposed to actually counting the respiratory rate? I have seen a patient with normal vitals die quickly and seen others with abnormal vital signs linger for close to a month. I often will recommend to nursing staff and families that the numbers are not what we are monitoring or even treating- it's the patient.—**AJR**

- Any head injury patient or any patient with spinal cord damage should prompt you to think, "Is there any possibility of autonomic dysfunction?" If there is, a prolonged period of hemodynamic monitoring may be warranted. We've seen more than one patient come back to the rehab floor too soon.—**CFB**

- Remember that autonomic dysregulation in spinal cord injury (SCI) patients is not just one thing. It can manifest as autonomic hyperreflexia, orthostatic hypotension, and bradycardia.—**CM**

- But SCI patients can also manifest autonomic dysregulation as postural orthostatic tachycardia syndrome (POTS). Please take extra precautions when changing the OR table position for patients with POTS. If you are not careful, you will inadvertently give them a tilt-table challenge.—**CM and CFB**

- Remember that the vital signs are not just there for us to fight them, they are the roadmap of homeostasis, but not homeostasis itself. And they are there to help us. I'll never forget a physiology professor who used to say the vital signs exist to help us "eschew the blue"—meaning get the oxygen delivered to the tissues.—**CM**

***Note from the Editors:** We appreciate the color blue where we can find it but not on patients (Figs. 153.2 and 153.3).

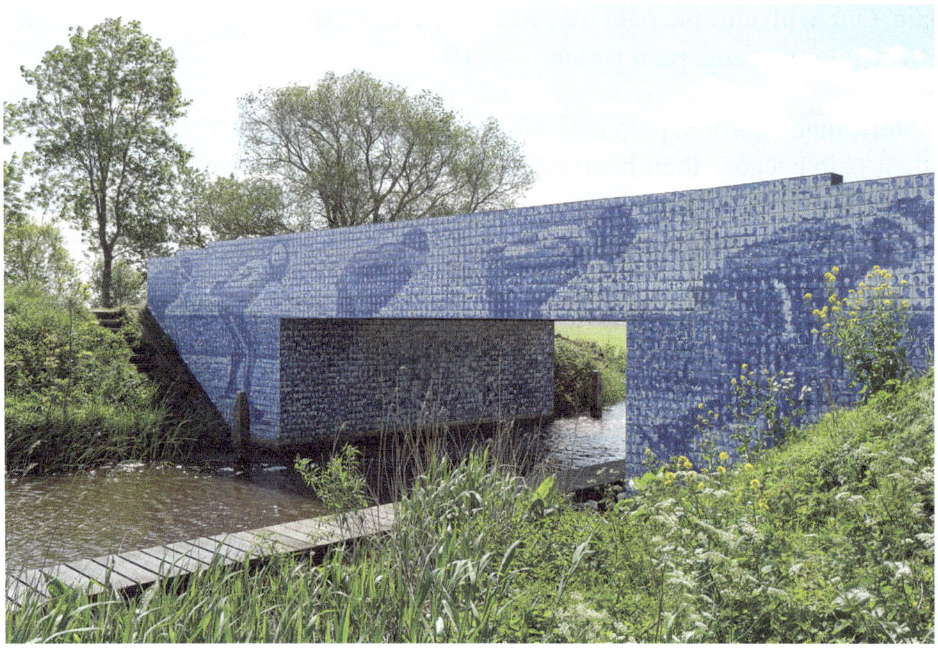

Fig. 153.2 An unusual blue tiled bridge in Holland. Photo: Harry Wedzinga; image used under license from iStock.com

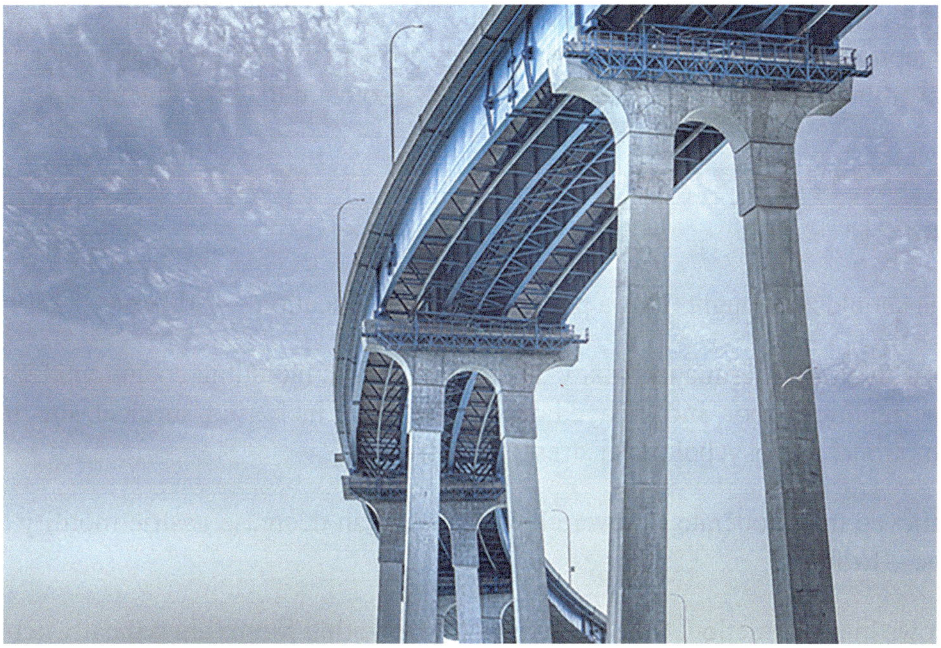

Fig. 153.3 A blue bridge against the blue sky near Sand Diego, CA. Photo: Martina Birnbaum; image used under license from iStock.com

Hypertension in Pediatric Patients

- *Never* ignore hypertension in kids—it's real until proven otherwise. You must seek and find the pathophysiology and etiology of any elevated blood pressure reading.—**KL**
- The top three culprits are obesity, obesity, and obesity!—**KL**
- Secondary causes include renal diseases, coarctation, and Williams syndrome.—**KL**
- Neurosurgical pediatric patients can present with hypertension due to intracranial hypertension or space-occupying pathologies like neuroblastoma.—**KL**
- Endocrine causes include hyperthyroid, pheochromocytoma, Cushing's, and primary aldosteronism (Conn's syndrome).—**KL**
- Hyperthyroidism is also a great imitator and could be deadly if general anesthesia is administered.—**KL**
- In 20 years, I have helped our nephrologists "diagnose" two pheochromocytomas when I refused to do anesthesia for an angiogram because they had hypertension of unknown origin and had not had their urinalysis and plasma labs for vanillylmandelic acid/pheo to be ruled out. Phew!—**KL**
- In the PACU, hypertension is pain until ruled out! And full bladder (same as for adults, discussed more below).—**KL**

- Last but not least, injection of local with epinephrine by the surgeons can produce it, as well. You would think the surgeons would let you know every time they do it but they don't. Every senior anesthesiologist has looked over the drapes and said, "Did you just inject something with epinephrine in it?"—**KL**

Hypothermia

- Hypothermia should be thought of as a perioperative complication.—**Editors**

- We now know that hypothermia has many deleterious effects including coagulopathies, cardiac conduction abnormalities, poor and delayed wound healing, increased surgical site infections, and increased emotional and psychological stress.—**Editors**

- It is now believed that moderate to severe hypothermia can decrease gastric motility to the point of clinical ileus.—**Editors**

- Heat only flows in one direction, from warm to cold. Operating rooms are typically kept on the cooler side so preventing hypothermia in the operating room setting is challenging.—**ANP**

- The hypothalamus does most of the thermoregulation in humans with some temperature at the spinal cord level.—**Editors**

- Remember that hypothermia can also occur during sedation cases as well. The degree may be somewhat less but is offset by the distress of shivering.—**Editors**

- Regional anesthesia is also characterized by heat loss.—**Editors**

- Know the physical mechanisms of heat transfer—radiation, conduction, evaporation, and convection. All of these mechanisms are relevant to how patients may lose heat during an operation, and there are simple ways to minimize heat loss from each mechanism.—**ANP**

- About 60% of heat loss from surgical patients is by radiation. The heat gradient is from the core tissues through the blood to the superficial tissues. Radiation loss is in the form of infrared waves. This is the basis of the familiar technology used to sense and identify persons in buildings or other locations.—**Editors**

- Evaporation heat losses occur because energy in the form of heat is consumed in the process of vaporization of water. Evaporation losses occur from all body surfaces, not just during sweating. About 22–25% of heat loss in the OR occurs by evaporation, particularly if there is a large wound.—**Editors**

- Conduction is the process by which there is loss of kinetic energy from molecular motion in skin tissues to the surrounding air.—**Editors**

- Convection occurs when heated air is moved away from the body in currents. This is why the cooling effect of wind is felt. In the OR, the laminar flow that is designed as part of the environment to minimize bacterial contamination is also the source of the convective flow that carries heat away from the body.—**Editors**

- Conduction and convection cause about 15% of heat loss.—**Editors**
- When I was a trainee, I knew the four methods of heat loss and I knew and used all the active and passive methods of ameliorating hypothermia. Honestly, though, I don't think I could have told an oral board examiner exactly what technique prevented what type of heat loss without a moment's hesitation. Here's a summary for you.—**CM**
  - Convection heat loss: Air warming blankets, forced air warming systems
  - Conduction heat loss: Fluid warmers, hot packs, heated air mattress, circulating water garments
  - Evaporative heat loss: Humidified gases, drapes placed over open wounds
  - Radiant heat loss: Ambient air temperature
- Forced-air warmers are effective, and they work most efficiently when they are used intelligently. The forced air blankets are designed to be placed *directly* on the patient's skin. Cloth blankets insulate in both directions, so if you place a cloth blanket between the forced-air warming blanket and the patient you have substantially limited the amount of heat you can transfer top the patient- not what you should do.—**ANP**
- The greatest decline in body temperature occurs in the first half hour or so after induction of general anesthesia, due to vasodilation and depression of the hypothalamus.—**Editors**
- One of the most important and simplest things to do is keep the thermoset temperature of the operating at least 25 °C for the first hour of the case.—**Editors**
- Hypothermia occurs not only by passive loss of heat but by active cooling due to infusion of fluids and blood components. Remember that blood leaves the blood bank refrigerator at a temperature that may not legally exceed 6 °C.—**Editors**
- Any fluid run at a rate greater than 500 ml/h should be warmed. This includes crystalloid, colloids, or blood.—**Editors**
- Prevention of hypothermia starts as early as 1–2 hours before initiation of anesthesia.—**Editors**
- An effective way to prevent a substantial redistribution of heat from the core to the periphery after induction of general anesthesia is to pre-warm the extremities. This will limit the heat that flows from the core to the typically cooler extremities and minimize the drop in core temperature.—**ANP**
- Remember that skin surface warming doesn't increase core temperature. You are not trying to increase temperature, just prevent redistribution.—**Editors**
- Also, patients don't like it when their necks get cold. Think about it, there was a reason the scarf was invented, right? It makes sense, all of those large vessels so near the surface.—**Editors**
- Surgical environments can help prevent heat loss (general realization that burn ORs must be kept warmer) or be considered to encourage heat loss (endovascular radiology suites with cooling for the fluoroscopy tubes coupled with surgical restrictions on warming devices).—**ANP**

- Don't give control of the operating room thermostat to the nurses in contradiction to the directives of the anesthesia team members who have the responsibility for the patient's vital signs and intraoperative warming.—**Editors**

- Use every standard of warming for OB patients, especially those undergoing operative delivery. We have found it that it isn't always done and there is no reason for this.—**CM**

Hyperthermia

- Hyperthermia is encountered much less frequently than hypothermia. Your differential diagnosis should include the following:—**ANP**
  - Heat stroke, which would be a presenting condition that should not cause diagnostic confusion.
  - Malignant hyperthermia is usually not a subtle diagnosis. Metabolic production of CO_2 is significantly increased, so there will be a need to ventilate aggressively that will probably not maintain normocarbia. Your next step should include sending an arterial blood gas while simultaneously initiating treatment.
  - Infection/sepsis would be the other likely cause of hyperthermia intraoperatively and, in most cases, would not need specific treatment.
  - Thyroid storm will be accompanied by sympathetic overactivity.
  - A much more innocent cause of hyperthermia is iatrogenic in etiology. Examples include excessive warming with radiant or forced air warmers or excellent insulation of a patient having orthopedic surgery distal to a tourniquet, so the only part of the patient's body exposed to ambient temperature is not perfused.

- Serotonin syndrome is also associated with increased temperature. Don't miss this. Always be aware of the serotonergic medications are on before you start the case. These include SSRIs, triptans (migraine meds), tramadol, and buspirone.—**Editors**

- Don't let multiple sclerosis patients get hyperthermic! They will be very displeased with you. And the neurologists, too.—**EAU**

Sleep

- Managing the perioperative period is about managing the physiology of sleep deprivation. This is nowhere truer than in the ICU but it's also true for regular OR patients. How many of them would you estimate get a full and restful night's sleep before their OR cases? Approximately zero.—**Editors**

- What are the basic physiologic issues of short-term sleep restriction?
  - Reduced glucose tolerance
  - Increased blood pressure
  - Sympathetic nervous system activation
  - Increased inflammatory markers
  - Reduced leptin levels
- There's a reason that sleep medicine is an anesthesia subspecialty.—**Editors**
- I had an attending that said that our true goal is to get the patient safely home to a good night's sleep in their own bed.—**CM**
- Natural sleep and general anesthesia aren't the same thing, of course, but could you tell a patient the similarities and differences in six sentences?—**Editors**
- Both sleep and surgical anesthesia rely on GABA-mediated inhibition of arousal-promoting brain nuclei. There is some similarity in the anesthetized state and non-REM sleep on EEG.—**Editors**
- However, anesthesia is characterized by a characteristic burst suppression pattern and sleep involves cycling between REM and non-REM states.—**Editors**
- The exact nature of anesthesia is dose-dependent and agent-specific.—**Editors**
- Sleep is endogenously and actively generated in the brain. It is not characterized by the anxiolysis or lack of nociceptive response that the anesthetic state is.—**Editors**
- Sleep is self-limiting and subject to a refractory period.—**Editors**
- The anesthetic agent that has a mode of action most similar to sleep structure and architecture is dexmedetomidine, especially with its effects on the locus coeruleus and mimicry of NREM Stage 3 sleep.—**Editors**

***Note from the Editors:** Who needs sleep more than students; so, we knew we wanted another student bridge (there are several others in this book). We went searching for a sturdy bridge on a nearby school campus and found this pedestrian bridge on the campus of Towson University (Fig. 153.4). It's not fancy, but it gets the students where they need to be. Recently, we drove underneath this very bridge at 7:50 in the morning and saw a group of kids dashing across it to 8 AM exam finals in sweatshirts and pajama bottoms.

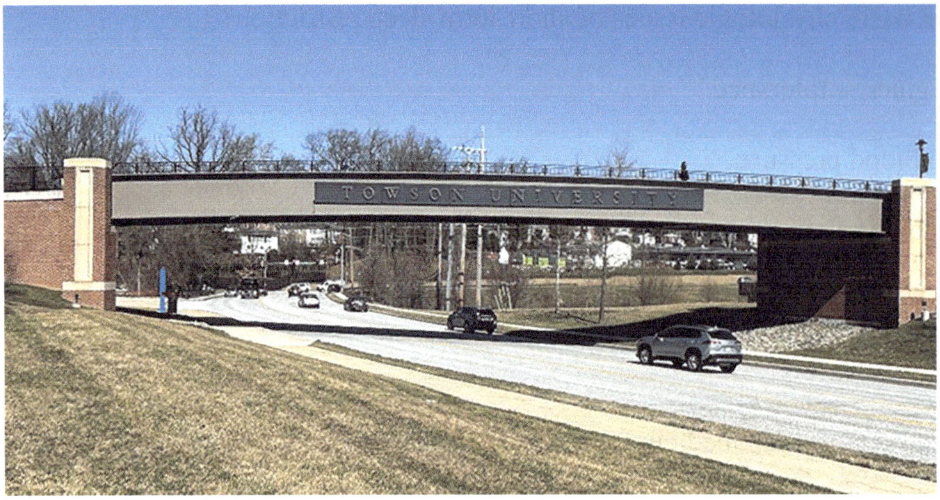

Fig. 153.4 The walkway from the dormitories near the Sheppard Pratt hospital property to the main campus of Towson University in Towson, MD. Photo: Eli Wright

Pulmonary

- Imposing the physiology of mechanical ventilation on patient is among the weirdest things we do. We completely turn the normal process of spontaneous ventilation 180 degrees when we convert ventilation to a positive pressure maneuver. The changes imposed by mechanical ventilation are second only to the changes in the brain due to induction of general anesthesia—**Editors**
- Pulmonary physiology is fascinating because neither ventilation nor perfusion to the lungs is uniform or static in either spontaneous or mechanically ventilated patients. In the upright patient there are the effects of gravity. In the prone and supine positions, there are different effects of gravity.—**Editors**
- Remember that, in general, in order for there to be alveolar ventilation, the alveolar pressure must exceed the pleural pressure.—**Editors**
- Prone positioning is beneficial in ARDS, and the changes are easily characterized radiographically, but may not hugely impact mortality.—**Editors**
- Know the five causes of hypoxemia—low FiO_2, shunt, dead space, hypoventilation, diffusion impairment. Think in these terms and you won't get lost, but they aren't always single issues.—**JCB**
- Don't focus just on the respiratory rate or the pulse oximeter reading when evaluating what is going on with the pulmonary physiology and circuit at any given time. Think about it—does the heart rate tell you the complete physiological state of the heart? Of course not.—**Editors**
- We forget that the lungs are very active metabolic organs. Remember that it is now understood they use more glucose than the kidneys, heart, and brain.—**Editors**
- Remember that significant atelectasis will occur in up to 90% of patients under general anesthesia.—**Editors**

- Atelectasis is not a benign process! It plays a significant role in abnormalities of gas exchange. It also has role in perturbations in static lung compliance that contribute to acute lung injury.—**Editors**

- Atelectasis does not have just one simple etiology. It is thought to occur via compression of the lung, absorption of air, and impairment of surfactant function. These deleterious effects are caused by the complicated mechanics of general anesthesia, especially with positive pressure ventilation—cephalad displacement of the diaphragm, shift of thoracic blood into the abdomen, trapping of gas in alveolar pockets, changes in the normal alveolar FiO_2, and anesthetic agent induced changes in the alveolar-capillary barrier.—**Editors**

- We have worked in academic departments where the anesthesiologists gave didactics on the above mechanisms to the pulmonologists, who were known to take copious notes. They might know more about the lungs under normal spontaneous ventilation than we do, but not about the ventilated lung. If the pulmonology and anesthesiology departments at your institution don't lecture to each other, it might be time to change that.—**Editors**

- Inhaled nitric oxide (iNO) improves V/Q mismatch. It also vasodilates by increasing cellular cGMP. The dose is 20–40 ppm. Rapid discontinuation of iNO = rebound pulmonary HTN. Tachyphylaxis and thrombocytopenia can develop!—**EAU**

- A garbage pulse ox wave form is exactly that—garbage.—**EAU**

- I once was told to never underestimate the power of PEEP. Remember that 5 cm H_2O is "normal."—**EAU**

- If a patient is requiring higher PEEP levels to oxygenate, then those PEEP levels should also be used during transport. Either add a PEEP valve to your AMBU bag, or transport with a portable ventilator.—**RGG**

- Remember that an anesthesia ventilator is designed to *deliver anesthesia*. Don't ever hesitate to get an ICU ventilator if yours isn't cutting it.—**EAU**

- Inhaled epoprostenol—iEpo (stimulates adenyl cyclase) is way cheaper than iNO.—**EAU**

- Don't forget to be careful if you have pulmonary venous hypertension—pulmonary artery vasodilators can make your right ventricle worse!—**EAU**

- You will always have to know the management of gradual hypoxemia on one lung ventilation. Here's the sequence.—**EAU**

  - FiO_2 100%
  - Confirm airway device position
  - Recruitment
  - Positive end-expiratory pressure (PEEP) application on the dependent lung

  - Continues positive airway pressure (CPAP) for the nondependent lung
  - Eliminate volatile anesthesia (hypoxic vasoconstriction inhibitors)
  - Resume two lung ventilation temporarily
  - Pulmonary artery clamp

- Understand pulmonary hypertension and how to manage it. Be knowledgeable enough to discuss the clinical situation and therapies in detail with the pulmonologists but also learn how to present it in an elevator pitch to the surgeons.—**RSB and editors**

- Intubated patients often have altered pulmonary mechanics that impact tidal volume as well as respiratory rate (RR). A restrictive pulmonary pathology (including positioning) causes shallow breathing that occur faster than the usual 12–16 breaths per minute. If this high RR is diagnosed as pain, titrating opioids to achieve a 'normal' RR will lead to hypercapnia and hypersomnolence.—**BTG**

- Alternatively, PSV with a high support pressure will trigger large breaths and a low RR regardless of patient comfort. In any case, the patient's brainstem senses $PaCO_2$ to determine respiration rate. Therefore, as long as the capnogram levels off at end-expiration, $EtCO_2$, combined with the knowledge of their baseline bicarbonate level can be a more accurate estimate of patient comfort and allow safe titration of opiates.—**BTG**

- It is a best practice to send an ABG for any patient with an arterial line and to subsequently calculate the $P_{A\text{-}a}O_2$ gradient. A gradient greater than ~180 mmHg implies that the patient will require an FiO_2>0.4 to maintain a PaO_2>60mmHg, which equals an SpO_2>90%. Online $P_{A\text{-}a}O_2$ gradient calculators will ask for elevation or atmospheric pressure. At an elevation of 1000 m above sea level, your $P_{A\text{-}a}O_2$ gradient is reduced by about 30–35 mmHg. Towns in the United States with an elevation above 1000 m are in the Rocky Mountains from New Mexico to Wyoming or are ski resorts and proudly display the elevation on their welcome sign.—**BTG**

- Remember that CO_2 has its own MAC! You can definitely have a patient who has hypercarbia to the point of sedation. We have seen hypo-ventilating patients wake up with a bit of bag-mask ventilatory assist.—**Editors**

- If you highly suspect a tension pneumothorax in your patient, any palpable rib space will do. Some patients have adipose tissue above the second intercostal space. Just make sure to stay above the rib.—**BB**

- It is quite likely that as a community we have overstated the risks of anesthetic induction and conversion to mechanical ventilation with most anterior mediastinal masses. The most recent studies support a standard approach to airway management in most circumstances, rather than awake intubation with maintenance of spontaneous ventilation throughout. I am *not* suggesting an incautious approach, just that many patients with anterior mediastinal masses will do very well with IV induction/intubation/mechanical ventilation.—**ANP**

- Low cervical spinal cord injury is one area where the patient will breathe better in the supine position rather than sitting upright unless you bind the abdomen.—**RVN**

- *Never* try to extubate a patient with an open abdomen or an open chest.—**EAU**

- Remember that ARDS is not a one-organ disease. The oxygenation and ventilation difficulties that are so familiar to us are just the pulmonary window into a really complicated and systemic pathology.—**CM**

- What's really interesting about the lungs in ARDS is that heterogeneity of the pathology—there are areas of relatively normal lung parenchymal adjacent to areas of dense consolidation and atelectasis. And techniques such as low tidal volumes and high levels of PEEP don't completely solve the problems.—**CM**

- Prone positioning is beneficial in ARDS (and the changes are easily characterized radiographically) but should be instituted early to impact mortality.—**CM**

- Pulmonary labs offer a lot of research opportunities to academically minded anesthesiologists but keep in mind that a lot of the basic science is worked out with animal models. If you will have trouble doing dog experiments, just know that about yourself, and keep searching for your niche.—**CM**

***Note from the Editors:** You might have thought there would be no way to find a "thoracic outlet bridge" on the Internet, and you would be wrong! We laughed when we saw this bridge and thought it would be perfect for this section (Fig. 153.5).

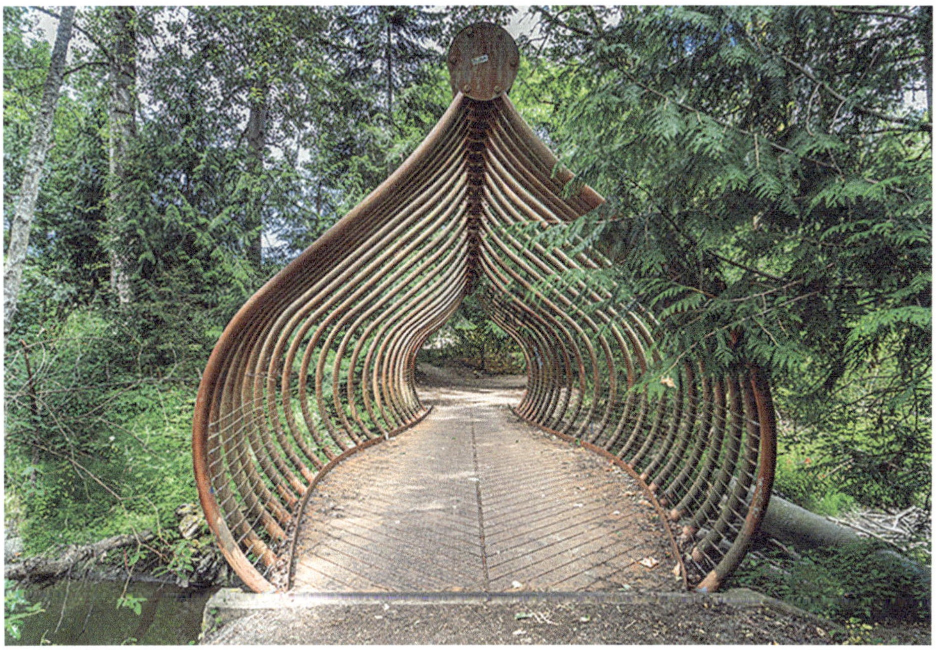

Fig. 153.5 The Salmon Bone Bridge is a pedestrian bridge over Longfellow Creek near Seattle. It was designed by an artist rather than an architect or engineer. Photo: gmc3101; image used under license from iStock.com

Cardiac

- Autonomic innervation affecting cardiac physiology: β1 (contractility, consumption), β2 (vasodilation), α1 (vasoconstriction).—**EAU**

- Right ventricular failure is underdiagnosed, undermanaged, and leads to significant increases in morbidity and mortality.—**DIA**

- Acute RV failure has an in-hospital mortality of 5–17%, increases hospital length of stay by 50%, and is associated with a 6-fold increase in perioperative major adverse cardiac events. Always think of the right heart.—**DIA**

- Pulmonary artery pulsatility index accounts for contractile power of the RV, ability for the RV to manage blood return, and is more predictive of mortality than other measurements available.—**DIA**

- The cycle of acute perioperative RV failure begins with an acute event that decreases RV perfusion. Focus on increasing the perfusion pressure of the RV in order to temporize until you can fix the underlying issue.—**DIA**

- Right ventricular failure is a complex, multifaceted issue that requires significantly more study and respect than we give it.—**DIA**

- The heart functions as a combined unit, neither ventricle can thrive without the other.—**DIA**

- Preoperative evaluation and postoperative care of patients with RVF requires astute physical exam skills and proactive management.—**DIA**

- A cardiac anesthesiologist once told me, "You really have to respect the right heart. Would you want to deal with the pulmonary circuit? I am sure the left heart feels it got off relatively easy.—**CM**

- The three 3-word phrases that scare me the most are "severe pulmonary hypertension", "severe mitral stenosis", and "acute aortic insufficiency" and if they don't scare you, they should! The first two deal with respecting the right ventricle and the potential to inadequately fill the left ventricle no matter what inotropy/physical support (including CPR) is used. In acute aortic insufficiency, patients have an acute large volume overload that the left ventricle cannot compensate for.—**BB**

- Aortic dissection patients should be hypertensive on arrival. Hypotension is an ominous sign in these cases. One of four things is happening: 1. tamponade, 2. dissection of a coronary artery, 3. tearing of an aortic leaflet causing acute aortic insufficiency, 4. there is a dissection flap protruding through the aortic valve causing severe aortic insufficiency. You need to think about and be afraid of all of these things.—**BB**

- Regardless of what the textbooks tell you about heart rate and SVR for certain valve lesions, keep the patient "where they live." They are already compensated unless they are presenting for emergent cardiac surgery. <u>Case in point:</u> a patient with very severe mitral stenosis may need a rapid heart rate because no amount of filling time will achieve an adequate end diastolic volume/stroke volume.—**BB**

- Lusitropy. Unless it is super acute, a low ejection fraction is much better tolerated than severe diastolic dysfunction. No one talks about it because you can't fix it, but is much scarier, for both reasons.—**JCB**

- For a patient with a significant arrhythmia, the best *AND* safest drug is electricity. The burns on the skin will heal.—**JKG**

- The physiology of every chamber of the heart in atrial fibrillation is disrupted. For one thing, the right atrium is stiff and relatively ischemic, compared to baseline. Don't think it necessarily needs a blood transfusion. The most important therapeutic intervention is to restore sinus rhythm, of course.—**Editors**

- Many patients develop some post-induction hypotension. Many are treated immediately with fluids and vasopressors. Other interventions I have found helpful are to improve venous return with some gentle Trendelenburg positioning, and if the hypotension is severe to decrease intrathoracic pressure by ceasing mechanical ventilation and opening the popoff valve, which will increase venous return even more.—**ANP**

- Normal SvO_2 is 60-80%. SvO_2 can be affected by a simple little *CHAT*:—**EAU**

  - Cardiac output
  - Hemoglobin
  - Arterial oxygenation
  - Tissue O_2 consumption

- There's no way to make this fun….just remember it!—**EAU**

  - Normal central venous pressure (CVP) waveform – **a -> c -> x -> v -> y**

    - **a** = RA contraction
    - **c** = RV contraction
    - **x** = RV relaxation
    - **v** = passive RA filling during *systole*
    - **y** = passive RA emptying via tricuspid valve

- Tamponade will cause an equalization of all four chambers during diastole. Remember to maintain sympathetic tone, avoid bradycardia, and minimize positive pressure ventilation. And remember to always have a high clinical suspicion for it.—**EAU**

- Arrhythmia assessment: EKG (12 lead), Holter monitor (continuous 24 hours), echocardiography (structural assessment), loop recorder (long term assessment less than years). Unstable arrhythmias should be treated with defibrillation.—**EAU**

- Myocardium extracts ~80% of O_2 in a resting state. Think about your liver during a dinner with your in-laws extracting all the alcohol you need to survive, same concept.—**EAU**

- Acute coronary syndrome (ACS) pearls—remember that a normal EKG does not rule out ACS!—**EAU**

  - ST depressions ≥0.5 mm is indicative of myocardial ischemia.

  - ST elevations in two contiguous leads measuring ≥ 1.5 mm in women and ≥2.0 mm in men is an STEMI.

  - Troponins are highly sensitive with a high negative predictive value.

  - Diagnosis can be assisted with echocardiogram, cardiac CT, and nuclear studies.

  - Indications for catheterization: STEMI, unstable angina, and stable ischemic heart disease.

- Remember that a stenosed coronary artery is already maximally dilated. There will likely be a constant pressure drop across that stenosis since the parameters of the flow system are fixed.—**Editors**

- Why is there less oxygen delivery at higher hematocrits in coronary artery disease? Here a possible answer: higher hematocrit means higher viscosity. At higher viscosity, flow rate decreases as viscosity increases at constant pressure drop.—**MDG and CM**

- Defibrillation only in patients who arrest on central VA ECMO. Chest compressions will make a bad day for you, the patient, and everyone within a 6-foot radius.—**EAU**

- If your Woods Units is >2, you might not make it out of the woods without a little help for your RV. Like Aretha said, R-E-S-P-E-C-T!—**EAU**

- Any chronic lesion in the heart is usually survivable in the OR. Any acute lesion? Buckle up.—**EAU**

Renal/Water/Bladder

- A patient with limited access to water due to immobility, or limited water intake due to dysphagia with or without an alternative feeding method (NG Tube, G-Tube or TPN) will often present with a reduced level of total body water. The same applies to patients who have 'messy' urinary issues (ostomy, briefs, significant BPH) or requires assistance to ambulate to the toilet as they will avoid having to make urine. Such patients often have events that increase their urinary, GI, or insensible losses and they never fully rehydrate themselves.—**BTG**

- Postoperative kidney injury causes real suffering that anesthesiologists often don't directly see.—**MPH**

- Acute kidney injury has the potential to progress silently to chronic kidney disease (CKD); this process can occur after apparent resolution of the elevated creatinine, over months, not years.—**MPH**
- Because postoperative kidney injury can cause CKD—CKD can be a long-term outcome of anesthetic management.—**MPH**
- Intraoperative urine output (UOP) *does not* predict development of acute kidney injury (AKI).—**MPH**
- Maintenance of adequate mean arterial pressure in the OR is likely the most important aspect of anesthetic management for kidney care.—**MPH**
- Kidney tubule pump/receptors are important. We don't often think of them in terms of "receptors", but thiazides and loops diuretics manipulate physiology very interestingly.—**JCB**
- MELD scores will trick you as it relates to renal dysfunction. Make sure to remember both ends of this curve, especially in patients with abnormal kidneys a priori.—**JCB**
- When on cardiopulmonary bypass, your kidneys show the largest proportional decrease in blood flow. Keep those beans perfused as much as you can!—**EAU**
- Make sure you always keep your patient warm—hypothermia can cause an increase in renal vascular resistance! It also makes it harder for your kidneys to handle glucose.—**EAU**
- Adrenal cortex = aldosterone, cortisol, androgens. The patient will be much more difficult to manage if this is not preserved. And remember that "cortex" is derived from the Latin word for bark. Plants (organic matter) don't do well without healthy bark.—**EAU**
- Aldosterone allows renal sodium reabsorption. It is released in response to Na/K balance and depends on the renin-angiotensin system.—**EAU**
- Don't forget that an acute AKI increases perioperative morbidity and mortality. Do whatever you can to protect the beans and remember that your drugs may work very differently.—**EAU**
- Never ignore an empty foley!—**EAU**
- Never be lulled into complacency by a full Foley!—**Editors**
- Remember that an empty Foley bag may indicate a catheter that is not properly placed. It may also indicate some I's and O's that were not properly charted or signed out.—**RGG**
- Renal dysfunction can cause coagulopathy—don't forget to check a TEG to evaluate platelet function. DDAVP—3μcg/kg can help!—**EAU**
- Bad kidneys = low erythropoietin = anemia.—**EAU**
- Dialysis patients always have the potential to be a difficult IV access. Give yourself a little bit of time (and maybe grab an ultrasound) to obtain IV access for them.—**EAU**

- Acidemia and hyperkalemia are real in renal failure patients, but most of them are well compensated. Remember their "normal" is different than your "normal". Always know their baseline EKG.—**EAU**

- Can you get through surgery with a patient who needs dialysis? Sure. But should you?—**EAU**

- Patients on peritoneal dialysis can have altered respiratory mechanics and increased intra-abdominal pressure.—**EAU**

- Offsite anesthesia for cystoscopy can be some of the simplest, yet dangerous anesthetics that you will provide. Any disruption in the plumbing circuity of the body is a disruption in the basic physiology. And remember that the bladder is not but a giant reflex mechanism.—**EAU and CM**

- Intractable hypertension in the PACU? Check the bladder and empty with whatever means necessary.—**Editors**

- The above happened to me once but with an additional twist. The patient had a Foley with a typical urine output but still complained of abdominal pain and was persistently hypertensive. We finally did an ultrasound and found that the bladder was significantly distended. Fortunately, I was on good terms with the urology service and one of the residents came up and took the Foley out and replaced it with an immediate output of almost a liter of urine. Hypertension resolved over the course of a couple of minutes, as well.—**CM**

Head Versus Heart and Kidneys Versus Everything

- This is why we come to work, to consider these questions, and make the right decisions. We can't give universal specific advice, except to say you have to understand where you are with the patient's physiology and where you are going. Each clinical situation depends on how you look at it.—**Editors**

- These issues are not just questions of perfusion as measured by a blood pressure cuff. Think about the patient's microcirculation always, always, always.—**CM and MDG**

- We will say that, you know, cardiac ischemia is more survivable than brain ischemia. There are cardiac assist devices but no brain-assist devices. And there is no such thing as a brain transplant.—**Editors**

- A mentor of mine used to say that every anesthetic is a neuro-anesthetic even though the surgery may not be a neurosurgery. In other words, with every anesthetic we are putting the brain and nervous system under, not the heart, unless it's a circulatory arrest case.—**CM**

- Remember that the head also includes the eye. Perioperative visual loss is a devastating complication. For every case, you have to think, are the eyes okay?—**Editors**

- Why should the kidneys get prime consideration when you are making risk/benefit decisions? Because even a little perioperative dysfunction has big implications for morbidity and mortality.—**MPH and Editors**

- Make sure you have a *clear* indication for the cases that deliberately put the baseline mean arterial pressure at risk. There may be indications but don't agree to give up one mmHg of perfusion pressure that you don't have to.—**Editors**

***Note from the Editors:** We searched high and low for a bridge that was purposely constructed without symmetry. An old school friend finally found this charming example in Hanover, PA, for us (Fig. 153.6a, b). Sometimes what you see is entirely relative to which direction you're facing.

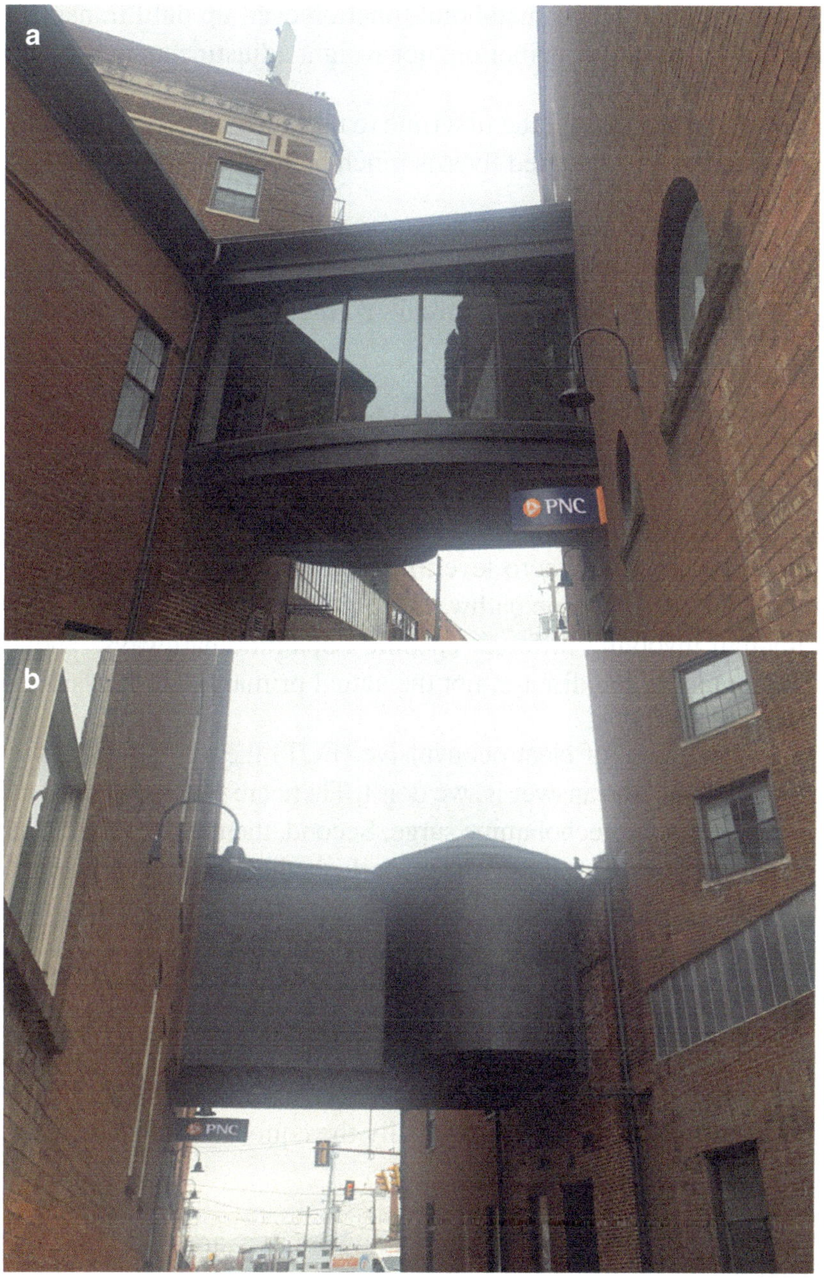

Fig. 153.6 (**a**) A walkway between two historic brick buildings in downtown Hanover, PA. The windows look toward the main street of the business district. (Photo: LouAnn Kopenhaver). (**b**) The same walkway bridge viewed from the alleyway. There are no windows on this side of the bridge and a funny little cupola. We're not sure why. Photo: LouAnn Kopenhaver

Other Disease States

- We'd prefer to take care of a stab wound to the abdomen with a perforated bowel any day over mesenteric ischemia, especially if the ischemia has been at all prolonged. Ischemic bowel is a dreadful disease. The mediators released cause awful morbidity. Just awful.—**Editors**

- Advanced liver disease = every system is diseased.—**EAU**

- A liver will retain some amount of its metabolic function even up until transplant. Do not count out enzymatic degradation, volume of distribution, nor weight adjustments in these patients.—**JCB**

- If you don't believe the above, you will the first time to take an anhepatic patient to the OR for retransplant. We agree with Dr. Briggs—a failed liver is much better than no liver.—**Editors**

- And the most difficult management problem in anhepatic patients isn't the coagulopathy, it's managing the unstable and labile hemodynamics. Go figure. But, thinking about it, for starters, there are no hepatic sinusoids attached to the portal vein circuit, so there is increased blood flow into the inferior vena cava.—**CM**

- If you do not think about true hepatopulmonary syndrome, you will never remember it. That is a scary shunt.—**JCB**

- It is overly simplistic to think of schizophrenia as a disease of psychosis or thought disorder, although it is often be defined as that at the macro level. It is now understood to involve complicated pathophysiology at the level of the dopamine pathways. In this way, it's analogous to the Parkinson's family of diseases, although involving different specific dopamine pathways. The altered mentation in schizophrenia is a symptom of the disease, not the actual primary pathophysiology.—**NBS**

- Ever think about the physiology of electroconvulsive (ECT) therapy? We see the seizure, but do we know what is really going on? The answer is, we don't. There are two recognized perturbations in baseline physiology. First, there is a catecholamine surge. Second, there is a transient increased permeability of the blood-brain barrier. However, it is not understood whether these perturbations in baseline physiology actually represent therapeutically effective aspects of the treatment.—**NBS and CM**

- Isn't it weird that ECT has been a recognized modality for 80 years or so (although not so benign in the early years) and psychiatrists still don't know exactly what happens or why it works? We think that most anesthesiologists don't think about the physiological derangements of ECT beyond doing the short mask airway. You are looking for the seizure but not thinking about the huge catecholamine surge. But a day working in the ECT suite is actually the equivalent of a day of injecting epinephrine into patients.—**NBS and CM**

- Always be mindful of varices and AVMs, no matter where they are.—**EAU**

- You can always assume that big vascular calcifications mean little vascular calcifications.—**EAU**

- The two anesthesia subspecialties that are totally—*TOTALLY*—based on physiology are OB and peds cardiac. Kids are just little bags of physiology without much reserve. With OB patients, you have the physiology of the parturient and then the physiology of the fetus and of course they are not exactly the same. It's very hard to offset or counteract the pregnancy-related physiological changes that have occurred in the mother, mostly you are just dealing with what's there. Studying both these areas of subspeciality practice for the boards is just a matter of knowing a few names and terms and having the physiology down cold.—**Editors**

- Pregnant patients can decompensate quicker than you think! Always think one, then two, steps ahead.—**EAU**

- If a parturient hemodynamically collapses, it's an amniotic fluid embolism. Don't think twice about it—call for ECMO and start to resuscitate. The sooner they get on ECMO, the sooner their brain gets oxygen again.—**EAU**

- You will never regret placing extra access in a parturient. It gives you a few extra seconds to get the physiology under management.—**EAU and editors**

- Don't miss malignant neuroleptic syndrome (NMS) and don't confuse it with the other malignant syndromes such as malignant hyperthermia and serotonin syndrome. For one thing, distinguishing between these acute and life-threatening clinical conditions is often on the boards.—**NBS and CM**

- NMS occurs with the administration of D2 blocking medications, such as the antipsychotics. It is characterized by fever, confusion, labile vital signs, and muscle rigidity. It does not take huge doses or greatly elevated blood levels. For example, it can occur with repeated, but not excessive doses of haloperidol in the ICU.—**NBS and CM**

- Even more than malignant hyperthermia, the initial occurrence of NMS does not imply breach of the standard of care. Failing to recognize it does. The treatment is cessation of the offending medication and supportive care. Bromocriptine and dantrolene have also been suggested as therapeutic modalities.—**NBS and CM**

- Don't let other specialists' lack of knowledge affect your management. *You are the gatekeeper.*—**EAU**

More Physiology Wisdom from *Avoiding Common Anesthesia Errors, 2nd Edition*

There is a wealth of additional tips, teaching tidbits, and overall physiology wisdom in our previous book, which is nicknamed "Green2." *Please* check out this information and remember that every single penny of royalties goes to FAER in perpetuity!

Green2 Chapters with More Physiology Wisdom

- To PEEP or Not to PEEP—That Is the Question
- Non-invasive Blood Pressure Management—It's Not Just a Piece of Nylon Around the Arm
- Avoid Errors in Blood Pressure Management
- How, Why, and When to Use Brain Function Monitors
- Malignant Hyperthermia: If You Get to the Point Where You See an Elevated Temperature, It's Already Happening
- Good Old-Fashioned Basic Perioperative Blood Pressure Control
- Protect the Kidneys, Not the "UOP"
- Avoid a 70% Mortality Rate: Do Everything You Can to Prevent Perioperative Renal Failure
- Do Not Use Urine Output as an Indicator of Volume Status in Hypothermic Patients
- Seek Out Hypercapnia in the PACU and Remember That an Acceptable Pulse Oximeter Reading is *Not* Assurance of Adequate Ventilation
- The Neurophysiology You Learned in Medical School Is Always Relevant—Get a Grip on It and Don't Let Go
- Don't Forget There's No Such Thing as a Brain Transplant—Preventing Perioperative Stroke
- What to Do and What Not to Do for Your Patients with Hypertrophic Obstructive Cardiomyopathy
- The Right Heart Should Never Play Second Fiddle to the Left Heart—What to Do When the Right Heart Just Really Ain't Right at All

Authors

Elizabeth Ungerman is an anesthesiologist and assistant program director in the UPMC system. She urges any anesthesiologist studying for any exam at any level to start with an in-depth review of the pertinent physiology, as there is no sense in just giving a question away.

Dan Asher is a cardiac anesthesiologist at Case Western/University Hospitals. He cares about other organ systems besides the heart, he really does, especially if they are misbehaving and making the pump run difficult.

Raj Nathwani is a trauma anesthesiologist at Harborview Medical Center in the University of Washington system. He has been known to grab a few minutes of physiology review time while the coffee machine and tea kettle are firing up in the morning.

Cathy Marcucci is a senior anesthesiologist who loves physiology and is never surprised to run into other engineers among her anesthesia colleagues.

154 Pharmacology Wisdom: Principles and Receptors

Sarah N. Fribance, Konstantinos Alfaras-Melainas, Rajen V. Nathwani, Catherine Marcucci, and Logan M. Olson

Contributors:

Edwin G. Avery IV, MD (EGA)

Ronald S. Bank, MD (RSB)

John C. Briggs, MD (JCB)

Harley S. Geller, MD (HSG)

Brian T. Gierl, MD (BTG)

Richard A. Jaffe, MD PhD (RAJ)

Amy J. Robbins, MD MBA (AJR)

Neil B. Sandson, MD (NBS)

Brant M. Wagener, MD PhD (BMW)

S. N. Fribance (✉)
Department of Anesthesiology and Perioperative Medicine, University of Pittsburgh School of Medicine, Pittsburgh, PA, USA
e-mail: fibrances@upmc.edu

K. Alfaras-Melainas (✉)
Department of Anesthesiology and Perioperative Medicine, University of Pittsburgh, Pittsburgh, PA, USA
e-mail: alfarasmelainisk@upmc.edu

R. V. Nathwani
Department of Anesthesiology and Pain Medicine, University of Washington School of Medicine, Harborview Medical Center, Seattle, WA, USA

C. Marcucci
Department of Transfusion Medicine Clinical Center, National Institutes of Health, Bethesda, MD, USA

L. M. Olson
Department of Pharmacy, Nebraska Medicine, Omaha, NE, USA

S. Mohamed et al. (eds.), *Anesthesia Bridges*, https://doi.org/10.1007/978-3-032-08294-7_154

Introduction

At Temple Med, back in the 1980s, the senior faculty and dean's office really did not want to write letters for med students going into anesthesiology if they had not received at least a high pass in pharmacology. One advisor said at the time, "We're not interested in having our students go into that specialty because it's the hot thing right now and then flop. We see pharmacology as a *sine qua non* for a successful anesthesiology career. We are hoping to send people out to the anesthesiology community that have a true interest in and affinity for pharmacology. Can't make the anesthesiology omelet without the pharmacology eggs!"

Basic Principles

- Although they are constantly used interchangeably, the terms "drug" and "medication" are actually not the same. Both drugs and medicines, when administered to the body, will have physiological effects. ***Medications*** generally used to treat disease or relieve pain are a subset of the drug pharmacopoeia. A ***drug*** is actually defined by the US Food and Drug Administration in the Food, Drug, and Cosmetic Act as:
  - A substance recognized in an official pharmacopeia or formulary
  - A substance intended for use in the diagnosis, cure, mitigation, treatment, or prevention of disease
  - A substance other than food intended to affect the structure or function of the body
  - A substance intended for use as a component of a medicine but not a device or a component, part, or accessory of a device
- Drugs are used as medications but also for spiritual, religious, and recreational purposes.—**Editors**
- Here are two of our favorite pharmacology quotes.—**KAM and Editors**
  - Pharmacology is benefitted by the prepared mind. You need to know what you are looking for.
  - Soon we will treat disease with a cell, not a pill.—**Siddhartha Mukherjee**
- We say this in every book we do—an anesthesiologist gets up in the morning to give powerful and even dangerous drugs in a precise manner. Or perhaps the father of toxicology said it best way back in the sixteenth century:
  - All things are poison, and nothing is without poison; the dosage alone makes it so a thing is not a poison.—**Paracelsus**
- This is often condensed to: "*The dose makes the poison*" or in Latin, *"Sola dosis facit venenum."*—**Editors**
- But it's also true that the application of the specific medication makes the poison. Remember that among the worst complications in the perioperative period are when an otherwise "benign" drug is

administered in the wrong place – such as into the arterial line or subarachnoid space. The effects can be catastrophic and the morbidity permanent. Everybody has heard of a horror story or two.—**Editors**

- We now understand that the pharmacokinetics and pharmacodynamics of a drug can vary from person to person based on genetic variations in drug metabolizing enzymes, transporters, and receptors.—**KAM**

- If you want to get into an interesting area of research, start delving into pharmacogenetics.—**Editors**

- From Mark Udall: Any doctor will admit that any drug can have side effects, and that writing a prescription involves weighing the potential benefits against the risks.—**KAM**

- Do not give a medication if you do not know what it does or how it works.—**KAM**

- You always have the option to administer more, but once a substance has been given, it cannot be taken back.—**KAM**

- The four modes of pharmacokinetic drug handling are: absorption, metabolism, distribution, and excretion.—**NBS and LMO**

- Another way to think of pharmacokinetics is to divide the administration of a drug into a time course. Intake is the time course involved in the movement of a drug from the site of introduction or absorption to the site of measurement, usually the blood. Disposition involves the time course of drug distribution and elimination from the site of measurement.—**Editors**

- Most everybody in anesthesia struggles a bit with the concept of volume of distribution of a drug. It's helpful to remember two things – it's a theoretical value and is predicated on the concept of the body as a simplified tank of fluid into which a drug is placed. This is because it's very difficult to actually measure the total volume of body fluids.—**Editors**

- Drugs with a high apparent volume of distribution are indicative of drugs that leave the plasma readily and redistribute to the tissues. The measured plasma concentration is therefore lower, as if a unit dose was dissolved in a larger theoretical homogeneous tank of fluid.—**Editors**

- *Quick memory aid:* lower measured plasma concentration for a unit dose of a drug means higher apparent volume of distribution and higher tissue absorption.—**LMO**

- Phase 1 drug metabolism generally involves oxidation. For most drugs, Phase 1 oxidation represents the main deactivation step for metabolism of pharmacotherapies. Metabolites are generally less active or inactive than parent compounds, except for prodrugs.—**NBS**

- Phase 2 metabolism is generally conjugative.—**NBS**

- Understanding the lipophilicity or hydrophilicity of a drug can help guide you to the most appropriate weight to use for dosing.—**LMO**

- Look up *every* medication the patient is on before you take them to the OR – at least what class of pharmacological agent the medication is in and its basic action. We are managers of the perioperative pharmacopoeia, and you don't want to have a nurse or surgeon ask you what the drug is and have to say, "Actually, I don't know."—**Editors**

- Ideal body weight was developed for insurance purposes, not for drug dosing.—**KAM**

- Make sure to have the OR Pharmacy phone number close at hand.—**LMO**

- The mechanism of action provides a great deal of insight into how a drug should be used. For some reason, people always seem to know agonists better than antagonists.—**LMO**

- We still do not have a complete understanding of the mechanism of action for many essential anesthesia drugs. For example, the exact mechanism of action for inhaled anesthetics remains mostly unknown.—**KAM**

- Even the mechanisms of action for well-known medications that we believe we have uncovered may be more complex than initially thought. A prominent example is the opioid receptors, which can form homo-and heterodimeric complexes, resulting in the creation of new receptors with distinct properties and pathways.—**KAM**

- Know the main adverse reactions and side effects of your medications! If we asked you the difference, could you tell us without having to think for even five seconds?—**KAM**

- *Side effects* are expected and known effects of a medication that is not the intended therapeutic outcome. They often occur because it is very difficult to design medications that have extremely specific effects at the receptor level.—**LMO**

- *Adverse outcomes* are unintended and deleterious effects that are not universally expected. They are often immune-mediated or gene-mediated such as allergic reactions or malignant hyperthermia. They can also be situational, such as deleterious adverse drug effects when a drug-drug interaction occurs.—**LMO**

- Remember, a patient cannot be in the pharmacologic state of withdrawal and overdose at the same time.—**NBS**

- Keep in mind the concept of context-sensitive half-life when employing continuous drips for extended periods.—**KAM**

- The context-sensitive half-life indicates how long it takes for the concentration of a drug in the bloodstream to decrease by 50% after stopping an infusion.—**KAM**

- While a drug given in a single dose might have a brief half-life, administering the same drug through an infusion could result in a prolonged half-life.—**KAM**

- For example, while propofol experiences a slight yet noticeable extension in half-life during prolonged infusions, midazolam and fentanyl swiftly elevate their half-lives even with brief periods of infusion.—**KAM**

- When instructing patients to *add* a medication to their regimen, I've found that they will often *switch* to the medication. Unless you are very explicit, patients get confused about adding a drug *vs.* substituting a drug. It is important to spell the plan out in clear and unambiguous terms.—**NBS**

- When the editors trained, the cost and supply chain of a drug weren't big issues. But they certainly are today and perhaps rightfully so! At any rate, mastering these concerns is part of mastering the drugs and it will remain that way. Find out the cost of the drugs you use and *teach* this information to your students and team members.—**Editors**

***Note from the Editors:** We canvassed our friends for photos of bridges with strong architecture since the following section is all about receptor structure. The small but dramatic suspension bridge is in the Boyce Thompson Arboretum near Superior, Arizona (Fig. 154.1).

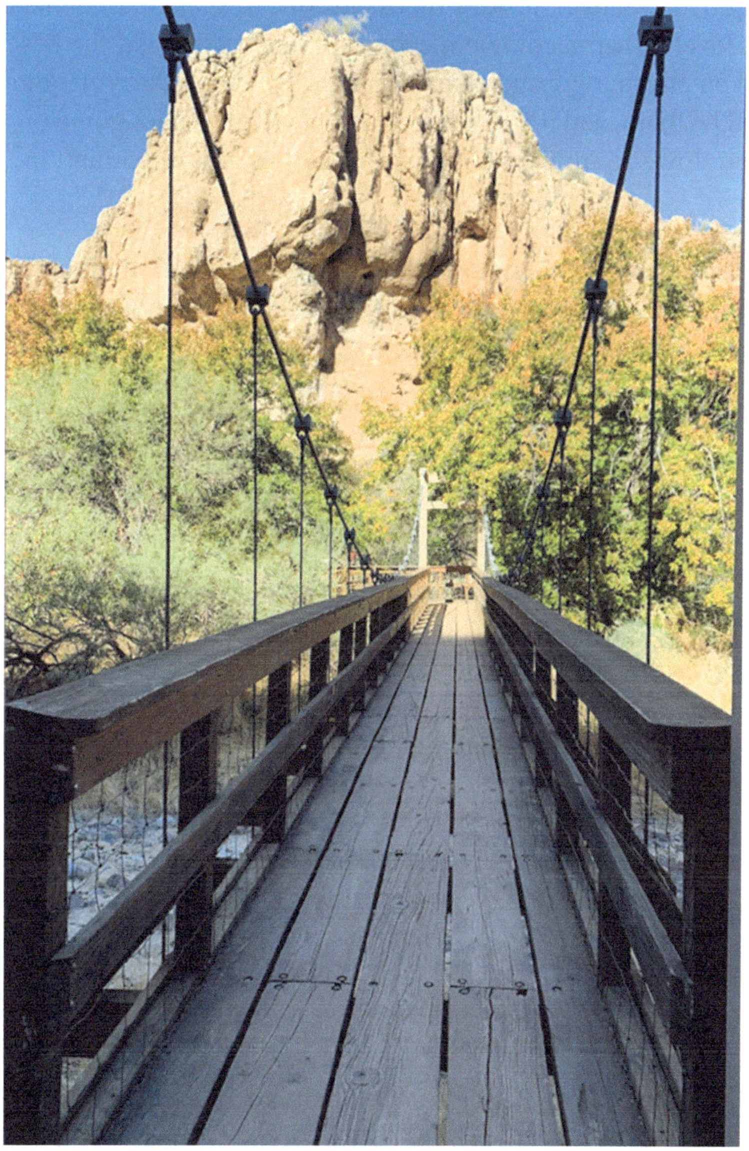

Fig. 154.1 Great natural and man-made architecture in Sedona, AZ, a great wonderful place to enjoy nature. Photo: Hailey James

Receptors

- Understanding a drug—really understanding what it is and how to use it most effectively—is impossible without understanding the pharmacokinetics and pharmacodynamics at the receptor level.—**Editors**

- Drugs and medications have therapeutic efficacy through the intended manipulation of the ligand/receptor interaction. Some medications alter the amount of naturally occurring ligand, others act to block the receptor. Side effects occur because of unintended or unavoidable ligand/receptor interactions. It's okay to remind your students and trainees of this every once in a while. It's easy to get caught up in the minutiae of a medication and lose track of the most basic principles.—**Editors**

- On the other hand, it takes some reading and a few cases to appreciate the beauty of a lovely pharmacologic or physiologic mechanism. It takes thousands of cases and faith in the best medical literature to appreciate that a lovely pharmacologic mechanism might not yield the best result for the patient. Don't be so focused on physiologic and pharmacologic principles that you ignore good evidence. The mechanism may still be there, and it's still important, but there is a lot going on in a human being, and the mechanism you love to think about might not be as important in the moment as you think.—**LMO**

- Anesthesiologists working in the operating room can get away with thinking about receptor physiology superficially, at least in the short term. *However*, a thorough understanding of receptors is really what separates our community and practice from that of other licensed independent providers.—**Editors**

- Don't assume that your team members understand receptor physiology and the choice of medications based on considerations thereof unless you yourself have discussed it with them. A lot of non-physician clinicians prescribe medications empirically and/or algorithmically based on symptoms.—**Editors**

- *Pharmacology is about the chemistry*, especially when considering receptors.—**SNF and editors**

- Mastering a receptor starts with understanding the ligand! Ligands are simply molecules that bind a specific (or a few) receptors. They can be proteins, hydrophobic molecules such as steroids, or gases such as nitric oxide.—**Editors**

- Once you've got the ligand down, then work on the overall effect of the receptor system, then the individual receptors. Don't forget to review where the receptor is found in the body!—**Editors**

- Don't just remember the name of the receptor but also the type and how it works.—**Editors**

- So, what are the basics that you should know? Just for fun, we put together a brief primer for teaching and review.—**SNF and CM**

- A receptor describes a macromolecule that chemically binds a ligand.—**SNF and CM**

- Ligand affinity is dictated by the strength of the chemical bond between the ligand and receptor, and these bonds can be covalent, ionic, hydrogen, or hydrophobic.
- Ligands are ***agonists*** (binding produces a biological response) or ***antagonists*** (binding does not produce any biological response).

- There are four major types of receptors.—**SNF**
  - Transmembrane ion-channel receptors
  - Transmembrane G protein-coupled receptors (GPCRs)
  - Transmembrane receptors with a cytosolic domain
  - Intracellular (cytoplasm or nucleus) receptors
- Transmembrane ion-channel receptors are very important for anesthesiology practice (Fig. 154.2).—**SNF**

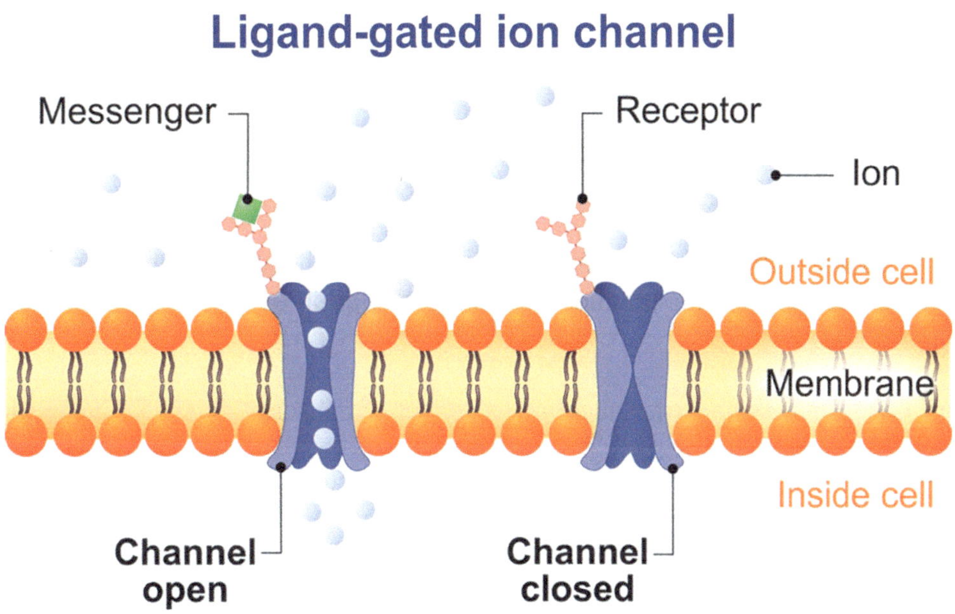

Fig. 154.2 Transmembrane ion channel depicting two different ligand states. Illustration: Image used under standard license from iStock.com

  - Ligand binding causes conformational changes of the receptor and ion channel
  - Leads to rapid cellular response to receptor activation
  - Examples are nicotinic acetylcholine (nACh) receptors and GABA receptors

- Transmembrane G-protein coupled receptors (GPCRs) are the most abundant type of drug receptor.—**SNF and editors**
  - The 2012 Nobel prize in Chemistry was awarded to Lefkowitz and Kobilka for their work on GPCRs.
  - These receptors transduce signals via activation of intracellular G-protein.
  - A single ligand can bind multiple types of GPCRs, meaning a single ligand can activate a variety of transduction pathways.
  - A receptor is defined by the ligand that binds it as well as the second messenger system it activates.
  - Examples are biogenic amines (acetylcholine, noradrenalin, serotonin), amino acid neurotransmitters (glutamate, glycine), and peptide hormones (angiotensin II, somatostatin).
- Many odorant or scent receptors are GPCRs, and there are hundreds of different types in the body, each for its own particular scent. This makes sense given the highly evolved nature of the sense of smell in most mammals.—**SNF**
  - Transmembrane receptors with cytosolic domain have several variants.
  - The intracellular domain is either enzymatically active (catalytic receptors) or bound to specific enzymes in the cytosol (enzyme coupled receptors).
  - They are associated with protein kinase activity, and phosphorylation of intracellular proteins by these receptors can lead to ion channel opening, modulation of gene expression, or activation of signal transducers.
- Examples are Janus kinase/signal transducer and activator of transcription (JAK/STAT) pathway.—**SNF**
  - Intracellular receptors are either in the cytoplasm or nucleus.
  - Ligands are mostly lipid-soluble and can pass through the cell membrane.
  - Ligand binding leads to receptor translocation to the nucleus in order to bind to specific DNA sequences to modulate gene expression.
  - Leads to slow but long-acting signal transduction
- Remember that acetylcholine binds to both muscarinic and nicotinic receptors, of course. Muscarine is an agonist that is not normally found in the body; it is a quaternary ammonium salt found naturally in mushrooms. It is one of the compounds that can make certain mushrooms deadly to ingest due to poisoning from cholinergic overdrive.—**Editors**
- Muscarinic ACh receptors are G-protein coupled receptors.—**Editors**

- Nicotinic ACh receptors are ligand-gated ion channel receptors.—**Editors**

- When you are first starting out as an anesthesiologist, it seems a bit incredible that the exact mechanism of general anesthesia is still not completely known. But this actually makes sense. We are still a fairly new specialty. And the physiologic state of general anesthesia is one of the most complicated and profound of all medical interventions. It involves four components—*amnesia, unconsciousness, analgesia, and immobility*—each component is most likely mediated by one or more receptors and neuronal pathways in different parts of the brain. And the light and heavy planes of each component are also probably mediated by different pathways and receptors.—**Editors**

- GABA is important because people screw with it, such as with benzodiazepines, and it causes a lot of delirium in the ICU. Also, it is the source of alcohol withdrawal and anxiety, and many of our anesthetics modulate it.—**BMW**

- So, we know that GABA receptors, particularly the $GABA_A$ subunit, likely play a major role in general anesthesia, but how? Most anesthetic agents potentiate GABA-mediated conductance, with the exception of nitrous oxide, xenon, and ketamine, which act at the NMDA receptor.—**CM**

- The NMDA receptors mediate excitatory neurotransmission in the nervous system. Tramadol and methadone act at both the NMDA and opioid receptors.—**Editors**

- Clinicians also often are a little fuzzy about medications that have a mixed agonist-antagonist profile at various receptors. They can tell you that but often aren't that clear about the receptors, mechanisms, and proportions of agonism and antagonism. One of the most important of these drugs for our community is buprenorphine. More about this important opioid in the next chapter.—**Editors**

- Don't forget that the dopamine receptor is part of the sympathetic nervous system. We tend to focus on the alpha and beta receptors and their agonists and antagonists but forget about the "third" receptor.**—Editors**

- Dopamine is a monoamine catecholamine neurotransmitter and hormone.**—Editors**

- There are at least five types of dopamine receptors and numerous subtypes. The action of dopamine is mostly in the central nervous system, and it has many, many functions, depending on the subreceptor. The D2 receptor is particularly important to psychiatrists, where antagonism has anti-psychotic effects.—**NBS**

- In terms of under-appreciated receptors, I would say serotonin receptor physiology.—**JCB**

- Serotonin is the naturally occurring monoamine ligand for the family of 5-hydroxytryptamine (5-HT) receptors. But can you name where it is produced in the body off the top of your head? The majority is made in the intestine and a small amount in the raphe nuclei (think back to med school) in the brain stem.—**Editors**

- 5-HT receptors are both GPCRs and ligand-gated receptors.—**Editors**

- Serotonin is correctly thought of as neuropsychiatric transmitter and serotonin receptors and important target for psychiatric and neurology drugs, but all 15 subtypes of 5-HT receptors are found outside the CNS. The biology is still being worked out, but serotonin plays a role in important perioperative issues including cardiovascular function, bowel motility, and possibly even platelet aggregation. Serotonin released from the gut binds to the 5-HT3 receptor to promote nausea and vomiting.—**NBS and CM**

- Serotonin syndrome should be familiar to all anesthesiologists, and especially chronic pain physicians. It most often occurs with the co-administration of two or more serotonergic medications, often but not always psych medications.—**NBS and CM**

- Signs and symptoms of serotonin syndrome include elevated blood pressure and heart rate, muscle rigidity, shivering, agitation, restlessness, mydriasis, loss of muscle coordination, twitching, headache, and confusion. It can range from mild and self-limited to fatal. The most reliable course of treatment is to discontinue the offending medications and then supportive therapy.—**NBS and CM**

- One of our senior colleagues once had a case of serotonin syndrome when methylene blue was injected into the scalp of a patient on fluoxetine [1]. Fluoxetine is a selective serotonin reuptake inhibitor (SSRI) and methylene blue is a competitive monoamine oxidase inhibitor (MAOi). It is recommended that SSRIs be discontinued prior to surgeries where methylene blue or other MAOi meds will be used.—**CM and editors**

- If you don't love pharmacology, which necessarily means loving receptor physiology and you don't love studying the receptors in the heart – all of them – then get out of anesthesiology as soon as you can.—**JCB, CM, LMO, and editors**

***Note from the Editors:** One of our favorite bridges captures the point above perfectly (Fig. 154.3).

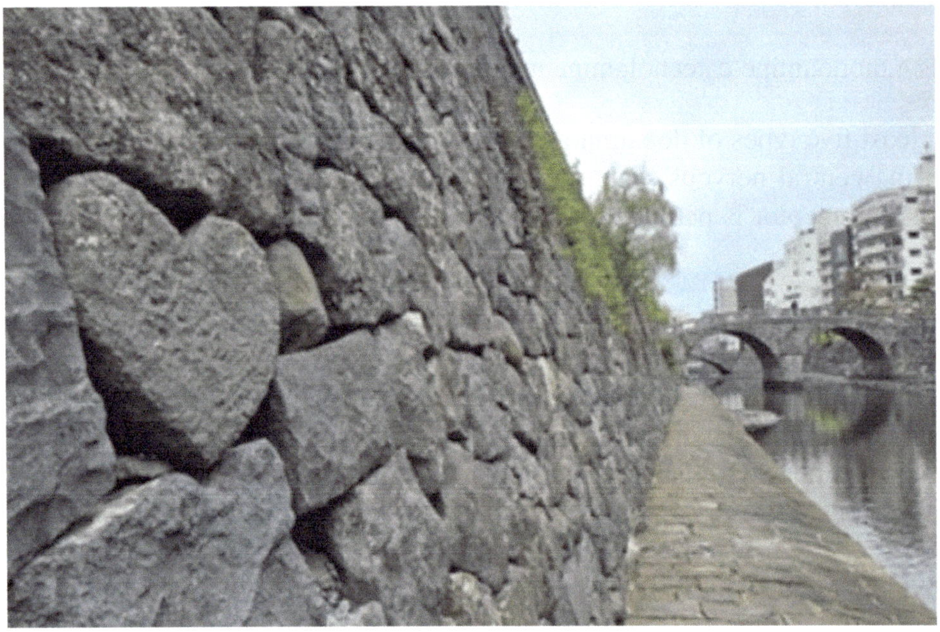

Fig. 154.3 This is an old stone wall and bridge in Europe. Photo: Image used under standard license from shutterstock.com

- I would also include the vasopressin receptors (V1 and V2), especially in cardiac patients, as particularly important but not that familiar to us.—**JCB**

- We did an informal poll and found that quite a few senior anesthesiologists did not have a good working knowledge of the vasopressin receptor basics. The ICU docs did the best, the working OR folks not so well. So, we pulled a few points together below, just for fun and reference, because raising blood pressure is what we do for a living.—**SNF and CM**

- Vasopressin (also known as antidiuretic hormone) is synthesized in the hypothalamus and is released with increased plasma osmolality, decreased arterial pressure, and reduction in cardiac volume.—**SNF and CM**

- The vasopressin system is one of three vasopressor systems in the body. The other two are the sympathetic nervous system (which we tend to have pretty good knowledge of) and the renin-angiotensin system.—**SNF and CM**

- We call the human hormone arginine vasopressin (AVP) because it contains arginine unlike other analogs such as desmopressin and terlipressin.—**SNF and CM**

- AVP has action at three subtypes of receptors, which are all G-protein coupled receptors.—**Editors**

- The V1 receptor stimulates vascular smooth muscle contraction.—**SNF and CM**

- V1 receptors are also found in myocardium leading to myocardial hypertrophy, hepatocytes causing glycogenolysis, platelets resulting in platelet aggregation, and in the myometrium causing uterine contraction. None of this is important to the practice of anesthesiology said no one ever!—**SNF and CM**

- So how does the V1 receptor work? Activation of the receptor stimulates phospholipase C. This mediates hydrolysis of inositol 4,5-bisphosphoate to inositol 1,4,5-triphosphate and diacylglycerol.—**SNF and editors**

- V1 second messengers activate enzymes, such as protein kinase C, and mobilize intracellular calcium stored in the endoplasmic reticulum. Emptying of calcium stores activates cationic channels that allow extracellular calcium to enter the cells.—**SNF and CM**

- The V1b receptor, also called V3 acts in the central nervous system (receptors mainly located in anterior pituitary) to modulate corticotropin secretion.—**SNF and editors**

- The V2 sub-receptor acts in the renal collecting tubule of the kidney. It increases free water absorption as a response to osmolarity and volume.—**SNF and JCB**

- Activation of V2 receptors leads to generation of cyclic adenosine monophosphate as a second messenger, which stimulates protein kinase and causes insertion of aquaporin-2 into the luminal wall of collecting ducts in the kidney.—**SNF and editors**

- Are you going to know these exact facts about the vasopressin receptors every single second of your working day? Probably not. But you should know that a decent amount about the V1 receptor and how it works and that the V2 receptor acts in the kidney. Lock that in at the very least.—**JCB and CM**

***Note from the Editors:** As stated above, mastering receptor physiology means studying detail. Just make up your mind to buckle down and do it. One of our favorite bridges captures the point above perfectly (Fig. 154.4).

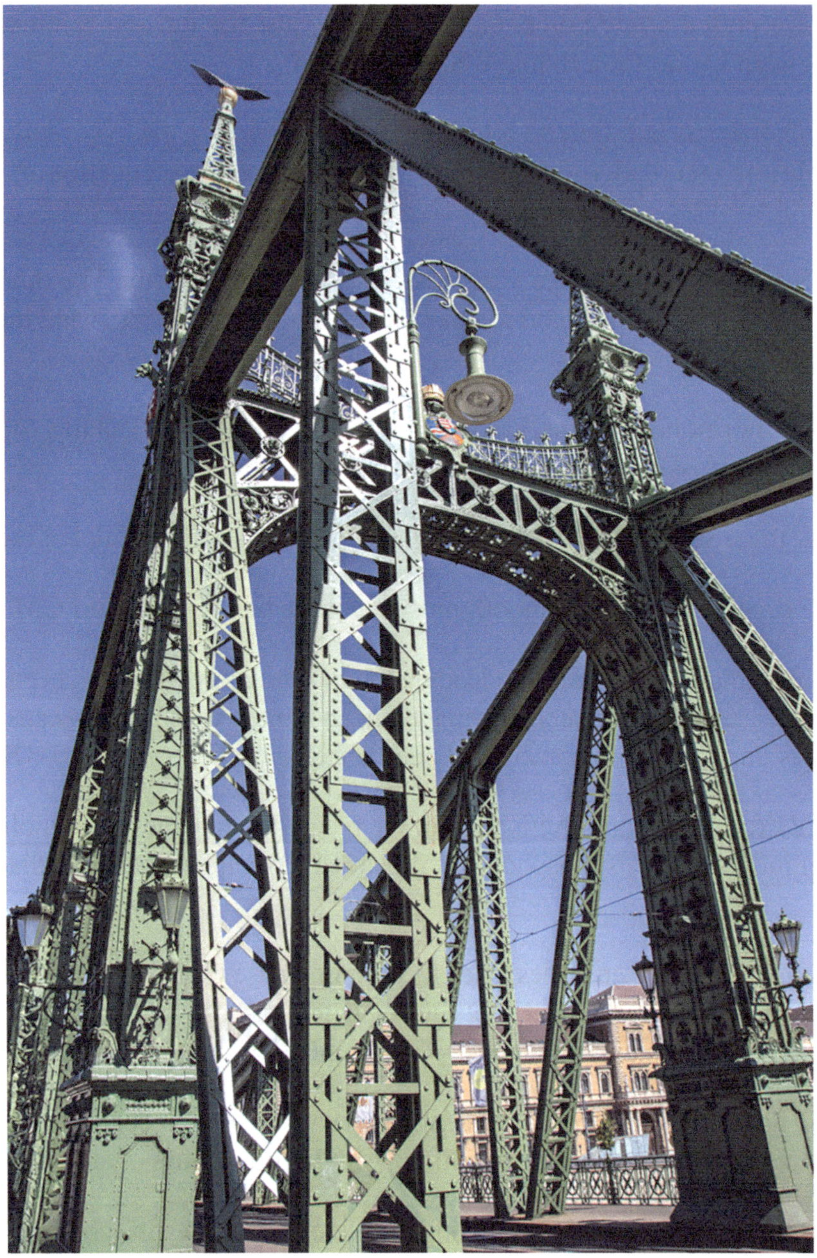

Fig. 154.4 The Liberty Bridge in Budapest, Hungary, is known for its decorative ironwork and architectural detail. Photo: Edward Shtern; image used under license from iStock.com

- Keep up on "emerging" receptors. I went through my entire residency, fellowship, and early career without once saying or writing "cannabinoid receptor." Nobody even ever really thought about it, as I recall. Not anymore.—**CM**

- Of course, cannabinoid receptors didn't just evolve because humans starting smoking plants. They are activated by endocannabinoids (endogenous cannabinoids), phyto- cannabinoids (plant-derived, for example THC), and synthetic cannabinoids.—**SNF and editors**

- There are two subtypes of cannabinoid receptors: CB1 and CB2, both G-protein coupled receptors, leading to a cascade of events that causes modulation of ion channels.—**SNF**

- The CB1 receptor is very potent in several brain regions, also found in peripheral nervous system and other peripheral tissues. It is often concentrated on presynaptic terminals which leads to suppression of neuronal excitability and inhibition of neurotransmission – likely playing a major role in neuronal plasticity.—**SNF and KAM**

- The CB1 receptors are associated with the psychoactive effects of cannabinoids.—**SNF**

- The CB2 receptor is found in immune cells (i.e. microglia, osteoclasts, osteoblasts) and a few neurons.—**SNF and editors**

- The CB2 receptor has been much less studied but is thought to be connected to immune modulation and likely plays a role in suppression of immune function. Researchers are investigating CB2 agonists as a potential treatment of inflammation and pain without the psychoactive side effects associated with CB1 receptor activation.—**SNF and editors**

- It's easy to see how the CB receptors could impact the practice of anesthesia – think chronic pain and sepsis.—**Editors**

- Watch what the palliative medicine anesthesiologists do in their prescribing practices. We've noticed that they have the most complete understanding of the receptor-medication interactions and consider them constantly in their clinical practice.**—Editors**

- Veterinary medicine uses some receptor pharmacology that we, unfortunately, do not. It can also be a question of money and patents. See the interesting example of atipamezole below.—**Editors**

- Although not misunderstood or misused, atipamezole is a very unfortunate drug. Atipamezole is a selective competitive alpha-2 receptor antagonist widely used in veterinary practice to promptly reverse the effects of dexmedetomidine [2, 3]. Although it has been shown to be safe and effective as a reversal agent in dexmedetomidine sedated humans, the FDA has not approved it for that purpose.—**RAJ**

- What is truly unfortunate is that the patent on atipamezole has long expired. This means that a drug company would need to invest several million dollars to get FDA approval with no way of recouping those costs. Without patent protection other drug companies would be free to produce and sell atipamezole at a significantly lower price. Result: no atipamezole.—**RAJ**

More Pharmacology Wisdom from A Case Approach to Perioperative Drug–Drug Interactions

There is a wealth of additional pharmacology wisdom as well as valuable teaching tidbits in our previous Springer book, which is nicknamed the "Blue Book." *Please* get a copy and check out this information as the introductory chapters were carefully written to be a concise and accessible refresher on basic pharmacology principles. As with all of our books, every single penny of royalties goes to FAER in perpetuity!

Blue Book Chapters with More Pharmacology Principles

- Pharmacodynamic Interactions: Core Concepts
- Pharmacokinetic Interactions: Core Concepts
- A Brief Treatise on the Area Under the Curve

References

1. Bojanic K, Sprung J, et al. Chapter 97: Wish we knew then what we know now – a case of serotonin syndrome in the operating room. In: Marcucci C, Gierl BT, Kirsch JR, editors. Avoiding common anesthesia errors. 2nd ed. New York: Springer; 2018.
2. Karhuvaara S, Kallio A, Scheinin M, Anthill M, Salonen JS, Scheinin H. Pharmacological effects and pharmacokinetics of atipamezole, a novel alpha 2-adrenoceptor antagonist–a randomized, double-blind cross-over study in healthy male volunteers. Br J Clin Pharmacol. 1990;30:97–106.
3. Karhuvaara S, Kallio A, Salonen M, Tuominen J, Scheinin M. Rapid reversal of alpha 2-adrenoceptor agonist effects by atipamezole in human volunteers. Br J Clin Pharmacol. 1991;31:160–5.

Authors

Sarah Fribance is an anesthesiology resident at UPMC. She grew up in Northampton, PA, and got her medical degree from UVA thanks to an abundance of support from her parents and siblings. She enjoys taking her dog on hikes and playing pick-up soccer with friends.

Stan Alfaras-Melainas is an anesthesiologist and assistant program director at UPMC. His favorite role in life, though, is being a busy family man and enjoying his time at home with his young family.

Raj Nathwani is a trauma anesthesiologist at Harborview Medical Center in the University of Washington healthcare system. He is of the firm belief that the success of the truly emergent case relies on mastery of the basic pharmacology and medication safety principles.

Cathy Marcucci is a senior anesthesiologist and transfusion medicine physician. Besides the day-to-day anesthesia drugs, she is most interested in psychiatric and neuropsychiatric drugs and sometimes even scores better than the psychiatry residents when playing Psychiatric Drug Jeopardy during Neil Sandson's psychopharmacology lectures.

Logan Olson practices in the medical and cardiovascular ICUs as a board-certified critical care pharmacist at Nebraska Medicine in Omaha, Nebraska. He received his Doctor of Pharmacy from North Dakota State University and then trained at Mayo Clinic in Rochester, Minnesota, for Post Graduate Year 1 and The Ohio State University Wexner Medical Center for Post Graduate Year 2. He enjoys going to the zoo with his wife and kids and taking on home improvement projects that are better left for professionals.

Pharmacology Wisdom: Clinical Practice

155

Konstantinos Alfaras-Melainas, Brandon M. Togioka, Rajen V. Nathwani, Anthony Passannante, Logan M. Olson, and Catherine Marcucci

Contributors:

Edwin G. Avery IV, MD (EGA)

Ronald S. Bank, MD (RSB)

Carol F. Bodenheimer, MD (CFB)

Herbert Chen, MD (HC)

Benjamin C. Conner, MD PhD*

Steven M. Frank, MD (SMF)

Sarah N. Fribance, MD (SNF)

Harley S. Geller, MD (HSG)

Brian T. Gierl, MD (BTG)

Vincent L. Hoellerich, MD (VLH)

Evan D. Kharasch, MD PhD

K. Alfaras-Melainas (✉)
Department of Anesthesiology, Perioperative Medicine, and Critical Care Medicine, University of Pittsburgh, Pittsburgh, PA, USA
e-mail: alfarasmelainisk@upmc.edu

B. M. Togioka
Department of Anesthesiology and Perioperative Medicine, School of Medicine, Oregon Health & Science University, Portland, OR, USA

R. V. Nathwani
Department of Anesthesiology and Pain Medicine, University of Washington School of Medicine, Harborview Medical Center, Seattle, WA, USA

A. Passannante
Department of Anesthesiology, University of North Carolina at Chapel Hill, Chapel Hill, NC, USA

L. M. Olson
Department of Pharmacy, Nebraska Medicine, Omaha, NE, USA

C. Marcucci
Department of Transfusion Medicine, Clinical Center, National Institutes of Health, Bethesda, MD, USA

S. Mohamed et al. (eds.), *Anesthesia Bridges*, https://doi.org/10.1007/978-3-032-08294-7_155

Daniel J. McCoy, MD '26 (DJM)

Mark Nelson, MD MEd (MN)

Alejandra Pelayo, BS (AP)

Amy J. Robbins, MD MBA (AJR)

Neil B. Sandson, MD (NBS)

Charles J. Yeo, MD (CJY)

Introduction

Clinical pharmacology in the perioperative period is the other *sine qua non* for being an anesthesiologist. It's impossible to be a good anesthesiologist without a deep and abiding interest in clinical pharmacology and the discipline and drive to work constantly to make your medication knowledge and practices better. We could fill an entire book just with pharmacology teaching tips and wisdom; below are only a few pearls from our collected wisdom.

Basics

- Anesthesiology entails the skillful manipulation of drug interactions to therapeutic benefit: Using desirable interactions to maximum advantage, converting undesirable interactions to desirable interactions, and attenuating or avoiding undesirable or dangerous drug interactions.—**Editors**

- Titrate (almost) everything! We give drugs and we see what happens. That's what we do.—**Editors**

- When the editors trained, the cost and supply chain of a drug weren't big issues. But they certainly are today and perhaps rightfully so! At any rate, mastering these concerns is part of mastering the drugs and it will remain that way.—**Editors**

- Don't discount the old-fashioned or old-timer medications and always think about what you would use if you were doing the case during a medical mission trip. Sometimes what's old becomes new again. Examples are ketamine, naltrexone, and methadone. Even nitrous oxide didn't die completely before it got a new look for OB patients.—**Editors**

- And consider good old lidocaine—it can be used for topical, intravenous, spinal, epidural, and regional anesthesia. Don't forget that you can nebulize it for the airway and put it into the cuff of the endotracheal tube. Lidocaine has probably done more good in the history of anesthesiology than any other medication, maybe? It would be such a mistake to underestimate it.—**AJR, CM, and Editors**

- Many medications we use are made synthetically but it's still good to know the origins of them. At one point, ephedrine was made from the low grassy shrubs of the *Ephreda* family. The plants are still widely used for medicinal and illicit purposes in some parts of the world.—**Editors**

***Note from the Editors:** There aren't *Ephedra* plants growing on this creek bank in Asia, as the plants flourish in drier locations, but they look just as ordinary as these grassy weeds and shrubs. In China, *Ephedra* species has been used as a folk remedy for asthma and other ailments for about 5000 years (Fig. 155.1).

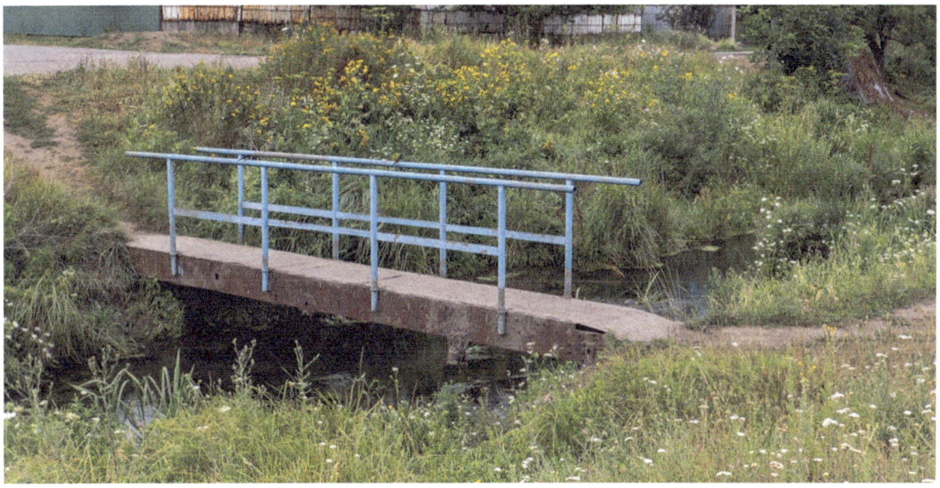

Fig. 155.1 A utilitarian bridge spans a weedy creekside landscape. Photo: Image used under standard license from stock.adobe.com

- In palliative medicine, we use so many of the old meds that have come back on trend—such as oral ketamine for outpatient cancer pain management and phenobarbital compounded suppositories for terminal agitation in the end-of-life patient. The stereotypical patients requiring phenobarbital are middle-aged formerly robust males with lung cancer who cannot be calmed through any other means, and it works great. Haldol, of course, is a palliative mainstay drug that has been in clinical use since FDA approval in 1967.—**AJR**

- Also, be aware that anesthesia drugs do go through periods of being "in style." Don't over-use the latest medication paradigm and don't under-use it.—**Editors**

- The OR pharmacist wants you to call even if you're just thinking about giving something out of the ordinary. Dispensing takes time.—**LMO**

- Being an expert in a subject means being a bit knowledgeable about the history of that subject. It's worth just a bit of time to read up on the history of anesthesia pharmacology, if only because you learn why what we have now is better. For example, copper kettles were important because they allowed the anesthesiologist could control the concentration of the volatile anesthetic being delivered to the patient. And did you know that "ether" isn't completely gone? Codeine is actually the methyl ether of morphine.—**Editors**

- Drugs are expensive—polypharmacy even more so. Does that patient really need that drug?—**RVN**

- Short acting medications are preferred, for example, captopril instead of lisinopril and NPH insulin instead of glargine. They can be held to prevent prolonged effects if clinical status changes and can also titrate up faster.—**RVN**

- We *never were* big fans of shooting medications into 1-liter IV bags. Not at all. Okay, we did put Anectine (powdered succinylcholine) into bags of crystalloid, because that's how you do a succinylcholine drip. But putting ketamine and propofol into 1-liter or 500 cc bags and then controlling the "drip" with the Cair clamp? Nah, don't think so. That's not precision administration of powerful drugs. You would think this is no longer done, but we have disturbing information to the contrary. A lot of senior docs have a policy to change the IV bags when they take over a case.—**Editors**

- Be really careful about new radical paradigm shifts in medication management. And the studies that purport to support them—because there is always more work to be done. I've learned that most fundamental practice changes in medication management swing a bit too far to the other side. Remember that the most effective and reliable anti-depressant of all time is cocaine—in an 8-week trial.—**NBS and Editors**

- Studying for a big test? Make sure you understand the differences in all the new versions of older drugs in a single drug class. For instance, in our day, there tended to be lots of questions on the differences between halothane, isoflurane, sevoflurane, and desflurane. And between mivacurium and atracurium. And of course, all the local anesthetics.—**Editors**

- Whenever you encounter a medication that you aren't so familiar with, work through all the clinical scenarios. How would you use the drug and what is the pharmacology with a "regular" adult patient, with a pregnant patient, in the pediatric population, in the cold patient, in the neurosurgical patient, in trauma patients, and so forth.—**Editors**

- The best medication is the one you don't have to give because you've avoided the problem. And sometimes a simple anesthetic delivered with minimal medications can be the most eloquent.—**Editors**

- The blood–brain barrier will be broached in the not-too-distant future. What is going to do it are the *RBC-hitchhiking* technologies. This involves using red blood cells to transport medications and nanotechnology, including to the brain. It is one of the most fascinating areas of pharmacology and certainly worth keeping an eye on [1].—**CM**

- The other area of pharmacology that is rapidly coming down the pike is personalized and genomic medicine or pharmacogenetics. It's already somewhat here but will be more and more relevant in the future, so start reading and learning about it now. There is already quite a lot of knowledge about genetic variability in drug metabolism. This knowledge base will continue to expand as the clinical correlations come on board [2].—**CM and NBS**

- We *always* suggest that anesthesiologists be familiar with Phase I metabolism of perioperative medications along with the genetic differences seen with the CYP450 super-family of (mostly) liver enzymes.—**NBS and CM**

- But it is important to recognize that inborn metabolism variation also occurs with the Phase 2 metabolic enzymes such as glutathione S-transferases (GSTs), sulphotransferases (SULTs), UDP-glucuronosyltransferases (UGTs), and NAD(P)H:quinone oxidoreductase (NQO1).—**NBS and CM**

- And remember that the basic mechanism of propofol action involves its interaction with an ionotropic receptor GABAA, inhibiting transfer of nerve impulses. Molecular studies have shown that polymorphic changes in the GABRG2 receptor gene turn out to be important in propofol anesthesia [2].—**CM and NBS**

- About 60% of your thinking and teaching should be on the pharmacology of anesthesia and about 40% on the physiology, which also includes the pertinent anatomy. We don't control the physiology; it exists before we assume care of the patient and resumes after the patient leaves our care. We also don't control the surgery. The pharmacology is the only thing we have complete control of and responsibility for—so it is worthy of the majority of our attention.—**Editors**

- I once had an interesting conversation with a medical malpractice plaintiff's attorney who had purchased a copy of the drug–drug interaction book that I had done with Neil Sandson and a number of the *Anesthesia Bridges* editors and authors. He did not wish to be named but did give me permission to paraphrase the conversation. His memorable line to me was, *"You don't sue on the physiology."* I asked what he meant, and he said that an anesthesiologist is much more vulnerable on medication issues than physiology issues.—**CM**

- This lawyer explained that it's much easier to go through a chart, looking for specific medications and doses than to abstract the underlying pathophysiology at work. What he told me was that people who are not physicians—litigants, lawyers, judges, and juries—do not understand the physiology well enough to litigate on it, and so the physicians always have the upper hand, which is not what the lawyers want. He also said, "As plaintiff's lawyers, we look for papers and short, simple case reports that easily illustrate the points we want to make, and the medical information in the *Journal of Applied Physiology* isn't going to be accessible to anybody but the doctors. That material is too hard for us to explain.—**CM**

- And then Mr. Malpractice Lawyer said, "But every medication has a fact sheet that lists complications and doses, and these are much easier to litigate with. For one thing, a superficial reading of medication complications sound pretty concerning. And you can find lots of case reports about every drug there is with lots of applications and doses quoted. And this is easy for judges and juries to understand. If the physician being sued gave a different dose for a different reason, then they have to explain it and it becomes their job to try to explain why, not ours." Scary, isn't it?—**CM**

- The operating room and the ICU are the only places in medicine where the patient is completely submerged in a medication river. Think about what's streaming to and around the patient—oxygen, IV fluids, anesthetic gases, TIVA, and so forth. Because the medications don't facilitate your case, they <u>ARE</u> the case. Somebody once told us that we are not pilots flying an airplane, we are in a canoe, trying to steer, while the patient is submerged in the water tethered to the maneuvers we make.—**Editors**

***Note from the Editors:** We like aqueducts for the same reason—the water is essentially the bridge (Fig. 155.2). To illustrate this, Amy Robbins sent us her personal photo of the famous Aqueduct of Segovia.

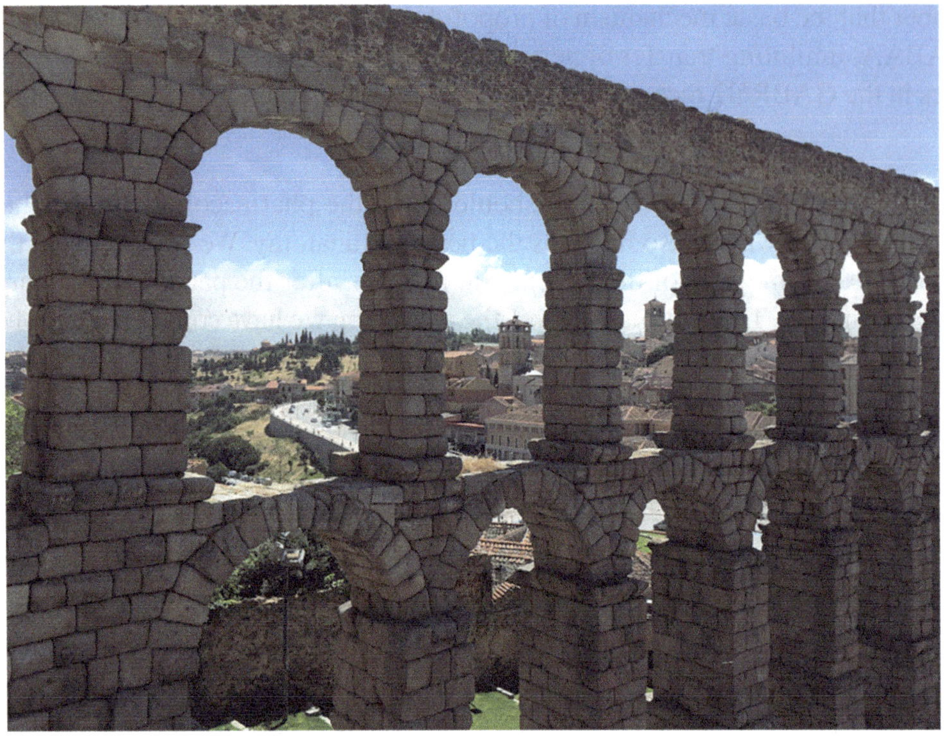

Fig. 155.2 The Aqueduct of Segovia. Built in the second half of the first century AD, it was carefully restored throughout the centuries and remained in excellent overall condition. It carried water to Segovia's public fountains and private houses until 1973. Contrary to popular myth, it was not affected by traffic vibrations but eventually fell prey to air pollution. It is now a UNESCO World Heritage Site. Photo: Amy Robbins

Medication Safety

- Teaching the specialty of anesthesiology means teaching the pharmacology of the anesthesia medications. And that in turns means teaching the safety of the medications.—**Editors**

- There is no recognized acceptable occurrence of medication error. It's not a complication, it's just a mistake, plain and simple. It will never be excused as something to be expected or overlooked by a quality assurance committee or risk management or plaintiff's attorney. If a serious medication error happens to you, you and the patient might get lucky but it's never going to be okay.—**Editors and CM**

- The key to drug and medication safety, as with any safety issue, is knowledge. You have to care enough and know enough to prevent the unforced errors. We all care enough, for sure, so then it comes down to knowledge. Do you know the look-alike medications, the black box warnings, the potential drug–drug interactions, and what drugs should be held in the perioperative period?—**Editors**

- But there is nothing wrong with not initially knowing the answer—it provides an opportunity for lifelong learning, as long as you are humble enough to admit it. Just don't guess. Knowing what you don't know is half the battle.—**RVN**

- Don't assume the pharmacist will always catch medication errors for you. Everybody involved in the chain of prescribing from the physician to the patient are responsible for checking the prescription—drug, dose, and route.—**RVN**

- Always work on the premise that the person who is actually administering the medication to the patient has the final and greatest responsibility for making sure it isn't a mistake or mishap. *You gave it, you own it.*—**Editors**

- There are three checkpoints to controlling anesthesia medications—in the vial, in the syringe, and in the drip. Each checkpoint is very amenable to visual inspection and confirmation, especially when signing over a case.—**Editors**

- *Always* double check medication drug vial content and dates each time you draw up a drug.—**EGA**

- Use the military method when drawing up drugs. "Is esmolol the drug I want to draw up? Am I drawing up esmolol now? Did I just draw up esmolol?" If you do this enough, it feels comforting not cumbersome.—**AJR, CM, and Editors**

- Label everything. Almost all drugs are clear, and interruptions happen. Tape the vial to the syringe if you're in an absolute pinch.—**LMO**

- Most drug errors I have witnessed occurred because someone glanced at the color of the label instead of reading it. Being color blind, I have to read the label. *Pretend you are color blind, read the label.*—**HSG**

- When I was a resident, I had an attending that would not accept an unlabeled syringe. There was no handing her an unlabeled syringe and saying, "this is the morphine." It went right in the trash. A pretty good safety practice, all things considered. Over the years, this had to have saved more than one medication error.—**CM**

- During transport—especially in highly pressor-dependent patients—be sure to anchor the IV lines to the bed with your hand so that if the poles were to fall over the line won't come out. This sequence of events has occurred and has resulted in fatalities.—**RSB**

- *Always* remember to program the infusion pump with a volume to be infused such that the pump will alarm in time for you to get more medication and with enough volume left in the tubing so that you don't have to reprime the giving set.—**RSB**

- Although annoying at times, please take a moment to read the medical record alerts. If it saves one serious error in your whole career, it's worth it.—**RVN**

  - Drug-interactions—if they are confusing or concerning just call the pharmacy and ask to speak with a pharmacist

  - Duplicate orders—review and discontinue

  - Therapeutic interchange—the substitution of a chemically different medication within the same class that is thought to have equivalent efficacy but lower cost

- We have mentioned this elsewhere in this book, but *don't talk when you are drawing up your drugs* in the morning! Jeff Kirsch was our program director, and he would sometimes stop by our rooms in the early mornings to discuss the various issues of the day. If you were drawing up meds or making drips, he would ask you to pause a moment while talking to him. It's a great policy. Just put all syringes and vials down for a minute. This also keeps the conversations necessarily short.—**CM, AJR, and RSB**

- Morning mantra on your way to work: *Right drug in right syringe injected into the right place in the right situation.*—**Editors**

- We were talking about the fact that medication errors were particularly dangerous because you don't often recognize right away what is going on. The patient arrests and you don't quite know why. This is in contrast to an airway mishap, where you usually know more quickly what the problem is.—**Editors**

***Note from the Editors:** We asked Ben Conner to send us a photo to accompany his important advice on the medicinal value of movement and he sent us a beautiful picture of the Grand Canyon (Fig. 155.3). Ben is just starting his career as a rehab medicine physician, and coordinated and participated in a 12-day adaptive rafting trip through the canyon while he was in medical school.

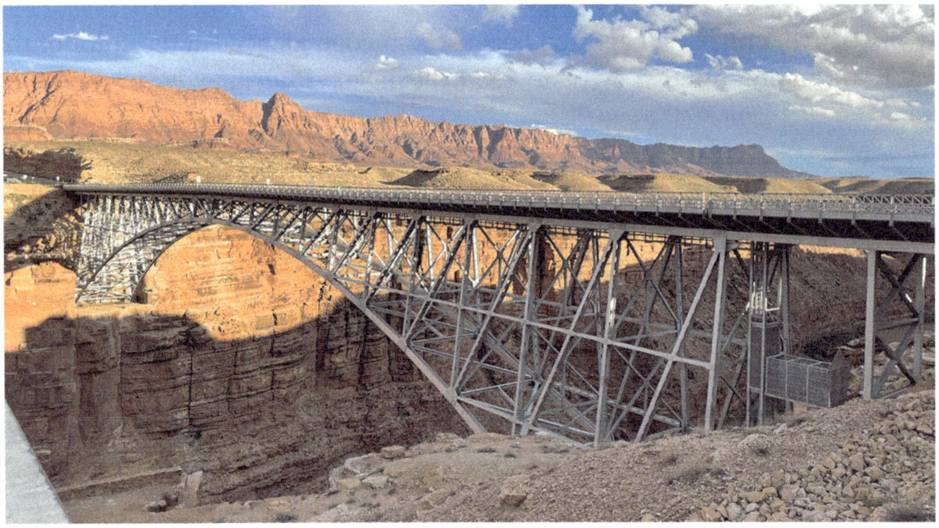

Fig. 155.3 Marble Canyon near Lees Ferry, the rafting put-in point of the Grand Canyon. That bridge takes you from the north to the south rim. Photo: Ben Conner

- *The things you do* during anesthesia should be done *quickly* and smoothly—inductions, emergence, extubation, and procedures. *The things you give*—medications—should be done *slowly* and smoothly.—**CM**

- Don't allow anybody on your team (resident or non-physician provider) to give large boluses of anesthetics/analgesics, except an induction agent and neuromuscular blocker (NMB). I once heard somebody (not a physician provider) mention he was going to "fire in" a medication—I think it was morphine. The anesthesiologist stopped him and said, "We are not cowboys, and this syringe is not a gun. We don't ever fire in anything to the patient, ever."—**CM**

- Pay extra attention to the NMBs and the drips during a case. These are the medications that you can lose control of. Think about it. You might give a bit too much or a bit too little opioid but that probably won't put the patient in serious jeopardy. Losing track of how many twitches your patient has and extubating a weak patient or mistakenly giving a NMB or a mistake with a drip with a powerful vasoactive substance is a different story.—**CM**

- *Don't forget the possibility of paradoxical drug effects.* Medication safety isn't just about labels and correct drug in the syringe. It also requires knowledge of pharmacology and receptor morphology and genetics, so please take the time to read up and study. The drugs of interest in anesthesia practice that can manifest paradoxical effects include opioids, barbiturates, benzodiazepines, propofol, and inhalational anesthetics and they can occur in both the OR and the ICU [3]. These may be associated with structural deviations with the $GABA_A$ receptors.—**LMO**

- In general, paradoxical drug effects involving mental status and unexpected excitation are known to occur somewhat more frequently in the elderly (especially with dementia) and patients with ADHD.—**Editors**

- Even the oldest and most basic drugs in our armamentarium can display paradoxical effects. Don't forget that prolonged exposure to morphine may cause pain in regions unaffected by the initial pain complaint [4]. This is not a question of the patient being difficult or drug-seeking. It is real.—**Editors**

- Vasoactive meds can also have paradoxical effects and so just assume that there are going to be some atropine questions on your exams. The dose-dependent paradoxical effects of atropine, especially in morbidly obese patients, may be due to the wide and rapid distribution in tissues. At very low doses, a central vagotonic effect on the sino-atrial node may predominate which can lead to bradycardia and AV block [5].—**Editors**

Preoperative Pharmacology

- Always, always, always ask patients and/or families what non-prescription and herbal medications they have been taking. And how much. Patients with serious medical problems can and do put themselves on all sorts of regimens, including medications and substances from their countries of origins. A good question to ask is, "What medications are you taking that you got off the internet or from a family member? How long have you been taking them?"— **Editors**

- It's not only what patients have started taking in the preoperative period, but also what they have stopped taking.—**Editors**

- More often than you would think, when you intend to *add* a medication, the patient assumes that they are supposed to *switch* medications, and they stop taking the first med.—**NBS**

- Don't always trust the home medication lists, as they are not always up to date. If the family or patient is unable to confirm home medications and the medical history hasn't been completed, you can look at the patient's dispense history to confirm home medications.—**RVN**

- If your patient has an insulin pump, ask them for a quick demo.—**KAM**

- If someone tells you they quit smoking, make sure they don't mean since yesterday.—**KAM**

- When patients stop smoking in the preoperative period, they are not only altering their physiology, but their pharmacology as well. Smoked tobacco is a clinically relevant CYP1A2 inducer. Smoking cessation, therefore, represents removal of induction of metabolism. In the succeeding, the blood levels of multiple 1A2 substrates can rise, including clozapine, cyclobenzaprine, theophylline, and warfarin. Smoking also induces CYP2E1, which is the main enzyme that metabolizes the inhalational anesthetics.—**NBS**

- Amphetamine and methamphetamine are the most commonly reported false positives on a urine drug screen.—**Editors**

- False-positive results are also possible for methadone and other opioids, barbiturates, cannabinoids, benzodiazepines, and phencyclidine.—**Editors**

- Medications that can cause false-positive drug screens include bupropion, chlorpromazine, clomipramine, dextromethorphan, diphenhydramine, ibuprofen, naproxen, promethazine, quetiapine, quinolones, such as ofloxacin and gatifloxacin, ranitidine, sertraline, thioridazine, trazodone, venlafaxine, verapamil.—**Editors**

- There is really no such thing as a false positive toxicology screen for cocaine. Current cocaine assays test for benzoylecgonine (BE), one of the three major cocaine metabolites and the longest lasting. Unlike other drug assays, the cocaine assay is relatively sensitive and specific for BE. False negatives can occur if there has not been time for the metabolite to accumulate in the blood, but false positives have not been reported, with the possible exception of drinking large quantities of Coca tea, which contains small amounts of cocaine, but is illegal in the US. *Note:* None of the clinically available local anesthetics will cause a false positive tox screen for cocaine.—**Editors**

Cannabis

- Cannabis is a really interesting medication and drug because it is used legally as a smoked product and as an edible for both medical and recreational purposes.—**Editors**

- So, as everybody knows, there has been a lot of political and legal movement concerning marijuana. Once society goes there, it often takes decades to go back, if that can ever be done. It is what it is. For our working careers, legal cannabis is here to stay.—**Editors**

- The explosion in cannabis is being driven by cultural forces, not science. There is ongoing research into the pertinent receptors and CBD clinical applications, and that is good, but the real question is how many people are going to get hurt with the widespread legal use of smoked and edible marijuana. We are career public health docs, and we think a *lot* of people will be hurt.—**NBS and CM**

- Foremost in terms of marijuana health hazards, children can and will get their hands on it. In addition to the risks of acute poisoning from little kids getting ahold of edibles, it is a terrible drug for teenagers. Of course, it blunts motivation, that has been well understood for the last thousand years. But we now know that cannabis also unmasks and/or creates persistent psychotic states, and the risk persists through the late teenage years.—**NBS and CM**

- Many states allow medical marijuana use, without any age restrictions. Although states that allow legal recreational use stipulate a minimum age of 21 for "purchase, possession, or use", we say please be serious! How successful has society been at preventing underage drinking? We think the potential for a mental health crisis in teens who use cannabis regularly is tragically very real.—**NBS and CM**

- The problem is that there is often an enormous amount of crossover between smoked "medical" cannabis use and recreational use.—**NBS**

- If you ask us, it's insane that people think it's worth smoking something to get a medicinal effect. There is no substance in existence that is worth the detrimental health effects incurred with smoking it.—**NBS and CM**

- The question is not whether marijuana is a gateway drug, *the point is that it has been* for a lot of people. It's not smart to assume that regular cannabis users are using only that.—**NBS**

- Addiction, at its core functional definition, is about people deranging their lives in harmful in order to keep using. And in this sense, marijuana is absolutely addicting, and any psychiatrist will tell you that.—**NBS**

- It is now known that *there is a cannabis withdrawal syndrome* seen in chronic heavy users that is characterized by irritability, anxiety, marijuana craving, decreased quantity and quality of sleep, and decreased food intake.—**NBS**

- Wondering why your extubated patient just doesn't seem to be turning the corner in the ICU or participating in acute postoperative rehab and mobilization protocols? Think about whether they are regular marijuana users and might be in withdrawal. Remember that for a patient to qualify for inpatient rehab, they must agree to (and be able to) actively participate in three hours of rehab per day, such physical, speech, or occupational therapies. This constellation of symptoms would make it really difficult for them to effectively engage and would likely need to be addressed for maximizing rehab outcomes.—**BCC, CFB, and CM**

- We have noticed that while patients make valiant attempts to "stop smoking" tobacco before surgery, this doesn't always seem to apply to cannabis. It's so ironic —public health officials have been waging an anti-tobacco war for decades at the same time there has been a huge societal push for decriminalizing and de-stigmatizing smoked cannabis.—**CM and NBS**

- Marijuana smoke is a strong irritant to the entire airway, especially because it is usually smoked with a long and deep inhalation and a respiratory pause, which deposits tar compounds and volatile chemicals in the lungs.—**Editors**

- Marijuana smoke contains numerous carcinogenic combustion products including about 50% more benzoprene and 75% more benzanthracene than tobacco smoke. Large, population-wide studies that definitively demonstrate a cancer effect from marijuana smoking may still be lacking but let's use our common sense here. Marijuana smoke also has more phenols, vinyl chloride, and nitrosamines than tobacco smoke. We'll see how the data develop but I certainly know which way I am betting.—**CM**

- We've had patients who have reported to surgery having smoked cannabis on the way to the hospital to calm their nerves, since they couldn't eat breakfast. We now have this specific question in our preop conversation checklist—"Did you smoke weed this morning?" We've had patients reply, "Yes, I did. They said I could take my regular medications. And since I couldn't eat, I figured I'd smoke double."—**Editors**

- The metabolism of the cannabinoids is truly complex and depends on how it is ingested. We are going to have to learn it as so many patients are likely to be using these compounds, either medicinally or recreationally or both. If you are interested in perioperative pharmacology, you are going to need an interest in the perioperative pharmacology of cannabinoids. There will be a lot of information coming out on cannabis-related drug–drug interactions that is certain.—**Editors**

- Cannabidiol (CBD)is an active component that is derived from cannabis but does not cause a high and is not addictive. has many potential therapeutic effects without intoxication and has the strongest P450 interactions [6]. It is metabolized by 2C9, 2C19, and 3A4. It acts as an inducer of 1A2, 2B6, and 3A4. A variety of studies have suggested inhibition of 2C9, 2C19, 2D6, and 3A.—**NBS and CM**

- Tetrahydrocannabinol (THC) is the psychoactive component of marijuana. It may act as an inhibitor of 1A2, 2B6, 2C9, 2C19, 2D6, 2E1, and 2J2 [6]. It may also induce 1A1 and 2C9.—**CM and NBS**

Intraoperative

- Keep an open but questioning mind about new protocols. They are not always optimized despite being adopted into widespread clinical use. For instance, when the early ERAS protocols were new, it felt like the patients were getting a basketful of extra meds. So many, honestly, that patients sometimes looked a little drunk in the PACU. I agree with the other *Anesthesia Bridges* authors who have suggested the need for ongoing evaluations—are these the best meds in the best doses to achieve ERAS? No need to be overly stubborn and obstruct progress in patient care but also don't be afraid to ask focused and necessary questions concerning changes in practice standards.—**VLH**

- There has been a significant increase in the proportion of general anesthetics administered without utilizing volatile anesthetics. There are many good reasons for this, but there are a couple of observations worth mentioning. The pharmacokinetics and pharmacodynamics of volatile anesthetic administration is very well described. The pharmacokinetics and pharmacodynamics of propofol and the commonly used opioid infusions are each well described individually, not so well in coadministration. I frequently observe concomitant propofol, opioid, ketamine, and dexmedetomidine infusions. While the individual pharmacokinetic parameters of each drug are likely only minimally affected by coadministration, exactly what happens pharmacodynamically is way beyond my, or anyone else's, ability to predict. I am not at all certain that this type of polypharmacy represents an advance.—**ANP**

- That said, everybody needs to know how to do a competent TIVA without thinking about it with a nanosecond of hesitation. For one thing, you may have a patient on buprenorphine present acutely.—**Editors**

- When we were all first doing TIVAs, the natural concern was that the patient would be too light. Actually, I saw a fair number of patients who had TIVA with an anesthetic plane that was too deep, including one patient who almost arrested and required norepinephrine to restore blood pressure.—**Anonymous**

- The most unusual TIVA I ever saw was with lidocaine! I kid you not. One of the legendary old guard at Hopkins (Dr. Donham) used that technique when the patient had true, documented malignant hyperthermia at a time when we didn't always have propofol readily available. I remember being astonished.—**CM**

- Remember that "Hang on, Mr. Johnson, they're almost done" is not an anesthesia technique or drug. Reassurance that the pain is almost over should never substitute for the appropriate use of an agent. Truly, "hang on" is not a phrase you should ever hear yourself say. Ever.—**Editors**

- It seems trite to say this, but the more cardiovascular illness present in your patient, the more consequence there is to anesthetic overdose. In patients with heart failure/poor left ventricular function, sympathetic tone is typically increased. Induction of anesthesia will have direct effects on individual organs such as the heart (reduced contractility), and indirect effects mediated by both the nervous system (decreased sympathetic tone), and the likely respiratory system effects of endotracheal intubation and mechanical ventilation (reduced venous return), our typical next steps. While we often talk about all of these changes in isolation, they all occur very close in time to each other.—**ANP**

- With difficult inductions in patients with cardiovascular disease, I prefer to use very small opioid doses, significant intravenous lidocaine doses, and modest intravenous propofol doses. Give the opioid time to work (4 minutes for fentanyl), choose your modest propofol dose, and give it a chance to work. In a sick patient walk away from the stopcock and give more time for the slow circulation to work before giving an additional dose, your patience will usually be rewarded with an unconscious patient who has not been overdosed.—**ANP**

- If TIVA is utilized, it is important to ensure that you have reliable primary access and a backup access in case of any complications or issues.—**KAM**

- Inhaled anesthetics are potent greenhouse gases, whereas TIVA generates large amounts of plastic waste and has the potential for significant impact on water resources.—**KAM**

- If a patient has risk factors for intraoperative awareness with recall and their physiology allows, it can be a good idea to use a processed EKG and/or give higher doses of midazolam and ketamine, especially if a TIVA is planned.—**BTG**

Postoperative

- Ask yourself daily if certain medications can be reduced/made PRN each day, usual meds to think about are CNS depressants but consider quetiapine (if used for delirium/sleep), hydroxyzine, benzodiazepines, opioids, methylnatrexone, naloxegol.—**RVN**

- De-escalating medications especially before the patient is discharged home avoids polypharmacy—if you start a drug, think about putting a stop date on it.—**RVN**

- On admission, some home meds should be restarted but not all of them—consider how sick the patient is and how their physiology is different to when they were at home.—**RVN**

- Patients have considerable confusion at discharge as to what their med regimen will be. Give very clear instructions on what to stop, what to start, and what to continue. Have the patient or other responsible person repeat it to you.—**AJR**

- For high-cost medications (especially chemotherapy / IVIG) work with your pharmacist to see if it needs approval from the Medication Stewardship Team. This review can take time so start the paperwork early. And remember that health insurance pharmacy coverage constraints can play a big row these days on what is covered/not covered for patients.—**RVN and AJR**

- No need for IV medications if patient taking PO or has feeding tube (e.g., steroids, PPIs, antiepileptic maintenance doses)—PO meds are typically cheaper and safer for the patient.—**RVN**

- Try to clean up ED and PACU orders to avoid duplicate opioids and benzodiazepines.—**RVN**

***Note from the Editors:** Ben Conner also sent us this interesting photo of another bridge across the bottom of the Grand Canyon (Fig. 155.4).

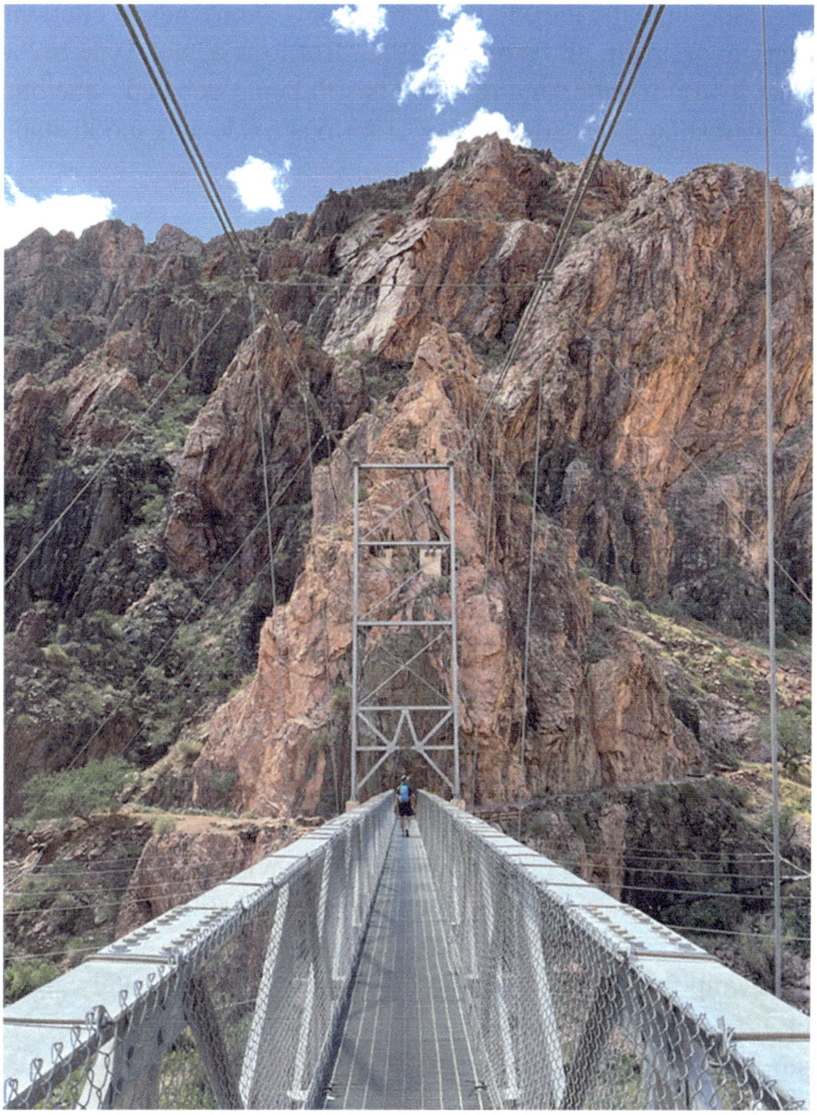

Fig. 155.4 The bridge at the bottom of the Grand Canyon, near Phantom Ranch. It is interesting how the architecture of the bridge's suspension system blends in with the surrounding geology. Photo: Ben Conner

Inhalational Agents

Nitrous Oxide

- Nitrous oxide was discovered in 1793 by Joseph Priestly. It has been in widespread clinical use for over 150 years. It remains in common use in dental suites. In recent years, it has also been in widespread use in countries, such as India. N_2O is a greenhouse gas that has been present in the atmosphere for more than a hundred years. The environmental impact of nitrous oxide can be calculated in CO_2 equivalents.—**Editors**

- As a fun exercise, we decided to see what would happen if we asked several of our senior colleagues about their professional history with N_2O. We got a range of answers, and their advice and wisdom demonstrate the value of talking to as many experienced people as possible. Substitute any drug for N_2O and start chatting with the senior docs.—**Editors**

- If you type "nitrous oxide" into the PubMed search window, thousands of citations will pop up. Yeah, yeah you might think to yourself, all from like 1985. But look again. Type in "nitrous oxide 2021" and you will see that its use in labor and delivery is still being debated—the question is not settled yet—and there are interesting papers on the use of nitrous oxide as a mood stabilizer. What's old is new again.—**Editors**

- I still use N_2O for inhalation inductions in children but really have no other use for it. I am doing TIVAs for general anesthesia (no gas) more often these days.—**VLH**

- I now do not use nitrous oxide at all and I teach all my residents that it is not needed (except in ED / obstetrics for sedation / analgesia). Healthcare is such a massive environmental polluter, and much of it in the name of "minimizing the risk to the patient," without ever considering the monetary or environmental cost which ultimately will kill millions of people (don't get me on my soap box!!).—**RVN**

- The University of Washington hospitals are in the process / aiming to disconnect all pipelines of nitrous oxide and then leave cylinders which can be attached to the anesthesia machines if needed.—**RVN**

- As an anesthesia agent, I loved it, and it was used in nearly every case when I was training. But clearly, it is an environmental disaster, and I honestly don't think the wake up is that much quicker and so we need to move on.—**RVN**

- I have never liked N_2O much during GETA, but it does provide amnesia, analgesia, and anxiolysis. Once I came into my room and the resident—for some reason I still can't fathom—had turned off the vaporizers at the end of the case while the NMB was still on board. We immediately put the patient on N_2O while we drew up fresh propofol and other maneuvers. Fortunately, the patient did not have recall. I also think it's good, easy, and cheap for brief, very stimulating interventions, like having K-wires pulled out.—**CM**

- From my OB lens, I have seen nitrous oxide make a comeback. Nitrous oxide has been used for labor analgesia for centuries throughout the UK; however, only recently did it gain traction in the U.S. Epidurals clearly provide the best labor analgesia, but satisfaction with the labor process includes more than labor pain control. Pregnant women seem to appreciate the anxiolysis, the control that nitrous oxide provides them, and perhaps the euphoria. In this manner, nitrous oxide has been associated with improved coping scores as well as improved satisfaction with the birth process. Therefore, I think it serves a role on labor and delivery for women that desire to avoid neuraxial anesthesia.—**BMT**

- The concern has been irreversible inhibition of methionine synthetase, which can occur after as little as a few hours of exposure to nitrous oxide. Elderly patients and raw food vegans tend to be lower in vitamin B12, which exacerbates the effect of nitrous oxide on methionine synthetase. Methionine synthetase is important for DNA synthesis, when it is impaired patients may be at increased risk of megaloblastic anemia, immune suppression, and possibly postoperative myocardial ischemia due to increased homocysteine concentrations.—**BMT**

- Many of my colleagues also avoid nitrous oxide because it is a greenhouse gas and because it is associated with PONV. However, short exposure to nitrous oxide does not seem to significantly increase

PONV and other agents that may be used in place of nitrous oxide, such as fluorinated agents and opioids are also associated with PONV.—**BMT**

- Personally, I use nitrous oxide in healthy patients without high risk of PONV having short surgery where a fast wake up would be helpful. I believe nitrous leads to a generally calmer wake up and that it has benefit for decreasing postoperative pain and reducing risk of hyperalgesia through its NMDA antagonism.—**BMT**

Volatile and Other Inhalational Agents

- One of the enduring and existential mysteries of our specialty is not so much that you give volatile and people go to and stay asleep, it's that you turn them off and they wake up.—**Editors**

- Remember that Dr. Ted Eger, who did the early landmark work on the volatile anesthetic agents was a chemist and mathematician by education. Sometimes the "math" of the volatile agents gets forgotten a bit (see below).—**Editors**

- Each additional 0.1 above or below 1.0 MAC is equal to one standard deviation in dose. So, if 50% of patients will not move at 1.0 MAC, then the percent is 68% at 1.1 MAC, 95% at 1.2 MAC, and 99.7% at 1.3 MAC.—**Editors**

- Inhaled anesthetics are potent greenhouse gases. Desflurane has the highest global warming potential—more than five times higher than isoflurane.—**KAM**

- For heaven's sake, don't miss any questions on inhalational anesthetics, especially isoflurane and sevoflurane, on your board exams. Just accept that before you take the medical test pertaining to these meds, you have to wade through the "chemistry test." Chemical structures, partial pressures, vapor pressures, MAC values, solubilities, metabolism, and metabolites. And the chemistry of the CO_2 canister! You have to be able to rank order every inhalational in terms of these parameters. There's going to be the ubiquitous high-altitude question, of course.—**Editors**

- And then you start the medical/clinical test—which inhalational anesthetic to use in the anesthesia subspecialty areas and why. There are so many review books and online quiz decks about the inhalational anesthetics. Force yourself to do/review every question until you know it cold. You can knock these subjects out quickly on the exams, giving you a bit more time to ponder the questions that aren't so straightforward like the peds cardiac or chronic pain questions.—**Editors**

- The thinking about everyday vasopressors for pregnant patients has gone through an interesting evolution. Initial studies showed greater vasoconstriction of blood vessels feeding the placenta with phenylephrine, compared to ephedrine. This led clinicians to preferentially use ephedrine. The next round of studies assessed fetal pH. These studies found the beta agonist effect on the fetus led to greater fetal metabolic requirement and lower umbilical artery pH at birth. Thus, clinician practice shifted to phenylephrine over ephedrine. The next round of studies is investigating norepinephrine. I don't suspect norepinephrine will become the standard because it really should be administered through a central line.—**BMT**

- Don't forget about heliox! It is usually an 80:20 mix of helium and oxygen. Helium is an odorless, tasteless gas that increases laminar flow. This make the heliox a great inhalational agent to deliver oxygen in the clinical situation of certain compromised airways. Sometimes in the airway rooms it will be continually available in the piped gas systems. If not, work with the respiratory therapists to come up to speed on the specialized equipment needed to use it. It has saved the day for our my patients several times.—**Editors**

Opioids

- First things first—the opioid pendulum may have swung too far! We strongly advise that everybody reads or rereads a great editorial in *Anesthesiology* in April 2021 titled, "Opioid-free anesthesia: Time to regain our balance" [7]. The very senior anesthesiologists who authored the editorial refer to two articles within that issue. The editorial itself refers the antecedents and precedents for the drive to develop opioid-free or low-opioid anesthetic regimens in the public health context of the opioid (fentanyl!) crisis. The authors present compelling data on unintended opioid overdoses and state the following.—**EDK and Editors**

- *The Point Is This*: Notably absent from this entire historical narrative is any mention of, association with, or causal attribution of the opioid crisis to intraoperative and immediate postoperative use of opioids to treat moderate-severe surgical pain.—**Editors**

- Similarly, it is a great and unfounded leap to say that there is an opioid crisis and therefore we must stop using opioids for surgery.—**Editors**

- Kharasch and Martin also discuss the issues of opioid-sparing vs opioid eradication and enhanced recovery after surgery and opioids. There is no doubt that many of the ERAS principles are good ones and the continued deployment of strategies for multi-modal acute and chronic pain management are worthwhile—no one is arguing otherwise. But as they state, "It is time to regain our balance in anesthesia. Opioid-free anesthesia may be *feasible*. Nevertheless, it appears neither logical nor beneficial to patients." The authors' editorial conclusion is relevant and succinct:

> Optimal postoperative analgesia will only be achieved by using the available tools in a manner tailored to the specific needs of individual patients. Our preoccupation with opioid-free anesthesia and analgesia distracts us from this challenge.
> What is clear is that our current analgesic pharmacologic armamentarium is inadequate to the task of providing adequate pain relief with minimal side effects, and it has not materially changed in decades.
> While academia and industry regroup after years of failures, hopefully new molecular, cellular, and systems-based approaches will help us to discover novel approaches to analgesia.
> In the meantime, we can work on using existing tools more effectively. We have not defined the optimal components of multimodal analgesic pathways, nor have we developed tailored approaches consistent with the goals of precision medicine. Rather than toss aside opioids, some of our most powerful tools, we should focus on defining the optimal use of these important drugs.

- *Always* guard your narcotics closely and *never* leave them unattended. I take mine with me when I go to pick up the patient or go to the PACU. You have to knock yourself out to avoid drug discrepancies with your opioids and understand that any lapses might/can/will be used against you.—**Anonymous**

- I am aware of at least two cases when nefarious actors were trying to find a way to drum up charges against anesthesiologists by finding opioid discrepancies. One of these cases involved administration not acting in good faith and picking through hundreds of back charts, looking for the tiniest gap in opioid charting to use against a junior anesthesiologist (which they didn't find). The other case involved a senior anesthesiologist who spoke an inconvenient truth to the powers-that-were and was threatened with an opioid surveillance action if he didn't retract and stand down. He subsequently resigned. I wish this all wasn't true, but unfortunately, it is.—**Anonymous**

- Methadone is an excellent and valuable pain medicine for cancer patients and chronic pain; however, it should be respected because of its very unique pharmacokinetic and pharmacodynamic properties.—**AJR**

- Remember that methadone can be used in conjunction with local anesthetics in blocks! For example, low dose methadone (0.2 mg/kg) added as multi-modal analgesia in transversus thoracic plane block for median sternotomy and has efficacy in improving ventilator time and ICU time metrics.—**Editors**

- We see more and more patients on buprenorphine, which can make their pain management challenging. Due to its long duration of action and high affinity for opioid receptors, it can interfere with the effectiveness of other opioids. Therefore, it is important to consider appropriate strategies to manage anesthesia during surgical procedures. This may involve adjusting the anesthesia plan, using alternative pain management strategies, or temporarily discontinuing buprenorphine prior to the procedure.—**KAM**

- Remember that buprenorphine is an opioid agonist! Some recommend that it be continued throughout the perioperative period.—**Editors**

- I wouldn't discontinue buprenorphine without consulting the pain docs.—**CM**

- Everybody should keep abreast of the recommendations for anesthesiologists to take a role in initiating postoperative buprenorphine therapy for patients with opioid use disorder. It can be lifesaving, but I have definitely worked in practice settings where there weren't the time, circumstances, or follow-up capabilities for an over-worked anesthesiologist to do that. I barely had time (on the order of minutes) to write my notes and see my next patient, much less assume responsibility to consider the management of opioid use disorder. Plus, my patients were signed out of the PACU via nursing protocol and the acute pain management wasn't routinely done by anesthesiologists. Just no way to do it.—**Anonymous**

- Think that postoperative respiratory depression from opioids is rare? It's not. Continuous post-operative capnography monitoring has shown that it occurs in up to 40% or more of patients on the general surgical floors. We know opioid-associated postoperative respiratory depression extends the duration of hospital stay and increases total costs of hospitalizations, but we don't know yet about many (or most) other outcomes metrics, including patient survival and other critical events. We don't even completely understand exactly who should get monitoring and for how long. We do a pretty good job making anesthesia safe overall and these are rare events so it would require a study with perhaps 10,000–20,000 subjects to be adequately powered. Maybe some of the machine learning applications will help us in the near future.—**Editors**

- When it is feasible, the utilization of regional anesthesia in conjunction with multimodal analgesia can provide potential advantages. This approach has the potential to enhance patient comfort and potentially mitigate the risks associated with opioid usage.—**KAM**

- If there is one table that needs to be committed to memory, it's the opioid equivalencies. It's not a huge amount of information, but there is no way to reason it out. You just have to be familiar enough to know it forwards and backwards.—**AJR**

- We have gone from routinely administering large doses of opioids to a majority of patients in the belief that adequately treating their pain during the anesthetic would result in better postoperative pain control, to a world in which opioid dosing is very parsimonious, and patients are complaining less of postoperative pain. This is partly due to effective application of complementary multimodal analgesics and regional techniques, and partly due to a revolution in thinking about the effect of intraoperatively administered opioids. Remifentanil showed us that short-term mu receptor stimulation causes hyperalgesia, and this effect is not limited to remifentanil. An extreme interpretation of what has been learned is that intraoperative opioids are not necessary if unconsciousness is maintained by other drugs, and we should aim for a modest opioid effect on emergence to give the patient analgesia as consciousness returns.—**ANP**

- Pain may be the fifth vital sign, but pain medications come with side effects. Rather than a fentanyl or hydromorphone infusion use intermittent boluses.—**RVN**

- Unless you have done a lot of time in chronic pain, we have noticed that anesthesiologists often don't have a ton of in-depth knowledge about the common outpatient pain meds. So, at the risk of being a little handbook-y, we thought we'd pull together some concise information for you (Table 155.1). Know what's really interesting, though, when you see it summarized like this? All of the common outpatient PO opioids have black box warnings!—**AP and CM**

Table 155.1 Common outpatient pain medication dosages

Drug (Brand)	Duration of action	Standard dosing	Half-life	Active metabolites	Black box warning (yes or no)
Oxycodone (OxyContin)	3–4 h	5-15 (mg) As needed	4.5–6.5 h	Noroxycodone Oxymorphone	Yes
Oxycodone Acetaminophen (Percoset)	4–6 h	2.5-10 (mg) Oxycodone 325–650 (mg) acetaminophen	3–5 h	Noroxycodone Oxymorphone NAPQI	Yes
Tramadol (Ultram)	6 h	50–100 (mg) every 4–6 h	7 h	O-desmethyltramadol	Yes
Hydrocodone (Vicodin)	4–6 h	10 (mg) every 12 h	3.8 h	Hydromorphone Norhydrocodone	Yes
Gabapentin (Neurontin)		900–1800 (mg) per day	5–7 h		Yes

- Immediate release gabapentin for neuropathic pain is usually dosed TID.—**BMT**

- We don't regularly adjust the weight-based dose of opioids for pregnant status. We do limit access to fentanyl in labor due to effects on the fetus. Patients can receive a maximum of 100 mcg fentanyl per hour and we stop offering this if we believe delivery will occur within 1–2 hours.—**BMT**

- Think carefully about all opioid use in pregnant women. For versions, we use a lipophilic opioid in the spinal but no systemic opioids as patients are usually worried about the effects on the baby.—**BMT**

- Remember that certain patients can be sensitive to the narcotic effects of opioids. This includes patients with previous or current traumatic brain injury and Trisomy 21. I once saw a teenager with this condition become obtunded for several hours with 50 micrograms of fentanyl.—**CM**

- Patients remember and evaluate their anesthetic based largely on only two aspects of the overall anesthetic plan, assuming they don't wake up paralyzed or very weak. Absent residual NMB, what stays with patients is their pain management and emesis management plans. They might recall just a bit that the propofol burned as they were going to sleep, but they have no memory and don't care how long emergence took. But every patient will know for sure whether they had pain, and if so, how much, and whether or not they had postoperative nausea and vomiting. So, it has to be of primary importance to you because it is of primary importance to the patients.—**CM and AJR**

Other Analgesics

- A fun thing to do is ask the old guard what their "must have" drug is and why. It's just a thought experiment, but you will hear some great anecdotes. My "go to" drug is ketamine because it is so densely analgesic. Also, you can use it in both peds and adult cases and in the delivery room.—**CM**

- There is really no analgesic medication that is FDA-approved for short-term use that isn't being used chronically. The promising new non-opioid pain medication suzetrigine is intended for acute, in-hospital use only. We think it won't be long until patients find a way to extend that. You heard it here first.—**NBS, CM, and DJM**

- The proliferation of ERAS protocols has been an excellent way to get clinicians working together to provide more optimal patient care. Preoperative acetaminophen has few downsides, and preoperative celecoxib is very safe in most circumstances. I think the anesthesiology community, in hindsight, was too eager to include gabapentinoids, such as pregabalin (Lyrica) and gabapentin in commonly administered preoperative bundles. I would recommend removing the gabapentinoids from routine preoperative order bundles and using this drug class more selectively. There has been no clinically significant reduction in pain with preop gabapentinoid administration, and significant sedation in some patients.—**ANP**

- Use multimodal analgesia and don't forget to optimize pain before increasing sedation (e.g., don't have post-op spine patients only on propofol).—**RVN**

- It is important to note that dexmedetomidine functions as an analgesic and adjunctive analgesic through multiple mechanisms across all stages of the perioperative period.—**KAM**

- There is good evidence that perioperative ketamine use decreases postoperative pain scores and opioid requirements through various different receptors and channels.—**KAM**

- Be aware of the psychomotor effects of ketamine. Also, be careful administering ketamine on patients with catecholamine depletion.—**KAM**

Neuromuscular Blocking Agents

- NMBs are also challenging because they are among the few drugs we give that are actively reversed, not just discontinued. Every senior anesthesiologist has learned that a large part of emergence and extubation difficulties are due to residual NMB. And remember that a "full" set of train-of-four switches does not mean the NMB is completely resolved. So many people lose track of this.—**CM**

- Medication mishaps concerning neuromuscular blocking drugs are among the worst. For one thing, NMBs are not titrated ml by ml at intubation. If you put a strong vasopressor into a syringe that is labelled fentanyl, that's bad. But you are probably not going to give an entire syringe of "fentanyl" at once. If you put the same vasopressor into a syringe that you think is your NMB for intubation, you have a much bigger problem.—**ANP**

- On induction, early paralysis is advisable. It will allow for early and easy mask ventilation. Remember hypercarbia is not your friend.—**MN**

- Make sure you don't lose track of how to do neuromuscular blockade the old-fashioned way and don't get dependent on sugammadex. I practice at several locations where sugammadex is not available or requires justification for use, due to its cost. Always imagine in the back of your mind what you would do if it was fifteen years ago—don't let go of the techniques and drugs from the "previous generation" that were used to reverse neuromuscular blockade.—**VLH**

- If succinylcholine has been used and the patient is not recovering quickly, pseudocholinesterase deficiency should be top of mind.—**LMO**

- And also, don't lose track of how to use succinylcholine! At one of Vince Hoellerich's practice locations, there is a surgeon who can routinely do a cholecystectomy in 15 minutes. So, Vince intubates with sux and then give several small doses to finish the case.—**Editors and VLH**

- I had the interesting experience of a patient who frequently came in for bronchial dilatation. The surgeons needed general anesthesia and significant neuromuscular blockade for about four minutes, but that was all—there was no incision and no real need for pain meds. I always did the case with a succinylcholine drip using succinylcholine powder to make the drip. Of course, repeated doses of sux mandate the use of twitch monitor to make sure that you don't get into Phase 2 blockade—if you titrate your drip or mini-doses to one twitch, it works great. But the most important thing was that it really allowed me to understand how succinylcholine works.—**CM**

- Got yourself into a Phase 2 blockade with succinylcholine? You have to wait! There is no alternative.—**Editors**

- Be mindful of the side effects of sugammadex. Those can be real!—**KAM**

- R(apid)-O(nset)-curonium.—**KAM**

- NMBs, such as atracurium and rocuronium are identified as the category of anesthetic drugs *most prone to causing anaphylaxis.*—**KAM**

- There is no reason to administer two different intermediate acting neuromuscular blockers during a case so pick one drug and stick to it. Mixing intermediate acting neuromuscular blockers will lead to potentiation of block, and it is not necessary. The difference between mixing drugs of a different class and of the same class is a matter of degree of potentiation.—**ANP**

- I have observed what I would describe as very sloppy practice with regards to rocuronium maintenance dosing since the introduction of sugammadex. The average maintenance doses administered in our practice have increased. What this does is increase the duration of relatively deep neuromuscular blockade and make it more likely that larger doses of sugammadex will be required for antagonism of deeper block.—**ANP**

- Best practice is to use a reliable method to measure depth of blockade, preferentially EMG monitoring, and administer rocuronium in recommended maintenance doses (0.1–0.2 mg/kg) as twitches return. This will lead to a better understanding of the pharmacokinetics of rocuronium, and reduced administration of both rocuronium and sugammadex for your health system. Reduced drug cost will follow better anesthetic practice, with the only downside being more frequent maintenance doses of rocuronium. Achieving equivalent or better outcomes at less cost is a win for our health systems.—**ANP**

- Regarding neuromuscular blocking agents, remember that most OB patients will be pretty weak after surgery if they have been getting magnesium. Based upon limited experience, even appropriate dosing of reversal agents may not prevent patients from having residual paralysis when they are on magnesium.—**BMT**

- When I was a trainee and then a young attending doing a lot of OB anesthesia, we would often get through the entire operative case just with the intubating doses of neuromuscular blockers (NMB). You just really want to be careful about this. The patient will retain her "pregnant physiology" postpartum for quite a while and you don't want to stress this physiology and put her at extra risk by being weak. And *nobody* wants to have to reintubate a post-section patient.—**CM**

***Note from the Editors:** Herb and Harriet Chen have been good friends of the anesthesia community for many years. Harriet is a professional photographer who is most interested in the interplay of light and color in the composition of her photographs. She graciously searched her portfolio for us and donated several photos, including this one of a bridge in Boston, MA (Fig. 155.5).

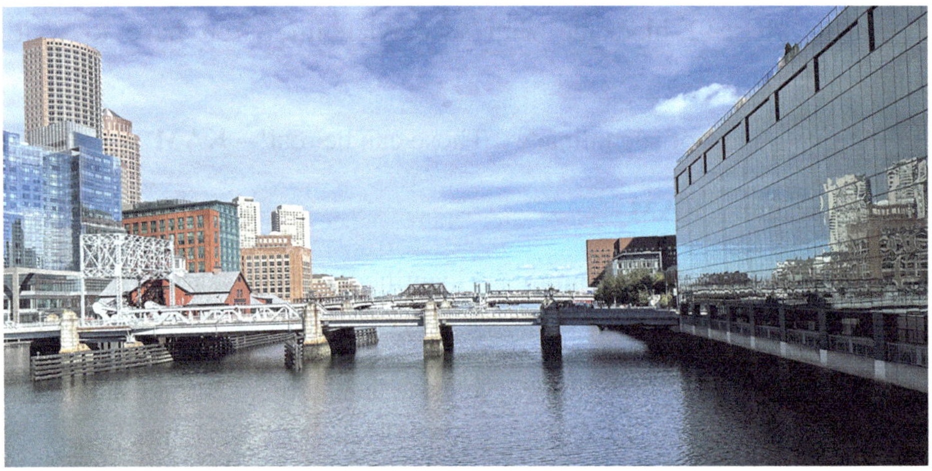

Fig. 155.5 This lovely photo illustrates that this small bridge in Boston serves not only to connect the two banks of the river but also delineates the river from the sky. Photo: Harriet Little Chen

Benzodiazepines and Other Sedatives

- Remember that midazolam can be used as an induction agent! And it doesn't always take that much. A friend of mine (surgeon!) who didn't drink any alcohol at all related to me that she essentially became apneic with the 2 mg of midazolam that she got on arriving to the OR. Monitors weren't even on yet and the anesthesia team realized they had essentially induced their patient.—**CM**

- Give IV benzodiazepine for a patient who is in active alcohol withdrawal to the point of seizing. If they are not actually seizing, then PO or IM benzodiazepines are preferred over parenteral agents due to the extended half-life. Which po benzodiazepine to give is a somewhat nuanced question and depends on the pharmacokinetic profile of the drug and the patient's medical state. If the patient doesn't have liver failure or encephalopathy consider metabolite-rich and agents

Table 155.2 All have black box warning as of 2020 https://www.fda.gov/drugs/drug-safety-and-availability/fda-requiring-boxed-warning-updated-improve-safe-use-benzodiazepine-drug-class

Drug (Brand)	Duration of action	Standard dosing	Half-life	Active metabolites	Black box warning (yes or no)
Diazepam (Valium)	12+ h	2–10 (mg) 2–4 times a day	20–80 h	Desmethlydiazepam Temazepam Oxazepam	Yes
Lorazepam (Ativan)	6–8 h	2–6 (mg) Divided doses	10–20 h	Lorazepam-glucuronide	Yes
Clonazepam (Klonapin)	6–12 h	1(mg) per day	18–50 h	7-aminoclonazepam	Yes

with half-lives of greater than 24 hours like diazepam (Valium) and chlordiazepoxide (Librium), typically Valium 5–10 mg and Librium 25 mg or 50 mg. If the patient does have liver failure/encephalopathy, consider Ativan or Serax, which have half-lives of about 6 hours and do not undergo Phase 1 metabolism.—**NBS and Editors**

- All the commonly available PO benzos will have efficacy to treat, however, selection should be more nuanced—for instance, if the patient has a degree of liver failure or is encephalopathic, you will want to select a benzo that does not rely on Phase 1 metabolism and has a comparatively shorter half-life, such as lorazepam (Ativan) or oxazepam (Serax).—**NBS**

- Several common diazepines also have black box warnings (Table 155.2).—**AP and CM**

Benzodiazepines

- Remember, haldoperidol is a D2 blocker and a relatively "clean acting" sedative. When given to delirious patients, it sedates the agitated behavior but *does not* treat the delirium per se. The only way to treat delirium is to treat the underlying cause.—**NBS**

- Don't ever let a patient suffer the consequences of alcohol withdrawal. It's one of the most straightforward single-agent withdrawal situations yet is so dangerous for the patient. There are at least six drugs/medications that can be used to treat it.—**Editors**

- Phenobarbital is an effective and safe option for the treatment and management of alcohol withdrawal. A recent retrospective study concluded that front-loaded phenobarbital dosing, when compared to low-intermittent phenobarbital dosing, for benzodiazepine-resistant alcohol withdrawal was associated with significantly lower mechanical ventilation incidence and continuous sedative use [8].—**KAM and CM**

- Mild to moderate alcohol withdrawal can be effectively treated with symptom-triggered benzodiazepines (typically lorazepam), but consider pre-emptive therapy for severe withdrawal, such as phenobarbital loading. It has the advantage of a longer half-life, avoidance rather than treatment of symptoms, and facilitates GABA-A channel opening, rather than increasing GABA-A receptor affinity for GABA [9].—**LMO**

- Consider utilizing the PAWSS (Prediction of Alcohol Withdrawal Severity Scale) to predict alcohol withdrawal severity.—**LMO**

- Alcohol is also an effective option for the treatment and management of alcohol withdrawal.—**NBS**

- Other alcohol withdrawal therapies that have been suggested or utilized in the literature include continuous infusion of GABA agonists, dexmedetomidine, antiepileptics, and antipsychotics. We admit that this introduces a significant amount of variability into clinical practice and there is a lack of uniformity and recommendations for the treatment of severe refractory patients. If your patient is in severe withdrawal, consider escalating care with adjunctive therapies.—**Editors**

Spinal Meds

- Some of the worst morbidity we have ever seen has been when there was a medication mishap that involved injection of the wrong medication into the spinal fluid. It is not unusual to see the word "catastrophic" in reports describing these events—**Editors**

- If you are young enough to not have seen this yet, go read a case report about accidental injection of vincristine into the subarachnoid space. It will scare the living daylights out of you. Vinca alkaloids are almost always fatal if giving into the intrathecal space or, if not, they cause a severe ascending paralysis. People have initially been convicted of manslaughter due to this drug error (the conviction was later voided).—**Editors**

- Jeff Kirsch was an incredibly supportive program director. He knew and understood all the nuances of clinical decisions that have to be made in the OR. But the one thing he made clear right at the start of training was that he would not support an off-label spinal medication injection. Even if you gave the medication and dose you intended to give and there was not an adverse outcome, if it was not on-label for intrathecal injection, he would not support that anesthetic plan.—**AJR, RSB, and CM**

- Keep a zone of safety around the meds on your spinal tray. Insist on personally verifying every single medication that crosses into that zone of safety.—**Editors**

- Remember that spinal medications are among the oldest of the anesthetic agents. Spinals anesthetics are at least a hundred years old. The local anesthetic agents came into widespread clinical use without rigorous neurotoxicity testing. Cauda equina syndrome and TNS are not that rare. It has been suggested that it is not the concentration of the local anesthetic on the label of the bottle that counts, it's the concentration in the perineural space.—**Editors**

- If you are working in a room where a spinal is given, you have to assume that it is possible that any medication given for that type of case can and in that room can end up in the intrathecal space. There are case reports describing magnesium sulfate ending up in the spinal.—**Editors**

- Opioids, especially lipophilic opioids, in spinals remain under-utilized! They can cause pruritis but have so much efficacy.—**Editors**

Vasopressors

- We still do not have complete understanding of our everyday basic "purple drugs"—*phenylephrine* and *ephedrine,* although we use them every day, often without a thought. But intra-op phenylephrine may be less benign that we think.—**Editors**

- Junior anesthesia and non-physician providers tend to think that giving ephedrine and phenylephrine "solves" their low blood pressure problems. Wrong. All those drugs do is give you a few moments *to begin to think about* what is going on. Solving the problem involves figuring out the source of the low blood pressure—hypovolemia, too much anesthesia, etc.—and fixing that.—**CM**

- The pressors work better together. Ephedrine+phenylephrine for serious hypotension. Epinephrine is your friend.—**SMF**

- Speaking of epinepherine, if you trained at Hopkins during the 1980s and 1990s (and a lot of the *Anesthesia Bridges* editors and authors did!), you were taught that your standard of array of "purple" drugs included phenylephrine 100 mcg/cc, ephredrine, and two dilutions of epinephrine, 10 mcg/cc and 100 mcg/cc. The phenylephrine and ephredrine came pre-mixed in your drug bag but you had to mix up the epinephrine syringes on your own. We can remember a particular faculty member telling us "As you go through your practice years, you might encounter people who don't routinely draw up epi and who don't think you should draw up epi for every case. I advise against this lapse—you may find that you only need it once every two years, but when you need it, you need that and only that and you need it in two seconds."—**Editors**

- I am one of those Hopkins trainees and I agree! "Peds epi" (10 ug/cc) is an extremely useful medication.—**RSB**

- However, I don't draw it up for every case. Instead, I check before every case to be sure that the epi and atropine boxes (with the bristojets) are in the cart and thus immediately available.—**RSB**

- Phenylephrine and ephedrine can also cover up a multitude of early severe problems—occult bleeding, anaphylaxis, pulmonary embolism, and so forth. So, if you are going to be in your other room, set some limits on how much your team members can give before calling you.—**Editors**

- When I was a new trainee, I had an attending that wanted to be notified if I felt I would need to give more than 300 mcg of phenylephrine in quick succession. I asked why, and they related a story of when a previous resident years earlier had given an entire syringe without realizing the patient had developed a tension pneumothorax.—**CM**

- Avoid excessive phenylephrine because it has a ceiling effect. When you've reached it, you may be too late to find a syringe of more powerful meditation like norepinephrine.—**MN**

- Phenylephrine is not that benign a drug in all circumstances! It has been associated with post-op AKI, and the detrimental effect seems to be dose-related in terms of both the amount and duration of phenylephrine administration, especially when given in an infusion. We understand that some of the ERAS protocols called for fluid restriction but don't take that too far. Hypotension is a risk factor for all sorts of poor outcomes, and if you can't lighten the anesthesia plane, sometimes you just need volume.—**Editors**

- Norepinephrine is your friend always. Balances the effects of anesthesia on the cardiovascular system. Great for the right heart when perfusion pressure is critical. Increase contractility and after load. This means life!—**MN**

- Acidosis can impair the β-adrenergic response to β agonists. On a contrary, vasopressin has been reported to retain vasoconstrictive activity in the setting of acidemia.—**KAM**

- Don't forget that calcium has inotropic and vasopressor effects.—**KAM**

- Be aware of new agents! One very useful one in particular is Giapreza (angiotensin II) for refractory vasoplegic shock—**RSB**

- The thinking about everyday vasopressors for pregnant patients has undergone an interesting evolution. Initial studies showed greater vasoconstriction of blood vessels feeding the placenta with phenylephrine, compared to ephedrine. This led clinicians to preferentially use ephedrine. The next round of studies assessed fetal pH. These studies found the beta agonist effect on the fetus led to greater fetal metabolic requirement and lower umbilical artery pH at birth. Thus, clinician practice shifted to phenylephrine over ephedrine. The next round of studies is investigating norepinephrine. I don't suspect norepinephrine will become the standard because it really should be administered through a central line.—**BMT**

Antihypertensive Agents

- Know the true baseline BP of your patient before any surgery.—**KAM**

- Hypertensive patients can be thought of as functionally volume contracted. Under anesthesia, the vascular capacity changes, and of course the patients can get very, very hypotensive. Don't overcorrect with meds and get into chasing the numbers up and down. Every senior anesthesiologist will have a philosophy on how much and how fast to treat hypertension. You don't have to practice very long before you understand that hypotension can cause as much acute trouble and perioperative morbidity as hypertension.—**Editors**

- One of my mentors wasn't too big on labetalol. Her point was if you want alpha blockade, give an alpha blocker; if you want beta blockade, give a beta blocker. She was primarily a cardiac anesthesiologist, so this makes sense.—**CM**

- Be cognizant of fluid from nicardipine and esmolol drips (e.g., nicardipine 15 mg/h = 150 mL/h). Start oral blood pressure medications sooner to wean these agents.—**RVN**

- Common blood pressure medications tips: captopril:lisinopril is 5:1 so would recommend starting at least 12.5 mg TID. Amlodipine can take at least 24 hours to see a clinical effect.—**RVN**

- Taking care of a hypertensive pregnant patient for non-OB surgery? Don't be shy about calling up your OB anesthesia colleagues for a quick review of what they would use before initiating care. There is no reason to be abashed by doing this. Do it if you need to!—**CM and BMT**

- For parturients who are hypertensive we transition to labetalol and hydralazine as soon as they are admitted to the hospital. Typically, poor blood pressure control is an indication for induction, so these patients don't sit at home with poorly controlled hypertension very long. Home antihypertensive treatment is typically oral labetalol, nifedipine, or hydralazine.—**BMT**

- ACEIs and ARBs are contraindicated in pregnancy. Methyldopa was previously used but is not as efficacious. Atenolol and propranolol are usually avoided. Beta-2 agonists provide tocolysis. Therefore, beta blockade may promote uterine irritability. Thiazide and loop diuretics are usually not used due to concern they will alter maternal physiology and decrease placental perfusion. The exception is loop diuretics for parturients with heart failure.—**BMT**

- Of all the serious medication mishaps I have seen, it feels like about half of them were with sodium nitroprusside, either given from a syringe or due to failure to control the drip. I had attendings who didn't allow it to be drawn up until needed.—**CM**

- I once saw such a bottoming-out of blood pressure due to sodium nitroprusside that CPR had to be done to get some circulation. I've also seen inadvertent sodium nitroprusside administration chased by too much epinephrine and the patient develop cardiac ischemia. Remember, it's a short-acting drug. Give just enough to temporize and then apply tincture of time.—**CM**

- Remember, nitroprusside for pregnant patients is not used due to the concern of fetal cyanide toxicity.—**BMT**

***Note from the Editors:** Here is another beautiful photograph that shows the structure not only bridging the water but also bridging the marsh and the sky (Fig. 155.6).

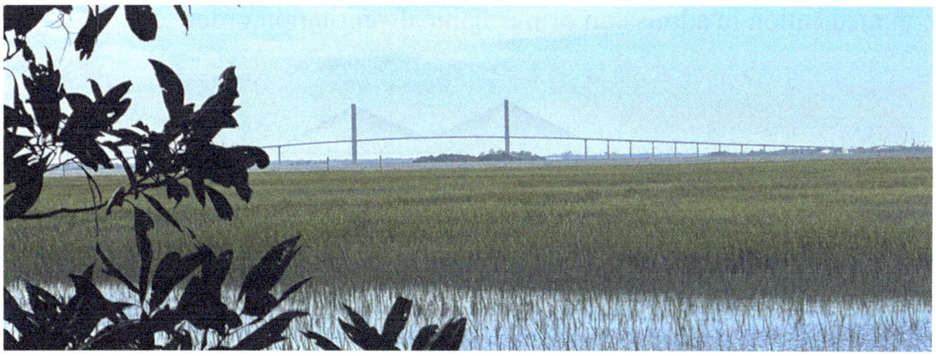

Fig. 155.6 The bridge at Jekyll Island, Georgia spans the Brunswick River and is officially named the Sidney Lanier Bridge. Photo: Harriet Little Chen

Antibiotics

- Remember that antibiotics were often initially developed as chemotherapy agents and the other way around. Makes sense, right? It's all about killing cells. These are incredibly potent and even dangerous drugs, which we tend to lose sight of because they have been around a long time and are in such widespread use. You are using them only because the problem you are trying to address is even more dangerous to the patient than the antibiotics are.—**CM**
- Choosing the initial antibiotics and dosing can be challenging—institutional guidance may be helpful. Otherwise, reach out to the pharmacy for help.—**RVN**
- Communicate with the surgeon for the appropriate timing of initial antibiotic dosing, especially if cultures are needed first.—**KAM**
- Don't forget to appropriately re-dose your antibiotics intraop.—**KAM**
- Stopping antimicrobials is just as important as starting them.—**RVN**
- Don't forget to start postop antibiotics and add stop dates to antibiotics.—**RVN**
- Cefazolin and vancomycin is not always the correct answer.—**KAM**

Stress Ulcer Prophylaxis

- Consider the risks of proton pump inhibitors. Could trickle feeding provide the protection instead?—**RVN**
- Stress ulcer prophylaxis is not needed on every newly admitted patient on mechanical ventilation, although it is often ordered on admission order sets.—**RVN**
- Be careful not to add a histamine-2 receptor blocker, for example, famotidine, ranitidine, and/or cimetidine, to a patient's home proton pump inhibitor for stress ulcer prophylaxis. As noted by RVN, it is a common medication in admission or mechanical ventilation order sets.—**LMO**

Miscellaneous Medications

- Oxygen is a medication! It's the most important and powerful medication we have. What other medication does (almost) every single patient get?—**Editors**
- Blood is the other most important medication we have! It has tremendous consequences and implications as a pharmaceutical, including immunological and potential infectious effects.—**CM**

- We noticed that anesthesiologists generally have command of our medications that have dosages, routes of administration, side effects, etc. But we don't have such great command of perioperative medications that have their own "physics"—such as oxygen, helium, and nitrous oxide.—**Editors**

- Then there are the medications that are ions—calcium, potassium, sodium, magnesium, and lithium are ones that you will regularly encounter in the perioperative period. Do you have a spot for each on your study spreadsheet? You should!—**Editors**

- We have noticed that parents will put their kids on just about any "medication" regimen if the child has something really serious or otherwise not curable or treatable. Who can blame them? These parents are panicked and desperate. Never show blame or judgment, but make it clear that you do need to know.—**Editors**

- Right now, there are about 150 monoclonal antibody (MAb) medications that have been approved by the FDA. It's a gigantic drug class. We advise you to know the ones that increasing numbers of people are on. For instance, MAbs including rituximab, reactivate hepatitis B in chronic carriers or patients with previous exposure and significant liver damage including fulminant hepatic failure has been seen [10]. This might be relevant information to perioperative provides both in the OR and the ICU.—**Editors**

- Street drug abuse, encompassing a diverse spectrum of substances, constitutes a pandemic. Managing anesthesia under these circumstances can indeed present a significant challenge.—**KAM**

- The more complicated the "regimen" of street drugs the patient is on, the less complicated your regimen should be. It might be out of fashion now, but I think this is a situation that calls for an opioid-based anesthetic plan with a short postoperative period of intubation. The opioids smooth out the hemodynamics, treat the pain issues that the chronic users of multiple substances often have, and help facilitate tolerance of the ETT while still intubated. I admit, maybe a bit out of style, but I've done it successfully hundreds of times. I don't think this the time to do a complicated regional technique on a heavily intoxicated patient. The only time I ever saw an anesthesiologist assaulted by a patient was when somebody was trying to do a block on a patient who was toxic due to methamphetamine use. The answer, in that case was the fentanyl syringe, I think. Allows time to sleep off the street drugs.—**CM**

- Regarding tox screens, they should be objectively determined based upon *a priori* rules for testing based upon risk factors. This can be an area where implicit bias comes into play and you have guard against this.—**BMT**

- I am rarely involved in neonatal resuscitation. Intoxicated mothers are definitely more likely to have a depressed fetus at birth, higher risk of abruption, fetal drug transfer, and usually placental insufficiency.—**BMT**

- However, I have had to resuscitate and intubate several newborns when the NICU team couldn't do it. Drunk mother, drunk baby.—**CM**

- Higher doses of antiepileptics are not always the best choice (for 2g of levetiracetam). At some point, you need to add another agent.—**RVN**
- Prostacyclin infusions for pulmonary hypertension are very dose /patient specific. Do not guess!—**RVN**
- Anticipate future insulin needs when starting insulin. Don't be afraid to start an insulin drip. A sliding scale won't be enough in a diabetic patient with glucose in 200s and just starting tube feeds.—**RVN**
- DVT prophylaxis is important—dose according to risk, patient weight and local policy and start as early as possible. If there is overwhelming, worry about bleeding risk, run a heparin infusion and monitor anti-Xa levels.—**RVN**
- When starting warfarin, use an online calculator or discuss with pharmacy—whatever you do—don't guess.—**RVN**
- Know the medications that can interfere with oral contraceptives (OCs) and warn the patients if you administered them. OCs are CYP 3A4 substrates and their therapeutic actions will be decreased if a 3A4 inducer is added to the medication regimen such as phenytoin, carbamazepine, or St. John's wort. Sugammadex and aprepitant will also lower the effectiveness of OCs.—**KAM**
- Everyone is on GLP-1 agonists. Be aware of the latest ASA recommendations for the NPO status.—**KAM**
- Administering anesthesia to a breastfeeding mother can raise concerns. It's important to be mindful of medications that should be avoided or used cautiously in this context.—**KAM**
- Which are two of the most interesting drugs in all of anesthesia? Methylene blue and Rhogam. But why? Because they are the only drugs where the cause of the problem is the antidote.—**Editors**
- Once you have true mastery of our drugs, start thinking about everybody else's because we are supposed to be perioperative experts, right? I asked Carol Bodenheimer what two messages she wanted to send to the anesthesia community and here they are—first, so many of our rehab patients who are on baclofen just have listed as "muscle relaxation." But remember that the peripheral effects are due to baclofen acting as a GABA analogue at the central GABA receptors in the brain.—**CFB and CM**
- Second, for any anesthesiologist, who works in intensive care, or intensivist in general, I see so often that gabapentin is completely stopped in renal failure patients or even CKD. But if you read the recommendations, clearly, they state that the limitations of gabapentin based on GFR are "consensus" opinion. But abruptly stopping gabapentin can have significant mental health consequences. It also can precipitate seizures. Our practice is to cut gabapentin dosing by 50% and monitor for signs and symptoms of too high dose, such as somnolence or cognitive changes.—**CFB and CM**
- We asked Herb Chen, a long-time and steadfast friend of the anesthesiology community, what were his "favorite" drugs? His answers were calcium and calcitriol. He is an endocrine surgeon so that

makes sense, of course. I admit that I went to the internet to do a quick review on calcitriol—hadn't reviewed the vitamin D analogs in some time. And then I was all prepared when a family friend called the next day to ask questions about (the anesthesia for) her upcoming parathyroid surgery. Of course, she wanted to go over all types of hyperparathyroidism and the associated medications. So thanks to Herb for his prompt answer back to us.—**HC and CM**

Memorable Medication Mishaps

- Almost 40 million patients in the US receive anesthesia every year. The average surgical patient receives at least 10 individual medication doses per case by the anesthesia team, and many patients receive many more, of course. This totals up to hundreds of millions, if not billions, of times that drugs are given by an anesthesiologist or other anesthesia provider per year. *The vast majority are given correctly, accurately, and safely*.—**Editors**

- That said, serious medication mistakes can happen at any time in an astonishing number of ways. If you can think of a way to make a mistake, it can happen.—**Editors**

- We asked our contributors to go into their memory banks to tell us the most memorable medication mishaps that they have ever seen or heard of. Keep in mind that the examples below are the aggregate knowledge of many senior anesthesiologists, occurring over many decades. These are not every-day occurrences. We hope they shock you a bit and motivate you to continue to develop, deploy, and teach every conceivable strategy for medication safety.—**Editors**

  - Cis-atracurium drip for OR was delivered to a patient's bedside in the preoperative area and almost hung by a nurse (near miss).

  - Ketamine 500 mg/ml was given rather than 10 mg/mL in a trauma rapid sequence intubation—the patient coded.

  - We also know of a different case when an entire bag of ketamine containing 500 mg was accidentally bolused.

  - Augmentin IV was given rather than thyopentone IV for rapid sequence induction in a C-section with resulting overt awareness

  - Heparin 40 cc was given on induction of anesthesia for a CABG instead of 40 cc of fentanyl. Coagulation nightmare.

  - Pushing epinephrine at induction instead of lidocaine.

  - The bedside provider started succinylcholine infusion before the induction drugs were given (in those days we used sux infusions for tonsillectomies). Of course, awareness ensued.

  - Similarly, too large a dose of "defasciculating" rocuronium was given before succinylcholine, with rapid onset of loss of control of upper airway and panic by patient. Have learned to keep these doses to 3 mg or at most 4 mg.

- Rocuronium was used instead of succinylcholine for ECT.
- Sodium nitroprusside infusion 50 mg bag was left in open position during induction. Unresponsive hypotension (until the bag ran dry).
- A nurse was taking care of sedating a patient for an MRI without an anesthesia team. This was a nurse-sedation case, not monitored anesthesia care. She pulled vecuronium instead of Versed (do not know how) from a Pyxis. The patient died in the MRI machine.
- Rocuronium was pushed instead of lidocaine during a sedation in endoscopy.
- Sodium pentothal was injected into an epidural catheter. This had no effect.
- Digoxin was injected into an intrathecal catheter. This has been reported more than once and fortunately, this patient survived.
- A resident gave tranexamic acid into a spinal instead of hyperbaric bupivacaine. This complication was relayed as second-hand information. Apparently, the patient experienced seizures, required intubation, and ICU admission.
- Cefazolin was given through the epidural catheter instead of local anesthesia.
- Dobutamine was confused for lidocaine with epi and injected epidurally. The glass vials look similar and a tech had restocked the dobutamine into a box labeled lido/epi with other vials of lido/epi.
- The worst medication mistake, of which I am aware, was a medical malpractice case in which I acted as a plaintiff expert. It was a 24-year-old who got an epidural for labor analgesia. The anesthesiologist placed the catheter intrathecally and then proceeded to inject sodium bicarbonate into the intrathecal catheter. As I recall, he didn't do a test dose, he didn't aspirate the catheter, and when she screamed upon bicarbonate injection, he didn't stop. In this era (1992), bupivacaine 0.25% and bicarbonate came in 50 mL syringes, which looked similar except that one had a yellow label, and the other was green. At any rate, the bicarbonate left the women a quadriplegic.
- Instead of giving 50 mcg of nitroglycerin, the resident gave 50 mg. The problem lies in the fact that the nitroglycerin was kept in 50 mg vials. The patient's blood pressure dropped precipitously, but amazingly, they did not code.
- A patient received an entire dose of vancomycin as a push, which immediately produced severe hypotension, rigid chest, and inability to ventilate. Epinephrine boluses were required to correct the problems and avoid serious harm.
- A second case of a new resident told to "give antibiotic" who mixed powdered vancomycin in a 10 mL syringe and gave it in one push. It certainly appears that extra and careful teaching is warranted around perioperative vancomycin.
- Someone didn't dilute the esmolol by 100 and the patient arrested.
- I had a CRNA hang a bag of heparin instead of hetastarch during a bowel resection.

- A junior anesthesia resident asked the pharmacy to send up oxytocin (Pitocin) instead of octreotide during an abdominal endocrine case and hung it while the attending was inducing in his other room.
- A large syringe of a prostaglandin medication was almost accidentally given instead of protamine during a cardiac case.
- When a very new CA-1, I gave a vial of naloxone to a 25-year-old man (I didn't know it had to be diluted). He did not have a single issue from it but I wanted to die when I found out.
- Administering medications to the arterial line instead of percutaneous central venous line.
- The norepinephrine drip in the ICU was increased to 0.8 mcg/kg/min rather than starting a second agent.
- Norepinephrine hung instead of aminocaproic acid and run at 210 ml/hr before a heart case
- Three people were setting up for an emergency heart. One set up the drip, another programmed the pump, and third attached drip and opened the stopcock … without putting the drip into the pump and ran in the whole bag.
- A bivalirudin infusion was running during the cardiac case. A single IMED-style pump was behind the IV pole with six pumps mounted on the side facing the anesthesia team. There were several attending and staff handoffs during the case, and the single pump "got lost" behind the other pumps. There was profound coagulopathy post bypass, obviously never resolved. With the drapes down, the bivalirudin pump was discovered, but the patient died.
- Protamine was mistakenly given on cardiopulmonary bypass and guaranteed death. There are anesthesiologists who do not even allow it to be in the room while the patient is on bypass.
- Potassium infusion administered unchecked in a 5-year-old during heart surgery with anticipated cardiac rhythm result.
- Phenylephrine 2400 mcg plus glycopyrrolate 0.6 mg instead of 3 mg neostigmine in a 16-year-old patient. BP >300 mmHg and post-operative MI.
- Decadron infusion was given to an awake patient without warning and lighting their genitals on fire.
- An anesthesiology resident was intubating on the floor and put his syringes on the bed. The patient coughed and raised his head and shoulders for just a moment. The meds all rolled under the patient. An embarrassing delay ensued while he had to get help to lift the patient back up while the intubating meds were retrieved.
- I have seen every single severe succinylcholine event described. When I was a junior resident, my attending was doing a request case—the young adult son of a surgeon. The patient had a bradycardic arrest on administration of the sux. One second the heart rate was 60, then the next second 30, then 15, then zero. I'll never forget seeing the EKG tracing slide down to a flat line. Chest

compressions were done and fortunately he was young and healthy, and his heart started right back up. But later, one of my mentors was debriefing the case for me and said, always remember, just five little milliliters in that syringe rendered a perfectly healthy young man *not just paralyzed but dead.* This happened very early in my CA-1 year and was the event that really gave respect for the power and responsibility of using our drugs. We were in the OR but what if the patient had been given sux for an intubation in the ER?

– I have also seen a hyperkalemic arrest with succinylcholine as well. The EKG tracing on the monitor changed acutely and in the classic pattern and the patient arrested. Serum potassium was found to be 6.9. Subsequently, even when intubating on the floor with sux, I always asked what the most recent potassium was and if the patient had any degree of renal failure.

***Note from the Editors:** This interesting photo shows the integration of the architecture of a famous bridge in Portugal into the cityscape (Fig. 155.7).

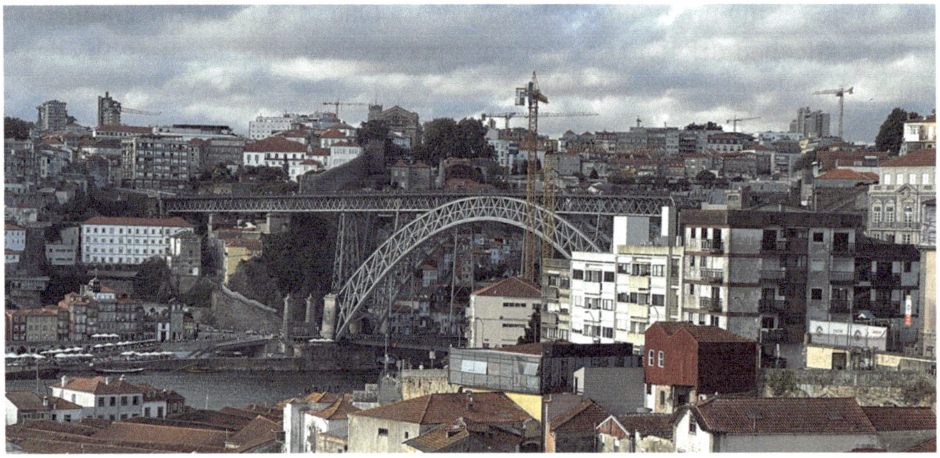

Fig. 155.7 A picturesque bridge over the Douro River in Porto, Portugal. Photo: Harriet Little Chen

Anesthesia Pharmacology for Medical Students —Issues and Opportunities

- Here are some thoughts for anesthesia educators when thinking about program development for the medical students. They are our future.—**Editors**

- As an early anesthesia trainee, I am intimidated by learning all of the pharmacology that we need for the OR, ICU, and pain and preop clinics, much more than the physiology knowledge that is necessary.—**SNF**

- We definitely did not have a lot of exposure to anesthesia drugs during my classroom portion of medical school. I remember a pharmacology lecture or two during our CV block that covered vasoactive agents, but nothing anesthesia-oriented at all. This seems sort of crazy, considering that around 30 million patients a year in the US undergo anesthesia for surgery or deliver babies with epidurals.—**SNF and Editors**

- During anesthesia rotations it was largely dependent on the resident/attending you were assigned to for the day and how much they were willing to teach, so it was pretty hit or miss. We didn't have any formal didactic sessions. We had an anesthesia interest group at my school that wasn't very active. It was mostly focused on helping students that had already decided to pursue anesthesia residency (application help, mentor connections) and less on introducing the anesthesia field to undecided students.—**SNF**

- Earlier exposure to anesthesiology in the classroom would've been great, but it is probably more realistic to intervene on the anesthesiology rotation. I think it would be beneficial if med schools would set up a didactic portion to the anesthesiology rotations. Even if that included some prerecorded lectures instead of live ones. That might make it easier to solidify some basic concepts in a more organized manner rather than only learning a couple scattered topics a day in the OR.—**SNF**

- At my med school, we were given outside reading resources to supplement what we were seeing in the OR but a regular didactic session would've been nice to have a space to ask more complicated questions than the OR setting would allow. Or even if we had been allowed to attend some of the already existing resident didactic sessions.—**SNF**

- Beyond just getting down all of the basic mechanisms, I am most interested in mastering the more specific indications for the drugs, such as the thought process of choosing between vasopressor agents. I would also appreciate help with common side effects we can expect after administration of the typical anesthesia agents.—**SNF**

Final Thoughts

- Remember that *movement is medicine.* There are countless and well-documented benefits of a physically active lifestyle that you have undoubtedly preached to your patients, but these are often overlooked by the same, busy, and often exhausted clinician that has touted its importance. Unfortunately, inactivity and its detrimental side effects will not discriminate between patient and provider.—**BCC and CFB**

- Exercise can and will look different for everyone, and there are numerous online videos and apps that allow even the busiest clinician to physically exert themselves for 20–30 minutes at a time, several times a week. Prioritize your own health by taking advantage of one of the most potent and easily accessible medicines on the market: *movement.*—**BCC and CFB**

More Pharmacology Wisdom from *Avoiding Common Anesthesia Errors, 2nd Edition*

There is a wealth of additional tips, teaching tidbits, and overall pharmacology wisdom in our previous book, which is nicknamed "Green2." *Please* check out this book and information and remember that every single penny of royalties goes to FAER in perpetuity!

Green2 Chapters with More Pharmacology Wisdom

- What Just Happened! What You Need to Know About Medication Errors
- Make Sure You Understand the Complex Medical and Legal Issues Surrounding Off-Label Drug Use
- Perioperative Beta-Blocker Therapy for High-Risk Patients Having Noncardiac Surgery—New Data, New Recommendations
- Should I Withhold or Continue Angiotensin Receptor Blockers in the Perioperative Period?
- Stop Metformin Before Elective Surgery or Intravascular Contrast Dye Study to Decrease the Risk of Lactic Acidosis
- Should I Administer Steroids in the Perioperative Period?
- Beware of the Bowel Prep
- What Drugs Require Slow Administration?
- Ketamine—Use It Well
- TIVA—What You Need to Understand to Do It Well
- Dexmedetomidine: Is There Such a Thing as a Free Lunch?
- Consider Chloroprocaine in Emergency Situations—It Is a Rapid-Onset Local Anesthetic With Low Systemic Toxicity
- Use Bicarbonate as a Buffer to Local Anesthetics—Especially for Skin Infiltration
- The Hows, Whys, Ins, and Outs of Succinylcholine
- Don't Get Burned by Incomplete Reversal of Neuromuscular Blockade
- Opioid Conversations—It's Not Only About the Table
- Not All Patients Are Naïve—Management of Perioperative Pain in Opioid-Dependent Patients
- The Basal Infusion Mode in Patient-Controlled Analgesia Is Both Friend and Foe
- Keep Discussing the Use of Ketorolac With Your Surgical Team Before the Need Arises and Keep Your Eye on the Literature
- Cardiovascular Vasoactive Drugs That Pump You Up
- Milrinone—the Not-So-Kidney-Friendly Intraaortic Balloon Pump in a Bottle

- Amiodarone and Alternative Anti-Arrhythmics—Double-Edged Swords for the Treatment of Atrial and Ventricular Fibrillation
- Ondansetron Is a Great Drug, We All Use It, But Watch Out for Headache and QT Prolongation
- A Word About Haloperidol in the Perioperative Period
- Remember That Not All Blue-Colored Compounds Are the Same
- Clonidine Considerations
- Drug–Drug Interactions Are Now Necessary Knowledge for the Anesthesia Provider and We Can Help
- The Six Patterns of Cytochrome P450 Drug–Drug Interactions Relevant to the Perioperative Clinician
- Don't Spend Time Rereading Tom Clancy Novels Until You Have Mastered These Basic Drug–Drug Interactions
- Drug–Drug Interactions and the P-glycoprotein Pump—Be Vigilant With the Patients on Digoxin
- Can You Name Six Drug–Drug Interactions That Involve Oral Contraceptives? Okay, You Can Now!
- Wish We Knew Then What We Know Now—A Case of Serotonin Syndrome in the Operating Room

References

1. Brenner JS, Mitragotri S, et al. Red blood cell hitchhiking: a novel approach for vascular delivery of nanocarriers. Annu Rev Biomed Eng. 2021;13(23):225–48.
2. Mikstacki A, Skrzypczak-Zielinska M, et al. The impact of genetic factors on response to anaesthetics. Med Sci. 2013;58(1):9–14.
3. Mottard N, Boulay G, et al. Paradoxical reaction to hypnotics in the ICU. Tanaffos. 2021;20(3):284–6.
4. King T, Ossipov MH, et al. Is paradoxical pain induced by sustained opioid exposure an underlying mechanism of opioid antinociceptive tolerance? Neurosignals. 2005;14(4):194–205.
5. Carron M, Veronese S. Atropine sulfate for treatment of bradycardia in a patient with morbid obesity: what may happen when you least expect it. BMJ Case Rep. 2015. epub 2015 Jan 29.
6. Smith RT, Gruber SA. Contemplating cannabis? The complex relationship between cannabinoids and hepatic metabolism resulting in the potential for drug-drug interactions. Front Psychiatry. 2023;13:1055481.
7. Kharasch ED, Clark JD. Opioid-free anesthesia: time to regain our balance. Anesthesiology. 2021;134(4):509–14.
8. Shah P, Stegner-Smith KL, et al. Front-loaded versus low-intermittent phenobarbital dosing for benzodiazepine-resistant severe alcohol withdrawal syndrome. J Med Toxicol. 2022;18(3):198–204.
9. Kessel KM, Olson LM, et al. Phenobarbital versus benzodiazepines for the treatment of severe alcohol withdrawal. Ann Pharmacother. 2024; Epub ahead of print
10. De Pauli S, Grando M, et al. Hepatitis B virus reactivation in patients treated with monoclonal antibodies. World J Virol. 2024;13(1):884–7.

Authors

Stan Alfaras-Melainas believes that as an anesthesiologist, you cannot excel in your craft without understanding the intricacies of pharmacology. As a mentor once told him, if you don't know the mechanism of action of a medication, it's best not to administer it. You must not only comprehend the dosage but also be aware of its peak effect, duration, interaction with other medications, and major side effects.

Brandon Togioka is a senior anesthesiologist at OHSU. He reads the pharmacology literature religiously and advises all anesthesia residents and trainees to learn the obstetric implications of the anesthesia medications *before* presenting to the labor and delivery deck.

Raj Nathwani is a senior trauma anesthesiologist at Harborview Medical Center, a hospital in the University of Washington system. He thinks a lot about pharmacology for his patient cohort, often while cycling the roads and hills of Seattle.

Tony Passannante has been at UNC Chapel Hill for 33 years as a clinical anesthesiologist working with vascular patients. He is married to Mary, who has also worked in one practice her entire career, and they have three children and two grandchildren. He wonders how such a basically logical person can remain a devoted New York Jets fan, despite empiric evidence.

Logan Olson practices in the medical and cardiovascular ICUs as a board-certified critical care pharmacist at Nebraska Medicine in Omaha, Nebraska. He received his Doctor of Pharmacy from North Dakota State University and then trained at Mayo Clinic in Rochester, Minnesota, for Post Graduate Year 1 and The Ohio State University Wexner Medical Center for Post Graduate Year 2. He and his wife are beyond busy with their three young children but get to the zoo as often as they can.

Cathy Marcucci is a senior anesthesiologist and transfusion medicine physician. Her favorite go-to medication has always been ketamine, but all the blood components are now tied for a close second. Her other favorite pharmacology fun fact is that she first met co-author Dr. Olson in an Uber heading away from Omaha's world-famous Henry Doorly Zoo.

Wisdom on General Clinical Practice and Clinical Excellence

156

Catherine Cooper, Mark Nelson, Ronald S. Bank, and Catherine Marcucci

Contributors:

Konstantinos Alfaras-Melainas MD MSc (KAM)

Daniel I. Asher, MD (DIA)

Edwin G. Avery IV, MD (EGA)

Michael S. Axley, MD (MSA)

Denis L. Bourke, MD (DLB)

John C. Briggs, MD (JCB)

Marlee Chamberlain, MD'26 (MC)*

Rose Christopherson, MD PhD (RC)

Benjamin C. Conner, MD PhD (BCC)

Niloofer Dalal, MD (ND)

Beth Darnall, PhD (BD)

Steven M. Frank, MD (SMF)

Many thanks to our (anonymous) colleagues who took the time to send us accounts of memorable positioning mishaps that they had seen or heard about.

C. Cooper · M. Nelson (✉)
Department of Anesthesiology, Virginia Commonwealth University, Richmond, VA, USA
e-mail: mark.nelson@vcuhealth.org

R. S. Bank
Department of Anesthesiology, INOVA Fairfax Hospital, UVA School of Medicine, INOVA Campus, Falls Church, VA, USA

C. Marcucci
Department of Transfusion Medicine, Clinical Center, National Institutes of Health, Bethesda, MD, USA

S. Mohamed et al. (eds.), *Anesthesia Bridges*, https://doi.org/10.1007/978-3-032-08294-7_156

Brian T. Gierl, MD (BTG)

Allan Gottschalk, MD PhD (AG)

Raymond G. Graber, MD (RGG)

Vincent L. Hoellerich, MD (VLH)

Theodore C. Houk, MD (TCH)

Deb Waterman Johns, BS (DWJ)

Caroline C. Koloski, BA (CCK)*

Kirk Lalwani, MD (KL)

Mark J. Lema, MD PhD (MJL)

Rajen V. Nathwani, MBBS BSc (RVN)

Logan M. Olson PharmD BCCCP (LMO)

Steven L. Orebaugh, MD (SLO)

Marcelo Quezado, MD (MQ)

LeeAnn A. Rhodes, MD (LAR)

Amy J. Robbins, MD (AJR)

Lisa L. Sandson, BArch (LLS)

Neil B. Sandson, MD (NBS)

Joseph M. Schwartz, MD (JMS)

Cobin Soelberg, MD JD (CS)

Brandon M. Togioka, MD (BMT)

Christopher A. Troianos, MD (CAT)

David Wallace, DO (DW)

Jonathan H. Waters, MD (JHW)

Jeanine Wiener-Kronish, MD (JWK)

Toby N. Weingarten, MD (TNW)

Bradford D. Winters, MD PhD (BDW)

Jessica Zvara, MD (JZ)

Jordan S. Zunder MBBS MSc (JSZ)

Introduction

The practice of anesthesiology continues to grow and evolve, and thus education in the art and science of our specialty must be a life-long process. There is an ongoing tension between wanting to make the case go as perfectly as humanly possible and allowing trainees to learn. We will all make mistakes in clinical judgment, management strategies, and even how we interact with our colleagues—and it is important to learn from these incidents and pass these lessons on to the people we mentor. An excellent clinician is one who understands the pathophysiology of his/her patient, has a well thought out plan, and can amend that plan on the fly as conditions change. The authors have compiled just a few additional tidbits to help both the student, and the teacher grow in clinical wisdom.

Basics

- Patients want state-of-the-art services, assured competency, altruistic intentions, integrity, accountability, honesty, objectivity, and compassion. In other words, treat them like you would want someone to treat your mother, grandmother, spouse or children. We are the ultimate service profession.—**MJL**

- **ALWAYS** have plan A, B, and C at minimum in your mind anytime that you undertake any critical clinical action, especially airway management. Have all of the resources needed for each plan available before you undertake the action.—**RSB**

- **VIGILANCE ALWAYS!** What gets people into trouble is that they aren't careful. And they fail to recognize system issues that compound into poor patient outcomes.—**Editors**

- Anesthesiologists are pretty smart. I don't think I've ever met or even heard of an anesthesiologist who wasn't bright. Cases go awry but I personally don't believe it's because people didn't know what to do. I think it's the lack of *something* but not the lack of knowledge that gets people into trouble.—**CM**

- I think trouble occurs because things run out or aren't available or aren't administered. You need a syringe of something critical, and you drop it on the floor and don't have a backup. Or you don't take an AMBU bag with you to the postoperative location. Or you look up and all the IV bags are empty. Or the CO2 scrubber is exhausted, or the sevoflurane isn't on when you thought it was. Or you think about putting in the second IV but then think you'll be okay without it. Or you really need a longer spinal needle but don't have one. There is a movement to eliminate waste and minimize costs in the OR and rightfully so, but this should be only up to a point. If you get a flash of intuition about something you need, believe what your experience is telling you and go get it or do it.—**CM**

- The best mantra I ever heard on what constitutes a successful anesthesiology practice: At the end of the day, *everybody* goes home safely It's not just the patient you are getting through a difficult case, it's also yourself.—**JZ and CM**

- Two things that need to be prioritized ahead of any therapeutic intervention. The first is safety—any safety consideration. The second thing to consider are what are the patient behaviors, characteristics, or other circumstances that will undermine an otherwise appropriate therapeutic. **JMS and Editors**

- Pick your battles! It's kind of like parenting and dealing with a spousal relationship. You don't need to fight about every little thing; you need to choose the most important aspects of patient care and stand your ground with a surgeon or the nurses. For things that do not harm the patient and patient care and the outcome—step down, let the surgeon or staff have the bone.—**AJR**

- Remember that you can collaborate, instruct, teach, and guide but you can't make somebody be a better or more careful clinician than they want to be.—**CM**

- When faced with a clinical decision that has a more and a less conservative option, chose the more conservative one.—**RSB**

- Don't be lax in following protocols and guidelines, be they ASA or institutional ones. Be consistent. You don't want to be the one that the surgeons, RNs, and everybody else goes to doctor-shop knowing that you'll bend NPO or other important policies.—**RSB**

- There are two kinds of anesthesiologists. Those that know and care about what is happening on the other side of the drapes, and those that don't. The first kind delivers better care. Which kind are you?—**SMF and Editors**

- Sometimes you will be pressured by the OR staff to proceed with a case. In those situations, I remember that the decisions I make can change someone's life forever. That thought makes me at ease to say no.—**MQ**

- When taking care of patients, look for ways to be efficient in your care. Turn the oxygen on first so that you start delivering oxygen as you apply the mask instead of applying the mask and then turn on the oxygen. Turn the monitor on first, to allow it to boot up, as you are connecting the monitoring devices so that it can start collecting data sooner.—**DW**

- Do not try to minimize or "sweep under the rug" clinical errors which you may have committed, accept them as learning opportunities. And don't be afraid to share mishandled clinical situations you have been involved in during your career with your trainees or junior staff, as these narratives can be very helpful learning tools.—**EGA**

- Have the same basic set up for every single case and just build on it depending on the complexity of the case. Have a mnemonic so that you don't forget anything. Don't shortchange yourself (and by extension your patient), especially for that quick remote case far from the OR and far from trained help. By doing so, in an emergency, you'll know just where to reach for what you need and, if alone in a remote case, you can just point to what's needed and ask the staff to hand it to you instead of their trying to search for something in your cart.—**RSB**

- Assure yourself that your vaporizers are completely filled at the start of every day. It's the money in your anesthetic bank.—**Editors**

- A colleague of mine once said (when challenged on something clinical), "I had a difficult decision to make, and I made it." In other words, we are paid for our judgment under stress. Don't be afraid to use it. It's what you trained for and what you spend your career developing and refining.—**CM**

- We all make mistakes, and errors will happen. Start learning how to deal with both by understanding and studying the difference. Mistakes are decisions that turn later to be wrong, especially when you are not satisfied with the outcome of these decisions. Errors occur when your decisions are compared to a set of rules. Remember that simulators were invented to teach decision science, grab ALL the time there that you can.—**Editors and EGA**

- If the PACU and ICU nurses are jockeying a bit to get your patients, you are probably doing a pretty good job.—**SMF**

- Always realize that anesthesia is a very humbling field. Don't get cocky. Don't get complacent. The risk that you take is not your risk, but that of your patient.—**RSB**

- Don't try to make history. You are not going to Stockholm, so don't even try. Just simplify the basics to the point that you can do them safely and reliably for the patient and everybody else.—**Editors and MC**

- Truth is like the sun. You can shut it out for a time, but it ain't going away.—**Elvis Presley**

- This is the only book in the history of anesthesiology to quote Elvis Presley. But what he said is true. **The truth always comes out**. Never hide or try to obscure a clinical fact or something that happened. *Never* alter the medical record, it's wrong to do that and is usually found out. Never portray a situation, patient, person, or yourself as more or less or better or worse than is really the case. Look directly at the facts and tell the truth. In clinical care, there is no fake it 'til you make it. That's a recipe for bad things happening to the patient. Plus, anesthesiology is too small a community for that type of shenanigans in either the personal or professional levels.—**Editors**

- It's not what you can "get away" with, it's what you can defend.—**RSB**

- *Work is for the details and home is for the big picture*. Meaning, focus on the small things and details at work but only the big things at night when you get home. During the case, concentrate on whether there might be ketones or glucose in all that nice clear urine and whether the IVs are in the right place to make it easy for the ICU nurses and whether you can get the patient extubated not even one minute later than you want. But once you are home, you have to let all that go and concentrate on the big picture. Was the patient stable in the PACU and was the case free of all major and nearly all minor complications? That's what really counts. Because there are more cases tomorrow.—**Editors and JZ**

***Note from the Editors:** Speaking of focusing on the basics and the big things when you are home, this is our favorite photo in the whole book (Fig. 156.1)! Jessica Zvara is in the habit of taking her kids and her good boy Hobbes out to get a regular dose of nature and splash around in the creek by their house. Have you ever seen a more adorable dog getting in touch with his playful side?

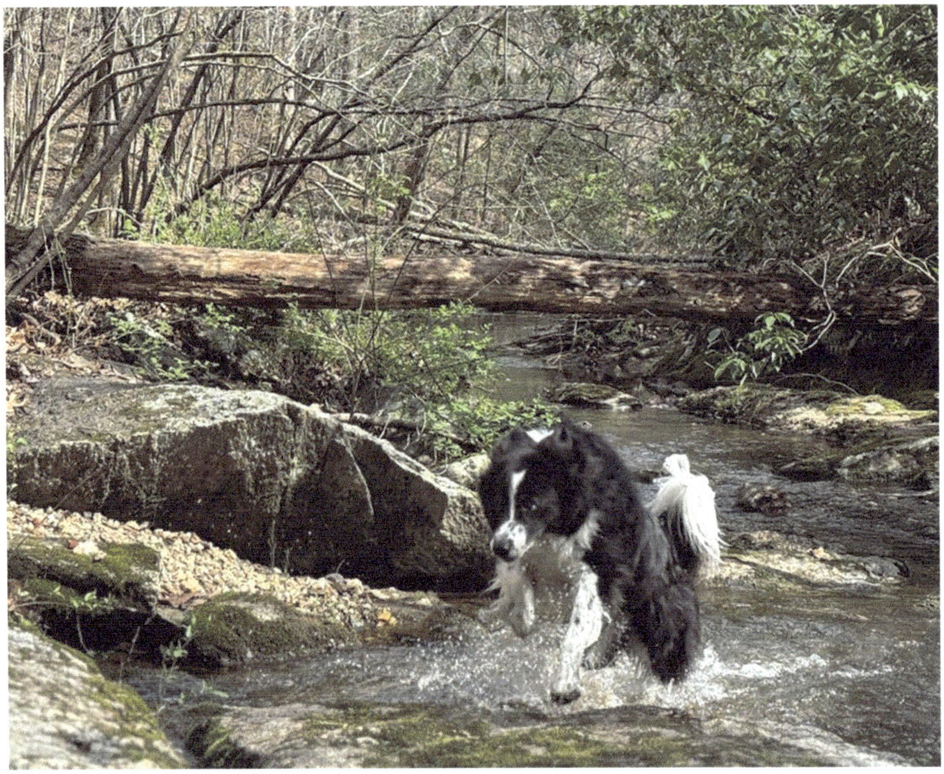

Fig. 156.1 We have titled this photo "Natural Log Bridge over Creek with Exuberant Dog." Hobbes joined the family when he was rescued from a shelter. Photo: Jessica Zvara

- Good information leads to good decisions. So don't just guess, suppose, or assume. And once you have made your decision, don't start disagreeing with yourself. That often leads to a second-best course of action—**Editors**

- Got a problem or a possible area of conflict? Always look to shed light, not heat. If you do have to shed some heat on something important, don't allow yourself to use an angry tone of voice. And always say "thank you" at the end of whatever difficult statement you have just had to make.—**NBS and CK**

- Make all parts of the case match each other. Surgeons have a big case; you have a big case. Big vascular surgery means big vascular access. Slow (difficult) to intubate means slow (careful) to extubate. Think the patient may have had cardiac ischemia? They need a formal rule-out postop.—**CM**

- Remember that tolerance is not the same as acceptance. You are surely going to have to tolerate some things in any job and practice location but that does not in any way mean to have to accept and adopt it. As it says in the song, don't confuse what you do with what you do to survive.—**NBS**

- To paraphrase the country music song, the operating room ain't a beer hall and it ain't a church. Do the very best you can do while you are there but don't lose sight of the fact that the goal, for everybody, is to get the case over with (safely) as soon as possible. No need for fanciness just for the sake of being fancy.—**Editors**

- Sometimes, the hardest thing to do is to do nothing.—**KAM**

- Seems like we review this for colleagues just about every other day, but it bears repeating—competence and capacity are not the same thing! The words are sometimes used interchangeably with each other and also are confused with the term consent, but they should not be.—**NBS and CM**

- Competence is a legal entity. Competency is assumed, it must be disapproved rather than proved, but never by a medical provider. It is a global decision determined by the courts and pertains to the legal right to make any decision on one's own behalf.—**NBS**

- Capacity is the possession of and ability to deploy the four key components of clinical decision-making. These are understanding, appreciation, reasoning, and expression of a choice. Capacity is what a valid consent is predicated on (with the assumption of a standing of legal competence) and always pertains to an individual decision. It is possible to have the capacity to consent for one procedure and not the next. Capacity to consent to surgery does not guarantee capacity to consent to anesthesia.—**CM and NBS**

- Review your institution's policy and descending list for substituted consent. And remember that consent does not always have to be given by a blood relative. Way down on the substituted consent list of the VA health care system is something along the lines of "concerned friend or neighbor." Not joking.—**CM**

- By definition, children, unless they are emancipated minors, never give consent. Rather they give assent.—**NBS**

- Evidently, still in this day and age, up to 30% of patients in the US aren't sure if anesthesiologists are physicians, roughly the same percentage of uncertainty for patients in Ghana and Saudi Arabia. Let's do everything we can to change that everywhere!—**Editors**

- "We don't get paid a lot of money to put patients to sleep, we get paid a lot of money to wake them up."—**David Sherer, MD**

- Remember that we are the last defense for the patient.—**KAM**

***Note from the Editors:** Speaking of defense, the bridge shown below is a 1950s reconstruction of the Old North Bridge in Concord, MA (Fig. 156.2). The bridge spans the Concord River. This is the location where the first shots of the American Revolution were fired on April 19, 1775, as the British guarded the river crossing and the colonists' militia advanced to guard their homeland. There have been at least eight reconstructions and restoration of the bridge in four different centuries. The current bridge approximates the 1775 bridge as close as records and drawings made possible.

Clinical Excellence

- Be a pilot. Be certain you can fly the airplane. There is an abundance of instrumentation in the cockpit, but none is more important than the skill of the pilot. Learn to use your instruments, but never become dependent on them to replace your vigilance, problem-solving skills, dexterity, intuition, and vision. Be a pilot.—**MN**

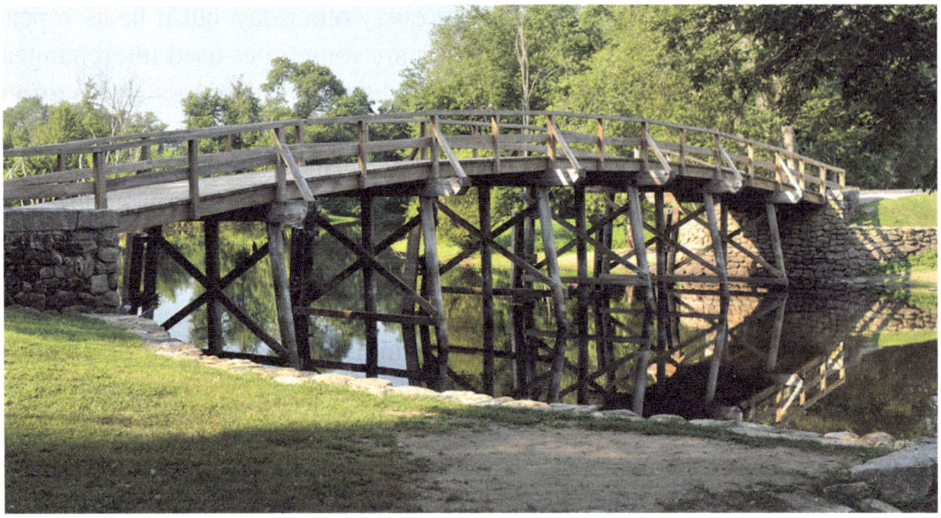

Fig. 156.2 Reconstruction of the Old North Bridge, Concord MA. It is not known who, or even which side, fired the first shot. Photo: nps.gov

- Be an artist. After all, we practice the art of medicine. Being able to read music doesn't necessarily mean you can play it. Be an artist.—**MN**
- Be the navigator who gets everybody through the shoals and around the sandbars.—**Editors**
- It's not how hard you work at increasing what you know and can do that counts; it's how hard you work at decreasing what you don't know and can't do.**—Editors**
- Being an excellent anesthesiologist first and foremost means being an excellent physician. And being an excellent physician means *being like* other excellent physicians and *being unlike* less excellent clinicians. And all excellent physicians work hard on retaining their basic medical knowledge. Never let the basic stuff in your first textbooks go, even if you let the textbooks themselves go and move your learning online.—**DLB**
- Excellence is a better teacher than mediocrity. The lessons of the ordinary are everywhere. Truly profound and original insights are to be found only in studying the exemplary.—**Warren Bennis**
- Excellence is never finished.—**Editors and MC**
- We've never known an excellent physician who wasn't an excellent communicator and a really decent person. Because we take care of acute and chronic patients from the cradle to the end of life, it takes a while to build a really robust anesthesiology knowledge base. While you are taking the time to learn our scope of practice, you can get yourself halfway to excellence by immediately commencing good communication and good person practices.—**NBS and CM**
- So, the basics of the practice of anesthesiology, such as basic airway management, including intubations and giving the everyday drugs, are not that hard to learn. Lots of people do it—nurses, assistants, paramedics, respiratory therapists, people in the ED, and even some military corpsmen and medics. However, we as physicians, can distinguish ourselves by not just the performance of these

clinical tasks but by our ongoing scholarly interests in them, our competence in managing the most advanced and complex issues and cases, and by continuing to strengthen our role as perioperative providers and consultants.—**RSB and VLH**

- The distances between specialties in medicine are decreasing and will continue to do so even as medicine becomes more complex. For example, medical and surgical oncology are getting closer in scope. Rehab medicine is moving into the ICUs. Anesthesia drugs are being evaluated and used for treatment-resistant states in psychiatry. Think about this when planning your career and research. I myself have a personal mission to merge my own two specialties—anesthesiology and transfusion medicine.—**CM**

- Lean into these trends, it is where our training as physicians counts the most. Stay up and brush up on the physiology, pharmacology, immunology, and genetics that underlie advancements in our specialty and others. See as many complex patients and do as many advanced cases as you can or keep abreast of the literature. Physicians need to be able to talk about medical and scientific topics that overlap with physicians in other specialties. Be available and front and center for our colleagues.—**Editors**

- I agree with the above advice! Psychiatrists talk to a lot of services, but I especially enjoy consulting with the anesthesiologists in my hospital system. They tend not to guess at things. They often send me their well-thought-out answer with a citation to a paper or the link to something in the ASA guidelines or APSF website. They not only tell us what to do but why. I am only half-joking when I say this should become the unofficial motto for anesthesiologists: "*We Tell You Why*".—**NBS**

- <u>Case in point:</u> I am a psychiatrist, and I have a lot of patients with PTSD and on prazosin. I had a patient who was concerned about taking their psych meds before going to the OR and how that would affect the anesthesia plan. So, I asked, the anesthesiologist who lives in my house. First, she reminded me who gave us the pharmacology lecture on alpha-1-antagonists in med school in 1988. Then she discussed that prazosin acts post-synaptically in the periphery and crosses the blood-brain barrier to act centrally. It is highly protein bound and exhibits a high first-pass effect. Kinetics may be altered in liver failure, renal, and heart failure. She recalled a few patients on it for pheochromocytoma instead of phenoxybenzamine but didn't think of it as the strongest available anti-hypertensive which is why people can take it for BPH and bad dreams and not pass out.—**NBS**

- <u>Case in point, continued:</u> Cathy was the medical director of her preoperative evaluation center for many years so she told me what questions she would have the preoperative clinic ask the patient (palpitations, chest pain, dizziness) and what she would use in the OR for hypotension or hypertension, depending on when the last dose was, given the short half-life of around 2–3 hours.—**NBS**

- <u>Case in point, final:</u> She also *absolutely insisted* that this depth of pharmacology knowledge is not special or unusual in her field for a five-day-a-week working clinical doc—and that any anesthesiologist who did not have this knowledge top of mind would be more than willing to review it and discuss at the soonest opportunity. Finally, she reminded me that sometimes what was old is new again in the pharmacopeia. Need I say more?—**NBS**

- Being an excellent physician comes down to simply putting the patient first. It's that simple. Everything else really follows from that.—**JCB, SMF, CM, NBS**

- Once a highly respected surgeon where I trained was talking about the best anesthesiologist he had ever seen. The lady he was referring to was not in a notable leadership position in the anesthesiology community. She had been educated and trained in China and was working at the old Loch Raven VA in Baltimore. I was highly curious about why this surgeon had such a great opinion of her. He said, "Because there was just no fooling around. Every word she said and every action she took was to in some way advance the case and the patient's well-being."—**CM**

- There are no small arteries.—**Editors**

- Don't tolerate corruption of the clinical standards any longer than you have to. If you see the clinical standards being mis-used or weaponized—rogue or malicious peer reviews and the like—start making plans to get yourself out of that situation. You don't have to die on that hill that instant but if the powers-that-be do it to somebody else, they'll do it to you. Sometimes you take a stand for clinical excellence by voting with your feet.—**Editors**

- Self-praise is no recommendation.—**Editors**

- If you do not stay humble, somebody else will do it for you.—**JCB**

- The trick is to be an excellent anesthesiologist and clinician without making your family and loved ones pay for it. If you can't be a good anesthesiologist without becoming a burdened, haunted, or troubled person, it's time to do something else.—**AJR and CM**

- The best physicians and anesthesiologists that we have known, and we have known quite a few, wear the mantle of their clinical excellence lightly. It's not a standard that they struggle to uphold and maintain. It's who they are, the way they go through life.—**CM and AJR**

- Concerned about that not-so-excellent clinician in your practice location? Of the 1.1 million professionally active physicians in the US, only about 4000–5000 undergo any type of state board action each year and many fewer actually lose or suffer suspension of their license. As a former peer reviewer for the state Board of Physicians, you will find that your "average or below" colleague will generally find a way to move forward, continue, and even flourish in their career and life, regardless of what you think and how much you shake your head. I advise young physicians to stay professional and courteous, don't comment unless directly asked or in the case of physician impairment or imminent patient harm, and look to their own practice, which is all they really control anyway.—**NBS**

- The always interesting existential question is whether it is better to be lucky than good—in both professional and personal life. This is actually a false dilemma between false equivalencies, as being good is volitional and being lucky is not. And it's not an either/or/than dilemma anyway. The real question is how often one or the other must prevail to be successful when both situations occur. Conduct your affairs such that it is only very occasionally necessary that you must be more lucky than good, but it is always the case that you are good when you are not lucky.—**JCB, NBS, and CM**

- What are the bricks of your bridge? Words? Publications? Teaching?—**Editors**
- We are a secret society. Enjoy the camaraderie because we've earned it.—**CM**
- Let your work sell you instead of you selling your work.—**CM**
- Always look far into the future. Your future happiness has so much to do with you and so little to do with what you are leaving behind.—**Editors**
- If you want to achieve (excellence) stop asking for permission**.—Unknown**
- Looking for a great practice location? Chase the vision, not the money.—**Editors**
- Patients pay their physicians for their trouble, for kindness they remain always in debt.—**Seneca**
- Need a little jolt of motivation to be excellent? Spend just five minutes reading the Wikipedia entries on these inspiring physicians that you need to know more about:
  - **Avicenna**—described as the father of early modern medicine, he was an Aristotelian disciple and wrote *The Book of Healing* and *The Canon of Medicine*
  - **Rabbi Moses Maimonides**—chief physician to the sultan of Egypt in the twelfth century, he wrote some of the most influential medical texts of all time including treatises on anatomy, physiology, diagnosis of disease, fever, surgery, asthma, diet, exercise, and lifestyle
  - **Rebecca Lee Crumpler, MD**—first African American woman to become a physician in the US, she faced crushing racism and sexism in the 1860s (Fig. 156.3). She practiced in Boston and Richmond focusing on the care of women and children in the African American community who could not otherwise obtain medical care or services.
  - **Dr. Samuel Freeman Miller**—practicing physician appointed to the Supreme Court by Abraham Lincoln in 1862. He lived in a devastating time and didn't always get it right. In the end, his best judicial action was authoring the unanimous decision in *Ex Parte Yarborough* that held that the federal government had broad authority to protect voters of color from violence.
  - **Walter Reed, MD**—lead the team that confirmed that yellow fever was transmitted by mosquitoes; he always refused to accept the accolade of "beating yellow fever", correctly crediting Cuban physician Carlos Finlay for theorizing that yellow fever is transmitted by a mosquito species.
  - **Dr. Gerty Cori—**first US woman to win the Nobel Prize in Physiology or Medicine for her work on glycogen metabolism; in spite of her groundbreaking work, she was sometimes offered positions as a laboratory assistant by the institutions that employed her husband.
  - **C. Henry Kempe, MD**—Holocaust-era and *kindertransport* survivor and US immigrant, he was the first to formally identify, recognize, and describe child abuse, publishing *The Battered Child* in 1962.

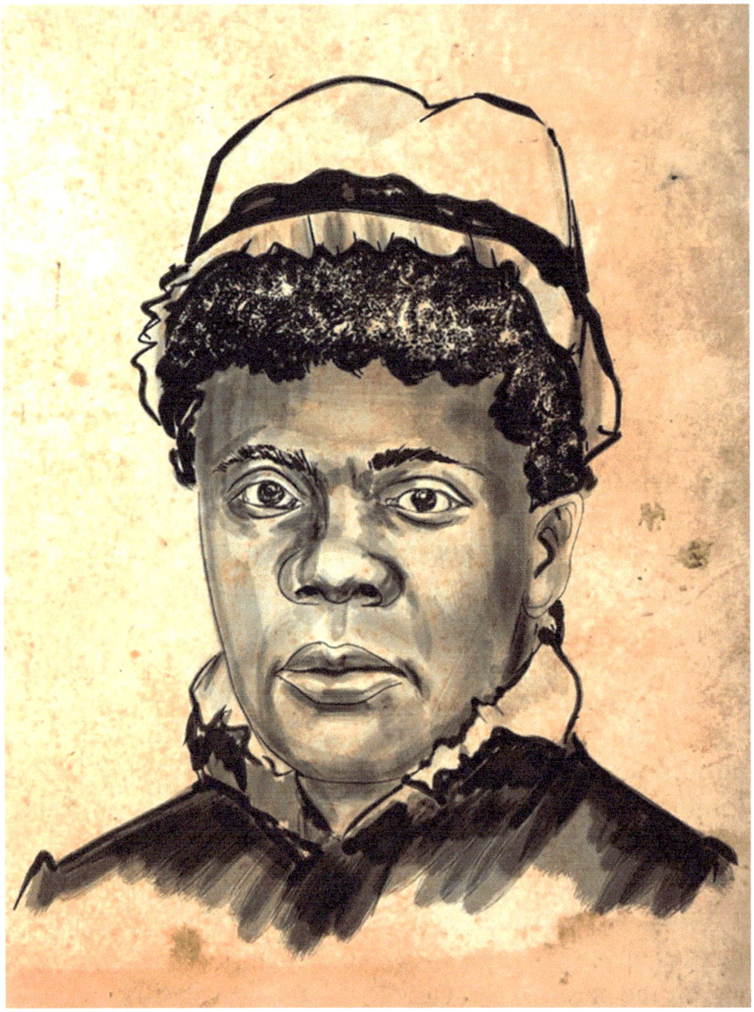

Fig. 156.3 Rebecca Lee Crumpler, MD graduated from New England Female Medicine College in 1864, which later became the Boston University School of Medicine. She was one of the strongest and most stalwart physicians in the history of American medicine. There are no known photographs or acknowledged portraits of her, but she was known for her intelligent eyes and direct gaze and probably looked a lot like the great-looking lady above. Photo: Image used under standard license from Shutterstock.com

Day-to-Day Clinical Life

- It is every physician's and anesthesiologist's job to protect the patient from the other consultants, himself, and us.—**TCH and Editors**
- It is rare to see a proper or effective mask airway done by anybody but the anesthesia team. If you arrive at a clinical situation where the providers have supposedly been masking a patient, just assume they haven't.—**CM**
- In the delivery room, watch out for neonatal "resuffocation"—when the pediatricians smother the newborn with the mask.—**CC**
- The cords are (almost) always up there in the middle somewhere.—**CC**
- If you put the endotracheal tube in the esophagus in the ED, leave it in and aim it someone else.—**CC**

- After a failed intubation, you can mask the first time and maybe the second, but you'll be very lucky to mask the third time.—**CC**

- Avoid tonsillar pillar pithing with Glidescope at every opportunity. Visualize and keep the stylet midline next to the blade until you see it on the screen.—**CC**

- Before extubation coughing is not breathing, after extubation, it is.—**CC**

- Spend some time listening to the sounds of and looking at the shape of vital signs. You will begin to recognize patterns that will alert you of an upcoming issue before that issue happens. I call this tapping into the AI in your brain.—**DIA**

- Don't ever assume that any bad physiologic data is an artifact. Be certain that it's not before believing that it is.—**RSB**

- In other words, always believe the monitor until you prove it wrong.—**CC**

- Bad sign in the EP lab or anywhere: BMI greater than EF.—**CC**

- If the lips are blue, the brain is too.—**CC**

- Perioperative delirium is the new perioperative renal failure or perioperative hyperglycemia. We mention delirium several places in the book, such as for pediatric patients or in the ICU, but the true incidence may be as high as 10% of all patients. It is associated with significant decrements in outcome, although still uncharacterized. Understanding, controlling, and minimizing delirium in patients receiving anesthesia is a great clinical and research area to become expert in.—**Editors**

- Excitement in anesthesiology is only good in someone else's room.—**CC**

- You know you're in a big case when you wonder if the blood on your hand is your own or someone else's.—**CC**

- You know you work in the OR when all your holiday decorations at home are packed in cardiopulmonary bypass pump boxes with handles.—**CC**

- Our job is to make sure the patient looks like a million bucks in PACU, even if they've looked like twenty cents for the whole case. You've done a good job if all they are talking about is the tape. You've done a great job if they are not even talking about that.—**CC and Editors**

- Anesthesia technique for apnea-prone 156 kg patient: "A little sedation and a lotta love." It's really true that we can be as soothing as what's in the syringe—**CC**

- Never hurry to extubate an obese patient. That extra 10 minutes you take could save not only the patient's life but years of litigation for you.—**KAM**

- Sometimes it is harder to cancel a case than it is to do it.—**KAM**

- If it's important to do, it's important to do right.—**CC**

- Learn from *OTHER'S* mistakes!! Read about bad outcomes and carefully review all articles that summarize data from the ASA Closed Claims Database.—**RSB**

- One of my partners frequently said: "Remember, you're coming to work. Your patient is coming to a major life event."—**RSB**

- "Sex, drugs, and billing fraud"—what a hospital lawyer said when asked what gets doctors in serious career-ending legal trouble.—**CC**

- Insanity is doing the same thing over and over and expecting different results! Each intervention or attempt should optimize over the previous.—**RVN**

- Keep the chatter to a minimum in the OR. I think it's a mistake to stand and the head of the bed and social chat with the surgeons during the case. Or even talk too much amongst the anesthesia team. Just about every time I ever saw a patient buck due to too little NMB was when there was talking going on, and this includes the daily anesthesia teaching lesson. Remember from Mitch Robbins' essay in Chap. 120 that pilots very rarely sit in the cockpit and chat.—**CM**

- One of *the best* ways to rapidly treat hypotension or hypertension is bed position—Trendelenburg or reverse Trendelenburg. It's effective, quick and immediately reversible.—**RSB**

- No IV or arterial line that you place in should ever come out accidentally—even if it gets hooked on the bed while moving. Learn how to properly secure your lines and *always* do so.—**RSB**

- You can administer IV fluids without giving any medications but not (usually) the other way around unless we are talking about medications in a block or spraying the airway. Therefore, practice scrupulous attention to what's in the bags and how it is given. Every bag visible, every bag labelled, every bag de-aired, no throwing the bags on the floor and counting them up later. That small 1-liter bag and intravenous line is what's keeping all 100 kg of your patient alive. You have to respect that.—**RSB**

- Knowing when to stop is as important as knowing what to do.—**RC**

- The smaller the patient, the larger the vigilance.—**KL**

- We once asked a senior faculty if he thought it was more important for beginning anesthesiologists to concentrate on mastering the heart or the lungs first. His answer was, "Neither! *First master the neck!*" Because, think about it, there is a lot going on for the anesthesiologist in that very small amount of anatomic real estate.—**Editors**

- *The neck* is where the airway is and where the emergency surgical airways happen (which we should all know how to do). It's where the most important block for an awake intubation happens—the transtracheal block. It's where we do most of our central access. It's *the front door for the heart*, remember that in the old days, physicians diagnosed heart pathology by watching the waves in the jugular vein. It's also important for preventing heat loss and keeping the patient warm. Small amounts of trouble can have big consequences—a small amount of bleeding or subcutaneous air or even edema is a different thing than if the bleeding is on an extremity. It's critically important in positioning—it's the one way to move a trauma patient in the field and kill them. Then there are the sleep apnea issues, which we feel are underdiagnosed and underappreciated. The editors thank Luke Graber for donating his beautiful drawings to *Anesthesia Bridges* (Fig. 156.4).—**Editors**

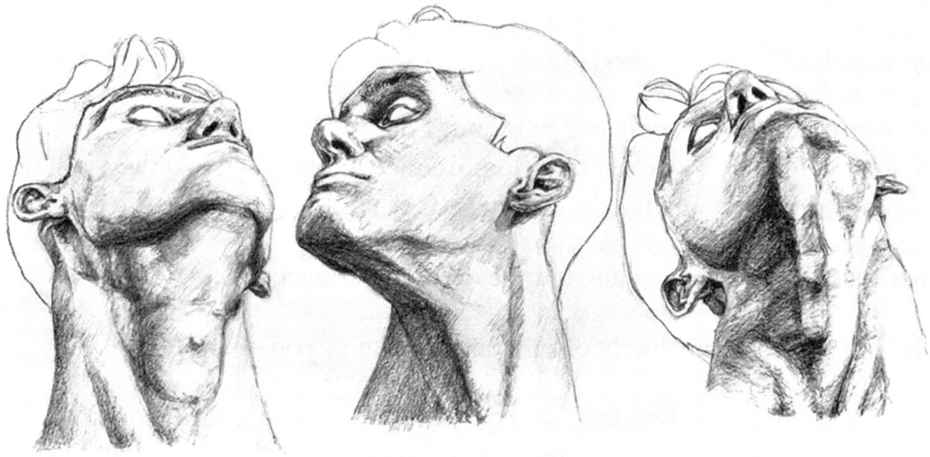

Fig. 156.4 These stunning and dramatic drawings of the human neck were done by *Luke Graber* in a figure drawing class during his BFA coursework

- The only people with more medicine than internal medicine are our friends in transfusion medicine.—**CC**

- The smaller the patient, the larger the vigilance has to be.—**KL and Editors**

- Pain service director on phone about request to the pain service: "I think it will be a lot easier to do it than to try not to do it." Moral—sometimes it's wisest not to delay or deny.—**CC and Editors**

- Report all needlesticks! Needlesticks in the health care setting have been associated with up to 20 different bloodborne pathogens. And incredibly, under-reporting continues to be a problem. If the number to report a needlestick isn't in your phone right now, get it before you leave work today.—**Editors**

- It is ironic because hepatitis B viral (HBV) transmission is now a greater risk to health care workers, even with an effective HBV vaccine, than hepatitis C virus. We are all HBV-vaccinated now, but there is a role for postexposure prophylaxis with hepatitis B immune globulin in decreasing the needlestick transmission rate. This is incredibly important as a number of the most important monoclonal antibody therapies, such as rituximab, are problematic in patients with a previous HBV seroconversion due to the possibility of viral reactivation and acute, even fulminate, hepatitis.—**Editors**

- I worked for many years in the VA health care system, where we certainly faced our challenges. My boss was Denny Bourke, and he told us that we could each pick one issue to try to fix and he would steadfastly support that. There were always 6–8 physicians in the group so in aggregate we had a pretty broad improvement portfolio but no one person was identified as a troublesome rocker of the boat. The public health systems are indeed like aircraft carriers, gigantic and a world unto themselves. And you can only redirect them one degree in either direction. Over time, that course change gets you to an entirely new longitude and latitude.—**CM and DLB**

- It's important to have a thorough knowledge of the literature, not so much to use it as a weapon but to have it on hand as a defensive strategy against attacks. Maybe carry one or two of the most important papers with you?—**DLB**
- I believe whole-heartedly in the evidence base, but I don't think it's possible to be a really excellent clinician or teacher without the spoken tradition. Be nice to everybody so they will be willing to collaborate and confer and tell you what they know.—**CM**
- And remember that people believe data, but they remember anecdotes.—**CM**
- If a case report happened to somebody else, it can happen to you.—**Editors**
- Do not go into private practice thinking that you will see less complicated patients than in academic practice. I recently did the anesthesia for a knee replacement in a patient who had a BMI of 50.—**VLH**
- There are quite a few sick people in community hospitals. For one, many recent immigrants who have settled in less populated areas lack basic health care, and need surgery and obstetrical care and they often present with all kinds of untreated conditions.—**VLH**
- I will say that transitioning to private practice will mean that you will have to go faster than in academic settings, and especially if you are coming from the public health systems. That common thinking is definitely true.—**VLH**
- *All surgical fires are considered to be a never event.* Unfortunately, there are still around 500 surgical fires a year in the US, approximately the same number as wrong-site surgery. Several people die each year from OR fires and burns. About 85% of these tragedies involve the head and neck.—**Editors**
- Surgical fires require the presence of something that can burn, a source of oxygen or an oxidizing agent, and an ignition source.—**Editors**
- Can you name 22 fire substrates that can act as a fuel source? Degreasers, prepping agents, drapes, towels, sponges, dressings, tapes, gowns, hoods, masks, ointments, benzoin, aerosols, alcohol, mattress, pillows, blankets, ECG electrodes, hoses, tissue, GI gases, and bone cement.—**CM** [1, 2]
- Oxidizing agents include oxygen, nitrous oxide, heliox, and methane/GI gases.—**Editors**
- There's a good recent primer on surgical fires by The Joint Commission online [3]. The title is *Updated Surgical Fire Prevention for the twenty-first Century,* but there is really nothing new suggested that is not already known. The human factors pros tell us that personal vigilance should not substitute for systems improvement in eliminating bad outcomes, but in this case, it kind of does. Sigh.—**CM**
- Some studies show there is a binomial distribution for patients who litigate surgical fires and burns, less than 18 years of age and 40–50 [1]. We once talked to a malpractice attorney who said he really

dislikes defending these cases as "being set on fire is a club nobody wants to be in and my only job then becomes to argue the monetary value of the degree of disfigurement and disability." He recalled having to once argue that a badly burned child would still be able to ride a bike and how that contrasted with his youthful idealism in law school. Successful tort actions in these cases are almost always in the six figures.—**Editors**

- The same malpractice attorney, who wants to remain anonymous, told me that positioning injuries, while they may result in large monetary awards, are easier to defend in some ways. Nobody is ever okay to leave the OR with weakness or paralysis but there are lots of neurological conditions that arise "naturally" as diseases. For example, strokes are common in society, as well as multiple sclerosis and Parkinson's disease. People also understand that they might be weaker with age and to suffer some degree of visual loss. Burns are always a result of trauma—and nobody ever expects to be a burn patient.—**CM**

- Always leave the OR with volume available. Moving the patient can result in reduced preload from redistribution of intravascular volume.—**DIA**

- What to do about the tattoos and piercings? Chidi Ani and Andrew Neice did a great little chapter summarizing the issues for *Avoiding Common Anesthesia Errors, 2nd Edition.* I've gone back and forth but finally got to the point where tattoos were something I dealt with and piercings I didn't. You avoid tattoos when possible but if that's where you need to put your needle, that's what you do. I ended up fairly strict about removing all jewelry including body jewelry. I do wish people would consider their health and possible future health needs when they get these very large tattoos. I just recently saw an article that implicates tattoos in an increased incidence of lymphoma [4].—**CM**

- Try to learn or review one new thing every day, even when you are in the thick of the busiest part of your practice. Alternate between esoteric and every day anesthesia issues or between anesthesia and general medicine topics. Remember that we still have not solved a whole bunch of big things—anxiety, PONV, and pain. In Chap. 120, we described the differences in training that pilots undergo, an analogy for us to quickly review complicated material is "differences study." You are looking for the exceptions. So, what did I review today? Morphine is the opioid that undergoes metabolism a bit differently. Unlike the opioids that undergo Phase 1 oxidative metabolism by hepatic CYP450 enzymes, morphine undergoes Phase 2 hepatic glucuronidation metabolism by UGT enzymes.—**CM**

- Or if you only have 2 minutes to study or review, look at a single aspect of an ongoing clinical question. For example, ketamine vs. etomidate for induction and intubation of unstable patients is a topic open to robust debate. But does one predict for greater 7-day survival? According to a prospective study done in UT Southwestern's ICU, it appears it might be ketamine [5].—**CM**

- The best thing I ever published was to be a middle author on a piece in *Avoiding Common Anesthesia Errors, 2nd Edition,* Chap. 281. It concerns strategy and tactics if you should ever find yourself in a chart war that you haven't started. Cobin Soelberg and Jeff Kirsch were the brains behind the little essay because it tells you what to actually do. If you only go and read one thing in that book, read this.—**CM**

- Rule for remote cases—the most valuable resource you can take is another anesthesia provider, even if it's a case that is usually done with one person. If you can't double up on people, double up on the basic portable emergency equipment. The further away you are from the home location, the more important it is that you will be able to keep your patient safe with the really simple stuff—an AMBU bag, a red rubber bougie, propofol ready to draw up into syringes. Never overestimate how quickly somebody will be able to come help you if there is a failure with the anesthesia machine.—**Editors**

- The best anesthesiologists will tell you that they still hear the voice of their most important clinical mentors in their head every day. Whose voice do you hear? Call them up sometime and tell them.—**Editors**

- People who design anything—protocols, systems, fabrics, buildings, furniture—know that you start with the white or blank or open spaces or volumes and construct a frame around it. The white space in our work is the time between intubation and extubation. Everybody is focused and understands the challenges of those critical times. But it's the time *during* the case and what you do with it that is really important and keeps the patient safe. It can also be is a dangerous time because it's when breaks are given and what are breaks but miniature sign outs and handovers? The scariest serious events happen during the middle of cases—airway fires, pulmonary embolism, bad transfusion reactions or events, power outages, and medication errors. *If these things happen before induction, don't start the case!* When they happen during the case, you have no choice but to continue the anesthetic while dealing with the emergency.—**DWJ, LLS, CM, and Editors**

- This is also why most experienced anesthesiologists are not terribly big on reading in the OR. Please refer to *Avoiding Common Anesthesia Errors, 2nd Edition* Chap. 282 for more information on the subject. It's a more complicated than you might think. Keep in mind that reading generally falls under the category of "anesthetizing while distracted." Reading per se has not been shown to be a gigantic factor in anesthesia malpractice cases, but we know that minor distractions can have be a big factor in poor outcomes, not all reading is the same, and online activity can and will be tracked. Always be aware of what your practice location and/or insurer may prohibit. Our best advice? Read quickly if there is a need to know but never for recreation or personal convenience.—**MSA, CM, and Editors**

Preoperative Anxiety

- Anxiety is terrible for caregivers and providers to deal with. Anger fades, pain often resolves, but anxiety can continue to persist and percolate. And it can colors every experience and all perceptions. It makes decisions and compliance more difficult, and pain more severe. It's even transmissible, especially from parents to children. Think deeply on this subject and take a robust approach to mitigate it with every single patient.—**CCK, NBS, and Editors**

- Research has shown that 60–80% of patients experience preoperative anxiety. And an even greater percentage of patients have *perioperative* anxiety.—**CCK and NBS**

- There is nothing straightforward about the anxiety of surgical patients. First of all, the receptor profile and physiology are complicated. GABA and serotonin receptors play a major role, and glycine pathways and receptors play a major inhibitory role but there are multiple directing effects and cascading indirect effects.—**CCK and NBS**

- But it's important to realize that anxiety is actually a cluster of illnesses. What we lump together in two words as "perioperative anxiety" can actually be a result of or reflective of chronic generalized anxiety disorder, phobias, PTSD, panic disorder, agoraphobia, guilt, embarrassment, and shame.—**NBS and CM**

- Specific situational anxieties can be derived from fear of language and communication barriers in both pediatric and adult patients, needles, loud noises, pain, cold, loss of control, nakedness, intubation, neuromuscular blockade, cardiopulmonary bypass, intraoperative complications including awareness, being left unattended in the OR, being ridiculed while under anesthesia, transfusion, poor outcome,or unfavorable diagnosis, and a sense of letting down or abandoning family through illness or absence.—**CM and NBS**

- Patients very, very often feel guilt and shame about their weight and their teeth. Take pains to reassure the patient that they are not presenting you with anything out of the ordinary and that you aren't comfortable with. One nice thing to say is, "It's okay, you did the best you could" even if that is not strictly true.—**NBS and CM**

- Most patients can tolerate some distress and discomfort, what generally causes or increases difficulties with anxiety is *uncertainty*.—**NBS**

- Honestly, I've reached the point where I tell friends and patients that going into the operating room can be a bit like going into a busy commercial kitchen—a lot of noise and bright lights and people bustling about and high-grade stainless steel and metal equipment.—**CM**

- **Neil Sandson** once remarked to me that you could practically develop a psychiatric fellowship on the treatment perioperative anxiety, that is how multi-factorial it is—involving personal history, interpersonal and family dynamics, medication panels, talk therapy, and complementary and alternative medicine. But this is good in a way, it gives us a lot of areas from which to approach treatment. But the psychiatrists also tell us that we are unlikely to "solve" perioperative anxiety without solving some of the downstream causes—pain, PONV, etc.—**CM**

- Set aside the notation that any degree of perioperative anxiety is inappropriate. There is no situation in medicine where the patient is required to place as much trust in a care provider that they have never previously met.—**Editors**

- Anxiety is fluid throughout the perioperative period. What a patient is anxious about in the weeks and days before surgery is different from the preoperative area. Patients may also voice corridor concerns when they are no longer in the presence of family. Postoperatively, patients may become anxious about the surgical findings or result and the necessity of waiting for a diagnosis. Almost every anesthesiologist that I have talked to worries about being an easy and uncomplicated case. Twenty-eight years ago, I apparently was quite agitated on emergence and extubation after an infertility surgery and (I guess) basically tried to get off the table, although I have zero memories of it. I still feel bad and a bit embarrassed about it.—**Editors**

- We ourselves know that anesthesia is safer than ever and also that it is not completely safe. I've had anesthesia a bunch of times and I'm never too happy the night before even when the anesthesiologist is somebody that I've trained with and I know them to be an excellent physician. I once took care of a senior physician (surgeon) who broke down and sobbed in the preoperative area over the stress of assuming the patient role.—**CM**

- The early studies that "established" that a calm and reassuring anesthesiologist is the most effective factor in mitigating preoperative anxiety were methodologically flawed, but it's probably true, nonetheless.—**Editors**

- That said, it's very important for everybody to address preop anxiety as much as possible before the OR. And remember, patients who go to sleep crying, wake up crying.—**Editors**

- Everybody has their own style, but one approach is not to make the patient make their own diagnosis. Rather than saying, "Are you anxious?" ask them, "What strategies have you been using to decrease nerves?" Also *always* ask what meds—theirs and others'—they may have taken preop. This includes alcohol and cannabis.—**Editors**

- When I was working in the VA health care system, where there is more time, I would give my patients a checklist of the nervous-making situations listed above and have them tell me which ones were particularly bothersome for them. Sometimes the families would pull me aside and tell me what their view was.—**CM**

- An OR nurse told me once that she and her colleagues requested particular anesthesiologists for themselves and their loved ones based on how kind and calm and reassuring the anesthesia docs were, not how technically brilliant.—**CM**

- Most patients should, can, and do perceive preoperative benzodiazepines. Caution is warranted, though, and you should not just give everybody the same number of milligrams of midazolam. Remember that the very patients who may be most agitated preoperatively and pre-induction may be the most sensitive to the sedating effects, airway obstruction, and respiratory depression, especially patients of any age with cognitive deficits.—**CM**

- Benzodiazepines are metabolized by **CYP 3A4**. The list of 3A4 inhibitors is well-characterized—protease inhibitors, some macrolide antibiotics, ketoconazole, itraconazole, and verapamil. You would hope the possibility of prolonged benzodiazepines.—**CM**

- The complementary and alternative modalities—such as music, games, meditation, aromatherapy, massage, yoga, acupuncture—for perioperative anxiety are really interesting and quite efficacious. The trick is to determine what will work best for the patient—distraction vs mindfulness and self-centering.—**Editors**

- Don't forget to give the parents a way through their anxiety when their child is in the OR. Kids always pick up on their parents' emotional states when they are reunited postop.—**Editors**

- Anxious patients don't rehab well. Especially those with anxiety surrounding the injury/condition they are rehabbing for, as it will negatively impact their self-efficacy for improvement.—**BCC and Editors**

- Start postoperative anxiolysis in the PACU. I have been known to give benzodiazepines when I felt that only that would do the trick. Not often, but I have done it.—**Editors**

***Note from the Editors:** Our young friend and *Anesthesia Bridges* contributor Caroline Koloski was a psychology major, health studies minor, and pre-med student at North Carolina State University. She is now busy getting ready to apply to med schools. We asked her to find us a bridge that demonstrated serenity. She chose this lovely scene of sun, sky, and water, and shot the photo in the evening of the longest day of the year (Fig. 156.5). We love how the architecture of the bridge and reflection in the water is also mirrored by the curve of the railing.

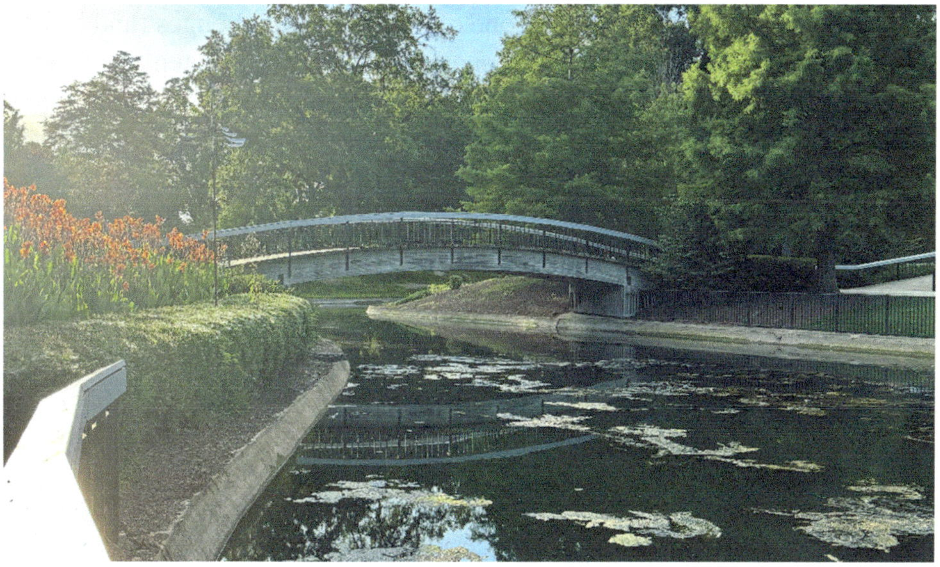

Fig. 156.5 A bridge reflection in still water in Pullen Park in Raleigh, NC, adjacent to the campus of NC State University. Photo: Caroline Koloski

Nausea and Vomiting

- Postoperative nausea and vomiting (PONV) are two of the most interesting perioperative physiologic responses we deal with in the perioperative period. Vomiting is a protective brainstem reflex experienced by most not all mammals. It is tremendously primitive as well as complicated and highly evolved at the same time.—**Editors**

- Vomiting is (almost) universally dreaded (and remembered). This is a bit weird because patients don't experience other protective mechanisms—sneezing, shivering, and even fever—with the psychological aversion that people have for vomiting. Pathological fear of vomiting is called emetophobia.—**NBS**

- As we mention elsewhere, PONV is one of the two things that everybody remembers about their surgery and perioperative experience. It is the "big little problem" of perioperative care.—**Editors**

- It's also hugely expensive. One small study in an outpatient setting determined the cost of PONV to be $1055 per patient. Even a one-hour delay in discharge from the PACU costs the US health care system hundreds of millions of dollars per year.—**Editors**

- Vomiting is extremely complex and is mediated by both somatic and autonomic nervous systems. There are two main areas of the brain that are involved—the vomiting center and the chemoreceptor trigger zone.—**AJR**

- Afferent pathways very often involve the gut but a wide variety of stimuli such as visual images, odors, motion, medications, and changes in body position.—**Editors**

- Remember that N/V can also be caused by occlusion of the coronary arteries, which are actually nothing if not tiny hollow viscera, correct? The first question to ask yourself when you have a nauseated or vomiting patient should be, "is this patient experiencing cardiac ischemia?"—**Editors**

- For my patients, the most important nausea and vomiting the serotonin and dopamine receptors have prime importance. But in palliative medicine, one of the biggest challenges (and learning points) is to figure out what is the cause of nausea. Is it a chemo drug? Bowel distension from constipation or tumor? We find the cause first then try to figure out the medicine that will hit it based on that. I advise a similar approach for all anesthesiologists.—**AJR**

- The efferent pathways involve the phrenic nerve to the diaphragm, the spinal nerves to the abdominal and intercostal muscles, efferent visceral autonomic nerves to the gut, and the efferent nerves to voluntary muscles of the pharynx and larynx. There is a prodromal relaxation and retrograde peristalsis followed by retching and expulsion of gastric contents.—**AJR**

- Nervous equals nausea! There is a huge emotional and psychological component to postoperative nausea and vomiting. Prevention starts before the patients goes to sleep.—**Editors**

- Prevention also means crafting an anesthetic plan that avoids medications highly associated with nausea and vomiting like nitrous oxide. Propofol has been suggested to mitigate the nausea effects of the volatile anesthetics. Remember that PONV also stands for "Propofol Overcomes Nausea and Vomiting."—**Editors**

- Multi-modal drug therapy can sometimes seem a bit kitchen sink-y. But treatment of PONV is one situation in which it is truly indicated. There are so many points to hit in the multi-factorial genesis.—**Editors**

- We recommend a rule of six for treatment of PONV—meds for 2–3 receptors, 1–2 complementary medicine techniques, the P6 acupuncture point, and the anesthesiologist's calm personality. I used to teach it as the "six for sicks" strategy.—**CM**

- Your medication options include anticholinergics, phenothiazines, antihistamines, butyrophenones, benzamides, serotonin receptor antagonists, steroids, pain control, anxiolysis, and adequate hydration. A single prophylactic does of dexamethasone may decrease PONV considerably, but it is not a risk-free drug.—**Editors**

- The P6 acupuncture is located in the center of the soft tissue between the thumb and forefinger. You can do it as acupressure or acupuncture either before, during, or after the case. It works quite well for some obstetric patients.—**CM**

- The complementary medicine strategies for PONV are really fascinating because they are inexpensive and have virtually no side effects. My favorites include meditation, visualization, breathing, peppermint, and music [6].—**CM**

Advanced and Emergent Care

- ICU management is a team sport—you can't win the game on your own. Use the expertise of those around you to get the best outcome for your patient.—**RVN**

- In a critical situation, *CALL FOR HELP EARLY*!!!! Your colleague(s) who are not as emotionally invested in the case as you will look with fresh and unbiased eyes and see things that you missed. Don't be threatened by this. They will also lend critically needed trained hands.—**RSB**

- Don't get lost in complex, critical care cases. The keys are, knowing and setting the correct priorities, anticipation, and compulsivity.—**RSB**

- All emergent patients need intensive care. That means that you need to plan to provide intensive care in addition to the usual anesthetic care, regardless of the amount of time that they have spent in one or more Emergency Departments. The same is true for inpatients and outpatients who are ASA 3 or 4.—**BTG**

- A pre-set series of treatments for an emergent patient can be helpful. A new clinician might start with a plan to place a central venous line, arterial line, and fiberoptic intubation—all while awake—while simultaneously infusing whole blood and appropriate vasopressors to support cardiac output. From that extreme, you can de-escalate according to the circumstances and be less likely to undertreat someone.—**BTG**

- An ASA 1 patient with a bad pathology can be very well compensated preoperatively and totally decompensate upon induction or during the case; don't overestimate the ability of a healthy patient with a dead gut, bowel obstruction and distention, an abscess, a crush injury, etc. to compensate due to induction or the evil humors released during surgery.—**BTG**

- The worst minute of being an anesthesiologist: push an amp of epi and nothing happens except your own heart rate and blood pressure increase.—**CC**

- Never draw a blood gas when the patient is purple. You already know what's going on and what you need to do *now*.—**CC and Editors**

- You know you're in the trauma rooms at night when you dash to the restroom at 3 am, wash your hands, and then drink water out of the sink faucet like a dog.—**CC**

- When Mike Tyson was asked by a reporter whether he was worried about another boxer's fight plan, he answered, "Everyone has a plan until they get punched in the mouth." This is really an update of an old military adage: "No plan survives first contact with the enemy." Why is this significant in our practices? The answer is that the unexpected can and will happen. You may be providing a text book anesthetic with railroad vital signs when a surgeon ruptures an aorta. So yes, it is important to have an anesthetic plan, but also to be able to quickly go to plan B and call for help if needed. And no, I am *not* saying surgeons are our enemies!—**RGG**

- The best monitor for severe hemodynamic instability is the trans-esophageal echocardiogram (TEE). If your institution has TEE, invest the time and effort to get the basic certification in it.—**RSB**

- In trauma or other mass transfusion cases, immediately check the lines to be sure that small bore connector tubing is not attached to your large bore volume line(s).—**RSB**

- Don't confuse a triple lumen catheter (TLC) with a volume line.—**RSB**

- In big cases, bad things happen when you are chasing something else, especially heart rate and blood pressure. It's so common to over-correct and give too much. Always anticipate which critical infusions might run out and have more immediately available, even if it makes the case slightly more expensive to do. Have a back-up bag for your most critical drip made up and ready to go.—**RSB**

- Bad sign: ECMO EtCO2 reads 666.—**CC**

- I'm a little leery of trying to characterize certain care paradigms based on blood loss, such as the questions of trying to determine which large blood cases are medically futile. We still don't even know the most reliable and accurate method to determine blood loss in a case, although the methods have been debated since the 1960s. I've done my share of massive cases, and I often could only estimate what the blood loss was to an accuracy of +/− five liters. All you can really do is work as hard as you can towards reasonable central filling pressures (one reason I like TEE for big non-cardiac cases), a reasonably low serum lactic acid, and a hematocrit somewhere in the middle. With not too much decrement in PaO2.—**CM**

- Think really carefully before your put your least experienced people in the eye room. They can be the easiest days but also the hardest days.—**Editors**

- The most difficult patient issue I ever had was with a patient who had a cataract and the person staffing the room decided to see how the patient would do with not one molecule of anything from a syringe. The patient was furious postop, and as the attending, I became responsible for handling the complaints, letters, and queries that went back and forth for weeks. And then secondly, eye cases are one of the very few places where routine surgical maneuvers can result in an instantaneous flatline cardiac arrest. Most other untoward surgical events result in bleeding that everybody can see and that gives you at least a few minutes to respond, not immediate death. I know of a colleague who was reading in an eye case and looked up and the monitor was flat lined. The surgeons were still operating unaware, thinking it was nice the patient wasn't moving much.—**CM**

Disease States

- Attributed to Osler; "Let me interview the patient; let the medical student conduct the physical exam; discard the lab results and I will give you the diagnosis. In other words, if you take time to listen to the patient *AND* you are well-formed on the matters of medicine *AND* if you ask the right questions, the physical exam and lab results should simply confirm your diagnosis.—**MJL**

- *Face your fears!* Admit (if only to yourself) what case worries you the most and buckle down and start figuring out how you will approach such a case if it presents itself to your OR. Our ability to handle the sickest and most unusual perioperative clinical situations is what distinguishes us from our non-physician colleagues.—**RSB and Editors**

- There are two types of disease states to deal with—those you know about and those you don't. *Always consider what the patient might have that isn't on the preoperative evaluation.* I myself have picked up significant aortic stenosis several times. Once, based on my preop exam, the patient went for a new valve instead of abdominal surgery. Another time, a junior person found an uncharacterized machinery murmur. He asked me for advice; I advised cancelling for a workup and new valve if necessary. The younger person decided to go ahead the next day. The patient died in the OR.—**Anonymous**

- Talk to your colleagues ahead of time about your own personal hypothetical scariest case. Your goal is to reduce scary to wary.—**CM**

- For me, the biggest concern has always been and will always be airway, airway, airway! When you lose it, it is often in the people who are least able to tolerate the loss and for whom its reacquisition is most difficult.—**AG**

- The one that scares me the most is any emergency when we potentially will be unable to secure airway (even surgical) and may require ECMO, because we don't have this readily available in my hospital. This includes really bad tracheal stenosis, bad mediastinal mass, and so forth.—**KAM**

- I am very wary of right heart failure and pulmonary hypertension. And both of those together! That is a day to bring your best game.—**JWK**

- Primary pulmonary hypertension. I have had a few women die shortly after delivery.—**BMT**

- Nothing scares me but I think long and hard about severe pulmonary hypertension.—**BDW**

- Probably pulmonary hypertension/right ventricular failure, especially in trauma—hypovolemia = arrest in these patients and they are all hypovolemic.—**JSZ**

- Hmmm…**Jeanine Wiener-Kronish, Brandon Togioka, Jordan Zunder,** and **Brad Winters** all picked pulmonary hypertension as the disease state that concerns them greatly. An uber-experienced pulmonologist/anesthesiologist, OB anesthesiologist, trauma anesthesiologist, and intensivist. If you are already worried about it, you are in very good company. If you are not afraid, you should be.—**Editors**

- Speaking of which, the elucidation of the role of nitric oxide in smooth muscle relaxation was of such seminal importance that the investigators were awarded the 1998 Nobel Prize in Medicine or Physiology. One of the laureates, Dr. Louis Ignarro, is married to anesthesiologist Sharon Williams MD, who trained with us at Hopkins in 1997–1998 before she finished her residency at UCLA.—**CM**

- Are you able to access nitric oxide for therapeutic use at your institution? Make sure you understand your available resources.—**Editors**

- Undiagnosed or unquantified heart disease, there are many patients walking around out there with unrecognized low EF.—**ND**

- I'll go with the old classic, aortic stenosis! And mitral stenosis, too, but it's much less common.—**CAT**

- The anesthetic plan for a patient with tight aortic or mitral stenosis certainly depends on the type of case you are doing, and out-patient vs in-patient. But in general, I don't think you need to do these cases with high opioid administration, as long as you manage the hemodynamics appropriately. I might insert an arterial line and manage hemodynamics using esmolol/etomidate instead of high opioids.—**CAT**

- What concern me greatly are patients with severe (as in Pickwickian) obstructive sleep apnea in very large people. Difficult for sedation, challenging airways, frustrating wake ups, no easy answers. Regional helps, but the sedation process is still fraught.—**SLO**

- We are I am also always very concerned with obesity. It is a medical condition that significantly alters the patient's physiology, mandates dose changes in anesthesia, makes airway management and access more difficult, increases risk in just about every category of perioperative complication especially in pregnant patients and parturients, and often makes the surgery more difficult.—**Editors**

- Let us repeat what we said above. Never hurry to extubate and obese patients. Because up to 20% of ICU patients may be obese, this also applies to the perioperative period, not just the OR.—**KAM**

- Remember that oxygen consumption for obese patients in the resting state is 1.5 times that for the non-obese patient due to increased tissue requirements and increased work of breathing. Mechanical ventilation while supine doesn't help matters either due to exacerbation of atelectasis.—**Editors**

- Junior anesthesiologists won't remember this but when we were first doing bariatric cases, we tended to think that everybody needed an awake intubation. Then we figured out this wasn't the case. However, it remains true that obese patients have a greater risk of difficult intubation (15% vs 6%), and stridor after extubation (15% vs 3%) [7].—**Editors**

- There is up to a 15% risk of reintubation of obese patients within 96 hours of extubation. Post-extubation strategies, such as high-flow nasal cannula and non-invasive ventilation may help decrease that rate significantly. Are you up on these techniques and does your practice location use them? [7]—**Editors**

- Be very careful before sending an obese patient with OSA home on the day of surgery. I Always personally check carefully for potential DDIs that could prolong the action of sedative and opioid medications. It's not hard to find deaths for this type of patient in the literature with the expected resulting litigation.—**Editors**

- Anesthesia technique for apnea-prone 156 kg patient—a little sedation and a lotta love.—**CC**

- The most I've been scared for the patients in recent years was by severe Covid. I had a 33-year-old patient who was 34 weeks pregnant with Covid and respiratory distress. I intubated her and could not get her O2 sat up above 50% for an hour. We delivered the baby but she went on to spending 3 months in the ICU getting pronated and ultimately was taken off life support. Severe bronchospasm can give you a similar sense of doom.—**JHW**

- Trauma × obstetrics—two patients at risk, mom has reserve until she doesn't, rapid hypoxia with any delay in airway or decrease in O2 carrying capacity.—**JSZ**

- To me, a really challenging case would be a baby with a traumatic brain injury who is bleeding. And this type of case is unfortunately not that rare. There are still many children riding unrestrained in cars, suffering from GSW or NAI and we know that falls remain a major public health risk for children. You approach such a patient by knowing and simultaneously applying the fundamental bedrock principle for each main issue—a pediatric patient, a TBI patient, and a bleeding patient—while first looking for commonalities in the clinical approach. For instance, is there a ventilation management strategy or an approach to access that works for all three circumstances? Sometimes in a difficult case tradeoffs have to be established but first figure out what aspects of the case don't have to be compromised.—**RVN and Editors**

- The ones that are scariest (but not for me) are the ones that where time is "of the essence" and the patient's diagnosis is missed. One that comes to mind is last year I saw a 36-year-old woman who was having worsening abdominal pain. For several months, she was passed from her primary care to GI, but she wasn't scanned. Turns out she had pancreatic cancer and although she had a poor prognosis to begin with, a lot of time had been missed.—**LAR**

- Other pain conditions that I am always very concerned about are headaches that may also have increased intracranial pressure due to a mass, temporal arteritis, and multiple sclerosis that is presenting as a radiculopathy. Since I have had a history of doing anesthesia, I really try to make a decent differential diagnosis and also make sure I do a good review of systems to look for any red flags.—**LAR**

- Severe heart failure in a patient with end stage kidney disease. You are going to hit one of the organ systems no matter how you care for the patient.—**CS**

- Other things that spring to mind are airway issues—doing an EGD in a patient with a mandibulectomy or laryngectomy. These cases are often urgent or emergent and finding imaging, or a surgical note, is often impossible.—**CS**

- Neuroendocrine tumors aren't terrifying per se, but the cases are exhausting. Even when you are prepared with central lines and arterial lines, pressers and such, the case is all over the map and changes second to second.—**CS**

- I don't really get scared about perioperative patients much since the Covid Delta surge. Some patients I think are likely to survive, and others not, but I am actually not very good at being right about this judgement anyway. So I am content with doing my best.—**MPH**

- Here's what happened to me the first time when I was an intern here at the Portland VA. The ICU nurses ganged up on me on Monday prerounds—"you are torturing this guy, he's gonna die, make him comfort care." I thought they were right and presented him that way to the attending. The attending said, "It was a beautiful sunny day yesterday and I played 2 rounds of great golf, and there is no way I am withdrawing care on this patient today." Next day, patient a little better. Three weeks later, he walked out the front door of the hospital.—**MPH**

- At work, I'm also scared of active shooters and any other person who has or might have a gun. But I must stress that the police have always been courteous and professional in our interactions.—**MPH**

- Best kind of 4 AM bleeding tonsil—the one that isn't bleeding at the moment.—**CC**
- For bleeding tonsil, let the patient sit up and hold their own suction during induction.—**CC**
- Bad sign: preoperative medicine consult says, "Do you have to?"—**CC**
- There is no such thing as a little bit of hyperthyroidism. Grave's disease is a fairly common cause of hyperthyroidism and those patients should be determined to be compliant with meds and clinically and biochemically euthyroid before proceeding with any case that is not emergent. If patients are medication avoidant or non-compliant, then they are at risk for thyroid storm. Remember that induction of anesthesia and manipulation of the neck and thyroid can precipitate thyrotoxicosis.—**Editors**
- If I could wave a magic wand and cure one disease which would also mean it would be banished forever from the palliative medicine universe, it would be ovarian cancer. Ovarian cancer is just an awful disease. Patients are typically on the younger side for end of life, they face sudden diagnoses of advanced cancer, pain, nausea, abdominal distension, and edema. It is extremely difficult for patients and difficult to control the symptoms. We rarely see a cure or remission.—**AJR**
- Like every anesthesiology resident, I was always hoping that there would not be a middle of the night perirectal abscess case. Couldn't it wait until morning? Until one awful night I saw a case of Fournier's gangrene. It was one of four times in my entire 30-year career when I was completely flummoxed and all I could do was think, "*What happened to this patient?*"—**CM**
- Accept that there are going to be several cases that stay with you forever, the cases that look back at you from the mirror in the middle of the night. Resolve that you will be part of the solution and never part of the problem for these cases. The specifics of the most bothersome are different for each physician. Sometimes the patients do okay, sometimes there is nothing that anybody can do. The other three cases for me were a case of fulminant bacterial meningitis in a young college student who turned black and died over the course of just a couple of hours (just *awful* if you have never seen one), a case of severe transfusion-associated graft-vs-host disease in a young male patient who had received platelets, and a case of advanced cutaneous T-cell lymphoma.—**CM**
- I would include with the advice above the additional point that it is certainly possible to develop a degree of PTSD from our day-to-day practices. Memorable and/or sad cases are one thing, but rumination to the point that our lives and care of other patients are compromised is another. Do not allow this situation to continue. There is simply no shame in getting professional help coping with the distressing aspects of what we do. Every decent-sized city will have psychiatrists who specialize in the care of other physicians. Seek them out. Often, a short, goal-directed course of therapy can do wonders to avert burnout or maladaptive coping behaviors.—**NBS**
- Remember Sandson's Law: An actively psychotic patient is capable of anything at any time. Occasionally, a borderline or sociopathic patient will also raise a ruckus with complaints or threats or try to steal medications and supplies.—**NBS**
- If you realize you are dealing with a patient with significant delusions or derangements in thought content, do not hesitate to call the psychiatric consultation and liaison service.—**NBS**

- Although it is common to worry about psychiatric patients being disruptive and causing harm to staff, it is more often that the patient is harmed, although completely inadvertently.—**NBS**

- It is folklore in the psych community that acute medical disease is somewhat organizing for the seriously mentally ill and that folklore is likely true. But underneath the acute illness is often serious chronic illness—smoking, addiction and alcohol use disorders, metabolic disease, malnutrition, poor dental health, inadequate vaccination status, and the like. A major hospitalization predicts a significant 2-year mortality rate for schizophrenic patients.—**NBS**

- I am always concerned about psychiatric patients who enter the perioperative period on drugs with a narrow therapeutic index such as lithium, tricyclics, any anti-depressants, and anti-convulsants. These medications exhibit drugs levels that can be deranged through cascading interactions. Examples are paroxetine, phenytoin, and carbamazepine.—**NBS**

- If your patient is on lithium, order daily 12-hour trough levels since perioperative fluid shifts can definitely affect lithium levels. And remember that NSAIDS (except for aspirin and sulindac) raise lithium levels.—**NBS**

- If there was one cardiac condition, besides the basics, that we could completely master it would be the important clinical issue of QT prolongation as torsades de pointes can be the result. Who is at risk is not always straightforward so this would be a great subject for grand rounds with the cardiologists.—**Editors**

- All halogenated volatile anesthetics prolong the QT interval, sevoflurane the most. Sevoflurane has been implicated in cases of ventricular arrhythmias.—**LMO**

- Monitor QT interval and QT prolongation for patients on tricyclic antidepressants! Especially in the ICU. This is not a theoretical concern.—**NBS**

- Other drug classes associated with QT prolongation are antiarrhythmics (of course), antihistamines, antimicrobials, neuroleptics, and prokinetics.—**Editors**

- QT prolongation is more serious and the patient is at greater risk of malignant ventricular arrhythmias when the heart is *low and slow*—low electrolytes such as hypokalemia, hypomagnesemia or both, and sinus bradycardia or any degree of heart block.—**Editors**

- Treatment of torsades de pointes is first defibrillation if necessary, keeping the heart rate fast, and intravenous magnesium.—**Editors**

- Has it become your job to institute new policies get more out of our workday miniature universe? More cases, more efficiency, more throughput? First consider the Lucas principle, named after Robert Lucas, who won the Nobel Memorial Prize in Economic Sciences—all action is individual behavior and people are rational creatures who will respond to policies in rational ways, even policies designed to fool them.—**Editors**

- Next, if you are trying to increase anything that represents an imposed cost, apply the wisdom of Jean-Baptiste Colbert, finance minister to Louis XIV.—**Editors**

The art of taxation consists in so plucking the goose as to obtain the largest possible amount of feathers with the smallest possible amount of hissing.

- Every person has to decide how to spend their lifetime allotment of career goodwill. Do you want to be the tax collector?—**Editors**

- Don't make the nurses or junior staff be the bearer of bad news and make the phone calls you don't want to make. If you must cancel or delay or a case, get on the phone yourself.—**CM**

***Note from the Editors:** We asked OHSU medical student Marlee Chamberlain to find us a bridge that reflects the complexity of the of the modern-day practice of anesthesiology. She sent the perfect illustration! This bridge is adjacent to the medical school campus, and she crosses it every day (Fig. 156.6).

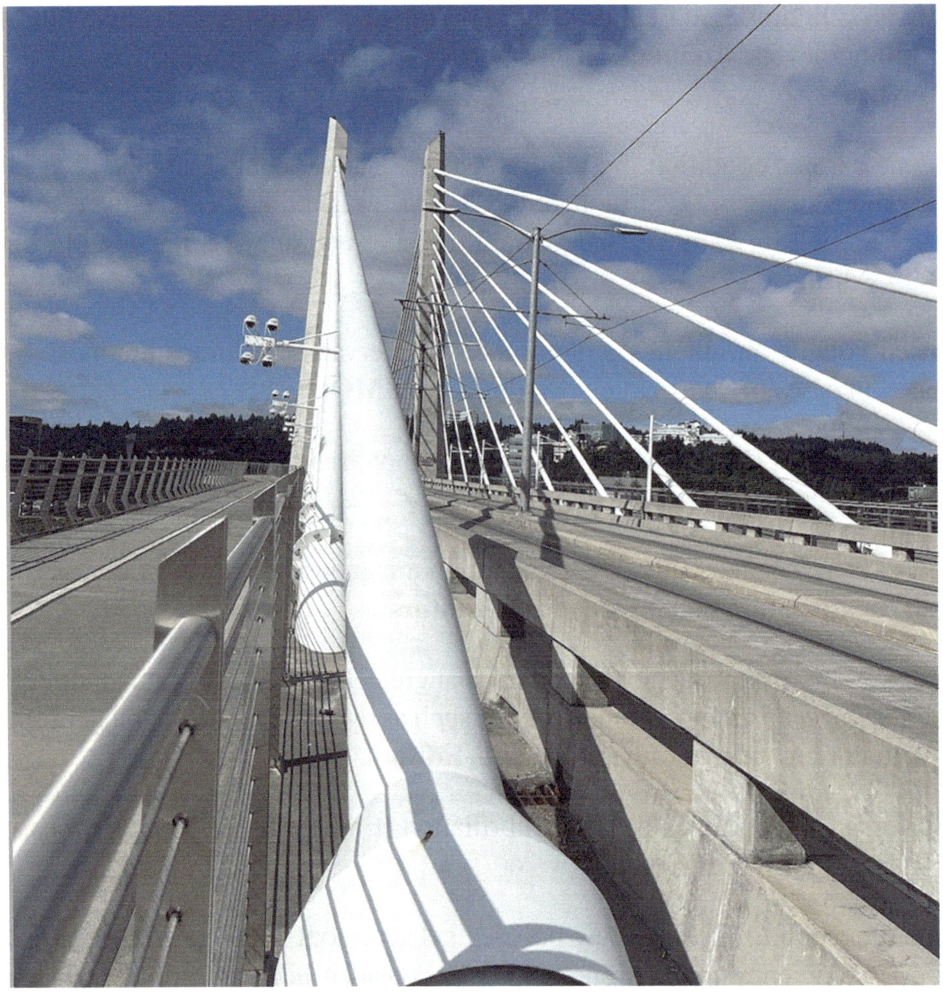

Fig. 156.6 The Tilikum crossing in Portland, OR. Photo: Marlee Chamberlain

Positioning—General

- Positioning for a patient is a lot like doing the pharmacology for the anesthetic plan. It's basically all on us. The patient comes into the OR in a neutral position. We then effect the perturbations of body planes and placement of body parts (except for issues like putting the patient's head in pins). We therefore have all the responsibility and liability if something goes wrong.—**Editors**

- Positioning injuries are not a gigantic percentage of the closed claims, but we have found that they can be really devastating to patients because they always involve pain, paresis, or paralysis. No patient expects to go into an OR as an intact functioning person but not come out that way. Positioning injuries are also really distressing to the anesthesia providers. We know of at least one anesthesiologist who left practice after a successful lawsuit for a serious positioning injury.—**Editors**

- Positioning patients is like doing the airway—never let anybody rush you. There is no defense against doing a rushed patient positioning.—**Editors**

- Always take just a few seconds to stand back after a patient has been positioned and do a visual survey of the situation. Does the patient look to be in a neutral situation? Could you imagine yourself in this position for however many hours?—**CM**

- The best advice I can give is to always be mindful about the common post-vaginal delivery complication of meralgia paresthetica, lateral femoral cutaneous nerve compression. I tell my residents that we did not cause it, but it would not have occurred without an epidural. The epidural blocks pain sensation and impairs motor strength so the patient is unable to protect themselves from over flexing the hip and compressing the nerve under the inguinal ligament.—**BMT**

- Positioning injuries happen. They are one reason that postoperative visits and notes are important. If somebody reports a possible positioning injury we advise that you *never deny and always document*.—**Editors**

- The best positioning injury is the one you avoid.—**Editors**

Positioning Mishaps—Falling Limbs and Falling Patients

We asked our (anonymous) colleagues to share some of the most dramatic positioning mishaps they have seen or heard about. One thing that will jump out at you is that *patients or body parts falling off the table* is unfortunately not really a rare event. Just a few of the positioning mishaps we know of are below and we thank everybody for sharing.—**Editors**

- Arms falling off table under drapes!

- New resident—first day in a room alone, robotic pelvic case, we got the patient intubated and then I had to go to my other room. When I came back the patient was positioned, and the case had started. At the end of the case, I saw one arm was tucked with the wrist hanging down. The patient definitely had a nerve palsy the next day. Fortunately resolved.

- I know about an ex-lap case that was for at least 3–4 hours, and at some point after the procedure was started, the left leg was hanging out from the bed. No one noticed for hours, until they removed the drapes. Patient ended up with severe permanent neuropathy on that leg.

- This happened to a colleague, not me! An elderly woman in OR in stirrups for gyn procedure, her legs weren't secure and flopped down and broke both her femurs. Not sure it was a positioning thing or an equipment failure—but still.......

- As a resident, I had a patient fall off the OR table mid-procedure. We were in the angio suite doing a fem-pop bypass. The patient was moved to the far right of the bed, the surgical leg (right leg) was frog-legged, and he had a BKA on the left side. When I tilted the bed five degrees, the patient started moving and continued sliding right off the table. I had just administered heparin as well! I kept thinking, "This is *NOT* happening." and also, "Don't let his head hit the floor!" Somehow, he remained intubated...

- Interscalene nerve block/catheter placed for a very large man having shoulder arthroplasty (BMI 42). After induction, I went upstairs for the next nerve block and was interrupted by a stat call to OR. I arrived to find that the ortho fellow had requested the table be tilted for positioning, but stability of the patient was not ensured. The man began sliding and no one could stop him! As he went to the floor, the CRNA grabbed his head and neck and stabilized the ETT. By some miracle, it did not come out. We had to call a trauma alert. The trauma team came to the OR to help us place him on a backboard and in a C-Collar. We awakened him to check his neck-he was enraged! It took almost two hours to send him, on the board, to the CT scanner and then bring him back to induce anesthesia. Neck cleared! He underwent the arthroplasty without further incident.

- I've had multiple patients in OB fall off the table when they were wedged and their bellies were so large that they toppled over.

- This didn't happen in the OR, but we took care of this patient many times for various procedures. The patient had earlier been grievously injured when he sat up for an albuterol breathing treatment in the ED. He fell face-first off the gurney, fractured his cervical spine, and became quadriplegic.

- The *WORST*..... not mine, but a colleague. Robotic prostate. Steep Trendelenburg. Morbidly obese patient. You can see where there this is headed..... patient slid off the table. While the robot was docked. Fortunately, no catastrophic injury but was terrible, terrible, terrible. I am neurotic about steep T-berg cases now!

- My sister was placed in a seated position for her labor epidural, but nobody was holding the other side of the Mayo stand. The anesthesiologist palpated her back so forcefully that he pushed her off the bed and onto her knees in the space between the labor bed and the wall. The worst part was hitting her chin on the stand as she went down and chipping her front tooth.

Positioning Mishaps—Prone

If there is one position that requires extra vigilance, it's the prone position. It's one reason why I have always been happy to do vascular and transplant cases—the patient is usually supine. I wonder how the people who work in the spine rooms tolerate the stress day in and day out.—**CM**

- What are five complications of prone positioning? You must know these cold!
- Complications include:

  1. Hemodynamic changes resulting in hypoperfusion including arterial compression.
  2. Central nervous system lesions and peripheral nerve compression injuries.
  3. A range of ophthalmologic conditions. Try to get through your entire career without one of these eye injuries. They are so devastating for patient and provider.
  4. Compartment syndromes and pressure ulcers.
  5. Airway edema—we've seen airways lost because the anesthesia team was too impatient to hold up on extubating. Sometimes 15 minutes back in the supine position or deflating the cuff and checking for a leak makes all the difference.

- Flipping a patient prone when the head and body weren't turned at the same time. The patient's neck made a terrible cracking sound, just like those terrifying chiropractor videos that you see online. We decided to turn the patient back supine and do a wake-up test to make sure they were moving all extremities. We then put the patient back to sleep and got the case done as it wasn't something that was really elective. The reviews and QA discussions went on for weeks and the surgeons were really frosted.
- Very bruised breasts in a prone patient who wasn't positioned properly.
- Flipping the patient prone in a face pillow without taping their eyes. My understanding is that it looked like something out of the Game of Thrones.
- I heard about a patient who basically needed to have their chin debrided and a flap pulled up because of an injury while prone during a spine case.
- I've seen *neuropraxia* several times from abducted shoulders when prone.
- Flipping patient from prone back to their bed, the bed slipped away from the table EVEN THOUGH IT WAS LOCKED because the floor was slippery. Caught the (very large) patient's head and shoulders with one hand and it was just enough to keep them in the air.
- *Remember* that the prone position and resulting shift of the weight of the visceral organs can be advantageous for oxygenation and gas exchange, especially in situations such as ARDS. Lung/alveolar recruitment is increased, there is decreased atelectrauma, and improved V/Q mismatch. For these reasons, the benefits of prone position in the ICU can outweigh the risks, but you have to be careful!—**CM**

Positioning Mishaps—Miscellaneous

- Left ulnar palsy during knee replacement. Affected arm was padded and positioned across the chest.
- My most memorable positioning event was something that happened to me when I was very junior. To this day, I feel that I had properly padded and positioned the arm but apparently not up to the standards of the infamously difficult and grumpy attending. He proceeded to dig his bony fingers into my ulnar groove while yelling to the entire room, "How do you like *THAT*, Johnson?!" My fourth and fifth fingers tingled until the next morning. *Note:* my name isn't Johnson.
- I watched a 250 lb. male orthopedic surgeon straddle an elderly woman on the OR table as he tried to relocate her hip. He was three feet off the ground, grabbing her leg, pulling upwards, trying to pop in back in the joint. It was a sight. Our thought? It wasn't our place to pull the surgeon off the lady, but it's probably not the best thing to do to have somebody climb on top of the patient.
- I did a tonsillectomy in a child years ago and the head was hyper flexed for the surgeon's view. She was a new attending, as was I. After surgery, the patient was slow to wake. Immobile, showing no signs of return of function. I mentioned, off hand, "The neck was hyper extended. I hope it wasn't too much." She freaked out, thinking that we caused a spinal cord injury and paralysis. There was a tremendous amount of anxiety for about 3 minutes when the gas wore off and the patient woke up normal as could be.
- I saw an infant get a total spinal and go into cardiac arrest when her little lower body was raised to put on a diaper.
- When I was an early resident, we were doing an elbow surgery and patient had arm propped up with forearm hanging down. Ortho attending kept yelling at me that we were not relaxed. I showed as I gave more roc and showed her the twitches. She then looked and realized the stand holding the arm was placed too distally and that is why the elbow could not achieve full flexion for her surgery. Had to take the whole enchilada down, unscrub, reposition patient, and basically start over.
- The patient's head slipped out of Mayfield pins—requiring plastic closure.
- I've seen several instances of flexing or rotating the head and then immediate *airway obstruction*—both in MAC and GA/ETT cases.
- Dental damage due to improperly placed oral airway during ECT—a bunch of times.
- Lower extremity compartment syndrome during a short case in lithotomy position—scary how fast it happened.
- Elderly patient with decades of steroid therapy. Classic tissue paper skin. Assistant helped the patient up in bed holding her by her forearms and sheared off all of her skin on the forearm.
- Not positioning per se but have definitely seen the accidental tourniquet left on after an IV placement—not good!

- The resident was trying to start an IV on the patient's foot when somebody at the head of the bed said, "I've got a decent IV up here." The resident immediately moved onto the next task without taking the tourniquet off. The patient ended up with severe CRPS in that lower extremity, which ended his professional career as a firefighter. He sued and ended up with a large settlement.

- The patient was having an aneurysm repaired in a seated position and the surgeons requested tight blood pressure control. The OR table was raised but the transducer wasn't. The anesthesia team member started a nitroprusside drip to control the falsely elevated blood pressure readings. The neurosurgery was successful, but the patient woke up with visual loss.

Our Surgical Colleagues

- Rest assured that the surgeons know who the really excellent anesthesiologists are. And they know who the less excellent ones are, too. But they tend not to really think about specific problems that we may have in our cases, or so we have been told.—**Editors**

- Be the best yourself. Be prepared on their case as well as your case.—**MN**

- The biggest wishful thinking statement in surgery: "This will only take 20 minutes."—**CC**

- The second biggest promise in surgery that might require a bit of salt, "I'll be there in ten minutes."—**CC**

- If the question is "Can we do this in the bed?", the answer is "no."—**CC**

- Something a surgeon told us once after two beers: "Every surgeon fetish is born from a screw-up."—**Editors and CC**

- Minimally invasive surgery = maximally annoying for anesthesia?—**CC**

- It's been said that high maintenance behavior in a surgeon is inversely proportional to skill level. Not sure if this is true, but we have wondered about it from time to time.—**CC**

- Realize that those who are aggressive are truly afraid.—**MN**

- Realize that the surgeons often really do not know any more than you do if you've prepared.—**MN**

- If you have to delay the start of the case to get some additional preop evaluation, try to emphasize it is not for the purposes of cancelling the case but rather so that the case can *proceed* on a more appropriate basis.—**Editors**

- It may very well be that the surgeons try to portray any issues that need further evaluation as an indication that you can't handle the big or complex cases or the sick patients. It never feels great when that happens but so be it. Don't respond to that type of comment in the moment, just ignore it. Keep the discussion focused on the patient's situation.—**Editors**

- Have some sympathy for them, they generally take the brunt of the responsibility for the outcome with the family.—**MN**

- Sometimes tempted to conclude that the surgeons aren't as good as they think they are? Neither are we.—**Editors**

- If there is an untoward outcome *always* attend the first meeting with the family, even if it means having your colleague cover your room for a time.—**MN**

- Never act aggressively toward anyone. Just look at them if they are inappropriate. Your eyes will say all that needs to be said.—**MN**

- Realize we all bring our personal lives with us to the OR no matter how much we try not to. For better or worse.—**MN**

- Every once in a while, it requires "prison mentality" realizing that your kindness can be mistaken for weakness.—**MN**

- If you want the discussion to remain between you and them, have it behind closed doors. Then be thoroughly honest.—**MN**

- Remember "controlled warfare" is what we seek. We do not want to see even our worst adversaries injured.—**MN**

***Note from the Editors:** To further honor Dr. Crumpler, who practiced in Richmond VA, we went looking for a cool bridge in that city (Fig. 156.7).

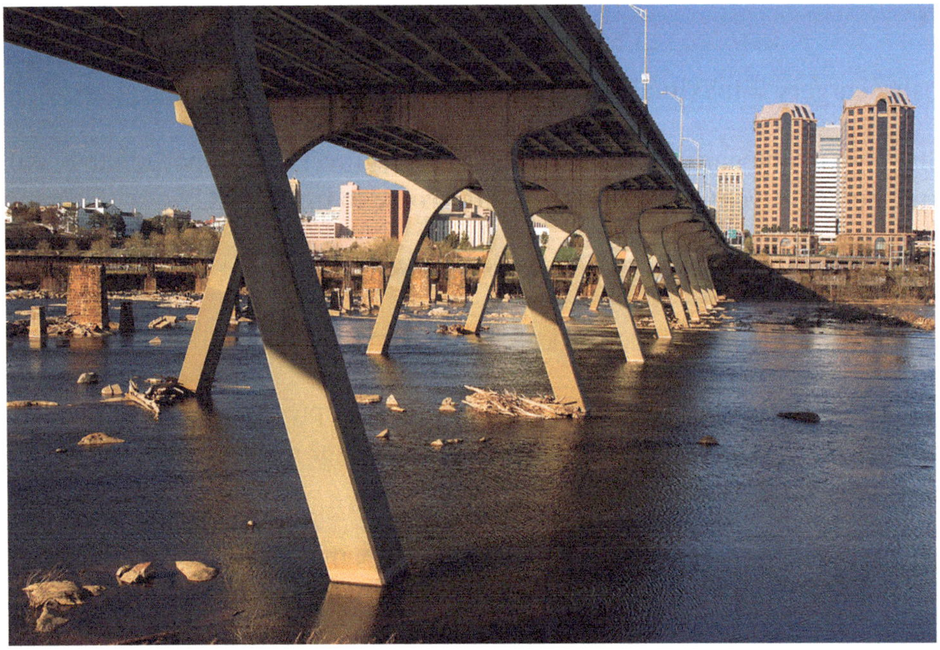

Fig. 156.7 A bridge with very simple but great architecture spanning the James River in Richmond, VA. Photo: Kirkikis, image used under license from iStock.com

Integrating Clinical Care and Academic Efforts; Looking to the Future

- Always be on the lookout for publishable events and issues. Don't be a knowledge hog! If you are practicing anesthesia, you should be reading the literature. And if you are reading the literature, you should be contributing to the literature, whenever and in whatever way you can. It doesn't take that long to write up a letter to the editor.—**Editors**

- If you are in private practice, the volume of cases that you and your colleagues will be doing means that you will be seeing some interesting and unusual clinical events. Jot down the specifics and call the program director where you trained and say you possibly have an interesting case report and letter to the editor, and does anybody still need to work on their scholarly activity project? Let the resident be first author as that is usually required to complete credit for the academic effort, you are the senior author, and maybe somebody helping to coordinate and push things along is the middle author?—**Editors**

- You know who I think should win the danged Nobel Prize? Karen Domino and her colleagues! With their careful and continuing analysis of closed tort actions, they have shown us where to look forward by looking back. Their abstract presentation at Euroanesthesia 2020 highlighted that up to 20% of closed claims are due to "failure to rescue." This is such important work. As we point out earlier in this chapter, in the perioperative period trouble happens not only because of what we do but also because of what we don't do, fail to recognize, or fail to inform. A more detailed description of Karen's presentation is online [8].—**CM**

- Transport and handoffs are both transition points in perioperative case that are very critical to patient safety and a successful outcome. There are many ways to develop your protocols for sign outs,and we are only half-facetious when we say don't take any action that doesn't apply the "S is for sign outs" rule—safety and stability, standardized (Six Sigma?), senior, supplies, and sacred. This is catchy and easy to remember.—**Editors**

- What does *"S is for sign out"* mean for teaching purposes? Don't leave the OR if you have any major maneuvers left to do! Apply a standardized protocol to sign out—the Six Sigma paradigm has been described to work. Don't send your junior person unaccompanied to do the transports or handoffs, this is a critical event and is worthy of the attendance of a senior person. Make sure you have the supplies you need—drugs, airway equipment, monitor. Never, ever, ever make a dash for it. And finally keep the process sacred—no interruptions, no discussion about any other patients or cases, just concentrate on the one patient in front of you.—**CM**

- Ever heard the simplistic statement that guidelines are only as good as the data upon which they are based? *Anesthesia Bridges* Editor Brandon Togioka sent us the additional valued and nuanced information below.—**BMT and Editors**

- I just completed a presentation that required me to look up this data. About 50% of guidelines are based upon level C evidence and < 25% of all professional society guidelines are based upon level A evidence. Does this mean all guidelines are no good? Not necessarily, I'm not sure we want to send that message. And remember that a considerable amount of clinical practice is based on checklists. I personally rely on guidelines quite a bit in practice, research, and as an expert witness. Here are three pertinent citations:

1. Fararoff AC. JAMA. 2019. 321:1069.

2. Jhawar N. Mayo Clinc Proceedings. 2023. 7:262.

3. Laserna A. Anesthesiology. 2021. 135:31.

- Remember that rejection is part of the academic and research process. Even senior mentors and giants in the field had their fair share of rejection of manuscripts and grants. Seek counsel. Find the way forward to realize your passion. Realize that sometimes you have to write the paper that's in the reviewer's head, not the paper in your head.—**BD**

- You can create security for yourself by diversifying both your research and clinical expertise portfolios. Have a few different lines of effort and expertise. Side projects and small pilots can supply critical preliminary data in the event you need to pivot or put in another grant or develop other areas of clinical expertise.—**BD and Editors**

- Infrastructure and environment are crucial to major academic success. If you do not have close colleagues in your department to collaborate with, investigate your broader options. Securing a strong research environment can sometimes mean changing institutions. The exact same principles are true for clinical work. Look for jobs where there is a robust and ongoing effort to coordinate and strengthen the practice location.—**BD and Editors**

- To bolster collaborative opportunities, demonstrate your value. Actively offer to help colleagues on projects, manuscripts, quality initiatives, and clinical subjects in valuable ways. Offer to do more than asked, and you will stand out as a collaborator that people will want to invite onto the next big project.—**BD and Editors**

- I can't remember the exact quote for the following, but it is along these lines: Finding your passion and special calling in both scholarly and clinical work is like walking around a party and listening to conversations. Wherever you find yourself standing is your area of interest. You speak when you think there is a knowledge gap in the conversation that you can fill. Therefore, read the literature (this is the conversation listening phase), seek out the knowledge gap, then speak up by publishing.—**BMT**

- I think it's a mistake to discount the lowly case report. I have always done a lot of teaching on equipment issues and mishaps from the recent case report literature because there aren't a lot of large, highly powered studies on some of the auxiliary anesthesia equipment but there can be significant clinical consequences if something goes wrong.—**CM**

- When I began training in transfusion medicine, I said to one of the senior physicians, "I feel like an immunologist." And he said, "In the future, we will all be immunologists. This is the way medicine is going. Common sense tells you that."—**CM**

- Soon we will treat disease with a cell, not a pill.—*Siddhartha Mukherjee*

- After spending two years at the NIH, I can assure everybody that cancer care for just about every kind of cancer will become multi-modal in the not-too-distant future. Surgical oncology isn't going to go away any time soon, but it will be closely coupled with the emerging cellular medicine applications, which are often predicated on the collection of stem cells by an apheresis procedure for chimeric antigen receptor therapy. Immune checkpoint inhibitor cancer therapies can be associated with atypical myasthenia gravis requiring plasmapheresis. I believe that we will see increased numbers of patients who have undergone apheresis in the immediate preoperative period.—**CM**

- There is a really great, short overview of apheresis basics for the anesthesiologist in *Anesthesiology* [9]. It's not a new article but I couldn't find anybody who could recall reading it. I highly advise everybody to go review it as it's quite short. Remember that plasmapheresis is a therapy for acute thyrotoxicosis.—**CM**

- The most common complications of apheresis are symptomatic hypocalcemia (up to 30% of patients) and citrate toxicity, which are fortunately easily treated, if you know what to watch for. Patients may be hypovolemic or hypervolemic.—**CM**

- If the replacement fluid is albumin as opposed to plasma, there may certainly be depletion of clotting factors. Fibrinogen may take up to 4 days to normalize and platelet counts can decrease as much as 30% with a single apheresis run.—**CM**

- The alteration of pharmacokinetics of the basic anesthesia drugs is still not fully characterized, especially opioid pharmacokinetics. Hydrophilic agents with high protein binding are readily removed. Lipid-soluble agents, such as propofol, the volatile anesthetics, and the benzodiazepines are probably less effected. Decreased levels of pseudocholinesterase leading to prolonged succinylcholine neuromuscular blockade are to be expected and have been reported.—**CM**

- Is there any reason why anesthesiologists shouldn't become the primary experts in the perioperative pharmacogenomics field? Evan Kharasch laid down a lot of great tread with his landmark work on the cytochrome P450 enzyme systems and the ensuing identification of drug–drug interactions. Remember that there is no genotypical CYP 3A4 metabolizer status, but there can still be up to a 30-fold variation in phenotypic metabolic efficiency. And the psychiatrists are already looking at the pharmacogenomics of ketamine for use in treatment resistant depression [10]. We should not let ourselves get behind the curve. There is a short chapter summarizing the current knowledge on pharmacogenomics in anesthesia in the Springer book *Pharmacogenomics in Clinical Medicine* (Fig. 156.8). It's a great place to start.—**CM**

- I saw this interesting article online about five emerging medical specialties: cancer immunologist, nocturnist, lifestyle medicine physician, clinical informatics, medical virtualist (telemedicine) [11].

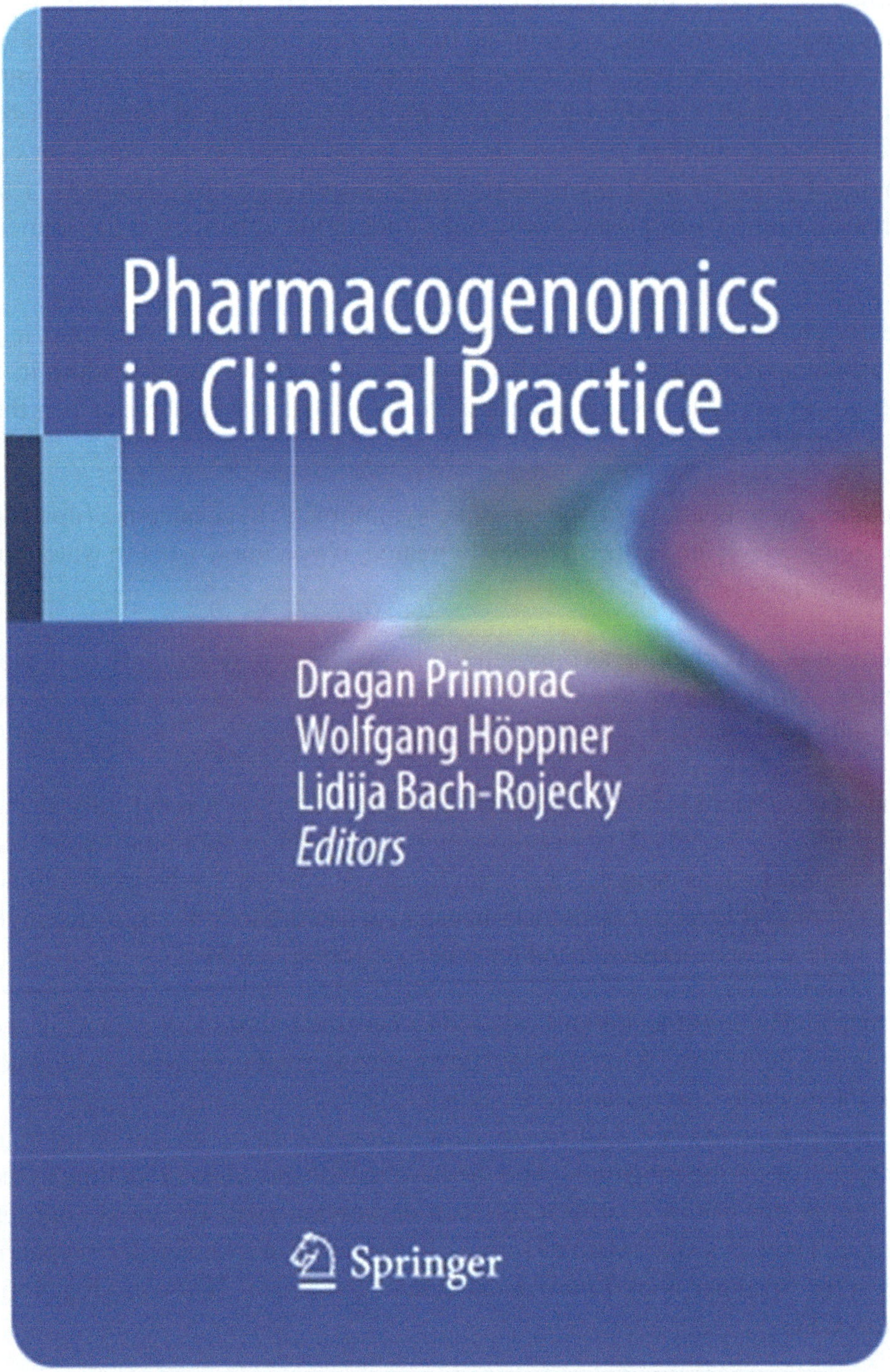

Fig. 156.8. A timely and informative Springer textbook. Photo: Courtesy of Springer, Inc.

What on this list can we research and incorporate? What can we do to optimize the preoperative immunological status of people having cancer operations? What would we see if we could develop a lifestyle program for the 5 days before surgery? If we could figure out a way to get people to sleep the night before surgery? Could preoperative telemedicine appointments be expanded and done with the rehab medicine folks to include more optimization and behavior modification as well as evaluation? Would that be a great professional niche for later-career or retired anesthesiologists?—**CM**

- We already know that a course of preoperative acupuncture has efficacy in improving outcomes. What if first-time patients could be given an in-person or virtual tour of an actual OR? I can't tell the hours I have spent trying to describe to friends what it's like to go into an operating room. Finally, transfusion medicine already has formal combined fellowship training programs that combine clinical blood banking and stem cell medicine and training in clinical informatics—can we do the same in anesthesiology at the resident level? There is magic everywhere, we need to lean in!—**CM**

- You do research to educate yourself.—**TNW**

- We will admit that academic output, quality assurance efforts, and innovation outreach aren't the lowest path of resistance in a busy career. I've had several great mentors who published a lot. Brett Simon used to say that you always get to the point with every manuscript where you are starting in with the scraps of paper. I myself always have reached the point when I want to put every project in the trash. Including this one! It can be frustrating and tough to push through and finish papers and projects. But Denny Bourke always used to tell me, "Look at it this way. You are choosing to suffer now so patients in the future can suffer less." —**CM and DLB**

- You have to get over your personal fear of making a mistake in your manuscripts. Once I was struggling with concerns that there was something in a manuscript that was going to be found to be not true in the fullness of time and I was therefore misleading the readers. I remember that Denny Bourke said to me, "It might be that your discussion section in subsequent papers is formulated a bit differently. But if you can't find anything wrong in the paper right now and the reviewers can't find anything wrong, then probably it's okay for this moment in time. The progress of knowledge base revises everybody's work in time. So you gotta let it go."—**CM and DLB**

- When you are driving home after work, thinking about your cases that day, also try to formulate one or two key clinical teaching points for the junior people who are coming up behind you. Try to come up with how you would explain and teach the days' challenges at the resident level and the medical student level. And remember, you don't really understand something if you can't teach it.—**CM, CCK, and MC**

- **Vigilance Always** isn't just for the past and present, it's also for the future.—**Editors**

More General Clinical Wisdom from *Avoiding Common Anesthesia Errors, 2nd Edition*

There is a wealth of additional tips, teaching tidbits, and overall general clinical wisdom in our previous book, which is nicknamed "Green2." *Please* check out this book and information and remember that every single penny of royalties goes to FAER in perpetuity!

Green2 Chapters with More General Clinical Wisdom

- Never, Ever Fire
- Good Old-Fashioned Basic Perioperative Blood Pressure Control
- Some Additional Thoughts on Blood Pressure Management Techniques—What We Believe, How We Do IT, and Where We Think the Science Is Going
- Protect the Kidneys, Not the "UOP"
- Avoid a 70% Mortality Rate: Do Everything You Can to Prevent Perioperative Renal Failure
- Do Not Use Urine Output as an Indicator of Volume Status in Hypothermic Patients
- Perioperative Hyperglycemia Is Associated with Poorer Clinical Outcomes So Consider Insulin Therapy for Both Diabetic and Nondiabetic Patients with Elevated Blood Glucose
- Seven Ways to Treat Hyperkalemia in the Perioperative Period
- Laparoscopic Procedures: Managing the Risks and Physiologic Effects During Camera Placement, CO2 Insufflation, and Vertical Positioning
- Could This Be Methemoglobinemia, Maybe?
- The Eye Room—Is This the Easiest of Days? Or the Hardest of Days? Regardless, Vigilance Is Key
- My Eye Hurts! Prevention, Diagnosis, and Treatment of Corneal Injuries After Anesthesia
- Never Forget That Patient Transport Within the Hospital Is One of the Most Dangerous Intervals in the Perioperative Period
- Seek Out Hypercapnia in the PACU and Remember That an Acceptable Pulse Oximeter Reading Is Not Assurance of Adequate Ventilation
- Let's Go Over It Again: Avoid Residual Neuromuscular Blockade in the PACU!
- Give the Intensivist the Best Handover to Improve Patient Outcomes

- Don't Miss Out on Ultrasound-Which ICU Techniques Are Helpful for the Anesthesiologist?
- Don't Overlook the Potential of Perioperative Acupuncture
- Consider Acupuncture as an Adjunct for the Prophylaxis and Treatment of Postoperative Nausea and Vomiting
- Don't Warm Up a Cardiac Arrest Patient Unless They Are Dying of Hemorrhage!
- What to Do If You Get a Needlestick Injury
- Understanding the Human Factor
- Minimize Errors in Anesthesia: Lessons Learned from Aviation
- Eliminate Communication Errors by Using a Spelling Alphabet and Spoken Digits
- Don't Ignore Your Intuition
- Ethics in Anesthesiology Practice
- Know When to Stop—Anesthesia Providers Have Got to Know Their Limitations
- Before You Press Play, Let's Talk About Music in the OR
- Never Rush Through a Signout
- Don't Ignore the Folklore—It Can Be a Powerful Ally in Your Clinical Practice
- Don't Underestimate the Role of Spirituality in Patients' Perception of Disease and Healing, and Remember to Uphold the Right to Self-Determination
- What's in a Name?
- We Are Not the Only People Who Care About the Patients
- Working in the OR—Sometimes the Staff Gets Sick or Injured, Too
- The Physician as Patient—What I Learned During the Last Five Times I Went to the OR on the Stretcher Instead of Pushing It
- A Primer on Simulation in Anesthesiology—Definitions and Concepts
- What Makes a Great Anesthesia Resident
- A Brief on the Legal Process
- How Not to End Up in a Closed Claims File—Lessons Learned From the ASA Closed Claims Project

- The Anesthesia Closed Claims Project—What's Trending Now
- A Careful and Complete Anesthesia Record Is the Best Defense Against a Lawsuit
- Document Disputes in the Medical Record—How to Avoid a Chart War and How to Survive One
- Reading in the Operating Room: Is It Worth the Risk?
- Going to the Operating Room with a Do-Not-Resuscitate Patient
- Refusal to Do a Case on Moral or Ethical Grounds: More Practical Navigation Through Choppy Waters
- Dental Injuries—Document Carefully and Do Not Overpromise
- Apologizing to Patients After an Adverse Event Is the Ethical Thing To Do and Just Might Keep You Out of Court
- What to Do About the Tattoos and Body Jewelry
- The Dao of Positioning
- The Supine Position—Complications Can Still Arise

References

1. Hart SR, Yajnik A, Ashford J, Springer R, Harvey S. Operating room fire safety. Ochsner J. 2011;11(1):37–42.
2. Leonovicz O, Cohen-Rosenblum A, et al. Operating room fire during total knee arthroplasty tibial impaction: a case report and review of the literature. Arthroplast Today. 2022;16:164–6.
3. The Joint Commission Issues Sentinel Event Alert on Surgical Fire Prevention [Internet]. Jointcommissionorg 2023 [cited 2025 Jul 27]. Available from: https://www.jointcommission.org/en-us/knowledge-library/news/2023-10-the-joint-commission-issues-sentinel-event-alert-on-surgical-fire-prevention.
4. Nielsen C, Jerkeman M, et al. Tattoos as a risk factor for malignant lymphoma: a population-based case control study. eClinicalMedicine (Lancet). 2024;72:102649. epub May 21, 2024.
5. Matchett G, Gasanova I, Riccio CA, et al. Etomidate versus ketamine for emergency endotracheal intubation: a randomized clinical trial. Intensive Care Med. 2022;48(1):78–91.
6. Centinkaya F. The effects of listening to music on the postoperative nausea and vomiting. Complement Ther Med. 2019;35:278–83.
7. Ge Y, Zhenxuan L, et al. Effect of high-flow nasal cannula versus non-invasive ventilation after extubation on successful extubation in obese patients: a retrospective analysis of the MIMIC-IV database. BMJ Open Respir Res. 2023;10(1):e001737.
8. News OM. Anesthesia malpractice claims failure rescue [Internet]. Ormanagementnet. 2025 [cited 2025 Jul 27]. Available from: https://www.ormanagement.net/Web-Only/Article/09-21/One-Fifth-of-Anesthesia-Malpractice-Claims-Are-for-Failure-to-Rescue/64958.
9. Youngblood SC, Deng Y, et al. Perioperative therapeutic plasmapheresis. Anesthesiology. 2013;118:722–8.
10. Meshkat S, Rodrigues NB, et al. Pharmacogenomics of ketamine: a systematic review. J Psychiatr Res. 2021;145:27–34.
11. Five emerging medical specialties you've never heard of — until now [Internet]. AAMC. Available from: https://www.aamc.org/news/five-emerging-medical-specialties-you-ve-never-heard-until-now.

Authors

Catherine Cooper is a senior anesthesiologist at VCU who spent many years doing cases in the liver transplant rooms. She is known for her extensive compilation of wise and witty sayings, which she generously shared with us.

Mark Nelson is a senior cardiac anesthesiologist at VCU. Although originally from Tacoma, Washington, his favorite sports team is the Dallas Cowboys. He is also an audiophile, so sound is one of his favorite things in life. He loves dogs, especially Dobermans and rat terriers.

Ron Bank is a senior cardiac and trauma anesthesiologist at INOVA. There is no area of the practice of anesthesiology that does not capture his interest. Besides spending time with his family, he loves SCUBA, travel, and baseball.

Cathy Marcucci is a senior anesthesiologist and transfusion medicine physician who has practiced in the Hopkins, University of Maryland, University of Pennsylvania, Department of Veterans Affairs, and NIH systems. She views teaching and academic publishing as two sides of the same coin.

157 Wisdom on Sepsis and Trauma

Jordan S. Zunder, Shawn Jia, John C. Briggs,
Catherine Marcucci, and Rajen V. Nathwani

Contributors:

Andrew B. Barker, MD (ABB)

Carol F. Bodenheimer, MD (CFB)

Introduction

Sepsis and trauma are two particularly fascinating areas of clinical anesthesia practice, both in the OR and the ICU. Doing them well requires a deep understanding and appreciation of the pertinent physiology, skillful deployment of our pharmacological resources, and great teamwork. It also requires forward thinking as well—we still don't have anywhere near all the answers with regard to either of these clinical emergencies. The opinions below are based on close observations. We hope and think that they will soon be established to be correct.

J. S. Zunder (✉)
Department of Anesthesiology and Pain Medicine (former), Harborview Hospital Center, University of Washington, Seattle, WA, USA

Department of Anesthesiology and Pain Medicine (current), University of Ottawa, Ottawa, ON, Canada
e-mail: jzunder@toh.ca

S. Jia
Department of Anesthesiology, The University of North Carolina at Chapel Hill, Chapel Hill, NC, USA

J. C. Briggs
Department of Anesthesiology and Perioperative Medicine, University of Alabama—Birmingham, Birmingham, AL, USA

C. Marcucci
Department of Transfusion Medicine, Clinical Center, National Institutes of Health, Bethesda, MD, USA

R. V. Nathwani
Department of Anesthesiology and Pain Medicine, University of Washington School of Medicine, Harborview Medical Center, Seattle, WA, USA

S. Mohamed et al. (eds.), *Anesthesia Bridges*, https://doi.org/10.1007/978-3-032-08294-7_157

Sepsis

Pathophysiology and Diagnosis

- Early recognition is important. Not just because they need volume or pressors but because the dominoes got knocked over. The longer you wait, the more organ systems you will lose. This is related to antibiotics, source control, inflammatory reactions, and secondary injury.—**JCB**

- Utilize hospital-wide screening tools (like MEWS) so that potentially septic patients are identified early and build a program that will respond to these alerts and work the patient up. ICU nurses, STAT nurses, rapid response teams….they are great for these.—**RVN**

- The body's systems are taught in silos. Even in "system based" models the attempt to fully capture aspects of physiology and pathology are lost. The manifestation of "sepsis" still remains an amalgamation of bad humors with much more fancy names. The interplay of body systems, genes, and pathophysiologic insult can result in so much dysfunction that a better question is what system isn't impacted.—**JCB**

- The most important physiology is the interconnectedness of the organ systems. Don't piss off the kidneys.—**ABB**

- Shock in sepsis may be a mixed picture. Central venous oxygen saturation trends, left ventricular outflow tract velocity time integral, and cardiac output monitor trends can all be helpful in sepsis management.—**RVN**

- Research regarding pro-inflammatory vs. anti-inflammatory states, steroid responsive vs. non-responsive, and all other presentations and interventions may all be correct, simultaneously. A willingness to ask and be wrong will define the next generation of pathophysiology. Understanding gene predisposition, host response, insult, and downstream response are only now being able to be assessed.—**JCB**

- Sepsis is *always* on the differential in the ICU. —**RVN**

- A low temperature is probably worse than an elevated temperature as a marker for severe sepsis.—**RVN**

- Assessing fluid status in a critically ill septic patient hinges on your ability to analyze data from multiple sources. Take advantage of all the information you have at your disposal to formulate a hypothesis of what's going on with the patient. This may include blood pressure, capillary refill time, urine output, lactate clearance, point of care ultrasound, pulse wave analysis, central venous pressure (CVP), central venous oxygen saturation (ScvO2), and the list goes on and on.—**SYJ**

- While some fluid status metrics may provide more insight than others, each contributes to a fuller picture. Relying solely on a single data point increases the likelihood of making an incorrect conclusion. The more data points you consider, the more accurate your assessment of the patient's fluid status is likely to be.—**SYJ**

- Two sets of blood cultures do not guarantee 100% sensitivity. Bacteremia is often transient. To improve sensitivity or to rule out a bloodstream infection more confidently, take additional sets of blood cultures at varied times.—**SYJ**

- Capillary refill time and respiratory rate are simple and very effective tests to identify sick patients—make it part of your examination every time.—**RVN**

- If you can't figure out the source of infection, aggressive imaging often provides the answer (i.e., CT chest abdomen pelvis).—**SYJ**

- A thorough history and exam is vital to work out where the infection is—a CT scan doesn't answer everything.—**RVN**

- If the patient has sufficient mental acuity, ask them if they are having any "unexpected" pain. One of our family members was a chest trauma patient and kept having positive blood cultures. They kept changing out her neck lines. She also kept complaining of significant thigh and leg pain, which was initially sort of ignored. Finally, somebody put it together and figured out that she had a septic knee joint.—**Editors**

- Also, don't forget to survey the head and neck for occult infections that might be the source of fevers and/or sepsis. I know of two patients who had unrecognized dental abscesses that were causing a lot of difficulty for the ICU team, until they figured out what was going on. Remember that coverage for dental flora sometimes requires very specific antibiotic coverage.—**CM**

- In the immunocompromised, you have to really hunt further and deeper for the sepsis source.—**RVN**

- The young otherwise healthy patient may not be symptomatic until near hemodynamic collapse.—**ABB**

- The chronically critically ill patient will not be able to demonstrate that they are becoming ill (think chronic necrotizing pancreatitis with a new sepsis)—they can become unusually hemodynamically labile, their white count decreases, they have high parasympathetic tone, or their blood sugar becomes challenging to manage where it hasn't been before.—**ABB**

- Septic cardiomyopathy may be the reason the patient is in shock—get the echo probe and take a look.—**RVN**

- I agree completely with the wisdom above. More than just septic shock may be at play. So allow us to repeat: *don't forget about the heart*. Septic/stress cardiomyopathy might be contributing, and RV dysfunction often accompanies ARDS. To know for sure, perform a point-of-care cardiac ultrasound or order a TTE for anyone with septic shock. You might find the patient has depressed cardiac function and could benefit from an inotrope. You might even stumble upon something totally unexpected, such as a big pericardial effusion or dynamic outflow obstruction.—**SYJ**

- If an ICU patient starts having a profoundly elevated white blood cell count that is disproportionate to their clinical severity of illness, think about C. diff.—**SYJ**

- Lactate levels, and lactate clearance may help identify if you are winning the sepsis fight.—**RVN**

***Note from the Editors:** Because sepsis is such a complex disease that must be viewed and understood from multiple perspectives, we asked a friend who is trained both in architecture and civil engineering if he could send us a bridge photo to act as a good visual metaphor. This stunning and visually complex photograph was taken of the C & O canal in metropolitan Washington, DC (Fig. 157.1).

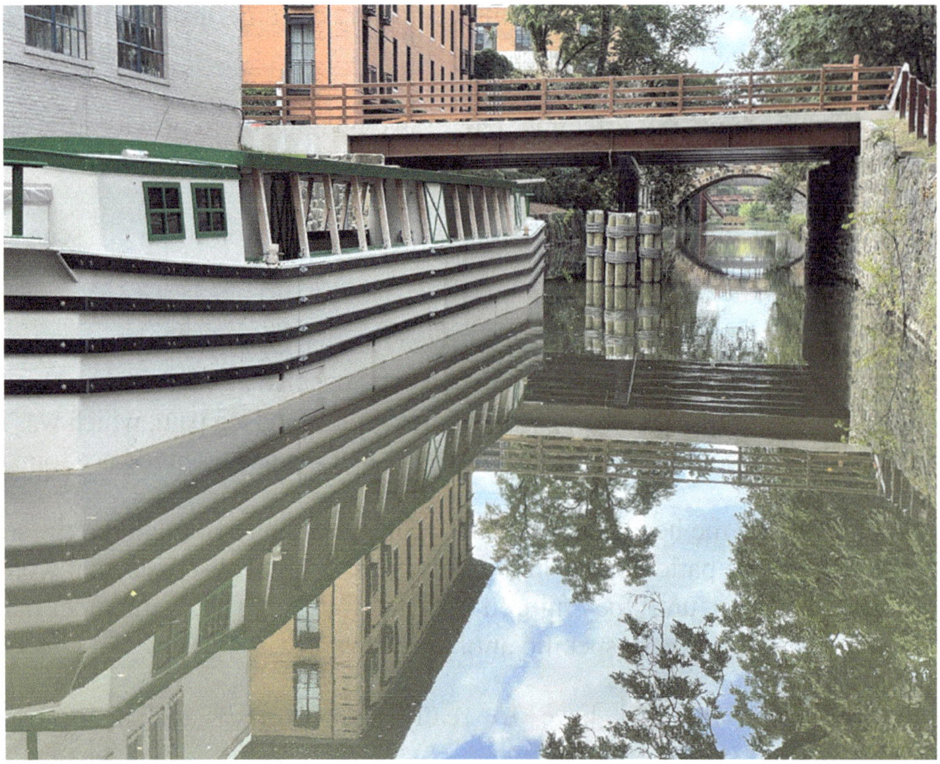

Fig. 157.1 A beautiful C & O canal bridge in a stunning cityscape with beautiful reflections in Washington, DC. Photo: Bo Johns-Hennessey

Clinical Approach to Sepsis and Therapies

- Build sepsis bundles for your hospital and audit regularly—antibiotics within one hour, up to 30 ml/kg fluid resuscitation in the first three hours, ICU admission within six hours……..easy to do, easy to track, and shows where the problems are in your system.—**RVN**

- Sepsis bundles are bundles—everything needs to be done to get the effect. Undertake regular audit cycles to make sure the basics are being done correctly.—**RVN**

- But steer clear of overly rigid, one-size-fits-all approach to fluid resuscitation in sepsis. Septic shock can coexist with conditions, such as congestive heart failure, severe ARDS, and right heart dysfunction. The initial 30 ml/kg of IV fluids recommended by "Surviving Sepsis" guidelines may actually be harmful for these patients. Always think about whether *the patient in front of you* patient truly needs the fluid and how they will tolerate the additional volume. If just following an algorithm was good enough, we wouldn't need those six years of post-graduate training, right?—**SYJ and CM**

- Do the simple things well before doing the expensive things, which often don't work. Keep your bed occupancy rates ideally below 95%, space out your patients, ideally in single occupancy rooms. Wash your hands, use hand sanitizer regularly, avoid cross contamination between patients. Many countries practice "bare below the elbows"—no lanyards, no ties, no white coats. Make sure staff quarantine at home when they are unwell, educate, and empower your nursing staff to manage sepsis.—**RVN**

- Many sepsis guidelines are based on limited evidence. For example, we think that filling the tank is a central component to maintaining organ perfusion in sepsis but remember that fluids increased mortality in the FEAST study in septic African children. Be willing to think out of the box.—**RVN**

- Balanced crystalloids are the fluid of choice in sepsis.—**RVN**

- You know what predicts fluid responsiveness? The fluid you just gave! If your last fluid bolus didn't even transiently improve the blood pressure or pressor requirement what makes you think the next one is going to? If you order a fluid bolus, make sure you follow up to see how the patient responded to it.—**SYJ**

- When administering a fluid bolus, opt for smaller volumes (250-500 ml) infused rapidly. Make your bolus both therapeutic and diagnostic. Following the bolus, observe its impact on blood pressure or, if available, on calculated cardiac output via some form of cardiac output monitoring.—**SYJ**

- Use POCUS and dynamic endpoints to guide fluid therapy. A passive straight leg raise may provide more information than another 500 ml fluid challenge.—**RVN**

- Blood pressure increase during a passive leg raise can provide a useful data point for fluid responsiveness. This can be particularly helpful in those who might be adversely affected by additional fluid, such as those with severe ARDS or heart failure. This method tends to be more *sensitive* if done when the initial mean arterial pressure (MAP) is low and when the MAP can be accurately measured using invasive arterial pressure monitoring. It is likely to be more *specific* in sedated patients, as lifting their legs does not cause them discomfort.—**SYJ**

- Don't have the energy to lift the patient's legs up? Putting the patient's bed in steep Trendelenburg position accomplishes something similar.—**SYJ**

- Have a hypotensive septic patient? Start the norepinephrine infusion, via peripheral IV, if necessary, at the same time that you're giving your fluid bolus. Should your patient's blood pressure improve with fluid resuscitation, just wean the pressors off. Don't let a patient sit with a MAP in the 50's while you're waiting for your fluid bolus to finish. Your patient's nephrons will thank you.—**SYJ**

- Low to moderate dose vasopressor infusions are safe through peripheral IVs for short durations—generally 24 hours or less. Use an IV that you're confident about. Monitor the IV insertion site frequently for signs of infiltration. If the pressor dose is increasing or you anticipate the patient is going to need pressors for a while, put in the central line.—**RVN and SYJ**

- When treating blood pressure, waiting for methylene blue and angiotensin-2 as last-ditch efforts may be counterproductive. Early use likely benefits some patients, the question is when and who, not if so.—**JCB**

- For a patient in septic shock on moderate to high dose vasopressors, consider giving stress dose steroids. This is a recommendation in the Surviving Sepsis guidelines. The literature shows IV corticosteroids reduce vasopressor requirements, even in patients without lab evidence of adrenal insufficiency, and may reduce mortality.—**SYJ**

- Don't discount a fever. Treat a fever but be mindful of using medication that mask fevers.—**ABB**

- And because continuous renal replacement therapy (CRRT) affects body temperature, detecting infections is especially challenging. A large study at the Mayo Clinic looked at 587 patients on CRRT, of whom 365 had infections and 222 did not.1 There was no statistical difference in body temperature while on CRRT between the groups. While not on CRRT, the infection group had significantly higher body temperatures.—**ABB**

- Start broad antibiotics early—delay increases mortality. Take cultures, and you can always stop antibiotics if cultures come back negative or narrow them to target the infection better.—**RVN**

- Microbiologists on an ICU team are worth their weight in gold. They will target the infection better, think of diagnoses that may have been missed, and provide antimicrobial stewardship.—**RVN**

- Bugs are clever; so you need to be fast and smart to outclass them. Remember they have been killing things far longer than humans have been around!—**RVN**

- Learn about your local antibiogram and make sure your antimicrobial choices change as resistance patterns change.—**RVN**

- Antimicrobials do not penetrate pus—you need a surgeon's knife to penetrate for you. Source control is vital for sepsis management.—**RVN**

- Critically ill septic patients often need MRSA antibiotic coverage. This patient population also often goes on to develop AKI. While vancomycin is the usual go-to antibiotic for MRSA, it's a known *nephrotoxin.* Consider using linezolid as your first line empiric MRSA coverage in critically ill patients.—**SYJ**

- But remember that linezolid is a weak reversible monoamine oxidase inhibitor! Be very careful when adding this drug to a medication regimen if the patient is also on antidepressant as current antidepressants exert effects through biogenic amine pathways. Drug interactions may include central serotonin syndrome or hypertensive episodes. Extreme caution is warranted in using beta-blockers to treat linezolid-associated hypertension as paradoxical increased hypertension may result due to unopposed alpha effects.**—CM and NBS**

- Cut back on antibiotics that aren't helping. Follow up your culture data daily for speciation and antibiotic sensitivity. Order your antibiotics with an end date!—**SYJ**

- Consider drug resistance when your antimicrobials don't seem to be working.—**RVN**

- Remember that the anti-microbials are implicated in some of the most predictable and clinically relevant drug-drug interactions. These drug–drug interactions (DDIs) are well-described at this point, so buckle down and accept that the standard of care involves mastering them.—**CM and NBS**

- Significant and clinically relevant DDIs involving ciprofloxacin, levofloxacin, erythromycin, the "azole' antifungals, and rifampin have all been clearly documented.—**CM and NBS**

- Continue anti-endotoxin antibiotics for at least 72 hours in NSTI.—**RVN**

- De-escalation of antimicrobials is just as important as escalation. Anti-microbials cause harm often at the population level with increasing resistance patterns. Also remember that many anti-microbials started life a chemotherapy agents and vice versa. They are strong and even somewhat dangerous drugs if not given for a firm clinical indication.—**RVN and CM**

- IVIG is an option in necrotizing soft tissue infections (NSTI) with toxic shock syndrome or in group A strep; but also may be beneficial in NSTI with profound vasoplegia even though source control has already been achieved.—**RVN**

- Low molecular weight heparin is advisable to decrease VTE risk in sepsis. It may also provide anti-inflammatory effects, anti-complemental activation, and the modulation of various proteases and decrease the risk of pulmonary hypertension by interrupting neutrophil adhesion to the lung membrane.—**RVN**

- Consider bicarb therapy with bicarb <5 mEq/L and/or pH < 7.1 or AKI stage 2/3.—**RVN**

- When patients are clearly dying, bring in palliative care teams and have early goals of care discussions.—**RVN**

- Taking care of sepsis patients is an ongoing series of ups and downs. Experienced intensivists know that the goal is to go get out of the latest valley.—**Editors**

***Note from the Editors:** This dramatic and memorable photo of the Arlington Memorial Bridge shows the approach across the Potomac River to the Lincoln Memorial and the National Mall (Fig. 157.2).

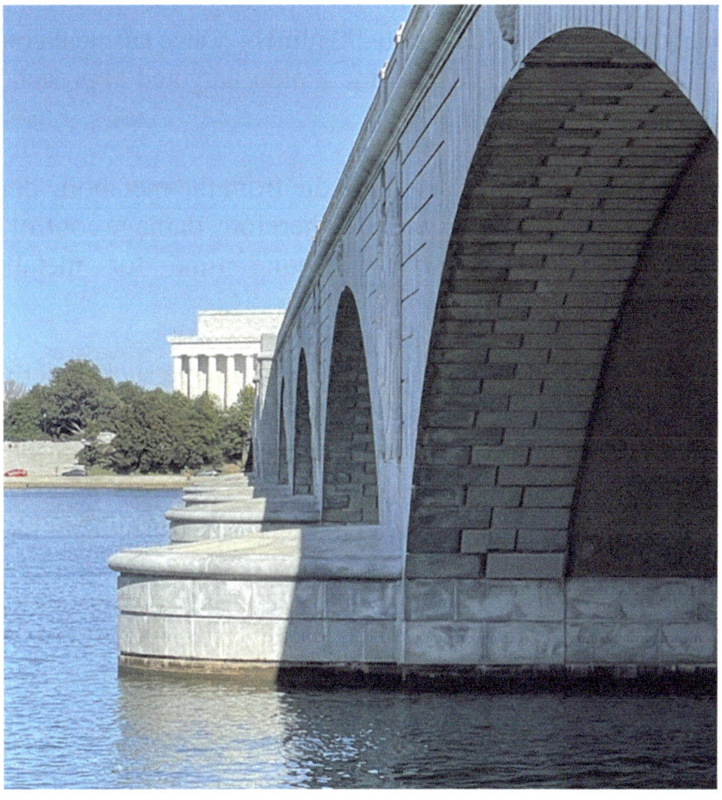

Fig. 157.2 The Arlington Memorial Bridge leads to Arlington National Cemetery on the Virginia side of the river and opened in 1932. Photo: Bo Johns-Hennessey

Trauma

Hemorrhage and Hormonal Considerations

- There are at least four basic kinds of trauma patients—patients who are in danger of bleeding to death overtly, patients who are in danger of bleeding to death covertly, orthopedic trauma patients (including hand trauma), and burn patients. Each has a different approach to both acute and chronic care. And understand that in a long-term ICU trauma patient, the acute and chronic care periods overlap.—**Editors**

- Working in the trauma field means following the decisions, advances, and outcomes in the military trauma community. No way around it.—**Editors**

- Hemorrhage is the leading preventable cause of death following traumatic injury. Intervention should be aimed at providing damage control resuscitation, such as permissive hypotension, hemostatic resuscitation, and damage control surgery.—**JSZ and RVN**

- In a real massive transfusion, having *reliable* IV access is better than what's theoretically optimal. While it's accurate that large-bore peripheral IVs typically offer faster flow rates compared to central lines, the risk of infiltration with peripheral IVs, especially when under pressure infusion, is high. In an unstable hemorrhaging patient losing IV access could be catastrophic. Therefore, obtaining dependable central access, with a preference for larger-sized introducers and catheters, should be a high priority during large-volume resuscitations.—**SYJ**

- Hemostatic resuscitation prior to surgical control of bleeding should consist of ratio-based administration of blood products targeting an SBP of 80–90 mmHg. Once surgical control has been achieved, laboratory and POCT testing can be used to guide a more targeted approach to resuscitation.—**JSZ and RVN**

- Severely injured trauma patients are more likely to die from the metabolic derangements induced by their injuries than incomplete surgical intervention. Therefore, damage control surgery aims to address immediately life-threatening injuries while allowing time for metabolic and physiologic optimization.—**JSZ and RVN**

- The body has evolved many compensatory mechanisms to trauma such as activation of hypothalamic-pituitary-adrenal axis, sympathetic nervous system, rennin-angio-tensin aldosterone system, complement system, hemostatic mechanisms. These mechanisms attempt to return the body to homeostasis and minimize volume loss. These should be supported, but over-resuscitation, especially with crystalloids, can overwhelm these mechanisms and lead to increased morbidity.—**JSZ and RVN**

- Restoration of normal or even supranormal blood pressures during resuscitation of the trauma patient may reflect the early phase of sympathetic stimulation rather than adequate resuscitation. The patient may still be significantly acidotic and hypovolemic. Normalization of base excess and lactate is a marker of meaningful resuscitation.—**JSZ and RVN**

- Severe trauma patients are often surviving by maximal catecholamine outflow. Therefore any vasodilation from medication, such as induction of general anesthesia, may precipitate cardiovascular collapse. Be judicious with drug doses, even ones like ketamine and etomidate, that are meant to be cardio stable. —**JCB**

- Damage control resuscitation—permissive hypotension, hemostatic resuscitation, and damage control surgery—aims to intervene on the lethal triad (acidosis, hypothermia, coagulopathy) thereby minimizing blood loss and optimizing tissue oxygenation.—**JSZ and RVN**

- Permissive hypotension aims to strike a balance between tissue perfusion to vital organs and minimizing clot disruption based on the notion that the "first clot is the best clot." However, there is a lack of evidence for improved outcomes with permissive hypotension, particularly in patients with blunt trauma injuries.—**JSZ and RVN**

- Hypothermia is one of the vertices of the lethal triad and is a significant contributor to morbidity and mortality in the trauma patient. Every effort should be made to return the patient to a state of normothermia. Forced air warmers are most effective for this purpose, but a warmed OR, fluid and blood warmers, warming blankets, and underbody warmers are useful adjuncts.—**JSZ and RVN**

- Hypocalcemia induced by the citrate load of massive transfusion inhibits the hemostatic effects of platelets and fibrin. Calcium should be administered every four units of RBCs or FFPs and ionized calcium levels should be monitored regularly.—**JSZ and RVN**

- Data show administration of tranexamic acid within three hours of injury decreases morbidity and mortality by inhibiting the exaggerated fibrinolysis induced by traumatic injury. Administration after three hours is associated with increased mortality.—**JSZ and RVN**

- Be extra careful of the very young and the old—their physiological limits can easily be overwhelmed in trauma.—**JSZ and RVN**

Shock

- The pathophysiology of traumatic shock is complex and involves an early sympatho-excitatory phase and a sympatho-inhibitory phase. A nuanced understanding of this pathology is critical to providing appropriate resuscitation and hemodynamic support.—**JSZ and RVN**

- Hemorrhagic shock is the most common form following traumatic injury. However, any form of shock (cardiogenic, obstructive, and neurogenic) may co-present in the trauma patient. Hypotension should have a broad differential diagnosis in order to provide the most appropriate treatment.—**JSZ and RVN**

- Multiple shock types may coexist. Hemorrhagic and neurogenic shock require similar treatment, but when coexisting, the volume requirement may overwhelm the capacitance. Low dose epi/norepi goes a long way in this situation. As mentioned, in the ongoing blood loss context, a normal blood pressure is not necessarily good. Keep this in mind when competing organ systems are malfunctioning.—**JCB**

- Using small dose opioids to unmask compensatory sympathetic tone is helpful when gauging the above point. Additional vasodilating agents may also mask true problems. The best approach isn't "always this" or "never that" but must be questioned for every patient.—**JCB**

- Shock index (HR/SBP) is a surrogate for resuscitation but can be confounded in young, healthy, or chronically medicated patients. Pay attention to labs, trend the big picture, and don't forget to ask why something seems abnormal if it is.—**JCB**

- The early phase of traumatic shock is characterized by vasoconstriction mediated by the sympathetic nervous system, leading to increased SVR and heart rate which maintains arterial blood pressure in the face of a decrease in cardiac output as a result of ongoing blood loss. This response is largely mediated by angiotensin-II (AT-II), vasopressin (AVP), norepinephrine and epinephrine.—**JSZ and RVN**

- The neurohormonal responses that maintain blood pressure during the early phase of traumatic shock (particularly increased arginine vasopressin, as well as angiotensin-II and norepinephrine) may become exhausted with ongoing blood loss in the late phase, contributing to a loss of vascular tone. Therefore, volume resuscitation in the late phase may be ineffective at restoring arterial blood pressure and exogenous supplementation of these hormones/neurotransmitters may be required. There is some evidence to suggest vasopressin infusions started early may decrease morbidity in severe penetrating trauma.—**JSZ and RVN**

- If you intubate a hypotensive patient in hypovolemic shock without resuscitating them first, there is a good chance you'll be doing CPR. The patient's spontaneous respirations generating negative intrathoracic pressure are the only thing sustaining their venous return. Try to hold off on intubating until you've restored at least some of their circulating volume.—**SYJ**

- The intact vascular endothelium is integral in maintaining vasomotor tone, permeability, patency and transport of oxygen and nutrients. Disruption of the endothelium as a result of either direct tissue injury or accumulation of inflammatory products may contribute to the tissue edema, vasoplegia, and trauma-induced coagulopathy of the distributive late phase of traumatic shock.—**JSZ and RVN**

- The late phase of traumatic shock is characterized by a vasodilatory shock that presents similarly to other forms of distributive shock. Vascular hyporeactivity results from a decrease in sympathetic tone, arterial vasodilation, and bradycardia, despite increased adrenal production of epinephrine and norepinephrine.—**JSZ and RVN**

- You don't really "cure" sepsis or trauma—the best you can aim for is to solve the puzzle. And sometimes that means minimizing interventions to only those absolutely necessary until you see which way the patients are going and how the heck you can best help them get home.—**Editors**

***Note from the Editors:** This very famous housing structure in Montreal is a great illustration of transitions, bridges, a complex puzzle, and home (Fig. 157.3). It is one of *Anesthesia Bridges* illustrator Lisa Sandson's favorite buildings.

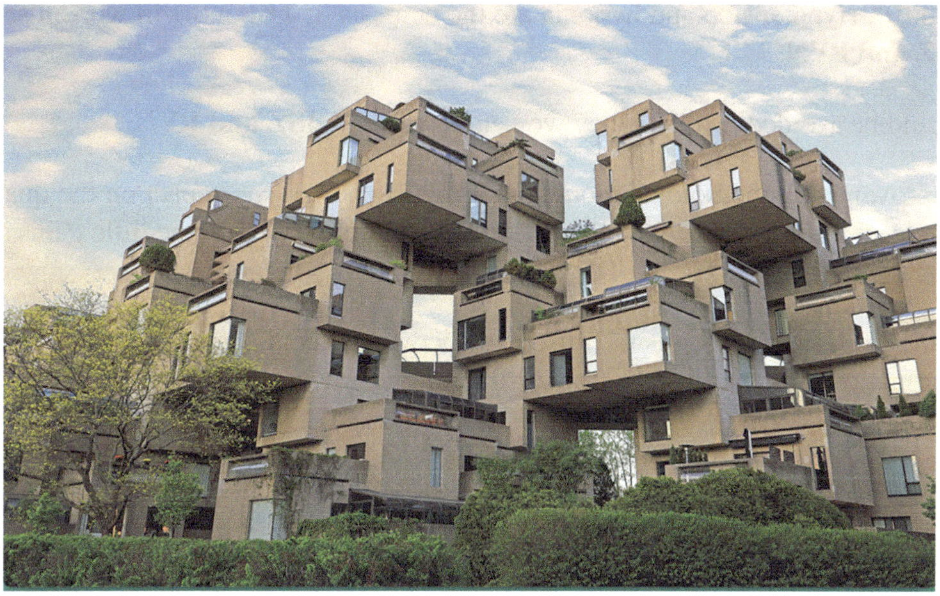

Fig. 157.3 Habitat 67 in Montreal, designed by Moshe Safdie. The design began as his thesis project. Each unit has a private landscaped terrace. There are covered bridge walkways between sections of the housing project but they are obscured by the dramatic configuration of the complex. Instead, the structure itself is the bridge. Photo: Vladone, image used under license from iStock.com

Brain and Spinal Cord Injury in Trauma

- Remember that patients with head trauma can have deadly bleeding without exsanguinating. Even 50 mL of blood loss in the head can have a devastating outcome.—**Editors**

- The most critical blood component for head, brain, and spinal cord trauma patients is *platelets*. Thrombocytopenia may be a risk factor for the occurrence and severity of bleeding in the central nervous system and may also be an outcome predictor. Check platelet counts early and often.—**CM**

- Patients with spinal cord injury are at significant risk of secondary injury from hypotension and hypoxia. Aim for MAPs >85 and normoxia, as long as they are not hemorrhaging.—**JSZ and RVN**

- Neurogenic shock in the acute setting is a diagnosis of exclusion—hemorrhage, tension pneumothorax, and tamponade/cardiac dysfunction must be ruled out first.—**JSZ and RVN**

- Neurogenic shock is secondary to loss of sympathetic thoraco-lumbar outflow. Treatment for neurogenic shock involves adequate fluid/blood resuscitation and vasopressors with alpha agonists. If the injury is above the level of the cardiac accelerator fibers (T1-T4), the patient may also need inotropy with beta-1 agonism. Therefore, often norepinephrine is used as the pressor of choice, with alpha- and beta-adrenergic action.—**JSZ and RVN**

- Isolated traumatic brain injury (TBI) patients should have higher SBP goals as per the World Federation of Neurosurgical Societies (WFNS) guidelines in mm Hg (18-49 yrs. >110, 50–69 years >100,

>70 years >110). Hypotension and hypoxia are the nemesis of TBI and will worsen secondary brain injury.—**JSZ and RVN**

- Steroids should be avoided in TBI—they worsen outcome.—**JSZ and RVN**

- A minor improvement in neurological outcome can have a massive impact on the quality of life the patient can expect forever more. Not all small gains are equal but often the little gains are synergistic and important.—**JSZ, RVN, and CFB**

- Time is brain, time is spine, time is the difference between life and death in trauma. The quicker you can get information and act on it, the better the outcome. But the actions must be controlled and careful.—**JSZ and RVN**

You and the Trauma Team

- Trauma is a team sport—for the patient to survive, every person in the team, from the prehospital paramedics through the rehab staff, needs to pull their weight, and work together.—**JSZ and RVN**

- Remember that the families can be very efficient, helpful, and effective trauma team members. We've had lots of people say, "I had to pull through for my kids." But nobody ever said that about the ICU physicians and nurses. And many, many times we have seen unresponsive patients suddenly respond to the voice or touch of a loved one.—**Editors**

- Trauma cases are very dramatic. We've found that they tend to stay with people -patients and caregivers both, for many years. Another reason to make sure they go as well as you can make them go.—**Editors**

- On the other hand, don't permit any family drama at the trauma bedside. Be firm about this if you have to.—**Editors**

- Trauma patients can easily decompensate when left alone in the ED—keep an eye on them.—**JSZ and RVN**

- Just because a trauma patient was stable when they came into the ED, doesn't mean they are now. Repeat exams and tests regularly. Do a primary, secondary, and tertiary survey so that injuries are not missed.—**JSZ and RVN**

- The anesthesiologist should (at least outwardly) be the calmest person during a crisis. Your response will set the tone in the OR and help the rest of the team remain calm, cool, and collected.—**JSZ and RVN**

- An apocryphal maxim states that a good surgeon deserves a good anesthesiologist; a bad surgeon deserves a great one. In truth, a favorable outcome for the patient relies on effective communication and team dynamics as much as on clinical acumen. Mutual respect and teamwork go a long way.—**JSZ and RVN**

- Make sure someone on the trauma team—surgeons or ICU—places a consult with the rehab medicine service as soon as is practically possible, especially for hand trauma or limb reattachment surgeries. The affected joint or joints may need to be immobilized, but the function in the remaining and proximal joints and maintenance of the proximal muscle mass and memory is an important principle in trauma rehabilitation. If your institution has a dedicated hand or upper extremity occupational therapist, early intervention by that service is also important for the best possible outcomes.—**CFB and CM**

- Be aware, however, that emotional and psychological recovery after trauma does not correlate directly with physical and functional recovery. Be sensitive to this when dealing with the trauma patients and their families. The correlation exists but is not linear and straightforward. Factors such as pre-morbid resilience may also be important determinants for recovery after trauma.—**CFB and CM**

- Organize your workspace as much as possible to decrease cognitive load so you can focus on providing clinical care. Discard used syringes, have a dedicated area for administered fluids and blood products, untangle, and label lines and monitoring cables. Deciphering which line goes where should not be an impediment to expeditious intervention. Remember that someone is going to have to come into this situation and give you a break at some point and you want to make things easier for those people. Neatness and organization will also make transport to ICU a simpler process.—**JSZ and RVN**

- In the OR, command and control is essential. Use your team effectively and keep on top of what is happening to the pt. Delegation is vital.—**JSZ and RVN**

- Have a plan A, B, C, D...........Z if needed. Trauma patients are unpredictable.—**JSZ and RVN**

- Concise and accurate closed loop communication is the only way.—**JSZ and RVN**

- Think *10 every 10*—take 10 seconds every 10 minutes to find out where the surgeons are and update them about where the resuscitation effort is.—**JSZ and RVN**

- While advanced trauma life support works in a sequential manner, the reality is, in modern trauma centers, everything happens at the same time—deal with the life-threatening stuff first but move quickly and move forward.—**JSZ and RVN**

- Learn to put in landmark based central lines, even if you have to actively seek the opportunity to do so. They may save your patient one day.—**JSZ and RVN**

- An arterial line is not a therapeutic procedure. Do not delay surgical control of bleeding for arterial blood pressure monitoring. The NIBP can be cycled q1min while you work on invasive BP access under the drapes.—**JSZ and RVN**

- CT scanners don't have to be a doughnut of death—you just need to keep resuscitating in the scanner. The information they provide can be lifesaving.—**JSZ and RVN**

- When the situation has stabilized, take a breath to recenter yourself. Check in with all members of the team and remind them that they are doing great work. Be the cheerleader and the coach.—**JSZ and RVN**

- When taking a trauma patient from the ICU back to the OR after an initial surgery, don't assume anything. The endotracheal tube may be endobronchial, lines may be interstitial, injuries may have evolved, or there may have been initial injuries that have gone unrecognized, and there may be occult blood loss. Always do your own examination. Just because an ICU case may seem like "plug and play" doesn't mean it is not complex and things can't go wrong.—**JSZ and RVN**

- Speaking to the families of trauma victims can be particularly challenging. Be truthful; do not sugarcoat the facts. Offer information in easily digestible chunks. Avoid jargon, humor, jocularity, and disapproval. Be sympathetic and allow the family to ask questions. Don't feel the need to fill the silence.—**JSZ, CM, and RVN**

- Distance yourself from any "social" aspects of the trauma case. Concentrate only on the technical details of the case before you. You must accept that at some point you may be taking care of the person who committed the crime or the drunk person who was driving the car. This is sometimes very hard, but you have to do it, or you cannot deliver the best care. Remember that you are not the social worker, the police, the judge, or the jury.—**Editors**

- Remember that when the case is over you are going home to dinner and bed. For the patients and families, the worst period in their life may just be starting.—**Editors and RVN**

- Burnout threatens to cut short the longevity of even the most resilient clinicians. After a difficult case, make sure you take time to look after your own well-being: have a good meal with family or friends, exercise, read a book unrelated to medicine, and listen to music. Do things that "fill your cup" so you can return to work refreshed and ready to take on new challenges.—**JSZ and RVN**

- Death is unfortunately part and parcel of trauma care—look out for your team and support each other. Those deaths help form who you are as a clinician, and they can make you or break you.—**JSZ and RVN**

- Trauma medicine is inextricably linked with transplant medicine, of course, for the near and probably distant future. Many institutions prefer to keep some separation between these teams and the ensuing discussion with families, for understandable reasons. Keep abreast on what's going in the transplant fields but also follow your hospital's policies for how the transplant donor issues are handled to the exact letter.—**Editors**

- Pursuing a non-ACGME accredited fellowship in trauma anesthesiology allows the fellow to customize training to their interests and focus exposure to better fit their long-term career goals. The breadth of clinical trauma training, including vascular, neurosurgical, regional, POCUS, ICU, transfusion, and pre-hospital issues, prepares graduates to offer value to a variety of departments and subspeciality groups, while experience in broader interconnected systems of care affords a unique insight into the functioning of complex trauma systems.—**JSZ and RVN**

- A fellowship may not be needed for your future job, but learning from experienced clinicians is a sure way to improve your care model.—**JSZ and RVN**

- Learn where your weaknesses are and train to deal with them—nobody is an expert at everything, but you can always get better.—**JSZ and RVN**

Final Advice!

- Sepsis, trauma, and shock all know each other. The close study of one of these clinical emergencies will benefit you in caring for the other, both in the OR and in the ICU.
- Here is one last tidbit that can apply to sepsis or trauma or *any* critically ill patient:
  - *Never* dismiss the intuition of an experienced ICU nurse, especially when it comes to sepsis. They're the ones in the thick of it, keeping a close eye on patients around the clock. When they raise a concern, telling you something doesn't seem right, it's a clear signal to go assess the situation. And if they come to you saying a patient "looks bad"? Things are about to get real serious, real fast.

Acknowledgment: The authors thank Amy Robbins for her careful review and helpful suggestions for this chapter.

Reference

1. Challener DW, Gao X, et al. Body temperature and infection in critically ill patients on continuous kidney replacement therapy. BMC Nephrol. 2023;24(1):161.

Authors

Jordan Zunder was an anesthesiologist and trauma fellow at Harborview Medical Center in Seattle. At present, he is a staff anesthesiologist at the University of Ottawa in Ottawa, Canada. His clinical interests include transfusion practices and POCUS in trauma. He is also an enthusiastic supporter of medical education, teaching medical students and residents at all levels. When not in the OR he enjoys trying to keep up with his wife and dog as they hike, bike, and run well past him.

Shawn Jia is an anesthesiologist and critical care medicine physician at UNC-Chapel Hill. His interests include critical care ultrasound, medical education, and perioperative quality improvement. He enjoys short rounds, shorter notes, and smooth inductions.

John Briggs is an anesthesiologist and critical care physician at the University of Alabama at Birmingham, where he is honored to be able to teach learners of all levels and continue to be humbled by the art and science of medicine. When not working, he is thankful for the love of family and graces bestowed.

Cathy Marcucci is a senior anesthesiologist who has done many trauma cases that lasted well into the next day. She has often wondered if any of these patients ever even knew her name and has finally accepted that they did not.

Raj Nathwani is now the lead for trauma anesthesiology and the program director for the anesthesiology trauma fellowship at Harborview Medical Center, a level one trauma center in Seattle. Experiencing excellent trauma care for soldiers and civilians wounded in Afghanistan has shown him what can be done with a focused well-practiced team—predicted non-survivors can survive!

Resuscitation Wisdom: Access and Fluids

158

Andrew B. Barker, Rajen V. Nathwani, Brant M. Wagener, Brian P. Barrick, Konstantinos Alfaras-Melainas, and Catherine Marcucci

Contributors:

David W. Barbara, MD (DWB)

John C. Briggs, MD (JCB)

Austin Brown (AB)

Catherine Cooper, MD (CC)

Abigail J. Crawford (AJC)

Brian T. Gierl, MD (BTG)

Patrick J. Forte, MD (PJF)

Albert Liao, LAc (AL)

Kristin King Liao, LAc (KKL)

Amy J. Robbins, MD (AJR)

A. B. Barker
Department of Anesthesiology and Perioperative Medicine, Heersink School of Medicine, University of Alabama at Birmingham, Birmingham, AL, USA

B. M. Wagener
Division of Critical Care Medicine, Division of Molecular and Translational Biomedicine, Birmingham, AL, USA

Department of Anesthesiology and Perioperative Medicine, Heersink School of Medicine, The University of at Birmingham, Birmingham, AL, USA

R. V. Nathwani
Department of Anesthesiology and Pain Medicine, Harborview Medical Center, University of Washington, Seattle, WA, USA

B. P. Barrick
Department of Anesthesiology, University of North Carolina – Chapel Hill, Chapel Hill, NC, USA

K. Alfaras-Melainas
Department of Anesthesiology and Perioperative Medicine, University of Pittsburgh, Pittsburgh, PA, USA

C. Marcucci (✉)
Department of Transfusion Medicine, Clinical Center, National Institutes of Health, Bethesda, MD, USA

S. Mohamed et al. (eds.), *Anesthesia Bridges*, https://doi.org/10.1007/978-3-032-08294-7_158

Juraj Sprung, MD PhD (JS)

Paul A. Tripi, MD (PAT)

Elizabeth A. Ungerman, MD (EAU)

Toby N. Weingarten, MD (TNW)

Charles J. Yeo, MD (CJY)

Introduction

Resuscitation questions—what to give, how much to give, and when to give it—are some of the most intriguing questions in anesthesiology. Over the years, the recommendations have gone back and forth quite a bit, even though we still don't know the definitive answers. This is what makes this subject so interesting and important.

Access

Basics

- "*Focus on doing the basics well*" is nowhere truer than with obtaining, securing, and maintaining vascular access. Our own mentors reminded us often that loss of IV access has probably resulted in more morbidity and even mortality than any other anesthesia event with the exception of loss of the airway.—**Editors**

- If you think you need more access, you do. You will not regret extra access.—**EAU and Editors**

- The access you secure keeps your patient alive every bit as much the airway.—**CM**

- There is nothing wrong with having a reasonable dose of caution about any line you yourself have not put in. Is it really where the person who put it in thinks it was? I was taught to also unhook every IV that I have "inherited" from another service, even the ICU, and make sure there is the appropriate venous (and not arterial backflow) backflow.—**CM**

- It's always possible to poke the needle out the back of any hollow structure.—**Editors**

- You organize your lines by organizing your thinking. Don't just hope and guess whether you will have enough access. Think it through! What access does the patient have now? Will you use that for the case? What line will you induce with? Where are the volume lines going? What lines do you need for monitoring? What about drips? Where is the backup site if any of these lines fail? —**CM**

- When teaching, do yourself and your trainee a favor and be very clear about how many attempts they are going to get before handing it over to somebody else.—**Editors**

- Not every level of trainee has to get a try at every vascular access procedure. And if it's a must-get on the first try, it's okay every once in a while, to just do it yourself. Use your social skills to settle any potentially ruffled feathers, "Do you mind if I take a crack at this one myself? That way if I blow it, you can be mad at me, and I can be mad at me."—**Editors**

- Ultrasound can be your true friend in a difficult IV access. But a big mistake beginners make is using ultrasound as a vessel finder rather than using it to augment their view of the anatomy.—**BMW and KAM**

- Don't make purse handles with the IV or arterial line tubing! Make a small loop with the tubing and *put the entire radius of that loop* under tape or a clear dressing.—**CM**

- Refresher! The gauge size of an IV needle/catheter indicates what the diameter of the lumen of the needle is, not a dimension of the actual IV catheter, itself. The larger the gauge, the smaller the lumen.—**Editors**

- Larger catheters and sheaths are measured in French (F). *1F = 1/3 mm and 0.013 inch.* This question was on my boards.—**Editors**

- When doing arterial lines and central venous lines, new trainees always put the wire somewhere silly—then, when they get blood return, they move around a lot and lose the flow before they can get the wire in.—**BMW**

- Organize your lines and stopcocks for transport! Get everything organized by the patient's head and neck. Get just one volume line with a set of stopcocks on top of a clean OR towel. Put the stopcock for the arterial under the clean OR towel or in some very out of the way location. You aren't going to be drawing a blood gas in the hallway. Also, make sure the transducer is at the level of the heart.—**CM**

- Remove lines and catheters (and drains) as soon as they are no longer needed—all act as an infectious focus.—**RVN**

- About 2% of claims in the ASA Closed Claims database involve line mishaps.—**Editors**

Venous Access

- Don't forget that an IV catheter is a piece of anesthesia equipment! They can crack and split and be subject to all sorts of malfunctions just like every other type of equipment we use. See below.—**CM**

- In my own personal peds experience, far and away the most common and potentially very dangerous "equipment" failures have been related to intravenous lines. I once attempted a rapid sequence induction in an infant with pyloric stenosis, only to discover the line became completely occluded. The infant was only partially induced with no circulating muscle relaxant, so we had to convert to a mask induction. All went well, but it was quite a challenge. I have seen several near compartment syndromes in failed IVs, mostly in infants.—**PAT**

- Remember that IV access may be the only preoperative "procedure" on the day of surgery that an adult patient may be wide awake for. I have had hundreds of people say to me, "They couldn't get the IV started." And then go on to describe their travails in great detail. It really is true that the IV start is your first chance to make a good impression.—**CM**

- This is so simple—don't try to start an IV hunched over an OR stretcher—sit down if it will be even slightly more ergonomic.—**Editors**

- When putting in an IV, you should be sitting, and your patient should not. Because once you've seen a patient just slide out of their chair and hit the floor in a faint when getting an IV started, you'll institute a new personal policy of not starting an IV unless the patient is on a stretcher. And watch out for the young guys who work out a lot, they can faint in two seconds. I once had a young man, a former Navy special forces, say "I feel woozy" and faint when I took the IV out of the package.—**CM**

- When starting IVs, new trainees like to remove the needle when they get flash rather than advancing the catheter. We think it's instinct, maybe? We know that the flash can occur when just part of the opening on the bevel of the needle is in the vein, but maybe the junior people aren't really aware of that. So, remember to impress on your students that the needle isn't withdrawn until the catheter is fully advanced into the vein.—**BMW**

- This is a bit of a casual statement, but IV mishaps—infiltration and loss of the IV—tend to happen to more junior anesthesiologists. Once you have a serious mishap, you tend to get a bit compulsive about IV insertion and integrity.—**Editors**

- UPMC published a survey study a few years back with respondents reporting that up to 7% of infiltrated IVs required medical attention [1].—**AJC and EAU**

- This study also found that there is a significant gap between what is understood to be "best practice" with infiltrated IVs—and what actually happens. Best practice would be things like checking compartment pressures, elevation, warm compresses, chart documentation and follow-up, and QA tracking. Does your department have guidelines on this clinical complication? If not, why not consider writing some?—**AJC and KAM**

- I put two IVs in most everybody who is getting a general anesthetic. I have been glad of that extra IV many, many times and have never once regretted it. I have also never had a serious IV complication.—**CM**

- A 16-g in the vein beats a 14-g in the imagination.—**CC**

- Don't bother to look for the vein before the tourniquet is on.—**CC**

- The issue in getting an IV in somebody "with bad veins" is first getting blood into the vein *before* you try to put the needle there. Do yourself a favor and exercise the arm against resistance five times, then put the arm and hand in a dependent position, *then* put the tourniquet on. Even a few minutes of strong isometric exercise will increase the local blood flow by a factor of 10 (at least). Try it, you won't be disappointed.—**Editors**

- Don't argue with people who use drugs intravenously about where the most likely place to get access is and where you won't get access. They already know for sure.—**Editors**

- Also don't argue with patients who don't use intravenous drugs but still state that they have bad veins. Sometimes this is because a phlebotomist had difficulty with a blood draw, or they previously had trouble getting an IV in a radiology suite. We have found that people are weirdly invested in the special difficulty of their veins, even when there are ropes popping out at you. Just nod gently and say, "Yes, I can see that they are very delicate."—**Editors**

- Remember to remind your trainees to start distally when putting IVs in! This seems so basic, but it can cause such trouble if you are not in the room when your (junior) team member is doing the access. It is so frustrating to blow an antecubital vein, put an IV in distal to that in the hand, and just have the crystalloid run out the hole in the vein higher up. If you are in another room, just tell your team to make sure to leave you at least one proximal vein as a backup IV site.—**Editors**

- If struggling with IV access, especially in pediatrics, go for intraosseous access to enable rapid drug/fluid resuscitation whilst further access is gained. Intraosseous access is one of the procedures that few people know how to do and everybody should. Military medics are particularly good at this technique.—**RVN and Editors**

- To avoid placing a central line in patients with challenging IV access, I've inserted a 12 cm 20 G catheter into the basilic vein, resembling a midline.—**KAM**

- IVs that infiltrate before induction are not always obvious. If it extravasates into loose adipose tissue, the IV may flow freely and "push" easily. It's when the patient is still awake after your subcutaneous depot of propofol and paralytic that you panic.—**BPB**

- We have seen almost an entire liter of fluid given into an infiltrated IV!—**Editors**

- Always investigate closely if somebody says to you in sign-out, "The IV in the arm isn't working that well." Or if an IV suddenly becomes "positional."—**Editors**

- When is 20 +20 not greater than 16? When it's the gauge of your IVs! In other words, two small IV catheters are not a greater value—and do not even equal—one big IV that runs well.—**CM**

- IVs get dislodged when patients are turned. Always put one person in charge of surveillance of the lines during the turns. This person is responsible for getting any disconnected IVs reconnected immediately after the turn.—**Editors**

- Interestingly, we cannot make any recommendations or give advice about putting IVs in extremities that are afflicted with paresis or paralysis. Common sense would tell us not to do it, but our rehab medicine friends told us that there is really little definitive information in the literature or widely accepted consensus in that community as to what is going on with lymphatic drainage in paralyzed limbs and so forth.—**Editors**

- Don't induce anesthesia with an IV you can't see the entire length of, including the point of entry into the skin.—**Editors**

***Note from the Editors:** Speaking of seeing the entire length of something, our young friend Danny Walker sent us a wonderful photo of a long plank bridge over a small stream outside of Sitka, Alaska (Fig. 158.1). Danny spends his summers on the F/V Aljac, fishing with his grandfather John Moore, a well-known commercial fisherman in Alaska who has an in-depth knowledge of the southeastern part of the state. As a result, Danny has amassed a huge portfolio of photographs of bridges in the beautiful Alaskan deciduous forests.

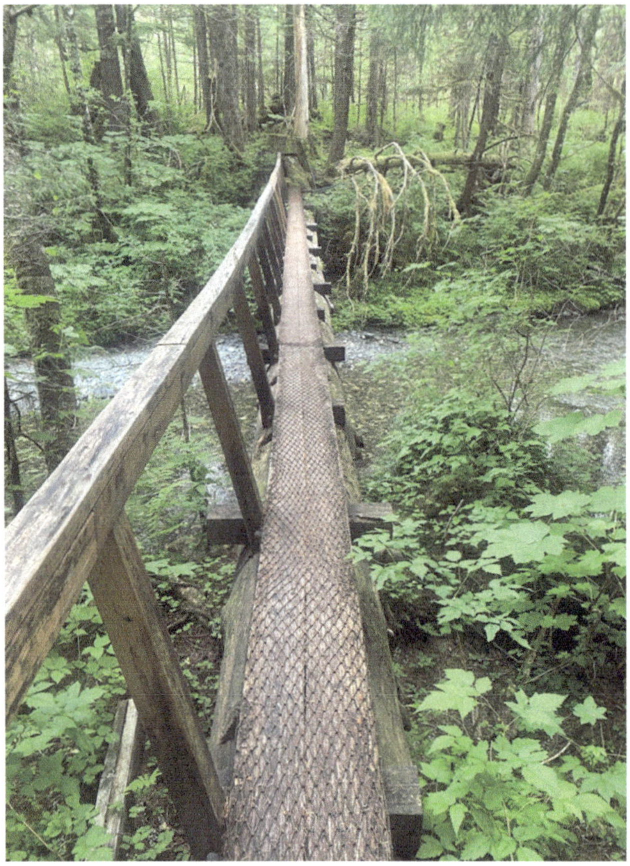

Fig. 158.1 Narrow wooden footbridge near Sitka, Alaska. Photo: Daniel Walker

Central Lines

- Don't confuse a triple lumen catheter (TLC) with a volume line.—**RSB**
- You do not want to be the person associated with central line-associated bloodstream infection (CLABSI). There are even anesthesia departments that have been known to post providers' names on a central line infection wall of shame. Most cases are preventable with proper aseptic techniques.—**KAM**
- As many as 28,000 patients per year die of CLABSI! It is one of the most morbid and mortal of all perioperative complications!—**Editors**
- Always remember to use Biopatch™ with your central lines. And how *exactly* is this dressing manufactured? It's made with a hydrophilic polyurethane foam that absorbs up to eight times the weight of the foam. The foam is impregnated with chlorhexidine gluconate to inhibit bacterial growth under the dressing.—**KAM and Editors**
- Subclavian access is associated with a lower risk for infection, followed by internal jugular (IJ), and then femoral.—**KAM**

- Venous femoral lines are associated with higher risk of thrombotic complications.—**KAM**

- In patients with chronic kidney disease, if possible, try to avoid subclavian venous access due to the potential complications such as deep vein thrombosis and venous stenosis, which can affect future hemodialysis arteriovenous access.—**KAM**

- If you are going to place a central line for volume, place an actual "volume line" such as an introducer. An 8 Fr double lumen is the equivalent of having two 18-g IVs. Hook them up to a rapid infuser and you will find that out to your dismay.—**BPB**

- Rose Christopherson always taught that the wire in central line placement should advance like butter. There should be no resistance or "threadiness" at all. Think about it. The diameter of the IJ is about 8–9 mm in the upper neck, about 10–11 mm in the middle neck, and about 12.5 mm in the lower neck. And it's filled with fluid traveling in the direction that you want to advance the wire. So, the wire should be basically whisked down the flowing tube of blood like you are doing the Class III rapids on the lower Youghiogheny. There should *never* be a "pop" of any kind. If there is, your case just got postponed until you figure out what happened. Even if that requires imaging.—**CM and AJR**

- We have had multiple cases of losing the central line wire—one that was even found months after during a follow up! We have also had cases of the wire being stuck and the patient had to go to the OR for cut down and vessel repair.—**KAM**

- I always tell my trainees that you can never let go of the wire from your hand, and you can never force the wire. Also, every time you advance your catheter, you need to check that your wire still moves. As soon as the catheter is in, I need to see the entire wire outside the patient and that it is intact, before I let them continue with the procedure. Finally, if you feel a lot of resistance and you cannot thread the wire, you need to remove your wire with your needle together, so the needle won't shred the wire.—**KAM**

- Here is something else—I always do manometry for IJ because we had a case that the wire went from the right IJ to right subclavian artery, and they only discovered when they did TEE. Unfortunately, they hadn't done manometry, and even though they used US for line placement, the arterial entry was lower, so they didn't see it.—**KAM**

- If you are a student reading this, here is what we mean by "doing manometry." To perform this procedure, an angiocatheter is threaded over a wire, and once in place, the wire is removed. Then, the included extension set for the central venous catheter is attached and held upright in the air. As the column of blood slowly fills the extension tubing, a meniscus is formed. If the angiocatheter is correctly positioned in the venous system, the meniscus should plateau, indicating proper placement."—**KAM**

- Learn to put in landmark subclavian lines—1 day it may save a life.—**RVN**

- In trauma or other mass transfusion cases, immediately check the lines to be sure that small-bore connector tubing is not attached to your large-bore volume line(s).—**RSB**

- When dilating a space for CVL placement, new trainees don't put their hands close to the skin while gripping the dilator; rather they put them further back. This puts a lot of force on the dilator and increases the opportunity for dilating out the back wall of the vessel. I haven't seen this personally, but I have seen it discussed in a morbidity and mortality conference.—**BMW**

- We have seen anesthesiologists take as long to suture in a line as it took to place the line in the first place! This needlessly slows down getting other access and turning the patient over to the surgeons. For anesthesiologists, the best and simplest knot to secure lines is the two-handed technique with three throws of a square knot. There are videos online or ask a surgical resident to show you how they do it, then practice until you are comfortable and efficient.—**Editors and CJY**

- Do *not* forget a wire in a patient. The wire stories are among everybody's most regretted complications. They are not fun presenting at morbidity and mortality conference.—**KAM**

- One common mistake I often observe is not making a sufficient skin incision, leading to unsuccessful dilation. On the other hand, you don't want to bag the vein. Once again, as with all of anesthesia practice, just enough and not too much.—**KAM and Editors**

- Large left IJ central lines, particularly introducers, can cause tearing of the left brachiocephalic vein or left mammary vein. If I'm relegated to placing one due to patient factors, I tell the resident, "Don't be offended if I almost literally hold your hand through it."—**BPB**

- Left IJ volume lines should be shorter than those on the right side.—**Editors**

- You can put lines in both sides of the neck, even volume lines, if you have to in order to save the patient's life. I have done it many times in liver transplants. However, you must be very careful not to venous pack the head. It is much better to use the left IJ line for pressors and drips only, if you can get your case done that way. Better yet, one volume line centrally and a short volume line in the antecubital fossa.—**Editors**

- Always pay attention to what an awake patient is telling you during and after central line insertion. I've had a few central lines myself, and once a nurse practitioner was trying to put a PICC line in, but the tip ended up high in my RIJ. The guy kept flushing it and telling me it was in the right place. I kept saying, "No, it's not. It's in my head." Finally, he said, "What makes you so sure?" And I said, "I can hear the injections in my right ear." Similarly, once I placed a central line that somehow got doubled back on itself and the patient said, "I think I can hear the thing swishing about."—**CM**

- If an awake patient who is getting a line suddenly starts trying to swallow or has difficulty talking, or saying they can't breathe, take those drapes down immediately! There's another central line kit in the workroom. Don't try to evaluate what's going on with the airway from the top side of the drape.—**Editors**

- Follow the current guidelines and thinking about changing out and removing central lines to the letter. No deviations. It's not defensible if you don't. Of course, the ICU people stay on top of this, so confer with your colleagues.—**Editors**

- Are the people who trained at Hopkins back in the day alone in thinking that drips and infusions—especially pressors—deserve a dedicated central line? I once picked a patient up from the (M)ICU who had—get this—four stopcocks in a row with all kinds of infusions hooked up to a 20-g peripheral IV. Oof.—**CM**

- External jugular (EJ) central lines are the discount store of lines. Know how when you go into one of those stores, there are bins of very inexpensive holiday and seasonal items on bins and racks right up front by the door? Every once in a while, you can find something there that works but usually, despite the easy accessibility and low expense, it's not really what you want. Pretty spot-on analogy for EJ lines.—**CM and RGG**

- And sometimes the accessibility of an EJ line isn't that great. We were taught to do them like a peripheral IV, with an 18-g IV catheter inserted first. Somebody else should apply some pressure distal to the insertion site to fill the vein. You have to position the needle and catheter almost parallel to the skin, otherwise you will poke right through someplace on the vein that you don't want. If you use a long 18-g catheter, you can just leave that in, or try to change it to a CVP catheter over a wire through the 18-g catheter. Sometimes the wire gets a bit hung up at the juncture and won't pass in which case you put some gentle downward traction on the shoulder and arm but if it doesn't slip easily in, that's it. Your "central" line isn't going central today. *NEVER* force the wire.—**Editors**

- I think EJs are a good line when you can't get a reasonable peripheral IV and you need something sooner rather than later. However, I don't particularly like them or trust them. They are positional, and I've seen them blow with resultant neck hematoma. They are not a reliable floor access when the patient is turning their head and moving around. I'd much rather place an IJ if you will need longer-term access.—**RGG**

- "Stuck carotids tend to show up in case reviews and, worse yet, litigation. Even if that's not what the primary case was about. People are funny about their carotid arteries." Said a hospital risk management attorney once upon a time to our residency class. So, if, in spite of every precaution and the diligent use of ultrasound, you stick the carotid artery, make sure you do the *FULL* remediation, whatever that is at the time and at your location. Back in the day, before US was used for central line placement, you had to hold continual pressure for 30 minutes. And that meant a full 30 minutes, not 22 minutes. Sometimes everybody would go on break but one other anesthesia person, and there you would be, holding pressure while everybody else ate lunch.—**CM**

- If you do put a good-sized introducer into a carotid artery, discuss this with your cardiac or vascular surgeon first before you pull the introducer. Early in my career, I saw a cardiac surgeon elect to prep the area, dissect down around the introducer, and stitch the hole shut. We then woke the patient up, to make sure she was neurologically intact. The case was postponed until the next day and went well.—**RGG**

- And don't think this can't happen, either. The use of ultra-sound may have decreased the incidence of central line complications, but it hasn't eliminated any entire categories of mishaps. There are still emergencies and people rushing and so forth.—**RGG and CM**

- In terms of lines in burn patients—we try to avoid placing IV over the burned area, but if we have too, we will. Our surgeons are really good in communicating if they need the site free for skin grafting, but in the really big ones, also many times they use artificial and cadaver integument. We try to change central line sites approximately every 14 days. Also depending on the burn surgeon in service, some patients may get PICC lines. We never get IV access with cut down.—**KAM**

- As always, watch what you say! We once knew somebody who was in the habit of speaking of "throwing in the lines." This person was actually a decent clinician but liked to affect the tough guy, cowboy image. Maybe that was to counteract the surgeons, who knows. At any rate, in the fullness of time, there was some sort of malpractice issue that included a central line complication and—we kid you not—this language was brought up by the opposing attorney in a deposition. Said cowboy-anesthesiologist prevailed in the case, if memory serves correct, but remained bitter that somebody he worked with had let that leak. Final message: you "place the lines" or "put the lines in", you never think or speak cavalierly about them.—**Editors**

- The posterior approach to the IJ isn't as easy in terms of ultrasound visualization but it's still valid in some situations. How do you do it? Identify the point of insertion for the introducer needle along the posterior edge of the sternocleidomastoid at the level just superior to where the EJV crosses the muscle. This is typically one-third of the distance between the mastoid and the clavicle. Most senior anesthesiologists have done a fair number, so ask around for someone to show you if you haven't done many.—**Editors**

- Remember that arterial blood does not always look that red. But if you are doing a central line and somebody says to you, "that looks red" *never* brush them off. We have seen senior anesthesiologists shush their techs and regret it a few moments later.—**Editors**

- I was once asked, at a party, what central line catheters are made of. I happened to be a plastics engineer before I went to med school, so I knew (either polyurethane or silicone rubber). My friend said she had previously asked at least six physicians and no one else was completely sure. So, always make sure that you know *the basics* about any equipment you use. For parties, if nothing else.—**CM**

***Note from the Editors:** *An Anesthesia Bridges* editor was recently in Albuquerque and was struck by the dramatic design of the access roads to Interstate 25 (Fig. 158.2).

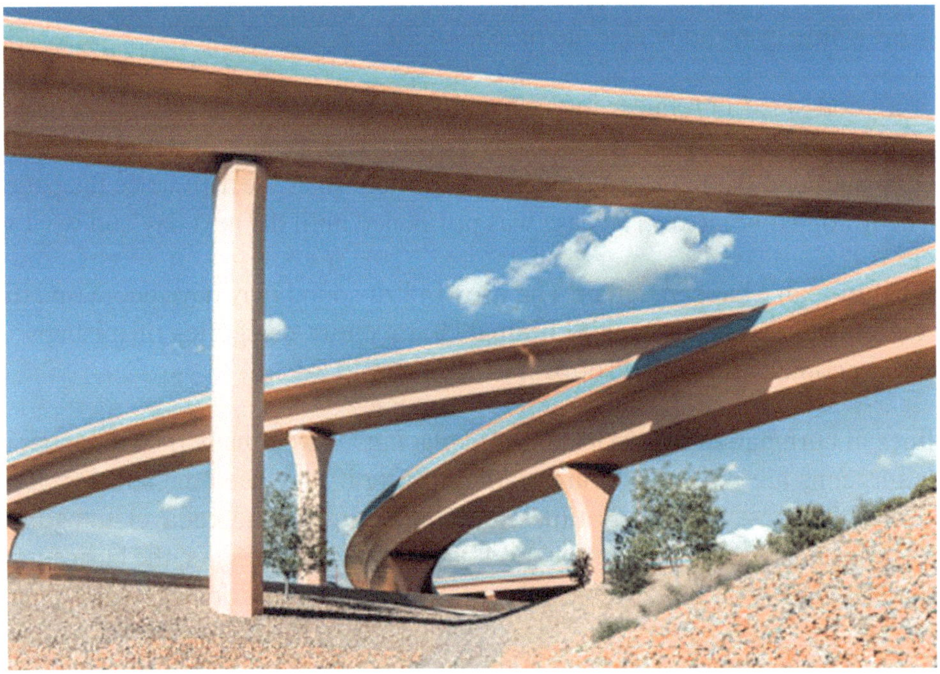

Fig. 158.2 Access ramps to I-25 in Albuquerque, NM. Beautiful colors! Photo: Cathy Marcucci

Arterial Access and Monitoring

- If you're "on the fence" remember I've never regretted placing a radial arterial line. I've regretted not having one. Also, if your gut is telling you to place an arterial line preinduction, do it.—**BPB**

- Don't loop the pressure tubing for an arterial line around the thumb! Why would you make a tourniquet, even a loose one, around the most important digit?—**CM**

- *Don't overflush the art line*. It has been shown that the volume of the arterial tree from the radial artery to the vertebral artery is only about 6–7 mL. Dr. Schauble (Hopkins old guard) used to say, "No need to retrograde flush the brain, it's perfectly capable of regulating its own blood supply."—**Editors**

- Arterial continuous flush devices deliver flush fluid at a high pressure, as high as 300 mmHg. —**Editors**

- It is well-established that increased flush volume and rate, and smaller patient size increase the risk of air embolization into the central circulation.—**Editors**

- Don't power flush the arterial line by hand at a rate greater than 1 mL/sec.—**Editors**

- Don't ignore respiratory variation on the arterial line tracing. If you see it, your patient is volume depleted.—**Editors**

- Always keep the art line stopcock on the plate. Never just have it sitting on the OR sheets or just hanging in the air.—**Editors**

- The incidence of iatrogenic complication from accidental intra-arterial (IA) injection isn't definitely known, probably due to reporting issues. It may be as low as 1:5000 anesthetics administered.—**Editors**

- One risk factor for inadvertent IA injection is the presence of vascular anomalies that are mistaken for venous structures that are mistakenly cannulated. Besides arterial malformations in the arm and hand, there are the situations where the veins and arteries are superficial and in close proximity—the antecubital fossa which contains the brachial artery and median basilic vein, and the groin, which contains the femoral artery and vein. You would *hope* that a trained anesthetic practitioner would recognize the difference, but it has happened.—**Editors**

- IA injection mistakes tend to happen in patients who already have pre-existing arterial and venous lines who present for urgent resuscitation, such as trauma patients and patients who need urgent/emergent reoperation.—**Editors**

- Put a piece of tape around the art line stopcock to prevent inadvertent injections, especially during transport! All the better if the tape is red, know what I'm saying? When I was a resident and fellow and was doing a lot of cases with a gazillion lines, I had a roll of labels made that said, "Arterial line" and I would label the entire arterial line pressure tubing at 12-inch intervals.—**CM**

- Clinical sequelae from IA injection range from "no adverse effects reported" to severe gangrene, necrosis, vascular occlusion, and amputation. Unfortunately, some of the worst offenders are the antibiotics.—**DWB, TNW, and JS**

- The initial pathophysiologic mechanism varies from crystallization and mechanical blockage to direct endothelial damage. The grievous common endpoint is usually thrombosis.—**DWB, TNW, and JS**
- Please go to Chap. 35, page 128 in *Avoiding Common Anesthesia Errors, second Edition* without delay and clip or copy the recommendations for treatment options in the awful event of an IA injection.—**Editors**
- What you do if you have an IA injection depends on what has been injected but one piece of advice—don't take the catheter out! After discontinuing the offending agent, aspirate or allow back flow to try to minimize any remaining agent in the vascular tree. It is generally agreed that administration of heparin is the initial treatment of IA injections.—**DWB, TNW, JS**
- IA injection is a true intraoperative emergency, so you will need to prioritize this care, including consulting the vascular surgery, plastic surgery, and radiology consultants, if necessary. The presence or absence of these factors seem to be predictive of outcome: cyanosis, cool extremity, delayed capillary refill, and sensory deficit.—**DWB, TNW, and JS**
- Symptomatic relief has also been shown to be helpful to a more favorable outcome—analgesics, elevation, massage, and passive motion devices.—**DWB, TNW, and JS**
- For some reason, most of the events that we have heard about when something has been put into the art line that doesn't belong there occurred during transport. We have even seen IV fluids and even blood components hooked up to the art line stopcock.—**Editors**
- Arterial lines are a great procedure to teach med students. They're both dramatic and fairly easy for a junior person to do. Satisfying for both teacher and student.—**Editors**

Acupuncture for Adverse Access Events

- We have to state right up front that we could not find any studies looking at the use of acupuncture as an adjunctive therapy in cases where there has been a serious intravenous or arterial line complication. We are hoping that this changes in the future. But we think that a badly infiltrated IV or inadvertent arterial line injection is at least *worth a consult* to your hospital acupuncture consult service, if you have one.—**CM, AL, and KKL**
- Acupuncture is now well-understood to have efficacy for swelling and/or edema.—**CM**
- In traditional Chinese Medicine (TCM), an infiltrated IV would be treated as a traumatically induced stagnation of blood. Points that move blood include Spleen 10, which we would use in our approach to this type of clinical complication, especially if there was a post-IV ecchymosis. We would also treat the soft tissue areas that are near, but not on, the affected area. Remember that the arm meridians, except two, are bilateral, so we would also consider treating the other arm or hand in the therapeutic approach to a postoperative subcutaneous collection of blood or fluid.—**AL and KKL**
- Not everybody "responds" equally to acupuncture, so there is the possibility that acupuncture would not be efficacious. However, the clinically significant risks of acupuncture, used on an upper extrem-

ity to treat IV infiltration and the accompanying edema and ecchymosis, would be extremely low.—**KKL, AL, and CM**

- In the absence of robust research, we are *not* advocating acupuncture for arterial line complications at this time. We are advocating that you start to consider what additional modalities may be found to be of efficacy for this very serious perioperative complication and that you watch the literature.—**CM, AL, and KKL**

- Acupuncture dilates blood vessels. In our private practice, if we were consulted for the problem of a comprised or constricted arterial lumen, our therapeutic approach would likely start with several major meridian points—Spleen 6, Stomach 36, Large Intestine 4, and Liver 3. Of course, an acutely thrombosed radial artery due to an inadvertent injection is not exactly analogous. The point is that there is an approach in TCM to the compromised blood vessel, including arteries, that has the potential to be adapted to related clinical settings.—**KKL, AL, and CM**

- Remember, the evidence of the anti-inflammatory nature of acupuncture is accumulating steadily [2, 3].—**CM**

Fluids

- Fluids are a drug and therefore should be thought of in the same way with risks and benefits considered—if you leave the hospital fluid loaded after an ICU stay, you have increased mortality.—**RVN**

- I had an attending who always replaced all the IV fluid bags when transporting a patient from the ICU. He used to say, "What if somebody accidentally put some heparin or sodium nitroprusside in that bag one second before we arrived to get the patient? We weren't there when that crystalloid was spiked, we don't know what's in that bag. Patients going to the OR deserve a fresh bag of OR crystalloid. Plus, it's easier to chart if our case starts with full bags."—**CM**

- A bag of crystalloid is <u>NOT</u> a hot water bottle. Do not heat them up and put them on the patient. Ever.—**Editors**

- Keep in mind that the IV bags are right at the eye level of the surgeons when they glance over the drapes towards the head of the table. One of the most embarrassing moments of my entire anesthesia career was when I was a very, very junior resident and the attending surgeon said quietly, "Cathy, I can't help noticing that both of the IV bags are empty." Gah. Made a vow not to do *that* again.—**CM**

- Never mix a calcium-containing product, such as lactated Ringer's, in the same line as blood products—it may result in a big blood clot.—**RVN**

- Don't forget that Plasma-Lyte is also FDA approved for use with banked blood! And there are transfusion medicine physicians who think it should be the standard of care.—**CM**

- Here's a great article online that goes over some of the normal saline issues.—**CM**

  "0.9% NaCl (Normal Saline)—Perhaps not so normal after all?" [4]

Colloids vs. Crystalloid

- The eternal lactated ringer's vs normal saline debate—I choose LR always as it is isotonic, and NS leads to more acute kidney injury.—**ABB**

- Our institution uses way, way too much albumin for routine resuscitation where crystalloid would be adequate.—**Editor**

- We are all pretty much a product of our training programs when it comes to fluid administration (and everything else, for better or worse). I came up when albumin was not in favor and so just really do not use it. But the opposite is true with hypertonic saline. I have used it with good efficacy—of course where appropriate and judiciously and following serum sodium carefully. I do feel that it has made a positive difference in open bowel cases through the years, especially in terms of total fluid given and safety and ease of extubation.—**CM**

- Several years back, my group did a randomized controlled trial looking at volume and type fluid administered to patients undergoing pancreaticoduodenectomy [5]. One arm of the study received 3% hypertonic saline (HYS) with a restrictive fluid therapy and had a significantly reduced fluid balance (65 vs. 91 mL/kg.) After adjusting for a number of factors including age, weight, and pancreatic texture, we were able to conclude that a moderately restrictive fluid regimen with HYS resulted in a statistically significant 25% reduction in complications.—**CJY**

- The most common hypertonic saline is 3%, but it can range much higher, as high as 29%. Remember that hypertonic does much more than expand plasma volume. There are also vasoregulatory, immunologic, and neurochemical effects. These include attenuating leukocyte-endothelial interactions, depressing neutrophil margination, and attenuating excitatory neurotransmitters. Like said above, IV fluids are medications!—**PJF**

- I like albumin. In the OR it works well, but the reason (in my opinion) the difference between fluid has never been shown is because it eventually equilibrates and there is no difference over days and weeks, but there is over hours… it would be interesting to see radiolabeled albumin in human trauma patients and neurotrauma. I digress…—**JCB**

- I almost never use NS outside of neuro/neurotrauma. The chloride is almost always problematic, and people end up chasing it.—**JCB**

- For burn patients, we either use LR or plasmalyte. We don't use albumin so much in ICU, we use FFP instead. But we do use albumin intraop, especially since the OR never happens within the first 24 hours of the initial burn injury. There are many reasons for usage of colloids in burn patients, including the lower hypoalbuminemia and to use less crystalloids that can have many deleterious effects, like increased intraabdominal pressures.—**KA**

***Note from the Editors:** Pre-med student and *Anesthesia Bridges* contributor Marilyn Walker was kind enough to review this chapter for readability and send us the photo below. Little Island at Pier 55 is a series of supported structures that is an artificial island park in the Hudson River at the intersection of West Street and West 13th Street in the Meatpacking and Chelsea Districts in New York City (Fig. 158.3). Sometimes the bridge *is* the destination.

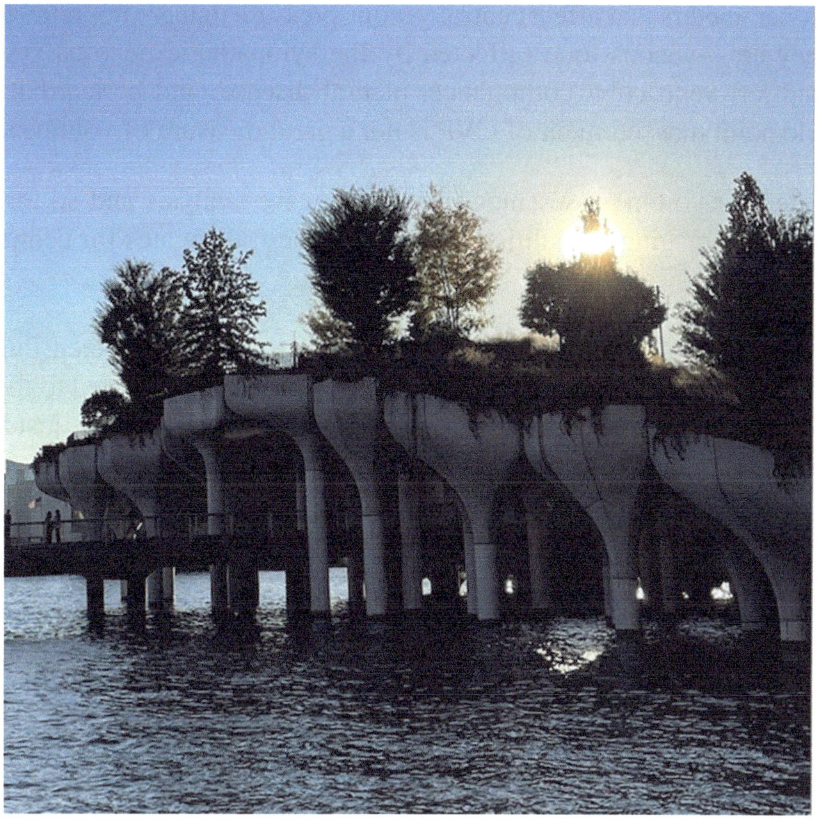

Fig. 158.3 Little Island at Pier 55, New York City. It opened in 2021 to fanfare and has picnic locations. Photo: Marilyn Walker

Volume Status and Resuscitation

Philosophy

- The Dao of resuscitation: We are all a bag of water, and we all bleed blood.—**AB and CM**

- If someone could come up with the truest way to decipher a patient's *volume status*, they would be heading to Stockholm with their formal wear. It's a vexing problem and nobody has it completely figured out. Keep in mind that (right now) volume assessment is just an estimate based on some indirect measurements and your experience. And the more senior you get, the more you become willing to admit that volume resuscitation remains entirely a clinical decision based on acute and chronic medical conditions, presentation of illness, and most recent medical history.—**ABB and Editors**

- The best explanation and summary of volume and preload is by Simon Gelman: "I think in most instances the truth of management in resuscitation lies somewhere in between a little pressor and a little volume."—**ABB**

- Our own simplest advice on goal-directed fluid therapy? You could call it the Goldilocks philosophy of volume repletion—give the patients the just right amount of fluid, and not too much and not too little.—**Editors**

- Can you name six parameters that affect central venous pressure that are not reflective of intravascular volume? Here they are—venous tone (affected by the sympathetic nervous system), intrathoracic pressure, right and left ventricular compliance, pleural disease, and pericardial disease. For these reasons, any single point measurement of CVP is *not* a great measure of volume status!—**CM**

- Most tools marketed for volume assessment like pulse wave analysis and so forth are best used as negative predictors. All imaging modalities are mostly fancy surrogates for central venous pressure. —**ABB**

- In other words, competent anesthesiologists have always used goal-directed fluid therapy — even before it was called that. Fluid management should always be individualized to the patient. We really disagree with and do not use algorithms where every patient gets X ml/hour., just because that's what the guidelines say.—**RVN and Editors**

- Goal-directed resuscitation is a way to conceptually put many people on the same page and create a pragmatic approach to fluid administration. I think it is common sense, however, there seems to be a vast deficit of that these days. Ultimately, I think it's a way to ingrain the concept of fluids as medications with indications and endpoints.—**ABB**

- My father was a trauma surgeon, and he created the negative pressure dressing in temporary abdominal closure for damage control laparotomy (The Barker Vac-Pack). He and I always discussed what he called "damage control resuscitation", which is resuscitate to a mean arterial pressure of around 60 mmHg, no more and no less, and replace blood loss with blood product. By the way, he stopped asking me when I was going to be a real doctor (a surgeon) when my brother decided to do anesthesia also.—**ABB**

- As for goal-directed fluid therapy—I use it and think it's valuable because we are able to monitor it now. I can look at stroke volume variation and left ventricular outflow tract velocity time integral and calculate fluid responses. While the principle may have existed before, it was not easily monitored. I think this is reflected in the fluid restriction in ARDS and sepsis and bowel ischemia and so on.—**JCB**

- It's the simple things that trip people up—like losing sight of the fact that hemoglobin and hematocrit are volume-based lab values. I once took over a case where the hemoglobin was reported as 9.8 gm/dL. Unfortunately, the patient was extremely under-resuscitated. With restoration of only about half the volume deficit, the repeat hemoglobin was 5.9 gm/dL. Needless to say, the rest of the resuscitation included with blood and blood components.—**CM**

- There were no airway questions on my oral exam, but just about every question somehow touched on volume status and resuscitation. The first stem case was an aortic aneurysm repair. The questions were about access, blood loss, the physiology of hypovolemia and hypotension, clamping the aorta, unclamping the aorta, and the physiology of resuscitation. I remember that the junior examiner asked me what the third space was. The second stem case was an OB patient with placenta accreta, with all the questions you would expect. The supplementary questions were all about resuscitating OB patients with various (serious) bleeding and hypotensive complications. They also wanted to talk about the hypertensive volume-contracted conditions. The junior examiner in that room said to me, "But can a volume-deficient patient be hypertensive?"—**CM**

Clinical Practice

- Resuscitation is a question of how much volume patients have lost before presenting to the OR, how much they will lose under your care while in the OR, and how you can get the patient optimized for the postoperative period. Always think in terms of before, during, and after.—**Editors**

- Remember that NPO guidelines are much different now (thank heavens) and an afternoon patient no longer comes to the OR with no fluid intake of any kind for 12+ hours. Fewer open cases are done nowadays, and patients are often sent home same day where they can normalize their fluid intake to meet their needs more reliably than we ever could.—**Editors**

- However, a patient with limited access to water due to immobility, or limited water intake due to dysphagia with or without an alternative feeding method (NG Tube, G-Tube or TPN) will often present with a reduced level of total body water. The same applies to patients who have 'messy' urinary issues (ostomy, briefs, significant benign prostatic hypertrophy) or requires assistance to ambulate to the toilet as they will avoid having to make urine. Such patients often have events that increase their urinary, GI, or insensible losses and they never fully rehydrate themselves. —**BTG**

- Also, bowel preps aren't as common as they used to be but still should not be overlooked in the fluid calculations for a case. Assume one to three liters of volume depletion for the standard bowel prep, and I think it represents true fluid loss. And remember that the effects of a bowel prep can be magnified in elderly patients. We've seen older patients with regurgitant valve lesions and bowel preps decompensate on induction of anesthesia.—**Editors**

- Resuscitate your OR patients in consultation with the postoperative team. I used to plan my fluids based on who the surgeons and the ICU docs were. Nothing wrong with being on the same page as the rest of the perioperative team. You can look at it that they are not continuing your resuscitation; you are initiating theirs.—**CM**

- Large bore (>18G) short peripheral IV cannulas are good for resuscitation. Remember that "resuscitation" can involve giving fluids to replace intraoperative losses. It doesn't always mean the Belmont. —**RVN and CM**

- Rapid infusion catheters (RIC) and sheath introducers/MAC introducers/ are even better for resuscitation—of course the risks also increase. That's student-level anesthesia practice. Work toward a deeper understanding of the larger lines. For example, sheath introducers are 6–8.5 French. When attached to a rapid transfuser, they can deliver about 25% more volume than a 14-g catheter.—**RVN and Editors**

- And a short sheath introducer can definitely go into a large antecubital vein—I used to do it all the time in liver transplants. You have to first put an 18-g catheter in, then change it out over a wire for the introducer. An antecubital introducer is safer than one in the neck, especially if the patient is a bit coagulopathic. For one, it's much easier to hold pressure if the placement goes awry.—**CM**

- Don't fully trust a volume line that you can't see (such as one in a tucked arm). You can easily squeeze several hundred milliliters of fluid into an extravasated line and cause compartment syndrome. Have a low threshold to place a central line in a case where you expect volume resuscitation.—**BPB**

- Sodium is what causes edema, not just water load—therefore normal saline is far from normal.—**RVN**

- To enable goal-directed therapy, we need to have goals, and therefore an ability to measure that goal. Some goals—dynamic variables such as stroke volume variation, pulse pressure variation, and cardiac output variability—are better than other static measures such as urine output, CVP, or PCWP. But use what you have.—**RVN and Editors**

- Hypotension needs a differential that we work through and not just another fluid challenge.—**RVN**

- Over-resuscitation can result in post-operative hypertension as well and should be on the PACU differential for "unexplained" elevated blood pressure.—**Editors**

- Just because somebody is fluid tolerant and fluid responsive, doesn't mean they need more fluid. Most of us at work are dehydrated but survive to the evening just fine!—**RVN**

- Of course, the advice above is a contextual statement. The situation is different for patients who aren't eating and who have drains and/or ongoing blood loss.—**Editors**

- Renal failure from venous congestion is probably under recognized—and maybe we should all be looking at VEXUS scans.—**RVN**

- Patients who get resuscitated when unwell need 'deresuscitating' when they get better (and they may need help achieving this).—**RVN**

- With respect to the advice right above—when Cathy Marcucci was doing a lot of our big and long open abdomen cases back in the day, she saw several patients suffer significant morbidity when the urine output went to zero the first night after surgery. She was also an early believer in inadequate perioperative renal perfusion as an independent and negative outcome variable. Her patients were decently, even robustly, resuscitated, and she used hypertonic saline whenever appropriate. We appreciated that the patients were never "shocky" in the morning. We were also in the habit of giving those patients a small dose of Lasix (10 mg) on POD #2. The point is that it's dynamic—the entire perioperative team should manage the fluid resuscitation for the point in the clinical course that you are at. One or two days makes a difference in what you are doing.**—CJY and Editors**

- Burn resuscitation for total body surface area above 20% can be very complex and challenging. There are multiple different formulas and protocols, make sure you are aware of the one that is used by your institution.—**KAM**

- In the UPMC system, the initial burn resuscitation protocol is with LR, with the *Rule of TEN*. Multiply % TBSA of the burn × 10 = initial fluid rate in mL/hr. (for adult patients weighing 40 kg to 80 kg). For every 10 kg above 80 kg, add 100 mL/hr. to the rate. And then we adjust it also according to UOP, CVP, and labs. If it's a difficult resuscitation, we will also add FFP.—**KAM**

- It never hurts to be prepared and ready for the worst during excision and grafting of those big burns—arterial line, central line, and blood in the room —**KAM**

- It still surprises me how much blood can be lost within a matter of few minutes during those procedures. And unfortunately, there is not an easy or accurate way to calculate blood loss.—**KAM**

- We live in the twenty-first century and we have an array of tools at our disposal—CVP, TEG, ABG, lactate, Vigileo monitor. Try to use them for guidance of challenging burn resuscitation in conjunction with your traditional ones, such as monitoring of blood pressure, heart rate, and urine output.—**KAM**

- Always use fluid warmers when resuscitating burns with TBSA above 20%.—**KAM**

- For difficult burn resuscitation, it is okay to give FFP for volume expansion. Colloids are okay after the first 24 hours of the initial burn injury.—**KAM**

- In a heart failure patient, mannitol and hypertonic saline can increase volume status and lead to intravascular fluid overload and pulmonary edema.—**BTG**

- Liver transplant—it's always volume!—**CC**

- As patients improve, actively de-resuscitate and remove the accumulated body water and sodium load.—**RVN**

- I once saw a senior attending spend <u>30</u> minutes de-airing the lines and infusions for a pediatric cardiac surgery case. That's not a typo. Not three minutes - <u>thirty</u> minutes.—**CM**

- I always de-air my IV fluid bags when I spike them, knowing that there is a 25–30% prevalence of PFO in general populations.—**KAM**

- I also de-air and burp every fluid bag and line, even for adult patients.—**RSB**

- Do not *EVER* inject a medication into a 1-liter bag of crystalloid to make a crude type of drip. We have seen people die that way.—**CM**

- Many IV infusions, for example nicardipine, will provide a large volume of fluid to the patient—be aware of this.—**RVN**

- If you want to go to the next level of understanding of how to hydrate a patient, talk to our colleagues who are also trained in palliative care medicine (PCM). The hydration questions are really complicated and interesting and the effects on every organ system must be considered. If you are starting a PCM rotation or fellowship, there are several articles that provide an excellent overview of the issues [6, 7].—**AJR and CM**

- "It is better to die dry than die wet." [8] This, of course, is a *general* statement. It depends on the specific clinical context, and there are some downsides to this approach. However, what the authors are trying to convey is that hydration for hospice and end-of-life patients should be given only to address specific problems and not for the vaguely defined purpose of "extending life."—**Editors and AJR**

- However, hydration that results in excessive fluid in the lungs is really to be avoided in every hospice and palliative care patient. Nobody should die with wet lungs if it can be reasonably avoided, that we can say for sure.—**Editors and AJR**

- The balancing of the fluid act in palliative medicine also involves the preferences of the dying end-of-life patient, their life expectancy and current symptomatology, and also the preferences of the close family members if that individual has not selected hydration preferences for the end of their life in advance. If there is ever conflict, or argument, it is imperative to know not only the pros and cons of end of life clinically provided hydration, but also important to know and advocate for the patient.—**AJR**

- Final piece of advice—what is true for the PCM patient is true for any patient remember when you undertake a resuscitation paradigm, you are balancing the resuscitation concerns of just about every organ system. If you don't find these issues compelling and interesting, perhaps it is time to consider a different line of work.—**Editors**

***Note from the Editors:** Water is incredibly important to the pueblo nations in New Mexico, and they maintain rigorous ground water and wetlands management programs. This shot shows a stream and bridge against the backdrop of the Sandia Mountains (Fig. 158.4).

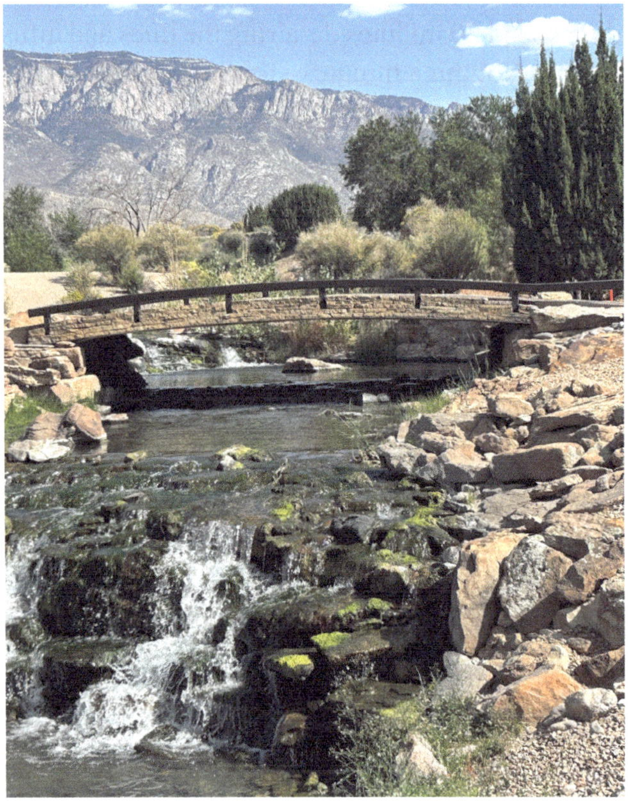

Fig. 158.4 Natural and manmade landscapes on the Sandia pueblo in New Mexico just north of Albuquerque. Photo: Catherine Marcucci

More Wisdom on Access and Resuscitation from *Avoiding Common Anesthesia Errors, 2nd Edition*

- There are many additional tips, teaching tidbits, and a lot of overall wisdom on access, fluids, and resuscitation in our previous book, which is nicknamed "Green2." We get this book out and reread these chapters frequently ourselves. So, please check out this information and remember that every single penny of royalties from our previous book goes to FAER in perpetuity!

Green2 Chapters with More Wisdom on Vascular Access, Fluids, and Resuscitation

- Crystalloid Fluids: More Than Just a Dash of Salt.
- Hypertonic Saline? Still the "Solution" to the Solution Problem?
- Synthetic Colloid Solutions Have Distinct Properties and Risk/Benefit Ratios That Require Your Attention!
- Do Not Use CVP to Guide Fluid Resuscitation.
- Protect the Kidneys, Not the "UOP".
- Do Not Use Urine Output as an Indicator of Volume Status.
- Inadvertent Intra-Arterial Injection Can Result in Severe Patient Injury.

References

1. Ball RD, Henao JP, et al. Peripheral intravenous catheter infiltration: anesthesia providers do not adhere to their own ideas of best practice. J Clin Anesth. 2013;25(2):115–20. Published online 2013 Jan 17.
2. Yu W-L, Park J-Y, et al. Changes of local microenvironment and systemic immunity after acupuncture stimulation during inflammation: a literature review of animal studies. Front Neurol. 2023;13:1086195.
3. Bai H, Xu S, et al. Clinical events associated with acupuncture intervention for the treatment of chronic inflammation associated disorders. Mediat Inflamm. 2020;27:2020.
4. Blumberg N, Cholette JM, et al. 0.9% NaCl (Normal saline)—perhaps not so normal after all? Transfus Apher Sci. 2018;57(1):127–31.
5. Lavu H, Sell NM, et al. The HYSLAR trial: a prospective randomized controlled trial of the use of a restrictive fluid regimen with 3% hypertonic saline versus lactated Ringers in patients undergoing pancreaticoduodenectomy. Ann Surg. 2014;260(3):445–53.
6. Bear AJ, Bukowy EA, et al. Artificial hydration at the end of life. Nutr Clin Pract. 2017;32(5):628–32.
7. Care of Dying Adults in the Last Days of Life. NICE Guideline, No. 31, National Institute for Health and Care Excellence (NICE); 2015 Dec. 16.
8. Ali H. Does hospice do IV fluids? [Internet] Melodia Care Hospice 2021. Available from: https://www.melodiacare.com/does-hospice-do-iv-fluids/.

Authors

Andrew Barker is an anesthesiologist at UAB who wrote to us when Green2 was published, with suggestions on how to present the subject of intravenous fluids in future books. So, guess who was nominated to do just that for this book! Please see Dr. Barker's excellent fluids summary in Chap. 125.

Raj Nathwani is the lead trauma anesthesiologist at Harborview Medical Center—UW Medicine. He rarely goes a day without considering these issues.

Brant Wagener is an anesthesiologist and intensivist at UAB. He is the director of clinical research and holds the Simon Gelman endowed chair.

Brian Barrick is a senior anesthesiologist at UNC—Chapel Hill and the director of thoracic anesthesiology. It is his firm position that there is no organ system that needs more consideration of the dangers of over-resuscitation than the lungs.

Stan Alfaras-Melainas is an anesthesiologist in the UPMC system. His clinical interests include the clinical management and fluid resuscitation strategies of burn patients.

Cathy Marcucci is a senior anesthesiologist and is also trained in transfusion medicine. Resuscitating patients is her favorite clinical problem to solve.

Resuscitation Wisdom: Blood Components and Blood Transfusion

159

Steven M. Frank, Robert J. Christian, Rajen V. Nathwani, Elizabeth A. Ungerman, Konstantinos Alfaras-Melainas, and Catherine Marcucci

Contributors:

Edwin G. Avery IV, MD (EGA)

Carol F. Bodenheimer, MD (CFB)

Leonard Chen, MD PhD (LC)

Xiaopo Cheng, PhD (XC)

Catherine Cooper, MD (CC)

Abigail J. Crawford*, MD '28 (AJC)

Willy A. Flegel, MD (WAF)

Brian T. Gierl, MD (BTG)

Raymond G. Graber, MD (RGG)

Michael D. Graham, PhD (MDG)

Tymoteusz J. Kajstura, MD PhD (TJK)

Kirk Lalwani, MD (KL)

S. M. Frank
Department of Anesthesiology and Critical Care Medicine, Johns Hopkins University, Baltimore, MD, USA

R. J. Christian
Department of Laboratory Medicine and Pathology, University of Washington, Seattle, WA, USA

R. V. Nathwani
Department of Anesthesiology and Pain Medicine, University of Washington School of Medicine, Harborview Medical Center, Seattle, WA, USA

E. A. Ungerman · K. Alfaras-Melainas
Department of Anesthesiology and Perioperative Medicine, University of Pittsburgh School of Medicine, Pittsburgh, PA, USA

C. Marcucci (✉)
Department of Transfusion Medicine, Clinical Center, National Institutes of Health, Bethesda, MD, USA

S. Mohamed et al. (eds.), *Anesthesia Bridges*, https://doi.org/10.1007/978-3-032-08294-7_159

Patricia Lee, MD (PL)

Yafet T. Mamo, MD (YTM)

Herleen Rai, MD (HR)

Tsung-lin Tsai, MD PhD (TLT)

John R. Walker (JRW)*

Jonathan H. Waters, MD (JHW)

Introduction

Up to half of all transfusions given in the country every year are given by the anesthesia teams in the OR and the ICU. Just like any therapy, there are risks and benefits and financial costs to administering blood and blood products. Since blood products are a donated, expensive, and sometimes scarce resource, we must use them wisely. Here are some thoughts and collected wisdom that may help educate you and guide your practice.

Blood Basics

- Blood is the only thing we give that is a medication, a fluid, and a transplant. Therefore, it is worthy of *triple* the study time and clinical attention.—**Editors**

- When I first went into blood banking, I just couldn't figure out what the basic core bedrock principles were. What would the blood banking equivalent of "Vigilance Always" be? Then one fine day I caught it. The core issues really come down to, "Keep the antibodies away from the antigens (except for diagnostic purposes), and what's in the soup?"—**CM**

- Blood saves lives when you need it but increases risks and costs when you don't.—**TJK and SMF**

- One unit of packed red blood cells will raise the hemoglobin by approximately 1 g/dL. If you get a greater bump than this, consider the fact that your patient is otherwise volume depleted.—**RVN**

- The price of blood and blood components floats. The "typical" cost of a unit of packed red blood cells to a hospital is in the low hundreds of dollars. But a rare donor unit, or a unit for a sickle cell patient, can be many more times than that. It is not unusual to have a single unit of red blood cells that has cost the hospital $1000. And that is just the purchase price for the unit itself. That doesn't include the overhead cost of the blood bank laboratory, the testing reagents, and the technologist time."—**Editors**

- The blood bank inventory is one of the most expensive and dynamic in an entire hospital. It is not unusual for a large hospital, especially if there is a busy trauma service, to spend $20–30 million per year buying blood and blood components. There is the ever-pressing issue of not having enough blood, but transfusion medicine departments also face the issue of having blood and components outdate, which is a very big no-no for blood banks. All of this fluidity in the blood inventory means that there is a gigantic opportunity for research and optimization.—**CM and SMF**

- There's a certain kind of agony associated with transfusion medicine: literally everyone you work with studied medicine, and they all know just enough about your job to think they know everything about your job.—**WAF and CM**

- The less the blood bank hears from the anesthesia people, the better, in a weird sort of way. It means that the OR team was happy with the blood bank's work and provided maximal help to the patient. But a quick thank you when the clinical acuity is over is always appreciated by the transfusion medicine staff.—**WAF and CM**

- Remember that, even in times of great national, regional, or local use of blood, the problem is not always that the blood supply is critically short; rather, it is that the blood supply is unstable. It is much more important for the overall and longitudinal public health that blood donors give predictably and reliably than that an enormous number of donors flood blood donation venues in times of emergency.—**WAF**

- Because transfusion is one of the most common "procedures" in the acute medical setting, it's relatively easy to power outcome studies.—**Editors**

Blood Rheology

- A decent number of anesthesiologists are also engineers, we've noticed through the years, especially chemical and biomedical engineers. It's time to dust off those engineering credentials! The solutions to the blood and bleeding problems are through engineered blood components and the biologicals, such as the collagen-based blood stasis products. There is just not going to be any other way to do it. Thinking about goal-directed therapies is ultimately thinking about delivering blood to the tissues. So, it is imperative to think deeply about the fluid mechanics of blood.—**CM and RGG**

- The bio-products will be modeled, analyzed, and evaluated against the standard of "real" blood and it is important to understand how blood functions as a fluid in order to do that. We think that there is a huge opportunity for anesthesiologists in doing translational research with the engineers. You heard it here first.—**CM and RGG**

- We are grateful to **Xiaopo Cheng** and **Mike Graham,** from the Department of Chemical and Biological Engineering at the University of Wisconsin (top national program!), for sending us a few basic principles to start to think about the physical and fluid properties of blood.**—CM and RGG**

- First, blood is a multiphase non-Newtonian viscoelastic fluid, and its biological roles are closely tied to its physical nature.—**XC and MDG**

- A non-Newtonian fluid is one for which the viscosity is dependent on the applied shear stress. Remember that ketchup is the classic non-Newtonian fluid. It becomes runnier when you shake the bottle.—**CM**

- In larger arteries and veins, blood can be treated as a single-phase fluid, exhibiting high-Reynolds number flow phenomena like turbulence and vortices. These factors are crucial in cardiovascular health. In fluid mechanics, the Reynolds number is a calculated dimensionless number that helps predict flow patterns in various situations, such as the transition from laminar to turbulent flow.—**XC, MDG, and CM**

- However, at smaller scales, where the size of blood vessels approaches the size of blood cells, its multiphase nature becomes important.—**XC and MDG**

- Blood shows shear-thinning behavior with a yield stress. The yield stress arises from aggregation effects and the shear-thinning and viscoelastic properties of blood are mainly due to the deformability of red blood cells under flow.—**XC and MDG**

- In the microcirculation, red blood cells (RBCs) migrate toward the blood vessel center, leaving an RBC-depleted cell-free layer near vessel walls. In contrast, white blood cells and platelets tend to reside in these layers, a flow-induced segregation phenomenon termed margination.—**XC and MDG**

- The segregation behavior during blood flow is substantially dictated by the contrasts in the cellular properties, such as shape, size, and deformability. Stiff and small cells marginate toward vascular walls, while flexible and large cells enrich around the vessel center. The segregation results from the competition mechanism between two cross-stream fluxes: wall-induced migration, and hydrodynamic pair collisions between blood cells.—**XC and MDG**

- Fåhræus and Lindqvist discovered that blood apparent viscosity at shear rate above certain values in capillary depends strongly on tube diameter. For diameters between 10 and 1000 μm, the apparent viscosity substantially decreases with decreasing tube size, before sharply increasing for tubes smaller than 10 μm. This behavior arises from the presence of the cell-free layer.—**XC and MDG**

- The Fåhræus effect states that measured "tube hematocrit" can be lower than inferred "discharge hematocrit." This difference lies in the combination of the nonuniform red cell concentration profile and the velocity profile in the in a blood vessel. — **XC and MDG**

- The Zweifach-Fung effect is the observation that in an asymmetric bifurcation, the outlet branch with higher flow rate has a greater hematocrit than the lower flow branch. This is mainly caused by the nonuniform cell distribution in the inlet branch, where the presence of a cell-free layer strongly impacts distribution in the outlet branches.—**XC and MDG**

- The renal tubules and the blood–brain barrier have nothing on the micro-circulation in terms of fascinating and complex physiology. It all starts with the deformability of the RBC. Keep in mind that a 7 μm RBC has to somehow get through a capillary that is 5–10 μm in diameter. A tricky engineering problem for our oxygen-carrying friends (Fig. 159.1).—**SMF and CM**

- From my perspective as a clinician, I find the above information important and relevant. The microcirculation works differently than the macrocirculation! All of our hemodynamic measures assess the macrocirculation which may explain why many of the transfusion trigger studies show no difference between a restrictive versus liberal strategy. At the microcirculation, the macro measure of hemoglobin is different.—**JHW**

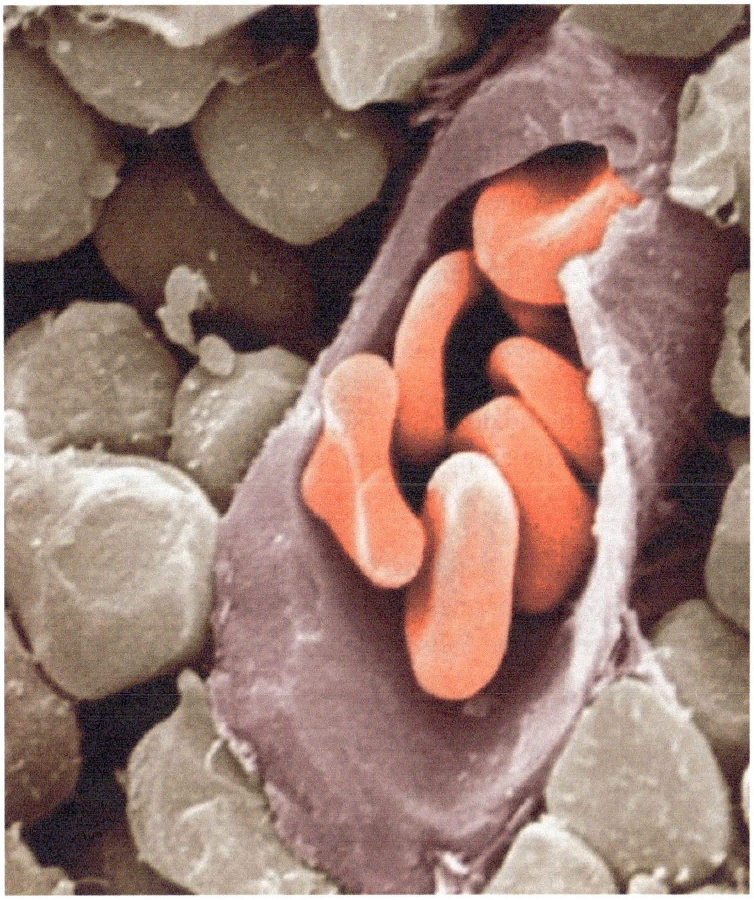

Fig. 159.1 RBCs in the microvasculature doing their delivery thing. Photo: courtesy of Steven M. Frank, MD

Blood Components and Transfusion Reactions

- Plasma should *never* be given solely as a volume expander.—**CM**
- Remember that transfused plasma has about 20,000 plasma protein in it, all the way from tiny amounts of troponins to albumin, by far the largest protein component of human plasma. The question really isn't why so many patients get transfusion reactions, it's why so few do.—**CM**
- If you want to automatically become the subject of laughing in the blood bank, order plasma to correct an INR of 1.6. This is because the INR of the plasma itself is about 1.1 to 1.3 but the relationship of INR and clotting factors in the bloos is not linear. Also, most patients with an INR < 2.0 are at low risk of clinical bleeding.—**CM**
- Platelets are the most expensive and have the shortest shelf life of all (surgical) blood components, so give them judiciously.—**SMF**
- The component with the overall shortest shelf life, measured in hours, is granulocytes. They are sometimes given in intractable cases of fungal infection when other therapies have failed, so ICU staff should be aware of this blood component. They are a very expensive blood component that requires a directed apheresis donation with some risk to the donor.—**CM**

- For all blood components, treat the whole patient, not just the lab value.—**SMF**

- Don't forget that blood components (except most platelets) are or were cold! Packed RBCs are stored at a temperature not to exceed 6 °C (42.8 °F). The majority of the plasma that you will use is probably going to be fresh frozen plasma. It has been thawed for 30 minutes at 37 °C. If you received plasma that was previously thawed, it will come from the blood bank refrigerator without warming.—**CM**

- Send the 'type and screen' early—often this involves two independently verified/separate samples, after which the blood bank will rapidly be able to electronically crossmatch blood products. This is safer for the patient and saves expensive/limited resources, like O negative blood.—**Editors**

- Something to keep in mind: most blood donors in the United States are Caucasian. If your patients are from a different ethnic group, finding compatible products for those rare blood types becomes more difficult.—**RJC and TLT**

- There are over 600 named blood group antigens. Many of these arise from rare genetic variants. The blood groups that are most important for anesthesiologists are ABO, Rh, Kell, Kidd, and Duffy. Keep in mind that the routine unit of red blood cells from the blood bank has been phenotyped *only* for the ABO and Rh antigens.—**CM and TLT**

- The antigens of the ABO blood group are not there just to frustrate blood bankers. They are complex carbohydrates on the surface of RBCs but are also strongly expressed on epithelium, sensory neurons, platelets, and the vascular endothelium.—**CM**

- Did you know that ABO blood type is linked to variable disease risk factors? For example, a number of clinical studies and systematic reviews have documented a positive association between non-O blood type and the risk of developing both venous and arterial thrombotic events [1]. The exact mechanisms aren't known but ABO-related thrombosis may be mediated by ABO carbohydrate modifications of von Willebrand factor (VWF) that cause impaired proteolysis and higher levels of VWF and then higher Factor VIII plasma levels.—**CM**

- The vast majority of platelet products are now apheresis platelets. We don't really think in terms of "pooled platelets" as the platelet product is from a single donor. Platelets may come in plasma (more useful in trauma/massive hemorrhage) or in platelet additive solution (less useful).—**RVN**

- An apheresis platelet product will have about one unit of plasma in the bag as well. That's quite a bit of volume, especially if you are transfusing more than one platelet product. We have seen a clinical service insist on transfusing three platelet products in rapid succession and put the patient into transfusion-related circulatory overload (TACO).—**CM and TLT**

- Major causes of refractoriness to platelet transfusion are non-immune mediated. The main culprits are splenomegaly, infection, fever, and DIC.—**YTM and LC**

- If unsure about the cause of refractoriness, assess adequate response to platelet transfusion by performing a CCI (corrected count increment) calculation. If 1-hour post-transfusion CCI shows adequate response, cause is most likely non-immune mediated. If 1-hour post-transfusion CCI is not adequate, then the cause of refractoriness is most likely either immune-mediated or splenic sequestration. Platelet refractoriness is generally defined as a CCI of <5000 after two sequential transfusions.—**PL and LC**

- The CCI is not so relevant to blood resuscitation in the OR or in an MTP that is taking place anywhere. However, remember that "resuscitation" can take place in the ICU over days or even weeks (think of the burn ICU or transplant patients). We have more than once heard complaints that "the platelet count won't bump" for patients who are going through long and stormy post-op ICU stays and requiring blood products on a daily basis. In this case, consideration of the CCI might be helpful in guiding clinical care.—**CM and TLT**

- The CCI is calculated by multiplying the difference between the post- and pre-transfusion platelet counts by the patient's body surface area and dividing that product by the number of platelets transfused. The post-transfusion platelet count sample should be collected within 60 minutes of transfusion completion. If the exact platelet count is unavailable, use 3×10^{11}.—**YTM and LC**

- A quicker way to estimate the CCI is to compare the pre-transfusion count with the 1-hour post-transfusion platelet count. The patient is refractory if the increase is less than 10,000/uL.—**PL and LC**

- Immune-mediated causes of refractoriness are caused by HLA class I antibodies and rarely, by HPA-antibodies formed by the patient. If HLA/HPA antibody screen is positive, the patient should receive crossmatch compatible platelets or HLA/HPA-compatible platelets. ABO-compatible platelets should be used when HLA/HPA-matched platelets are unavailable.—**YTM and LC**

- ABO compatible platelets might be worth trying when HLA-matched platelets are not available.—**PL and LC**

- MHC Class I antibody screen is sufficient to evaluate whether patient's immune platelet refractoriness is due to HLA alloimmunization since platelets do not express class II antigens.—**YTM and LC**

- It's rather surprising that anesthesiologists don't know more about transfusion reactions (TR). Just a couple basics will help. First, we need to be concerned about the immune-mediated reactions—which are caused by mismatch or incompatibility between the recipient and donor product.—**CM**

- The two types of immune-mediated TRs are acute hemolytic and delayed. Acute reactions occur within 24 hours of transfusion, and delayed reactions occur after 24 hours and usually about two weeks later but can occur up to 30 days after.—**CM**

- Acute hemolytic reactions are most common with red blood cells but can occur with any blood component. The typical etiology is with a mismatch within the ABO blood group but can occur with other antigens such as Duffy and Kell.—**CM**

- Acute hemolytic reactions involve the fixation of complement and intravascular hemolysis. People often don't understand this. The Rh blood antigen is gigantic and complicated, you would think all those potential sites of immunological activity would cause acute life-threatening hemolytic transfusion reactions. But nope—doesn't fix complement.—**CM**

- Delayed hemolytic reactions are typically characterized by extravascular hemolysis and do not involve the fixation of complement. The implicated antigens include Rh, Kidd, Duffy, Kell, and the MNS antigens. Note that Duffy and Kell antigens can be involved in either acute or delayed hemolysis.—**CM**

- Want to impress the heck out of the blood bank? We live in an increasingly diverse world, so learn a little bit about the rare blood types of your different patient cohorts. Table 159.1 gives just a tiny sample of important rare blood types for several racial and ethnic groups.—**JRW and CM**

- Remember that the trouble occurs when an individual who needs blood is negative for a high-prevalence antigen—this is never a good thing—because most donor units will have the antigen that the recipient doesn't. This means that there is an increased potential to form antibodies against the antigens you might get that you yourself don't have. You want the same antigens on your RBCs that the rest of the population has on theirs.—**JRW and CM**

- And what does all the alphabet soup in Table 159.1 mean? Here's your glossary. You don't have to memorize it, but it's good to be familiar with the terms.—**JRW and CM**

  Di—Diego blood group, most individuals have the Di(b) antigen. Antibodies can cause moderate to severe delayed transfusion reactions.

  U—High-frequency antigen in the MNS blood group system. About 2% of African Americans lack this antigen and can form anti-U antibodies, which are been implicated in severe hemolytic transfusion reactions and hemolytic disease of the fetus and newborn.

  Fy—Duffy blood group, antibodies can cause transfusion reactions ranging from mild to severe; usually but not always delayed reactions.

  Rz—Rare haplotypes in the complex Rh blood group system.

  Jk—Kidd blood group. These antibodies are dangerous because they can be difficult to detect in routine cross match. They are a common cause of delayed transfusion reactions. "*Kidd hides*."

  Dr—An antigen in the Cromer blood group system that is implicated in regulation of the coagulation cascade.

  Kp—The K antigen is one of the most clinically significant in the Kell blood group. Anti-K antibodies have been implicated in significant transfusion reactions and hemolytic disease of the fetus and newborn. Know what blood bankers say about this blood group antigen? "*Kell kills*!"

  Vel—A vexatious blood group antigen for many reasons! Not the least of which is that anti-Vel antibodies will readily hemolyze Vel + RBCs. These antibodies are important and have caused severe transfusion reactions.

Table 159.1 The rare blood types associated with several racial and ethnic groups

Some rare blood types by Ethnic/Racial group	
Ethnic group	Rare blood type
Hispanic	Di (b−)
Black/African American	U−, Fy (a−b−)
Native American, Alaskan Native	RzRz
Pacific Island, Asian	Jk (a−b−)
East European/Russian Jews	Dr (a−)
White	Kp (b−), Vel−

- Always ask about previous blood transfusions and transfusion reactions when doing a pre-operative evaluation. I blush to admit how many times I haven't done this.—**CM**

- Don't dismiss reports of a previous transfusion reaction, even if it occurred at another hospital. Blood banks have a responsive and close network and information can be exchanged quickly. If you catch the suggestion of a transfusion reaction in the patient's history, get your own transfusion service involved as soon as possible.—**CM and AJC**

- The CDC defines 13 classifications of transfusion reactions. There's a great online resource.—**CM**

  - https://www.cdc.gov/nhsn/pdfs/biovigilance/bv-hv-protocol-current.pdf

- <u>One of the best clinical pick-ups</u> I ever saw was by Jeff Kirsch when I was a junior resident. We were doing a case in Room 1 in the old GOR at Hopkins and about halfway through the case, the blood in the Foley just became the slightest bit blood tinged. It was a busy mid-level trauma case; we'd given a decent amount of blood for sure. He came into the room, and I mentioned that there was just a tiny bit of blood in the Foley bag. He immediately said to me, "Call the blood bank, and tell them we need to rule out a hemolytic transfusion reaction."—**CM**

- <u>Best clinical pick-up, continued:</u> There were no other signs of transfusion reaction that I could see, I thought, "Really? It's probably from the urgent Foley placement, or maybe the patient is a bit cold and coagulopathic." We sent the requested blood samples down to the blood bank, and danged if it wasn't a genuine hemolytic transfusion reaction. It really was! I asked Jeff how in the world he picked that up. I will always remember him telling me, "Well, first of all, this is what hemolysis looks like in anesthetized patients. They're not able to sit up and tell you about it. Second, in a trauma case there's a lot of possible hemodynamic collapse and extensive hemorrhage going on—that's the shouting. But it's important that you also pick up the whispers that something bad is happening and you are losing red blood cells in a different way but still serious way."—**CM**

***Note from the Editors:** *Anesthesia Bridges* contributor and pre-med student John Walker was out and about in Philadelphia recently and sent us this photo of a beautiful bridge with iron railings that reminded him of the bi-concave shape of a red blood cell (Fig. 159.2).

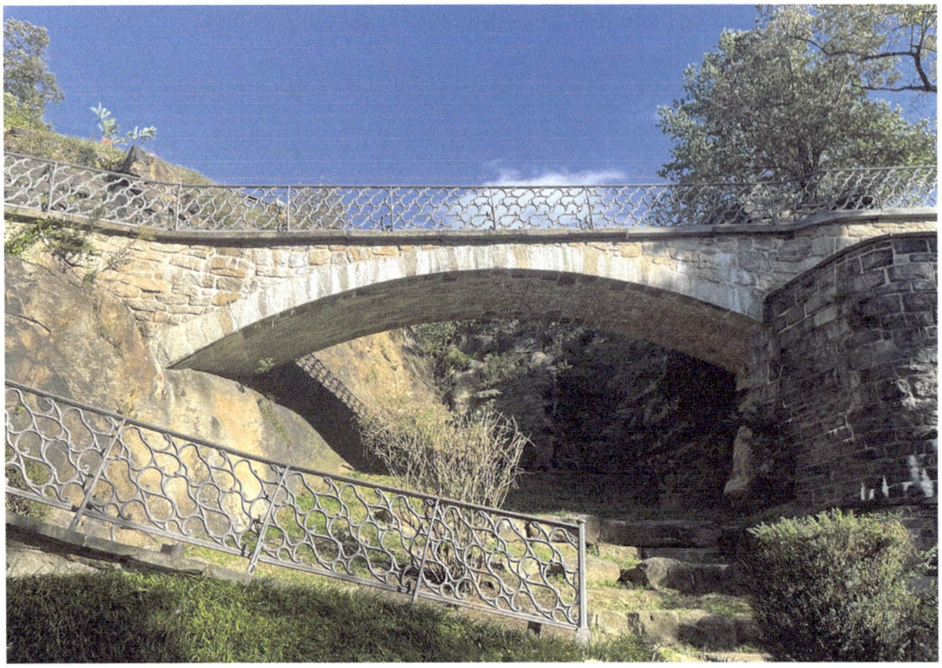

Fig. 159.2 A beautiful bridge in Fairmont Park in Philadelphia, PA. Look at the railings! Photo: John Walker

- TACO vs. TRALI—the eternal debate—these are incredibly important transfusion reactions, especially for ICU teams. Patients die every year from both these reactions, which must be reported to the FDA.—**RJC and TLT**

- TACO stands for transfusion-associated circulatory overload. Since blood is a colloid, it doesn't distribute into the extracellular compartment easily. So, if your patient can't handle the extra fluid—for example, pediatric and elderly patients, those with cardiac or renal issues—then they are at risk of circulatory overload. With all the fluids patients get, it's easy to overlook this fact, and TACO tends to be under-reported. TACO is also the leading cause of transfusion-associated deaths. So, always transfuse as slowly as possible, especially in patients at risk.—**RJC and TLT**

- TRALI stands for transfusion-related acute lung injury. It's thought to be mainly due to HLA or HNA (human neutrophil antigen) antibodies present in blood products, which activate neutrophils sequestered in the lungs, which then leads to the lung injury and pulmonary edema. The blood donation world has put strategies in place to reduce the risk of having these antibodies present in blood components, so the risk of TRALI has dramatically decreased. That being said, it still occurs, and it can happen with any type of blood product, not just plasma, and there is no method to predict which patients will get TRALI.—**RJC and TLT**

- Clinically, TACO and TRALI present similarly as they both cause pulmonary edema, but TACO is way more common, about 1–3 per 100 transfusions, compared to TRALI, about 1 per 10,000 transfusions. TACO is also responsible for more transfusion-related deaths than TRALI.—**RJC and TLT**

- Once you think you have a case of TACO or TRALI, stop the transfusion and alert the blood bank. Both are treated with respiratory support. TACO should respond to diuretics. TRALI won't respond to diuretics and will likely require oxygen supplementation and may need vasopressors. The blood bank will tell you exactly what to order, such as a B-natriuretic peptide test, which has a sensitivity and specificity of 81% and 89% in TACO and can help with the hemovigilance evaluation.—**RJC and TLT**

- Blood is wasted every day. There is an enormous wastage of autologous units in the blood bank. Here are a few of the things we've seen in the operating rooms.—**RGG and CM**

  - Blood and FFP are meant to stay cool. If you aren't immediately transfusing, these products should be *left in a blood cooler under ice*. If you return blood and FFP to the blood bank, and the blood temperature is out of range, they will discard these.

  - *Repeat*—blood *under* the ice! This is really important in that little understanding exists of this need. I like to say that its opposite to where one would put their beer. In college, the ice was placed under the beer cans.—**JHW**

  - Platelets and cryoprecipitate are meant to stay warm. If these are returned to the blood bank, and they are in a cooler, the blood bank will discard these.

  - *Make sure* at the end of the case that someone takes responsibility to return unused products and coolers to the blood bank. I know of several occasions where a cooler spent the night in an operating room and was discovered the next day by morning staff.

  - The above points should be part of the continuing education of anyone who touches blood products in the operating room—both nursing and anesthesia staff.

  - Don't electively order cryoprecipitate unless you are sure you are going to give it. It is probably the most expensive blood product we commonly use from the blood bank. If returned to the blood bank, it can be re-allocated to another patient but must be given within several hours, otherwise the unit is wasted.

Transfusion Thresholds

- The subject of transfusion thresholds—when to start and when to stop—is gigantically complex. It is a common misconception that the transfusion medicine/blood bank aims to restrict the use of blood products altogether. *Not true*. Transfusion practices are designed to optimize patient clinical outcomes while avoiding unnecessary transfusions.—**HR and SMF**

- The development of transfusion practice guidelines should be a *collaborative* effort between interdisciplinary teams and the blood bank laboratory, always with the ultimate goal of optimizing patient care [2–5]. The guidelines are not set in stone. And they are just that—guidelines.—**HR and Editors**

- Nobody has a greater interest in getting transfusion guidelines and thresholds right than our blood bank colleagues. The AABB (formerly known as the American Association of Blood Banks) maintains interdisciplinary committees of subject matter experts to scrutinize the entirety of available data and update guidelines accordingly.—**HR and CM**

- The blood bank is not a dispensary! There are physicians and professional staff down there who are responsible for justifying every blood component that gets released. If they call you to discuss the reason for a transfusion, it's because they have a true need to know. Please do not let your professionalism lapse.—**CM and AJC**

- That said, I once gave a lecture to experienced blood bank staff on the disproportionate amount of liability that is shouldered by the anesthesiologists if there is either morbidity or mortality due to bleeding or under-resuscitation, based on data in the Closed Claim File. My transfusion medicine audience had not had a previous comprehensive understanding of our legal risks and were a bit aghast on our behalf when learning about it.—**CM**

- Various factors are considered when formulating recommendations for red blood cell (RBC) transfusion thresholds. These recommendations are based on the premise that patients highly value avoiding the rare but potentially life-threatening adverse events associated with transfusion. In other words, patients prefer to avert adverse reactions, and clinicians prefer not to have to manage them if avoidable. The common restrictive transfusion threshold is a hemoglobin value of 7–8 g/dL. A liberal transfusion threshold is usually 9–10 g/dL.—**HR and Editors**

- Restrictive transfusion thresholds have demonstrated non-inferiority compared to liberal thresholds in many situations.—**HR and Editors**

- And in some situations, restrictive thresholds may actually be superior. For example, in neonates with severe thrombocytopenia, those randomly assigned a threshold of 50,000 platelets/mm^3 had a higher rate of death or major bleeding compared to those assigned a threshold of 25,000 platelets/mm^3 [6].—**RJC and TLT**

- The decision to transfuse a patient with RBCs should not be solely determined by Hb levels. The transfusion approach should be holistic, considering not only Hb levels but also the patient's hemodynamic stability, the rate of Hb decline, and the presence of associated symptoms—such as shortness of breath, chest pain of cardiac origin, and hypotension. But keep in mind that a post-transfusion hemoglobin of 14 gm/dL is as unwanted as a pre-transfusion of 4 gm/dL.—**HR and CM**

- Hemodynamically stable hospitalized patients, including those in critical care units, may be transfused using a restrictive threshold (Hb $\leq$7 g/dL). *However*, there may be some need to revise this if the rehab medicine team feels that the anemia is limiting the ability to complete rehabilitative therapies. There aren't conclusive data for required hemoglobin levels for acute in-patient rehab, so this will be on a case-by-case basis. You will need to be willing to discuss issues that might come up in rehabilitation including dizziness and tachycardia that do not resolve quickly or extreme fatigue during therapy. The question will be whether these might be ameliorated with transfusion to increase intravascular volume and oxygen-carrying capacity.—**HR, CFB, and Editors**

- A restrictive threshold (Hb $\leq$8 g/dL) is suitable for patients undergoing orthopedic surgery, cardiac surgery, and those with preexisting cardiovascular disease.—**HR and Editors**

- Remember that patients always set their own transfusion guidelines! In other words, consideration of the physiology and clinical status is paramount. The recommendations regarding restrictive vs. liberal transfusion strategies do *NOT* universally apply to specific patient subgroups in clinical care settings such as acute coronary syndrome and severe thrombocytopenia with a risk for bleeding.—**HR and Editors**

- Once when I was a vascular anesthesia fellow, I was in an extremely complex vascular case. This was back in the days when aortic surgery was always open. I remember my attending saying to me, "Okay, this patient is going to bleed and try to go over the cliff for the entire case. We need to give him and the surgeons a decent distance from the edge of that hemodynamic precipice. So, we are going to do the rule of 10's today. I have to go start my other room but when I come back, I want the CVP to be 10, the PCWP to be 10, and the hemoglobin to be 10. Any time the patient gets off this spot, we are going to tap him back towards 10." This was good advice then and it's good advice now. It was goal-directed transfusion before we used that term. You resuscitate for the situation.—**CM**

- Then there is tricky problem of platelet transfusion thresholds. This is also evaluated on a continual basis by the transfusion medicine community [7].—**Editors**

- It's a bit surprising how low-quality a lot of the evidence is for specific platelet thresholds. Guidelines have been established but in general, there are few strong recommendations. Here are just a couple.—**Editors**

  - One unit of prophylactic platelet transfusion if the platelet count is less than 10×10^9 cells/L to reduce the risk of spontaneous bleeding.

  - Prophylactic platelet transfusion for placement of central access if the platelet count is less than 20×10^9 cells/L.

  - Prophylactic platelet transfusion for elective lumbar puncture or major elective non-neuraxial surgery if the platelet count is less than 50×10^9 cells/L.

- If you need to give platelets before a planned procedure, there is no need to start the night before. Depending on how low the platelet count is, perhaps one platelet product on the morning of the procedure with a unit dripping in during the procedure. Remember, there is a lot of plasma volume and/or platelet additive solution in those platelet bags.—**CM**

- The transfusion medicine community is starting to look at ability to complete both inpatient and outpatient rehab as an outcome measure for transfusion efficacy, so we should as well.—**CM and CFB**

Bleeding, Transfusion, and Patient Blood Management

- Patient blood management (PBM) is about doing the "right" thing.—*SMF*

Right dose—Right product—Right patient—Right time!

- So, the cool thing about PBM is that everybody wins if the patients only get the blood they need and don't get blood they don't need. It's best for the patients since blood transfusion has risks. It's best for the hospital and blood bank not to have to procure and manage that expensive resource. And it's best for the overall public health and the blood supply if unnecessary transfusions are avoided since the donor supply chain is not robust.—**TJK, CM, and SMF**

- Patient blood management is a team sport! At Hopkins, there are caregiver team members in at least 15 different departments, from the hospital executives on down.**—TMJ and SMF**

- The other really cool thing about patient blood management is that it can be approached in so many ways and at so many points.—**SMF**

  * Anemia treatment—preop and postop.

  * Surgical techniques—less invasive and careful attention to control of bleeding.

  * Topical hemostatics and newer cautery.

  * Cell salvage—an incredibly important component of PBM.

  * Minimize phlebotomy.

  * Computerized provider order entry with clinician decision support.

  * Antifibrinolytics—tranexamic acid and aminocaproic acid (Amicar).

  * Point of care testing—TEG and rapid turnaround.

  * Audits with feedback.

  * Education!

- To add to Steve Frank's list, there are a few other techniques may help reduce the need for transfusion.—**RGG**

  * Controlled hypotension—lowering systemic blood pressure has been shown to reduce blood loss in orthopedic procedures such as total hip replacement. It can be done with multiple techniques—including spinal or epidural anesthesia, vasodilators, remifentanil, and dexmedetomidine.

  * Acute normovolemic hemodilution—this technique includes the removal of whole blood from a patient shortly after induction of anesthesia, with maintenance of normovolemia using crystalloid and/or colloid replacement. The amount of blood removed typically varies between 1 and 3 units, depending on the starting hemoglobin level of the patient. This whole blood is then reinfused later when the patient's hemoglobin level has dropped to the point that they need transfusion. This techniques works best when the patient has a high starting hemoglobin level, and 2–3 units of blood are removed at the start. This technique has a modest effect on reducing the need for non-autologous transfusion.

- Remember, four dollars of iron tablets can avoid $400 worth of blood. This is especially true for young menstruating females. —**SMF**

- Preop autologous donation is a nice way to induce anemia before surgery, subject the red cells to cold storage, then have them thrown in the trash in a substantial number of cases, since they cannot be used for other patients. This happened to me with my lumbar fusion in 2006 and I was billed $1000 because it was not covered by insurance. I paid *cash* to be rendered anemic before my surgery.—**SMF**

- If a patient declines allogenic transfusion and there is time before surgery, the first priority should be to optimize the red cell mass with iron and erythropoietic medications.—**TJK and SMF**

- The goal of perioperative management of patients for whom transfusion is not an option can be most simply summarized as: *keep the blood in the patient.* Every additional effort from minimizing blood draws to maintaining perioperative normothermia helps.—**TJK and SMF**

- Daily blood draws in the ICU can be as much as 1% of total blood volume if you are not careful about it. This is enough to cancel out erythropoiesis.—**TJK and SMF**

- Remember that even mild hypothermia of less than 1 °C will increase bleeding by 16%.—**SMF and CM**

- Blood loss is indirectly proportional to how hard the surgeons try. The Six "P" s for surgical bleeding are: pressure, patience, prayer, prolene, plasma, and platelets.—**TJK and SMF**

- If the surgeon says the patient's not bleeding, suggest they take the suctions out for 5 minutes.—**CC**

- There are three types of major blood loss cases—arterial bleeding with the prototypical case being repair of the aorta, venous bleeding with the prototypical case being liver transplant with veno-veno bypass (in the older days) or any case involving any part of the vena cava, and cases with a mixed vascular pattern but in which hypothermia is a major and defining factor, such as trauma cases and circulatory arrest cases. Hemostasis and resuscitation are managed differently depending on what type of bleeding you have.—**Editors**

- Bleeding you see, hemorrhage you hear, exsanguination is silent.—**CC**

- Scalp lacerations can be the source of terrific blood loss.—**Editors**

- So, about IV access for blood and blood component transfusions. If you are just dripping a component in, including platelets for a procedure, an 18-g IV is fine. If you are going to put any type of pressure on the line to give the blood rapidly, I think you need at least a 16-g. I've seen people put a pressure bag on a unit of blood hooked up to an 18-g IV and I've also seen that blow a lot of peripheral IVs, especially in the hand—maybe not so much if the 18-g is in the antecubital fossa.—**CM**

- Don't forget about interosseous (IO) lines. A line that runs like a 16-g IV catheter can be achieved in about 3 seconds with an IO line.—**JHW**

- The thing about trying to establish guidelines on transfusion practice in response to bleeding is that it's not only how much blood has been lost or what the thresholds for transfusion or medical futility are. It's also about *what* is bleeding. Bleeding from a ruptured spleen is very different that bleeding from a fractured liver. And bleeding from the iliac vein is very different than bleeding from the cavernous sinus. Only we can make those calls (in consultation with the surgeons). The blood bank can't really make those decisions.—**CM**

- When evaluating the risk-benefit ratio of blood transfusion, we have to keep in mind that we just don't really know that much about the immunological consequences of blood transfusion in the grand scheme of things. We don't even completely understand who develops antibodies in response to transfusion. We do know that it can be very situation dependent and depend on age, gender, and rate the transfusion is given. The point is to be very aware, with every single unit of blood, that you are giving one of the most complex biologics imaginable. Remember that a unit of plasma has literally thousands of different serum proteins. So, let's repeat this: We have a decent start on understanding and controlling the infectious risks and complications of blood transfusion. We don't really have a clue to understanding and especially controlling the full immunological consequences. Not a clue.—**Editors**

- For instance, if you want to really get a bit weirded out, read Evan Bloch's paper on microchimerism [8]. As the paper cited states, "Microchimerism, the coexistence of genetically disparate populations of cells in a receptive host, is well described in both clinical and physiological settings, including transplantation and pregnancy. Microchimerism can also occur after allogeneic blood transfusion in traumatically injured patients, where donor cells have been observed decades after transfusion." It's not understood why it occurs in that clinical subset, but it's hypothesized to be linked to the immune disruptions that occur in severe trauma. It's been seen with transfusion of a variety of blood products and may possibly be linked to graft-vs-host disease. The only recognized risk factor to date is age of blood product with fresher products posing a greater risk.—**Editors**

- The question of favorable outcomes with the transfusion of new vs. old blood is interesting and it hasn't been completely settled yet. But there is one thing we know for sure about new blood. There isn't enough "brand new" blood for everybody to get it.—**Editors**

- If giving tranexamic acid (TXA), give it early (<3 hours from trauma). It may help, but probably does not harm if given early. It is cheap. Pre-hospital TXA is the ideal. Start with either 1 or 2 gm IV. The CRASH protocol is to then run 1 gm over 8 hours, but if the patient is massively hemorrhaging, they may need more.—**RVN**

- When the patient is bleeding or unstable for any reason, aim for Hb > 10 g/dL, platelets >100 K/microliter, INR < 1.5 and fibrinogen >200 mg/dL.—**RVN**

- Every time a lab test is drawn, blood is wasted, and adds to iatrogenic anemia and costs money.—**RVN**

- In fact, a typical number of labs drawn daily in the ICU is over 1% of a patient's blood volume and cancels out erythropoiesis. Order labs only when they are needed. So, consider whether the test is needed, and how often it needs to be repeated. Most labs can run tests on smaller tubes / samples—check with your lab.—**RVN, TJK, and SMF**

- TEE is a great way to rule out other causes of shock and monitor cardiac function and filling with ongoing resuscitation.—**RVN**

- In massive hemorrhage, maintain blood composition by replacing with 1:1:1 or whole blood until in control or labs available to guide resuscitation.—**RVN**

- Rapid turnaround is essential for labs to guide resuscitation—at a minimum, use an emergency hemorrhage panel (hemoglobin, hematocrit, platelet count, PT, APTT, fibrinogen), or bedside viscoelastic test with blood gases (for pH, lactate, potassium, ionized calcium). Keep a note of when in the resuscitation the sample was sent, for example after two units of packed red blood cells and two units of fresh frozen plasma.—**RVN**

- Don't be afraid to tell your cardiac or liver transplant surgical colleague that the thromboelastography is normal and surgical bleeding should be addressed.—**EA**

- Stop the tank from emptying whilst you refill the tank—in other words, control the hemorrhage simultaneously whilst resuscitating!—**RVN**

- If things are not in control, activate a massive transfusion protocol (MTP). It can always be cancelled later.—**RVN**

- If your hospital doesn't have a massive transfusion protocol (MTP), collaborate, and write one. If they do have one, monitor it, research it, and write it up (or at least the outcomes).—**RVN**

- The key to the successive deployment on an MTP is calmness and organization. And dare we say it? A certain amount of neatness. But not the kind of neatness that wastes time, the type that saves time and keeps you from mislabeling syringes. Your anesthesia workstation should stay neat and organized—yes, even in the thick of things—and don't throw empty bags onto the OR floor. They are a slip hazard, and you just have to pick them up at the end of the case anyway.—**Editors**

- Ask about the MTP when interviewing for anesthesia jobs. How many? Post-hoc reviews? Who is on the transfusion committee?—**Editors**

- Contact key personnel early to get control of the bleeding—surgeons, interventional radiology, gastroenterology team (for GI scope), blood bank (for products), hematologist (for complex coagulopathy or reversal of anti-coagulants/anti-platelet agents).—**RVN**

- In massive hemorrhage, maintain blood composition by replacing with 1:1:1 or whole blood until in control or labs available to guide resuscitation but remember that we don't know the whole story on whole right now.—**RVN and CM**

- Always keep track of when in a fast-moving resuscitation the sample was sent, for example, after two units of packed RBCs and 2 units of FFP.—**RVN**

- I've seen two very bad equipment mishaps with Level 1 transfusers—which highlights the risks with high pressure/blood transfusion, even though the equipment is also amazing when used properly.—**RVN**

- In Afghanistan, we had a local national come in post blast and/or gunshot wound. The patient was very unstable, got a subclavian large bore line, and was hooked up to the Level 1 transfuser. The patient promptly became difficult to ventilate, hypoxic, and suffered a PEA arrest. An emergent thoracotomy revealed a left chest *full* of blood (everything we had just put through the Level 1)—clearly had torn his subclavian vein and so products under pressure caused tamponade! He survived! Learning point:—major vessels can get injured during central line placement—there can be dilator injuries or a central line's lumens can be extravascular. If the patient is not responding properly to volume or meds being administered through a central line, think about these possibilities.—**RVN**

- Here is another Level 1 mishap—somebody hooks it onto a line with additional ports. Then gives a high dose of calcium whilst transfusing through level 1. Everything just turns into one very big clot, and the line gets obstructed. Learning point, have a dedicated line for the Level 1 and don't transfuse anything else apart from blood products through that line.—**RVN**

- Because blood components are so cold, be pedantic about keeping the patient normothermic —warm the fluids/blood products, use underbody and overbody forced air heaters, and cover the head with reflective cap and intravascular warming device if needed.—**RVN**

- Rapid infusion catheters (RIC) and Cordis /MAC introducers/PA sheaths are great for resuscitation. Learn to put in landmark subclavian lines—1 day it may save a life.—**RVN**

- Level 1 infusers (and better still) Belmonts are the ideal way to fluid/blood resuscitate, but always keep an eye on the infusion catheter—a leaking catheter can rapidly lead to compartment syndrome.—**RVN**

- Using a Belmont with a reservoir chamber allows you to stay ahead in the resuscitation.—**RVN**

- Designate staff to run the Belmont, check blood products, and keep a tally of what has been given.—**RVN**

- In an MTP, ask for a blood cooler from the blood bank so that items are only taken out when needed—cooled products can only be out for 30 minutes before they need to be used or discarded.—**RVN**

- When it comes to massive transfusion protocols, remember to warm the blood, give calcium, and *watch over the drapes to know when the bleeding has stopped.*—**TJK and SMF**

- When is a massive amount of transfused blood too much to survive and so continued transfusion is medically futile? Nobody knows the answer to that question at this time. Maybe it's even a false dilemma. But what trauma anesthesiologists are starting to look at is the point at which survivability begins to decrease. At Hopkins, we established the "50–50 rule." In other words, after 50 units of blood, we have about 50% survival. This will change of course, and we think one big factor that will impact this number is when happens in the pre-hospital resuscitation.—**TJK, SMF, and CM**

- We also know that rates of infection and thrombotic events start to increase significantly after about 10 units of transfused blood.—**SMF**

- Let's focus on <u>fibrinogen</u> for a minute. Our current sources of fibrinogen include FFP, cryoprecipitate, and fibrinogen concentrate. There is some controversy about what a target level of fibrinogen should be when a patient is actively bleeding. A reasonable goal with our current knowledge is 200 mg/dl. Here is some more in-depth info below.—**RGG**

  * Fibrinogen concentrate (RiaSTAP) comes in bottles of approximately 1000 mg (range 900–1300 mg). In an 80 kg patient, it takes about two bottles to raise fibrinogen level by 50 mg/dl. It is expensive—cost to the hospital is about $1000 per bottle. The pharmacy charges the patient $5000 per bottle. It can be mixed and ready to go in minutes.

  * Cryoprecipitate: a 1-unit volume of cryo contains a range of 150–300 mg of fibrinogen in 10–20 ml. As a rough estimate, 10 units of cryo will raise the fibrinogen level by about 50 mg/dl in an 80 kg patient. It also contains fibronectin, factor VIII, factor XIII, and von Willebrand factor (vWF). It takes about 45 minutes to prepare cryo once an order is received.

  * FFP: We don't routinely use FFP as a main treatment to raise fibrinogen, but it does have significant fibrinogen content. 1 unit of FFP typically contains 500 mg of fibrinogen per 250 ml bag of plasma, so four units of plasma will raise the fibrinogen level by 50 mg/dl.

- Here is a bit more advice.—**RGG and JHW**

  * Cryoprecipitate has the advantage of being cheaper than human fibrinogen concentrate (RiaSTAP), and also has other clotting factors. However, it has a long preparation time, and more donor exposure. So ideal use is when you know you will need fibrinogen placement, and have adequate time to order and prepare, for example, fibrinogen <200–225 mg/dL on pre-pump labs, dissections, and very long pump times.

  * RiaSTAP has the advantage of fast preparation time. So, if the patient is coagulopathic and actively bleeding, it has an advantage over cryoprecipitate.

  * FFP is generally not used to treat low fibrinogen due to the large amount of volume it contains, and also the time it takes to prepare it and administer it. However, it is nice to know you are giving some fibrinogen when you are giving FFP.

  * While FFP is generally a poor way of raising fibrinogen concentrations, FFP can be returned to the blood bank; whereas cryo is typically wasted if it's not used.

- It still surprises me how much blood can be lost within a matter of few minutes during skin grafting for a big burn. And unfortunately, there is not an easy or accurate way to calculate blood loss. Just be advised that they can and do turn into MTP cases.—**KAM**

- Young (pre-menopausal) Rh-negative women may need RhD IVIG if they have received O POS blood in the pre-hospital or perioperative periods. This is handled differently in different institutions, but the blood bank is the best place to start for guidance. Rh immunoglobulin is also usually recommended by SOP for patients who receive out of Rh group platelets although not always given.—**CM and Editors**

***Note from the Editors:** Just for fun, we asked *Anesthesia Bridges* contributor and med student Abigail Crawford if she could possibly find us a bridge that looked like the membrane of a red blood cell, complete with an antigen protruding from the cell membrane and she did it! (Fig. 159.3).

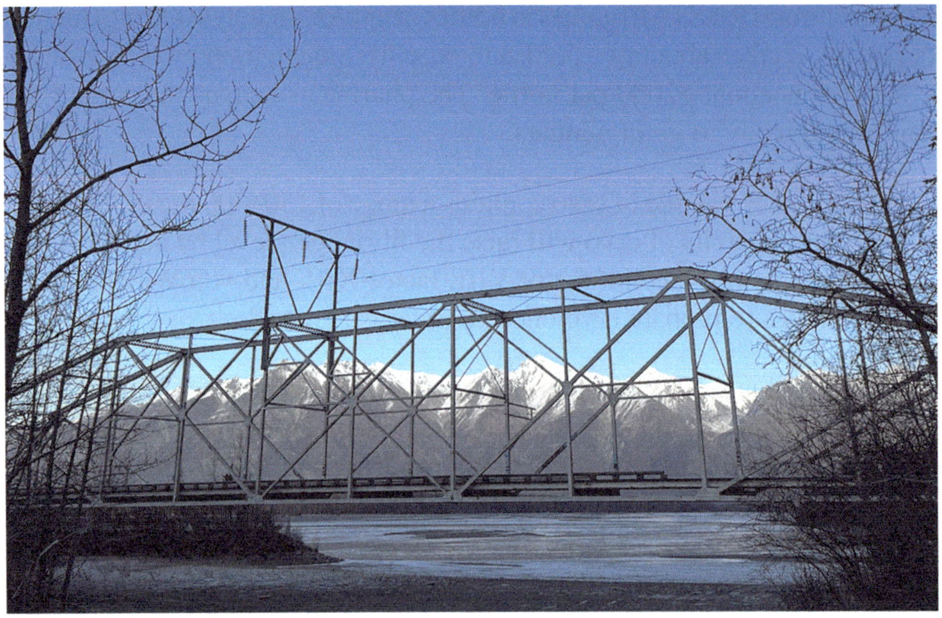

Fig. 159.3 A spare but stunning bridge scene in Alaska - look at that beautiful sky. Photo: Abigail J. Crawford

Pediatric Transfusion and Patient Blood Management

- Pediatric patients are not just small adults, especially when it comes to blood volumes. You don't want to "dilute" out your patient's platelets or clotting factors by giving a whole unit of red cells when an aliquot will work. There are several calculations out there to estimate blood volumes, so talk with your transfusion service about which ones your institution uses.—**RJC and TLT**

- For pediatric patients beyond the neonatal period (>4 months old), one main difference compared to adults is their blood volume—kids grow fast, and their blood volume changes along with that—again, there are ways to estimate blood volume, which can be useful during surgery or a massive transfusion.—**RJC and TLT**

- Kids also have an ability to tolerate blood loss—studies show that otherwise healthy pediatric patients may be able to tolerate lower hemoglobin levels than adults, especially when the anemia develops slowly.—**RJC and TLT**

- And a third difference involves the age-appropriate hemoglobin/hematocrit levels—levels continue to increase after the neonatal period but won't reach adult levels until after adolescence.—**RJC and TLT**

- Be careful about giving out-of-group plasma-containing products to small patients. Plasma-containing products have donor antibodies, for example, the plasma in a unit of platelets from an O donor has anti-A and anti-B antibodies. These have the potential to cause hemolysis when giving them to out-of-group recipients—such as giving type O platelets to a type A patient. This risk increases in patients with small blood volumes, and most institutions don't titer every plasma-containing unit.—**RJC and TLT**

- Neonates (patients younger than 4 months old) have special considerations when it comes to transfusion. If you don't routinely work with pediatric patients (and even if you do), it's a good idea to consult with your transfusion service about any special requirements and institution-specific policies. The last thing you want is a delay in getting blood products that could have been prevented.—**RJC and TLT**

- Institutions have their own policies for what is required for neonatal transfusion. It's a good idea to talk with your transfusion service about age cut-offs, irradiation requirements, additive solutions, volume reduction, what is considered a "fresh" unit, and so forth. The transfusion medicine team should be giving regular lectures on the current issues to the pediatric anesthesia and PICU teams.—**RJC and TLT**

- Because neonates have very small blood volumes, it is especially important that you try to minimize phlebotomy as much as possible. Talk with your transfusion service and clinical labs to see how much sample they need or if they can use a sample from the mother for transfusion testing.—**RJC and TLT**

- Neonates require irradiation of all cellular blood products (red cells, platelets) to prevent transfusion associated graft versus host disease. Talk with your transfusion service about this, especially if irradiation is not done on site, so you can get a sense of how long it will take to get blood products.—**RJC and TLT**

- Standard practice is to transfuse neonates with a relatively high doses (10–20 mL/kg), putting them at risk of circulatory overload. You should transfuse the product as slowly as possible, so the neonate has time to compensate.—**RJC and TLT**

- If you plan to volume resuscitate an infant or neonate, especially with blood, you will generally need a 22-g IV as the volume line.—**KL**

- Because maternal antibodies can cross the placenta, you need to consider both the transfusion needs of the infant and the mother's antibodies.—**RJC and TLT**

- Leukocyte-reduced blood products are considered CMV-safe, and studies evaluating this have found no transmission of CMV in patients receiving leukocyte-reduced components. In fact, the main source of CMV transmission in neonates was found to be breast milk from CMV-positive mothers.—**RJC and TLT**

- For routine, small-volume, simple transfusions in neonates, studies have shown that the different RBC additive solutions are equivalent in terms of safety and efficacy. If you transfuse slowly, the age of the RBCs doesn't have a large impact on serum potassium. This may not necessarily be the case for those getting larger volumes, like during surgery, exchange transfusion or ECMO, or those with transfusion-dependent chronic anemia.—**RJC and TLT**

- Whole blood is generally not licensed in neonates/young infants—clarify the lower cut off with your blood bank.—**RVN**

- Studies suggest that rates of transfusion reactions are higher in pediatric patients compared to adults, so be on the lookout for signs and symptoms of transfusion reactions.—**RJC and TLT**

- Perioperative RBC transfusions are independently associated with development of new or progressive postoperative venous thromboembolism in children, infants, and neonates. These findings need further validation in prospective studies and emphasize the need for evidence-based perioperative pediatric blood transfusion decisions.—**RJC and CM**

- In general (even outside of ECMO), for really small pediatric patients getting larger transfusions, washed cells may be preferred to minimize the storage lesion, such as increased potassium levels.—**RJC and TLT**

- However, potassium levels increase linearly over time with storage, so one can get around this with the use of fresher units (<5–7 days old).—**RJC and TLT**

- There really haven't been any good trials or anything looking at this in ECMO for kids though. For example, UCLA mentions washing on a case-by-case basis for ECMO, and in general just use fresher units to minimize tech time and wastage.—**RJC and TLT**

- The consensus recommendations put out by the Pediatric Critical Care Transfusion and Anemia Expertise Initiative only recommend washing for anaphylactic prophylaxis, and that future studies are needed to study the types of red cell manipulations and their impact on outcomes in ECMO kids. On top of that, individual institutions have their own SOPs on age/weight cutoffs for those who "require" washed red cells, so pediatric kids on ECMO by default may get washed red cells depending on the institution.—**RJC and TLT**

- All that to say there are varying practices throughout the country, and outcomes seem to be fairly similar between them. There really is no right answer right now, so each institution has to figure it out on their own.—**RJC and TLT**

- Don't forget that even tiny pediatric patients can require activation of an MTP. One of the most stressful blood resuscitations that I have ever done was a neonate in the PICU with a single ventricle who was on central ECMO with ongoing bleeding. The child was tiny (<2 kg) and having to manage minute volumes for an MTP made me definitely earn my pay. Overall, we transfused about 600mls of blood over 12-hour night shift.—**RVN**

***Note from the Editors:** In the summer of 2025, five towns in Rockland County, New York held a blood drive contest to see which municipality could collect the most blood. It was dubbed the Senator Weber Five Town Blood Challenge. To highlight the contest, the Tappan Zee bridge was lit in blood red light at night (Fig. 159.4). Clarkstown, NY took the prize for the most blood collected and the most new donors registered. Go Clarkstown!

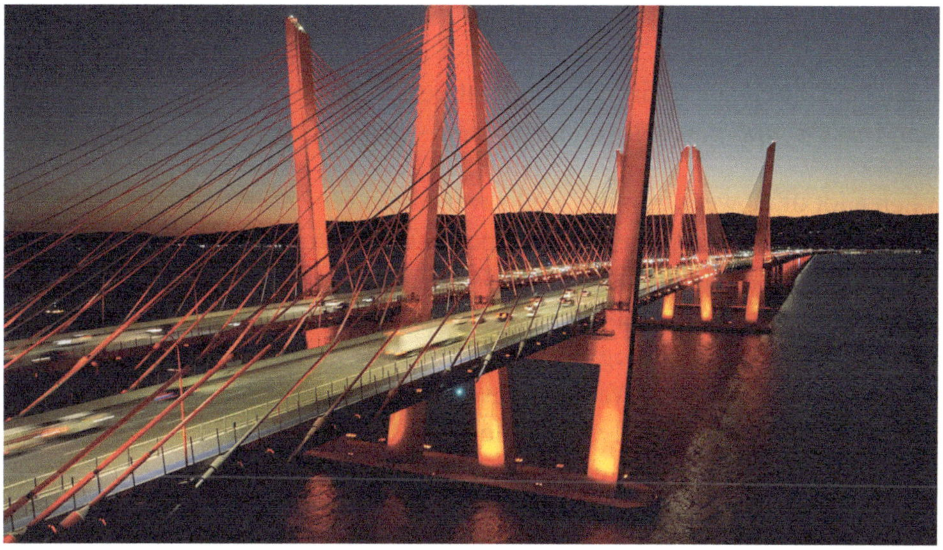

Fig. 159.4 The Tappan Zee bridge lit with blood-red floodlights to call attention to a competitive blood drive between five towns in Rockland County, New York. Photo: Image used under standard license stock.adobe.com

Sickle Cell Disease

- When it comes to patients with sickle cell disease (SCD), prevention is key. That can't be stressed enough, because not only do patients with SCD get exposed to more blood products, but also they are actually more prone to making antibodies to blood products. That means in emergent situations, you should try your best to hold off on transfusing until compatible blood can be found.—**RJC and TLT**

- Because patients with SCD are so prone to antibody formation, transfusion services will preemptively provide more extensive antigen-matched blood. So not only is the product ABO-Rh(D) matched, but also they are matched for C, c, E, e, and K. This means that getting those blood products will take additional time.—**RJC and TLT**

- Once a patient with SCD makes an antibody, transfusion services will do even more extended antigen matching, which can add even more time to finding matched units. **RJC and TLT**

- There are over 300 major antigens present on red cells, and we can't routinely test for all of them. But once antibodies are formed, we have to match for them. The more antibodies that are formed by the patient, the harder it is to find units that don't express those antigens. This means that it can take days or weeks to find a matched unit, and there may only be one unit available. Sometimes, it's impossible to find a completely matched unit and you may be stuck giving a unit that is at a higher risk of causing hemolysis. So bottom line: prevention, prevention, prevention!—**RJC and TLT**

Cell Salvage

- Cell salvage is also called cell saving, intraoperative blood salvage, and autotransfusion. There are four equipment makers who make the brands in use.—**EAU and JHW**

- Honestly? When a lot of us were training, cell saver blood was a bit of an afterthought. It was used in vascular cases but not commonly elsewhere. A perfusionist would come in at the end of the case and hand you a unit of cell saver blood that you didn't tremendously need at that point but found a way to give to the patient. We didn't consider of using cell salvage in trauma cases, a messy abdominal case, or, heaven forbid, in a surgical oncology case. I never once in all the time I spent in the delivery suite saw it used for operative deliveries. We never, ever washed surgical laps or sponges; I don't think we ever even considered it. This was really a terrible waste, literally and figuratively! Cell salvage is now an integral part of patient blood management strategies. And pretty much every way we did back in the old days has been improved upon!—**CM**

- Plus, common sense tells us that the necessity of cell salvage will only increase in clinical practice. The supply of donor blood components is tenuous and, unfortunately, isn't really strengthening. Clinical care of the bleeding patient is going to *have* to go towards the direction of increased deployment of autotransfusion. This is another clinical issue that there just isn't any way around. Fortunately, the research is pretty reassuring—there seems to be a number of situations and ways to safely incorporate cell salvage into an expanded range of cases.—**JHW and CM**

- Remember, each unit of packed red blood cells (1pRBC) contains 200 ml of RBCs, while 100 ml of salvaged blood carries 56 ml of RBCs.—**EAU and JHW**

- The obstacles to auto-transfusion are education, cost, and contradictions. There are emerging solutions for all three of these.—**KAM and JHW**

- Cost is probably the easiest to deal with as there are knowable costs for both cell salvage and allogeneic transfusion. In general, the fixed costs of a cell saver setup are approximately equal to the cost of crossmatching 2 units of red blood cells. In the UPMC system, we have tabulated the costs of the red blood cell units themselves and have found that the overall cost of cell salvage blood is equivalent to one unit of RBCs but significantly reduces costs with an increasing number of transfused RBC units.—**EAU and JHW**

- Few hospital practices are static and, as our world becomes more diverse, the population genetics of blood group antigens will also become more diverse. Any public health factor that makes it harder to find and crossmatch a unit of allogeneic blood will make that blood more expensive. It is not *that* unusual to need a unit of donated red blood cells that costs $500 or more. The best way to keep that cost down is to not need that expensive blood in the first place and using cell salvage for that patient can help with that a lot.—**LC and CM**

- So, consider using cell salvage *early*. And we mean "early" in several ways—it should automatically be part of the transfusion plan in a wide variety of cases. And it should also be given as early as possible in the resuscitation and/or surgery. A 2015 study looked at the effects of (essentially) autotransfusion of the chest tube blood resulting from hemothorax injuries. The study found that overall allogeneic red blood cell and platelet transfusions were reduced (with the attendant costs, of course) without differences seen with in-hospital complications, mortality, and 24-hour post-admission INR.—**RVN, EAU, and JHW**

- The first stage of cell salvage involves blood collection, anticoagulation, and filtration. The second stage is blood concentration, and the third stage is blood washing.—**KAM**

- There are really big clinical and research opportunities with the use of cell salvage in obstetrics. As we mention above, several decades ago, this was never done. However, today numerous US and UK organizations advocate for blood salvage during the peripartum period.—**KAM and JHW**

- The major issue with cell salvage for obstetrics of course is the problem of amniotic fluid embolism. It's a grievous disease with a mortality rate of 60–80% that also leaves only 25% of survivors neurologically intact. Fortunately, the incidence is extremely low-ranging from 1:8000 to 1:300,000. However, the low incidence requires a considerable number of participants for statistically reliable results when studying the use of blood salvage and amniotic fluid embolism.—**EAU and JHW**

- Safety protocols for applying cell salvage in obstetrics involve thorough washout of biochemical, cellular, and bacterial contaminants. A demonstrated adequate tissue factor washout has been demonstrated, and there is an exponential potassium decrease in platelets and potassium with increased wash volume of salvaged RBCs.—**KAM and JHW**

- We've been able to demonstrate a significant reduction in amniotic fluid markers (biochemical, cellular, and bacterial) with wash and filtration. This includes a 97% decrease in four types of bacteria.—**JHW and EAU**

- But what about cell salvage in oncology cases? The concern is that tumor cells will be concentrated and transfused back to the patient, leading to widespread metastases. Multiple researchers found that the presence or absence of circulating tumor cells holds little prognostic significance [9, 10]. Tumor cells circulate in the peripheral blood of all major carcinomas but not in healthy subjects.—**EAU and JHW**

- In immunocompromised mice, 70–90% of injected cancer cells survive and extravasate but only 0.1% form metastases [11].—**KAM and JHW**

- Leukocyte depletion filters effectively remove tumor cells.—**EAU and JHW**

- Several meta-analyses and systematic reviews found no significant difference in mortality with blood salvage in cancer surgeries.—**KAM and JHW**

- In trauma cases, autologous transfusion showed no statistically significant impact on survival rates, bloodstream infections, length of stay, other in-hospital complications, or INR differences. Autotransfusion of washed, culture-positive blood may not significantly increase the infection risk in severe abdominal injury patients.—**EAU and JHW**

- Additionally, various studies concluded that in abdominal or thoracic traumas, early autologous fresh whole blood transfusion reduces allogeneic transfusions, with no effect on mortality or postoperative infection.—**KAM and JHW**

- While blood contamination by bowel contents is typically considered an absolute contraindication to autotransfusion, in dogs reinfusion of contaminated blood minimally affects survival with 20–30% hemorrhage but significantly decreases survival with 40% hemorrhage. The use of antibiotics was deemed to eliminate the risk of autotransfusion.—**EAU and JHW**

- Allogeneic blood leads to immunomodulation, and surgeries often result in hematogenous dissemination of bacteria.—**EAU and JHW**

- Recommendations for cell salvage in dirty surgeries involve minimizing stool aspiration into the salvage system, washing blood with increased volume, and filtering it with a Pall RS leukocyte depletion filter.—**KAM and JHW**

ECMO

- ECMO is complicated, and so is transfusion medicine, so working regularly with your transfusion service is key. Your transfusion service is likely aware of the patients that are on ECMO, but if you haven't already started that conversation, you may want to start now. You definitely don't want your first interaction with your transfusion department to happen during an urgent case.—**RJC and TLT**

- While on ECMO, red blood cell loss can exceed normal red blood cell production by the patient.—**RJC and TLT**

- As whole blood travels through the ECMO circuit, the red cells, platelets, and coagulation factors are damaged/activated, leading to increased clearance.—**RJC and TLT**

- Patients on ECMO require more red cell transfusions than those not on ECMO.—**RJC and TLT**

- Almost all patients on ECMO will require a red blood cell transfusion, averaging between 1–2 units per day.—**RJC and TLT**

- There is no standard hemoglobin threshold at which to transfuse. There is quite a bit of data so far that suggests a more restrictive versus a more liberal threshold has no influence on patient outcomes. *But* the final answer probably isn't in yet.—**RJC and CM**

- Minimizing phlebotomy and duplicate testing on ECMO patients can result in fewer transfusions.—**RJC and TLT**

- Better anticoagulation monitoring during ECMO can lead to less phlebotomy draws, reduced testing, reduced circuit changes per ECMO day, and increased savings.—**RJC and TLT**

- Chromogenic anti-Xa assay is the best assay to monitor heparin levels while on ECMO, though increased free hemoglobin and bilirubin can cause falsely low results. PTT is second best but is sensitive to other coagulation factors and inhibitors (like lupus-like inhibitors which are common in ICU patients). Activated clotting time (ACT) is the least sensitive—at low heparin levels (like those used during ECMO) there is no correlation between ACT and heparin levels—it's basically a random number generator.—**RJC and TLT**

- Coagulation monitoring is pretty nuanced, and some facilities have even developed their own way of testing anticoagulation levels on ECMO patients, so you should have a low threshold when it comes to contacting the transfusion service/clinical laboratory about anti-coagulation monitoring.—**RJC and TLT**

- Unless the circuit is primed with red cells and plasma, there will be a dilution of blood components when ECMO is started. This dilution is more profound in patients with smaller blood volumes. Even when the circuit is primed with red cells/plasma, platelets will still get diluted initially, so expect your patient's platelet count to decrease, especially in smaller/pediatric patients.—**RJC and TLT**

- For adults, ECMO does not require washed red cells, freshness of the unit does not matter, and the additive solution of the red cell unit does not seem to impact patient outcomes. This is different for pediatric patients.—**RJC and TLT**

More Wisdom on Resuscitation Using Blood Components from *Avoiding Common Anesthesia Errors, 2nd Edition*

There is a wealth of additional tips, teaching tidbits, and overall wisdom on bleeding and blood components in our previous book, which is nicknamed "Green2." *Please* check out this information and remember that every single penny of royalties goes to FAER in perpetuity!

Green2 Chapters with More Wisdom on Bleeding, Blood, and Resuscitation

- Know What Screening Tests Are Performed on Volunteer Donor Blood.
- Red Blood Cell Primer.
- Type and Screen or Type and Crossmatch?
- Special Circumstances: Patients with Antibodies.
- Plasma—It's Not Just to Fix an Abnormal INR.
- Plasma Part II: Is This Plasma or Pea Soup?
- Remember That the "Universal" Donor Is Different for Red Cell and Plasma Products.
- Platelets—Often a Mystery!
- Cryoprecipitate—The Most Misunderstood Product in the Blood Bank.
- Washed Blood Products Are a Source of Confusion—Here's Some Help.
- This TEG Tracing Looks Like a Rorschach Blot… Is It Time for a Transfusapalooza?

- Transfusion Reactions.
- Transfusion Outcomes.
- Directed Donation Is Generally Not a Good Idea.
- Not All Acute Lung Injury After a Transfusion Is a Transfusion-Related Acute Lung Injury.
- Jehovah's Witnesses and Bloodless Medicine.
- The Ethics of Jehovah's Witnesses and Transfusion.

References

1. Goel R, Josephson CD, Flori HR, et al. Perioperative transfusions and venous thromboembolism. Pediatrics. 2020;145(4):e20193029.
2. Tobian AA, Heddle NM, Yazer MH, et al. Red blood cell transfusion: 2016 clinical practice guidelines from AABB. Transfusion. 2016;56(10):2627–30.
3. Carson JL, Stanworth SJ, Roubinian N, et al. Transfusion thresholds and other strategies for guiding allogeneic red blood cell transfusion. Cochrane Database Syst Rev. 2016;10:CD002042. Updated in: Cochrane Database Syst Rev. 2021;12:CD002042.
4. Carson JL, Grossman BJ, Kleinman S, et al. Red blood cell transfusion: a clinical practice guideline from the AABB. Ann Intern Med. 2012;157(1):49–58.
5. Carless PA, Henry DA, Moxey AJ, et al. Transfusion thresholds and other strategies for guiding allogeneic red blood cell transfusion. Cochrane Database Syst Rev. 2010;10:CD002042. Updated in: Cochrane Database Syst Rev. 2012;4:CD002042.
6. Curley A, Stanworth SJ, Willoughby K, et al. Randomized trial of platelet-transfusion thresholds in neonates. N Engl J Med. 2019;380:242–51.
7. Kaufman RM, Djulbegovic B, Gernsheimer T, et al. Platelet transfusion: a clinical practice guideline from the AABB. Ann Intern Med. 2015;162(3):205–13.
8. Bloch EM, Jackman RP, Lee TH, et al. Transfusion-associated microchimerism: the hybrid within. Transfus Med Rev. 2013;27(1):10–20.
9. Cole WH. Efforts to increase host resistance to cancer. Surg Gynecol Obstet. 1973;137:853.
10. Salsbury AJ. Immunologic aspects of transfusion and cancer. Cancer Treat Rev. 1975;2:55–72.
11. Chambers WH, Kondo M, Billings PR, et al. Immunologic consequences of blood transfusion. Adv Cancer Res. 2000;79:91–121.

Authors

Steve Frank is a senior anesthesiologist in Baltimore, Maryland. He is a nationally and internationally recognized expert in patient blood management. The most notable transfusion in his career was the lifesaving one he himself received when he was helicoptered to shock trauma for an emergency splenectomy after a bicycle vs. car head-on collision. His helmet and the blood saved his life.

Rob Christian did his transfusion medicine fellowship at the training program that is based at the University of Washington system, Bloodworks Northwest, and Seattle Children's Hospital. He is now back at OHSU as a board-certified transfusion medicine physician. In true Pacific Northwest fashion, he loves outdoor activities, especially hiking and kayaking. He also enjoys woodworking but claims he is not very good at it… yet.

Raj Nathwani is a trauma anesthesiologist who has thought deeply about every issue noted above. He is not a big believer in "should" or "must." Instead, it is his firm conviction that each resuscitation case must be evaluated on the unique circumstances of the case.

Elizabeth Ungerman is a cardiothoracic anesthesiologist in the UPMC system and the associate program director. She tries to teach her trainees the principles of bleeding hemostasis and resuscitation with each case, no matter how routine. She is a Pittsburgher by origin and roots for the expected teams, naturally.

Stan Alfaras-Melainas is an anesthesiologist and critical care physician at UPMC. He is also the assistant program director of the anesthesiology residency program. His true passion in the medical field is resuscitation of burn patients, something that can be extremely challenging, and many times involves the rapid transfuser. In his private life, he definitely prefers the sunshine of Greece over the clouds of Pittsburgh, but feels his patients are worth it.

Cathy Marcucci is a chemical engineer who is trained in both anesthesiology and transfusion medicine, so this topic is close to her heart in several different ways. The complex problems of resuscitation have always been her favorite area of anesthesiology practice.

Wisdom on Procedures and Equipment

160

Catherine Marcucci, Bradford D. Winters,
Brant M. Wagener, Amy J. Robbins, and Ronald S. Bank

Contributors:

Brian Adolph

Robert Adolph

Andrew B. Barker, MD (ABB)

Mark J. Baskerville, MD (MJB)

Meena Bhatia, MD (MB)

Carol F. Bodenheimer, MD (CFB)

Niloofer Dalal, MD (ND)

Raymond G. Graber, MD (RGG)

Allan Gottschalk, MD PhD (AG)

Ronald L. Harter, MD (RLH)

Kirk Lalwani, MD (KL)

C. Marcucci (✉)
Department of Transfusion Medicine, Clinical Center, National Institutes of Health, Bethesda, MD, USA

B. D. Winters
Department of Anesthesiology and Critical Care Medicine, Johns Hopkins University, Baltimore, MD, USA

B. M. Wagener
Division of Critical Care Medicine, Division of Molecular and Translational Biomedicine, Birmingham, AL, USA

Department of Anesthesiology and Perioperative Medicine, Heersink School of Medicine, The University of at Birmingham, Birmingham, AL, USA

A. J. Robbins
Stanson Health, a Premier Inc. Company, Charlotte, NC, USA

Atrium Health, Carolinas Palliative Care and Hospice Group, Charlotte, NC, USA

R. S. Bank
Department of Anesthesiology, INOVA Fairfax Hospital, UVA School of Medicine, INOVA Campus, Falls Church, VA, USA

S. Mohamed et al. (eds.), *Anesthesia Bridges*, https://doi.org/10.1007/978-3-032-08294-7_160

Lucas Meuchel, MD (LM)

Steven L. Orebaugh, MD (SLO)

Amy J. Robbins, MD MBA (AJR)

Charles H. Sandson, BS IME (CHS)

Neil B. Sandson, MD (NBS)

Cobin Soelberg, MD (CS)

Brandon M. Togioka, MD (BMT)

Joanna Walker, MD (JW)

Jenny Wang, MD MBA (JW)

David A. Zvara, MD (DAZ)

Introduction

The practice of anesthesiology continues to grow and evolve as new procedures and equipment are continually introduced in just about every area of our specialty. These innovations are what make anesthesiology so great. Becoming and remaining proficient in procedures and mastering the safe and effective deployment of equipment resources are crucial ways to provide exemplary care to our patients. The wisdom below is just a tiny fraction of the necessary knowledge, but we hope that it stimulates careful thought and the desire to keep learning.

Procedures—General Advice

- If mastery of physiology and pharmacology is half of being an excellent anesthesiologist, mastery of procedures and proficiency in use of our equipment is the other half. Think of every really great anesthesiologist you know of—they all will be known for their expertise (or at the very least solid competency) in procedures and equipment. And no really great anesthesiologist will be bad at these things.—**Editors**

- The operating room is a unique place as it is one of the only instances in all of medicine where major invasive procedures are always done sequentially by two services. The surgeons generally cannot start theirs until we finish ours. It's not surprising that they sometimes get impatient with the time we are taking —it's actually remarkable that it doesn't happen more often.—**Editors**

- In other words, one major component of procedures is time. No procedure that takes excessive amounts of time is going to be seen as successful by anybody. Never skimp on the time it takes for the local anesthesia to take effect but do work on efficient setups, patient positioning, and so forth. It will save time overall if the patient is correctly positioned the first time because it will mean fewer attempts. We had an attending at Hopkins who asked the senior residents to organize themselves such that performance of a major neuraxial procedure was not longer than induction of general anesthesia.—**Editors**

- The most important quality for the skilled proceduralist is empathy. Anesthesiologists will do more procedures and stick more needles in people than they will ever have stuck in them. Keep in mind that the average healthy person in the US receives an average of 165 needlesticks in their lifetime—and of course, often our patients aren't the average, healthy patient. Needle phobias are common and real—of all the recognized phobias, they seem to have the strongest genetic basis. They are also the only phobia that has a vasovagal component, which may be evolutionary. So, have compassion!—**CM, KL, and JW**

- Never do a procedure to the point of pain and exhaustion for the patient. You have got to know and understand when both you and the patient have tried hard enough. How do you know when you have reached this point? *Stop immediately*, if you can imagine your patient going home and saying, "The spinal was so, so painful!" or "They just couldn't get the catheter in. They tried and tried and couldn't get it!"—**Editors**

- Pay extreme attention to your internal reactions to doing procedures and be honest with yourself. The moment you realize that you are starting to avoid certain procedures is the moment that you must take definite and purposeful action to increase your confidence and skills on that procedure. If you don't, your career has started to decline right then and there, even if you don't want to admit it to yourself.—**Editors**

- Successful procedures are all about having soft hands and remembering that millimeters count! Name one invasive procedure in the whole practice of anesthesiology where 2 mm doesn't make a real difference?—**Editors**

- Being really good at procedures is also a matter of being able to visualize anatomic structures in three dimensions. Study atlases and models and 3D recreations. The ultrasound is there to confirm anatomy that you are already familiar with. It's more a question of "The such-and-such nerve should be visualized just lateral to this bony landmark" as opposed to "Where is the dang nerve?!"—**Editors**

- On the other hand, anatomic variations do occur. IJs can be small or occluded, carotids can be posterior to IJ veins, and the beauty of using technology such as ultrasound is that it allows you to safely adjust your technique.—**RG**

- When doing or teaching procedures, always think about what you want to happen *and* what you don't want to happen. And have a thorough understanding of the most common complication of any procedure and the most serious. Clearly enunciate these goals in your thinking and teaching.—**Editors**

- When picking up a patient in the ICU, get a sign-out on every procedure the patient has recently had—"Were there any problems with the placement of the feeding tube? Has the patient been bronched recently? How did the pacemaker placement go, and how is it pacing?"—and give a sign-out on everything when dropping the patient off as well.—**Editors**

- Recognize that we are dealing with a huge potential for professional liability. Excluding dental damage, "improper performance of anesthesia procedure" accounted for 27% of 2013–2018 claims in the Anesthesia Closed Claims Project.—**Editors**

- When evaluating the patients' baseline health for the risk-benefit ratio of a procedure, don't forget to factor in their mental health. Ask whether they have claustrophobia and/or agoraphobia. Agoraphobia means "fear of the marketplace", but the phobia is now understood to involve fears of threatening situations that the patient feels they cannot escape from—and procedures under drapes qualify.—**NBS and CM**

- *Only one procedure at a time in an awake patient*! It's distressing and not fair to a patient to have them stuck in several places at once. It also disadvantages the people doing the procedures.—**CM**

- Give the patient something to do during procedures if they are not going to be substantially sedated. Or even if they are. Ask them to count up or down or visualize their five favorite beaches to discuss with you when the procedure is done. If it doesn't disrupt your position, you can ask them to alternate wiggling the toes of each foot. You can also use touch or pressure on a different part of the body at the time of a needlestick or aromatherapy during a longer procedure such as a dressing change in the ICU. *The point is that distraction theory (or cognitive engagement) works. But only if you do it.*—**NBS and Editors**

- Borrow from sports and performance psychology. Before starting a procedure, take just a couple seconds and visualize or even pantomime each step. We tend to forget or miss things in a procedure that are not in our direct line of sight, so do a visual sweep of the environment before stepping into it to do the procedure.—**Editors**

- *Don't forget about the feet*! There's a wonderful drawing below (Fig. 160.1). More surgical procedures are done below the waist than above, especially if you count obstetrical deliveries. For example, in the last decade the most common surgeries were musculoskeletal procedures such as knee and hip arthroplasty, laminectomy, and spinal fusion. So, the surgeons tend to be more comfortable working on the lower trunk, legs, and feet than we are. They can be the site for both central and peripheral venous and arterial lines; in fact, dorsalis pedis art lines are surprisingly easy to do. The big toe is also a reasonable alternate site for pulse ox monitoring for a patient with Raynaud's (if you have that type of pulse ox probe). And please look at Chap. 145 on the ankle block.—**Editors**

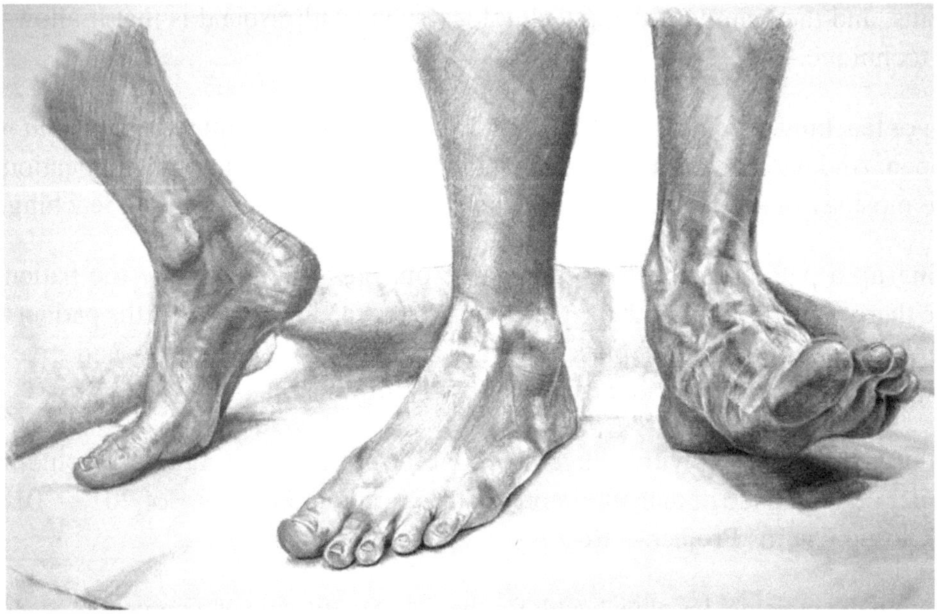

Fig. 160.1 The feet are the most architecturally interesting and sophisticated part of the human body, even more so than the hands because they are weight-bearing as shown in these beautiful anatomic drawings. Illustration: Luke Graber

- And whether or not you use the legs and feet for procedures or monitoring, don't forget to check them when you do your total body surveillance before, during, and after the surgery. Check for positioning, pressure points, padding, and making sure they won't fall off the OR table. Also check for forgotten tourniquets! We once saw a tourniquet left on the lower leg after an attempt at an IV placement, and it resulted in a ferocious case of chronic regional pain syndrome. Also, we believe that the risk to diabetic feet from needlesticks and so forth is real. We've seen it, and so we do avoid procedures and equipment in and on the feet for patients with diabetes, lower extremity edema, and peripheral vascular disease.—**Editors**

- Psychiatric patients should get the procedures they need! Do not *a priori* rule out entire classes of procedures for entire classes of patients. First, keep in mind that acute "medical" illness and hospitalization are often organized for patients with schizophrenia or thought disorders and these patients will often be calm and cooperative in the perioperative period. There is the slight possibility that procedures done on awake patients will be associated with the development of subsequent fixed delusions, but this is only one possible complication to be factored into the risk-benefit assessment and not an absolute contraindication. The psychiatric consultation and liaison service can help with assessment and consents.—**NBS**

- Be prepared with an answer when a patient asks you how many times you have done a procedure you are proposing to do. A good approach is to say, "I don't really know the exact number of times I've done this procedure, but I learned how to do it back in residency and have been doing it since then—about X number of years."—**Editors**

- Start learning about therapeutic apheresis and (especially) stem cell transplants. These procedures will become increasingly indicated for a large number of transplant and cancer patients. It won't be too long before stem cell transplants are surgical oncology are considered adjunctive therapies of each other. I just finished a two-year fellowship in stem cell medicine at the National Institutes of Health, so trust me on this one. There's a good primer on *Medscape.*—**CM**

- Invest in the highest quality of eyeglasses, including (perish the thought) reading glasses, graduated lenses, and bifocals! You may find it somewhat incredible to think about now, but there will come a time when you are doing an invasive procedure, and you will realize that you needed to have first put your glasses on or taken them off. But your hands are in your sterile gloves—so *now* what do you do? We know anesthesiologists who retired not because they felt that their knowledge, stamina, memory, or hands were declining but their eyesight wasn't quite what it was.—**Editors**

- Don't be surprised if you find you have unexpected difficulty doing procedures when pregnant, especially in the later months. You may not be able to get as close to the table and your hands might feel a bit stiff or swollen—remember that pregnant women sometimes can't even wear their wedding rings in the last weeks before delivery. But you don't want to do less than your usual excellent level of procedural performance, and you don't have to do the most complicated invasive procedures until the minute your own epidural goes in. It's better to do some weeks in the preop clinic in the weeks before you go out on maternity leave. And be patient with yourself, all those skills will still be there when you return from leave and your hands are back to their pre-pregnancy size.—**Editors**

Equipment

- First and foremost, develop and maintain a very expansive definition of "anesthesia equipment." Our equipment is really everything we use in the OR—everything in the anesthesia work room, all the scopes, everything in the OR, PACU, ICU, remote locations, and pain clinic. And it's not just what we can see and touch. It's also things like the software and the charting and patient records system.—**Editors**

- Not everyone will be supremely good at procedures, but anybody can be expert about the anesthesia equipment if they choose. It's a question of time, effort, and diligence devoted to the study of the machinery.—**Editors**

- No other specialty uses such a wide array of machines and equipment as prodigiously yet intimately as we do (Fig. 160.2). Think about it—the surgeons use equipment but mostly small hand-held instruments, except maybe the orthopedic surgeons (maybe). The cardiac surgeons are the beneficiaries of the cardiopulmonary bypass machine, but they are not themselves operating it or using it. The radiologists read films, but they don't actually use the radiographic equipment, their techs do it. We are actually hands-on with equipment from an IV set to a rapid transfuser, TEG or ROTEM equipment, ultrasound equipment, and the anesthesia machine. I think this is why there are so many engineers in our specialty. The ability to master not only the pharmacology and physiology, but also the equipment is what sets us apart from other perioperative physicians, maybe even more than airway management.—**CM and Editors**

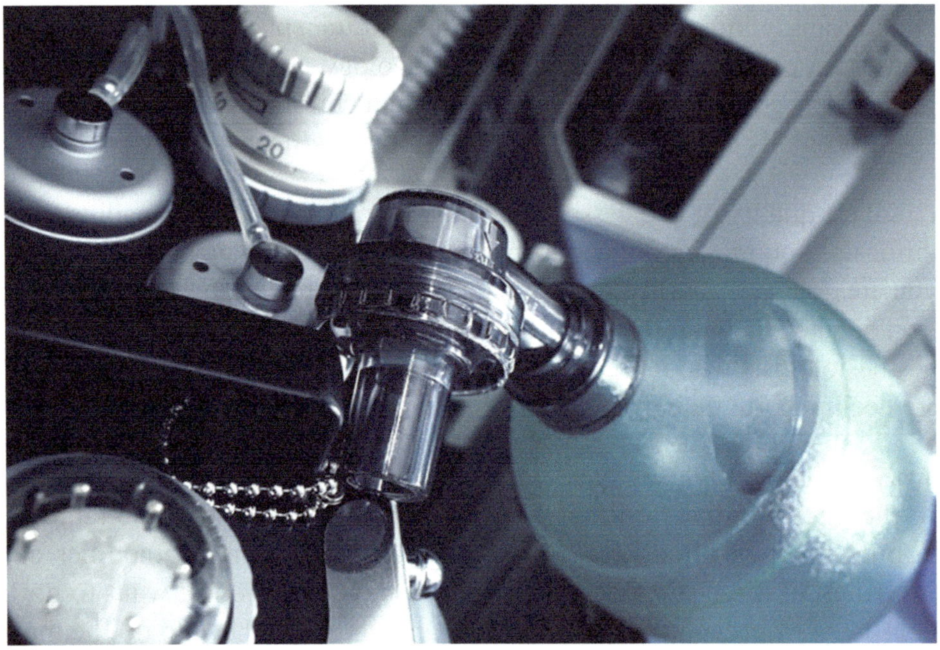

Fig. 160.2 How many of us have an AMBU at home? We bet Ron Bank does, and an array of other airway equipment as well. Photo: Image used under standard license from stock.adobe.com

- Just go ahead and invest the money in whatever you need to keep you up to date on your equipment knowledge and skills. It's just the price of making a living as an anesthesiologist. We think there is still reason to own a definitive equipment Bible. The *Anesthesia Bridges* authors and editors all trained with the classic *Understanding Anesthesia Equipment* by Jerry Dorsch and Susan Dorsch but there are others, such as *Anesthesia Equipment Principles and Applications* by Ehrenwerth, Eisenkraft, and Berry or *Anesthesia Equipment Simplified* by Rose and McLarney.—**Editors**

- Make up your mind that you will not miss any equipment questions on the board exams. According to the ABA website, you can expect 12–20 questions on equipment on the BASIC exam out of the 200 questions on the test. It would be such a shame to miss any of those questions when the information is so readily available and doesn't change very much over the years.—**Editors**

- When you are new in a hospital system or there is installation of a EPR software package, force yourself to learn every new nook and cranny of that software. We are aware of huge problems that ORs and ICUs have had with the installation of a certain common EPR as staff had difficulty scanning the patient's ID bracelet for the release of blood products in the blood bank. This resulted in the use of scarce emergency release red blood cell components when typed and crossmatched blood was sitting in the blood bank.—**Editors**

- The biggest and most expensive piece of anesthesia equipment is the entire simulator suite! Why would you not want to be truly accomplished in that space? Plus, it's a great area to develop a research career around. We have barely scratched the surface in understanding simulator applications to anesthesiology. Early on, the biggest simulator equipment error our community made was not truly accepting that simulator training was necessary, and that it could help make better and safer anesthesiologists. If you didn't jump on the simulator bandwagon early, promise yourself you will lead the pack with the next big thing in anesthesia equipment.—**Editors**

- Interface with your equipment not just as a user, but as an expert in the technology itself. What are the costs of using this equipment? Liabilities? Outcome studies? How is the technology issue managed in practice locations where this equipment remains unavailable?—**Editors**

- After the simulator suite, the second largest and most expensive piece of equipment is the anesthesia machine. After airway articles in the literature, this subject is what we would scan the literature and conference schedules for. There is still quite a bit of information coming out on problems and issues pertaining to anesthesia machines and the breathing circuit.—**Editors**

- Of course, when the *Anesthesia Bridges* editors and authors trained, we spoke of the "anesthesia machine." Now the concept is more of an "anesthesia workstation." But think about this—it's really one of the only industries that demand on-the-spot, critical thinking and action where a lot of the critical equipment (the vaporizers, the anesthesia cart, and drugs and so forth) are *behind* the operator. And if you at the head of the bed, working on the airway, there is no critical equipment in your line of sight. When the surgeons are operating, there is nothing in their line of sight except the surgical field, but they have somebody to hand them equipment. We often compare ourselves to pilots and the nuclear industry, but they are not turning around to work at their consoles or check their instruments and monitors. The industrial engineers and human factors experts tell us that there is a lot of research that can be done into optimizing the ergonomics of delivering anesthesia.—**CM, Editors, and CHS**

- Remember that anesthesia machine checkouts are based on FDA guidelines of *what* needs to be checked, not *how* to check it! There is no universal machine checkout protocol, it is manufacturer specific. If you need a refresher, there are a number of good and short review videos online. I watched them several times during my recent late-career second fellowship as I was not in the OR on a day-to-day basis.—**CM**

- We have found that one of the biggest overall issues in machine checkout is turning things on and *then not turning them off*. Also, if something gets missed or skipped, we have found that it tends to be the low-pressure leak test.—**Editors**

- Don't want to scare anybody, but once I was giving a deposition (was neither the plaintiff nor the defendant) and a hostile attorney first asked me whether I had passed both my written and oral boards on the first try and then asked me to tell him how to do an anesthesia machine checkout, which had nothing to do with the case at issue. I said only about a hundred words before the guy cut me off. A different attorney told me later that he was trying to see if I would get rattled.—**Editors**

- Anesthesia machine "failures" are as varied as the components of the machine. Pretty much everything has been reported in the literature. In general, though, they involve perturbations in pressure, including line failure, and not controlling the valves. Plus, empty vaporizers! **Editors**

- Just go over the vaporizer information forward and backward. Over and over again. Some form of vaporizer question is on every exam.—**Editor**

- We certainly all know about more about the anesthesia machine circuit after the recent pandemic than we did before. For example, Pham and Nguyen discussed anecdotal reports of inadvertent PEEP of up to 18 cm H_2O when waste-gas suction was not available or not properly connected. This is a great short paper; we recommend you read it [1].—**Editors**

- Also, when the anesthesia machine is used instead of an intensive care unit ventilator, it is important to keep the fresh gas flow at least equal to the minute ventilation to prevent excessive humidity in the circuit and to monitor condensation in the circuit and inspiratory carbon dioxide pressure.—**Editors**

- Watch the literature closely for outcome studies on equipment applications and optimization. Some will be immediately obvious—think of the pulse ox. Some, not so much. Do pulmonary artery catheters still deserve their place in our practice? Do patients benefit from early extubation and/or increased use of non-invasive ventilation strategies in the ICU? Can the use of cell salvage to decrease allogeneic transfusion be expanded to cancer surgeries? These studies will balance outcomes and application against cost and safety.—**Editors**

- You will get most of your journal learning about equipment failures or complications from case reports. You don't want to craft your entire practice of anesthesiology around anecdotal reports, but they have their place. For example, when video laryngoscopy first became available, there were reports of soft palate injuries during endotracheal tube insertion, which was a consequence of practitioners focusing on the video screen and not paying attention to how they were inserting the styletted tube through the oropharynx. These reports helped us improve our technique to reduce future complications.—**RGG and Editors**

- In gaming, there is always a basic question that is asked when someone is learning a new game—"How is it scored?" When learning new equipment, the question should always be, "What is the backup for each critical component?" For instance, what happens if the valve gets stuck or the power fails?—**Editors**

- Speaking of backup, consider the title of this case report, "Electrical failure during cardiopulmonary bypass: a critical moment." [2] This description of what happened when "the power went out" during a pump case is a great little review of what can happen and what to do and includes references to other articles. It makes the point that there are actually three ways for the power to fail—main line failure, generator failure, and uninterrupted power supply failure. The authors quote an expected power failure of 1/1000 in pump cases, which is rare, but not that rare. It discusses which lines need to be clamped, how to manage the reservoir, and notes, "If the aorta is clamped, *the only solution is hand-cranking*. Hand-cranking is effective in terms of restoring systemic perfusion, but the universally accepted time limit for a single person is 15 minutes, to prevent exhaustion. Even when hand-cranking was performed for only 1 minute, the flow rate achieved in the second half of that minute was not as high as desired." The case report also stresses that more proactive education on what to do in power failures is sometimes lacking but is the best way to get the patients through these events.—**Editors**

- We like the above-mentioned case report as it stimulates thinking. We don't all do pump cases, but we all do cases with critical equipment. When was the last time you attended a lecture on equipment failure or sat down and thought through what you would do?—**Editors**

- *Mastering your equipment means understanding the alarms. NEVER* reach up and hit the reset button or turn the alarm off without understanding why. *NEVER* use a piece of equipment if you have ascertained that the alarms "aren't working right." If the alarms are defective, then the equipment is defective and shouldn't be in use (Fig. 160.3).—**Editors**

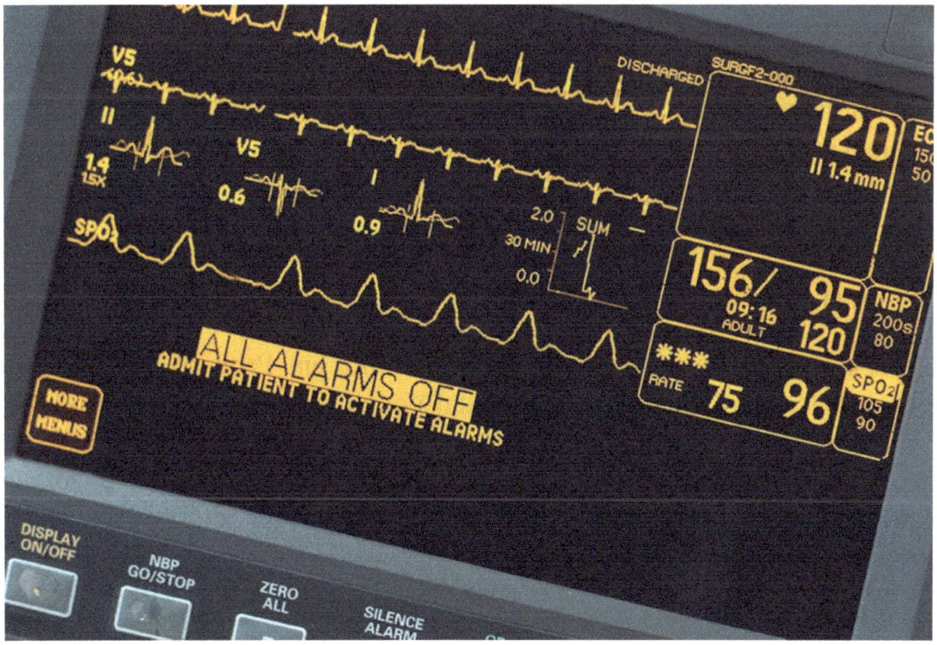

Fig. 160.3 What's wrong with this picture? The most important principle of medical alarms is that they have to be *ON*. Photo: Image purchased from shutterstock.com

- The science of alarm design is a fascinating one and relies a lot on human factors. Medical alarms are interesting because they are more auditory than alarms in other industries. They must alert the anesthesiologists but not disrupt the surgeons. Think of the flashing lights of a police or ambulance siren or even a forklift that is backing up—that type of visual alarm signal would not be acceptable in the OR. Anesthesiologists don't get a lot of direct training on alarm theory or science. If you are a young person, why not develop a lecture or teaching module on medical/anesthesiology alarms?—**Editors**

- Medical alarms are subject to strict regulations. An article published by Texas Instruments gives the some of the basics on medical alarms [3].—**Editors**

  - Medical alarms must be functional for all uses, as well as foreseeable misuses and identified single-fault conditions for the device.

  - Medical alarms are classified according to the low, medium, or high priority of an abnormality or failure event.

  - Standards are very specific for auditory alarms, defining the pulse frequency range, shape of the pulses, and pattern of the signal burst as well as a maximum amplitude difference between pulses. Alarms for equipment used in the ICU must also consider the difference between the first four harmonics, as measured in an anechoic chamber with a reflective floor, so that there are no spots in the ICU where the direct and reflected harmonics of the auditory alarm cancel each other.

  - Alarm sound levels differ in decibels as they relate to priority.

  - Physiological alarms (relating to patient conditions) are distinct from technical alarms related to equipment status.

  - Alarms may be "melody" based for various applications, including cardiac, ventilation, oxygenation, fluid/drug delivery, and equipment or supply failure.

- This does not take into account the human factors engineering to prevent alarm fatigue, which is a particular problem in the ICU. One study estimated that the average ICU patient generated 150–400 alerts per shift, of which 85–99% were false or "clinically insignificant." [4]—**Editors**

- Did you know that the ASA has a Statement on Principles on Alarm Management for Anesthesia Professionals? [5] Have you ever read it?—**Editors**

- The Statement specifies a certain Alarm Management Policy and Principles that is applicable to anesthesiology equipment, apart from general hospital equipment. Chief among the principles is that alarm system settings should be customizable, but clinicians should not indefinitely silence or disable alarms. Also, individual anesthesia professionals should not be able to change default settings.—**Editors**

- Don't use the laryngoscope like a crowbar!—**BMW**

- Machines may be less fallible than humans, but they are not infallible. They can fail. That being said, when an incompetent person uses a technology don't be surprised if you get poor outcomes (think Swan-Ganz catheter use).—**BDW**

- Pulse oximetry is an inherently racist technology. It is the only thing we have to easily non-invasively measure oxygenation, but it doesn't measure everyone equally.—**BDW**

- The pulse oximeters are sensitive to the electrical interference of the Medtronic stealth machine used for neurosurgery. We keep Purrelle hand sanitizing wipes in the OR—they have a thin bit of foil in the wrapper, and I usually open one end, take the wipe out, and insert the patients pulse ox/finger in the wrapper to shield the pulse ox from the interference. Works like a charm.—**ABB**

- The best monitor for severe hemodynamic instability is the TEE. If your institution has TEE, get a basic certification in it.—**RSB**

- There are several pieces of anesthesia equipment that often appear on board exams and in lectures. We believe that anesthesiologists—at all career stages—learn the fundamentals of the equipment (when they need to) but then tend to lose track of the basics. This equipment includes *the vaporizers, the CO_2 scrubbing cannister, and the line isolation monitor*. Make a study sheet or bookmark a video on your laptop and review them in rotation—just 10 minutes before you leave work for the weekend will keep knowledge of this basic anesthesia equipment at the top of your mind.—**Editors**

- For example, the line isolation monitor is not there to frustrate you. It's there to protect you! And your patient, of course.—**Editors**

- You would be surprised at the number of anesthesiologists who can repeat the mantra of, "Start unplugging equipment…" without being able to tell you at the detailed level why the line isolation monitor exists in the first place. This is because they are a bit shaky on the isolated circuit design of an operating room.—**Editors**

- Study of the line isolation monitor demonstrates that the first question, when mastering a piece of equipment is not what does this equipment do, it's why is this equipment needed?—**Editors**

- The overall goal is to keep the patient from becoming grounded in a potentially "wet" electrical environment. There is a special "safety" circuit design that isolates OR current (and the patient) from the main power circuit that is intended to accomplish this. And any time you have a safety design, you need a monitor to tell you if your safety device is not working—hence, the line isolation monitor (Fig. 160.4).—**Editors**

- If a faulty piece of equipment is connected to the isolated power system, it will convert the power system to a grounded system. Keep in mind that the faulty equipment will not necessarily shock the patient.—**Editors**

- The best way to master a circuit is to draw it (Fig. 160.4)! There are also multiple short tutorials on isolated power systems on the internet.—**Editors**

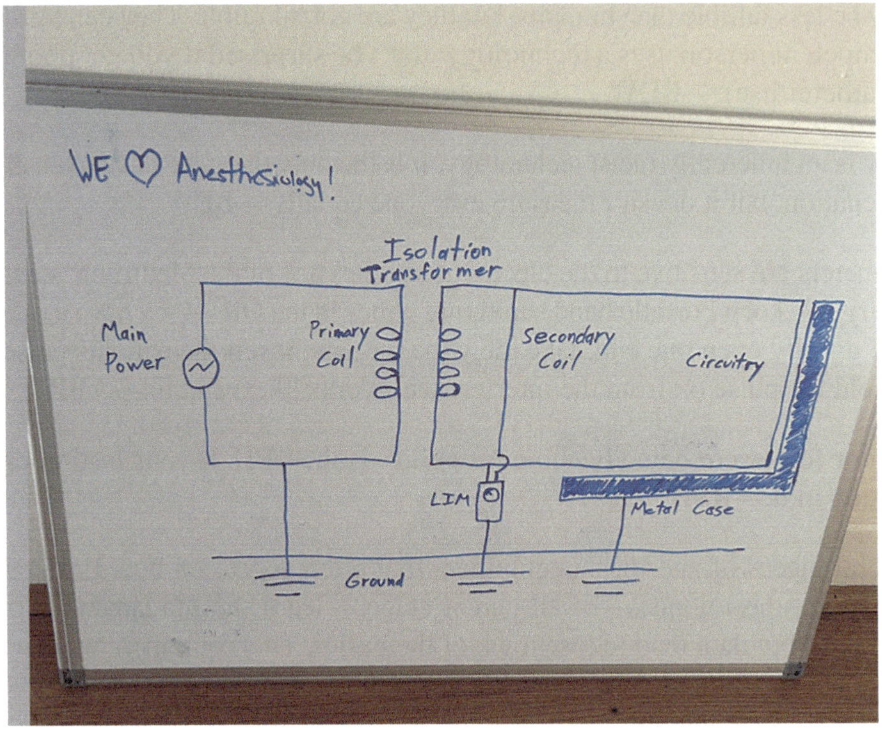

Fig. 160.4 We dare you to draw this cartoon diagram of the line isolation design of an operating room every night for two weeks and NOT understand it. Photo: Cathy Marcucci

- Remember that any source of electricity in an OR can be a source of heat. Any source of heat can be a source of burns or fire.—**Editors**

- As you are getting a patient ready to turn over to the surgeons and the surgeons are draping, you must think, "Are we in the process of building a fire?"—**Editors**

- You *will* see a fire in the OR at some point in your career. Or a patient who sustains an iatrogenic burn. I have seen fires/burns three times, including once when a surgeon set his own surgical gown on fire.—**CM**

- We have been told by the legal staff that an inadvertent iatrogenic burn is an automatic win on any type of claim by a patient, except possibly if sustained during an attempt to restart the electrical rhythm of the heart, as Jim Gilman notes elsewhere. Nobody expects to come to the hospital and be burned, and there is no way or place to assign culpability. The dermatologists and plastic surgeons tell us that even small burns on the face, hands, genitals, and feet cause patients a lot of pain and distress. Patients really do not take too kindly to this type of perioperative complication.—**Editors and JLW**

- A corollary to preventing burns and fires is to back up a step on your surveillance and always do a quick survey of all the *heat sources* in an OR. Are the surgeons using the correct electrocautery device for the case? Are you in firm control of your warming devices, and are they all devices being used as per the manufacturer's specifications? Remember—never improvise a warming device. There is no place for bags of hot IV fluids to warm a patient. Are there any errant OR lights? We have seen patients burned by OR lights that had had parts removed between cases. Not just read about it in case reports, we have actually seen it with our own eyes.—**Editors**

- A hospital risk management attorney once shared with us in confidence that they dread equipment-related litigation. Unlike litigation that involves questions of errors in judgment or recognized complications of a disease state or treatment plan, tort actions pertaining to equipment mishaps that could have been prevented are much easier for the plaintiff to pursue. It is a simple matter to get the manuals, and it is all there in black and white. The anesthesiologist is expected to know how it works and how to use it correctly and safely every time. There is little defense of "I didn't know or understand that" about iatrogenic equipment injuries.—**Editors**

- *Please use the prescribed personal safety equipment every time*! A lead thyroid shield and eye protection for *every* radiation case in the OR. And turn your radiation badges in or do the equivalent! To his eternal credit, Jeff Kirsch used to run around the Hopkins ORs making sure people had lead—I distinctly remember him bringing me thyroid shields. And if you missed handing your badge in, he or Lynda Miller would be on the phone to you the next month, reminding you. He was the PD of a huge residency program; I blush to think of the extra time and aggravation this caused him.—**CM**

- *Control your equipment at home*! Anesthesiologists are often active, gadget-owning people in their personal lives. On the rehab services, my colleagues and I have seen many more anesthesiologists who have been seriously injured than become seriously ill. Keep your planes, boats, cars, motorcycles, bicycles, camping equipment, skis, SCUBA, hunting, fishing, and other sports equipment in tiptop shape. If your patients deserve the utmost in equipment safety, so do you. Please think very carefully before using a lot of power tools, as well.—**CFB**

- There is a really interesting list of equipment events below. But I don't know that what has really made the biggest impression on me are the big screw ups. Mostly, I think it's the variety of common screwups that trainees (or people that think they are trained) make that cause risk and harm to the patients. It can be even trivial equipment issues that get you into trouble—you need a pair of scissors or a light source and don't have one. Or you forget to check the suction before starting on the airway. Or you start to put monitors on the patient and realize they have blood on them (always check the blood pressure cuff, EKG wires, and pulse ox after the cleaning staff has been through).—**BMW and Editors**

- Speaking of the suction cannisters—once we saw somebody kick a suction cannister in anger and get suspended without pay for a short interval. The hospital, location, and decade will remain unnamed, but we are not joking.—**Editors**

- Don't be a Luddite! The quickest way to outdate yourself in your career is to outdate yourself on the equipment.—**Editors**

- If you want to be a true expert on perioperative equipment, spend some time learning about the equipment used by the other perioperative services, especially critical equipment. Let's say you are getting ready to start a big case and wondering when the cooler of blood is coming up to the OR. You get a call that the machine that does the automated crossmatch is down. What does that mean? Have you ever even *seen* that machine? What do you tell the surgeons? Is there still a backup manual method for this critical step in a big OR case?—**Editors**

Answer:

** Yes, every blood bank that does machine crossmatch of blood product will be able to do an "old-fashioned" manual crossmatch, but it will take much longer to get the blood products ready. An uncomplicated machine crossmatch will take about 20 minutes (approximately). If you need multiple units of manually crossmatched blood, you are talking on the order of hours. If you've never seen either done, run down to the blood bank and ask to watch, just so you know what the terms mean and what the equipment looks like.

** And for another thing, we are often the last people to see the patient before the procedure starts and we have fielded lots of questions about the other equipment the patient will face. For example, do you know how much current is used in ECT treatments? Do you know the voltage? Do you know whether the blood in the blood bank is irradiated and if so, how? Do you know *why* blood is irradiated? Do you know how many air exchanges there are in an OR or how bright the OR lights are and what the basic parameters are for lighting in the operating room? Do you know the differences and reported complications of a Wilson frame vs. Jackson table? Do you know the incidence of trocar vs. Veress needle complications in laparoscopic surgery? You don't have to be an expert, but it is nice not to have to essentially say to the patient, "I have no idea." And it's a sign of professional excellence to be interested and a bit knowledgeable about other equipment that is used in the perioperative period.

Answers:

** Modern-day ECT typically uses just under 1 A of current, applied across 200–400 volts for about 6–8 s. The current traverses the brain either bilateral (temple to temple) or unilateral (from the front to the back of the head on one side of the brain.

** Only cellular products (red blood cells, platelets, and granulocytes) are irradiated and typically are exposed to about 25 Gy of irradiation. There are several types of irradiators used in blood banks—many radioactive isotope (cesium) irradiators are being switched to X-ray irradiation. Many people, even in the medical field, assume that irradiation of blood products is for pathogen reduction—nope. It's to decrease the incidence of graft vs. host disease. Not all cellular blood products are irradiated in the US but in countries, such as Japan where there are highly linked population genetics, all blood is irradiated.

** Airflow is the operating room is highly designed as it is potentially a significant source of surgical site infections. It's pretty complicated but generally an operating should have 20 air exchanges per hour with 4 exchanges of outside air and the laminar air flow patterns matter quite a bit. There's quite a bit in the surgical literature about air purification and additional laminar filters stationed next to the operating field on outcomes—is there anything we can borrow for the ICU and our procedure suites? [6] This would be a great area for teaching and research. And finally, remember, there are HVAC mechanical engineers who design only for hospitals and so there is a lot of information in the engineering literature and specifications.

** Operating room lighting design must consider multiple parameters—illumination, light patch diameter, volume of light, shadow management, color temperature, heat management, and safety. Generally speaking, OR lights are designed to approximate ambient light on a sunny day. The brightness of a surgical light is measured in Lux and typically is between 40,000 and 160,000 Lux. A surgical light head weighs about 45 kg.

** The Wilson frame is based on the simple geometry of the arch—this has been understood since the beginning of mathematics (Fig. 160.5). The frame is used when patients are positioned for lumbar surgeries. It can be used with any surgical table, but the patient is always prone The pads can be moved apart depending on the width of the chest and abdomen. They support and position the lumbar spine but not much else. They cost around $6000.

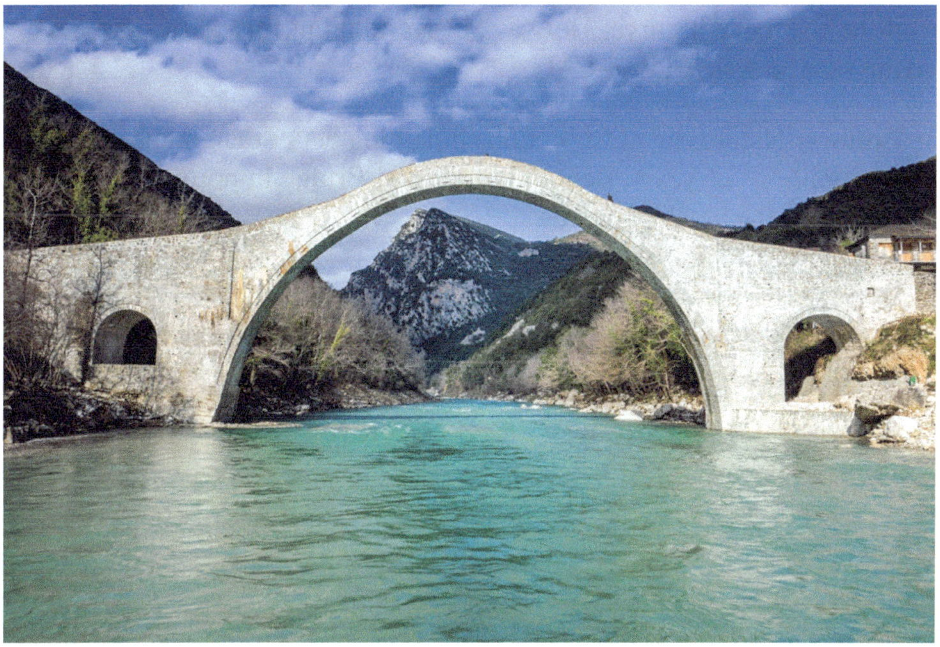

Fig. 160.5 Even the ancients understood how an arch distributes weight. Photo: Image used under standard license from stock.adobe.com

** The Jackson table is a rotatable table that is used for spinal fusion and instrumentation. It can be used for spine surgeries in the supine, prone, and lateral positions. The stated advantages include ease of position, particularly for obese patients and the ability to turn the patient prone and supine. However, there is no central table support, and it is difficult to easily identify when it is locked, and patients have been reported to have fallen off of it [7]. There are many versions available. A typical basic Jackson table is in the range of $60,000. They sometimes pop up on eBay for around $35,000.

** Trocar and needle insertion are still considered the most dangerous events in laparoscopic surgery and there are still severe injuries and deaths occurring every year. The anatomy is very relevant. The umbilicus is used as because the skin is attached to the fascia and anterior peritoneum with minimum intervening muscle or fat and the midline insertion point is avascular. Once the instrument is placed off the midline, there is the risk of hitting superior and inferior mesenteric arteries. Also, the distal aorta and right common iliac artery are particularly vulnerable to injury since the junction of these two vessels is directly below the umbilicus.

** There are still no conclusive data as to which approach to the abdomen is safest. Overall, Injury to the vasculature probably occurs in about 0.50% of cases and to the bowel in about 0.05–0.10%. The most important statistic is that *30–50% of the bowel injuries and 15–50% of the vascular injuries are not diagnosed at the time of injury*. This delay has contributed to mortality rates of 3–30% for bowel and vascular injuries.

- Elsewhere in this book, we give a shout-out to the late, great **Tommy Tung**—one of the best anesthesiologists our community ever had. Once I walked into the anesthesia control center and Tommy was in there with a stack of journal articles and an old-fashioned yellow highlighter. I asked him what he was reading, and he looked up with that smile of his and said, "Latest in transesophageal echo, don't want to get left behind." The thing was? He wasn't a cardiac anesthesiologist—he was a neuroanesthesiologist—and this was years before TEE was used widely outside the cardiac ORs. But he could foresee the wide applicability of TEE and also felt that pulmonary artery catheters were somewhat higher on the risk/benefit curve. He was always looking forward to the next best equipment thing and making sure he was ready.—**CM**

***Note from the Editors:** Nature can always build something better than humans can and that will last, not for years, but for millions of years. Behold the Natural Bridge in northwest Alabama (Fig. 160.6). We think it looks a bit like the brachial plexus.

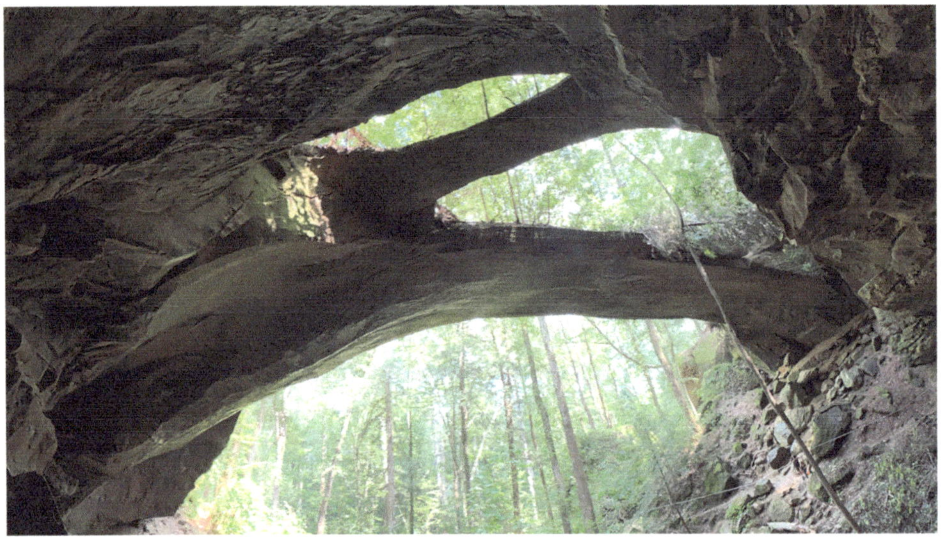

Fig. 160.6 The Natural Bridge dates back about two hundred million years. It is about 60 feet high, 148 feet long, and is composed of sandstone and iron ore. It is the longest natural arch bridge east of the Rockies. This stunning shot was taken from the nearby cave. The area was later inhabited by the Creek Indians, who almost certainly sheltered under and near the formation. Photo: Chloe L. Wagener

25 Equipment Events

We thought it would be illustrative to collect some personal stories and anecdotes on equipment failures and the lessons learned therein. The authors and editors listed below went out to their colleagues with the simple question, "What are the memorable equipment issues you were faced with?" What was interesting was how quickly people emailed us back and the level of detail they sent. Because our colleagues were frank and generous in sharing the problems they had seen and encountered, we decided not to name names or institutions.—**AJR, CM, RLH, MJB, BMT, ND, ABB, BMW, CS, SLO, DAZ, LM, AG, MB**

1. The biggest for me was an anesthesia-induced oxygen failure. We were providing anesthesia in the basement neuroradiology suite. As usual, the machine was set up for that case that day and was plugged into the wall oxygen supply with an extension. During the case, we suffered a loss of oxygen pressure.

   As with most events like this, several factors led to the event. First, there was a failure in the coupling between the anesthesia machine and the extension used to access the wall oxygen supply. One could plug the machine into the extension, but it did not always engage and open the supply to the wall oxygen source. Thus, there was the illusion of being coupled to the wall oxygen supply.

   Next, the person performing the machine checkout, as part of their "usual" checkout procedure, opened the spare oxygen tank to check the pressure, but left it open. The explanation, later on, was that this was so that they would not have to open the tank should the wall pressure fail. However, there never was any pressure in the oxygen line from the wall, and anesthesia proceeded uneventfully until there was no more oxygen left in the tank.

   Fortunately, an AMBU bag, a quick recognition that there was no pressure in the spare tank when the attending anesthesiologist sought to open it, and replacement of the tank resulted in no patient harm or interruption of the procedure. Shortly thereafter, the problem with the coupling was identified, and it was replaced. Even knowing after the fact that there was a problem with the coupling, it was still easy to convincingly engage the machine to the extension without oxygen flow. After a little more experimentation, it became clear how to engage it successfully, but nonetheless, the extension was replaced permanently after many years of use by us in that basement suite.

   Lesson: Always keep top of mind what you will do if you lose your oxygen supply and make sure you never lose the ability to quickly change a tank. And stay out of basements!

2. I'm sure this has haunted a few anesthesiologists. It relates to auscultation for tube placement. A few years ago, in the dead of the night, with a septic, multi-trauma patient for bring-back ex lap, we had ongoing difficulty with oxygenation at the end of the case. Not profound hypoxia, just annoyingly low, in high 80s, and somewhat lower than when she came down, on the same FiO_2.

   Peak airway pressures had been mildly elevated in ICU and hadn't really changed. It had been an uncomplicated washout/check for bleeding, so there was no real reason for this. The breath sounds were equal (we perceived) and so we spent half an hour or so ruling out tube obstruction, treating potential bronchospasm, suctioning, recruiting, checking for leaks, increasing the PEEP. Didn't seem to have much effect. We decided that this was simply her pulmonary dysfunction from trauma, circulating mediators, open abdomen with packing, etc. and transported back to ICU. Whereupon a CXR revealed the mainstem intubation. Reviewing the prior CXR, it was relatively close to the mainstem before transport to OR, and our moving her on and off the OR table likely allowed it to move another cm and therefore into the bronchus.

   Lesson: Don't just trust your ears because we have other equipment available! And the airway is something that is easily evaluated by sight as well as sound. So, put down a bronchoscope, get a CXR, or check the ultrasound for bilateral lung sliding early in the workup/management of an airway or ventilation issue. Don't let any available equipment go unused if there are airway or ventilation difficulties.

3. O2 central line failure. No oxygen! Scramble, scramble. As soon as the medical student stood up from his stool, O_2 returned like magic. One of the stool legs was on the O_2 line and occluded flow.

   Lesson: With the malfunction of any type of "line", start at the source and work towards the patient.

4. Induced anesthesia with a resident, went to squeeze the bag to ventilate. *NO BAG*! How in the world could have possibly happened?

   Lesson: Visually confirm the integrity of the circuit *on every case*.

5. Stuck exhalation valve. I unscrewed the valve apparatus, and was going to clean the valve (humidity, likely). The disk valve popped out of my hand like a tiddly wink, flew in the air, landed, and rolled somewhere under the operating room table in the middle of a craniotomy, somewhere around midnight. No help. No circuit. Yipes!!! I scrambled like mad on all fours searching, searching, hoping, and hoping… and I found it! Replaced it and thanked my lucky stars that it was a near miss and not a full crash.

   Lesson: Any piece of equipment that can be taken apart can be dropped. This is why auto mechanics use pans as they are disassembling something on a car. And anything that can be dropped can roll someplace inconvenient, dirty, or bloody.

6. I was a CA3 on call. We used to carry around those equipment bags—nylon fishing tackle bags with all our stuff in them. One night I got a call at 2 AM to go to the NICU, everyone else was in the ORs but me. I ran to the NICU; a small baby was in respiratory distress and the NICU people could not get him intubated. He was maybe 6–8 months old but a former preemie. They couldn't mask him, and he was in laryngospasm from multiple attempts. So, I get to the head of the table, assess, draw up whatever muscle relaxant I had—I think it was probably atropine and succinylcholine. The baby did have an IV, so I pushed the relaxant, the baby calmed down. I went to intubate and OOPS! I never pulled out my laryngoscope, it was in the bag on the floor. I rushed to it, grabbed whatever I could in small size, sweating and praying the light would go on. And it did. I intubated successfully and the saturation readings returned to normal. I thought I was going to die.

   Lesson: A version of this has happened to many, many experienced anesthesiologists. In this case, after we heard what had happened to our resident colleague, we all started putting our tackle bags right on a Mayo stand at the head of the bed when we arrived at an intubation. Also, a quick visualization exercise might help—take a second to imagine that you are getting ready to intubate in the OR.

7. I was the sole anesthesiologist (no residents, etc.) at a fairly newly opened free-standing ambulatory surgery center. Planned GETA that I couldn't intubate, this was well before video laryngoscopy. I attempted two sizes of LMA but could not get an adequate seal. Fortunately, I was able to effectively mask ventilate. I asked for the fiberoptic scope. They brought a shiny new fiberoptic scope, still in its lovely case. *No light source available*. I waved the white flag at that point and simply woke the patient up.

   Lesson: When opening a new site, confirm that you not only have the equipment you need but that it actually is immediately available to use.

8. Having a video laryngoscope or ultrasound machine turn off in the middle of a procedure because it was neither charged appropriately nor plugged in.

   Lesson: Can you still intubate the old-fashioned way—without a VL? You better make sure you can. Can you do a block or line without ultrasound? Do you want to? What is the current institutional and legal climate for continuing without the availability of ultrasound?

9. Always assume that the tip of anything you put in, rather than on, a patient can break off and be lost. This did not happen to me personally but once at my institution we had the tip of an LTA kit break off below the vocal cords. The ENT service had to come and fish it out for us. I rarely us the LTA kit anymore.

   Lesson: The end of anything can break off!

10. Once someone in my department used a nasal airway as an oral airway. Naturally, the patient swallowed it, because of course, and the surgeons had to scope it out of the stomach.

    Lesson: Only use things for their designed purpose. Anything that goes in the mouth can block the airway or be swallowed.

11. The foam within the humidity filter on the vent circuit was inhaled by a patient and lodged in their ETT when they took a very big breath.

    Lesson: As we were saying above about things ending up in the airway.

12. We were transporting a patient on VA ECMO in an elevator and when navigating the circuit over the ridges of the elevator entrance, the oxygenator got stuck and cracked in half as someone used force to try and push the bed forward. The patient lost half their blood volume… in the elevator. I still have nightmares about this.

    Lesson: Never apply force to any piece of equipment! And transport is one of the most dangerous times of the perioperative period. Can you *imagine* the hubbub this anesthesia care team found themselves in?! Gah. No wonder nightmares are still an issue.

13. This was many, many years ago but made an impression to last. Somehow when the cardiac patient was leaving the OR to make the trip to the CSICU, the neck cordis side port became disconnected, and the patient was bleeding from that open line into the bed. The patient had been covered up to the chin with a clean blanket for transport, so it wasn't noticed. But way back in that day, the transport involved going by the family waiting lounge, and it was common to stop for a few seconds so the families could catch a glimpse of their loved one, safely through surgery. In this case, an elderly spouse asked if she could give her husband the briefest air kiss on the cheek. She was in her 80 s and put her hand near his shoulder to steady herself as she bent down to blow him a kiss, of course putting her hand right on the puddle of blood, which squished up through the blanket. She said, "What's this red fl--" before slumping onto the stretcher and the patient in a cold faint. In the middle of the busy hallway to the ICU, in front of the main entrance to the family waiting room.

    Lesson: Any time you use or put a piece of equipment on a patient, even if it's only a blanket, you must think, "What other problems could I be causing or covering up with this?"

***Note from the Editors:** What you can see is always what it is easiest to be vigilant about and every engineer knows this (Fig. 160.7). So, start thinking about what you can't see and what the patient will never see. For example, the patient will never the machine checkout in the morning and how the fiber-optic scopes are cleaned but it is incredibly importantly that these equipment tasks be done correctly. Accept that part of "vigilance always" is the paradigm of, "What is going on that is not right in front of my eyes?"

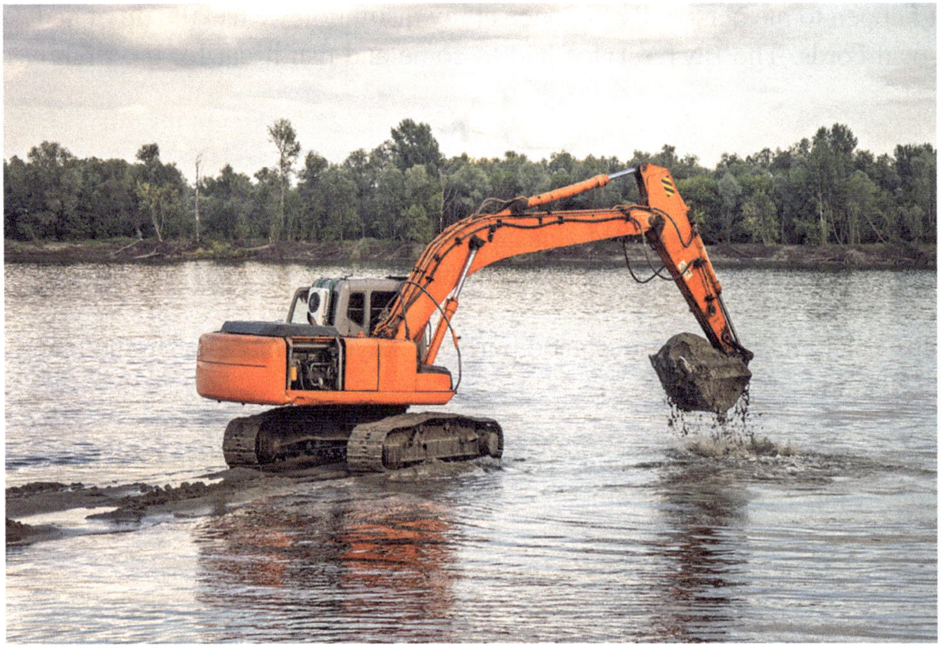

Fig. 160.7 The part of the bridge that is under the water is way more important that what's above in terms of engineering a margin of safety. Borrow from this principle liberally. Photo: Image used under standard license from stock.adobe.com

14. Here is a good one for any OB or regional anesthesiologist. One time we placed a combined spinal epidural for labor. Sometimes we defer the epidural test dose when these are placed. The block went perfectly and was completed quickly. We secured the epidural catheter to the patient's back. After taking down the drapes and positioning the patient supine we attempted to administer the epidural test dose. No matter how hard we pushed, the syringe plunger would not budge. We assessed the catheter connection and replaced the epidural cap. The plunger still would not move. We had the patient move into different positions thinking the catheter may be compressed between laminae. This also made no difference. Finally, we had to pull the epidural and replace it. When we looked at our single orifice catheter, we realized that the catheter had a defect, there was no opening.

    Lesson: Always look at the tip of an epidural catheter before and after placement. We also used to do a tiny test injection when we were setting up the tray to make sure the lumen is patent.

15. When transporting a cardiac patient from the OR on multiple pressors I had a full bank of IV pumps glitch and reset when we hit a bump. This also happened to me again going into the elevator.

Lesson: The dang infusion pumps! Who among us has not had a "pump event"—so frustrating! We were taught to "lift" the pump pole over bumps and the elevator door gap to prevent this. Also take a syringe of whatever is in your two most critical drips with you during transport and if you get into a really bad situation, titrate tiny doses by hand.

16. I have seen an epidural catheter connected to an alaris pump and *nitroglycerin infused into the epidural space*. The patient had a nitro infusion running and everything was unhooked to move from transport to ICU bed. All the luer lock sites are interchangeable so this was an unfortunate mishap.

    Lesson: Anything that *can* be mis-connected, will be. Anything in the room that could go into the epidural space will find its way there.

17. We once had an arterial line and CVC transducer flip flop in a crashing patient. Actually, not flip flopped initially, just art line cable attached to CVC transducer, so we had concern about the extremely low blood pressure readings and 'odd waveform'. And we also had A labor and delivery patient in the ICU crashed to OR for emergent section and the PAC transducer was connected to BP cable/outlet in OR.

    Lesson: Anything that can be connected to the wrong port or outlet will be at point in time. Learn to trace your lines from the monitor to the patient—don't just grab whatever cable is there on top of the blankets and plug it in without confirming what it is for. It might take a second or so to do that but it's quicker than trying to figure out how the wires (literally) got crossed.

18. Most recently we had a IABP that would just shut off because of some glitch in its electronics. The model is actually now under a recall status.

    Lesson: Always make a careful documentation of any equipment failure like this, including pictures if possible. Every one of these "shut off" events need to be reported immediately to the equipment and QA groups.

19. TIVA case. The propofol pump is not alarming, and unfortunately no propofol is being administered. Patient recall.

    Lesson: When you are delivering an anesthetic "by machine" always think and check—am I delivering the anesthesia that I think I am delivering? For example, review every possible mix up with the vaporizers.

20. One mistake is having the patient/table at the wrong height/angle for the proceduralist to do their job without making it harder or killing their back.

    Lesson: the equipment has been engineered and is there to make our job easier. Adjustable equipment is made to be adjusted.

21. However, once when I was a medical student, I saw a very tall anesthesiologist come into a room and insist that the OR table be raised while he put the arterial and several other lines in. I don't remember what the case was, but the patient was already asleep. I clearly remember him arrogantly repeating, "Raise the table as high as it goes! I need to be comfortable to put these lines in!" What he didn't

realize, and nobody else seemed to realize, was that somehow this trapped and pinched the patient's *other* arm under a Mayo stand to the point that the patient's skin was broken. I still remember, almost 35 years later, how mad the nurses were and that they got into a huddle and planned to file a patient safety incident report on the anesthesiologist.

Lesson: Do a quick visual scan of the whole patient any time you move them in any dimension to optimize placement of lines or a procedure. And don't be arrogant.

22. *And also…* the biggest equipment event that I've seen was when the OR table was being raised and caught the corner of the anesthesia machine. Eventually the anesthesia machine flipped over, ruining all the vaporizers! Can you imagine the cost of that easily avoidable equipment error?

    Lesson: Some of the biggest equipment mishaps involve the OR tables! If you think about it, it makes sense. On the flip of "adjustable" is that any large, heavy piece of equipment that is partially motorized and designed to be moved in more than one plane sets up the possibility of errors and events.

23. Another big, big fail was using an angio table with the patient not belted in. Only 5°–7° of lateral tilt was enough to help the patient slide off the table and on to the floor! Right after receiving 5000 units of heparin, no less!

    Lesson: Patients can and do end up on the floor. Don't think it can't happen to you. *It happens*. Hospital attorneys dread these events because they are indefensible.

24. One of the biggest events that I have seen happened when there was both a procedure and equipment "failure" and happened when a new fellow was training a new resident. They were placing a pig-tailed catheter for pneumothorax, and the wire got left in the patient's chest. Fortunately, it was also still in the catheter. I noticed something funny on the CXR and was able to get wire out. Radiology said the read was normal. Lots to say here!

    Lesson: If it's your resident and your fellow, it's your procedure, and you are ultimately responsible. Lost wires are actually not uncommon. When you are teaching, it is always okay to remind your trainee not to let go of the wire. Also, the best "radiology reads" are to confirm or provide details for what you already know, not to tell you the answer for something you don't know. The radiologists get things wrong from time to time, just as we do.

25. Once we discovered undiagnosed acromegaly in a patient because we could not get the pulse ox on his finger. He was just under 6 feet tall, about 200 pounds, and when we tried to figure out why, we noticed that his hands were about twice the size of a nurse who was about the same height and weight.

    Lesson: Equipment events aren't all bad! Play close attention to something that "isn't working."

***Note from the Editors:** This picture also comes from Natural Bridge Park in Alabama. While seeing their sister take a photograph of the natural bridge and feeling a bit envious, the Wagener brothers also wanted in on the action. They scouted around the park and took photographs of a man-made bridge that goes over a small stream formed by the tapping of a nearby artesian well (Fig.160.8). While not as impressive as the natural bridge, it serves a purpose, nonetheless.

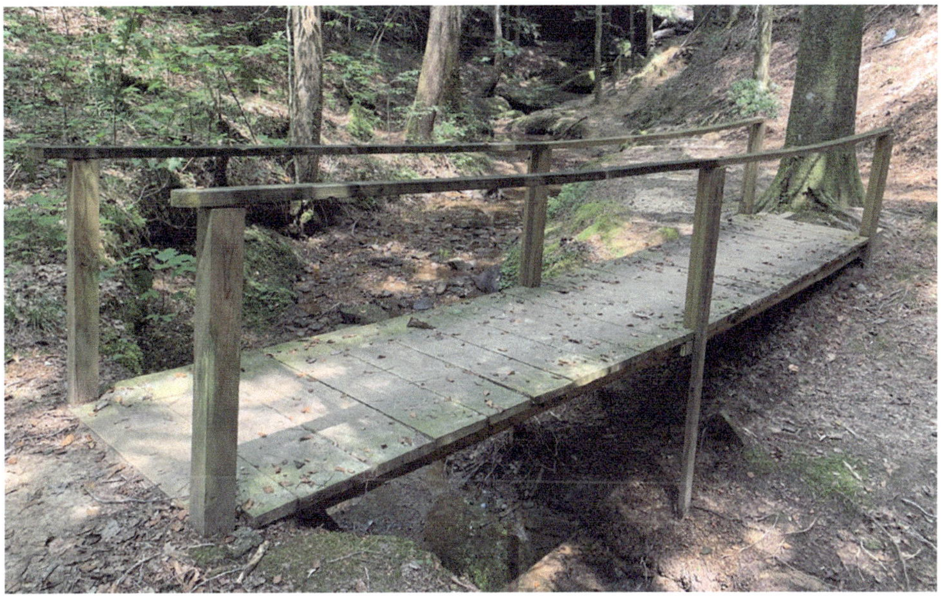

Fig. 160.8 A charming footbridge in Alabama's Natural Bridge Park. Photo: James Wyatt Wagener and Nathaniel Ryan Wagener

Bonus Content

While we were thinking about the Dao of anesthesia equipment, I just happened to have a conversation with Robert and Brian Adolph, uber-experienced auto mechanics and shop owners. A few of their thoughts apply to us, as well.

- The biggest mistake people make with equipment is not to think about it very much when it is working fine. The next mistake they make is to waste time in anger and frustration when something goes wrong and they have to fix it. A lesser but still important mistake is not to keep equipment cleaned.

- You should always remember that your equipment will only be as good to you as you are to it.

- Certain industries have engineered their equipment so users don't know very much about how the equipment actually operates? Have you ever seen the autoclave for the OR in use or seen an ICU ventilator cleaned before being stored?

- The most important thing for any successful equipment person to do is have a thorough knowledge of the owner's manual. That's how the best mechanics do their repairs - they work off detailed checklists. When is the last time you looked at the owner's manual for the infusion or the bypass circuit?

- The best auto mechanics do and think about nothing when they are at work but fixing cars. If it is not busy, they are on their computers but not watching news or sports or worse. They often don't think that much about fixing cars when they're not working because they don't have to. They've used their time wisely while on the job. They also seek every equipment certification that they are qualified for or is offered to them. How many of us start with qualifications in ECG and never stop?

- Finally, almost all equipment breaks a little before it breaks completely. Don't ignore whatever warning signs you see with your equipment - instead, consider it a gift from the equipment fairies.

More Wisdom on Anesthesia Equipment from *Avoiding Common Anesthesia Errors, 2nd Edition*

There is a wealth of additional tips, teaching tidbits, and overall wisdom on anesthesia equipment in our previous book, which is nicknamed "Green2." *Please* check out this information and remember that every single penny of royalties goes to FAER in perpetuity!

Green2 Chapters with More Wisdom on Anesthesia Equipment

- Pulse Oximetry: Perhaps You Need a Refresher?
- The End-tidal CO_2 Monitor Is More Than Just a Device to Tell You That the "Tube Is In the Airway".
- Noninvasive Blood Pressure Management—It's Not Just a Piece of Nylon Around the Arm.
- Avoid Errors in Invasive Blood Pressure Management.
- How, Why, and When to Use Brain Function Monitors.
- Do Not Improvise Techniques to Warm Patients—Use Warming Devices Only As Per Manufacturers' Recommendations.
- Transesophageal echocardiography: Contraindications, Complications, and Misinterpretations.
- Scavenging Waste Gases Is Perhaps the Only Action We Take That Benefits Us But Not the Patient.
- Carbon Dioxide Absorbers Save Gas and Moisture but Create the Potential for Mechanical Hazards.
- Infusion Pumps: Get Them Going and Keep Them Going.
- Don't Bring the Fiberoptic Scope into the MRI Scanner.
- Understanding the Operating Room Circuit and the Line Isolation Monitor—It's Really Pretty Simple.
- Cell phones in the Operating Room—Here Are the Issues.
- Don't Let the Tourniquet Cause Extra Pain or Complications.

References

1. Pham V, Nguyen L, et al. Coronavirus disease 2019: anesthesia machine circuit pressure during use as an improvised intensive care unit ventilator. Anesth Analg. 2021;132(5):1191–8.
2. Durukan AB, Gurbuz HA, et al. Electrical failure during cardiopulmonary bypass: a critical moment. Kardiochir Torakochirurgia Pol. 2016;13(2):143–4.
3. SSZT261 Technical article | TI.com [Internet]. Ticom 2020 [cited 2025 Jul 27]. Available from: https://e2e.ti.com/blogs_/b/industrial_strength/posts/demystifying-medical-alarm-designs-part-1-iec60601-1-8-standard-requirements.
4. Lewandowska K, Weisbrot M, et al. Imapct of alarm fatigue on the work of nurses in an intensive care environment - a systematic review. Int J Environ Res Public Health. 2020;17(22):8409.
5. Statement on Principles for Alarm Management for Anesthesia Professionals [Internet]. Asahq.org 2025 [cited 2025 Jul 27]. Available from: https://www.asahq.org/standards-and-practice-parameters/statement-on-principles-for-alarm-management-for-anesthesia-professionals.
6. Stawicki SP, Wolfe S, et al. The impact of comprehensive air purification on patient duration of stay, discharge outcomes, and health care economics: a retrospective cohort study. Surgery. 2020;168(5):968–74. https://doi.org/10.1016/j.surg.2020.07.021. Epub 2020 Sep 2.
7. Dauber MH, Roth S. Operating table failure: another hazard of spine surgery. Anesth Analg. 2009;108(3):904–5. https://doi.org/10.1213/ane.0b013e318195b7a9.

Authors

Cathy Marcucci is an engineer and anesthesiologist. Her favorite procedure is putting up the Christmas tree. Her favorite machine of all time is the Rube Goldberg she built in her high school physics class—with seven different types of motion and mechanization, mind you.

Brad Winters is an anesthesiologist and intensivist at Hopkins. His favorite procedure is adjusting the derailleurs. He considers it a total pain in the neck, but the results are beautiful. His favorite machines are bicycles (the most efficient machine humans ever designed) and locomotives.

Brant Wagener is an anesthesiologist and intensivist at the University of Alabama—Birmingham. His favorite procedure is making breakfast burritos on Saturday morning with real green chile from Hatch, NM. His favorite machine is Sonny, the robot that could violate the Three Laws of Robotics in "I, Robot" and Chat-GPT is also pretty cool. Model rockets with his boys go a long way, as well.

Amy Robbins is a palliative medicine anesthesiologist and medical executive in Charlotte, NC. Her favorite procedure is pruning roses in her new rose garden. Her favorite machine is her Breville air fryer, specifically used for French fries. And any plane her brother is flying.

Ron Bank is a cardiac anesthesiologist at INOVA Fairfax. His favorite procedure is popping the cork on a nice red wine on a Saturday night to watch a movie or show on a far-too-rare date night with Kathryn. His favorite equipment, hands down, is SCUBA equipment.

Wisdom on Airway Management: Basics, Devices, and Techniques

161

Steven L. Orebaugh, Kirk Lalwani, Sharon T. Kapulek, Harriet W. Hopf, Michael S. Axley, Brian T. Gierl, and Catherine Marcucci

Contributors:

Ronald S. Bank, MD (RSB)

Denis L. Bourke, MD (DLB)

Niloofer Dalal, MD (ND)

Edward J. Damrose, MD (EJD)

Charles W. Emala, MD (CWE)

Steven M. Frank, MD (SMF)

Daniel M. Frohwein, MD (DMF)

Deborah Gerson, MS CCC-SLP

Brian T. Gierl, MD (BTG)

Note: The *Anesthesia Bridges* senior editors are grateful to every author and contributor who sent us ideas and suggestions for this topic. They can all legitimately lay claim to being an airway expert—simply by being a working anesthesiologist. We thank them for taking the time to share their best clinical and teaching points.

S. L. Orebaugh
Department of Anesthesiology and Perioperative Medicine, University of Pittsburgh School of Medicine, Pittsburgh, PA, USA

K. Lalwani
Department of Anesthesiology and Perioperative Medicine, Oregon Health and Science University, Portland, OR, USA

S. T. Kapulek
Department of Anesthesiology, University of North Carolina at Chapel Hill, Chapel Hill, NC, USA

H. W. Hopf
Department of Anesthesiology, University of Utah, Salt Lake City, UT, USA

M. S. Axley
Oregon Anesthesiology Group, Portland, OR, USA

B. T. Gierl
Department of Anesthesiology & Perioperative Medicine, University of Pittsburgh Medical Center Presbyterian, Pittsburgh, PA, USA

C. Marcucci (✉)
Department of Transfusion Medicine, Clinical Center, National Institutes of Health, Bethesda, MD, USA

S. Mohamed et al. (eds.), *Anesthesia Bridges*, https://doi.org/10.1007/978-3-032-08294-7_161

Vincent L. Hoellerich, MD (VLH)

Michael P. Hutchens, MD (MPH)

Kirk Lalwani, MD (KL)

Andrew Mannes, MD (AM)

Frederick Mihm, MD (FM)

Anthony N. Passannante, MD (ANP)

John S. Rogoski, DO (JSR)

Brandon M. Togioka, MD (BMT)

Jennifer N. Tripi, MD (JNT)

Jennifer Tripi was at UNC—Chapel Hill when she found and edited the last crucial set of airway tips for the chapter and sent us a photograph of the UNC hospital walkway. She is now a busy attending at The Ohio State University.

John Rogoski was a senior anesthesiologist at The Ohio State University. He was the recognized airway go-to guy.

Introduction

The airway words of wisdom are the most valuable that we can pass on to our junior colleagues. Their importance is weighted by the gravity of the relevant clinical situations they pertain to, of course. The goal is to get through your entire career as an anesthesiologist without a single serious airway mishap. We hope the wise sayings that we ourselves were taught and now teach make that responsibility rest a little easier.

General Airway

The Basics

- The most important resource in all of airway management is oxygen! Consider it both airway equipment and an airway drug. If you get into airway trouble, put the patient on oxygen and then think.—**Editors**

- Airway management in the US is predicated on the ASA algorithm, which is formally called the ASA Practice Guidelines for Management of the Difficult Airway. *Get out the current version and look at it every month.* You may think, "Oh, I already know this, I don't need to do that." But you do. The bottom part of the document will get a little fuzzy to you because the average practitioner doesn't get down to that part of the algorithm with great regularity (it is certainly to be hoped). So, it does require regular, proactive review. Here's where it is: pubs.asahq.org/anesthesiology/article/136/1/31/117915/2022.—**Editors**

- Because you can learn a lot from comparing guidelines and because we are all citizens in the anesthesiology world, we also recommend that you become very familiar with the *Difficult Airway Society*. The DAS is based in the UK and the site has intubation, extubation, and pediatric guidelines, as well as courses and other educational materials for patients such as how to obtain a difficult airway "ALERT Card." The DAS is endorsing airway courses, as of 2022. It's a resource you should be aware of.—**Editors**

- The DAS link is at https://das.uk.com/guidelines.—**Editors**

- Similarly, we should all review and stay familiar with the "*Vortex Approach*" which is represented below (Fig. 161.1a, b). The original publication was published in the British Journal of Anaesthesia and titled, "The Vortex: A Universal High-Acuity Implementation Tool for Emergency Airway Management." [1] The most up-to-date information is on the vortexapproach.org website. It's a fascinating human factors model for delivering care in acute airway situations.—**Editors**

- The *Vortex Approach* provides a prompt for optimizing success at each of the three upper airway lifelines in order to enter the Green Zone (Fig. 161.1a). The Green Zone is described as, "any situation in which adequate alveolar oxygen delivery can be confirmed and the patient is no longer at imminent risk of critical hypoxia. This provides the clinical team with time to pause and consider the opportunities available to them before further instrumenting the airway. These opportunities include optimizing patient physiology, strategizing regarding further interventions, and mobilizing resources".—**Editors**

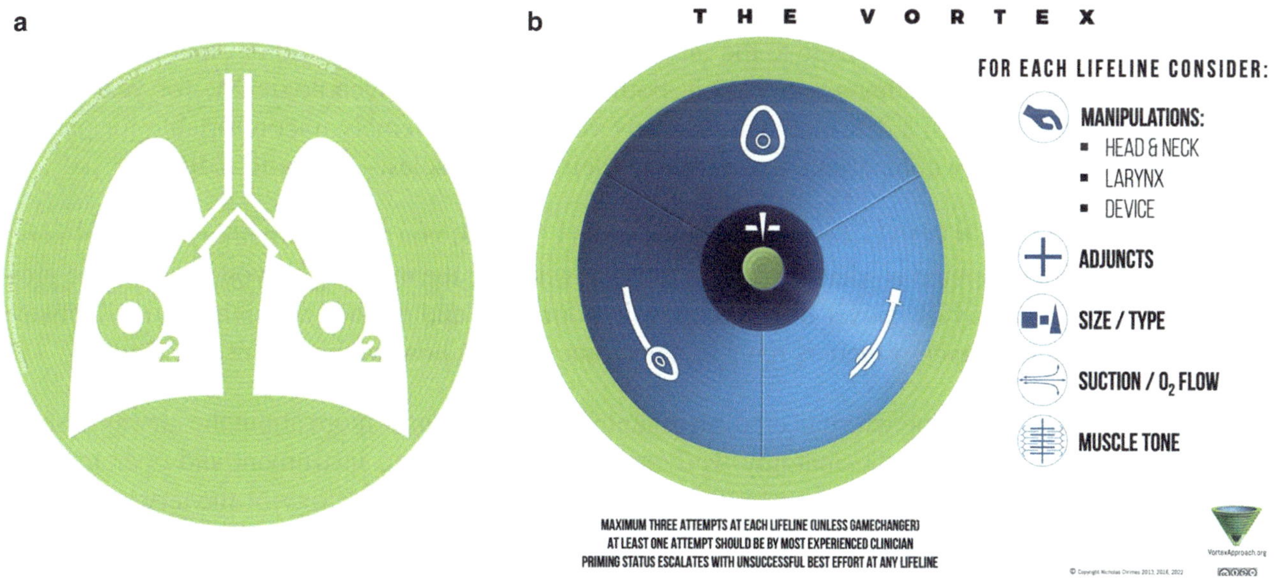

Fig. 161.1 (**a**) Identifying the Green Zone. The essential question to be answered to identify entry into the Green Zone is, "Can adequate alveolar oxygen delivery be confirmed?" Illustration: Image and caption used with permission of Nicholas Chrimes. (**b**) The Vortex Approach. Illustration: Images used with permission of Nicholas Chrimes, Vortexapproach.org

- Optimizations for each lifeline can be categorized under five general headings. It is expected that optimizations from multiple headings, rather than only one, would be expected to contribute to a best effort at any lifeline.—**Editors**

- Remember that "the airway" is not just the vocal cords! It is comprised of every anatomic structure that plays a part in transferring oxygen to the blood and carbon dioxide to the atmosphere. It starts at the lips and teeth and the distal nares and continues to the alveoli and pulmonary vasculature.—**Editors**

- Airway injury cases in the Anesthesia Closed Claims Database includes injuries not just to the vocal cords and trachea but also to the temporomandibular joint, the pharynx, and the esophagus. About 18% of closed claims pertained to esophageal injuries—much higher than you would think. With an esophageal intubation, we tend to think no harm has been done—"Nope, the endotracheal tube (ETT) is in the esophagus, let's try again, we'll just decompress the stomach after the airway is secured." But evidently that is not what happens when the issue gets to the lawyers.—**Editors**

- Always believe a history of a difficult airway!—**EJD**

- Always make every effort to send the patient home with the voice they came to the hospital with. Because a person's voice is a deep part of their identity—people are attached to their voices and so are their families. Never brush off mention of a voice change.—**DG and Editors**

- With this in mind, ask your patients on the day of surgery if they are in their regular voice and take pains to document postoperatively that their voice is at baseline. Have a plan to deal with both short-term and longer-term voice changes—make friends with the otolaryngologists at your practice location and develop a relationship with a speech and language pathologist. Usually, voice changes due to intubation will resolve over several days, but every once in a while, it takes longer or there has been true disruption of the anatomic structures.—**DG and Editors**

- Occasionally, there is nerve damage to the innervation of the larynx in thyroid or other neck surgery. Patients can struggle with this complication, both physically and psychologically, for years, especially if they are left with a deepened and/or raspy voice. It is extremely uncomfortable for patients when they involuntarily compensate by overusing their neck muscles.—**DG and Editors**

- Never let anyone—**ANYONE**—rush you on an airway or push you to do something you feel is not right. Airway management is what we do, it's why we get up in the morning. If you let someone pressure you into an airway maneuver that you know in your heart and mind is not right, you will always have regrets about it, even if there is not a bad outcome. Ask us how we know this.—**Editors**

- There is no one in medicine who can credibly maintain that they know more about the airway than we do. The ENT people know the anatomy well, and they know how to instrument and operate in the airway, but they don't routinely manage the physiology and pathophysiology of the airway down to the alveoli.—**Editors**

- The reverse is true of the pulmonologists. They know the lungs inside and out, but not the head and neck anatomy so much and they don't have the technical and manual experience that we have in intubating. And no specialty knows and uses the induction meds like we do. So, whoever wants to argue with you that you were too careful or lacked expertise with the overall management of an airway will most likely lose.—**Editors**

- And here is a corollary about airway management in private practice. We were told by a senior faculty, "If you go into private practice from residency, they are going to want you to go faster than you are used to going. And in some respects, you are going to have to do that. But never compromise your thorough and careful airway management in the name of going faster. Sooner or later, it will catch up to you, and that private practice isn't going to be lining up to take the responsibility (and the blame).—**Editors**

- Never hesitate to listen to advice from any nearby helper—technician, therapist, or nurse—they may see things or have suggestions that haven't occurred to you in the heat of the moment. As the anesthesiologist, don't be shy about making the final decisions but also don't hesitate to collaborate.—**VLH**

- We agree with Vince Hoellerich! Be humble and also consult with other physician providers. Retain the right to make the final airway decisions (because you bear the liability!) but also do not hesitate to consult with your colleagues who also might have knowledge of the airway. This especially includes the ENT surgeons. We have also found that the interventional pulmonologists can be very helpful with the airway.—**Editors**

- At the hospital where several of the editors trained, the surgeons were asked to standby in three ways—to do a rigid bronchoscopy, to do a suspension laryngoscopy, and to do a trach. We don't recall there ever being any pushback on a request for help. The thoracic surgeons often said that they felt it was remarkable that anesthesia didn't do our own rigid bronchoscopy—they felt it was well within our skills toolbox. Don't ever feel shy about asking for standby if necessary.—**Editors**

- Watch the National Health Service-produced video, "Just A Routine Operation"—every anesthesiologist should view this. It's on YouTube at the URL below. *Watch it.*—**RSB**

  https://www.youtube.com/watch?v=VndU2zap_Rg

- Always assume that a "established" airway—whether managed by endotracheal tube, supraglottic device, mask, or resumption of vocal cord reflexes and function and spontaneous ventilation—can become unsecured and/or unestablished in the blink of an eye. Never lose sight of the possible need to take definitive action if that occurs. What *exactly* would you do if faced in the next minute with loss of the airway from inadvertent extubation, vomiting and aspiration, or an airway fire? And remember that not everyone would consider a laryngeal mask airway (LMA) a "secure" airway in the first place.—**Editors**

- If the patient is going to be leaving the room with a tracheostomy, such as resection of head and neck cancer, make sure you tell them that they will not be able to talk. And spend some time discussing and agreeing with the patient how you will communicate with them after during and emergence. We've found that hand squeezes are effective and something that most patients can do.—**Editors**

- Looking for an area of clinical excellence to specialize in? The difficult airway team is a great team to get onto—difficult airways are relevant in every single segment of anesthesiology—pediatric, trauma, cardiac, neuro, obstetrical, and head and neck cancer, to name a few. And the ongoing airway research questions will never be exhausted.—**Editors**

- Read *EVERY* airway article or guideline you see, as long as the source is reputable. Attend every airway conference you can.—**Editors**

- Every anesthesiologist needs to invest in access a definitive airway atlas if your practice has not. For reference, if nothing else, and online if not in hardcopy. The editors all had Steve Orebaugh's wonderful book when it came out: *Atlas of Airway Management—Techniques and Tools*, which is now in a second edition with collaborator Paul Bigeleisen. I once had a patient come in and report that he had a difficult airway history but had been intubated using a technique on such-and-such page in Steve's book. Not joking. Needless to say, he was intubated a second time using that very technique as shown on that very page. Steve is a talented and prolific writer above and beyond the *Atlas* (Fig. 161.2).—**CM**

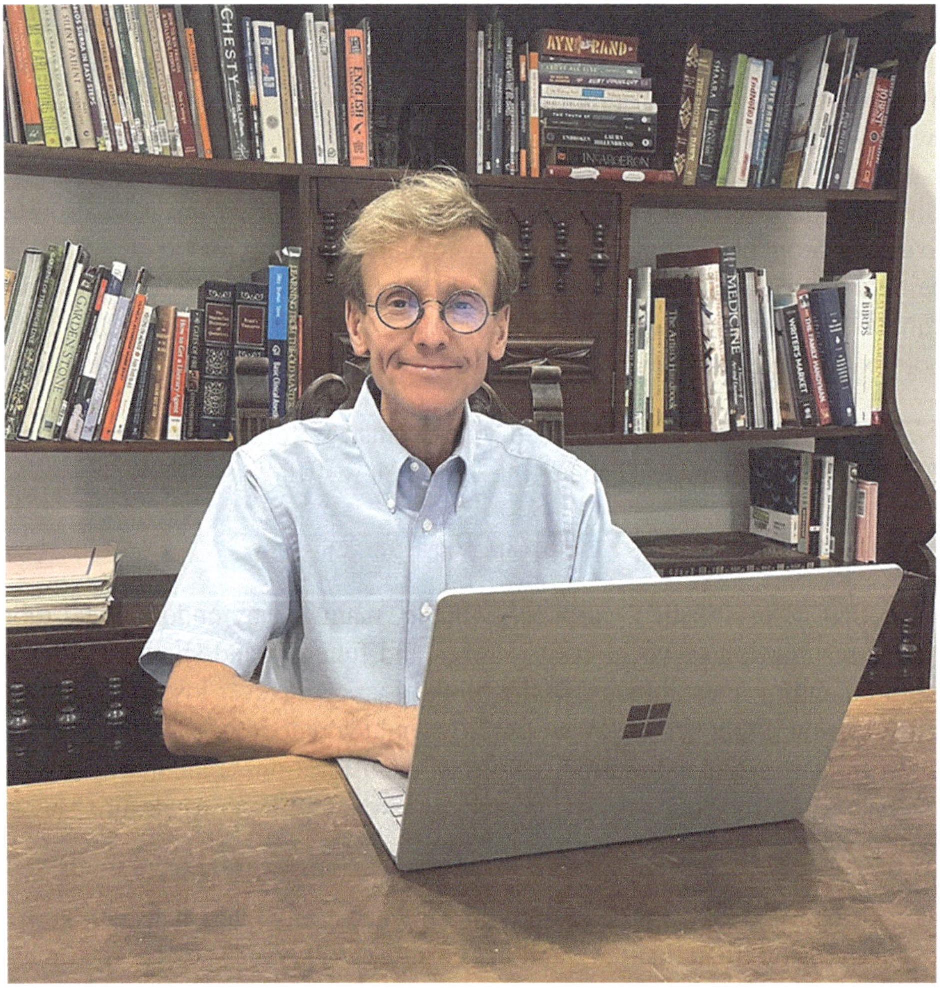

Fig. 161.2 Steve Orebaugh, behind his laptop as usual. Besides his famous airway atlas, he has published a patient education manual, two fantastic novels, magazine articles, and 75+ medical manuscripts including peer-reviewed journal articles, reviews, and book chapters. He's also an accomplished editor. Photo: Image used with permission of Steve Orebaugh at steveorebaugh.com

- Get involved in teaching pre-hospital providers. It's fun, rewarding, and helps you to think outside of the usual OR/hospital box. We're the airway experts. We should be teaching them. They appreciate it very much when we do. It is a great service to the community. Also, it could be you or your family's airways that they will someday manage.—**RSB**

- You establish and maintain control of your airway situation by maintaining control of your drugs—both at intubation and extubation. We have seen so, so, so many airway situations happen, both at intubation and extubation, because the anesthesiologist either couldn't stop giving drugs to try to facilitate intubate or failed to recognize the level of drug action still taking place at extubation.—**ANP and Editors**

- Remember that the larynx causes more coughing than the lungs, and even the pulmonologists have been known to admit this.—**Editors**

- Study long COVID! It's clinically significant and it's real and it's not just for the internists and rehab docs. It is now understood that severe viral infections knock out macrophage peroxisomes which can lead to severe scarring. Functionally, patients will present as diffusion-impaired restrictive lung disease.—**Editors**

Getting Ready for Airway Assessment and Management

- Do a very careful airway exam on every patient. Don't get burned and end up with an unanticipated difficult airway. In particular, don't confuse a patient's extension of their upper back and neck together with neck mobility.—**RSB**

- A thorough preoperative exam should include not only evaluation for ease of mask ventilation and laryngoscopy but also rescue techniques. You should be able predict a correct laryngoscopic view 90% of the time. The view should be better than predicted the remaining 10% of the time. If it is worse than predicted, you need to reevaluate your exam.—**STK**

- Bad things can happen quickly. It is imperative to have several well thought out backup plans to successfully secure the airway.—**STK and JNT**

- One of the things that tends to go by the wayside in the busy day-to-day practice of anesthesia is evaluation of aspiration risk. We are all aware of the risk associated with ascites and emergency cases. But how many of us think actively about it for every case, regardless of airway technique? Remember that sedated patients can also aspirate. We once saw a patient vomit and aspirate during a cataract case when the globe was tugged on. The patient later died of aspiration pneumonitis.—**RSB and CM**

- In addition to Ron's and Cathy's thoughts above, we think it is important to mention other etiologies of "full stomach", such as diabetes, weight-loss and diabetic medications, esophageal strictures, and *any* pregnant patient. Hepatomegaly and splenomegaly can also cause delayed gastric emptying. In these cases, consider point-of-care ultrasound (POCUS) to look at stomach contents.—**BTG and Editors**

- Always consider decompressing the stomach with a naso-gastric (NG) tube *prior* to induction of anesthesia in any patient at high risk of aspiration, for example bowel obstruction or acute abdomen. A full liter or more of gastric contents showing up in the patient's mouth after induction never ends well; think about how you will quickly respond in any case where this might occur.—**VLH**

- Patients often present with an NG tube. In which case, they can be a helpful anatomic guide on laryngoscopy to show where the esophagus is in all the folds of pink tissue. However, sometimes, the surgeons do not request them as they are not helpful to the situation, for example, in closed loop bowel obstruction. So, it's never a bad idea for a quick check with the surgeons about an NG tube.—**BTG and Editors**

- As a corollary, a senior anesthesiologist once told me, "It is nearly impossible to vomit when an NG tube is on suction."—**BMT**

- Early in my residency we were doing a rapid sequence for a full stomach. The attending thought I was about to squeeze the bag and took his hand off the cricoid to stop me. The patient aspirated and died several days later. *Lesson*: This doesn't definitively prove the efficacy of the Sellick maneuver, but the case definitely made a big impression on me early in my career.—**DLB**

- A patient that has emesis with an ETT in place should be checked and suctioned; you can still aspirate around an ETT cuff.—**BTG**

- *ALWAYS* be sure that there is an AMBU bag in your OR. And an Eschmann stylet. And a second appropriately sized face mask. This sounds so basic, so simple. Yet, you'll be amazed how often these simple redundant and rescue airway devices are needed and not there—**RSB and BTG**

- Elevate the head and the back in everyone. No one ever regretted ramping a patient. Ample literature now supports this, and it's not just for the obese patient.—**SLO**

- Adequate "sniffing" position should look just like that-as if the patient was pushing his head well forward to take a sniff of the morning air. Too often, our "sniffs" in the OR are a bare minimum of forward displacement on squishy foam donuts.—**SLO**

- The "sniffing position" is often essential when using a curved Macintosh blade but consider a more neutral position with neck extension when using a straight Miller blade.—**VLH**

- Remember that it takes about 3 minutes to fully preoxygenate a patient. It's really surprising how often this isn't done. But if you do it and use a short-acting neuromuscular blocker for your intubation, if you have a difficult airway, you have the same 3 minutes (or more) before you hear the awful sound of the pulse ox dropping.—**RSB and CM**

- Evaluate preoxygenation with EtO_2 and target a value >0.8. If you have difficulty measuring exhaled gases, disconnect the sampling line, place it inside the mask, and cover the now disconnected sampling port.—**BTG**

Devices and Techniques

Mask Airway

- I remember well my first week of anesthesia residency. My preceptor was the great **Dr. Srinivasa Raja** at Hopkins. Everybody else was learning how to use a laryngoscope. But Dr. Raja had Pete Pronovost and me doing mask airways in the very busy ECT suite for the first week. At the time, I must confess that I felt a little left out and left behind on the new CA-1 curve. By the end of the week, everybody else had "done" the airway on five or six patients. Pete and I had managed the airway of *forty patients*. Okay, it probably wasn't forty patients, but it seemed like it to us. It was such a wise way to start the live airway training of brand-new anesthesia residents.—**CM**

- I agree with the above! When I trained, we had to learn to do a mask airway for an hour. I fear that it is becoming a lost art, especially with the wide-spread use of LMAs. Remember, learning to be competent at the mask airway is not just about holding the mask on the face, it's how you really learn to feel the bag and understand lung compliance.—**ND**

- You keep patients alive by ventilation, not intubation.—**ND**

- If you are a petite person and your patient is not, there is no shame in starting the mask airway with both your hands on the mask—somebody else can do the bag. You want to avoid even one wasted breath or one squeeze of the bag that goes into the stomach. Keep in mind, though, that stomach insufflation is actually due to a good mask seal and poor positioning, not small hands per se.—**ND and BTG**

- Positioning the patient's head and neck for a mask airway is even more important than for intubation.—**Editors**

- And then, when you have the patient's head and neck correctly positioning, you draw the face up to the mask from the angle of the mandible, you don't compress subglottic tissue and squash the mask down. You really don't want to see pressure marks on the patient's face after a mask airway.—**Editors**

- If you have a *GOOD* mask airway, you have an airway! In a code situation, for example, don't feel any immediate pressure or intimidation to get the patient intubated as soon as possible. Take your time, prepare fully to allow for the best chance at first attempt success.—**VLH**

- When doing a mask airway, we were taught to visualize the column of oxygen/respired gases between the anesthesia circuit and the patient's lungs. Don't let your column collapse.—**Editors**

***Note from the Editors:** In honor of the *Anesthesia Bridges* editors, authors, and contributors from University of North Carolina at Chapel Hill, we thought we would include several views of the sky bridge to their main hospital (Figs. 161.3a, b). The goal is always to focus on *work* on the way in and on *home* on the way out, is it not?

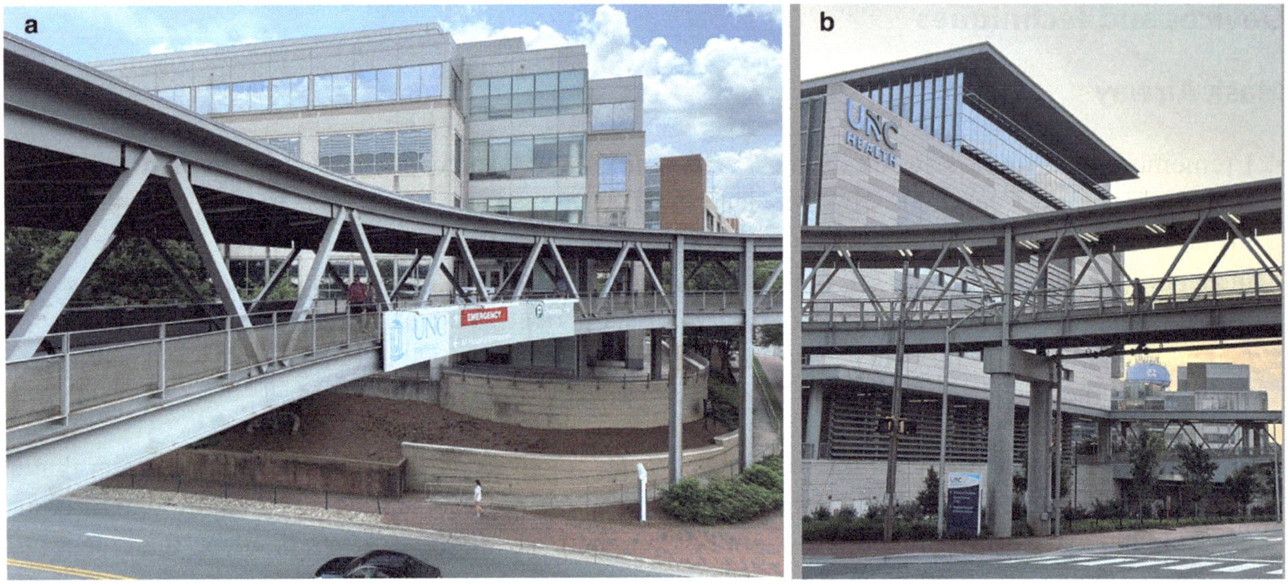

Fig. 161.3 (**a**) The view of the skyway, heading into the hospital. Not every bridge walkway has a view of a water tower in Carolina blue in the background. Photo: Jen Tripi (**b**) A view of the sky bridge walkway at the UNC-Chapel Hill university hospital, heading the other way. Photo: Anthony Passannante

Laryngeal Mask Airway (LMA)

- An LMA is essentially a mask airway that is placed around the glottis. When compared to an oral airway, they are better at preventing soft tissue from obstructing the airway, are less stimulating, and more effective at facilitating ventilation.—**STK**

- Keep supra-glottic airways (SGAs) handy and practice them as often as possible.—**SLO**

- The laryngeal mask airway has been used for several decades. It was designed to allow spontaneous ventilation during surgical procedures not requiring muscle relaxation. Over the years its use has evolved to include positive pressure ventilation and use in unconventional positions such as prone, lateral, and steep Trendelenburg. Although a very successful and frequently used device, it is not without risk. —**STK**

- A known risk associated with the LMA is aspiration. In my opinion, LMA stands for "*L*et *M*e *A*spirate."—**STK**

- Aspiration is also a risk with intubation—as in all techniques, careful selection and technique make it safe when used in the right patients. Many of us have used LMAs our entire careers without a serious aspiration complication.—**KL and Editors**

- LMAs do *not* protect the airway in patients with a full stomach, significant gastroparesis, or reflux.—**STK**

- You cannot necessarily tell if the LMA is mispositioned without confirming its position with a flexible scope.—**STK**

- Studies show that an improperly placed LMA may lead to gastric insufflation with excessive pressures. The peak inspiratory pressure and tidal volume achieved with the LMA is limited by the cuff leak pressure, body habitus and pulmonary compliance of the patient. Exceeding the leak pressure greatly increases the risk of gastric insufflation.—**STK and Editors**

- Historically, providers added more air to the cuff to increase the leak pressure when the real problem was mispositioning. The result was not necessarily a better seal, but overinflation of the cuff and risk of mucosal and nerve damage. Do not do this.—**STK**

- Yes, the LMA has been associated with lingual and recurrent laryngeal nerve damage. Newer LMAs have a pressure gauge or are self-pressurizing to avoid this risk.—**STK**

- The best approach to an LMA that is not adequately seated is to reposition it after ensuring the patient is adequately anesthetized. The better part of valor may be to replace the LMA with an endotracheal tube (ETT), which can then be used as an LMA but with a safer and secured airway. The point is to not limp through the case with only a partial airway.—**STK**

- LMAs are part of the ASA difficult airway algorithm. They can be a bridge to laryngoscopy when difficult mask ventilation is encountered. You can also intubate through the LMA if you suspect or know that laryngoscopy will be difficult. Take a moment to review that section of the algorithm.—**STK**

- LMAs can be a lifesaving adjunct in the can't ventilate, can't intubate scenario. Don't forget you can intubate through an LMA by placing a flexible scope and threading the ETT over the scope and through the LMA. In these situations, it is essential that the provider use an *intubating LMA*. They are shorter than non-intubating LMA's which allows more of the ETT to be advanced into the trachea. This minimizes the risk of dislodging the newly placed ETT as the LMA is removed.—**STK**

- LMAs have also saved lives when the patient is in other than the supine position and inadvertently becomes extubated. We've seen it and we've done it.—**Editors**

- Intubating LMA's are also designed to accommodate an adult ETT. Know what size ETT will fit through each size LMA before you begin. If the ETT will not fit through the LMA you will have to start over and may lose the airway on the next attempt. Use a smaller ETT than typically used, such as 7.0 vs 7.5 in an adult male, to minimize the chances of the tube getting stuck as you try to enter the larynx. Practice this technique on mannequins or patients with normal airways to become comfortable with the steps.—**STK**

- With the advent of disposable flexible scopes, a new intubation through LMA technique is possible. The scope enters the larynx through the LMA, the LMA is removed over the scope, then the scope is cut essentially turning it into a bougie. Next, the ETT is threaded over the cut scope. The advantage of this technique is that it does not matter whether you have an intubating or non-intubating LMA. In this situation, using a smaller ETT is still a good idea. Importantly, *you must have trauma shears* to cut the scope (they are inexpensive and easily bought online). It is also wise to insert a video laryngoscope to watch the ETT enter the glottic opening. This minimizes the chance of the ETT flipping the scope out of the larynx if you use excessive force. This technique is fast, effective, and may save a life. It is wise to practice on a normal patient to learn the steps.—**STK**

- Every physician in the chronic pain clinic should have airway drugs available and an LMA "within reach."—**AM**

Laryngoscopy and Endotracheal Intubation

- An attending told me once, "In some respects, intubation is quite simple. There are only four choices: The tube either goes in through the mouth or the nose, and it goes in either awake or asleep."—**DMF**

- A corollary to the above: There are actually two *other* choices—it ends up in the esophagus or the trachea.—**VLH**

- Don't do "quick looks." Laryngoscopy and intubation are two of the most profoundly invasive procedures done in all of medicine—you are taking complete control of one of the major organ systems of the body. Treat these procedures with the gravity they deserve. Be fully prepared—on your first attempt. We once saw a quick look on a Ludwig's angina patient, before the definitive airway equipment was in the room, result in the patient's death. Corollary to the above: In certain instances, nasopharyngoscopy is your friend.—**Editors**

- While the patient has spontaneous respiration make good use of this time. Pay attention to positioning (sniffing position, wedge placement, and table height), adequate pre-oxygenation etc. Make sure that all the equipment, including alternative or backup equipment such as bougie, supraglottic airway, and cricothyroidotomy kit are present. This should be your standard procedure when you set up your room for the day. There will be times that require immediate intervention, hopefully they will be rare, and you will be prepared. The goal is first pass intubation so take every advantage when you can while you can. Don't be rushed by production pressure or impatient colleagues.—**JSR**

- I don't use my fingers to scissor open the mouth for laryngoscopy. It can just as easily be done with a tongue depressor.—**CM**

- Sharp or jagged teeth can easily tear the ETT. It seems to happen to everybody at least once. Once it does, you learn to watch carefully for jagged dentition or broken crowns. You can even put a small, folded piece of gauze over any sharp edges, but not so small that you lose it in the oral pharynx.—**Editors**

- If you ever work with an anesthesiologist from a country with national dental benefits, they will be shocked by the overall poor state of American dentition. Every single US anesthesiologist at some point has had or seen teeth come loose, not a lot hopefully, but at least once. Do not feel superior if this hasn't happened to you yet, because it will. We have seen instances when thread or tape was tied around the tooth pre-induction so that it did not get lost in the airway when it got bumped out. Inadvertent tooth extraction becomes a very big issue if it ends up in the trachea or bronchial tree, which we've seen.—**CM**

- For new trainees, check your eye dominance if you are struggling. The laryngoscope in the left hand favors right eye dominance. If you are left eye dominant, you may be focusing on the scope and not the cords.—**JSR**

- When you can't get a good view during direct laryngoscopy, your first reflex should be to elevate the head, not crank it back into further extension (which, admittedly, is our first reflex). That is when teeth tend to get broken. —**SLO**

- Don't be reluctant to have helpers at the bedside assist with lifting the head-it's very hard to lift a human head with a laryngoscopy for more than a few seconds without becoming fatigued. Helpers can dramatically remove the stress on your arm.—**SLO**

- External laryngeal pressure, in which the right hand is used to manipulate the *thyroid* cartilage to improve the view, is helpful in at least half of cases. This should be a reflex developed through use in every easy case, so that it is automatic in the difficult ones. Remember, the right hand doesn't have much to do after the laryngoscope is inserted and the search for the glottis has begun, so it can be quite helpful in this regard. When the view is obtained, a helper must retain that thyroid cartilage pressure with the same force/direction, so the right hand can then accept the tube and place it in the glottis.—**SLO**

- Don't bend over and put your face close to the patient's mouth. Stand up straight so that your arm can be extended, and your motion will be to lift the patient's head, rather than to try to get the laryngoscope blade to go around the corner (natural motion if your elbow is bent).—**HWH**

- Wear your mask and eye protection both during intubation and, more importantly, during extubation. You are much more likely to get sprayed in the face during extubation and, although fairly rare, mouth and eye exposures have resulted in cases of viral hepatitis. <u>FYI</u>: Hospitals are required by law to provide appropriate eye protection gear.—**HWH and Editors**

- To reduce contamination of your workspace, wear two pairs of gloves for intubation. In an elective intubation that is going smoothly (easy, no desaturation), after the tube goes between the cords, and before you inflate the cuff, while still facing the patient, remove the outer gloves, leaving you a clean pair to finish the intubate with [2].—**HWH**

- Use half-inch tape to secure the ETT, because it makes it easier to avoid the vermillion border. If you are concerned about sticking, use a liquid adhesive or skin barrier prep. The second strip of tape should cross over the first, but most of it should be on separate skin, to provide additional security.—**HWH**

- Learn how to evaluate and assess for successful endotracheal intubation by physical exam alone —*not* end-tidal CO_2 monitor! You never know when you may have a monitor failure or not even have access to one—for example, mission trips in low-resource settings, on the battlefield, or helping a citizen on the street.—**VLH**

- If it doesn't sound right, it's probably not right (or something's wrong). Just listen over the stomach with the *first breath* (that's a Jon Benumof)! When listening for breath sounds, if you can't hear clear bilateral breath sounds after intubation, it's either become an esophageal intubation, a main-stem intubation, or there is severe bronchospasm (or maybe a defective stethoscope). In any case, your *immediate* intervention is required. Don't waste another 30 s trying to decide what you already know.—**VLH and BTG**

- As a corollary, you need *four* $ETCO_2$ breaths to confirm the tracheal position of the tube; the stomach always contains some CO_2. As a resident, we know this and do this. As you do your second ten thousand cases, sometimes this falls off a bit. Don't let that happen.—**BMT and Editors**

- But as a second corollary, know your patient's pathology before you intubate and plan your post-intubation auscultation accordingly. As a junior thoracic anesthesiologist, you learn quickly that a tumor in a mainstem bronchus is going to impact your clinical assessment. Once we saw a surgical resident, who was rotating on anesthesia, intubate a patient who had lung cancer in his left bronchus. The patient was in the OR for a bowel obstruction. The surgeon, who was focused on the GI issue, intubated the patient correctly (we think), used his left hand to auscultate the left chest (no breath sounds), and took the tube out before we could blink. Such a shame.—**Editors**

- The only reason *not* to give four breaths post-intubation is if you are in the esophagus. No need to ventilate the stomach four times! We had a senior faculty who used to say, "ain't no alveoli in the stomach, so figure it out quick." Again, listen over the stomach with one, initial breath.—**Editors and BTG**

- Recognize that you've entered the difficult airway algorithm the second you or someone on your team puts the ETT into the esophagus.—**Editors**

- Put the tape around the tube where you are going to say it is taped! Amazing how often this doesn't happen.—**HWH**

- Put the filter/heat and moisture exchanger (HME) between the ETT and the circuit. When you disconnect the circuit, leave the filter on the ETT and you will protect yourself from exposure to pathogens in the patient's lungs.—**HWH**

- The amount of air that you place in the ETT balloon can indicate tracheal size/stenosis and location. A tube with the balloon traversing the cords will require less air initially or will move up from the glottis and out of the mouth as you as you inflate it because modern balloons are cone shaped. These ETTs should be re-evaluated and advanced under direct laryngoscopy or fiberoptic bronchoscopy.—**BTG**

- Similarly, a recurrent leak that responds to more and more air placed into the cuff could be due to the cuff herniating upwards out of the cords. A new seal can be achieved by hyperinflating a cuff in the oropharynx, but this is a dangerous way to ventilate as there is a limited amount of pressure that can be delivered without a leak and simultaneous inflation of the stomach can lead to reflux and aspiration.—**BTG**

- The goal of inflating the ETT cuff is to create a seal but also avoid undue pressure on the tracheal mucosa. So, always feel the pilot balloon as you inflate—only to a pressure that provides a secure seal.—**VLH**

- And if you are teaching intubation and airway management, devise some type of ongoing protocol for monitoring the cuff pressure. Because think about this a minute. It's one of the few airway and intubation parameters (or any anesthesia parameter) that we can't actually see or visually assess—you can't reliably estimate the pressure in a cuff by looking at it. And cuff pressures are not routinely measured and charted.—**CM**

- And it's important, because a high endotracheal tube cuff pressure can cause quite a bit of mortality. When I was training, sometimes in July or August, two senior faculty would make surprise visits to your room with a small manometer—the "cuff police," as they called themselves. We are not sure if we recommend that, but perhaps every room could have a manometer in the anesthesia cart. Or maybe the supervising attending has one in her scrub pants pocket.—**CM**

***Note from the Editors:** The late *Anesthesia Bridges* contributor John Rogoski was a recognized airway expert at Ohio State for many years. We were in Columbus in March 2023 for the early rounds of the NCAA basketball tournament and snapped this picture of the wonderful foundations of a bridge in the downtown Riverwalk area adjacent to the Scioto River in his honor (Fig. 161.4).

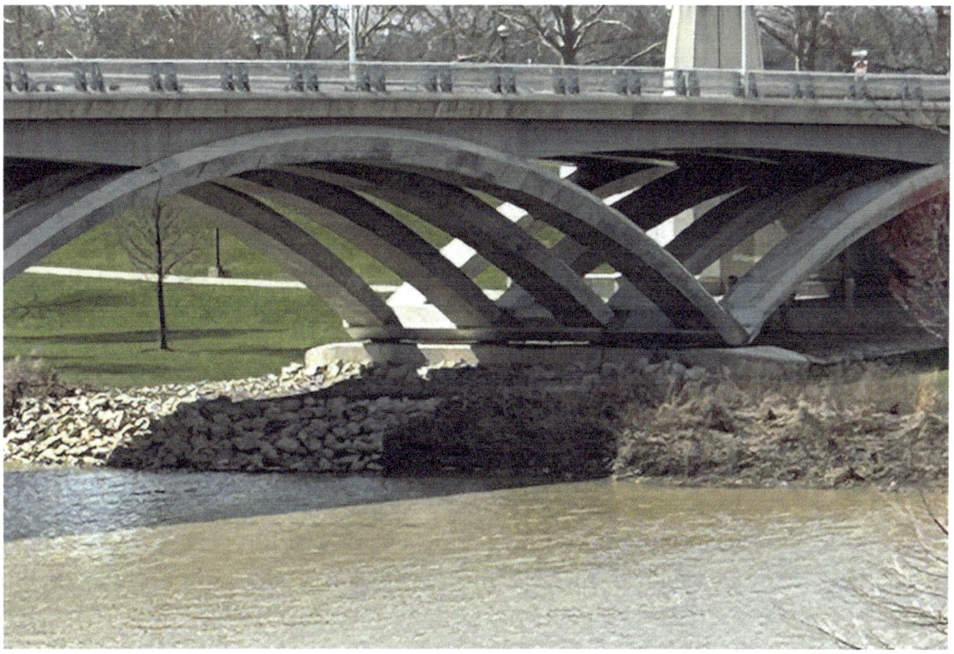

Fig. 161.4 The Rich Street Bridge in Columbus, Ohio. It was completed in 2012 and replaced the equally beautiful Town Street Bridge. The original anchor of the older bridge remains and was revitalized as The Prow, an observation platform in the Scioto Mile Promenade Park. Photo: Catherine Marcucci

Adjunct Airway Devices

- Never forget the utility, simplicity, and versatility of an Eschmann stylet (aka bougie)—this familiar, inexpensive, portable, low-tech device should be an important part of your armamentarium, and it's very easy to practice its use during routine cases.—**SLO**
- Develop and maintain a broad range of practical skills through practice whenever possible in "easy" cases: direct laryngoscopy with both curved and straight blades, supraglottic airway placement (even if it's just for ventilation before actual laryngoscopy), video-laryngoscopy with both Macintosh-type blades and hyper-acute blades, and fiberoptic techniques.—**SLO**
- The Aintree catheter is another device that should be used periodically to maintain familiarity and skills.—**SLO**
- Try to be expert in the latest airway device. We once saw **Ron Bank** do an amazing save with a light wand (this was back in the day) in the old ED at Hopkins. Most of us tried it a couple of times when the anesthesia department first got them but thought, "Nah, don't like it, too hard to keep midline." But Ron practiced and got really good at it. He used to carry one with him at all times on call when he was a senior resident. In this instance, it saved the patient from a tracheostomy… or worse.—**Editors**

Nasotracheal Intubations

- Nasal endotracheal tubes (NETT) are typically used in procedures involving the facial bones and dental structures.—**STK**
- A nasal Ring-Adair-Elwyn (RAE) tube is specially designed to direct the circuit away from the surgical field. They come with a preformed bend.—**STK**
- The most important consideration for selecting the correct size NETT is the height of the patient. Taller patients require a longer tube but may not have a large enough nasal cavity to accommodate a larger tube. Downsizing the tube is problematic because a smaller diameter tube is also shorter. In this situation, the cuff may be too close to the vocal cords and herniate above the cords with neck manipulation. Therefore, you must measure the distance from the tip of the tube to the bend as it emerges from the nose.—**STK**
- It is also important to look at the manufacturer of the nasal RAE since the bend is not standardized. For example, the Parker Flex Tip nasal tube has more length from tip to bend in each size. This allows you to use a smaller diameter tube and not sacrifice length compared to a Sheridan tube. A 6.0 Parker tube measures 28.5 cm at the bend versus a 7.0 Sheridan which is 28 cm at the bend. For additional reference, a 7.0 Sheridan nasal ETT is 26 cm at the bend.—**Editors**
- Don't assume you know. Look at the ETT!—**STK**
- If a tall patient's nose cannot accommodate a larger tube, try using a straight ETT instead. This is less convenient for the surgeon but may provide the additional length needed. Alternatively, use a micro

laryngoscopy tube. They come in 3 sizes: 4.0, 5.0, and 6.0 inner diameter. All have an adult cuff and measure 32 cm from the tip to the end of the tube.—**STK**

- Another option if an oral tube will interfere with the surgical procedure, is a submental intubation. In this situation, a wire reinforced flexible ETT is placed orally. A submental incision is then made and the ETT is pulled through to be connected to the circuit under the chin.—**STK**

- At the beginning of the case, the patient may desaturate prior to completing the intubation. If the NETT is in the oropharynx, you can close the mouth and pinch the other nostril with one hand while giving positive pressure via the attached circuit. This usually avoids the need to remove the tube and mask the patient. The NETT is effectively functioning as a nasal trumpet with attitude.—**STK**

- Likewise, at the end of the case when the patient is emerging, pull the NETT back to a trumpet length (usually 10–14 cm depending on patient height) and wait until you are absolutely sure it is safe to remove the tube. The advantage of this technique is it negates the need to insert a traditional nasal trumpet if the patient obstructs, it allows suctioning of the oropharynx when the mouth may be wired or banded, and it is less likely to collapse than a standard nasal trumpet; hence some call it a *nasal trombone*. It is very easy to send the patient to PACU with the tube taped to the face as your trumpet. It can be removed when no longer needed.—**STK**

- NETTs can cause significant bleeding on insertion. Tamponade the bleeding at the end of the case by pulling the ETT into the nasal pharynx and inflating the cuff. If you have already removed the ETT, pass a foley catheter through the nose and use the balloon to tamponade the nose.—**STK**

- Use the red rubber catheter (RRC) trick to minimize bleeding. Place the distal end of your nasal endotracheal tube (NETT) snugly into the proximal end of an appropriately sized RRC. Insert the RRC smoothly (and with no bleeding!) into the nose. Pull it out from the mouth using a Magill forceps while you gently allow it to pull the nasal ETT (whose tip is protected by the RRC) into the nose and airway. Pull the RRC/NETT junction out of the mouth, disconnect the RRC and let the nasal ETT flop back into the oral cavity, and then intubate in the usual fashion!—**KL**

- The above method was validated by a fellow of ours in Seattle using a double-blind study design [3]. It also saved a soldier with massive facial trauma who was intubated nasally by one of our ex-residents on the front line, and he wrote back to tell us how the trick "saved the day and impressed the military surgical team!"—**KL**

Video Laryngoscopes

- First and foremost —there is a critical concept that junior people or anesthesiologists who rarely use video laryngoscopes (VL) often miss. Visualizing the vocal cords with traditional laryngoscopy often means intubation will go smoothly. Hyper-angulated blades can alter anatomy such that intubation with a Cormack II or IIb view can be easier than intubation with a Cormack I view.—**BMT**

- If you have transitioned your practice to using a videoscope for all of your intubations, *make sure* you perform enough direct laryngoscopies with a laryngoscope to ensure that you can use it effectively should you need it as a back-up.—**MSA**

- I use the McGrath as do most of my partners. The techniques used for videoscopes versus laryngoscopes are considerably different. You would think there would be instantaneous competency using a videoscope, given the number of traditional laryngoscopies we've all done, there isn't.—**MSA**

- When first learning or teaching videoscope techniques remember *that is a camera*. The structures that you are trying to visualize—the vocal cords—are midline, so that is where you place the camera. It takes some time until you unlearn the instinct to sweep the tongue to the left.—**MSA and CM**

- I try to make as much room on the right side of the mouth as possible. Sometimes if I have a patient with a small mouth opening, I will have someone hook a finger into the angle of the mouth and pull.—**MSA**

- In order to successfully intubate with a videoscope one must use a stylet, and it must be rigid. I shape my ET tubes to resemble an ice hockey stick.—**MSA**

- I pass the endotracheal tube along the angle of the right side of the mouth into the retropharynx and rest the tip between the arytenoid cartilages. At this point in most cases, the tube will pass without withdrawing the stylet. If not, pull the stylet back two or three inches without pulling the tube back—often the tube will flex into place in the trachea. Taking the stylet out completely and twisting the tube as you advance it through the cords is also sometimes effective.—**MSA**

- I don't take the videoscope out of the mouth until I've visualized the tube between the cords with the balloon inflated. I've had tubes become dislodged in the time between removing the blade and inflating the cuff. This can be deceptive because the tube can wedge itself into place in the airway outlet while the cuff is still external to the vocal cords.—**MSA**

- Do not persist with a videoscope. If after two or three serious attempts you have failed to succeed, in my experience, you are unlikely to ultimately salvage the airway with this technique. Don't waste extra time trying to do it.—**MSA**

- When using the GlideScope with a hyper angulated (S) blade, always use the GlideScope stylet. There are two components to a VL intubation: seeing the vocal cords (VC) and passing the ETT. All too often, especially in "anterior airways"when using a hyper angulated blade with a regular, malleable stylet, the cords can be visualized but the ETT can't be passed through them as it can't make the correct angle without bending. The Glide stylets are made for such intubations. They are far superior to regular, malleable stylets.—**MSA**

- It's also important to understand that the optimal direct laryngoscopy and VL view are very different. With VL the optimal view is to see the epiglottis about half-way down the screen—the glottis/VCs don't fill the screen—so that one can more easily visualize and steer the styletted ETT to and thru the VCs.—**MSA**

- Also, remember that the best stylet may well be an fiberoptic bronchoscope (FOB)!! Using VL to distract the oropharynx while using the FOB as an active stylet—with or without actually using the FOB camera—is extremely effective!!—**Editors**

- When using a video laryngoscope, the stiff "J-shaped" stylet can actually be used to direct the tip of the ETT. By gently withdrawing the stylet while visualizing the airway, the tip of the ETT will flip up a bit (move anteriorly) and may help placing the ETT in the trachea. If you can't quite visualize, get a stylet, and play with it a bit—**VLH**

- As with other techniques, if you can't identify landmarks back up. If you can see the cords but can't reach them with your tube, try backing up the scope slightly, often times you are pushing the structures beyond your reach.—**JSR**

- To better preserve the curvature of the stylet, consider insertion at the 3 o'clock position and rotating up to 12 o'clock once you are around the tongue, this may preserve the curvature better than placing the tube straight in next to the blade.—**JSR**

- Rotating the ETT on a malleable rigid stylet so that is loaded with "reverse camber" or a reverse curvature of either 60° or 90° causes the ETT to leave the stylet at a different angle, which can allow it to be more easily maneuvered through the cords [4]. When inserting the stylet into the ETT, consider curving it in the opposite direction of the tube's natural curvature. You will find that this will often times provide for a smoother passage through the glottis. There are lots of pictures of reverse camber ETTs online or watch the Verathon video on GlideScopes that recommends this at https://www.verathon.com/video-laryngoscopes/—**JSR and BTG**

***Note from the Editors:** Speaking of reversing course, sometimes you have to stop and think about that a moment. Here is a young lady and her dog on a bridge, deciding which way to go (Fig. 161.5).

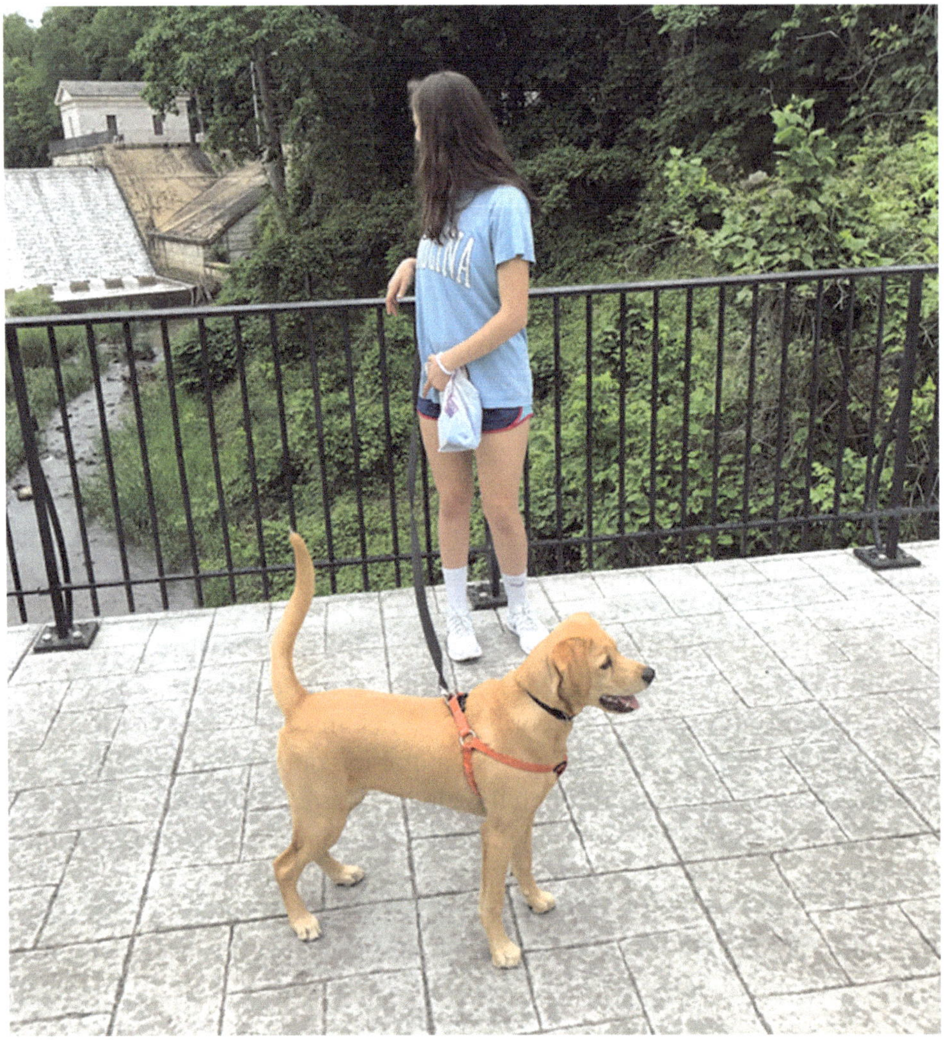

Fig. 161.5 The bridge by the dam at Lake Roland Park in Baltimore County, Maryland. Photo: Cathy Marcucci

Jet Ventilation

- Jet ventilation is used during surgical procedures involving the larynx. The jet is commonly used through a port on the rigid bronchoscope.—**STK**

- Jet ventilation is a must-know technique for the younger anesthesiologist (Fig. 161.6). It's weird how slow older people were to adopt it when the technique first came into widespread clinical use. There were some years when the people who knew how to do it and who liked doing these airways (and so did not avoid those cases!) were able to set themselves apart. If you are not getting enough of these cases in your training, seek them out, even if you have to stand and watch in somebody else's room. You don't want to leave training without being completely competent and confident.—**Editors**

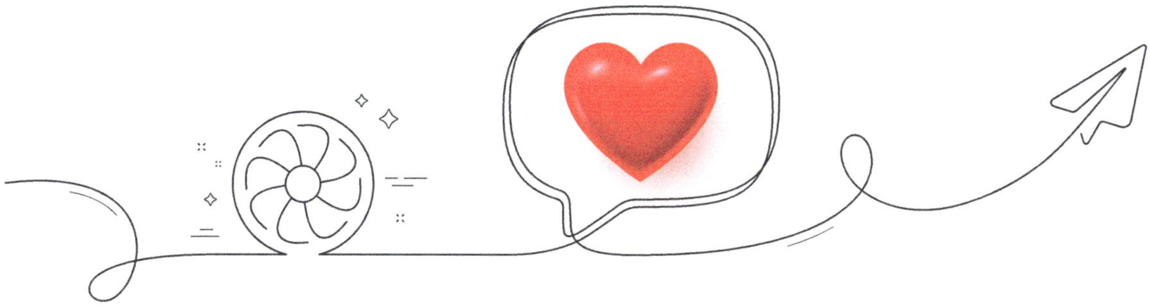

Fig. 161.6 We love this pictorial representation of jet flow! It perfectly captures that embracing and mastering this technique was true forward progress for patient and practitioner alike. Photo: Image used under standard license from shutterstock.com

- Keep in mind that the various techniques of jet ventilation arose because of clinical needs of both the patients, anesthesiologists, and surgeons. Advantages include improved visibility and surgical access, reduced peak airway pressures, less hemodynamic compromise than with conventional intermediate positive pressure ventilation, reduced ADH production and fluid retention, avoidance of endotracheal tube ignition during laser surgery, good in low resistance/large volume airway leak, and use in emergency trans tracheal airway management. What was there to be afraid of? We think maybe it was the physiology and physics. Elsewhere in this book, Brad Winters advised to never let you of your physics, and this is where that wisdom applies. Get on one of the YouTube sites if to to brush up.—**Editors**

- All techniques of jet ventilation are based on the same principles, which are really pretty simple: Jetstreams originating from high-pressure sources are cut by pneumatic or electronically controlled flow interruption devices; this generates a tidal volume that is supplemented by entrainment of gases at the jet nozzle. Expiration is dependent on passive lung and chest-wall recoil. The rest of the physiology and physics is generally dependent on whether the specific technique involves high or low frequency ventilation.—**Editors**

- But remember that there is a prodigious range of possibilities for barotrauma in a jet ventilation airway case: pneumothorax, pneumomediastinum, pneumopericardium, pneumoperitoneum, subcutaneous emphysema, gastric distension, and gastric rupture as well as dysrhythmias, necrotizing trachea-bronchitis, and necrotizing enterocolitis in neonates. I was taught that if a case with an airway that is being managed with jet ventilation goes south, it's a complication of the pulsed jet pressures until absolutely ruled out.—**CM**

- Since there is no ability to administer anesthetic gas via the jet, it is important to maintain general anesthesia with a total IV anesthetic. The patient does need to be paralyzed. Remifentanil is a great intraoperative adjunct—it has very rapid onset, short duration of action, and provides intense analgesia without prolonged respiratory depression.—**STK**

- The jet procedure itself is stimulating, but the patient typically does not have significant pain postoperatively. Minimizing longer acting narcotics is prudent. Spraying the larynx with 4% lidocaine at the end of these procedures can improve patient satisfaction and provide a better postoperative experience.—**STK**

- Jet ventilators typically connect to a pure oxygen source. Some are equipped with a mixer to allow air to dilute the O_2. But never forget the possibility of fire.—**STK**

- Remember: Adequate ventilation may not be obvious since CO_2 is not reliably measured. Watch the chest rise as you insufflate for a few seconds. Then make sure you give adequate time between breaths for the patient to exhale.—**STK**

- Jet ventilation for intratracheal lasering is best accomplished with a Hunsaker tube. This device is placed in the trachea distal to the operative site. The air jet is directed down the center of the trachea by a plastic cage which holds the jet tube in the center. This minimizes the chance of jet trauma to the trachea.—**STK**

- Jet ventilation for an emergency airway can be done with a 14-g angiocatheter (preferably Teflon—they reduce kinking) placed through the cricothyroid membrane in adults and an 18-gauge catheter in pediatric patients. These catheters allow for oxygenation only. They are too small for ventilation. They are only useful for ~45 minutes before the hypercarbia is no longer tolerated. A pressure of 50 cm H_2O is needed in an adult. Children do not require and do not tolerate 50 cm H_2O, so you may be able to get by with an AMBU bag.—**STK**

- Jet ventilation is not without risk, especially when using an IV catheter. These catheters tend to kink. They must always be held in place by a person because they are easily dislodged with the jet. This can cause immediate massive subcutaneous emphysema and loss of the airway. Because they are relatively short, the jet may be directed against the wall of the trachea. This can also result in mucosal perforation and subcutaneous emphysema.—**STK**

Airway Anesthesia—Awake and Fiberoptic Intubations

- Remember that awake and fiberoptic intubations are for when you can't find the airway. If you know where the airway is but it is narrow (like in tracheal stenosis), the correct technique may be an inhalational induction, depending upon the patient's physiology.—**Editors**

- I agree with the above. I learned to do adult inhalational inductions for cases where there was severe tracheal stenosis due to trauma or prolonged intubation but not for other anatomic difficulties.—**CM**

- If there are both tracheal stenosis and additional difficulties in airway anatomy and physiology, the best approach is the most conservative—a patient who is both awake (although perhaps sedated) and breathing spontaneously.—**BTG and Editors**

- Awake fiberoptic intubation (FOI) in the OR is becoming a lost art. Translating that skill to the ICU in a critically ill patient… more difficult, because we've stopped doing them in the OR, or we can only do the procedure with heavy sedation, something that might not be safe in the critically ill. You don't want to get into the position of avoiding awake FOI because you have no confidence in dealing with the patients' anatomy or FOI skills… rather, you want to be able to plan awake FOI because you have confidence that you can do it without torturing the patient, and without the procedure going sideways and failing.—**FM and Editors**

- There are patients with a "physiologically difficult airway" (such as pulmonary hypertension, anterior mediastinal mass, shock on pressors/inotropes, profound hypoxemia on HFO_2 or BIPAP) who should have an AFOI, because if done properly with topical anesthesia only, it is often the safest means of achieving intubation with the least hemodynamic or respiratory perturbations.—**FM**

- Learn and be very comfortable with awake intubation skills, especially awake fiberoptic intubation (AFOI) skills. Intubating while your patient maintains whatever spontaneous respiratory effort that they have provides a huge safety margin and is far less stressful. Don't take away their spontaneous effort unless you're SURE that you can take it over!—**RSB**

- First, of course, is a thorough history of all factors that would be relevant in an awake intubation—you'd be surprised how often this is rushed through. We've seen preop histories that were little more than asking patients for a strong nasal exhalation onto the shiny laryngoscope blade to see which nares causes more "fog." You should take a history of nasal trauma/congestion, cocaine use, gag reflex, previous airway history including dental history, intubations, surgeries, tracheostomy. And history of anxiety, phobias, and pain conditions. Then review current anatomy including radiographic studies. Then a thorough exam, paying extra attention to the neck.—**Editors**

- Make sure that the patient understands the risk-benefit ratio when doing an awake intubation. Reassure them that although they will not be intubated with general anesthesia onboard that does not mean that they will be intubated with NO anesthesia onboard; if you plan to use sedation, you might call it a 'twilight intubation,' as patients seem to understand the term twilight. Let them know that they will be sleepy and may actually wake up with less throat pain and coughing than patients who are intubated asleep.—**Editors**

- Preparation for awake fiberoptic intubation begins in the preoperative area with administration of anti-sialagogues. If planning a nasal intubation, don't forget nasal decongestants, and nasal anesthesia.—**STK**

- A dry airway is very important when performing an awake intubation. The goal is to minimize oral secretions which will otherwise interfere with visualization of structures and make the whole process much more complicated. Glycopyrrolate works well, but you must give it early enough to work effectively. It should be given at least 30 minutes (IV) or 60 minutes (SQ/IM) ahead of time. If you titrate in 0.1 mg IV every 5–10 minutes, you can achieve a dry airway without any significant change in heart rate. The anti-sialagogue effect will last for at least 4 hours, so you don't have to worry about it wearing off too soon.—**STK**

- Make sure to remember to give a nasal decongestant preoperatively if you are planning a nasal intubation. These medications take at least 15 minutes to work but stay effective for many hours.—**STK**

- Nasal decongestants work best to minimize nose bleeds in patients who have nasal congestion. They will not prevent bleeding as well if the nasal anatomy is difficult or there is the presence of spurs, septal deviation, or enlarged turbinate, because nasal ETT placement is traumatic on a good day. —**STK**

- Nasal decongestants are potent vasoconstrictors so be mindful of your dosing. They are meant to be sprayed or dropped, not squirted into the nose. The maximum dose for oxymetazoline is 3 sprays/nostril which equals a total of 0.6 mLs every 12 hours.—**STK**

- If a nasal intubation is planned, topicalize the nasal cavity preoperatively by placing pledgets with lidocaine along the floor of the nose or placing a pediatric nasal trumpet coated in 5% lido ointment into each naris. An alternative technique involves spraying lidocaine via an atomizer into each nostril once you are in the OR.—**STK**

- In cooperative patients, 3–5 mls of nebulized 4% lidocaine 15 minutes before the procedure with instructions for the patient to breathe deeply through their nose is very effective at topicalizing the entire tract you plan to traverse with your fiberoptic scope.—**KL**

- Always remember that the vagus nerve is running its own little universe in the neck (Fig. 161.7). We spend a lot of time visualizing the vocal cords and looking at the arytenoids, I think that sometimes it's easy to let go of a deep and intimate knowledge of the innervation of the airway structures and the branches of the vagus nerve. Try to aim to match the three-dimensional spatial appreciation of the airway that the head and neck surgeons have.—**CM and Editors**

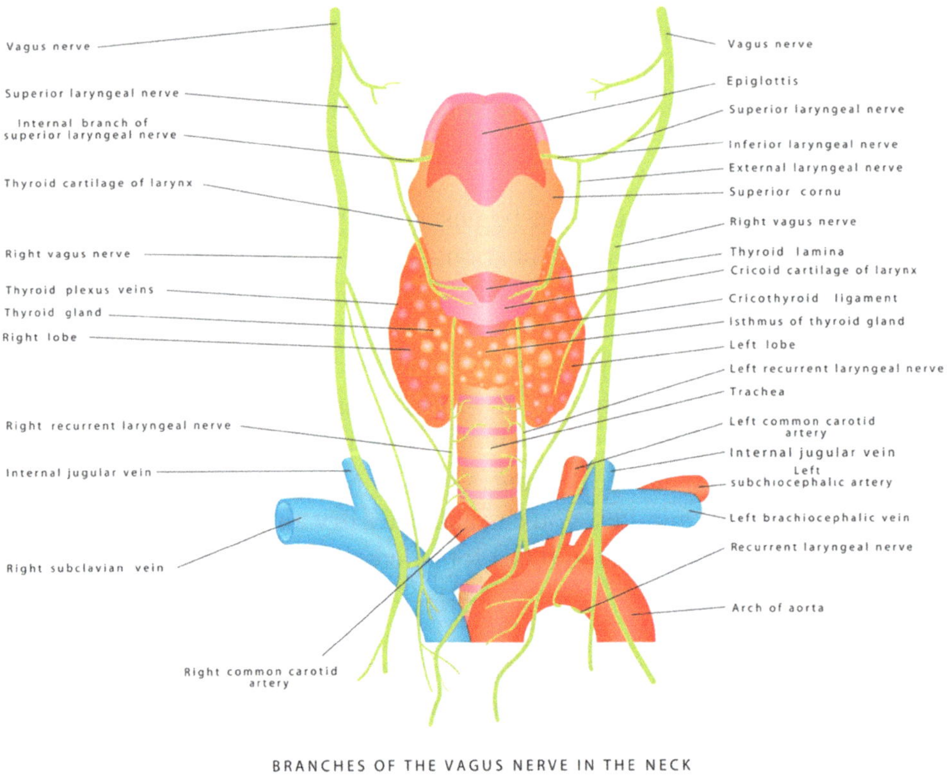

Fig. 161.7 The busy world of the vagus nerve in the neck. Review this anatomy frequently, it frequently crops up on exams and has been known to be a gotcha question in depositions (at least one of the *Anesthesia Bridges* editors was interrogated in this way). Photo: Image used under standard license from stock.adobe.com

- Topicalization is paramount for awake techniques; make certain that the superior laryngeal and recurrent laryngeal nerves are well-covered (Fig. 161.7). No amount of sedation (except too much sedation!) compensates for inadequate topicalization.—**SLO**

- The superior laryngeal nerve originates from the inferior vagal ganglion and divides into an internal and external branch. The internal branch of runs beneath or lateral to the greater horn of the hyoid and penetrates the thyrohyoid membrane to provide sensory innervation to the larynx. If you have time to make only one teaching point to the med student, it's that topicalization of the distribution of the internal branch of the superior laryngeal nerve is crucial to successful awake intubation.—**Editors**

- The tricky thing about the recurrent laryngeal nerve is that it is not always recurrent. There are clinically relevant anatomic variations—called "non-recurrent laryngeal nerve anatomy" —in about 0.7% of the population.—**Editors**

- Don't apply airway topicalization too early, you may have a delay and need to apply more topical anesthetic, this will increase the dose without additional benefit.—**JSR**

- The gag reflex can be controlled by blocking the glossopharyngeal nerve on either side of the mouth. You can place lidocaine pledgets in the gutter created by the tongue and molars preoperatively. Push the pledget up against the base of the palatoglossal pillar, and you will anesthetize the lingual branch of the glossopharyngeal nerve, which covers the base of the tongue. Alternatively, an injection of lidocaine can be made into the base of the pillar. Injection should only be done in the OR with full monitors. Be careful—the carotid artery is in close proximity!—**STK**

- I am a big fan of the transtracheal airway block for FOI. To me, it's one of the easiest airway blocks to do. The landmarks are readily apparent, and the bubbles tell you that you are in the airway. Make sure to tell the patient to expect to cough when you do the injection.—**CM**

- I agree with Cathy as above, but here's a tip. When doing a trans-tracheal injection (through the cricothyroid membrane) consider using an IV catheter for the injection and leave it in place until after intubation. It's safer to inject through a catheter than a metal needle (and the patient *is* going to cough), the catheter can be used to apply more topical, if necessary, it can also be used to pass a guidewire if needed emergently, it marks the trachea if an emergent cricothyrotomy is needed, and it is good practice to access the trachea if you ever need to perform emergent transtracheal jet ventilation.—**JSR**

- I agree with the above suggestions for the trans-tracheal block, but I feel it is important to teach and recommend a gauge for the needle. I like to use a 20-g, as the needle isn't long enough to penetrate the back wall. You don't want your trainees to someday try a 14-g needle, which seems dangerous.—**BTG**

- If you are going to do an airway block via the transoral approach, you had better check and document that you feel the carotid pulse in the usual position in the neck. Retropharyngeal position of the carotid arteries is well-described. I have seen a patient seize when lidocaine was injected directly into an artery during an airway block.—**CM**

- Placing a directing oral airway (Berman, Ovassapian, or Williams) is a good test of airway topicalization—the patient should tolerate insertion of this implement easily if he/she has been numbed appropriately.—**SLO**

- Remember that airway topicalization does not always even mean awake intubation. Sometimes it means just an awake look. Once I had a patient who came in for abdominal surgery. He was about 5′10″, 165 pounds since the age of 18. Good thyromental distance, Mallampati II. No history of head and neck pathology of any type. No sleep apnea. But he had all these capped teeth. When I asked about that he reported that, during a previous surgery 10 years ago, they had had trouble intubating him and had broken all his teeth. The patient asked me to go out and get the details from his wife. So, I trotted out to the family waiting room and she confirmed that "they had great difficulty putting the breathing tube down" and the dental repairs had cost a fortune.—**CM** (1 of 2)

- Normally I teach that you should never assume that you are any better or any worse than any other anesthesiologist when it comes to managing difficult airways. But, in this case, I just couldn't figure out what in the world had happened. I discussed with the patient that we would do thorough topical anesthesia on the airway and then I would do an awake look with a laryngoscope to see if I could see the vocal cords, which I could, easily. So, we just did a standard induction and the resident intubated without difficulty. After the case was over, I wrote a letter for the patient to carry with him to show to future anesthesia teams, which I later found out saved the patient a lot of trouble at subsequent hospitals. I never did find out what the trouble had been with the first "difficult" intubation.—**CM** (2 of 2)

- You can also do airway topicalization to decrease discomfort and airway reflexes in a case you plan to intubate and extubate routinely. I once had a patient who was a heavy cannabis smoker—I mean heavy—and who coughed himself blue at extubation. He coughed and coughed and coughed. He was actually hypoxemic. He came back to the OR the next week and we did airway anesthesia for him before intubating him for the case. Yes, we knew we were suppressing those reflexes and that might be an issue for handling secretions or vomiting but we applied the risk-benefit ratio.—**CM**

- I have also seen airway topical anesthesia and blocks done for a patient who had a planned intraoperative wake-up test in a neurosurgery back case. And we would like to emphasize the point that this topicalization should start with glycopyrrolate.—**CM and BTG**

- Finally, I sometimes have done some amount of airway topicalization in carotid endarterectomies to tamp down the hemodynamic overdrive, hypertension, and tachycardia or both when those patients wake up and cough. Often just a lidocaine nebulizer pre-induction blunts that big upswing in vital signs, which can be helpful if the patient is at risk for cardiac ischemia.—**CM**

- Sedation for an awake intubation is sort of a fine art. It really depends on the patient. You do want some anxiolysis, but also it is important to keep the patient cooperative and compliant. It is much easier to pass the endotracheal tube through the vocal cords if the patient is awake enough to take a deep inhalation on request. I have seen patients given droperidol which was kind of awful. They didn't move much or make a lot of noise but described the feeling of knowing what was happening and not being able to move or say anything as utterly terrifying. We don't think anybody uses high dose droperidol since the black box warning, but ketamine has some of the same issues, if you are not watching your trainees or staff closely to make sure that a benzodiazepine is carefully titrated in.—**CM**

- The other most important ingredient in the awake intubation is TIME. We are aware of patients who have suffered post-traumatic stress disorder due to awake intubations without proper topicalization of the airway or proper coaching; tell them that if they aren't comfortable, you'll stop and make them comfortable.—**Editors**

- And then, remember that awake intubation does not always mean FOI. The smoothest and quickest way is sometimes the blind nasal intubation. If you've done a lidocaine nebulizer and careful topicalization of the nares, the endotracheal turns the corner in the nasal pharynx and often ends up just above the vocal cords. You can sometimes even hear the respirations through the ETT as well as see fogging. You can then ask the patient to take a deep breath and *gently* advance the ETT 1–2 cm through the cords. This was actually the chosen method of intubation at emergencies and codes in the 1970s and 1980s, as it was feared that succinylcholine would lead to hyperkalemic arrest. The first time I saw this, I heard my attending say, "Mr. Johnson, are you okay?" The patient nodded. The ETT was advanced. "Mr. Johnson, are you intubated?" The patient gave us a thumbs up.—**CM**

- *Denny Bourke* has a similar story. When he was at Penn, way back in the day, he once had a patient who had an awake nasal intubation with really, really good airway anesthesia. Somehow, there was some sort of commotion in the hallway outside the OR and the patient was comfortable enough to get off the OR table and walk over to the doorway to see what was going on, just breathing through the nasal endotracheal tube like it was snorkeling gear.—**Editors**

- Keep the length of the fiberoptic cable taut to improve your ability to manipulate the tip of the scope, use small rotation of the wrist not gross movements of the shoulder or elbow, pass the scope carefully, if you cannot identify a landmark, back up until you are oriented, be efficient in your movements, sometimes the quickest way to achieve success is to slow down.—**JSR**

- Learn to use the supra glottic airway as a conduit for fiberoptic intubation; this is a handy skill which can be practiced in routine airway management.—**SLO**

- Keep good communication with your awake/sedated patient as their cooperation is an important part of the procedure. Speak to them directly and not "around them" as though they are not present. Use positive and reassuring language. If you show frustration or agitation, it will be multiplied in the patient and those present in the room.—**JSR**

- Keep available another ETT of the same size as you intend to use, this will supply you with an additional connector in case yours gets dropped and can't be found.—**JSR**

- When using a supraglottic airway as a fiberoptic intubation guide, resist the idea of altering a device (such as cutting elevator bars, etc.) to facilitate passage of a scope more easily or ETT. You will be assuming any and all liability when you alter a medical device should the device fail or cause a complication. Instead familiarize yourself with the use of the Aintree and other exchange catheters for their intended purpose.—**Editors**

- Have a plan in place for what you will do if you can't do the FOI. Seriously. What will you do?—**Editors**

Complications and Troubleshooting

- In elective settings, tape the eyes before you start mask ventilation, because ventilation and intubation present a higher risk of corneal injuries. Consider removing your badge, or tuck it away, so it is not the source of injury.—**HWH**

- And there are many other ways to scratch the corneas! We have seen corneal lacerations occur from bracelets, watches, and rings. Yes, even rings that are underneath gloves. We once saw a small pair of scissors fall out of the pocket of a scrub top and scratch a patient's eye. It's really best to come to the head of table to intubate without free of falling and pointed objects.—**Editors**

- In the face of decreasing O_2 saturation or difficulty or inability to oxygenate and or ventilate, if critical call for help immediately. Then, trouble shoot starting with the patient first, *then* the anesthesia machine and not vice versa. Simply disconnecting from the anesthesia machine and connecting the AMBU bag to the ETT immediately eliminates the tremendous complexity of the anesthesia machine from the equation—while you and the help that you called stabilize the patient.—**RSB**

- A nebulized anticholinergic, such as ipratropium, should always be considered in a patient with a reactive airway. It inhibits cholinergic-mediated bronchoconstriction and is synergistic with beta agonists.—**CWE**

- A common way to achieve a right-mainstem intubation is to put the patient into Trendelenburg with an endotracheal tube just above the carina. The intrathoracic contents shift cephalad, and an endotracheal tube that had been ventilating both lungs is now in the right mainstem bronchus. The ETT doesn't have to move much at all for this to happen.—**CWE**

- The best way to induce bronchospasm is to put an endotracheal tube at the carina. The carina is the most densely innervated region of the airway resulting in parasympathetically mediated irritant-induced bronchospasm.—**CWE**

- There are an astounding number of ways to inadvertently extubate a patient. I am aware of a case where the anesthesiologist accidentally extubated a patient putting an IV in a hand. Evidently, the tube was somehow in the way and was "just moved over" a little bit—right out of the larynx. Leaving the connection to the ETT a bit loose allows it to act as a safety disconnect; anyone in the OR can reconnect the circuit, reintubation can be difficult.—**CM**

- When thinking about airway fires, don't neglect the intra-thoracic space! During thoracic cases beware of any loss of volume in the circuit. It could be 100% O_2 leaking into the surgical field from the lungs. In thoracic surgery if there is a loss of volume from the circuit immediately think of this, tell the surgeon, stop using the cautery, and figure out what's going on. Use an FiO_2 of 0.3 for thoracic cases when possible and appropriate for just this reason.—**RSB**

- Secretions are the enemy—remove them—especially during emergence.—**SMF**

- An airway in the ICU is automatically one grade more difficult than the same airway on the operating table.—**MEH**

***Note from the Editors:** Speaking of complications and troubleshooting… this is the collapse of the Fern Hollow Bridge in Frick Park (Fig. 161.8).

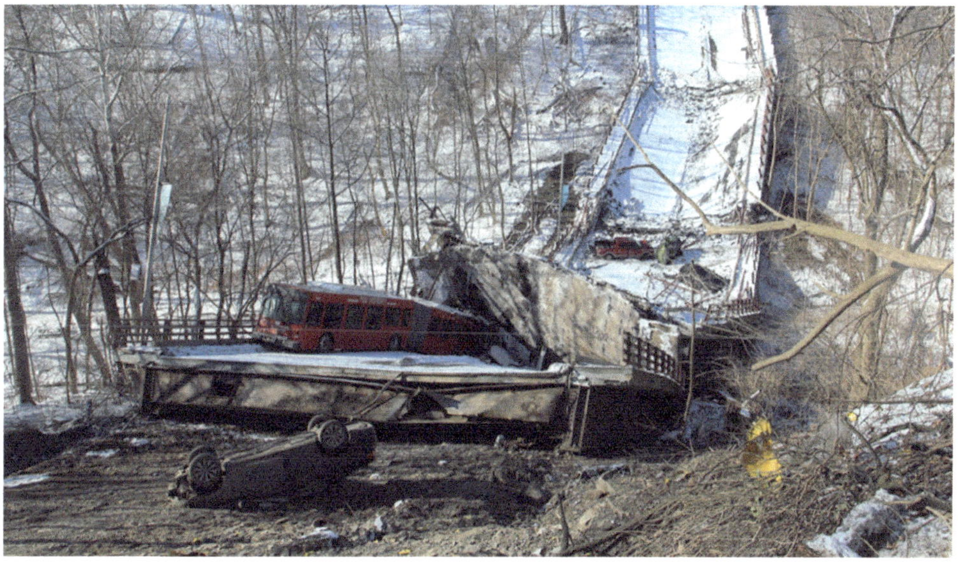

Fig. 161.8 This bridge in a Pittsburgh park collapsed on the same day that federal executives, including the President, were scheduled to visit the city to highlight the need for ongoing infrastructure rehabilitation. By the grace of the universe, there were no fatalities in this catastrophic bridge failure. Photo: Image from ntsb.gov (public domain) https://www.ntsb.gov/news/press-releases/Pages/NR20240221.aspx

Extubation

- The Difficult Airway Society mentioned above has guidelines for the Extubation of the Difficult Airway. Find them at https://das.uk.com/guidelines.—**Editors**
- If you needed a certain position to intubate a patient, you should place them in the same position for extubation in case you need to reintubate.—**SLO**
- Let's say it again—wear your mask and eye protection both during intubation and, more importantly, during extubation! You are much more likely to get sprayed in the face during extubation.—**HWH**
- Do not underestimate the possibility that the patient will cough up a mucous plug after extubation and obstruct the airway. I once had a patient who had a large upper abdominal tumor that was causing preoperative hypoinflation of the lungs. I extubated the patient without any difficulty after a very quick open-and-close case, but he was a heavy smoker, and he coughed on the stretcher before leaving the room. He completely obstructed his airway with a mucous plug and arrested. I had about 90 s to get him reintubated and suctioned enough to resuscitate. I remember that **Brad Winters** came over from the ICU to help me when he heard the stat call to the room.—**CM**
- There's really no reason for a "rocky" emergence and extubation. It happens when you are trying to do too much at once and when you have rapidly changing but mismatched levels, of anesthetic agent and neuromuscular blockade (NMB) at the same time. Just go into emergence and extubation with

a 20 ml syringe of propofol ready. If you are not going to make a smooth landing, give enough propofol so that you can reset your emergence and extubation conditions and make a second pass at the landing strip.—**CM**

- Think about it—if the patient still has some NMB onboard but not anesthesia, they will be flopping about, and a half induction dose will give you the amnesia and time for the patient to regain strength while you gently assist ventilation for a few minutes. If the patient has too much neuromuscular recovery for the inhalational anesthesia onboard and starts moving wildly when the drapes are still up, a half-induction dose of propofol will give you time to let the surgeons finish and get the volatile anesthetic onboard. Yes, it's going to add a bit of time to the case but it's better than one of those awful wakeups. My residents have always had fun teasing me about this, "Okay, Cathy, calling to let you know we're getting ready to extubate, I just drew up the propofol." But it works.—**CM**

- For a case that is more than several hours long or if the patient has been lateral or prone, always deflate the ETT cuff before extubating to make sure there is a leak and the absence of tracheal edema.—**Editors**

- About 1/3 of serious airway events happen when the patient has been successfully intubated at some point. This could involve an ETT change, an inadvertent extubation, or even a planned extubation. *Never* leave the OR if you think you might have to reintubate.—**Editors**

- The late **Dr. James Schauble**, who was one of the old guard at Hopkins, always used to say that a smooth, controlled, and quick but safe emergence and extubation was the hallmark of the expert anesthesiologist. As he said, "Lots of people are taught to intubate—emergency room physicians do it, respiratory therapists do it, technicians and corpsmen do it in the field. And you can really give almost anything to induce general anesthesia. Emergence and extubation are much more interesting and difficult to do well. And we are the only ones thinking about that and teaching it." And of course, he was totally correct about this.—**CM, AJR, and RSB**

Airway Wisdom in 200 Words

- Never stop learning about the airway and how to manage it. This includes simulator training and keeping your skills current on fiberoptic intubation.

- It is critically important that you keep up with Guidelines from the ASA, SPA, DAS, and ANZCA.

- Nobody completely keeps up with the journals. Everybody gets a bit behind and has to toss or delete unread stuff from time to time. But at least scan the abstracts of the airway articles. Attend the airway talks and workshops at conferences, even as you become a senior anesthesiologist.

- Peek into the critical care, military, and surgical journals every once in a while, for airway content and case series and reports.

- Use every airway device and do every awake intubation that you can. Seek them out. This is our particular area of expertise.

- Your first try is your best chance! Don't do "quick looks."
- The simple, old-fashioned red Eschmann stylet has saved thousands and thousands of airways. Ask any senior person. Never be without one in your airway kit.
- While you are querying the senior people, ask them to tell you about the biggest airway surprise they ever got into.
- ***Humility, always.***

More Basic Airway Wisdom from *Avoiding Common Anesthesia Errors, 2nd Edition*

There is a wealth of additional tips, teaching tidbits, and overall airway wisdom in our previous book, which is nicknamed "Green2." The above advice builds on the collected clinical pearls in that book. *Please* get a copy and check out this information as the airway chapters are especially packed full of valuable clinical points (if we do say so ourselves) and remember that every single penny of royalties from this book goes to FAER in perpetuity!

Green2 Chapters with More Basic Airway Wisdom

- Basics of Airway Management (Part I)—Always Keep in Mind Complications That Can Occur with Existing Endotracheal Tubes and Tracheal Extubation.
- Basics of Airway Management (Part 2)—(More Tips and Tidbits to Read on the Train).
- Optimize the Airway: Bag-Mask Ventilation.
- Optimize the Airway: Direct Laryngoscopy.
- Advantages and Disadvantages of the Laryngeal Mask Airway.
- Avoiding Challenges with Video Laryngoscopy.
- Do Not Overinflate the Cuff of the Endotracheal Tube.
- Consider the Use of Lidocaine in the Cuff of the Endotracheal Tube, But Beware the Risks and Alternatives.
- Anesthesia for Awake Intubations.
- Awake Intubations—Being Able to Do Them Comfortably and Safely for the Patient Is the Benchmark for the Airway Expert.

References

1. Chrimes N. The Vortex: a universal 'high-acuity implementation tool' for emergency airway management. Br J Anaesth. 2016;117(Suppl 1):i20–7.
2. Mecham EM, Hopf HW. A proposal to minimize work area contamination during induction. Anesthesiology. 2012;116(3):712.
3. Elwood T, Stillions DM, et al. Nasotracheal intubation: a randomized trial of two methods. Anesthesiology. 2002;96(1):51–3.
4. Jain D, Kumar R, et al. Tips and tricks to improve video laryngoscopy skills. Airway. 2021;4:163–7.

Authors

Steve Orebaugh is a senior anesthesiologist in the UPMC system where his career-long interests have been management of the difficult airway (true airway guru!) and regional anesthesia.

Kirk Lalwani is a senior pediatric anesthesiologist and pediatric airway expert at OHSU. He is known for his clinical acumen and calm and effective teaching style on the difficult airway (and everything else).

Sharon Kapulek is a senior anesthesiologist and the departmental airway expert at UNC—Chapel Hill. She has a particular interest in the laryngeal mask airway.

Harriet Hopf is a senior anesthesiologist at the University of Utah. She is a dedicated anesthesiology educator in all aspects of airway management.

Mike Axley is a senior anesthesiologist in private practice the Portland, OR area. He practiced and taught airway skills for many years at OHSU.

Brian Gierl is a senior neuro-anesthesiologist and fellowship director in the UPMC system in Pittsburgh, PA. He is particularly interested in the difficult airway in the acute neuro-anesthesiology and/or acute neurosurgery patient.

Cathy Marcucci is a senior anesthesiologist who has taught airway management techniques to residents and trainees in the Hopkins, University of Maryland, and Penn systems.

Wisdom on Advanced Airway Management: Pediatric and Obstetrical Airways, Double-Lumen Endotracheal Tubes, the Surgical Airway, and More

162

Kirk Lalwani, Brandon M. Togioka, Edward J. Damrose, and Catherine Marcucci

Contributors:

Ronald S. Bank, MD (RSB)

Brian T. Gierl, MD (BTG)

Vincent L. Hoellerich, MD (VLH)

Harriet W. Hopf, MD (HWH)

Sharon T. Kapulek, MD (STK)

David C. Mayer, MD (DCM)

Introduction

Anesthesiologists must master advanced airway techniques and management, as well as the basics. This requires a commitment to lifelong learning and an ongoing quest for ways to optimize airway management for pediatric and obstetrical patients and patients who require surgical airways or one-lung ventilation. Several experts share their collected wisdom below.

K. Lalwani
Department of Anesthesiology and Perioperative Medicine, Oregon Health and Science University, Portland, OR, USA

B. M. Togioka · E. J. Damrose
Department of Otolaryngology - Head and Neck Surgery, Department of Anesthesiology, Perioperative and Pain Medicine, Stanford University, Palo Alto, CA, USA

C. Marcucci (✉)
Department of Transfusion Medicine, Clinical Center, National Institutes of Health, Bethesda, MD, USA

S. Mohamed et al. (eds.), *Anesthesia Bridges*, https://doi.org/10.1007/978-3-032-08294-7_162

Pediatric Airway Management

Basics of the Pediatric Airway

- First, don't let your knowledge of the basic and crucial pediatric airway differences lapse! We study it for the boards and then sometimes sort of let them go out of our minds. We believe these should be on that electronic index card you look at every month when you pay your bills online. Here they are.—**KL**

  1. Neonates and infants have tiny mandibles and relatively big tongues compared to adults, so there's a lot less room in the mouth for airflow. For mask ventilation, your fingers should be on the edge of the mandible, not on the middle of the submental area, as that pushes the tongue up and can obstruct airflow.

  2. The larynx is higher and more anterior, so you will get a better view in neonates and young infants by bending down and looking along an upward axis rather than towering above and looking downwards. Many pediatric anesthesiologists raise the table and sit down to intubate these patients.

  3. The big tongue needs to be swept aside effectively for a view. Place your scope in the mouth starting in a sideways position, and as you straighten the scope out sweep the tongue off to the side.

  4. The floppy epiglottis loves to slip off your straight blade and obstruct your view, especially when you manipulate the larynx or apply cricoid pressure.

  5. Positioning the airway properly is half of your view. Slight cervical flexion (or at least not extension) with atlanto-occipital extension (sniffing position) makes a huge difference. This is easy to achieve with a roll of towel placed under the lower part of the neck.

  6. The subglottis is soft and collapsible in infants, so cricoid pressure often does one or two things: obstructs the airway so gentle ventilation is impossible, and often also pushes the larynx to one side so you have no view. These can be remedied by gently reducing the pressure on the larynx and moving your assistant's hand gently to the left or right until the larynx comes into view, respectively.

  7. The subglottis is the narrowest part of the pediatric airway. So always check the leak around the tube so it is not too tight (leaks at high pressure >25 cm H_2O or not at all), or too loose (leaks below 15 cm H_2O). The latter will get worse if there is a change in compliance, like laparoscopic surgery or the prone position, so if in doubt, use a bigger tube.

***Note from the Editors:** We went looking for a really tiny bridge since this section is all about the tiny airway (Fig. 162.1).

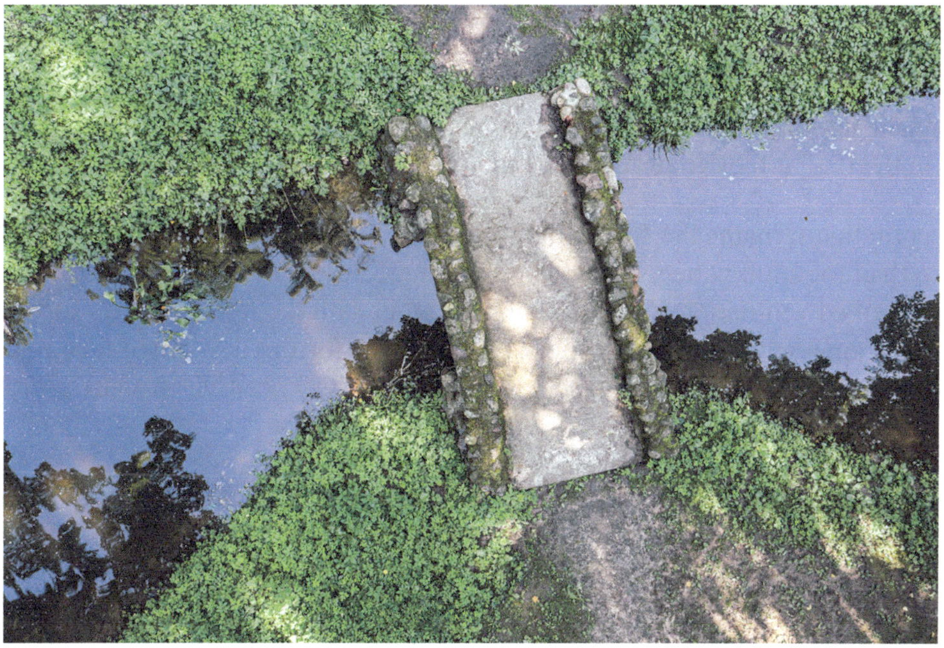

Fig. 162.1 A tiny bridge that is only one stepping stone long, reinforced with pebbles. Photo: Mr_Twister, image used under license from iStock.com

Endotracheal Tubes

- Here are the approximate sizes of endotracheal tubes (ETTs) for the kiddies:
  - Preemie: 2.5–3 uncuffed.
  - Neonate/term: 3.0 cuffed or 3.5 uncuffed.
  - 0–9 m: 3.5 cuffed
  - 9–18 m: 4.0 cuffed
  - 18 m–3y: 4.5 cuffed
  - 4y: 5.0 cuffed
  - 6–8y: 5.5 cuffed
  - All ranges approximate of course.
- A way to "calculate" pediatric ETT size is as follows: length of patient in centimeters/20 will give you a good estimate of the appropriate size. For example, a patient who is 110 cm long—110/20 = 5.5 ETT or for an 80 cm patient, 80 cm/20 = 4.0 ETT and so forth. If you don't know their length, you could also compare the EET diameter to the diameter of their ring finger.—**KL**

- It's so important to remember that you have less margin and less time when dealing with a kiddie airway, even a "normal" uncomplicated airway. Everything happens faster.—**Editors**

- Once, we saw an anesthesia team drop the mask during an extubation. The little patient coughed and desaturated in the time it took to turn around and get a new mask.—**Editors**

- Bag-mask ventilation remains the foundation of airway management for pediatric patients, perhaps even more so than for adult patients. There aren't a huge number of cases done these days with face masks and controlled ventilation for adults. Contrast this with the mask airways for general anesthesia done in the rooms with 20 myringotomy cases posted for the day. Also, face mask airways are used as airway interventions at times—such as the mask airway positive pressure used to break bronchospasm in a pediatric patient for general anesthesia.—**Editors**

- For the really little patients, two fingers on the mask and one finger on the mandible.—**Editors**

- Pediatric intubation is all about technique, not brute force. You should *not* have to use your forearm and arm muscles to lift the infant's head off the table to get a view (shudder!). To learn proper technique and prevent the aforementioned travesty, practice intubating while holding your laryngoscope near the blade base with your thumb and first 2 fingers only; this will prevent you from using the brute force of your limb muscles to levitate the child's head, and if your technique is good, allow you to intubate virtually all children with finesse and minimal force.—**KL**

- Tube getting stuck at the point of entry into the larynx during nasal, bougie or fiberoptic intubation (FOI)? It's the bevel. You can disengage the cords, rotate so that the bevel is oriented anteriorly and readvance, or rotate the ETT 360° for several turns (until the distal part eventually turns around), and it will pop right in.—**KL**

- Desaturation after intubation and definitely in the trachea? Assume right mainstem intubation unless proved otherwise. Remember, distances are small in infants, so even a perfectly placed tube with the head in extension may be right mainstem when you put the head in the neutral position. If head flexion is the plan for surgery, like a posterior fossa craniotomy, check the position of the tube with the head in a neutral position before taping it.—**KL**

- Neonates need a high initial pressure to open their tiny alveoli with the first couple of breaths during manual ventilation. After that, maintaining some PEEP keeps them open, but if you have difficulty seeing chest rise when you start positive pressure manual ventilation and are not inflating the stomach (use an airway!), continue with higher pressures until you open the air sacs up.—**KL**

- The best treatment for laryngospasm is… wait for it… *PREVENTION!* Extubate either fully awake or deeply anesthetized, not in between. Take your time. Babies take a while to wake up, sometimes prematurely (no pun intended) before they are actually ready to wake up. Plenty of repeated suction (palatoplasty and tonsillectomy patients merit gentle suction to a limited depth with a soft suction catheter) removes secretions that can fall on the cords and cause laryngospasm. Other common causes? Your patient is not deep enough, like a hefty teenager having an LMA placed with inadequate propofol dosage, and oral or nasal intubation with inadequate depth of anesthesia if not using a muscle relaxant.—**KL**

- If you do have laryngospasm, try conservative measures but don't wait too long!! Give the succinylcholine *before* the patient is rapidly desaturating and/or bradycardic. There's no shame in laryngospasm, only in failing to treat it soon enough.—**KL**

- The other editors emailed me to ask if I ever extubate a pediatric patient under the drapes or before the drapes are completely down. My answer was... *nope, never*. You'd be in a bad situation if the kid vomited or went into laryngospasm under the drapes!—**KL**

Pediatric Difficult Airways

- First and foremost, maintain the appropriate level of clinical vigilance and even suspicion. It's sometimes a bit of a shock to anesthesia trainees when they encounter their first pediatric difficult airway—**Editors**

- Remember, a significant percentage of congenital and genetic syndromes and malformations involve the head and neck. And syndromes that involve the connective tissue also often involve the head and neck.—**KL**

- Here are the conditions that are typically associated with difficult airways. This is important for board examinations, but of course also for real-life practice. These kids can be every bit as difficult to intubate as the hardest adult airway.—**Editors**

  * Pierre-Robin sequence (PRS).

  * Goldenhar syndrome.

  * Treacher-Collins syndrome.

  * Apert's, Pfeiffer's, other craniofacial syndromes.

  * Klippel-Feil syndrome.

  * Mucopolysaccharidoses—especially Hunter-Hurler and Morquio's syndrome.

  * Beckwith-Wiedemann syndrome.

  * Trisomy 21 (Down syndrome).

- There has been an interesting evolution in airway management for patients with Trisomy 21 over the last 30 years. Many of the editors and authors were taught that every patient should have a recent radiologic evaluation of the cervical neck before airway manipulation and management. This is often not possible within the constraints of the modern perioperative timeline. Generally, radiographic studies are only indicated in Trisomy 21 kids if they have symptoms of neck issues or neurologic signs. A simple neck radiographic study may be sufficiently sensitive if this is under consideration and there is some literature to support this practice change. This is actually important for all anesthesiologists since there are many adult Trisomy 21 patients presenting to the OR [4, 5].—**KL**

- Drooling is a very strong sign of a compromised airway. It indicates an inability to handle secretions. Very bad sign indeed.—**Editors**

- Don't try to alter the head and neck position of a child with a compromised airway. They have already reflexively put themselves into the position that best maintains airway patency—upright with head extended forward. And you can lose that airway if you try to change it. We have seen inexperienced anesthesiologists get into terrible situations when trying to get a patient to lie reclined for induction. We have also seen children with epiglottitis ride up from the ER, sitting bolt upright in their mother's lap, who was riding on the stretcher.—**Editors**

- Speaking of epiglottitis, it's not only a board's question. Normally, the epiglottis is something that we glance at as we move it out of the way (Fig. 162.1). But acute epiglottitis still happens from time to time. With widespread vaccinations against the inciting infectious agents, it is seen less commonly in young children and is now seen in older children and adults. The average age of patients admitted for epiglottitis is 45 years, although infants less than a year old and adults older than 85 years are considered to be at elevated risk, as well (Fig. 162.1). Around the year 2000, there were about 30 deaths per year in the US due to epiglottitis, although the exact number is not known.—**Editors**

- A patient with epiglottitis becomes one of the highest priority cases in the hospital until the airway is secured, so rally whatever anesthesia troops you can; there's no shame in asking for help.—**Editors**

- I can still remember having such a case come in emergently (is there any other way?) when I was a new attending. **Jim Fackler** is an experienced pediatric anesthesiologist and critical care attending and a great guy, and fortunately for the patient and myself, he was still in the PICU that night. I hadn't even had time to call him yet, but somehow, he heard about it and walked over to help me. I was never so happy to see an OR door swing open in my entire career. *Still grateful to Jim 25+ years later.*—**CM**

***Note from the Editors:** Jim Fackler went to Rush Medical College and so, in his honor, we wanted to include a Chicago bridge (Fig. 162.2).

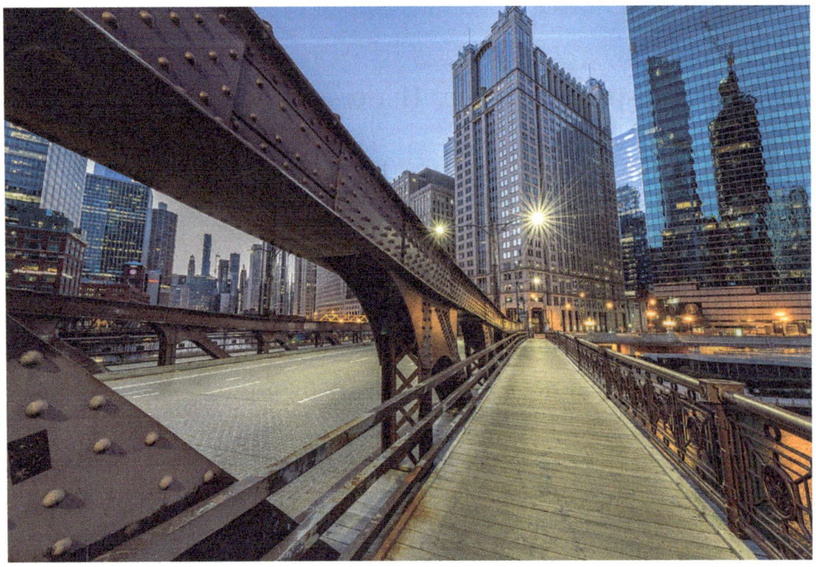

Fig. 162.2 A dramatic perspective view of the Chicago Riverwalk. Photo: Chris DeBasco, image used under standard license from iStock.com

- Be familiar with more recent findings from the *Pediatric Difficult Intubation Registry*. Use video laryngoscopy (VL) first rather than direct laryngoscopy (DL) for higher first-pass success rates; use high flow supplemental oxygen during attempts for apneic oxygenation that increase time to desaturation; more than two attempts result in higher complication rates, so follow the established principles and make your first attempt your best.—**KL**

- Learn how to intubate blind with a gum elastic bougie. Its simplicity is its strength. Practice electively on routine patients by dropping the epiglottis after DL to obscure the cords and arytenoids, then use a bougie with a hockey stick bend at the tip and probe above and behind the epiglottis while *rotating gently* from left to right, seeking out the elusive opening while keeping the esophageal opening in view. If you've practiced it a dozen times before, you're halfway to success already!—**KL**

- When you are just learning to intubate, you can work on your "blind" bougie placement by first doing a DL to distract the airway tissues a bit, just to get the feel of sliding the bougie though the cords. Put the anterior surface of the bougie on the posterior surface of the epiglottis. And then try the technique without direct laryngoscopy or with an intentionally poor DL view. Use your most gentle hands to avoid just fishing around in the back of the throat but don't psych yourself out, a whole lot of anesthetic technique is placing the tip of needles and catheters blindly.—**BTG and Editors**

- Fiberoptic intubation has no age limit! It can be performed in neonates and even premature babies (there are neonatal fiberoptic scopes that you can use with neonatal ETTs). One thing to remember is that you need to scale down movements of your scope to millimeters at a time, not centimeters, as you will rush past oropharyngeal structures like a speeding train into the esophagus and then be puzzled at how you got into this pink wonderland with no cords in sight. So, very, very minimal incremental advances of your scope will allow you to identify structures on your way in rather than going too far on your first attempt. Early glycopyrrolate is your friend for minimizing secretions and bradycardia.—**KL**

- Awake or lightly sedated FOI needs great topicalization if you don't want to induce general anesthesia beforehand. Don't forget nebulized lidocaine 4% in preop, as many kids will be comfortable with nebulizers and take to it quite happily from the parent, leaving you with a comfortably numb airway.—**KL**

- Don't be hesitant to use combined techniques. Too much lingual or oropharyngeal tissue collapsing your world view? Use a laryngoscope or video laryngoscope to lift the tissues out of the way and ask your friendly assistant to hold the scope while you now perform unencumbered FOI. Can't see past the oropharynx? Consider an LMA and then intubate through the LMA after ensuring your patient is deep enough and breathing spontaneously, giving you plenty of time. Goopy scope with obstructed view after going through nose boogers? Guide the scope out through the mouth, wipe clean, "anti-fog it," and slip back in and proceed. Difficulty with nasal intubation? Intubate orally first and secure the tube. Now take your time with the nasal and use the oral as a visual guide to make the switch when positioned near the vocal.—**KL**.

- Have a Plan A, B, and C for elective difficult airways using multiple strategies without causing trauma. Never hesitate to have an ENT colleague and a tracheostomy kit in the room and ready to go in critically difficult situations. Better to have them there early than trying to find one in extremis! —**KL**

Airways in the OB Suite and OB Airways for Non-Obstetrical Cases

- The incidence of aspiration pneumonia in pregnant women is very low. There are no randomized, controlled trials supporting the routine use of oral non-particulate antacids before cesarean delivery. Non-particulate antacids taste bad, and they cause nausea and vomiting. How then should one proceed? Most expert witnesses would testify that the use of nonparticulate antacids before Cesarean Section is the standard of care. There are no expert parturients to testify that it tastes bad.—**BMT**

- We onetime had a parturient who had reported eating shrimp scampi the night before to celebrate a special occasion. She vomited the entire undigested meal during delivery. This was an unforgettable illustration of "parturients are full stomachs *always*."—**Editors**

- It's a bit ironic, though—NPO status has a much greater impact upon our clinical decision making in obstetrics than asthma, but complications related to asthma are significantly more common. In the United States, bronchial asthma is the most common chronic disease of pregnancy, with an estimated prevalence of 8%. About half of these patients will experience an asthma attack during pregnancy. Carboprost is contraindicated in these patients.—**Editors**

- Remember the rule of one-thirds—a third of patients with bronchial asthma will improve during pregnancy, a third will experience no change in symptoms, and a third will experience a worsening of symptoms. It's not completely understood why, but it is likely a combination of factors, including an increased incidence of gastroesophageal reflux disease, undertreatment due to concern that asthma medications may impact fetal development, and a higher incidence of respiratory tract infections.—**Editors**

- Severity of asthma during pregnancy can be predicted by assessing pre-pregnancy asthma severity and planned compliance with pre-pregnancy asthma medications. Patients with severe pre-pregnancy asthma are much more likely to experience exacerbations requiring hospitalization or emergency department visits, compared to patients with mild intermittent asthma. Similarly, patients who remain on their pre-pregnancy asthma medications are much less likely to experience severe exacerbations.—**Editors**

- Some patients prefer to halt or decrease use of asthma medications during pregnancy out of concern for fetal well-being. Some studies have shown an association between chronic asthma medications and preterm births, low birth weight, and congenital malformations. However, it may be an exacerbation of asthma that is associated with malformation, not asthma treatment.—**Editors**

- In fact, we were facetiously taught that the last three questions of a preoperative interview, even if it is in the seconds before an emergent general anesthesia should be, "Do you have asthma, do you have asthma, do you have asthma?"—**CM**

- Consider all the patients that come through your labor and delivery suite each year. One out of 50 is a potential difficult intubation, and 1 out of 800 is a failed intubation. Early epidural analgesia allows you to avoid airway instrumentation in these patients.—**BMT**

- The best way to avoid general endotracheal anesthesia on the labor floor is regular communication with your obstetric colleagues and frequent assessment of your patients with epidural labor analgesia.—**BMT**

- If you have hypoxia after intubating a pregnant patient evaluate the position of the distal end of the endotracheal tube. It is easy to mainstem a pregnant patient. The gravid uterus can displace chest contents cephalad, shortening the distance from the teeth to the carina.—**BMT**

- Let's think about the use of LMAs in pregnant women and parturient. They are definitely not indicated for first-line airway management, but in an emergency, you take what you can get, and I would not hesitate to use one if a life-threatening situation were upon me.—**BMT**

- We recommend that, if you do get into a situation where you are relying on an LMA, you have somebody hold cricoid pressure while the LMA is in the airway.—**BMT and CM**

- If you have to use an LMA, you should be able to titrate the bag and your hands to avoid excessive pressures. Try to avoid high peak inspiratory pressures and keep a bit of pressure in the circuit at other times. Or better yet just gently assist spontaneous ventilation.—**Editors**

- Have a low threshold for controlling the airway in the case of an obstetrical emergency—this includes the bleeding emergencies and also the dreadful complications of air or amniotic fluid embolism. Sadly, maternal mortality still exists, and nobody should get to the point of being coded without a controlled airway.—**Editors**

- Remember that the delivery room has two patients who might need airway management. It's not unheard of for the OB anesthesiologist, at some point, to help manage the baby's airway, either to establish a mask airway or even to intubate. It's not a terrible idea to spend time with the pediatric anesthesiologists from time to time to keep your skills up on the tiny patients.—**Editors**

- I was taught that you learn emergency airway techniques to use them in the OB suite! Truly, you may need to use every single advanced airway skill you have in an emergency situation, and you must use them all, if necessary. Because there just is no emergency like an OB emergency. Don't believe us? Read the three patient anecdotes below!—**CM**

- Before we had readily available video laryngoscopes, I had a parturient that was unable to be intubated and unable to be mask-ventilated. We were also unable to ventilate through an LMA. The patient was on the table for an emergent cesarean delivery for fetal bradycardia. I performed a percutaneous needle cricothyroidotomy with a 14G angiocath and used jet ventilation until backup arrived. Ventilation was not fantastic in a pregnant woman in the supine position, but it kept her alive until a video laryngoscope arrived. A colleague used the video laryngoscope to intubate. I did not let the obstetricians cut the patient's skin until the patient was intubated. Amazingly, the baby ended up being ok.—**BMT**

- During fellowship (1991), where I was the sole anesthesiologist on call in L and D a patient needed an urgent C-section. Prior to my arrival on call, a resident had attempted a labor epidural but got a dural puncture, so the attending suggested threading an intrathecal catheter. It was so-so for labor, and she did not want it replaced. Dosing her spinal catheter failed to achieve a surgical block so GETA with rapid sequence induction was planned. The airway exam was not worrisome.—**DCM**(1 of 2)

- Unfortunately, I failed to see the vocal cords with two different blades. No LMA and no bougie or videoscopes at this time. Called for help from the main hospital. Mask ventilation was not successful, and the patient desaturated to 30% and severe bradycardia was present. I did a needle cricothyroidotomy with jet ventilation, and the heart rate and SpO_2 returned to normal. The patient was still not emerging, though. Fortunately, the fetal heart rate was still OK. During over-aggressive jet ventilation, the patient developed severe soft tissue crackles, and it was clear that some of the jet ventilation was going into soft tissues. The patient's neck enlarged so much that the 14 g catheter was no longer in airway. The SpO_2 dropped again, and patient went into ventricular tachycardia. The obstetrician and I started formal cricothyrotomy, but tissue edema made it nearly impossible. The general surgeon showed up just then and completed the trach successfully, and the patient did not code. In the ICU next day, she stated that they could not intubate her two years prior at another hospital.—**DCM** (2 of 2)

- The most difficult airway situation I ever had in the OB suite was when I was a CA-3. The patient weighed well over 200 kg and had extreme upper body and neck obesity. She came crashing back with some sort of bleeding emergency—I can't remember exactly what it was, but it was bad. There was a loud, chaotic scene. The patient was hysterical and uncooperative, and we couldn't get or keep an oxygen mask on her. She did have an IV, though. There wasn't time to do an awake FOB, and her BMI was too high, and she was too panicked, to do the case under local. My attending looked at me and said very, very quickly and softly, "This patient and the baby are probably going to die."—**CM** (1 of 2)

- I still don't know what made me do it, but I leaned over her on the OR table and said forcefully, "Brandi, open your mouth or you and the baby will die!" Which was absolutely true, but something I have never said to a patient before or since. At any rate, she opened her mouth, I did an awake direct laryngoscopy, saw the cords, and intubated awake before she knew what was happening. The attending grabbed a syringe, induced general anesthesia, the surgeons did an emergency section (and I think maybe hysterectomy?), and everybody lived. The baby was fine. I still have mixed feelings and some rueful regrets about what I did, intubating her completely awake like that, and also about what I said to stop the thrashing and get her to open her mouth. But we had no other option. We just had no other option. I distinctly remember that the OB sent me flowers several days later, but my mother (a non-medical person) was appalled when I told her about it. But, in truly emergent situations, you do what you have to do. Fortunately, the patient didn't remember much of even going back to the OR and left the hospital with a beautiful baby girl. Editor's note: Brandi isn't her real name.—**CM** (2 of 2)

***Note from the Editors:** There are several beautiful urban bridges featured in this chapter, but we still love green bridges in green gardens the best. Why, you may ask? Because in the US at least, that's the color of oxygen (Fig. 162.3).

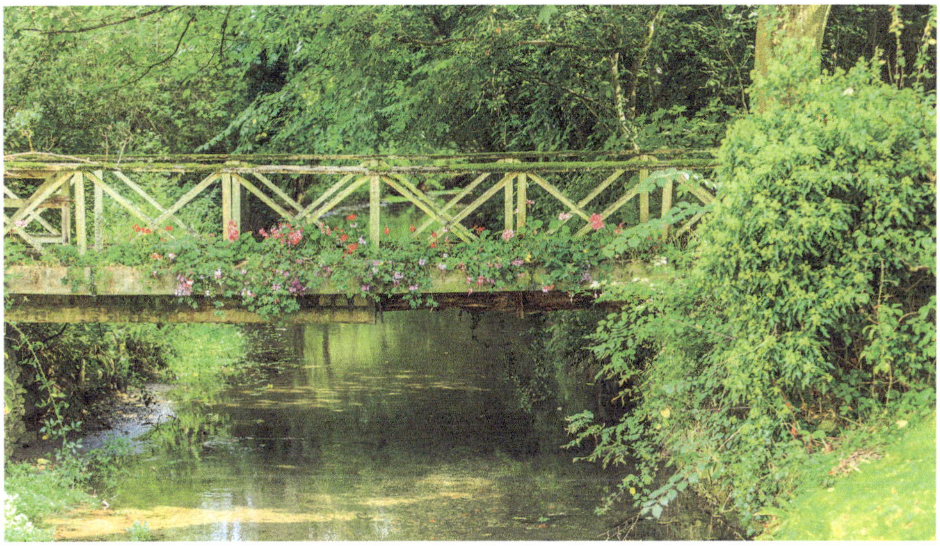

Fig. 162.3 A rustic bridge in a verdant pastoral landscape. This bridge is so green, it's got its own flower boxes. Photo: Image used under standard license from stock.adobe.com

General Airway Wisdom from Our ENT Surgical Colleagues

General Thoughts

- The value of the preoperative endoscopic airway assessment (PEAE) cannot be overemphasized. For your otolaryngologic patients, more often than not they have already undergone a fiberoptic laryngoscopy, which may already be videorecorded, or at least the findings documented somewhere in the medical record. Take a moment to review these preoperatively. If an exam has not been performed or documented, do it yourself—there is much knowledge to be gained by looking before you leap.—**EJD**

- Spend time with ENT colleagues in their clinics to gain experience with fiberoptic laryngoscopy if you feel your skills need brushing up.—**EJD**

- Stridor, even if faint or in a seemingly asymptomatic patient, is a red flag. These patients merit PEAE prior to consideration of general anesthesia.—**EJD**

- Likewise, the history of airway surgery/reconstruction is another red flag. The surgical changes that reconstructive surgery may induce can affect your anesthetic plan—consider PEAE prior to proceeding to surgery.—**EJD**

- Beware of the patient who has had prior anterior neck surgery—especially thyroidectomy or anterior cervical disk fusion—who presents for revision surgery. Recurrent laryngeal nerve injury and a concomitant unilateral vocal cord paralysis can be silent. A new injury on the side of the only working recurrent nerve will precipitate bilateral vocal cord paralysis, which may be appreciated for the first time once the patient is extubated. These patients can present with stridor in the OR or in the PACU and may need reintubation or tracheostomy.—**EJD**

- Beware of the "coroner's clot"—congealed blood that accumulates in the nasopharynx, especially after nasal surgeries such as septoplasty, endoscopic sinus surgery, or adenoidectomy. Suctioning of the oropharynx only may leave this mass of clot behind, whereupon extubation and the first deep breath by a patient, it may be aspirated into the distal airway, and result in asphyxiation. Make sure to suction the nasopharynx in these situations prior to extubation.—**EJD**

- Vocal cord paralysis can result from laryngeal mask airways, likely from overinflation of a poorly fitting device, or from endotracheal intubation with a cuff that sits in the subglottis. Take time to ensure your devices are positioned appropriately.—**EJD**

Other Potential Difficult Situations

Adult Trisomy 21 Patients

- Due to increased lifespans, it is estimated that there are now more adult Trisomy 21 patients than pediatric patients. Besides congenital laxity of the atlanto-axial ligaments, degenerative cervical spine disease occurs in up to 60% of adult patients. This can include cervical stenosis. Have a low threshold with flexion/extension radiographic studies with a neurological evaluation if any of the following are elucidated on preoperative exam: neck pain, abnormal neck posture, falls or stumbling, decrement in fine motor skills, hyperreflexia, or ataxia.—**Editors**

- As with pediatric Trisomy 21 patients, routine cervical imaging for asymptomatic individuals is not recommended, but cervical spine positioning precautions with in-line stabilization may be performed during intubation for all patients [1–3].—**Editors**

- Besides cervical spine issues, Trisomy 21 patients can have other airway issues, including a small oral opening, large anterior tongue, and supraglottic or subglottic stenosis, so both mask airway and intubation may be more technically difficult.—**Editors**

- In some studies, the incidence of obstructive sleep apnea is as high as 85% in adult Trisomy 21 patients. Body habitus and derangements in pulmonary physiology may predispose to more rapid apneic desaturation. Gastroesophageal reflux is also very common in this patient cohort.—**Editors**

Ludwig's Angina

- Ludwig's angina is septic cellulitis of the submandibular, submental, or sublingual spaces, almost always an extension of a peri-molar abscess of the second or third molars. It can happen pre-extraction or post-extraction of the offending tooth. The clinical situation can arise very rapidly, even in a matter of hours. This means that you will see Ludwig's angina patients during evening call hours. There is no "waiting until morning for these patients"—either at home, downstairs in the ED bay, or on the floor.—**Editors**

- Anesthesiologists are generally familiar with the head and neck manifestations, but must remember that in severe cases, the infection can extend into the thoracic cavity and pericardium and can also be the prime etiology of septic shock or pre-shock physiology. And don't be fooled by a lack of apparent large abscess on the alveolar ridge of the mouth because often the dentition and gums look fairly benign.—**Editors**

- It is imperative that the anesthesia team works with the surgical team from the time the patient arrives. The patient should never be left unattended.—**Editors**

- These patients should have the standard airway exam, but this is one of the situations when tongue mobility has clinical relevance. Tongue mobility is a fairly unique consideration in the Ludwig's patient, as the disease process itself involves the submandibular space, which may become edematous and hardened.—**Editors**

- This is one of the situations where the first attempt to secure the airway must include the ability to do a definitive airway—surgical, if necessary. *No "quick looks" in these patients while you are waiting for equipment or the surgeons to arrive.*—**Editors**

- Remember that topicalization of the airway can be challenging, as infected tissues are likely to be acidotic Local anesthetics have poor penetration through nerve membranes in acidotic tissue.—**Editors**

- An experienced surgeon must be at the bedside, ready to do an awake tracheostomy if necessary. For every Ludwig's angina patient that we have seen, this meant at the bedside, with the trach tray opened.—**CM and Editors**

- Take great care not to "crash induce" the patient once the airway is secured. The patient's hemodynamics might not support it.—**Editors**

- Ketamine is a good drug to consider for these patients. They can have small amounts titrated during an awake airway and then a careful induction.—**Editors**

- These patients also need a compassionate post-op visit to answer questions, especially if there was an awake airway. In general, we have found that the patients are okay with the conservative airway management they received. They knew and understood that they were in big trouble.—**Editors**

***Note from the Editors:** To show our appreciation for the *Anesthesia Bridges* editors, authors, and contributors who are in or love New York City, we asked several young friends to send us original photos of their favorite NYC bridges. This interesting structure is the High Line on Manhattan's West Side (Fig. 162.4).

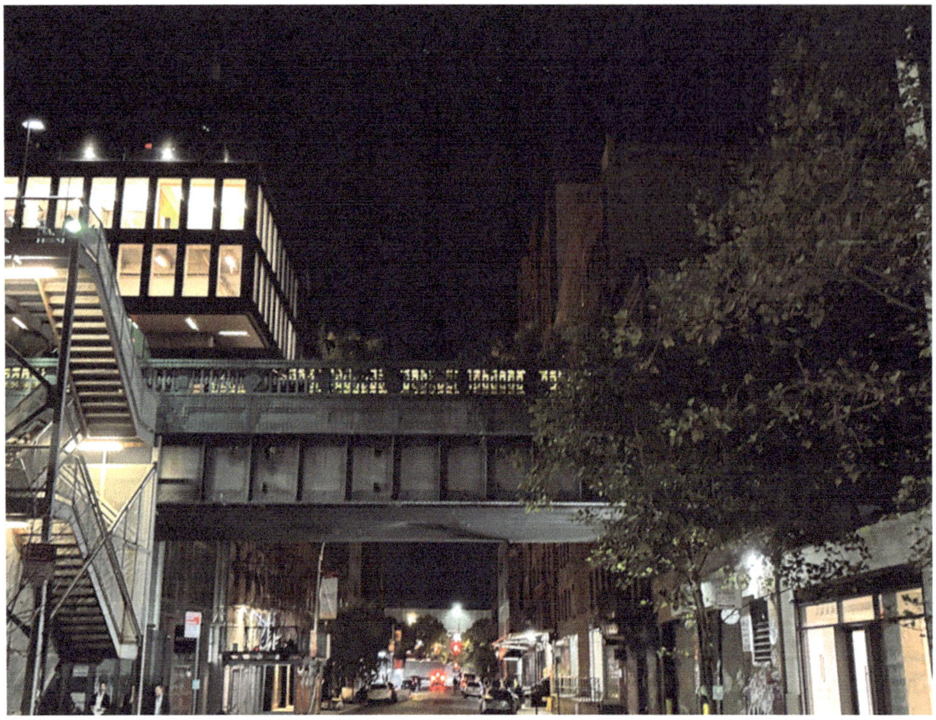

Fig. 162.4 A beautiful night view of the High Line in Manhattan. It is a former elevated freight line that is now a cherished public park two stories above the busy city streets. It is operated and maintained by the Friends of the High Line. We love the architectural quality of the stairs and the way the pattern in the railing mimics the design of the windows in the overlooking building. Photo: Josh Stich

Facial Hair

- Ask your preoperative evaluation people if they will consider "giving patients the option" to shave their facial hair before the day of surgery. Admittedly, this is a bit tricky because we don't want to give the impression that dealing with facial hair is beyond our basic competency levels. Older people are a bit set in their ways, but young people who wear facial hair often shave it and grow it back on a whim. Perhaps a good way to frame it is simply to say that many patients find that the tape pulls on their facial hair, which pulls on the skin and can cause the facial skin to feel abraded.—**Editors**

- We know of a colleague who keeps an electric razor kit in his lockers for the very instance of a patient who decides on the spur of the moment that the facial hair can go. To address hygiene concerns, he uses a razor with a new disposable head for each new patient. A bit expensive but he doesn't use it every day and it's cheaper than an avoidable airway complication.—**Editors**

- Cover beards with transparent film dressings, for example Tegaderm, to eliminate the leak with mask ventilation. You can use multiple small pieces (my preference) or one large piece with a slit for the mouth. Leave it in place until after you successfully extubate, in case the patient requires mask ventilation again.—**HWH**

- I second Harriet's advice above. And I would add "the bigger the beard, the more the Tegaderm." I have used this trick many times, and it has saved me many times, especially when intubating on the floors or in the ICU.—**BMT**

- In patients with beards or mustaches, incorporate a bit of the mustache into the tape around the ETT for greater security.—**HWH**

Prone Positioning

- Prone positioning requires the utmost careful consideration of the airway—every single time. You have to get through your entire career without losing a single prone (or other) airway. Some tips for the prone position are listed below—yes, you have already heard these, but please just remember that the trick is to make yourself do them every single time. —**Editors**
  - Glycopyrrolate 0.2 mg at the start of the case to reduce the secretions that may dissolve your tape's adhesive.
  - Tape and tie the endotracheal tube, kind of like using a belt and suspenders to keep your pants up.
  - Benzoin and mastisol to make the tape stick better then place transparent IV dressings over everything.

- Never have a situation where the circuit is not supported and pulling on the ET tube—but be careful about tying or taping the circuit to the bed frame to take the weight off the ET tube. The stylet can make a great hook that can be released with one hand if needed.—**Editors**

- You are going to get your patients and yourself into a lot of trouble if you don't think about laryngeal edema in every single prone patient. *At the very least*, you should do a cuff leak test before extubating on every single prone patient.—**Editors**

- We know that laryngeal edema occurs in almost half of *all* patients, although it is often asymptomatic or only minimally clinically relevant. Several independent risk factors are thought to include female gender, ratio of ETT to airway size, emergent intubation, and self-extubation. Interestingly, the length of intubation is not positively correlated with laryngeal edema. But prone and even lateral positioning *are* known risk factors.—**Editors**

- This a situation where a "restrictive" fluid plan is in order. A starting point in your clinical plan could be 3 mL/kg/hr. That said, you have to deal with bleeding that is actually occurring, and you have to keep the kidneys perfused and the eyes perfused. And we know that the purple drugs are not a true substitute for volume in keeping an adequate perfusion pressure. But this is what was used in a study that evaluated a restrictive resuscitation protocol vs. liberal resuscitation (5 mL/kg/hr. plus replacement of urine volume) [4].—**CM**

- Pay close attention to your initial visual and instinctual impression when you turn the patient supine and look at their face and eyes. As we discuss elsewhere, "instinctual" clinical judgement is actually built on experience. Generally, we advise that you don't have a junior trainee extubate somebody who was prone without taking a look at the patient and being present in the room. If you think, "Wow, really swollen!" *then put the patient's head up and leave the patient intubated!* You don't want to safely safeguard the ETT and airway while the patient is prone and then lose control of it at the end of the case. Everybody will get over it, and an hour may make a difference. The worst that will happen, if the patient is otherwise stable, is that you get a reputation for being a really cautious and careful airway manager. So be it.—**Editors**

Surgical Airway

- Know how to do a surgical airway!—**RSB**
- When I teach this, I usually say it exactly how I heard it at The Difficult Airway Course—Anesthesia, a few years back: "*Know when and know how*." This is so utterly critical in both respects. Too often, it's tried too late, if at all.—**RSB**
- I think that it's very important to practice front-of-neck airways (FONAs) with the exact equipment that one has at their institution on pig tracheas (or similar model) annually. I don't think that there is any better substitute for this. Under stress, one has to be familiar with the surgical equipment and how to do this technique. Despite the fact that we have 24/7 trauma surgery support to do FONAs at our institution, as well as a DAR (Difficult Airway Response) team (I was the lead on this), I still arrange for this training for my group on a Saturday morning in Jan or Feb. It's well attended.—**RSB**
- Preparation for that one lifesaving cricothyroidotomy you may have to perform over the course of your career begins with a thorough physical examination of each of your patients. It is essential to palpate or ultrasound every one of your patients' necks to improve your skill at identifying the cricothyroid membrane.—**STK**
- Once the patient is under general anesthesia, palpate the neck again. Head and neck position can change after induction and the previously noted landmarks may disappear. Determine how to position the neck quickly in the event of an emergency. Placement of a shoulder roll, pulling the chest skin down while pulling the neck skin under the mandible upwards, can optimize access to the surgical site, but only if you think to do so.—**STK**
- For an *adult* patient:
- Stand with your dominant hand in the cephalad position. Palpate the cricoid membrane—below the thyroid cartilage and above the cricoid cartilage—it is the exact location where the transtracheal lidocaine block is performed.
- If time, ask for a no. 15 blade if no time, any blade will do. Using your dominant hand, make a midline incision, moving from foot to head, about 4 cm long. Use enough pressure to reach the cricoid membrane in two passes of the blade.

- Palpate for the cricoid membrane. Once you find the membrane, use the scalpel poke through vertically.

- Once you have entered the airway, always maintain some type of instrument in the trachea until the airway is finally secured. If there is any ventilation taking place, you will hear burbling sounds and see bubbling in the field.

- Turn the blade 90° and widen the tracheotomy by 0.5 cm in each direction. Insert a rigid suction catheter into the site and remove the scalpel.

- "Intubate" the tracheotomy site with a 6.0 styletted ETT with the tip bent to a 75° angle with a curving motion towards the feet. Watch the cuff pass 1–2 cm below the caudal end of the incision.

- Gently inflate the cuff, remove the stylet, and check for adequate ventilation and CO_2 return. Use gentle ventilation. Aggressive ventilation if the ETT has been misplaced into a tissue plane in the neck can cause extreme worsening of the clinical emergency.

- Do not let go of the ETT until it has been sewn in place.

<u>Notes:</u> bleeding should be controlled with suctioning or pressure/packing only. Cautery should not be used due to the risk of airway fire. The patient should be seen as soon as possible by an otolaryngology for initial evaluation and assessment. Do not worry about aesthetics; this was a life-saving procedure. Scars can be repaired, and the surgeons have experience in reconstruction, if necessary.

- Many societies also recommend the scalpel-finger-bougie technique, so we wanted to give that a mention. This is the study behind it—everybody needs to read this paper [5]. Here are the thesis and conclusion of the paper:

Background: Surgical airway creation has a high potential for disaster. Conventional methods can be cumbersome and require special instruments. A simple method utilizing three steps and readily available equipment exists, but has yet to be adequately tested.

Conclusion: The three-step method, using an elastic bougie with an endotracheal tube, was shown to require fewer total hand movements, took less time to complete, resulted in more successful airway placement, and had fewer complications compared with traditional cricothyroidotomy.

***Note from the Editors:** A surgical airway is like traversing this treacherous bridge—you just have to get your patient and yourself to the other side (Fig. 162.5).

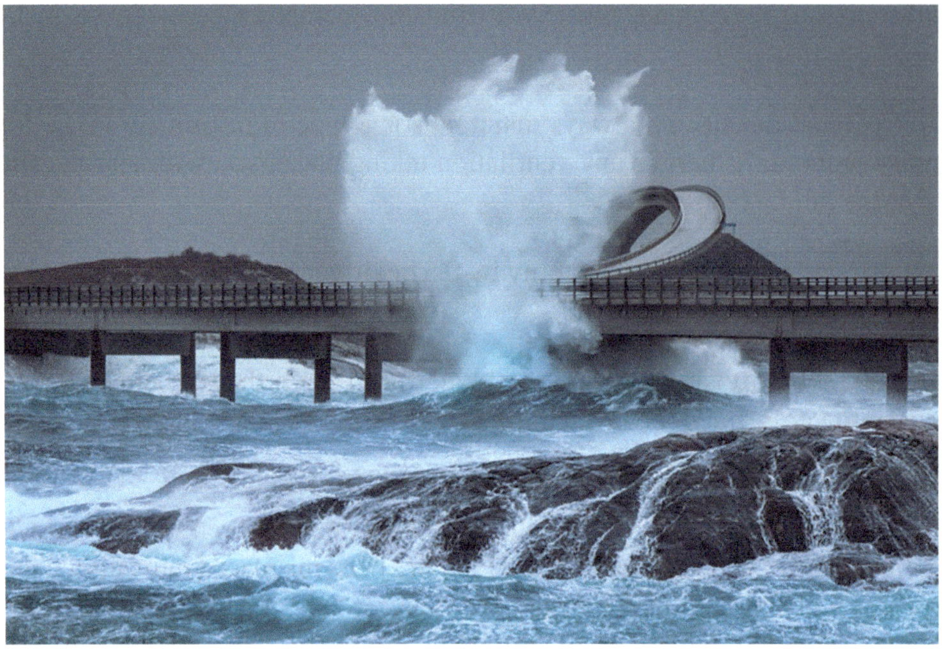

Fig. 162.5 The scary Storseisundet Bridge in Norway. Photo: Image used under standard license from iStock.com

Additional Wisdom on the Surgical Airway from Ed Damrose

- Practice front of neck access at least twice a year. You must be able to secure the airway as fast as possible, ideally in less than 60 seconds. Seek simulator training on these techniques if available at your institution or at conferences. Ask your ENT colleagues for help in getting this done.—**EJD and Editors**

- No patient should die from loss of the airway without an attempt at a cricothyrotomy—this is difficult to defend legally, and hard to explain to a patient's family when they ask if you did all you could do to save their loved one. And remember, people do it on airplanes. You are going to be expected to have knowledge and some level of expertise on these techniques.—**EJD**

- And *do not hesitate* to ask the ENT or OLHN surgeons to be in the room with a trach kit nearby (or even open!) if you feel that might be necessary. We truly don't mind and will break somebody out—even a senior resident—to standby. We'd much rather be there electively than called emergently.—**EJD**

- A knife is something to intubate and to ventilate with—carry one with you in your emergency airway pack!—**EJD**

- When performing emergency cricothyrotomy, the only thing that matters is speed. No survivor will care about their scar.—**EJD**

- When considering cricothyrotomy, remember there is nothing you could possibly do to the patient that is worse than anoxic brain injury or death. Every complication you can think of is fixable by your ENT colleagues. *Repair and reconstruction are much simpler than resurrection.* And remember that an anesthesiologist doing a surgical airway is the very definition of "emergency."—**EJD and Editors**

- When performing a cricothyrotomy, make big incisions—you have a higher likelihood of entering the airway at some point—even if it's not through the cricothyroid membrane. Remember the airway is mostly air—accessing anywhere inside of it is a win for the patient.—**EJD**

Laser Surgery

- You *must* have the proper endotracheal tube for laser surgery. No laser-appropriate ETT available—no laser surgery. The editors are aware of at least one case when the anesthesiologist was pressured to do a laser case without the appropriate ETT. An airway fire resulted with catastrophic results, including the patient's eventual death.—**Editors**

- Laser surgery should *not* be done with 100% inspired oxygen.—**Editors**

- We have seen surgeons set *themselves* on fire with the laser. Not joking!—**Editors**

Single Lung Ventilation

- First of all—use the precise terms. There is a tendency to use the terms "up" and "down" when talking about single-lung ventilation. But what is the "down" lung? Is it the collapsed lung that is not being ventilated or the dependent lung in the lateral position that is being ventilated? It's much more precise to use the terms "dependent lung" or "ventilated lung" or "isolated lung." After you clamp the bronchial lumen, the question to ask the surgeons is, "do you have adequate lung isolation?" instead of, "is the lung down?"—**CM**

- Thoracic cases are a good opportunity to review the physiology of PEEP and V/Q mismatch, which we do in Chap. 153.—**Editors**

- The first question you should ask when intubating with a double lumen endotracheal tube (DL ETT) isn't, "Do we have lung isolation?" The first question should be, "Is the ETT in the trachea, and if so, where is it in the trachea?"—**CM**

- People who do not place DL ETTs regularly often try to go for the complete placement all in one rapid, overly brisk thrust of the tube into the airway and then immediately clamp the bronchial lumen in the hopes that they nailed it on the first try. But it's too much distance in the multiverse, and there are too many variables to get the bronchial lumen from being held in your hand at the head of the bed to the correct position in the correct bronchus in one big swoop. It's better to do it gently and efficiently in two stages. So, when placing a left-sided DL ETT:

  - First, under direct laryngoscopy, intubate the trachea with the bronchial lumen, then the tracheal lumen until you see the tracheal cuff just go through the cords. Don't worry about getting the exact placement, just get it in the trachea. Bronchial cuff goes up, tracheal lumen gets clamped, where are your breath sounds? That tells you where your bronchial lumen is. If you have left-sided breath sounds only, you're basically done. This happens more than you think.

  - If you have bilateral breath sounds, then the bronchial lumen is still above the cords, and you have to advance and position the DL ETT a bit more.

  - Next, both cuffs down, under DL, rotate the DL ETT 90° towards the bronchial lumen side while advancing a moderate amount. People often under-rotate and over-advance. If you have to "exaggerate" any of the motions, over-rotate. Then, both cuffs up, where are your breath sounds? They should be bilateral. If not, then you've over-advanced and the tracheal lumen is at the carina or down the left bronchus. You'll have to withdraw a bit under DL. But if not, then, clamp the tracheal lumen—where are your breath sounds? If correctly placed, they should be on the left side only. Then, finally, both cuffs up, clamp the bronchial lumen, to reverse check. Should have right-sided breath sounds only.

  - This sequence allows you to check and correct proximal and distal location in the trachea, as well as placement of the bronchial lumen, just with auscultation.

- I was taught to confirm placement of the DL, ETT clinically, using auscultation only and then only use FOB to double-confirm placement by viewing the carina through the tracheal lumen and the cuff of the small lumen just below the carina.—**CM**

- You want to be able to confidently place a DL ETT even if you don't have FOB available. It's surprisingly difficult to use a FOB as a "stylet" to get the bronchial tube in place because often you don't know where the distal end of the FOB is located.—**CM**

- Generally, problems with achieving lung isolation on initial placement of the DL ETT happen because the tube is in too far. If you begin to have problems with high-pressure alarms and ventilating the dependent lung during the case, the usual problem is that the bronchial cuff is partially obstructing the carina.—**CM**

- But the problems with achieving lung isolation after the turn are also sometimes that the ETT has often pulled back a bit if not properly supported during the turn.—**CM**

- Be wary of over-taping a DL ETT. You need perhaps twice the amount of tape as for a SL ETT, not five times as much. Don't put so much tape on that you can't move the tube a millimeter or two without untaping; the tip of the DLT will move relative to the carina if the patient is moved for the procedure.—**CM**

- But, that said, be extremely careful about trying to seriously adjust or reposition a DL ETT after the patient is turned and positioned. I have seen so much trouble happen, including the extubation of the entire trachea. I agree that you should recheck by auscultation, not just by FOB, that you have lung separation after you turn but before the patient is secured on the armrest.—**CM**

- If you've lost lung isolation and feel you will need to reposition with the FOB, consider turning back to the supine position and working with the DL ETT that way. The surgeons are not going to be thrilled about it, but may prefer that to not having lung isolation. It's just too risky and difficult to try to untape the ETT and bronch the patient in a lateral position while bending and twisting your body to get in the plane of airway.—**CM**

- The above steps are ideal for teaching placement of a DL ETT, but the same basic principles hold true even when you are doing thoracic cases in a busy private practice. When positioning a double-lumen ETT, we still take time using the fiberoptic bronchoscope to ensure ideal position. When listening for bilateral and then unilateral breath sounds, if it doesn't sound right, it's probably not right. We do not hesitate to check again for proper positioning, both before and after turning the patient lateral, taking as much time as we need. The surgeons feel it's a good trade.—**VLH**

- I never was completely expert at placing a right-sided DL ETT and I did a two-year thoracic anesthesia fellowship and did *a lot* of thoracic cases for the first 5 years of my clinical practice, and then regularly have done chest cases for the balance. I did them, but was never as confident about it. Something about the take-off of the right main bronchus? Not sure. So, I just decided to get really good at using left-sided DL ETT with the opposite scheme of applying the clamps if we needed right lung isolation.—**CM**

- Be careful when you apply the clamp to the DL ETT for lung isolation! Once, I saw somebody absentmindedly pick up a pair of scissors instead of a clamp and cut the top of the DL ETT clean through.—**CM**

- If lung isolation doesn't happen, it doesn't happen. You want this to be a rare request, rare indeed, and it's not ideal, but the surgeons can pack the operative field with wet towels to deal with a lung that's partially inflating when it's not supposed to be. It's happened to me once or twice in my career. The surgeons were nice about it.—**CM**

- One trick is to place a suction catheter down the bronchial lumen to deal with slow insufflation of the isolated lung.—**CM**

- We are aware of the current thinking on not over-inflating the lungs during anesthesia, but feel there is still a place for ventilation strategies to minimize atelectasis in the dependent lung.—**Editors**

- *Respect the double lumen tube change!!!* Changing out a double lumen ETT to a single lumen ETT is one of the most dangerous things that we do. Have a good and consistent plan to do so. When I was in training, this was always done with two anesthesiologists in the room. Be sure that the room understands that you're performing a critical procedure.—**RSB**

- If the airway was difficult in the first place or if the airway is now significantly edematous or bloody, consider leaving the DL ETT in place. If it's not safe, it's not safe. The ICU may fuss a bit, but they will just have to deal with it. We have seen attempts to change the DL ETT result in emergent tracheostomies. The repair of the thoracic problem was a success, but the airway wasn't. *NOBODY* was very happy that day, instead of just the ICU being unhappy. Apologize and offer to buy them a double chocolate-chip cheesecake, and remember that we're all on the same team. They'll get over it. And you might get the patient back in the OR a day or so later to do the ETT change to a single lumen if prolonged intubation is planned.—**CM**

- You should work to become proficient in each "next-generation" or alternative technique for single lung ventilation, such as placement of an EZ-Blocker. Scott Mittman taught me a great pearl for using this approach to single lung ventilation. While the EZ-Blocker is not steerable, if the device can't be advanced to straddle the carina due to not being centered w/the carina, you can use external manual manipulation of the larynx to center the blocker over the carina. I've used this many times. It's a great technique. It also works well for not only the EZ Blocker but also for the Fuji Blocker and other similar devices.—**RSB**

***Note from the Editors:** To show our appreciation for the *Anesthesia Bridges* editors, authors, and contributors in Oregon, here is the Benson Bridge at Multnomah Falls (Fig. 162.6).

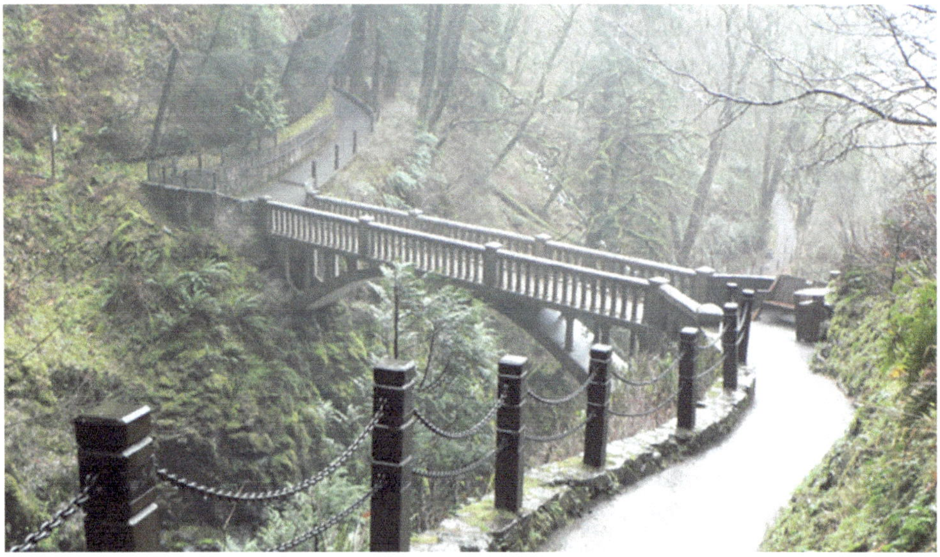

Fig. 162.6 The Benson Bridge, looking away from the waterfall. Photo: Emma Bailey, pinesnvines.com

Jet Ventilation

- We include this topic here not because it is inherently difficult per se, but you must know what you are doing as jet ventilation (JV) requires focused training. Seek these cases out in your training. Or if you are way past training and need brushing up, do that with airway courses and seminars on jet ventilation. Make sure you know how to do this case, one way or the other.—**Editors**

- Jet ventilation (JV) has a low risk/benefit ratio in the hands of experienced people but requires good communication with the surgeons. It is the ventilation technique of choice for a number of airway situations when it is advantageous to have access to the maximum space in the airway or if the clinical situation mandates limited ventilation-associated movement such as ablation of ectopic heartbeats or ablation of liver tumors.—**Editors**

- Jet ventilation cases are suitable only for total intravenous anesthesia. And every anesthetizing location where JV is used must have the capability for conventional ventilation. No exceptions to either of these.—**Editors**

- Remember that jet ventilation can be done via a standard endotracheal tube as long as the connection between the ETT and jet ventilator allows for passive extubation.—**Editors**

- Insufficient oxygenation with jet ventilation is something *that must be solved*. Remember that JV has been associated with acute pneumothorax, so that requires emergent management. Slow decreases in oxygenation can be addressed with increases in inspired oxygen concentration, moderate increases in jet ventilation driving pressures, repositioning to infra-glottic ventilation, intermittent positive pressure ventilation, or conversion to standard ventilation.—**Editors**

- Insufficient carbon dioxide elimination is usually addressed by increasing the driving pressure. You could theoretically increase the driving pressure to the pressure of the gas sources (about 55–65 psi), but <50 psi is generally considered the acceptable pressure limit. In general, the upper limit of acceptable $PaCO_2$ is about 1.5 times the baseline value. CO_2 should be corrected to baseline at the end of the case with conventional ventilation via ETT or LMA.—**Editors**

- Although there are definite indications for JV, there are some special consideration and complications of JV—insufficient expiratory time, barotrauma to the entire airway below the catheter, dislodging of foreign bodies or fracture of airway tumors, incomplete control of the airway, and limited methods to monitor gas exchange and pulmonary mechanics. You have to know these complications thoroughly and maintain high vigilance. JV is a specialized technique—even so, you aren't going to be able to claim lack of familiarity as a reason for not proactively dealing with the possibility or occurrence of these events.—**Editors**

- Kids can also undergo jet ventilation! Driving pressures should start at 5–10 psi and be increased gradually until chest rise and fall is noted or to a max <30 psi.—**Editors**

Airway Trauma

- This is not the situation to demonstrate how creative you are by doing anything needlessly complicated. The first and final goal is to figure out a way to get oxygen to the tissues. The simplest and fastest method is what is called for, even if that is an awake trach.—**Editors**

- The more complicated the airway trauma/damage, the simpler the intubating aids you will need. The fanciest fiberoptic scope isn't going to be much help if all you would be able to see is blood. We were taught that the really damaged airways are done as much by feel as by sight. And the things that help you are bougies and wires and so forth.—**Editors**

- If you think there is any likelihood of supra-laryngeal trauma or fracture, go straight to the low surgical airway.—**Editors**

- Airways for trauma patients are sometimes done with little or no anesthesia or neuromuscular blockade, depending on the clinical situation. That doesn't mean you don't give an amnestic agent later. We had a senior, legendary faculty member who often gave scopolamine 0.8 mg after the airway was secured if the patient was sufficiently stable. Of course, IV scopolamine is no longer available in the US (transdermal patches are), so this isn't an option today. The point is to at least think about amnesia—midazolam has been reported to cause retrograde amnesia, so that is one possibility.—**Editors**

- Head, neck, and chest crepitus indicate a fracture somewhere in the airway. *This is a true emergency airway situation.* Never underestimate the difficulty of securing such an airway. If you feel crepitus on the chest wall, assume that there is also involvement of the para-tracheal tissues.—**Editors**

- If you ever have exposure to people who have to intubate in the field or who have trained in developing countries, pump them for information as to what they have seen and done. Yes, we have advanced modern techniques to show them, but they have things to show us as well, so be polite and humble and soak up all the details you can.—**Editors**

- The military sometimes sends its special forces medical personnel to the Baltimore hospitals to observe hospital care of trauma cases and practice intubations. These soldiers have some incredible stories to tell, especially the Air Force pararescue teams. They do interosseous access as readily as we do venous access, and they intubate on the sides of mountains and while swinging from helicopters (not joking). Honestly, we have not been too proud to ask them exactly how they did that.—**Editors**

- We also have colleagues who have worked with visiting anesthesiologists from Afghanistan. These physicians can do retrograde wire-guided intubations for difficult airways with astonishing ease. Most US anesthesiologists have done few or no intubations using a retrograde wire. But the *possibility* of that technique is one reason to routinely do transtracheal lidocaine for awake intubations—just to remain comfortable with crossing the cricothyroid membrane.—**Editors**

Airway Cases

Putting it all together, here are two airway cases from **Ron Bank.**

Case 1: Neck Mass

About 10 years ago, I was asked to care for a woman who was a recent immigrant with no prior medical care. She presented with a huge goiter. Her trachea was compressed to a couple of millimeters.

I assembled a multi-disciplinary team consisting of anesthesia, ENT, trauma surgeons, respiratory therapy, and others. After much discussion, we decided that we'd do the thyroidectomy in the cardiovascular suite. Plan A was to place wires under local for veno-veno ECMO prior to an attempt at an awake FOB intubation. ENT was there with a rigid scope. The trauma surgeon was there for an emergent surgical airway although the goiter was so large that this would likely not be possible. We had heliox on the anesthesia machine. We had an interpreter for the patient present at all times.

After careful airway anesthesia, fortunately I was able to do an awake FOB with a small armored, ETT and all went well. It was very reassuring to have all of the people and equipment for plans B, C, and D in the room, on the same page. During the debrief, the common theme was how great a professional experience it was and how well all the departments worked together.

This was a great airway case to point out the value of thinking outside of the usual airway box to the point of having our cardiac surgical colleagues and ECMO team involved.

Editor's note: This is also the rare situation where an inhalational induction with a spontaneous breathing patient can be considered.

Case 2: Neck Fusion

I was asked to take care of a lady with ankylosing spondylitis who the team was unable to intubate at another area hospital. I saw that her neck was fused in extreme flexion such that an emergent surgical airway would not be possible. I was able to do an awake FOB, and the surgery went as planned. I took care of her for two subsequent surgeries via the same technique. For many years she kindly sent us a Christmas card and a note of appreciation. This was yet another case in which I was so grateful for the airway mentors of my residency imploring me to become adept at doing awake intubations.

Advanced Airway Wisdom in 200 Words

- The routine pediatric airway is about anatomy, gentle and sophisticated technique, and prevention—of bradycardia, laryngospasm, and everything else.
- The difficult pediatric airway is about recognizing who is at risk.
- Epiglottitis is now seen in adults as well as children!
- Managing the airway in obstetrical patients is about arranging the entire anesthetic plan to minimize the need for general anesthesia. And if you have to do an emergent or difficult airway, the prime goal is to *safely* get oxygen to the mother and baby. You must understand the physiology of the gravid patient and the implications for desaturation and ventilation.
- Consult and confer with the surgeons early and often—could you do a surgical airway today?
- You could get a request for one-lung ventilation at any time, especially if you do trauma cases. How comfortable would you be if you had to do one tomorrow? And remember, the most critical aspect of one-lung ventilation is making sure you get and keep the trachea intubated! Once you position your patient with a DLETT, you can't really substantially reposition it. Don't turn the patient over to the surgeons until you are comfortable with the placement.
- How you manage a difficult airway is not really about where or how you put the tube, it's really about how you manage the time in preparing to secure that airway. And always think about how you would explain it in a deposition. Why you did or could take the time to do certain preparation and maneuvers and why you didn't or couldn't.—**Editors**
- ***Vigilance (and humility), always!***

More Advanced Airway Wisdom from *Avoiding Common Anesthesia Errors, 2nd Edition*

There are many additional tips and teaching tidbits, and additional advanced airway wisdom in our previous book, which is also known as "Green2." Even the titles of the Green2 chapters can be read as individual clinical pearls. All royalties go to FAER in perpetuity, so please get a copy and check it out!

- The Child with a URI.
- Accept That You Will Have to Meet the Clinical Challenges of Obesity and Obstructive Sleep Apnea in Your Pediatric Patients.
- Double Down on Pediatric Airway Equipment.
- Optimizing Bag Mask Ventilation and Direct Laryngoscopy in Children.
- Why You Should Expect Hypoxemia During Induction and Emergence of the Pediatric Patient and What to Do About It.
- When Not to Extubate Deep! And If the Patient Is Already Coughing or Swallowing, It's Too Late Anyway.
- An Easy Intubation Does Not Guarantee an Easy Reintubation—Especially After a Carotid Endarterectomy or Cervical Spine Surgery.
- Plan for an Airway Fire with Every Head and Neck Case.
- There are Special Considerations Involved with Both Intubation and Chronic Airway Management of Burn Patients.
- This Is No Time for Wishful Thinking: Always Troubleshoot an Increase in Peak Airway Pressure.
- The Key to the Smooth and Skilled Placement and Use of Double-Lumen Endotracheal Tubes Is to Take It One Step at a Time.
- Airway Management in the ICU, Including the Dreaded Leaking Cuff—How to Bring Your Best Game.
- Ludwig's Angina.
- Jet Ventilation—How to Adequately Handle This Exotic Ventilation Technique and Earn the Admiration of Your Spectators.
- High-Frequency Jet Ventilation—the View from Philadelphia.

- Know How to Perform a Cricothyroidotomy.
- Don't Make the Mistake of Thinking That a Tracheostomy Is a Guaranteed Airway.
- Helium for the Compromised Airway—You Have to Understand the Principles and Properties but We've Seen Some Amazing Saves.

References

1. Bouchard M, Bauer JM, et al. An updated algorithm for radiographic screening of upper cervical instability in patients with Down syndrome. Spine Deform. 2019;7(6):950–6.
2. Hengartner AC, Whelan R, et al. Evaluation of 2011 AAP cervical spine screening guidelines for children with Down syndrome. Childs Nerv Syst. 2020;36(11):2609–14.
3. Malinzak EB. Perioperative care of adults with Down syndrome: a narrative review. Can J Anaesth. Published online 24 June 2021.
4. Jan R, Alahal A, et al. Effect of two regimens of fluid administration on airway edema in prone-position surgery. Anesth Essays Res. 2020;14(3):467–73.
5. Quick JA, MacIntyre AD, et al. Emergent surgical airway: comparison of the three-step method and conventional cricothyroidotomy utilizing high-fidelity simulation. J Emerg Med. 2014;46(2):304–7.

Authors

Kirk Lalwani is a senior pediatric anesthesiology at OHSU. His primary philosophies and techniques for the difficult pediatric airway are based on the principles of preemption and prevention.

Brandon Togioka is a senior OB anesthesiologist at OHSU. He firmly believes and teaches that there is no such thing as a "routine" airway in the OB suite.

Edward Damrose is a senior OLHN surgeon at Stanford with special interests and expertise in laryngeal surgery. We thank him for taking the time to send us airway wisdom and advice from the surgical side of the drapes.

Cathy Marcucci is a senior anesthesiologist who believes the best way to handle a difficult airway is to never be more than two minutes away from an awake, spontaneously breathing patient.

Wisdom on Regional Anesthesia and Pain Medicine

163

Steven L. Orebaugh, Raymond G. Graber, Rita B. Merman, Catherine Marcucci, and Anis Dizdarevic

Contributors:

Ronald S. Bank, MD (RSB)

Denis L. Bourke, MD (DLB)

Carol F. Bodenheimer, MD (CFB)

Anis Dizdarevic, MD (AD)

Dawn Dillman, MD

Charles W. Emala, MD (CWE)

Joel Feinstein, MD

Raymond G. Graber, MD (RGG)

Ron L. Harter, MD

Vincent L. Hoellerich, MD (VLH)

M. Concetta Lupa, MD

Rajen V. Nathwani, MBBS BSc (RVN)

Logan Olson, PharmD BCCCP (LO)

S. L. Orebaugh
Department of Anesthesiology and Perioperative Medicine, University of Pittsburgh School of Medicine, Pittsburgh, PA, USA

R. G. Graber · R. B. Merman
Department of Anesthesiology and Perioperative Medicine, University Hospitals of Cleveland, Cleveland, OH, USA

C. Marcucci
Department of Transfusion Medicine, Clinical Center, National Institutes of Health, Bethesda, MD, USA

A. Dizdarevic (✉)
Department of Anesthesiology, Columbia University, New York, NY, USA
e-mail: ad2689@cumc.columbia.edu

S. Mohamed et al. (eds.), *Anesthesia Bridges*, https://doi.org/10.1007/978-3-032-08294-7_163

Amy J. Robbins, MD MBA (AJR)

Brandon Togioka. MD (BMT)

Joanna L. Walker, MD (JLW)

David A. Zvara, MD* (DAZ)

Introduction

Regional anesthesia is one of the most exciting areas of anesthesiology. The evidence base is still being established with respect to individual techniques and clinical outcomes as new block techniques are being developed and refined. Working diligently to acquire new skills and maintain expertise is a great way to distinguish yourself in your career.

Regional Anesthesia

General

- Expertise and excellence in performing regional anesthesia (RA) is the same for all aspects of the practice of anesthesiology—knowing the basics and doing them well every time.—**Editors**

- The regional anesthesia websites are great—and experienced anesthesiologists visit them all the time. The American Society of Regional Anesthesia (ASRA) has guidelines on strategies for reducing complications and managing perioperative coagulation medications if RA is planned—these guidelines are periodically updated. The ASRA guidelines website is: www.asra.com/advisory-guidelines. The transfusion medicine service can also help with thoughts about the need for specific lab values and components before a RA procedure is done, as they follow the literature on this closely, because platelets.—**Editors**

- We also regularly review the NYSORA website—yep, even with our senior status. We only wish it had been in existence when we were training. The illustrations for the block techniques are particularly good. It's at NYSORA.com.—**CM**

- Don't avoid RA because the INR is 1.3 or 1.4! This lab value *does not* need to be corrected with fresh frozen plasma. The transfusion medicine folks, ASRA, and NYSORA generally agree that there is adequate perioperative hemostasis with an INR <1.5.—**CM**

- It takes a while before you understand that doing successful regional anesthesia (RA) really requires the buy-in of the nurses, surgeons, and most importantly, the patients—much more than general anesthesia does. RA should not take a lot more time than general anesthesia; if it does, you run the risk of losing the support of the surgeons. But even more important than speed is confidence and smoothness. We were taught that although we already "believe" in RA, we have to make sure everybody else does, as well.—**Editors**

- That said, it's a mistake to view and present regional anesthesia as an either/or situation for the patients. There's always a continuum between regional and intravenous anesthesia and analgesia. They are best used as adjunctive techniques to each other, and that's exactly what we say, "We are planning a combination of anesthesia techniques for you today. Sometimes patients need a bit more intravenous medication, and sometimes they need a bit less." In other words, nobody has "failed" if a competently performed block is done and the patient ends up with deep sedation or even an induction.—**Editors**

- Keep in mind that the regional anesthesia arena has seen a lot of seminal advancements in perioperative care in the last several decades. This includes the vastly increased use of ultrasound, the early recovery after surgery (ERAS) protocols including the incorporation of blocks into cardiac anesthesia, and the decrease in administration of perioperative opioids. No working anesthesiologist—at any career stage—can afford to not work towards increasing and maintaining expertise in regional anesthesia. But remember, no matter how fancy the technique, successful deployment is predicated on the rock-solid knowledge of the nerve and peri-neural anatomy, especially for the long-track nerves.—**Editors**

***Note from the Editors:** Speaking of long tracts, we can convince ourselves that the famous and scary Millau Viaduct has a faint semblance to nervous system architecture (Fig. 163.1).

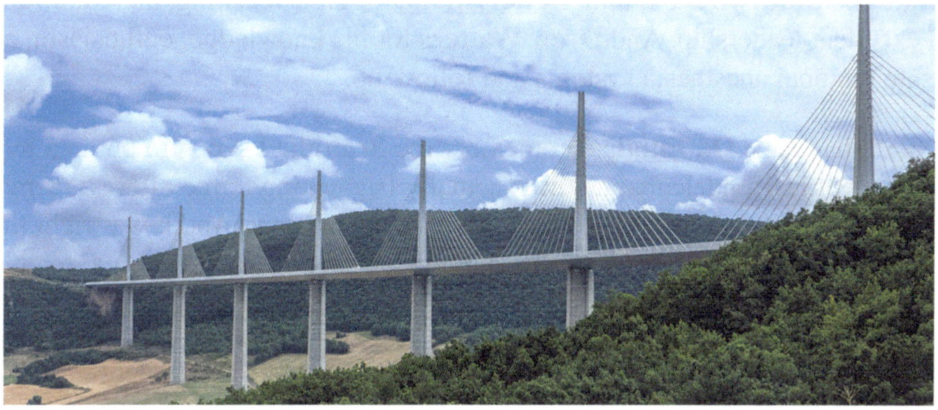

Fig. 163.1 The Millau Viaduct is a remarkable multi-span cable-stayed bridge in southern France. It was completed in 2004 and is the tallest bridge in the world. It carries heavy car traffic between France and Spain. Photo: David Taljat, image for editorial use non-fiction book from iStock.com

- Wrong-side procedures are clearly established by the Joint Commission and pretty much everybody else to be "never" events. It doesn't matter what the surgeons and patients say. If you do a block where there wasn't supposed to be one, accept that you have committed what is basically a legally indefensible act. Call your departmental leadership and risk management people immediately and do exactly what they say to do and nothing that they tell you not to do. The first big decision is whether it's safe to redo the intended block and proceed with the case. In some cases, it may be. You will not be making this decision by yourself. —**Editors**

- *Never* let a consultant dictate the performance or non-performance of regional anesthesia to you. There is no clearance for a specific anesthetic technique, and this includes regional anesthesia.—**Editors**

- As an anesthesiologist with regional technique skills, you may block any part of the body. Refresh your knowledge in anatomy and utilize block techniques whenever possible.—**RBM**

- Name one high-strung or excitable regional anesthesiologist? You can't!—**Editors**

- Have you ever noticed that the practice of regional anesthesia is also sort of mentor-driven? Ask any established anesthesiologist who the best regional anesthesiologist they ever saw was and why they were so great, and almost everybody has no trouble coming up with their answer. We asked the *Anesthesia Bridges* authors and editors this question and are very happy to give a shout-out to their mentors.—**Editors**

Chetta Lupa: Karen Boretsky. Never afraid to learn or teach a thing.

Dawn Dillman: Glenn Woodworth. Knows the anatomy down cold, so could point out and identify all of the things to help you know where you were and what to avoid.

Brandon Togioka: Glenn Woodworth again! No matter how obscured the image, he can always find his target and guide the resident-handled needle to the correct location with his words.

Raj Nathwani: There are two at our unit—**Paul Bhalla** for great teaching, incredible anatomy knowledge, and excellent leadership. And **Drew Walters** for his knowledge, enthusiasm, and use of tech to set up safe regional anesthesia systems and follow-up.

Amy Robbins: It has to be **Dr. Emala.** I remember the first time I saw him put in a hypobaric spinal and put the patient in Trendelenburg, it was actually frightening to me after so many times that we tilted the patient up with a hyperbaric spinal. I was in amazement. And it was right there that I realized the importance of knowing all the approaches and variations to a regional anesthesia technique

Chas Emala: (Srinivasa) Raja. Calm approach and excellent technical talent.

Cathy Marcucci: I agree that **Dr. Raja** was the best! What I also remember is how calm and quiet he was when doing a regional anesthetic technique. There was just no stress or fuss, ever. Even in the old days before the use of ultrasound, instead of a regional anesthesia procedure being something of a metaphorical ordeal, when you were working with Dr. Raja, you ended up thinking, "Hey, why aren't we doing RA for every single patient?"

Ron Harter: JW Chen. He was the department regional expert at Georgetown, where I trained. This was well before ultrasound-guided blocks, and he had a remarkably high success rate for his blocks, which was not easily achieved in that era. He seemed to have a three-dimensional picture in his head of where he needed the needle to go.

Anis Dizdarevic: Anthony Robin Brown. First, because of the passion and love he had for regional anesthesia, and secondly, because of his mentorship and the wisdom and inspiration he provided.

Ray Graber: Jack Fraser was an early mentor of mine—he was the chief at the Cleveland VA at the time. We specifically spent a lot of time working on paramedian spinal and epidural techniques, along with axillary blocks by trans-arterial technique. However, I was self-taught for many of the more recent blocks. I think a good RA doc needs to understand anatomy, know how to use (ultrasound) US effectively, and needs to be continuously learning because the field keeps evolving.

David Zvara: It's *ALL* of the newer generation skilled with ultrasound. A needle can go just about anywhere with extraordinary precision. It's not "who is great," but *Who*.

- We should be able to do the blocks that the surgeons do, with some notable exceptions. What blocks are in the nah-no-thanks category? Retrobulbar and peribulbar blocks, intra-articular lidocaine in knee capsules or other joint spaces, dental blocks done for oral-maxillo-facial surgeries, and transoral retropharyngeal blocks. Also, the circumcision penile block is usually not our domain. One chairperson that we consulted said, "Pudendal blocks. I'm out on that one, too."—**Editors**

- Don't forget the educational outreach! We do blocks for pain control and relief. The rehab medicine folks do blocks not only for pain, but for spasticity control, and functional optimization. We should be consulting and conferencing with our colleagues regularly.—**Editors and CFB**

- Here is an example: Decades, ago, I askedan an anesthesiologist if he thought it was appropriate to do a cervical epidural injection in an outpatient office setting. I was told, "Maybe, if whoever does it is prepared to monitor or even intubate the patient." I went back to my team to discuss our protocols a bit further!—**CFB**

- Expect evolution in your practice and be open and inquisitive to learning and communicating—see next!—**Editors**

- When I started my career in the late '80s, we were doing epidurals for total knees. We would administer epidural morphine to help out with postop analgesia, with the resultant side effects of urinary retention and nausea. Then we switched to epidural infusions for a day or two, but had to pull them out so postop DVT prophylaxis could start, and patients could ambulate. Our next evolution was to add a single-shot femoral nerve block to the intraoperative epidural and postop epidural infusion combo. This worked so well, we switched to spinals and femoral nerve blocks and got rid of the epidural infusion hassle.—**RGG**

- We then moved on to spinal and femoral nerve catheters. This worked really well, but ambulation and physical therapy were problematic. We eventually evolved to shorter spinals with adductor canal blocks, with surgeon infiltration of the joint capsule and through the posterior joint capsule to get the sciatic innervation. Our techniques had to evolve as surgical techniques and expectations changed. What was once an inpatient stay of 5–7 days is now frequently a same-day surgery. In your practice, don't be stagnant—be an evolver. Work with your surgeons as a team to identify goals and help them accomplish them.—**RGG**

- And continue to look for new applications throughout the perioperative period. Regional anesthesia is now used more extensively in the ORs and even burn ICUs for burn patients with improved outcomes.—**Editors**

- If a patient who has received regional anesthesia becomes hemodynamically unstable, the block has to be on the differential until clearly excluded. It's really surprising how often local anesthetic toxicity is missed.—**Editors**

- Local anesthetic toxicity isn't just peri-oral numbness and a metallic taste. It can also initially present as dizziness, drowsiness, dysarthria, dysphoria, agitation, confusion, tinnitus, and other auditory changes. Ask your senior colleagues which of these they have seen.—**Editors**

- Of course, later symptoms include seizure, coma, and hemodynamic (cardiac) collapse. We all pretty know that. What junior people don't realize is how fast local anesthetic toxicity can progress to severe complications and even arrest. I've seen it happen in a matter of minutes.—**CM**

- Back when it first came out, I gave intralipid to an ICU patient and saved them from an arrest (one of my most memorable cases to this day), even though it had to come up from the pharmacy. Today, I would not do regional anesthetic (with a few exceptions) if it wasn't on the block cart or very nearby. Start getting ready to use it at the very first sign of local anesthetic toxicity.—**CM**

- Here is the CYP-450 metabolism of the common anesthetics. Look for inducers and inhibitors of these hepatic enzymes before doing regional anesthesia.—**NBS**

  – <u>Lidocaine</u>—3A4 (primary) and 1A2 (secondary).

  – <u>Bupivacaine</u>—3A4 (primary) and 2D6 (secondary) and 2C19 (secondary).

  – <u>Mepivacaine</u>—1A2 (primary).

  – <u>Ropivacaine</u>—1A2 (primary) and 3A4 (secondary).

  – <u>Chloroprocaine</u>—pseudocholinesterases (plasma) and nonspecific esterases (ocular tissues).

- My favorite local anesthetic is chloroprocaine. It's really not possible to achieve a toxic level, so it can be used in liberal quantities in a "splash block."—**CM**

- Developing an anesthetic plan these days is not so much a question of intravenous anesthesia *or* regional anesthesia. It's more a question of intravenous anesthesia *and which* regional anesthesia. Remember, a patient who is on buprenorphine can roll into your OR at any time. You have to stay current on the latest additions to the basic roster of block techniques.—**Editors**

- Plan for block failure. I was taught to discuss and consent to the salvage blocks upfront. One of my mentors said that pretty everybody knows the basics of the basic blocks and how to get a patient through an anesthetic when the block is dense. What's really important is to demonstrate knowledge and competence (to the patients, surgeons, and board examiners) by a smoothly and expertly executed Plan B.—**CM**

- Follow the block! We are sorry to say we are aware of significantly bad complications and outcomes (in the last 10 years) after a block that perhaps could have been avoided if the patient had had a post-operative visit from the anesthesiologists. These are cases that got into the papers and the internet. Also, remember that chronic regional pain syndromes can develop after apparently uncomplicated regional anesthesia, especially on the extremities.—**Editors**

- Starting in about 2015, the desire for all hospitals to adopt a "system-ness" became the trend in healthcare. Expansion, acquisition, and collaboration of services across multiple hospitals, ambulatory surgical centers, and procedural areas. Suddenly, we weren't only spread out under one roof, we were spread out across dozens of miles. This meant that anesthesiologists had to have extraordinary regional anesthesia skills available in multiple locations, with varying degrees of support. This skill set became a driver for our hiring practice. Someone we "drop" into any location, and they could do it all on their own. This skill, and the ability to communicate to others what they need in the moment, was something we looked for in all our interviews. Today, with the emphasis on ERAS protocols and a de-emphasis on opioid-based anesthetics, RA skills are more important than ever. So don't waste time wondering if you need to get up to speed on the latest the new block—you do.—**DAZ and Editors**

- If the patient experiences significant pain during block placement, *stop the injection!* It seems so simple, but there are so many cases floating around out there of bad outcomes that started with a painful injection.—**Editors**

***Note from the Editors:** We were delighted that David Zvara sent us the picture below as a bonus when he sent us his advice about the importance of regional anesthesia skills in the hiring process (Fig. 163.2).

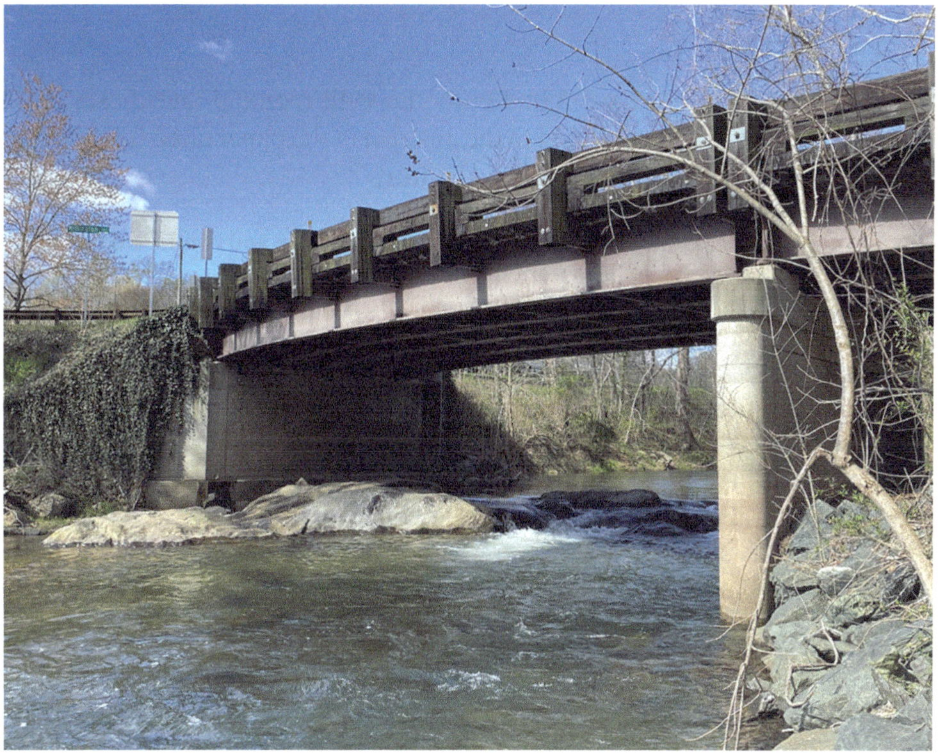

Fig. 163.2 A great photo of a bridge observed while traveling around North Carolina. Photo: David Zvara

- About half the pharmacology questions on my written boards were on local anesthetics. Fortunately, I had done 3 months of OB anesthesia right before finishing my residency and had had lots of time to talk to Chas Emala and Dr. Raja about these medications. They sat the senior residents down and helped us develop a study sheet of all the local anesthetics pertinents—doses, durations, the whole works. Their point was that these were the first anesthetic agents known, and it would be a moral offense to miss even one simple question about them. That sheet was handwritten of course since this was long ago, but I wish I still had it. They even insisted that we know the order of absorption of local anesthetics, we tried to insist back that there wouldn't be such a question on the test—but there was. So here it is.—**CM**

- *Rate of Local Anesthetic Systemic Absorption (Fastest to Slowest).*

  IV > Tracheal > Intercostal > Caudal > Epidural > Brachia Plexus > Lower Limb > Subcutaneous

Ultrasound-Guided Nerve Blocks

- First, the use of ultrasound in performing nerve blocks has been transformational. It is now the sine qua non for a lot of successful regional anesthesia.—**Editors**
- Has the use of US-made regional anesthesia safer? Early evidence showed that ultrasound guidance reduced the incidence of vascular injury, local anesthetic systemic toxicity, pneumothorax, and inadvertent phrenic nerve block. It took a little longer for data to show that acute nerve injury was decreased [1].—**Editors**
- There are still all kinds of ways to have a bad outcome with regional anesthesia, even if with ultrasound guidance. We agree with the statement in the abstract in the paper cited just above [1]. Ultrasound is literally the wand; we remain the magicians.—**Editors**

  > Ultrasound has revolutionized the way we approach regional anesthesia and contributed to patient safety. It is important to note that patient safety does not hinge on one single technology. Patient safety in regional anesthesia relies on a well-trained practitioner to pay meticulous attention to indication, block and patient selection, anatomy, pharmacology, equipment, and technique.

- The *Anesthesia Bridges* editors asked me for my own opinions/practice on use of US in RA in "regular" practice.—**AD**
  - Neuraxial/spinal/epidural certainly could be done without US.
  - Scalp blocks could be, but we often do use US to look for a blood vessel.
  - Intercostobrachial superficial nerve could be done without US, but we tend to use US for more precise injection.
  - Intercostal nerve could be done without US as well, but US makes it safer and more precise, so it is not done as much without.
  - Ankle block could be done without US, but we tend to use it for the tibial nerve block for better and safer injection.
  - Digital blocks and blocks for carpal tunnel could also be done without US, but we typically do not perform those.

- In a foreign and/or low-resource practice where US was not available, we could do the following blocks: ankle block, neuraxial blocks, intercostal blocks, femoral block, axillary block, paravertebral block, popliteal block. Of course, you would need a twitch monitor for some of these.—**AD**

- Without US, in this day and age, I would not do: interscalene, infra and supraclavicular, transversus abdominis plane (TAP) block, rectus block, quadratus lumborum block, PEC blocks, serratus plane block, and parasternal blocks.—**AD**

- When teaching regional anesthesia, start with a gel block for eye-hand coordination and "muscle memory." Learning on a phantom is a reasonable start. But students master this within a couple of minutes. Why is it more difficult to perform peripheral nerve blocks with US guidance in patients? I tell trainees this: people move. They breathe and shift. It's inevitable. You move, subtly, even as you try not to. Needles bend a bit as they traverse tissues and fascial planes. It takes only a fraction of a millimeter of deviation and the needle is no longer visible. The well-imaged needle is a constant pursuit, and it is not shameful to find yourself reacting continuously to the above alterations. "Show me your tip" is the mantra of anesthesiologists who train residents to do these blocks. It takes time and experience to get good at this, but even then, you often find yourself in pursuit of the fabled "needle in a haystack (tissue bed)."—**SLO**

- How then, to image the needle best: I like echogenic needles. I used to favor smooth needles, using them as a sort of "test" for residents. It is more challenging to see the smooth needles for deeper targets/steeper angles. But I've evolved. This is a visual technology. Why should we make it hard? If I truly believe that the best outcome and safety for the patient results from the optimum view of the needle tip as it draws near to the nerve, why would I downgrade this image by using a smooth needle. Others would argue with this, given a higher price for echogenic needles, but in educational circumstances, I think they are the right answer. This may be different in a private practice, and I am sensitive to that argument.—**SLO**

- Some other tips for optimal needle imaging: A less-steep angle of approach is helpful, meaning closer to parallel is best. This can be accomplished by using a longer needle and moving a bit further away from the transducer. Also, one can "heel" the transducer over, to create a greater degree of parallel alignment between the probe face and needle. This requires pressing into the soft tissue, which is usually possible and not painful, unless up against an osseous structure like the clavicle. And always remember that putting local anesthetic in the right place means first putting the needle in the right place. —**SLO**

- Aligning the needle across the long axis by eye, during insertion, is also helpful. Admittedly, probe covers make this difficult—smaller covers for the trans-vaginal probes work well and aren't so "baggy."—**SLO**

- In addition, rotation of the transducer can be very important—if you only see a section of the needle, rotate slowly to bring the entire needle into view. Look for the bevel at the tip, and also note that some echogenic needles are created to show two separate sections of echogenicity, and if you don't see both, look carefully with some rotation to find the second, so you do not lose the actual tip.—**SLO.**

- It is natural to "tilt" the transducer to capture the needle in the long axis when it deviates out of the plane of section. But a certain degree of tilt is often necessary for an optimal view of the underlying anatomy, including the nerve target. A significant change in this pre-established tilt, to see the needle, often degrades the anatomical view, and the operator is put in the uncomfortable position of having to shift the tilt of the transducer back and forth to see the needle and then the nerve, then back to the needle. A much better way to cope with the loss of the needle image from the plane of section is to translate the probe back and forth, across the path of the needle, without changing tilt. The needle will "flash" into view, allowing one to home in on the needle and then lock in on that image, at the same tilt as originally established for the optimum view of the nerve.—**SLO**

- On approaching a nerve, as the needle traverses the tissues, it is important to chart a course that is tangential to the neurologic structure. Connective tissues or fascial planes often surround the nerve, and as the needle approaches, their elastic nature allows for "tenting' which permits needle advance only grudgingly, holding the tip back, until enough force is applied to "pop" through the fascia. The needle tip is suddenly thrust forward, and if aligned with the nerve, it can easily impale it. If a tangential course is maintained, the needle tip will simply slide alongside the nerve, a far more desirable outcome.—**SLO**

- Our goal is to apply a layer of local anesthetic around the nerve's epineurium. This may require multiple needle re-directions, but sometimes fascial envelopes are quite practical for this purpose. For instance, placing a needle between the C5 and C6 nerve roots in the interscalene groove and then injecting 10 or 12 ml of local anesthetic is typically all that's necessary. The fascial lining of the middle and anterior scalene muscles along the groove permits the liquid to bathe the nerve elements without one having to place the needle above and below each one of them. If the nerves "bounce" with each aliquot of fluid injected, you can be pretty confident of a successful block.—**SLO**

- It's important to realize that local anesthetics must travel not only around the nerves but also *along them*, to provide a significant blockade of conduction. It is suggested that three nodes of Ranvier must be covered by the solution to suppress saltatory conduction. Moving the transducer proximally and distally, away from the point of injection, can help to establish that this longitudinal flow has occurred.—**SLO**

- Veins are pesky, compressible structures that can get us in trouble. It helps to "bob" up and down with transducer during the initial scanning, to find them. In addition, turning on the color Doppler can reveal unsuspected vessels. Finally, if there is no evidence of tissue spread during the injection of the initial 1–2 ml of solution, one should be wary. This is usually due to a tip that is out of plane, but it could also be due to an intravascular needle tip. A compressed vein will not "open up" when you inject into it; the vessel will conduct the injectate into and out of the screen (in the "z axis") where a 2D ultrasound image cannot capture it. Stop injecting and find the tip, and look for vessels at this point. Also, remember that a compressed vessel will often have a "negative" aspiration for blood.—**SLO**

- As noted, we seek to inject local anesthetic solution around the nerves, not into them. Given the vagaries of ultrasound, a tip may inadvertently find its way into a nerve, traversing the epineurium. But it takes very little solution to cause a nerve to expand on ultrasound imaging-if the first 1 ml of injectate results in expansion, pull back. The vast majority of intra-epineural injections are not within fascicles and will likely cause no harm. Some estimate that about 50% of pre-ultrasound injections for nerve blocks were intra-neural, and significant nerve injuries were quite unusual, even then.—**SLO**

Spinal Meds

- If somebody asked you at a party how many different medications could be given in a spinal, would you know? This happened to me, and I did not know. We advise taking the time to become truly expert and knowledge in the areas that border on anesthesia practice. It's enriching for us as practitioners and helps us be better knowledge ambassadors.—**CM**

- Obviously, anesthesiologists aren't giving a lot of intrathecal rituximab. But we dare say that every senior anesthesiologist who contributed to this book has been asked to "help out" with a spinal for another service in one way or another at some point, usually diagnostic taps, but not always. It's our thing; we do it the most and best of any other clinician. Why not just take a bit of time and study up on the matter so that when you are asked to help the oncologists get the tap, you know a bit about what they are planning on administering and so that you *can* answer questions at parties?—**Editors and LO**

- Just for your personal reference files, here is a reasonable spinal med list.—**LO.**

  – **Local anesthetics**.

    - bupivacaine,
    - lidocaine,
    - ropivacaine,
    - chloroprocaine,
    - mepivacaine,
    - tetracaine,

  – **Opioids**.

    - fentanyl,
    - morphine,
    - hydromorphone,
    - sufentanil,
    - buprenorphine,

- **Benzodiazepines**: midazolam.
- **Alpha2-adrenergic agonists**: clonidine and dexmedetomidine.
- **General anesthetic**: ketamine.
- **Steroids**: hydrocortisone.
- **Antibiotics**.
  - polymyxin B,
  - colistin,
  - vancomycin,
  - aminoglycosides (amikacin, gentamicin, tobramycin),
  - daptomycin,
  - tigecycline,
  - amphotericin B,
- **Muscle relaxants**: baclofen.
- **N-type calcium channel blocker**: ziconotide.
- **Chemotherapeutics**: cytarabine, methotrexate, rituximab, thiotepa, topotecan, trastuzumab, etoposide, interferon.
- **Antisense oligonucleotide**: nusinersen.

- We think that neuraxial opioids are under-used and underappreciated. But the itching and the potential for respiratory depression are real, especially with the water-soluble opioids.—**Editors**
- When I trained, any patient who received intrathecal morphine went to a monitored bed for 24 h. Today, there are different policies in place at various hospitals. These must be scrupulously attended to. This is an okay place in your clinical practice to be a bit conservative.—**CM**

***Note from the Editors:** We knew the day we started *Anesthesia Bridges* that this beautiful arched set of stairs would be in the book. This is the Dexter Avenue King Memorial Baptist Church in Montgomery, AL, where the Rev. Dr. Martin Luther King, Jr. began his first pastorship in 1954. The stairs form a bridge over the entrance to Dr. King's basement office (Fig. 163.3).

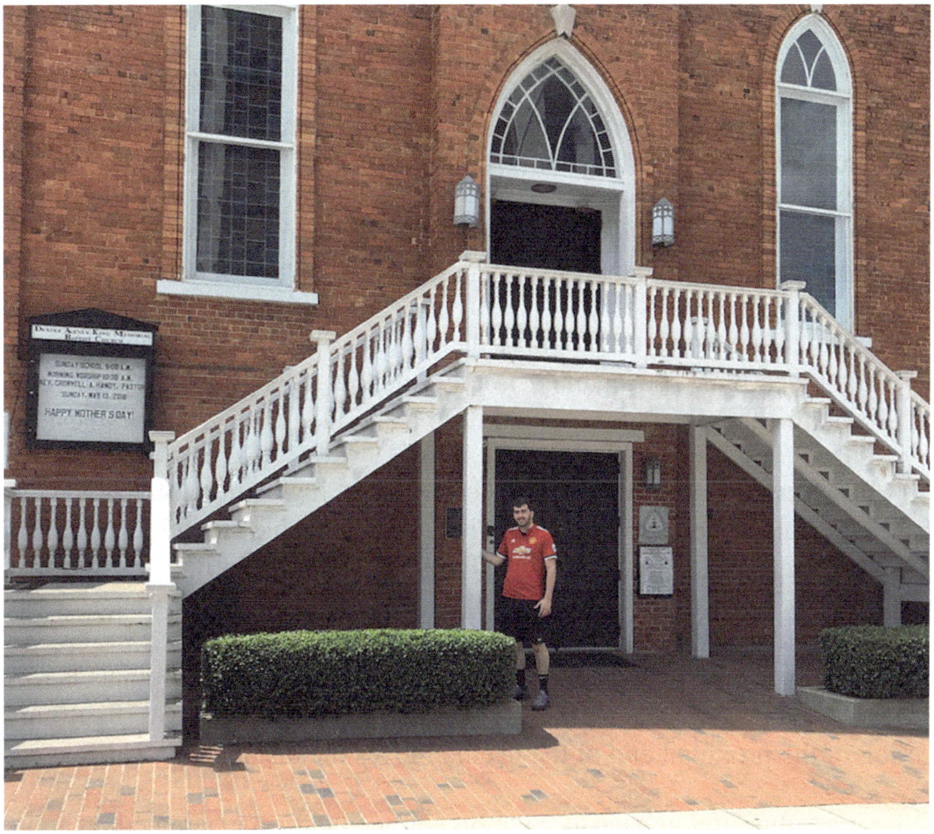

Fig. 163.3 The historic, beautiful, and inspiring Dexter Avenue Baptist Church, as it was called in the 1950s, when a very young Dr. King was the pastor. *Anesthesia Bridges* author Charlie Sandson visited in 2019. Photo: Cathy Marcucci

Central/Neuraxial Blocks

- I still think that positioning is important in neuraxial blocks, especially spinals, because you still have to open the spaces. If the patient is lateral, junior people who can't find the correct spaces are almost always too low, the soft tissue and midline dimple can sag a bit, and the bony structures are above the needle insertion site. Also, lateral patients tend to roll forward a bit, so a needle that you think might be perpendicular to the back isn't.—**Editors**

- Don't undersell the risks of neuraxial anesthesia in an attempt to oversell the benefits. Just because you have never had a patient who suffered serious neurological sequelae after a spinal doesn't mean the risk is zero. Risks to the spinal cord involve direct trauma, compression from hematoma, compression from abscess, neurotoxic effects of neuraxial drug delivery, spinal cord ischemia, and the effect of predisposing conditions. Plus the dreaded wrong-drug-in-syringe human error.—**Editors**

- The above issues don't have that much to do with visualization of the bony landmarks by ultrasound, so don't be lulled into a false sense of security that ultrasound guidance has made the risks essentially zero. It hasn't. Plus, we now have an appreciation of the possible long-term sequelae of post-dural puncture headaches. We know senior people who were taught to tell patients that spinal headaches could be uncomfortable were never dangerous. Oof. That is just so untrue.—**Editors**

- Don't hesitate to use a long spinal needle. It might make the difference between a quick and easy entry to the CSF vs. multiple needle passes.—**Editors**

- Don't think your patient's family won't look at the patient's back and count up the number of needle sticks they see evidence of because they will.—**Editors**

- Glycopyrrolate and/or ephedrine is *not* the treatment for symptomatic, severe bradycardia and hypotension post spinal placement—epinephrine is!!—**RSB**

- When you retire, spinals are what you will miss the most. Such a small amount of the right medication delivered to the right location—so elegantly simple. And that satisfying feel when you know you have entered the CSF and the backflow of the spinal fluid is unique to regional anesthesia.—**Editors**

- *Learn how to do paramedian spinals*. Every accomplished regional anesthesiologist is comfortable doing them. Practice on patients who are thin with easily palpable anatomy. This technique will frequently bail you out when a spinal is difficult. Partners will start calling *you* when they can't get a spinal.—**RGG**

- The best way to get more comfortable with the paramedian approach to spinals is to study an actual spine model and "practice" with an actual spinal needle on the model. Start getting a feel for how much redirection of the proximal end of the needle moves the distal end.—**Editors**

- Do not consider it a failure if you have to go to bigger needle for the paramedian approach. We don't teach that you necessarily will use a bigger needle, but the decision to use the paramedian approach is often dictated by an anticipation of increased technical difficulty in entering the CSF, thus a practitioner may have a lower threshold for choosing a larger gauge needle with the perception of a more difficult approach.—**CWE and RGG**

- As you are mastering the paramedian approach for spinals, work on the same approach to the epidural space. I do them often. I think my chronic pain background and use of X-ray-guided spine procedures helped me master the technique.—**AD**

- I do paramedian epidurals and like them but usually don't start with that approach. With nerve blocks and liposomal bupivacaine, we aren't doing as many epidurals these days.—**VLH**

- The paramedian approach is my first approach for thoracic epidurals. I only use that technique to approach the convex side of scoliosis for lumbar epidurals.—**BMT**

- I personally don't palpate most backs prior to starting my spinal procedure. Palpating before you have the patient properly positioned and prepped doesn't accomplish much because the patient will likely not be optimally positioned till you are actually performing the procedure. I prep, make sure the patient is optimally positioned, then palpate, with my skin wheal local anesthetic ready to go. I try to eliminate wasteful steps that don't contribute to a procedure.—**RGG**

- When performing nerve blocks, particularly spinals and epidurals, if you hit bone STOP. You just gained some information. Try to assess whether the needle is pointed left, right, too cephalad, or insufficiently cephalad. When you have decided, do not waste the information you have gained, withdraw the needle sufficiently to redirect, correct, and immediately advance the needle in the corrected direction.—**DLB**

- There are great online teaching tools now for neuraxial anesthesia but there is still nothing better to learn from than an actual scale model of the bony vertebral column. We had faculty back in the old days who always had one nearby when they were teaching spinals and epidurals to beginners. As Dr. Bourke says above, you haven't "missed" when you hit bone; if you've studied the anatomy at all, you've just made an identification for the needle's location.—**Editors**

- When using a 25-g needle, remember the needle's bevel may cause the needle to bend away from the bevel. So, if you hit bone and cannot decide which direction to correct, withdraw an inch or two, rotate the needle 180° and advance again. This often leads to success.—**DLB**

- Long gone are the days where we would do spinal anesthesia and not worry about how long the recovery period was. It is important to choose your local anesthetic and dose to facilitate throughput through the system and achieve goals such as early ambulation. This also will reduce the need for bladder catheterization.—**RGG**

- There are no hard and fast rules for which local anesthetic to use and expect some evolution in your practice. Also, if you are not regularly in the joint rooms, don't be a bit shy about asking your colleagues for their customary practice. For example, I now use mepivacaine for joint surgery (knees and hips) when the patient is planned for discharge on the same day. Tailored to the individual surgeon, of course. —**RGG**

- I have used a lot of 0.5% bupivacaine (which is mildly hypobaric) in spinal anesthetics for the hips. Since it tends to rise, you will get a denser block in the operative hip when you are in the lateral position. —**RGG**

- I personally have had three spinal anesthetics and an epidural. I had one epidural and two low-dose lidocaine/fentanyl spinals for my three knee scopes. I wanted to watch the knee scopes on the arthroscopy monitor, so I requested no sedation.—**RGG**

- From this personal experience, I learned a couple of things. *First*, a spinal is much more pleasant to have than an epidural—you really feel the pushing during the loss of resistance process. *Second*, the low-dose lidocaine/fentanyl was good for an hour case and wore off fast. *Third*, beware of excessive fluid loading a patient who is having a spinal without a foley. No fun having a full bladder waiting for the spinal to wear off! My third spinal was for an open appendectomy in the days before laparoscopic techniques. During that case, the spinal worked fine, but they gave me propofol sedation because I was talking too much.—**RGG**

- When I was doing a lot of neuraxial blocks in the VA health care system, it was common to use hyperbaric bupivacaine and then use lateral positioning to achieve a dense one-sided block. We didn't do any formal studies, but it seemed that the PACU recovery times for the block were faster, and the patients were able to ambulate more quickly. This was important because the patients and families often needed to be on the afternoon or early evening shuttle buses. —**CM**

- Don't dose an epidural immediately prior to transport!—**CM**

Peripheral Blocks

Upper Extremity

- No approach to brachial plexus blockade in the neck is free of diaphragm affect. If you are wary of adverse respiratory effects in a compromised patient, do not block the brachial plexus above the clavicle.—**SLO**

- As far as the block for upper extremity, phrenic nerve sparing blocks are performed not as often, as they require more expertise and more uncertainty with analgesia coverage. Suprascapular nerve block, superior trunk block can be utilized in this case, along with other supportive blocks (infraclavicular, axillary).—**AD**

- Realize that interscalene block (ISB), even with low volumes, has a very high chance of affecting the diaphragm, but most patients have no symptoms or significant change in oxygen saturation.—**SLO**

- If you strongly believe that your patient would be beneficial from the nerve block for shoulder surgery, but the patient has COPD, do not panic. You have another option than ISB. Consider the suprascapular nerve block. This block can be specifically targeted to provide shoulder analgesia with dramatically different effects on lung function. Perform this block, provide good postoperative analgesia, and surprise the surgeon.—**RBM**

- When anatomy or imaging is unfavorable at the level of interscalene block, a supraclavicular block can be utilized for shoulder surgery, but the effect on the C4 root (the supraclavicular nerves), which innervates the skin over the top of the shoulder, is less likely to be covered by the block. Check this sensation, along with deltoid function, if the block is expected to be surgical.—**SLO**

- Follow-up to Steve Orebaugh's point and reiterating what is mentioned just above—you can do a superficial cervical plexus block to supplement a supraclavicular block if you are concerned about inadequate coverage of the shoulder skin.—**RGG**

- Don't forget to advise hand/wrist surgery patients receiving supraclavicular block that "eyelids and diaphragm" could be affected.—**SLO**

- Lower volumes of local anesthetic solution, and distal movement of site of injection reduce the impact on the diaphragm.—**SLO**

- The infraclavicular approach to the brachial plexus can be frustrating: the needle angle is steep, the nerves are not well-demarcated, the chest wall is close, and the vessels are about. But a "periarterial" approach, with injection of local anesthetic solution around the artery seems to work well. This is also the idea place for a catheter since neither arm nor neck motion are likely to dislodge it.—**SLO**

- As with supraclavicular block, the pleura is close to site of injection in ICB… find it and keep it in your sites as you manipulate your needle.—**SLO.**

- Axillary block is in danger of being forgotten-it seems antiquated and clumsy, with more needle sticks and redirections, but keep it in your repertoire by at least studying the anatomy when you have the opportunity. This is a great escape block for larger people, when supraclavicular block seems daunting due to deep nerve levels and poor visualization, or those with severe pulmonary disease.—**SLO**

- Possible salvage techniques for the shoulder and upper extremity: superficial cervical plexus block, intercostobrachial supplementation, suprascapular nerve block, axillary nerve block, superficial skin supplemental for scope portal sites.—**Editors**

- For lower arm and hand, consider these salvage/supplementation techniques: individual nerve blocks of the ulnar, median, and radial nerves at the elbow; field blocks of the medial and lateral cutaneous nerves just below the elbow crease.—**Editors**

Lower Extremity

- Despite the flight to adductor canal block for painful knee surgery, the femoral block still has a few reasons for being, for example, above-knee amputation, and postop blocks after complex knee scope procedures, such as when a brace prevents access to the adductor canal.—**SLO**

- To add to Steve's list, femoral blocks are also helpful after patella tendon and quadriceps muscle rupture repairs, where the muscle relaxation prevents muscle spasm that would stress these repairs.—**RGG**

- Blocks at the mid-thigh, commonly conducted as "adductor canal blocks" are actually at the level of the distal femoral triangle, which is favorable for knee arthroplasty surgery, as the nerve to vastus medialis is likely to be affected by the injection.—**SLO**

- More distal injections, into the true adductor canal, are unlikely to affect the nerve to vastus medialis, and are best reserved for ankle/foot surgery in which the saphenous block alone is to be affected for postoperative analgesia.—**SLO**

- Blocks at the mid-thigh, into the distal femoral triangle, have minimal chance to spread distally into the popliteal fossa, to affect the popliteal plexus, which innervates the posterior aspect of the knee and most of its internal structures… so for knee arthroplasty, either a posterior block (such as the "iPACK" block) or directed local infiltration analgesia by the surgeon should accompany the adductor canal block.—**SLO**

- Sciatic blocks at the infragluteal level can be tricky: proximal hamstring tendons can look a lot like the sciatic nerve… use a stimulator for confirmation!—**SLO**

- Popliteal sciatic blocks can take a long time to set up, especially if the injectate is place around the sciatic nerve or around each of the branches… improved success rates and more rapid onset occur when the needle is placed between the tibial and peroneal nerves just as they bifurcate. Distal "halos" around the nerves are a reliable sign that the solution is inside the perineural sheath, which aids both circumferential spread and longitudinal spread, which are both essential for successful block.—**SLO**

- We do acknowledge that sciatic blocks have become less favored in the current era, as we have moved to avoid postoperative motor block. However, there are still situations in which this block can be quite useful. One is for either below-knee or above-knee amputations. Another is for femoral or tibial osteotomies, since the sciatic nerve innervates the posterior femur and much of the tibia and fibula. Pain for both of these surgeries can be addressed with a preoperative sciatic block, in combination with a femoral block.—**SLO**

- Also, it is not uncommon for patients to complain of deep or posterior knee pain after ACL reconstruction, despite the provision of a preoperative femoral or adductor canal block. This can be addressed with a postoperative sciatic block. In these situations, it is not usually essential for the patient to bear weight or walk within hours of the surgery, so the inevitable motor block is not an important adversity.—**SLO**

- Ultrasound can be used to improve the accuracy of ankle block: tibial nerve, sural nerve, and deep peroneal nerve blocks can be visually guided, reducing the inaccuracy of five "blind" injections.—**SLO**

- Salvage/supplemental techniques for the hip and lower extremity include lumbar plexus blocks (less favorable due to technical difficulty and serious complications), three-in-one blocks, lateral femoral cutaneous nerve block, single-shot sciatic block, obturator block, tibial and common peroneal block, and adductor canal or saphenous nerve block. These may seem old-fashioned and out of style, but you need to know the variety of approaches to a regional anesthesia clinical situation.—**Editors**

- Also, give your patients who have a lower extremity regional anesthetic as their primary anesthetic modality something to do with their hands and upper body. I've seen RA done so skillfully that the patient spent the case watching a movie or reading. Once we asked a patient if he wanted to read a magazine on sports, fishing, or national parks. The patient said, "Got anything about dogs?"—**Editors**

***Note from the Editors:** We didn't have any intraoperative reading material on man's best friend for this patient, unfortunately. But dogs do make everything and everybody better! Our good friend Elaine Matte Mut is a talented and award-winning recreational photographer, and she sent us two shots of the famous St. Louis landmark, one with a member of the Matte-Mut family and one without (Fig. 163.4). We all voted on which to use, and guess who won?

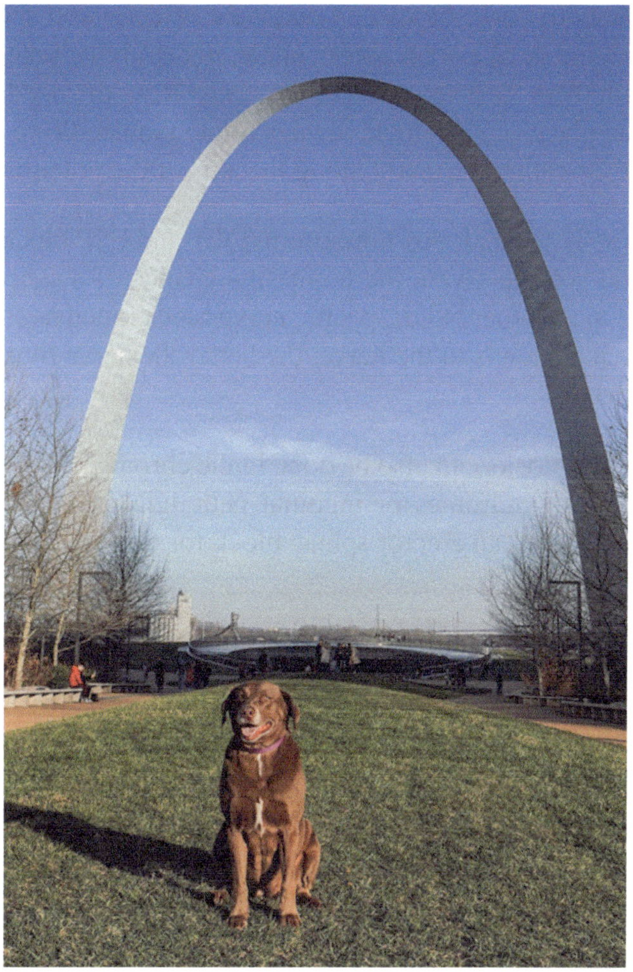

Fig. 163.4 The famous Arch in St. Louis, with good girl Honey helping to make the shot. Photo: Elaine Matte Mut

- I think the intercostal nerve block (ICNB) is one of the most under-used and underappreciated blocks. It's such an effective and versatile block and great rescue analgesia technique, but is rarely used by anesthesiologists, probably due to fear of side effects and injury to surrounding tissues.—**AD**

Fascial Plane Blocks

- Why fascial plane blocks (FPB) rather than epidurals? Let's compare two major parameters: pain relieve and complications. Recent evidence from meta-analyses and systematic reviews comparing the analgesic efficacy of epidural versus different fascial plane blocks—for example, paravertebral, quadratus lumborum, transversus abdominis plane—show that the analgesia was comparable and an epidural and FPB are equally effective in treating postoperative pain. Epidural blocks have many well-known sequelae, like epidural hematoma, spinal cord injury, post-operative neurologic deficits, post-dural puncture headache, hemodynamic instability, and loss of bladder control. You can avoid these with fascial plane blocks. Fascial plane blocks are easy to perform and can serve as a promising alternative to an epidural for postop pain management.—**RBM**

- When performing a continuous nerve block and placing a catheter you should know the bevel direction. The catheter will exit the needle at an obtuse angle, not straight. Take a clean 18G Tuohy needle and catheter and play with them. See how the catheter exits from the needle. For example, when you perform an erector spinae plane (ESP) block, always rotate the needle so that the bevel faces down. This will help you direct the catheter exactly along the axis of the potential ESP space.—**RBM**

- The plane blocks—such as TAP, quadratus lumborum (QL), and ESP blocks—are volume dependent. The more local anesthetic volume given, the higher the chance of a successful block—keep LAST syndrome in your mind. On the other hand, specific nerve blocks such as sciatic or femoral are distant dependent: the closer the injection is to the nerve, the better the nerve block—keep intraneural injection in your mind!—**RBM**

- Remember that fascial plane blocks can also be done in the chronic pain clinic. Think TAP blocks for abdominal nerve entrapment syndromes or inguinal neuralgia pains. Pec blocks can be done for chronic pain after mastectomy, or an erector spinae block for chest area pain.—**AD**

Other

- Don't forget about the cervical plexus block. It's one of the more interesting "old-fashioned" blocks since it can be used for a bunch of things—awake central lines, thyroidectomy and similar surgeries, carotid surgery, supplement for shoulder and clavicle surgeries, and so forth.—**AD**

- The thing is, thyroid and carotid surgeries are typically done under general anesthesia, and surgeons tend to do infiltration for these procedures. We do cervical plexus blocks routinely in shoulder surgery, along with interscalene. Having a committed and skilled team to perform them efficiently after induction of anesthesia, using US guidance, would certainly be beneficial.—**AD**

- We had an interesting group discussion about the need to maintain proficiency with Bier blocks. I recommended this in both editions of *Avoiding Common Anesthesia Errors*. My point being that they are easy to do—all you have to do is find the vein and control the tourniquet. This is one block where US is not needed.—**CM**

- However, several of our expert regional anesthesiologists felt that they are not used much these days and are quite fine with that. The thought is that given the variety of available regional blocks, short-acting local anesthetics, wrist and digital blocks, and technicalities involving the use of tourniquet and related discomfort, it has been coming out of favor.—**AD and Editors**

- We concluded that whether you do them has a lot to do with your patient cohort and they are not contraindicated in specific situations. I have always worked in situations where patients often came to the OR to have small sharp objects removed from the soft tissue of their hands and forearms—glass and metal pieces, including broken needles. The surgeons would often post a very short case and request a Bier block, so I am very comfortable doing them. It might be good for the younger generation to know how to do them for use in a low-resource setting.—**CM**

- Although they are not commonly done block, scalp blocks are very interesting for several reasons. First, they use a large volume of local anesthetic—up to 60 cc—so calculations for systemic toxicity and considerations of DDIs are especially important. Second, there are several parts of an awake craniotomy that are especially painful—insertion of pins, dissection of temporalis muscle and traction of the dura close to the middle meningeal artery. Adjunctive pain medications such as the short-acting opioids are used, but only in amounts that do not prohibit adequate EEG monitoring.—**Editors**

- Scalp blocks are done with a 22-g needle to place a circumferential band of local anesthetic from the glabella to the occiput. Can you name the nerves blocked and their locations?—**Editors**

  * *Supraorbital and supratrochlear nerves*—anterior scalp and superior to the block.

  * *Zygomaticotemporal and auriculotemporal nerves*—anterior scalp and inferior to the block.

  * *Greater occipital nerve*—posterior scalp and superior to the block.

  * *Lesser occipital nerve*—posterior scalp and inferior to the block.

- The scalp block can go in perfectly and be working, and patients commonly will have headaches ranging from mild to severe. That's what the fentanyl is for. It doesn't mean the block isn't working.—**Editors**

- Interestingly, although I am a regional anesthesiologist, I have never done scalp blocks. When I was an emergency medicine doc, I sewed up and stapled my share of scalps. What I remember: The scalp bleeds like crazy. Compression is helpful to reduce the hemorrhage. Bleeding should be pretty well controlled before sewing up to avoid a subgaleal hematoma. A layered closure helps as well. We always used lidocaine with epinephrine to provide vasoconstriction. I wish I'd known about blocks for the greater and lesser occipital nerves and the greater auricular nerve. Probably would have come in handy—that was way pre-ultrasound!—**SLO**

- There are a lot of opportunities and applications for regional anesthesia in the ICU. Potential pain targets are chest tube pain, thoracotomy pain, abdominal surgery pain, and ileus. Even if anticoagulation is needed so you cannot do epidurals, you can still consider intercostal blocks, rectus sheath blocks, and serratus plane blocks. Also, consider stellate ganglion blocks in the ICU for arrhythmias. —**AD**

Note: As *Anesthesia Bridges* went to press, Dr. Dizdarevic was putting together a review paper of ICU regional anesthesia. Make sure you head to the literature to read it.—**Editors**

Soft Tissue Regional Anesthesia

- Know who does soft tissue regional anesthesia better than anyone—and without sedation? The derm-onc folks for MOHS surgery. We asked Joanna Walker at Penn for some tips on how she trained on doing soft tissue anesthesia for surgery and what her advice is.—**Editors**

- For most of my cases, I use 0.45% or 0.9% lidocaine with epi, buffered with bicarbonate. I use this concentration on all body parts, except to limit the volume on the digits and penis. In some cases, MOHS surgeons will use bupivacaine to provide early post-operative pain (consider for nail procedures or large flaps).—**JLW**

- Residency training in dermatology provides didactics on different types of local, calculating maximum dosage, signs of toxicity. As we do biopsies and procedures in residency, we learn tips like bracing against the patient in case they move and keeping the needle pointed away from the eye.—**JLW**

- We spend considerable time in learning ways to make the injection less painful (a slow injection is much less painful)—inject into subcutaneous fat first and then anesthetize the skin, vs small aliquot into the skin and slowly inject more through already anesthetized skin, always re-introduce the needle into already anesthetized area, using smaller needles, and buffering solution to a more neutral pH.—**JLW**

- Fellowship provided more training such as nerve blocks and numbing proximal to distal in the path of a sensory nerve.—**JLW**

- If we need to establish a deep MOHS layer, we keep more lidocaine on hand and inject more into the sub fascial layers as we go… the needles aren't long enough to penetrate deeply from the skin surface.—**JLW**

- If we are operating on a very large surface area, we use tumescent lidocaine—injecting a large volume of normal saline and a small amount of lidocaine. —**JLW**

- We haven't seen the anesthesiology and derm-onc surgeons (or plastic surgeons for that matter) work together on training and projects but believe each specialty would be welcome at the other's conferences and clinical settings. Plus, multi-disciplinary studies and papers are the best.—**JLW and CM**

***Note from the Editors:** Joanna Walker's dermatology-oncology suburban practice location is in Radnor, PA, which is just outside Philadelphia. Patients on their way to see her there often stop to visit the Brandywine Battlefield Park and hike the nearby short trail along the Brandywine River (Fig. 163.5).

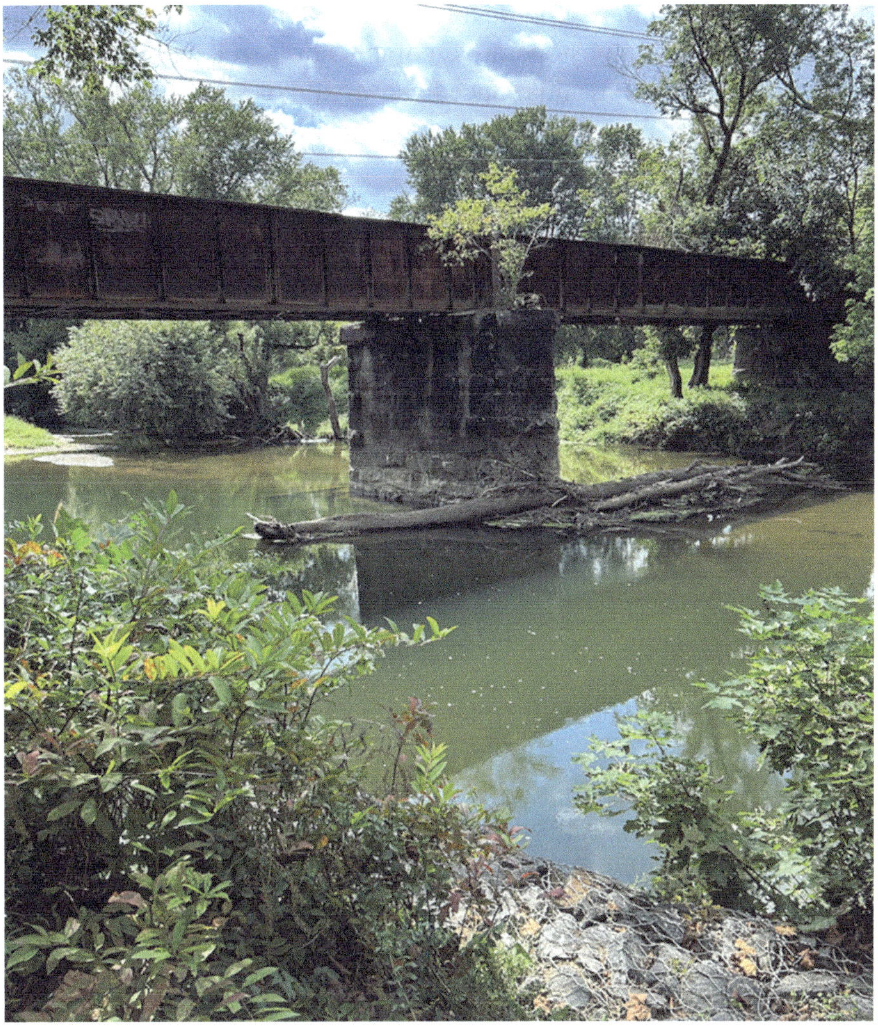

Fig. 163.5 The Brandywine River Valley is beautiful and historic. It was the site of an epic Revolutionary War Battle, as more than 30,000 British and American fought back and forth for an entire day across this small river. Washington and the Continental Army lost the battle but learned that they would have the strength and resilience to persist and win the war. The old railroad bridge that spans the river near the Brandywine River Museum is no longer in use. Photo: Cathy Marcucci

Pain Medicine—Some Thoughts

- Why do we need an acute pain service? Several factors, as listed below, have made this service critical.—**RBM and AD**
  - The opioid crisis: Over 8% of opioid naïve patients become chronic opioid users after initial exposure to opioids following surgery. Patients with opioid prescriptions after short-stay surgeries have a 44% increased risk of long-term use. Over 80% of patients receive opioids after low-risk surgeries.
  - Do we treat adequately postoperative pain? NO!!! Management of acute postoperative pain remains suboptimal and nearly 80% of patients report moderate to extreme pain following surgery.

- You as an acute pain specialist may provide improved postoperative pain control and comfort in the postoperative period, decreased postoperative complications related to pain, decreased length of stay, increased patient satisfaction, and reduced conversion of acute pain to the debilitating disease of chronic pain. For all these reasons, be an acute pain management doctor!
- Furthermore, for patients with complex pain history of surgeries resulting in severe pain, it can be very beneficial and informative to have a preoperative evaluation with a pain specialist to formulate a plan before, during, and after surgery, along with coordination with the acute pain service. And these benefits accrue not only for the patients but also for the entire perioperative team.

- *What staff do you need to make a block service work efficiently?*—**RBM**
  - **An attending (you!):** Ideally regional anesthesia and acute pain management fellowship trained. Tasks include supervising and performing nerve blocks, doing consults, rounding, billing, and teaching.
  - **Residents**: Ideally two residents—a senior and a junior, one on call 24/7. Tasks include performing blocks, participating in consults, and rounding on patients.
  - **Nurse practitioner**: Tasks include communication with nursing staff, nursing education, and pre-rounds on patients.
  - **Coordinator**: This is a must-have position. Tasks include reviewing OR schedule and updating daily work sheet, communicating with surgeons, coordinating patients coming to preop hold for blocks, review schedule for the following day, contact surgeons' offices to secure a consult for appropriate patients, maintain communication throughout the day with all relevant parties, order the drugs and monitor stock of supplies, prepare monthly statistics, etc.
- Many preoperative, intraoperative, and postoperative interventions and management strategies are available for reducing and managing postoperative pain: nerve blocks, multimodal analgesia, and surgeon injected local. A nerve block is a vital part of ERAS.—**RBM**
- An anesthesia pain service should survive due to its benefits of improving patient satisfaction and discharge times, but it is important to be cost-conscious. All supplies that the pain service uses have a cost. Wasting supplies and unnecessarily using more expensive ways to accomplish a procedure impact the profitability of the service. Close attention to the financial aspects of implementation, including projecting return on investment, is necessary in today's cost-conscious healthcare environment.—**RBM**
- Facilities in which surgery is performed should have an organizational structure to oversee the development, implementation, and evaluation of policies and practices to assure safe, evidence-based, and effective postoperative pain control. Whether through an existing quality improvement committee or a designated pain management team, the process should be interdisciplinary.—**RBM**
- Have *strong* guidelines for practice!—**RBM**

* Have written protocols for all types of blocks.

* Get consent for every procedure.

* Time outs prior to blocks are a key part of good acute pain service care. You cannot afford to have a wrong-sided block!

* Have high standards for teaching—including written-out goals and objectives.

- Make your life easier by establishing excellent surgeon-pain service relationships. If you can help make your patients and their families happy through your excellent care, this will go a long way towards establishing surgeon satisfaction, too. —**RBM**

- Remember that "pain" is the cortical processing of nerve signals from the periphery.—**Editors**

- You cannot tell a patient they are not in pain because you can't know what they are thinking and feeling. As we have mentioned elsewhere, apparently normal vital signs do not rule out a pain state.—**Editors**

- *All pain hurts*. That said, I have special empathy for patients with neuropathic pain. You cannot *believe* how much those pain syndromes hurt. They can be devastating emotionally, psychologically, and physically. We speak from personal experience.—**Editors**

- There are also variations in pain perceptions based on age, cultural, and gender differences. Be respectful of this. Also, do not assume that members or veterans of the armed services have high pain thresholds—they don't necessarily. —**Editors**

- Patients who live with autism-spectrum challenges have unexpected (often higher) pain thresholds.—**Editors**

- Also, be respectful of how a patient's emotional state impacts their pain perceptions and needs. We have seen this go both ways. For instance, we have seen pediatric patients who indicated no post-operative discomfort burst into tears when a stressed patients approaches the bedside. We have also seen young parents who needed to get back to caring for a family get up out of bed and get going home in literally 3 days after what would seem to be really extensive and painful traumatic injuries.—**Editors**

- Patients can have a lot of trouble even from the "minor" sources of pain. For instance, necklines and tape and surgical dressings can be uncomfortable to the point of pain. Same with vacuum wound healing devices. Also, chase down every pain complaint. A patient who develops inexplicable back pain may be lying on something. —**Editors**

- Beginning anesthesiologists often do not distinguish between pre-existing chronic pain, acute pain, and the tricky problem of acute-on-chronic pain. No matter which type of pain you are treating, always think about a comprehensive plan for the pain problem that's in front of you, *but also* how you can make the job easier for the anesthesiologists who are following you in the care of the patient. Your care plans sets up their care plans—it's a big circle.—**Editors**

- You also have to deal with the big subjects like treating depression and anxiety, speaking of circular etiologies.—**Editors**

- The practice of chronic pain management involves the art of ruling out as much as what you rule in. For example, for back pain, you must rule out facet arthropathy and trigger points before you initiate a lot of expensive and invasive imaging studies and maneuvers.—**Editors**

- Nobody should die in pain. —**Editors**

- Remember, a markedly aberrant pattern of patients with significantly under-treated pain can be an indicator of drug diversion. It's still happening in this day and age.—**Editors**

- *Finally, be humble*. Pain is the oldest and most primitive medical complaint—as old as the human condition. It was possibly the original symptom that drove the development of medicine—and we still really don't know that much about it, including how to definitively treat it.—**Editors**

More Regional Anesthesia Wisdom from *Avoiding Common Anesthesia Errors, 2nd Edition*

There is a wealth of additional tips, teaching tidbits, and overall physiology wisdom in our previous book, which is nicknamed "Green2." *Please* check out this information and remember that every single penny of royalties goes to FAER in perpetuity!

Green2 Chapters with More Regional Anesthesiology Wisdom

- Complications of Regional Anesthesia: Don't Touch the Needle Before You Know Them.

- Make Time for a Timeout Before Placing a Block—the Preprocedure Check.

- Chlorhexidine: Killing Bacteria… and Allergic Patients?

- What Is the Correct Brachial Plexus Block to Perform?

- Getting the Right Ultrasound Image.

- Interscalene Blocks—Preventing the Blues!

- The Old-Fashioned Bier Block Is Still Relevant—the Trick Is to Not Let the Surgeons Get Ahead of You.

- Remember the Low-Risk/High-Yield Blocks.

- Preparing to Fail: The Dynamics of a Failed Block.

- Salvage Techniques for Incomplete Lower Extremity Blocks.

- More Than a Stick and a Burn: Local Anesthetic Systemic Toxicity.
- Lipid Rescue—Where Are We Now?
- A Patient Who Is Planned for Spinal Anesthesia Asks, "Can This Paralyze Me?" What Are the Facts and What Do You Say?
- Spinals in the Lateral Position.
- Consider the Paramedian Approach for Spinal Anesthesia in the Hip Fracture Patient.
- When Is a Whisper a Cry for Help? When the Patient Has a High Block.
- Issues Related to Discharging the Post-Spinal Patient.
- Epidural or Truncal Block? Sorting It Out.
- Dang It! Wet Tap.
- Consider Continuous Paravertebral Block as Your Primary Analgesic Technique.
- Pneumothorax After Paravertebral, Supraclavicular, or Interscalene Block.
- Epidural Anesthesia for Mastectomy.
- What Is the Right Level for Postoperative Epidural Catheter Insertions Based on Type of Surgery?
- Know the Complications of Epidural Corticosteroid Injections.
- If You Are New to Neuraxial and Peripheral Nerve Block Infusions—a View from Both Academia and Private Practice.
- What to Do With a Prolonged Block.
- Regional Anesthesia in the ICU—What Should We Use and When Should We Use It?

More Wisdom on Local Anesthetic Drug–Drug Interactions from *A Case Approach to Perioperative Drug–Drug Interactions*

There are also many additional tips and teaching tidbits on local anesthetic drug-drug interactions (DDIs) in our *other* previous book, which is nicknamed the "Blue Book." *Please* check out this information and remember that every single penny of royalties goes to FAER in perpetuity!

Blue Book Chapters with More Wisdom on DDIs Pertaining to Local Anesthetics and Regional Anesthesiology Wisdom

- Comfortably Numb *(local anesthetics).*
- Naturally Occurring and Nasty *(cocaine, propranolol).*
- LOL-LOL: Little Old Lady—Lots of Lido *(lidocaine, bupivacaine).*
- The Spinal Countdown *(general anesthesia after spinal anesthesia).*
- Are Drug–Drug Interactions the Smoking Gun of Local Anesthetic Toxicity? Smoking Gun I *(ropivacaine, fluoxetine, CYP1A2, CYP3A4).*
- Are Drug–Drug Interactions the Smoking Gun of Local Anesthetic Toxicity? Smoking Gun II *(bupivacaine, methocarbamol).*
- A Perfect Storm? *(omeprazole, nicardipine, diltiazem, bupivacaine, CYP3A4, CYP2C19, CYP2D6).*
- Shake, Rattle, and Roll *(lidocaine, cimetidine, CYP3A4).*
- Hello, We Have a Patient With Acute Delirium, and We Need an Urgent Psych Consult *(lidocaine, metoprolol).*
- Fatal Pain Relief *(local anesthetics, intrathecal morphine).*
- Lipid Lifesaver *(local anesthetic, lipid emulsion).*

Reference

1. Barrington MJ, Uda Y. Did ultrasound fulfill the promise of safety in regional anesthesia? Curr Opin Anaesthesiol. 2018;31(5):649–55.

Authors

Steve Orebaugh is a professor of anesthesiology at the University of Pittsburgh Department of Anesthesiology. His area of greatest interest is regional anesthesia and educating residents in peripheral nerve blockade. He is most appreciative of the support of his wife, Jennifer, and daughter, Olivia, who support him with both patience and affection. He enjoys woodworking, gardening, and creative writing in his spare time.

Ray Graber serves as the vice chair for quality measures at University Hospitals Cleveland Medical. He has dual interests in cardiac and orthopedic anesthesia. During his 30+ year career, he has focused on process improvement, reduction of errors, and improving patient outcomes.

Rita Merman is the chief of the division for chronic pain management and the program director of the regional anesthesiology and acute pain medicine fellowship at University Hospitals Health System, Cleveland. She was one who stood at the origins of the acute pain service at University of Pittsburgh Department of Anesthesiology. And then went on to found the acute pain service and regional fellowship at UH Cleveland Medical. Nothing would be possible without the support from her family—her husband, Mark, and son, Yury.

Cathy Marcucci trained and was first on faculty at Hopkins. She has also been a senior anesthesiologist in the University of Pennsylvania and the University of Maryland systems. In spite of all the flashy new blocks available today, her favorite regional anesthetic technique to do and teach remains the good old-fashioned spinal.

Anis Dizdarevic is an associate professor of anesthesiology at Columbia University Irving Medical Center. He serves as Director of Regional and Orthopedic Anesthesia as well as Director of Anesthesiology Services at New York Presbyterian Allen Hospital/Och Spine Center. He has a background in chronic pain management, and special interests in perioperative pain, acute to chronic pain transition, minimally invasive anesthesia, and analgesia for critically ill patients

Wisdom on Acupuncture for Pain and Other Conditions

164

Joshua L. Stich, Marilyn X. Walker, Catherine Marcucci, and Scott D. Mist

Contributors:

Kristin King Liao, LAc (KKL)

Albert Liao, LAc (AL)

Amy J. Robbins, MD MBA (AJR)

Introduction

We are of the belief that acupuncture, when used as a complementary medicine modality, has a definite place in perioperative medicine. The accumulating evidence base supports our position. The best applications for acupuncture are those situations when there is a gap between Western medicine and wellness. Because this is an emerging huge area of clinical practice, there is still a lot of work to be done. Below are just a few pearls to stimulate your curiosity.

Basics

- Acupuncture is a key component, but just one practice, of Traditional Chinese Medicine (TCM), a system of healthcare and wellness beliefs and practices that is several thousand years old.—**KKL, AL and SDM**

J. L. Stich
Albert Einstein College of Medicine, New York, NY, USA

M. X. Walker
Marilyn X. Walker, BS (MXW), New York University, New York, NY, USA

C. Marcucci (✉)
Department of Transfusion Medicine, Clinical Center, National Institutes of Health, Bethesda, MD, USA

S. D. Mist
Department of Anesthesiology and Perioperative Medicine, Oregon Health and Science University, Portland, OR, USA

S. Mohamed et al. (eds.), *Anesthesia Bridges*, https://doi.org/10.1007/978-3-032-08294-7_164

- The origins of acupuncture are a bit shrouded in ancient history. The earliest references to acupuncture and acupuncture implements date back about 3000 years. Acupuncture texts were developed in China over several millennia. For example, detailed books of acupuncture date to 300-100 BCE with the Yellow Emperor's Classic of Internal Medicine. This was a book that was a compilation of other sources that were several hundred years old. Detailed acupuncture texts also exist from the Ming Dynasty period between the fourteenth and sixteenth centuries.—**SDM and CM**

- Acupuncture spread to Europe and America in the fifteenth through nineteenth centuries. Acupuncture has been practiced, debated, and researched in the West since that time.—**SDM**

- TCM (and acupuncture) are based on the concept of qi. This is translated as vital energy or vital force but literally means vapor, air, or breath. TCM therapeutic modalities are based on the flow of qi along specific meridians or channels that can be mapped anatomically onto the human body.—**CM, KKL, and AL**

- Acupuncture recognizes 365 "classic" points on the body that provide specific points for therapeutic access to the qi meridians. Various acupuncture texts will cite an additional 150 or so points. The disciplines of specialized hand and ear acupuncture add several hundred more points. Overall, there are probably less than 1000 recognized acupuncture points.—**SDM**

- In TCM, disease and/or unwellness occurs when the qi is blocked, causing unbalance between the yin and yang.—**CM, SDM, and AL**

- It is a misconception that acupuncture causes "turn-on/turn-off" responses in the body. Acupuncture is a treatment modality that balances the physiological homeostasis and healing mechanisms of the body.—**KKL and CM**

- There are five yin organs—heart, kidneys, liver, lung, and spleen. The overall health of these organs is of utmost importance in TCM. The five yang organs are small intestine, large intestine, gallbladder, urinary bladder, and the "triple heater" organ, which is not an anatomical location but pairs with the pericardium. The therapeutic approach in TCM acupuncture concerns achieving balance and wellness in the primary yin organs through treatment of the paired yang organs.—**AL and KKL**

- Interestingly, the brain is considered to be neither a yin nor yang organ. In TCM, the functions of the brain and mind are distributed and dispersed between the five yin organs and brain diseases of all types are considered to be systemic diseases. There is little or no differentiation between "physical heath" and "mental health" in TCM.—**CM and AL**

- Each of the yin organs also corresponds to one of the five basic emotions:

  * <u>Lung</u>—sadness and grief

  * <u>Heart</u>—joy

  * <u>Liver</u>—anger

  * Spleen—worry

  * Kidney—fear

- When I talk to my patients and the pain fellows, I am careful in discussing the organs, as it is understandable to think that we are actually working on the heart, lungs, liver, kidneys or spleen. Rather the organs are a short cut name for a relationship within the body.—**SDM**

- For example, when we talk about the liver, it has a couple of main functions that include promoting the smooth flow of qi, storing blood, and nourishing the tendons. If a person comes in with cirrhosis of the liver, we might or might not work on the Chinese liver. With symptoms like insomnia, fatigue, jaundice, abdominal distention, oftentimes they have problems that include the spleen, stomach, the governing and conception channels, and the gallbladder. Common points used in treatment include Stomach 36, Spleen 3, Gallbladder 34, Conception vessel 12, and Liver 3. From the TCM point of view, we are treating the liver, but we are not measuring ALT, AST, ALB, or TBIL. We are looking at the symptoms and if they still have cirrhosis but no signs or symptoms, we feel that the yin Liver organ is better.—**SDM**

- Other TCM practices include moxibustion, herbal medicine, Chinese massage called tui na, and practices such as tai chi and qi gong that combine exercise with meditation.—**Editors**

Physiology and Mechanisms

- Human neuroimaging data demonstrate that acupuncture stimulation modulates a wide network of brain regions. These areas include the primary somatosensory, secondary somatosensory anterior cingulate, prefrontal, and insular cortices, as well as the amygdala, hippocampus, hypothalamus, periaqueductal gray matter, rostral ventral medulla, and cerebellar vermis.—**MZW and SDM**

- It is noteworthy that the demonstrated central nervous system effects of acupuncture result from needle placement and stimulation along the peripheral organ meridians, supporting the concept of the brain and peripheral organs sharing qi.—**JLS and SDM**

- Stimulation of acupoints can produce pain relief primarily through activation of neurotransmitters. Although the mechanism is unclear, pain cessation likely relies heavily upon the endogenous opioid system.—**JLS and SDM**

- The endogenous opioid mechanisms triggered by electroacupuncture (EA) are contingent upon the acupoint and frequency used. Low-frequency EA induces the release of beta-endorphin, endomorphin, and met-enkephalin combined with μ- and δ-opioid to achieve pain management.—**JLS and SDM**

- Different types of research suggest that upregulation of serotonin (5-HT) receptors by EA can alleviate surgical pain.—**JLS and SDM**

- Human neuroimaging data indicate that opioidergic and/or monoaminergic neurotransmission can be modulated by acupuncture stimulation, with its effects impacting a wide network of brain regions. Functional magnetic resonance imaging (fMRI) deactivation in regions including the thalamus, insula, anterior cingulate cortex, and premotor cortex has been seen following acupuncture stimulation compared to a non-stimulation baseline.—**JLS and SDM**

- Both verum and sham acupuncture have been found to reduce fMRI pain responses in the thalamus and insula of fibromyalgia patients; PET data using carfentanil in this same population also support μ-opioid receptor involvement in acupuncture and/or sham analgesia [1].—**MZW and SDM**

- EEG studies have found that acupuncture modulates painful somatosensory evoked potential amplitude at both short and long latencies following stimulation, suggesting that acupuncture may have both humoral and neural mediated effects on pain.—**MZW and SDM**

- There are multiple acupuncture-evoked pathways for modulating both the innate and adaptive immune responses. Acupuncture will initiate a mechanical and thermal stimulus within acupoints. This causes electrical signals to be transmitted to the central nervous system, which produces distinct descending regulatory pathways.—**JLS and MZW**

- Cholinergic/anti-inflammatory and vagus/adrenal pathways may modulate the innate immune system, including macrophages and neutrophils.—**JLS**

- Acupuncture-stimulated spinal/sympathetic and brain/gut pathways may modulate the adaptive immune response.—**SDM**

- If all of the above is a bit complicated for you, just remember that the three main mechanisms of acupuncture occur through modulation of the autonomic nervous system, inflammatory responses, and the endocannabinoid system.—**CM and SDM**

***Note from the Editors:** Students and patients of Traditional Chinese Medicine often travel to China, a land of many beautiful bridges (Fig. 164.1).

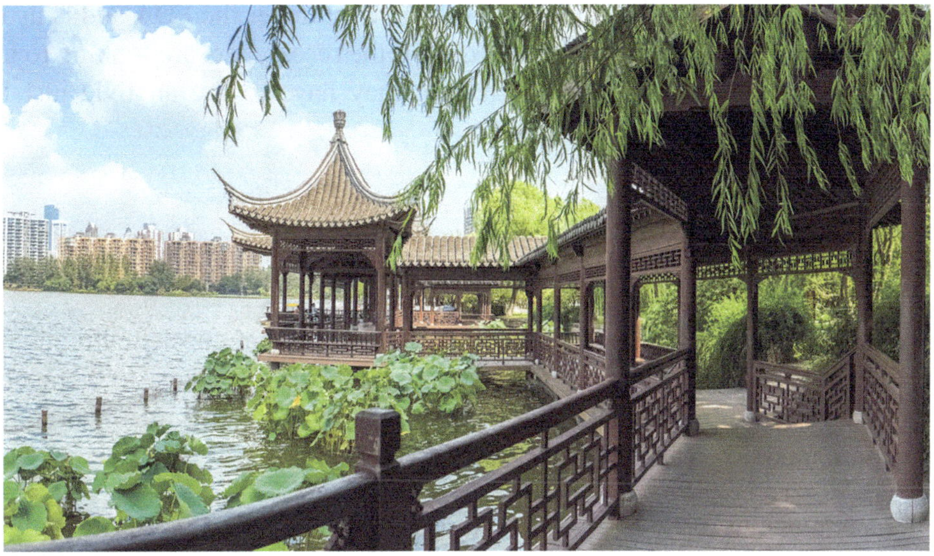

Fig. 164.1 A beautiful traditional corridor and bridge walkway over Lake Mochou in Nanjing, China. Photo: Image used under standard license from shutterstock.com

Acupuncture Research

- We've looked at a lot of the studies on acupuncture and would steer our readers towards results that are reported in PubMed. We probably wouldn't make any recommendations for changes to clinical practice based on anything in the lay press.—**CM and SDM**

- In many acupuncture studies, the control arm is not a true placebo control. The commonly used placebo control has very active mechanisms of increasing endogenous opioids in the system—even if it is short-lived. This is a likely explanation of why acupuncture and sham acupuncture are less differentiated [1].—**SDM**

- Variations in acupuncture methods and point selection are not necessarily sources of bias in acupuncture studies. Rather, they are different types of treatment that need studies to understand which protocol is most effective for which type of patient.—**MZW and SDM**

- A recent review of acupuncture research for palliative care patients reported, "While the evidence for use of acupuncture to treat symptoms in palliative care patients is relatively weak, the evidence base is growing. Experts worldwide are also increasingly recommending acupuncture as a treatment for symptoms in palliative care. Since acupuncture is a safe, nonpharmacological treatment but with small, clinically significant effects, these recommended uses appear as pragmatic efforts to bridge the gap of treatment options available to this patient group." [2]—**AJR**

- There is a lot of interesting research on acupuncture being done in Europe, especially Germany and the Scandinavian countries, so keep an eye on that literature. Those researchers have the advantage of having a lot of national health registries. Of course, a majority of studies are being done in Asia.—**Editors and SDM**

- Right now, any TCM research that includes herbs is covered under the FDA and is usually regulated under the food category. It is only regulated as a drug if the researchers are looking to have an indication for a specific formula or herb—in which case they have to file an IND just like any other pharmaceutical.—**SDM**

General Clinical Correlations

- In the last several hundred years, acupuncture has had a somewhat checkered reputation within the construct of Western medicine—ranging from pseudoscience and quackery to therapeutic communities dedicated to the goal of implementing acupuncture as an alternative treatment in the face of recognized therapeutic modalities.—**Editors**
- We believe that acupuncture is most reliably and responsibly used as a **complementary** therapeutic modality, especially when there is a gap between the limits of Western medicine and wellness.—**CM and SDM**
- Clinical trials have shown that acupuncture can control pain and inflammation in many diseases. The World Health Organization acknowledges **acupuncture as a viable treatment for forty-three diseases.—JLS and SDM**
- The Johns Hopkins Medicine (hopkinsmedicine.org) website states: "Studies have shown that acupuncture is effective alone or when used with conventional therapies to treat (a number of) conditions."—**CM**
- The Hopkins website lists the following conditions as being amenable to acupuncture therapy.—**CM**
  - Nausea caused by surgical anesthesia or chemotherapy
  - Dental pain after surgery
  - Addiction
  - Headaches
  - Menstrual cramps
  - Tennis elbow
  - Fibromyalgia
  - Myofascial pain

  - Osteoarthritis
  - Low back pain
  - Carpal tunnel syndrome
  - Asthma

- Individual acupuncture manipulations may have differential effects on blood perfusion.—**MZW and SDM**
- Acupuncture generally has a favorably low complication rate, with the large majority of complications involving superficial bleeding and/or bruising. More serious complications have been reported, but these have usually been found to result from inexperienced, poorly trained, or unlicensed practitioners.—**SDM**
- **Important:** It's not only a question of where you put the acupuncture needles but when. The answer to that question is that acupuncture has been shown to have efficacy throughout the entire perioperative period, as well as in the chronic pain clinic and in palliative and hospice care.—**SDM and CM**

Preoperative

- Acupuncture points at the Pericardium-6 (P-6; Nei Guan), Yintang (Extra 1), and Shenmen points are thought to have efficacy in mitigating preoperative anxiety. This has now been demonstrated across a range of patients including patients for elective surgery, adolescents, obstetrical patients, and surgical oncology patients.—**CM and SDM**
- The same results are found when preoperative acupuncture is given to decrease the incidence of postoperative nausea and vomiting (N/V). The results can be quite dramatic, decreasing the incidence of postoperative N/V in laparoscopic and gynecological surgery patients from as high as 30% to as low as 10%.—**CM and SDM**
- A small but interesting study looked at the effects of auricular acupuncture on preoperative blood pressure in a randomized controlled trial [3]. Preoperative treatment at the HX6 7i-Ear apex, TF4-Shen men, TF1-Superior triangular fossa, and CO15-Heart points showed statistically lower systolic and diastolic blood pressure in the cohort of study subjects who were 65-70 years old.—**Editors**

***Note from the Editors:** The Longevity Bridge in Repulse Bay near Hong Kong is part of the Kwun Yam Shrine complex. It is surrounded by many fanciful statues and creatures. Local folklore maintains that travelers who cross the bridge have three days added to their lives.

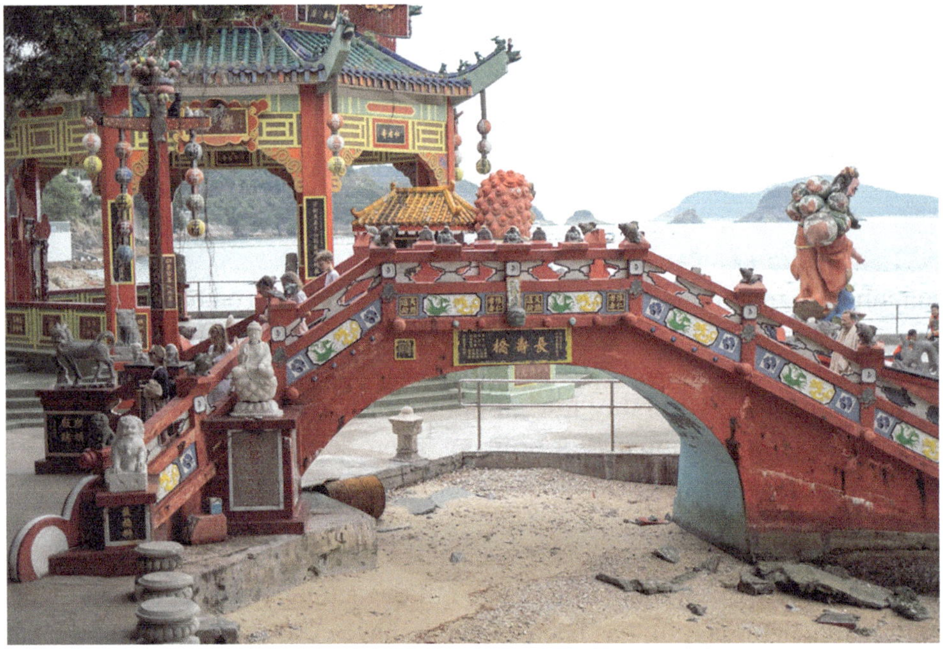

Fig. 164.2 The Longevity Bridge in Repulse Bay, near Hong Kong. Photo: Image used under standard license from adobestock.com

Perioperative and Intraoperative

- Preoperative and perioperative acupuncture dovetails closely with the concept of enhanced recovery after anesthesia. Fundamental to this treatment paradigm is mitigating the perioperative stress response. This is coming down the pike, so lean into this emerging area of clinical practice.—**CM and SDM**

- Several researchers in China have proposed a national acupuncture registry to facilitate acupuncture integration in perioperative care [4]. Their intention is to support data mining and the development of large, multi-center trials and research protocols, as well as to aid in the development of clinical guidelines. Surgical outcomes of interest to the authors include preoperative anxiety, intraoperative hemodynamic instability, postoperative pain, postoperative cognitive dysfunction, and postoperative nausea and vomiting in surgical patients.—**Editors**

- For example, while some applications of acupuncture can down-modulate autoimmune states, intraoperative acupuncture can also serve to reduce immune suppression [5].—**Editors and SDM**

- A 2016 meta-analysis published in *Laryngoscope* in 2016 looked at the outcomes after tonsillectomy of postoperative pain intensity, rescue analgesic consumption, and postoperative nausea and vomiting in patients who had received perioperative acupuncture versus patients who had received a pharmacologic pain control agent or sham acupuncture [6]. In the acupuncture group, 48-hour pain scores, postoperative need for analgesics, and nausea and vomiting were less. Importantly, no major adverse acupuncture effects were noted.—**Editors**

- Electro-acupuncture has some efficacy ameliorating cardiac ischemia-reperfusion injury after cardiopulmonary bypass as demonstrated in a randomized controlled trial [7]. Sixty patients were randomized to receive EA at bilateral Neiguan (PC 6), Lieque (LU 7), and Yunmen (LU 2) for 30 minutes each day for five consecutive days before surgery. Serum cardiac troponin I levels were decreased in the treatment arm for 24 hours. EA pretreatment also reduced the inotrope score at 12 hours, 24 hours, and 48 hours after the intensive care unit arrival and shortened intensive care unit stay time.—**Editors**
- Using the correlation of organ/mental state above, compression of the Spleen 6 point has been shown to be an effective complementary technique to ameliorate anxiety level and consumption of sedatives and analgesics during labor [8].—**SDM and AL**

Pain

- Compared with a single therapy, acupuncture combined with medical therapy is more effective than routine care in pain management.**—MZW and SDM**
- Acupuncture may play an essential role in formulating the analgesic treatment plan, effectively ensuring patients' quality of life and lowering the ratio of drug use.—**MZW and SDM**
- Acupuncture has great potential to not only relieve pain but also contribute to improving overall health by reducing patients' dependence on other, possibly more addicting drugs with adverse side effects.—**MZW and SDM**
- With a growing dependence on opioids and NSAIDs, acupuncture has emerged as a safer alternative. The pain relief derived from the release of endogenous opioids has a faster, longer-lasting action in acute pain analgesia. With a lower incidence of adverse events compared with drug therapy, acupuncture can be an effective alternative for better pain relief.—**JLS and SDM**
- With acupuncture, administration techniques and effectiveness tied to the practitioner's personal clinical experience, outcomes and treatment time courses are variable. Randomized controlled trials have suggested administration of EA three times weekly for eight weeks as likely to have the optimum effectiveness in knee osteoarthritis (KOA) pain reduction. Meta-analyses suggest that it takes five to eleven weeks to achieve EA maximum effect in limb pain.—**JLS and SDM**
- Don't forget that acupuncture has efficacy for preoperative pain as well as postoperative pain. One study compared acupuncture with femoral nerve block in elderly patients with femoral neck fracture [9]. There was no statistical difference in visual analog scale (VAS) scores, nursing quality scores, sleep quality scores, delirium numbers, and perioperative complications were collected and compared between the 2 groups. VAS scores were also similar on day 1 and day 2 after admission.—**Editors**
- The role of anticipation of pain in mediating pain relief has arisen as a possible explanation for placebo analgesia. Despite overlap between placebo and verum acupuncture networks, differences in

dorsolateral prefrontal cortex and rostral anterior cingulate cortex modulation may support non-specific pain expectancy while amygdala, insula, and hypothalamus modulation may demonstrate acupuncture specificity.—**JLS and SDM**

- While there have been a variety of studies investigating the effectiveness of acupuncture analgesia, limitations of these studies include experimental designs of the control group and the use of a placebo as a possible cause. As a result, further studies are required to explore the effectiveness of acupuncture.—**MZW, JLS, and SDM**

- Some experimental evidence has shown little difference between sham and true acupuncture; the placebo effect has called into question the validity of acupuncture as a pain treatment protocol. That being said, acupuncture in conjunction with traditional medical therapy has proven more effective than routine care by itself.—**JLS and SDM**

- The manipulation of acupuncture, especially for pain, closely relates to physicians' personal clinical experience, and it requires careful consideration to achieve standardization. Heterogeneity among practitioners may determine the analgesic effect.—**MZW and SDM**

- However, on the topic of differences among practitioners, in clinical studies, we have found ways of keeping the diagnostic aspects intact but then standardizing the treatment based on Chinese medicine diagnosis. This reduces the influence of practitioner difference [10, 11].—**SDM**

Final Thoughts

- In some training programs in physical medicine and rehabilitation, residents and fellows are offered the opportunity to take adjunctive training and certification in acupuncture. Wouldn't that be a great idea for anesthesiology training programs?—**CM**

References

1. Harris RE, Zubieta J, et al. Traditional Chinese acupuncture and placebo (sham) acupuncture are differentiated by their effects on mu-opioid receptors (MORs). Neuroimage. 2009;47(3):1077–85.
2. Birch S, Bovey M. Acupuncture as a treatment within integrative health for palliative care: a brief narrative review of evidence and recommendations. Complement Med. 2020;26(9):784–91.
3. Ma J, Zhang Y, et al. The effect of auricular acupuncture on preoperative blood pressure across age groups: a prospective randomized controlled trial. Clin Exp Hypertens. 2023;45(1):2169452.
4. Zhang W, Zhang H, et al. Perioperative acupuncture optimizes surgical outcomes: theory, clinical practice and future perspectives. Am J Chin Med. 2022;50(4):961–78.
5. Gliedt JA, Daniels CJ, et al. Narrative review of perioperative acupuncture for clinicians. J Acupunct Meridian. 2015; Epub ahead of print
6. Cho HK, Park IJ, et al. Can perioperative acupuncture reduce the pain and vomiting experienced after tonsillectomy? Laryngoscope. 2016;126(3):608–15.

7. Yang L, Yang J, et al. Cardioprotective effects of electroacupuncture pretreatment on patients undergoing heart valve replacement surgery: a randomized controlled trial. Ann Thorac Surg. 2010;89(3):781–6.
8. Samadi P, Alipour Z, et al. The effect of acupressure at Spleen 6 acupuncture point on the anxiety level and sedative and analgesics consumption of women during labor: a randomized, single-blind clinical trial. Iran J Nurs Midwifery Res. 2018;23(2):87–92.
9. Lu L, Hu J, et al. Comparison of femoral nerve block and acupuncture analgesia for acute preoperative pain in elderly patients with femoral neck fracture: a retrospective study. Am J Transl Res. 2022;14(2):1076–83.
10. Mist S, Ritenbaugh C, et al. Effects of questionnaire-based diagnosis and training on inter-rater reliability among practitioners of traditional Chinese medicine. J Altern Complement Med. 2009;15(7):703–9.
11. Mist SD, Wright C, et al. Traditional Chinese medicine diagnoses in a sample of women with fibromyalgia. Acupunct Med. 2011;29(4):266–9. Epub 2011 Oct 25

Authors

Josh Stich is a member of the Albert Einstein medical class of 2028, and anesthesiology is looking interesting to him at this point. His undergraduate major was in the neural sciences, so the mechanisms and clinical correlations of acupuncture make a lot of sense to him. He has plans to keep up a range of outside interests, even while in med school, and will be blogging about the Australian national parks in his spare time and on vacations.

Marilyn Walker is a pre-med student who recently graduated from NYU with a double major in chemistry and psychology. Before starting medical school, she plans to continue to pursue her passion for the sciences as an intern at the Sigurdsson neuroscience lab at NYU Langone. In her free time, she enjoys playing tennis and is currently training for a marathon.

Cathy Marcucci is a senior anesthesiologist who has a deep interest and belief in integrative medicine, especially acupuncture. She once underwent a course of acupuncture treatments and was completely cured of a bad case of chronic regional pain syndrome. She has the pictures to prove it.

Scott Mist is a pain researcher and an acupuncturist at the Oregon Health & Science University's Comprehensive Pain Center. Over the last couple of years, he has ventured back into the field of coaching boys' volleyball. Trying to keep up with teenage boys, Scott finally understands why he has an abiding interest in pain relief.

Wisdom on Pediatric Anesthesiology

165

Paul A. Tripi, M. Concetta Lupa, Oliver Karam,
Catherine Marcucci, and Kirk Lalwani

Contributors:

Miya Asato, MD (MA)

Harley S. Geller, MD (HSG)

Amy J. Robbins, MD MBA (AJR)

Jennifer N. Tripi, MD (JNT)

Introduction

The key to being a great pediatric anesthesiologist is understanding the differences between children and adults in anatomy, physiology, and psychology; mastering the art of supporting, relating to, and reassuring the families; and remaining calm and effective in emergencies. We thank our senior authors, **Paul Tripi**, **Kirk Lalwani**, **Concetta Lupa**, and **Oliver Karam**, and contributors **Harley Geller**, **Jen Tripi**, **Amy Robbins**, and **Miya Asato** for sending us their words of wisdom and best teaching tips.

There is additional clinical advice pertaining to pediatric anesthesiology in several other sections of this book. We also refer you to the excellent compilation of pediatric anesthesia clinical wisdom that Kirk Lalwani assembled for *Avoiding Common Anesthesia Errors, 2nd Edition*—all profits from that book are pledged to FAER in perpetuity. Finally, we were delighted when Dr. Lupa sent us the picture below of her gorgeous grandmother. She gave us a bit of family background:

P. A. Tripi
Rainbow Babies and Children's Hospital, University Hospitals Cleveland Medical Center, Case Western Reserve University School of Medicine, Cleveland, OH, USA

M. C. Lupa
Department of Anesthesiology, Department of Pediatrics, University of North Carolina at Chapel Hill, Chapel Hill, NC, USA

O. Karam
Department of Pediatrics, Yale New Haven Children's Hospital, New Haven, CT, USA

C. Marcucci (✉)
Department of Transfusion Medicine, Clinical Center, National Institutes of Health, Bethesda, MD, USA

K. Lalwani
Department of Anesthesiology and Perioperative Medicine, Oregon Health & Science University, Portland, OR, USA

S. Mohamed et al. (eds.), *Anesthesia Bridges*, https://doi.org/10.1007/978-3-032-08294-7_165

This is my Nonna, Maria Concetta DeCaria, who went by the nickname of Connie (Fig. 165.1). She was born in 1921 in Pittsburgh. She married my Nonno, who was from Calabria, Italy. They had 3 boys, my father being the youngest. Sadly, she and Nonno both died when my dad was only seven years old, and I never got to meet either of them, but I have always felt her presence in my life. It would have been unimaginable in her time for a woman to have had the career and support that I have been given. Love and family were of the utmost importance in her life and these values have been passed onto me and continue to be what I pass onto my own children.

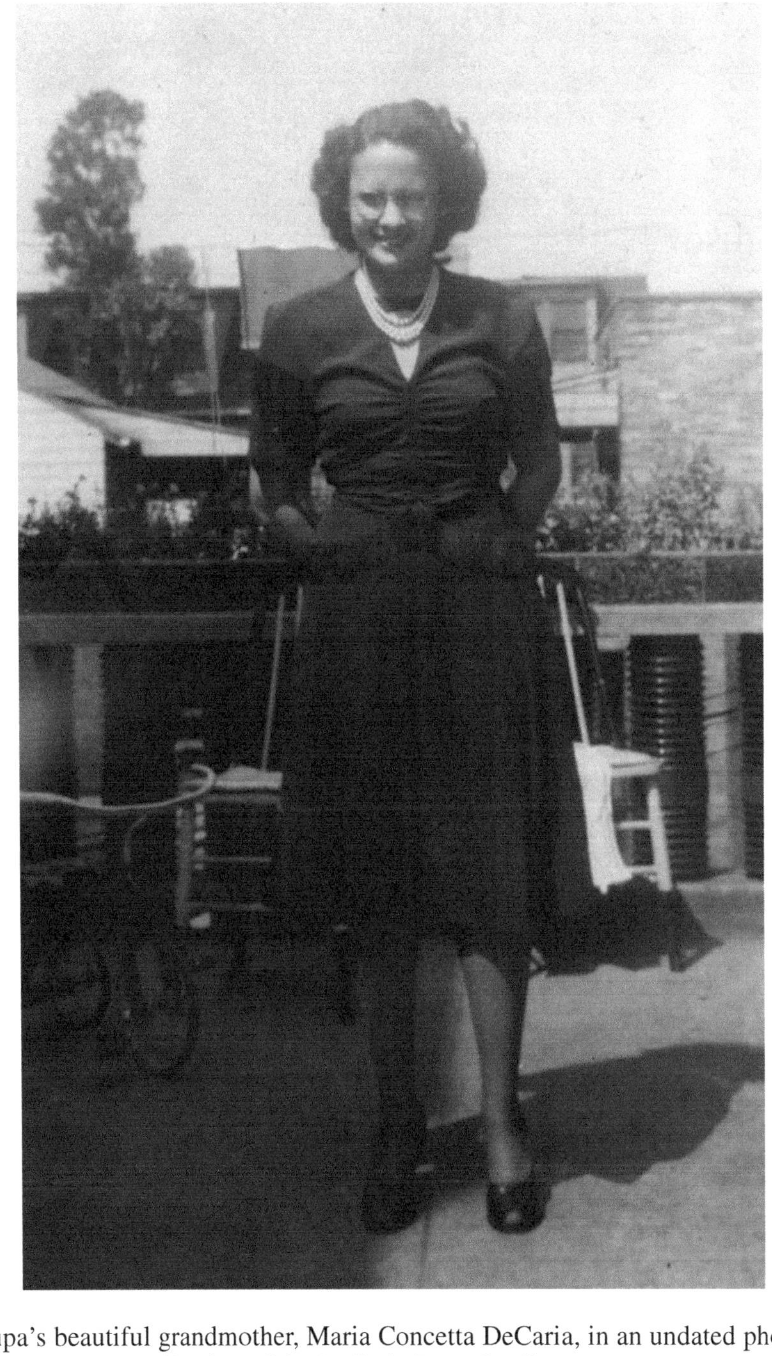

Fig. 165.1 Chetta Lupa's beautiful grandmother, Maria Concetta DeCaria, in an undated photo, probably in the late 1940s or very early 1950s. Photo: Collection of the DeCaria-Lupa family

General

- The first lesson is: Pediatric anesthesia teaches you attention to detail!—**KL**
- Every emergency that can happen with adults can happen with kids, only they happen more quickly.**—Editors**
- Never suggest or imply to parents that you know more about their child than they do. Instead, communicate that you do know more about how to keep them safe in the perioperative period. Emphasize the safety issues always.—**Editors**
- Parents fear the separation from their children most of all—that the little patient will be scared or in pain and they will not be there to comfort them. Whenever possible, but within the limits of common sense and good medical practice, minimize the physical and emotional distance between the child and the parents.—**Editors**
- Establish excellent relationships with your colleagues and always be willing to help them—because no matter how good you think you are, you will need their help.—**PAT**
- When discussing various matters with hospital administrators, patient safety is always your trump card to get your way.—**PAT**
- When facing a vexing clinical situation, always ask a colleague for help or input.—**PAT**
- When you feel defeated by a failed procedure or poor outcome, remember that you are not alone and use the experience as motivation to improve yourself in areas such as knowledge, skill set, or work habit that may provide a more positive outcome moving forward.—**PAT**
- In the course of your daily work, you will frequently encounter problems or questions without obvious answers. Write these down as quickly as feasible, as often they will provide the basis for an excellent research or QI project.—**PAT**
- Whenever feasible, complete all your work at the hospital, so when you go home you can be as good a parent to your own children as you are a doctor to your patients.—**PAT**
- To the degree possible and allowable, never dress like a doctor when caring for children!—**PAT**
- Always leave for work at least 15 minutes early.—**PAT**
- When finishing up your clinical workday and dealing with a variety of frustrations, relax if you can say to yourself that your patients did well. If you have a patient that is struggling, do everything you can to help that patient and thoroughly transfer the patient's care to another individual or team before going home.—**PAT**
- Don't live too close to the hospital, as the drive in and drive home are a good time to gather your thoughts for the coming day and clear your head of the events of the day. This is an important step in separating your work life from your family life.—**PAT**

- The most difficult pediatrics case I ever did was many decades ago. It wasn't a sick neonate or a complicated cardiac case. It was the elevation of a deeply depressed skull fracture in a little patient who came in with a divot in her skull the exact size and dimensions of the head of a hammer, although the parents reported it as "falling off the bed." The first thing the father said to me after the surgery wasn't, "Is she okay?" The first thing he said was, "Is anybody going to be able to tell?" The case bothers me to this day, over 30 years later. I remember discussing it with my attending, who said, "You will get this type of case again." And I did. I probably should have discussed these cases with a professional, just to process my anger, but I never did. Looking back, that was a mistake.—**CM**

- Place your PACU and OR nursing teams on a pedestal, as they often fly under the radar while providing essential, hands-on care to your patients. Their excellent work should be acknowledged frequently and authentically.—**PAT**

- Subspecialty certification in pediatric anesthesiology was offered starting in 2011 and it was high time. Of all the anesthesiology subspecialties, this is the one where a trainee, junior anesthesiologist, or occasional practitioner can should watch, study, and query the most experienced practitioners. —**JNT** and **Editors**

- Seriously! We recommend you emulate, borrow, and steal the techniques and skills of the senior pediatric anesthesiologists. It's really an art.—**Editors**

- Understand that the practice of pediatric anesthesia is institutionally dependent, especially for things like whether the parents are present for induction. Of course, it is always the attending anesthesiologist's final call, but if you change practice locations, be prepared for this. You may have to reconsider whether you want to, and would have support for, bucking the local practice culture.—**Editors**

- Also understand that pediatric anesthesia is always evolving. Since we have been in practice, we have seen revision and updating of the thinking on NPO status and regional anesthesia for children. Don't get stuck in the generation in which you trained, move with the research and times.—**Editors**

Education and Supervision

- Remember that trainees beginning their first rotation in pediatric anesthesiology are often fearful of having a bad outcome in an infant or child. Reassure them that this is a normal way to feel and encourage them to use this fear as motivation to be as prepared and attentive as possible.—**PAT**

- Provide close supervision to trainees with little or no experience caring for infants and children, preferably in a 1:1 teacher-to-student ratio.—**PAT**

- Trainees should be instructed to contact their supervisor immediately with any suspected problem, given that oxygen desaturation, bradycardia, and other vital signs disturbances can deteriorate rapidly in infants and children.—**PAT**

- Patient safety may sometimes trump a good educational experience. For example, a pediatric anesthesiologist, rather than the trainee, should replace a lost IV in a neonate with no access.—**PAT**

- For any given clinical case, focus on preferably one and a maximum of three learning points or themes for your trainee. Basic concepts can be replaced with more sophisticated teaching points as the trainee gains experience.—**PAT**

- When providing feedback, always start with what the learner did well, before providing constructive feedback for areas of improvement.—**PAT**

***Note from the Editors:** *Anesthesia Bridges* editor and author Kirk Lalwani has an appreciation for the Charles Bridge in Prague (Fig. 165.2). It is a medieval stone bridge across the Vltara River in the Czech Republic. Construction took several decades in the late fourteenth and early fifteenth centuries. Legend has it that the first stone was laid at exactly 5:31 on July 9, 1357, which formed a chronological palindrome: 1357-9-7531. King Charles IV felt this palindrome acted as a numerical bridge that would give the structure extra strength.

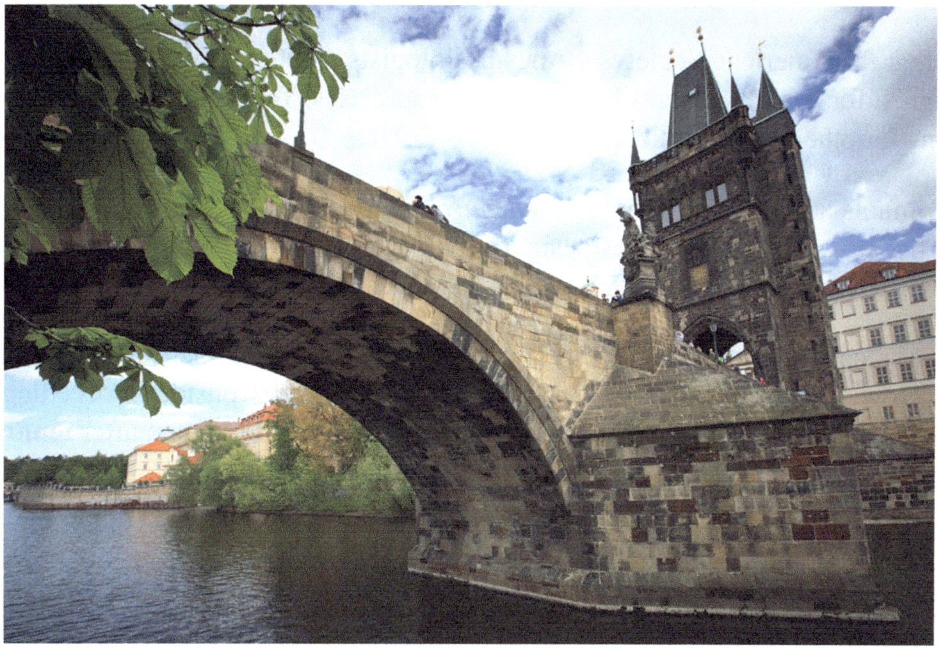

Fig. 165.2 The Charles Bridge in Prague, Czech Republic. In centuries past, it was the most important connection between Prague Castle and the Old Town section of the city. It is lined with an avenue of Baroque statuaries that were added in the 1700s. It has been subjected to numerous devastating floods and has undergone extensive renovation throughout the centuries. This is the view looking towards the Old Town. Photo: Image used under standard license from shutterstock.com

Post-Graduate Training to Be a Pediatric Anesthesiologist

- If you do not feel some trepidation when you decide on a career in pediatric anesthesiology, then choose a different subspecialty.—**PAT**
- You will have many "failures" during your training, but these are your best growth opportunities.—**PAT**
- Resist that feeling that you have come close to mastering all there is to know in this specialty, as you will be reminded time and time again that there is always much more to learn than you could ever assimilate.—**PAT**
- Always seek out the most challenging cases and always be willing to volunteer when extra help is needed at the end of the day. Along with helping an infant or child in need, such behavior is often rewarded in tangible and intangible ways.—**PAT**

Preoperative Fasting

- Remember that the American Society of Anesthesiologists practice guidelines for preoperative fasting are designed for healthy patients having elective surgeries. Your clinical judgment should dictate modifications for other patients.—**PAT**
- Families of infants and children should be *encouraged* to provide liberal clear liquids until 2 hours prior to elective procedures under anesthesia. Dehydrated infants and children are irritable and prone to hypotension on induction of general anesthesia.—**PAT**
- Do not cancel a case because a child is found to be chewing gum, otherwise you will be canceling many cases. However, do confirm no other ingestion has occurred. Consider proceeding once the gum is removed or pursue a more conservative approach of delaying for 2 hours after removal.—**PAT**
- During preoperative fasting, children generally prefer carbohydrate containing clear liquids to non-caloric clear liquids.—**PAT**
- Allow and encourage breastfeeding until 4 hours prior to an elective procedure.—**PAT**
- Parents will sometimes revise fasting history once realizing that a violation of guidelines may result in case cancellation. Always assume their first history is most accurate.—**PAT**

Preoperative Evaluation

- Observing the child play and interact with family members is the most critical part of your physical exam.—**PAT**
- When compared to standing, sitting during your evaluation makes you less threatening and empowers the patient and family.—**PAT**

- When agitated that a patient and family have arrived late for their surgery, please remember that children don't drive. To the extent possible, you should not penalize children for their parents' misbehavior.—**PAT**

- Give yourself extra time to perform your preoperative evaluations. This is your best opportunity to establish a relationship with your patients and their families, and to give them a favorable impression of you.—**PAT**

- When performing a preoperative evaluation, always take a few minutes to first meet the family and establish a connection. When hospital administrators or surgeons push back that you are spending too much time, calmly explain that this is an essential part of providing pediatric anesthesia.—**PAT**

- When presented with a neuro-atypical or very anxious child, it can be helpful to ascertain from parents what sensory stimuli are most challenging for them to handle. Utilize your child life specialists to help you assess what perioperative needs are helpful for all pediatric patients, but remember they can be especially useful for the anxious or sensory-sensitive child. Make sure the OR staff is aware that noises can be triggering. Consider turning down the lights in the room before entering. This can provide a visual clue that you are hoping to keep the environment calm and quiet.—**MCL**

- Be sure to know one good magic trick or other child-friendly activity, as this will help you connect with your patient and family. Your audience will always be changing, so a little talent goes a long way!—**PAT**

- Juggling is an excellent skill to acquire, as children enjoy watching it and they love to try it themselves.—**PAT**

- Respect the growing autonomy of your adolescent/teenage patients by directing much of your history-taking to them rather than the parents. Be sure to answer all their questions, along with their parents' questions.—**PAT**

- Insist that your hospital/surgery center have a written, unambiguous policy regarding preoperative pregnancy screening, testing, and reporting of results to minors and their families. Be aware that this policy will vary by institution and may reflect differences in state laws regarding emancipation of minors.—**PAT**

- The cliché that your first attempt at an intravenous line is your best chance to be successful is especially true in pediatric anesthesiology, as a child will become increasingly resistant to repeated attempts. Consider preoperative sedation or change your plan to inhalation induction before making repeated attempts.—**PAT**

- Never cancel a case without first having a discussion with the surgical team. This is a courtesy to the surgeon and allows for a united front when explaining the reason for the cancellation to the family.—**PAT**

- When dealing with an uncooperative child who is refusing to drink premedication, it is best to step away from the bed and allow the parents to use their usual routine to convince the child to drink medicine. Sometimes enlisting a child-life specialist for encouragement is a great help.—**PAT**

- If you are lucky enough to have child-life specialists on your staff, celebrate and appreciate the many ways they can improve your patients' experience. Don't waste this valuable resource.—**PAT**

- A kid is never going to tell you the full truth about illicit drug use, including alcohol and smoked substances, with the parents present. Even if they admit to the substance, they are not going to admit to the amount.—**Editors**

- Remember the 50th percentile of weight for a 1-year-old is 10 kg. Babies double their birthweight at 6 months and triple it at 1 year. A rough estimate of the weight trajectory for the first 5–6 years is that children will gain 2–3 kg per year after age one. This results in:

  - 1-year-old ~10 kg

  - 2-year-old ~12 kg

  - 3-year-old ~14 kg

  Therefore, if you see your next patient is a 3-year-old and the weight is listed as 28 KILOGRAMS, double-check that this hasn't been written in POUNDS before dosing based on weight! If it is indeed a 28 kg 3-year-old, consider grabbing the ultrasound and preparing for all the difficulties that can come with this body habitus!—**MCL**

Intraoperative Management

- Arrive early enough to fully prepare your operating room for the first case *and* subsequent scheduled cases. There is no worse way to start your day than to rush through this critical component of safe patient care.—**PAT**
- Transporting a child to the operating room from the preoperative area can result in significant patient anxiety and resistance. In most cases, you can avoid this problem by carefully assessing preoperative child anxiety and by providing sedation when necessary.—**PAT**

- If hospital policy allows it, parent presence during induction of anesthesia is most effective with a pairing of an anxious child and a calm parent. Anxious parents are generally not helpful, and calm children generally do well during induction without a parent present.—**PAT**

- A pediatric anesthesiologist told us once that the most challenging "anxious parent" situations are not when you are anesthetizing the children of other anesthesiologists but when you are caring for the children of physicians who are not anesthesiologists and other medical professionals. They have almost always read up on specific drugs and techniques and understand enough to ask reasonable questions, but don't have enough knowledge to really understand the care of a patient under anesthesia. Sometimes they even arrive with a proposed plan of care for their child.—**KL and Editors**

- If your own kid goes to the OR, consider not attending the induction. You already know your colleagues will be careful, and they don't need the extra stress of you being there. My own children went to the OR several times and did fine without me present at induction. At age five, my daughter created a sensation when she rode the stretcher back to the OR, got inside the room, and said, “Oh, so this is what my Mommy does!”—**CM**

- Always check the pre-existing IV before induction!—**KL**

- Always be very wary of the IV in the antecubital fossa.—**KL**

- Also, always be very wary of the “floor IV.” Just because you hear a report that a patient coming from the floor to the OR has access, doesn’t mean you have to believe it.—**Editors**

- Don’t forget about the saphenous vein! It’s a beauty. It lies directly anterior to the medial malleolus, and because it is not always visible, it is often left untouched. Tips for accessing this vein include pointing the big toe down and holding it there in a “ballet toe” position to extend the vein and keep it from moving away. Remember that this vein, and any vein in the lower extremity, can be especially nice to use when you have performed a caudal, because the child is less likely to be bothered by it, and therefore it may be undisturbed longer.—**MCL**

- Firmly fixate the vein when inserting an intravenous catheter. 24-g catheters are short and prone to kinking or falling out of the vein, so reserve these for infants or situations where obtaining intravenous access is difficult.—**PAT**

- If the tape and/or dressing used to secure an intravenous catheter becomes wet for any reason, remove the tape and dressing completely and dry the skin before reapplication. Whenever possible, perform this process *prior* to emergence from anesthesia. Thrashing infants and children will easily dislodge poorly secured catheters.—**PAT**

- The “three attempts” rule for establishing intravenous access does not apply to anesthetized patients without access. If there is any difficulty inserting the catheter, the most skilled and experienced provider should make subsequent attempts.—**PAT**

- Be mindful of your flushes. In neonates and small babies under 5 kg, it is critically important to be mindful of your fluid administration. For example, when caring for a 1.5 kg baby, the estimated blood volume is close to 135 mL. If you administer a 5 mL saline flush with medications five times throughout the anesthetic, you have given 16 mL/kg of volume and diluted your blood volume by 25 mL!—**MCL**

- Flush medications as close to the vein as possible and familiarize yourself with the dead space of every type of tubing attached to your patient in order to avoid overdosing volume in a patient. Similarly, minimize free flowing fluids in small patients to avoid an accidental overdose. Many hospitals utilize a buretrol, but I would caution against this. If the buretrol is filled to 50 mL, and that amount is given during the start of the case in this particular child, the child will receive over 30 mL/kg in fluid.—**MCL**

- Distraction is a powerful and important tool during mask inhalation induction of anesthesia in young children. Videos and video games are especially effective.—**PAT**

- Without exception, fully monitor infants prior to induction of anesthesia. Provide at least pulse oximetry monitoring to anxious children undergoing inhalation induction and immediately attach additional monitors once the child is anesthetized.—**PAT**

- When performing intravenous induction of anesthesia, verbalizing each medication and dose you are about to inject provides one last opportunity for you and other members of your team to recognize any errors in medication choice, sequence, or dosage.—**PAT**

- Bradycardia is hypoxia unless proved otherwise.—**KL**

- While we all recognize that bradycardia in children is caused by hypoxia until proven otherwise, I disdain the practice of using atropine to improve or pre-treat the heart—**HSG**

  ** The best way to know that the patient is hypoxemic is a dropping heart rate—atropine will mask this effect.

  ** The best way to know that you have improved hypoxemia is to see an increasing heart rate—atropine will mask this effect.

  ** The last thing that a hypoxemic heart needs is increased oxygen demand due to an increasing heart rate—atropine will exacerbate this problem.

- Because of their rapid oxygen consumption and ease of airway obstruction, infants and children can rapidly deteriorate from "pink and stable" to "blue and near arrest."—**PAT**

- From my now retired colleague Dr. Danny Robinson: *Oxygen is your only friend.* I had a T-shirt with this printed on it for his graduation party, as did all my other colleagues with his other sayings.—**KL**

- During an emergency, it is very difficult to calculate the proper dosing of medications. Always make these calculations before you start your anesthesia care.—**PAT**

- Certain medication errors are more common or severe in infants and young children due to their relatively small size compared to adults. For example, many medications are formulated based on adult dosing and require dilution for administration in these young patients. Ten-fold or even 100-fold dosing errors may occur. Stay totally focused and triple-check your calculations when preparing such medications.—**PAT**

- You can always give more drug, but you can't take any back.—**KL**

- Use of fiberoptic endoscopic intubation may be needed emergently when managing a patient with a "difficult airway," yet this technique is under-practiced. Never pass up an opportunity to utilize this technique in elective and controlled situations *when it is indicated*, even when alternative, more commonly performed techniques may be successful.—**PAT**

- Trainees should study and understand the differences between infant, child, and adult airway anatomy and physiology before performing airway intubation in infants and children.—**PAT**

- Ultrasound-guided nerve blocks in infants and children can be safely performed under general anesthesia.—**PAT**

- Topically applied or injected local anesthetics, ultrasound guided peripheral nerve blocks, or regional anesthetic techniques, either singly or in combination, provide excellent supplementation of general anesthesia for painful surgical procedures in infants and children.—**PAT**

- When faced with abnormal vital signs measurements, resist the temptation to blame the monitor. Always presume measurements are accurate until proven otherwise.—**PAT**

- Be extra vigilant when you are completing a case that has kept you overtime or frustrated you. You will be more prone to being careless or less attentive in such situations, especially during emergence from anesthesia and transport to PACU.—**PAT**

- Never let a pediatric patient fall off the table. There is as much risk of this (or more) at the end of the case as at the beginning. Somebody has to keep a hand on the baby at all times, and this is also true of bigger kids as well.—**KL**

- A child's arterial tracing can tell you a great deal in a glance. For example, the upstroke reflects contractility while the fullness of the wave describes volume status.—**HSG**

- Babies can bleed to death in their head.—**KL**

- Babies wake up thrice—extubate on the third wake up!—**KL**

- The best way to treat laryngospasm is to prevent it.—**KL**

- Never underestimate the power of a proper two-handed jaw thrust to prevent and alleviate laryngospasm—**KL**

- One of the biggest omissions that junior and senior pediatric anesthesiologists make is failing to keep up with the adult anesthesia literature. Pretty much everything that can happen to adults under anesthesia in the perioperative period can happen to pediatric patients *and then some*. Cardiac arrest, ventilatory failure, seizures, strokes, loss of airway, allergic reactions, transfusion reactions, aspiration, reactive airway events, sleep apnea, malignant hyperthermia, dental and soft tissue damage, and latex allergies. *Everything.* And they can present to the perioperative period pregnant and intoxicated on any number of substances, as well.—**Editors**

- I agree with the editors. As a clinician who did pediatric as well as adult cases, I think when you do the occasional pediatric anesthesia case, there is a tendency to put laser focus on the "smallness" of everything in peds cases—tiny lines, tiny ventilator volumes, tiny dosages of meds and fluids, getting all the tiny air bubbles out of everything and so forth, but you can lose focus that all of the "big" problems still occur—positioning injuries, eye injuries, medication errors, anesthesia machine issues, problems with the CO2 canisters, and so forth.—**AJR**

***Note from the Editors:** Paul Tripi's favorite bridge *by far* is the Lagoon Bridge in the Boston Public Garden (Fig. 165.3) and he told us why:

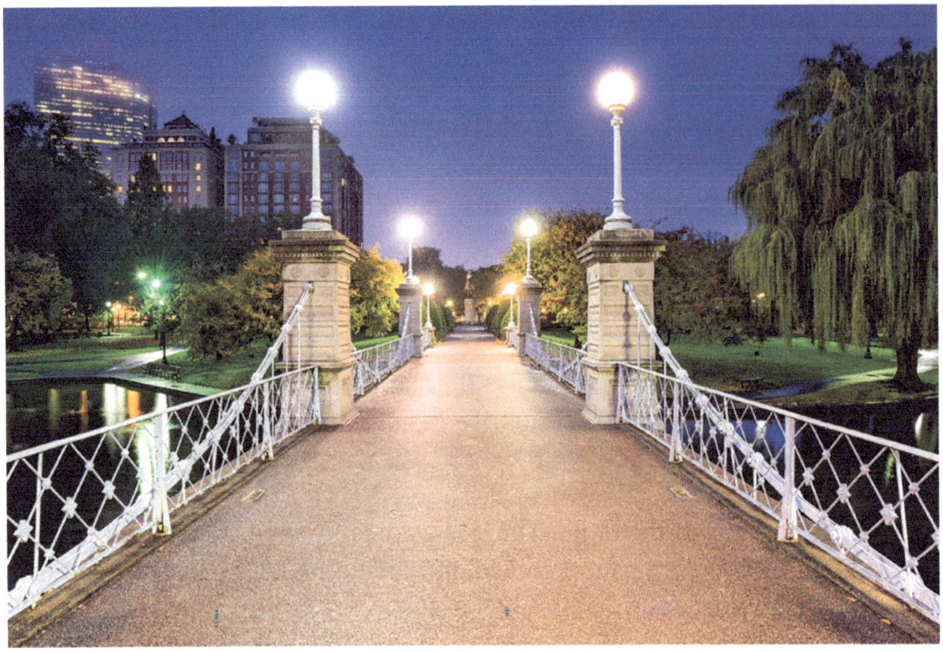

Fig. 165.3 The Boston Public Garden was established in 1837 and was America's first public botanical space. The Lagoon Bridge was completed in 1867 and was declared a National Historic Landmark in 1987. The bridge has been extensively restored and returned to its original appearance. However, for safety reasons, the entire structure of bridge now rests on girders and the charming wrought iron suspension system is now entirely decorative. Photo: Image used under standard license from shutterstock.com

I proposed to my wife on this bridge, right by one of the granite columns. It seemed like the perfect spot, given that she was born and raised near Boston and had visited many times, and I had crossed this bridge twice daily during my exercise routine as a medical student. The nice thing about proposing marriage in a place that's been there for almost two hundred years is that you know you will be able to go back to the exact spot to commemorate the occasion...which we have done many times!

Postoperative Transport

- When transporting a patient to PACU, always bring a t-piece with a bag and mask and an oxygen source, as it is not uncommon for an infant or child to develop an obstructed airway and hypoxemia. Keep your emergency drugs with you, along with propofol to rapidly manage emergence agitation.—**PAT**

- Be vigilant of the infant or child's airway patency and respiratory effort during transport, no matter how minor the procedure or minimal the sedation provided.—**PAT**

- When transferring care to the PACU nurses, always provide a thorough report and never leave the bedside unless you are fully satisfied the patient is in stable condition with a reliably patent airway.—**PAT**

- Following tonsillectomy and adenoidectomy, transport children in the lateral position, which allows for drainage of secretions and avoidance of airway obstruction from the tongue.—**PAT**

- We were taught, as others were, that there is almost no acute problem in the pediatric perioperative period that is easier to take care of in the PACU or PICU than in the OR. For one thing, the lights are better in the OR. Therefore, do not hesitate if the tonsils start bleeding or the patient develops stridor or the drain output greatly increases, to turn around and head back to the OR. One of my faculty at Hopkins always asked the room turnover people to wait a few moments before pulling off the circuit and breaking down the room.—**Editors**

PACU/Postoperative Management

- Do not disregard a parent's concern, no matter how trivial it might seem.—**PAT**

- Remember that the time until the parents can see their child after surgery is excruciating. Minimize it as much as possible, but avoid having the patients seeing a patient who is in significant distress.—**Editors**

- Persistent nausea/vomiting, pain, or respiratory distress despite treatment are vexing problems most safely managed with hospital admission. Discharging your patient to home after a long battle to improve such problems often results in your own uneasy drive home as you worry about your patient.—**PAT**

- Avoid standing orders for patient discharge from PACU or discharge to home unless you fully trust others to properly and safely interpret provided criteria for safe discharge.—**PAT**

- Regardless of hospital or departmental policy, make every effort to personally see every patient post-operatively. This allows you to reassure yourself the patient has done well and provides you with an excellent opportunity to hear any feedback from the patient and family.—**PAT**

- If a patient in PACU has presented significant clinical challenges and you are undecided about discharge to PICU versus the regular post-operative surgical ward, *choose the ICU.* You will rarely, or perhaps never, regret sending a patient to PICU out of an abundance of caution.—**PAT**

- Avoid codeine and tramadol for postoperative pain management in children due to variable activity of cytochrome P450 CYP2D6, which may result in apnea. This is absolute in children less than 12 years old.—**PAT**

- Parents are often terrified when observing emergence delirium in their children, so take extra time after treatment to offer reassurance and explain what occurred.—**PAT**

- There is really fascinating work going on in the pediatric anesthesia community regarding acupuncture and other complementary modalities. There are studies noting the efficacy in pediatrics receiving stem cell transplants, hemodialysis, oncology, and palliative care.[1, 2] Both families and nurses are training in human touch modalities such as Reiki. Time to incorporate some information from the studies and work towards increased clinical use in the pediatric PACU and the PICU? We think so.—**Editors**

- Take every precaution to avoid corneal abrasions in pediatric patients. They can cause great distress even for adult patients, and we have seen babies and tots cry and cry because of them. If a little patient seems inconsolable in the PACU, consider an evaluation. Also, be forewarned that parents really don't take this perioperative complication very easily.—**Editors**

Neonates and Preemies

- Never trust a preemie!—**KL**

- When providing general anesthesia to any premature infant under 60 weeks post-conceptual age, admit to the hospital for 24 hours for post-anesthesia apnea monitoring.—**PAT**

- A neonate is one big vagus nerve in a bag of water.—**KL**

- Neonatal ventilation often fails in inexperienced hands due to a lack of recognition of the need for a much higher airway pressure for the first breath that expands those collapsed alveoli. If you are teaching this case, make sure you discuss this with your trainee beforehand.—**KL**

- And you should be able to *see* the ventilation, not just hear it. If the chest isn't moving, you aren't ventilating.—**HSG**
- Neonates have an increased risk of toxicity to local anesthetics.—**PAT**

- A common mistake in caring for neonates is to allow them to become hypothermic. Take stringent measures to avoid heat loss in these patients.—**PAT**

- Neonates respond to painful stimuli, as neural pain transmission begins in development as early as 22 weeks gestational age.—**PAT**

- In neonates with "unprotected" airways, opioids and sedative medications must be carefully titrated in small doses. Be especially vigilant and conservative when transporting such patients to or from the operating room, and be certain you have all necessary equipment and emergency medications for bag-mask ventilation and airway intubation.—**PAT**

- When managing a neonatal emergency, be certain a cardiac evaluation has been performed, as many of these disorders may be associated with congenital heart disease.—**PAT**

PICU

- In the PICU, it is easier to take time to make a clinical decision than in the OR, because the physiological changes are less abrupt. There is frequently time to wait for labs before intervening, for example, to wait for hemoglobin levels before transfusing red blood cells, for lactates before increasing epinephrine, or a lung ultrasound before giving additional fluid boluses.—**OK**

- In the PICU, the long-term effects of sedatives and analgesics are still unknown. Some medications, such as benzodiazepines, are believed to increase the risk of delirium. Therefore, sedation and analgesia strategies should be adjusted for critically ill children.—**OK**

- PICU ventilators have different characteristics that warrant different settings than in the OR. For example, the PEPP and tidal volumes settings might differ, since the circuit compliances and the engineering designs are different. Some patients might need a lower setting on the PICU ventilators.—**OK**

- PICU electronic medical records are designed differently from anesthesia systems. For example, orders must be entered before the intervention can be charted. If a fluid bolus isn't prescribed, it will not be included in the fluid balance. If a dose of morphine isn't prescribed, it will not be recorded as given.—**OK**

- Communication in the PICU is more complex than in the OR as there are many more team members and consultants. Therefore, clear communication and handoffs are paramount to the safety of care.—**OK**

- As most PICUs are closed units, the pediatric intensivist is the final decision maker. They need to be aware of all suggestions; suggesting changes solely to the bedside nurse or the residents without making sure the intensivist is aware and agrees with the plan will lead to loss of information and confusion.—**OK**

- We should never order tests that will not lead to a decision.—**OK**

- As the patient's status might change slowly, for example, the FiO2 increased by a few percentage points each hour, or the lactate level increased minimally from one blood draw to the next, it is easy to miss the tipping point where the patient needs a new intervention, such as being intubated or the addition of a new vasopressor.—**OK**

- Just because you can doesn't mean you should. Have conversations with the families about their goals of care.—**OK**

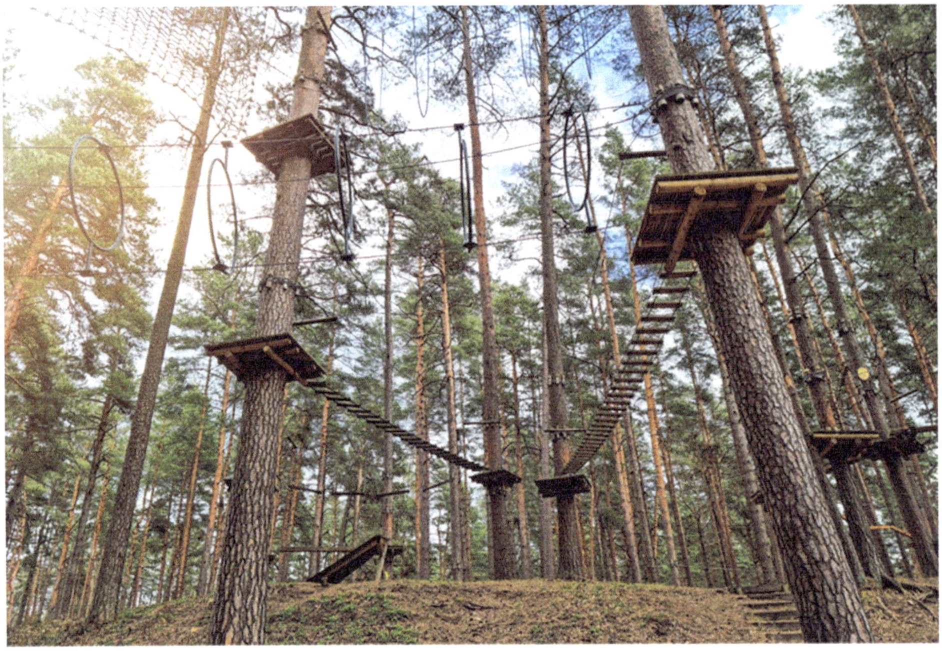

Fig. 165.4 The children of *Anesthesia Bridges* contributor Carolyn Metzler have done the Sandy Springs ropes course, which looks a lot like this, many times. Photo: Image used under standard license from adobestock.com

- A patient with decreasing urine output might not need a fluid bolus. SIADH is a frequent complication of critical illness; it would be treated with fluid restriction, not fluid boluses. It is easy to measure natremia and lactatemia and assess if the patient is in low cardiac output or is hyponatremic.—**OK**

***Note from the Editors:** Ropes courses and climbing bridges are very popular for kids of all ages. The occasional adult sometimes gets up the nerve as well (Fig. 165.4).

Out-of-OR Cases

- These cases require extra vigilance as often you are far from those who can help you when needed.—**PAT**
- Care providers who have ordered these studies/procedures often have not considered the anesthesia risk to the child entailed in successfully completing the study or procedure.—**PAT**
- You are a gatekeeper with these cases. Be sure the need for the study/procedure justifies the anesthesia risk for the child.—**PAT**
- Don't assume that sedation or general anesthesia is always needed. Occasionally, your services are not necessary, and you can encourage the patient/family to proceed without anesthesia care.—**PAT**
- When caring for children in MRI, be vigilant that no ferromagnetic objects are inadvertently brought near the scanner. Serious injuries and damage to equipment can occur. Be especially vigilant in an

emergency situation, when it may be most prudent to remove the patient from the scanner room.—**PAT**

- Stem cell medicine is a rapidly expanding area of clinical practice. Increasing numbers of children will undergo apheresis procedures for the collection of hematopoietic stem cells, either as autologous or allogeneic donors. This includes children under 4 years of age and with significant acute and chronic medical conditions and disabilities. The developing standard of care is to provide sedation for these procedures in a monitored care or ICU setting, as the procedures can last many hours. The sedation for the apheresis procedure, usually based on dexmedetomidine, is a continuation of the sedation provided in interventional radiology for placement of the apheresis lines. But be aware that this is an emerging out-of-the-OR practice opportunity and there will almost certainly be refinements in the clinical practice paradigms.—**CM**

Some Specific Disorders

- In patients being treated for malignancy, avoid routine use of corticosteroids for prophylaxis of nausea/vomiting, as it may violate a protocol being utilized for treatment. Contact the primary team prior to administration.—**PAT**
- In children with Williams-Beuren syndrome having general anesthesia, encourage ingestion of clear liquids until two hours prior to induction and provide intravenous hydration pre-induction if they have any evidence of dehydration during your preoperative assessment.—**PAT**
- Never administer succinylcholine to a patient with Duchenne muscular dystrophy due to the risk of hyperkalemic cardiac arrest. Be especially vigilant that this drug is removed from your emergency medications and that "breakers" are aware of the patient's diagnosis.—**PAT**
- A pyloromyotomy for correction of pyloric stenosis is *not* an emergency surgery. Confirm normalized blood electrolytes and adequate hydration prior to proceeding.—**PAT**
- Before proceeding with anesthetic care in children with congenital heart disease, be sure you fully understand the lesion and past interventions, and their physiologic and pharmacologic implications.—**PAT**
- In infants and children with unrepaired Tetralogy of Fallot, be fully prepared to manage sudden hypoxic episodes.—**PAT**
- Life-threatening bradycardia may occur in children with Trisomy 21 during induction of general anesthesia. This is especially dangerous during inhalation induction without intravenous access.—**PAT**

- In children presenting with symptoms of epiglottitis and pending airway obstruction, *DO NOT* instrument or invasively examine the airway outside of the operating room. Airway management is most safely provided under general anesthesia in a spontaneously breathing patient.—**PAT**

- Occulocardiac reflex induced bradycardia during strabismus surgery is common in children. Immediately inform the surgeon to stop the procedure until bradycardia resolves and consider treatment with an anticholinergic medication.—**PAT**

- When managing a child with an acute epidural hematoma, time is of the essence, so avoid delaying surgery for time-consuming placement of invasive lines.—**PAT**

- Beware of performing general anesthesia in a patient with an anterior mediastinal mass, especially if it is causing respiratory distress when supine. Full airway obstruction may occur under general anesthesia.—**PAT**

- In children with airway foreign bodies, slow inhalation induction of anesthesia and maintenance of spontaneous ventilation promote airway patency.—**PAT**

- In children undergoing airway surgeries, open and ongoing communication between the surgical and anesthesia teams is critical to smooth and successful outcomes.—**PAT**

- In infants with pyloric stenosis, always attempt to empty the gastric contents prior to induction of general anesthesia. Having done that, always assume the stomach is still full.—**PAT**

- Infants and children with traumatic injuries often become hypothermic, which exacerbates problems such as acidosis and bleeding. From the moment they arrive in the trauma bay, take steps to reestablish or maintain euthermia.—**PAT**

- Avoid thinking of upper endoscopy as a minor procedure in infants and children. This procedure usually requires general anesthesia with either a native or secure airway, and it often can result in challenging airway management and laryngospasm.—**PAT**

- When managing infants and children with sickle cell disease, remember to optimize or avoid these *five Hs* to avoid sickling and associated painful crises or acute chest syndrome: *H*ypotension, *H*ypoxemia, *H*ypothermia, p*H* (acidosis), and *H*ematocrit.—**PAT**

- Keep in mind that children in status epilepticus are incredibly medically fragile. Acute care of these patients does not only involve stopping the seizures and protecting the airway. Individual treatment strategies depend on the etiology of the seizures—if they are due to underlying infectious or ICP issues, stopping the seizures is only *the start* of definitive treatment. Mortality in status epilepticus is also closely related to cardiorespiratory or metabolic compromise (check blood glucose levels repeatedly!) as well as the side effects of therapy, such as hypotension caused by medications.—**MA** and **CM**

- Be mindful of the pediatric clinical scenarios that will re-present in adult patients—for example Tetralogy of Fallot, other genetic syndromes, and anomalies. You will be faced with these clinical challenges again in adult patients.—**AJR**

Summary

- *Never* be afraid to ask questions or call for help. Odds are your clinical instinct is correct!—**JNT**

- Pediatric patients will challenge you, and always have something to teach you. Stay humble and eager

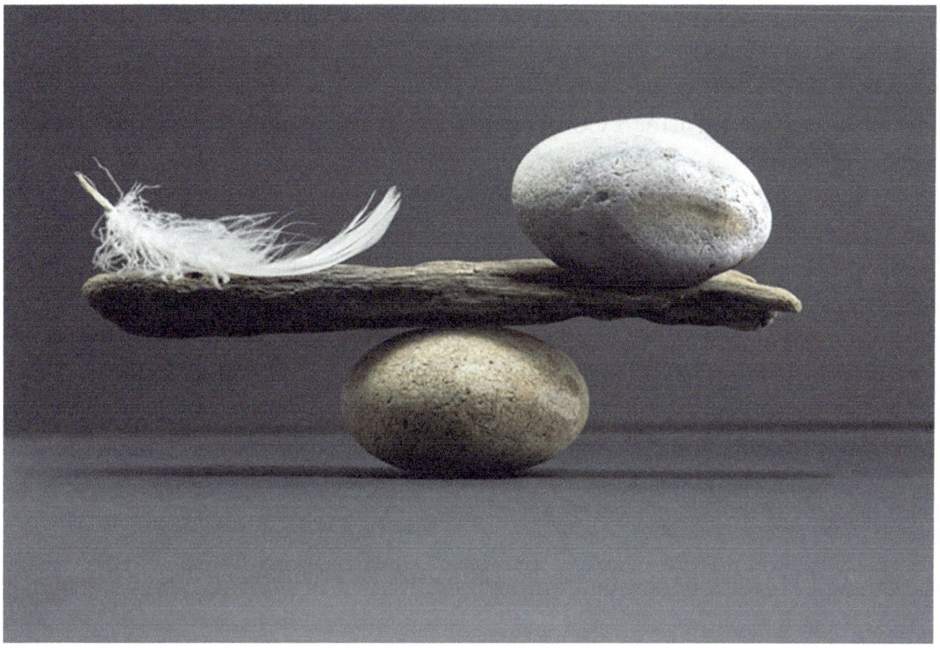

Fig. 165.5 This is the essence of pediatric anesthesiology. Photo: Image used under standard license from shutterstock.com

to learn.—**JNT**

- Pediatric anesthesiology is a team sport. Ensure you know your teammates and utilize your nursing and surgical colleagues to help provide the best care to your patient.—**JNT**

- Never forget that every second of every pediatric case is about managing anxiety—both those of the patients and their families. Even if you are mid-case and the parents are far away in the waiting area, what can you do this minute to decrease their stress hours from now?—**Editors**

- This little balance beam and bridge is the perfect metaphor for the practice of pediatric anesthesiology (Fig. 165.5). The pressures of your case might feel to you like the rock at times but your job is to make it look and feel like the feather to everybody else. Accept that you are in the middle, absorbing the static and dynamic stresses of the case.—**Editors**

Clinical Wisdom from *Avoiding Common Anesthesia Errors, 2nd Edition*

The *Anesthesia Bridges* editors thank *Kirk Lalwani* (the senior author of this chapter) for being a great academic pediatric anesthesiologist and a great colleague. He was a section editor for *Avoiding Common Anesthesia Errors, 2nd Edition,* nicknamed "Green2," and wrote and/or edited the following short chapters in that book that are each packed with additional clinical advice, tips, and wisdom. Many of the titles are teaching points in and of themselves. We highly recommend you check them out!

Green2 Pediatric Anesthesia Chapter Titles:

Assent, Consent, and Refusal: Informed Consent and Decision-Making for Adult and Pediatric Patients

- NPO Guidelines Made Easy—Always Maintain a Firm Hold on Current Principles, Best Practices, and Your Own Common Sense
- Aspiration and Food Injury—When Not to Extubate Deep
- Don't Underestimate the Power of Distraction During Separation and Induction of Anesthesia in Kids
- Parental Presence on Induction—It's Your Call and How to Do It
- The Child with a URI
- Accept That You Will Have to Meet the Clinical Challenges of Obesity and Obstructive Sleep Apnea in Your Pediatric Patient Cohort
- Neuromuscular Disease in Kids Can Be Very Challenging Because You Don't Always Have a Definitive Diagnosis—Here's How to Approach the Clinical Situations
- Pediatric Patients with Epilepsy: Considerations for Patients on a Ketogenic Diet and for Cortical Mapping
- Neonates Deserve Perioperative Analgesia, Too
- Anesthetic Considerations in Patients with Fontan Physiology Who Present for Noncardiac Surgery
- Anesthesia for Kids and Neurotoxicity: You Are Going to Be Asked, So Don't Be Surprised and Don't Act Uninformed
- Double Down on Pediatric Airway Equipment

- Optimizing Bag Mask Ventilation and Direct Laryngoscopy in Children
- Why You Should Expect Hypoxemia During Induction and Emergence of the Pediatric Patient and What to Do About It
- Why Air Bubbles and Air Emboli Can Be So Serious in Pediatric Patients and How to Safeguard Your Patients
- Pediatric Fluid Management
- Keeping Babies Warm in the Perioperative Period Is Important, Challenging, and at Times, Dangerous!
- Pediatric Arterial Access—and the Beat Goes On
- Pediatric Regional Anesthesia—The Karma of Caudals
- Avoiding the One-Hour Wake Up, or How to Save the Sanity of the Parents and Your Own Reputation at the Same Time
- When Not to Extubate Deep! And if the Patient is Already Coughing or Swallowing, It's Too Late, Anyway
- Emergency Delirium—Don't Undercall It, Don't Overcall It, and Don't Let It Happen
- Too Much, Too Little, Just Right: Avoiding Opioid Withdrawal in Pediatric Patients on Chronic Opioids
- Careful and Conservative Clinical Judgment Is Required Before Discharging a Pediatric Patient to Home
- Chronic Pediatric Pain: There's Always More Than Enough Pain for Everybody and It's Not About the Blocks!
- But It's Just an Herb! Avoiding Problems Resulting from Nontraditional Pain Medications in the Pediatric Population
- Okay, There are Herbals, but What About Those "Other Herbals?"
- Pitfalls in Pediatric Sedation
- Pitfalls of Pediatric Anesthesia for International Service Missions
- Pediatric Cardiac Arrest under Anesthesia—Predicting and Preventing the Most Devastating Complication of All

Avoiding Common Anesthesia Errors, 2nd Edition is available on Amazon and all the major medical book websites.

Note: The editors thank Drs. Asato and Karam for contributing to this chapter.

References

1. Zucchetti G, Candela F, et al. The power of Reiki: feasibility and efficacy of reducing pain in children with cancer undergoing hematopoietic stem cell transplantation. J Pediatr Oncol Nurs. 2019;36(5):361–8.
2. Thrane SE, Williams E, et al. Reiki therapy for very young hospitalized children receiving palliative care. J Pediatr Hematol Oncol Nurs. 2022;39(1):15–29.

Authors

Paul Tripi is currently semi-retired, enjoying his many hobbies and staying in touch with a long career in pediatric anesthesiology. All of his current activities center around his wife, Jayna, and his three daughters, who keep his life perpetually interesting and full of happiness. He has a wide array of hobbies, which include several favorites: Traveling, chess, personal finance, studying world history, and juggling. His daughters have occasionally encouraged him to hang up the stethoscope in favor of pursuing a career as a traveling juggler/magician.

Chetta Lupa is a professor of anesthesiology and pediatrics at the University of North Carolina at Chapel Hill. She is grateful always to her husband Chip and her daughters Anna and Emilia for their support in her career and forgiveness for not always being home to make dinner. Besides caring for children in the hospital, Concetta enjoys every minute making memories with her family, whether traveling, baking, or enjoying social outings with friends.

Oliver Karam is a professor of pediatrics and the chief of the pediatric intensive care unit at Yale. He is in eternal debt to his wife and children since they agreed to move from Geneva, Switzerland, to Montreal, Canada, back to Geneva, then to Richmond, Virginia, and now to New Haven, Connecticut. When he is not at work or answering emails, which is a rather infrequent occurrence, he likes to take aerial photos with a drone.

Cathy Marcucci is a senior academic anesthesiologist and inveterate anesthesiology educator. She is also fellowship-trained in transfusion medicine. When not taking care of patients and/or putting the latest book together, she dedicates her time to mentoring junior colleagues, writing copy for animal rescues, and travel.

Kirk Lalwani is a senior pediatric anesthesiologist at OHSU. Besides his patients and family, he is devoted to teaching and mentoring his trainees. The editors of this book have relied many times on his clinical experience and expertise, and his overall life wisdom when putting together content for the anesthesia community.

Wisdom on Obstetrical Anesthesiology

166

Brandon M. Togioka, David C. Mayer, Emily C. Rhinehart, and Catherine Marcucci

Contributors:

Raymond G. Graber, MD (RGG)

Introduction

Many anesthesiologists complete their training with OB anesthesia rotations with some relief and then take pains to avoid the service in their clinical practice careers as much as possible. We think this is a shame. As we mentioned below, the labor and delivery suite is the one place where practicing anesthesia helps a patient achieve a really joyful outcome. When done well, OB anesthesia is also very elegant—if you are interested in regional anesthesia and acute pain management, then OB anesthesia might be a good fit. Interestingly, on the labor deck, patients tend to assume the baby is okay and focus on what they are doing and how they are doing in getting through the stages of labor. In an operative delivery room, parturients assume they will be okay and not that worried with what is happening to them, but instead are focusing on how the baby is doing. We have found so many times, after an urgent or emergent or even planned operative delivery, the first thing the patient says is, "Is the baby okay?"

The Basics

It's been stated that the physiological changes of pregnancy are a bit tricky because while some changes influence normal biochemical values, other mimic the symptoms of a medical disease [1].

B. M. Togioka
Department of Anesthesiology and Perioperative Medicine, School of Medicine, Oregon Health & Science University, Portland, OR, USA

D. C. Mayer
Department of Anesthesiology, University of North Carolina at Chapel Hill, Chapel Hill, NC, USA

E. C. Rhinehart
University of Southern California, Los Angeles, CA, USA

C. Marcucci (✉)
Department of Transfusion Medicine, Clinical Center, National Institutes of Health, Bethesda, MD, USA

S. Mohamed et al. (eds.), *Anesthesia Bridges*, https://doi.org/10.1007/978-3-032-08294-7_166

These are principles that you should review every once in a while. No, on second thought—review them often. They are always on the in-training exams and the boards in some way, shape, or form. Even if you don't do OB anesthesia in your practice, pregnant patients come to the OR as trauma patients, cancer patients, and with acute appendicitis, to name just several surgical presentations.—**BMT**

- The physiologic changes in pregnancy affect every organ system. In some cases, they begin shortly after conception. For the anesthesiologist, the most important physiological changes in pregnancy occur in the hematologic, gastrointestinal, cardiac, and respiratory systems.

- As most of you are aware, the body prepares for blood loss by increasing maternal blood volume. For allowable blood loss calculations use 100 ml/kg instead of 65–70 ml/kg for maternal blood volume. Physiologic anemia of pregnancy occurs because plasma volume increases 50%, but red cell mass only increases 25%. Generally speaking, hemoglobin should not drop below 11 mg/dl. If it does, there is pathology beyond physiologic anemia—often it is iron deficiency anemia. The increase in red cell mass that occurs during pregnancy has been shown to vary based on iron reserve.

- White blood cell count typically increases during pregnancy, and it is normal for the white blood cell count to increase during labor, such that women with longer labor have higher white blood cell counts. Therefore, the isolated finding of an elevated white blood cell count on labor and delivery may not require investigation.

- Platelet count also falls during pregnancy to the low normal range. The platelet count commonly decreases 50,000/microliter by term. Very rarely (<1% of the time) does the platelet count drop below 100,000/microliter from gestational thrombocytopenia alone. Accordingly, the finding of a platelet count below 100,000 microliters should prompt an investigation into other etiologies.

- There is a physiological hypercoagulable state in preparation for hemostasis post-delivery. Factors II, VII, VIII, and X increase as do fibrinogen and von Willebrand factor levels. Factor IX does not reliably increase during pregnancy. This means patients with hemophilia A will have a natural bump in FVIII, but patients with hemophilia B may require factor replacement prior to delivery. Protein S, which helps reduce the risk of DVT and PE, decreases in almost all pregnant women. Consequently, pregnant patients are at risk for deep venous thrombosis from the first trimester to 12 weeks post-partum.

- Pregnant women are at increased risk for aspiration pneumonia due to having a higher incidence of significant gastroesophageal reflux, larger gastric volume, slower gastrointestinal throughput, and weaker gastroesophageal sphincters. It is common practice to administer some pharmacologic aspiration prophylaxis prior to cesarean delivery, including a nonparticulate antacid, metoclopramide, or an H2-blocker. *Similarly, it is considered standard of care to induce with a rapid sequence intubation for all pregnant women.*

- Cardiovascular changes begin to manifest shortly after conception, they peak from the early second to the early third trimester, thereafter they remain relatively constant until delivery. Compared to pre-pregnancy levels, cardiac output increases 30%, mean arterial pressure decreases 10%, and systemic vascular resistance decreases 30%. The initial increase in cardiac output is due an increase in stroke volume, whereas the increase in heart rate drives the increase in cardiac output during the third trimester. For parturients with maternal cardiac disease, it is important to consider how they are handling current cardiovascular changes, and how much additional change you expect prior to delivery.

- In addition to cardiovascular changes that occur during pregnancy, significant cardiovascular changes occur during the first and second stages of labor. Cardiac output increases an additional 25% during the active phase of the first stage of labor, and it is increased 50% above pre-labor levels during the second stage (the fetal expulsion stage). These changes can be lessened by the provision of epidural labor analgesia.

- Cardiac output is significantly affected by maternal position after 20-weeks gestation. Accordingly, all parturients carrying a greater than 20-week gestation fetus require left uterine displacement. Supine hypotension syndrome can occur when the gravid uterus compresses the inferior vena cava, decreasing cardiac preload and causing maternal hypotension. Just turning from lateral to supine may decrease cardiac output by 25%. Changes in maternal position can be significant enough to cause actual deleterious effects in placental perfusion without affecting upper extremity blood pressure. Supine hypotensive syndrome is characterized by an increase in maternal heart rate, a decrease in pulse pressure, and clinical symptoms such as dizziness, lightheadedness, nausea, pallor, and difficulty breathing.

- Interestingly, left ventricle mass increases during pregnancy. By the third trimester, the average left ventricle has become 1/3 larger.

- Dyspnea is extremely common during pregnancy. The etiology is unclear, as many women begin to experience dyspnea before the uterus reaches a large size. It is hypothesized that physiologic hyperventilation induced by progesterone may be the culprit. Minute ventilation at rest increases 50% by the third trimester—driven mostly by an increase in tidal volume. Progesterone stimulates hyperventilation, driving the partial pressure of carbon dioxide lower in the mother, which presumably helps the fetus clear carbon dioxide via the creation of a larger concentration gradient.

- It is well known that pregnant women desaturate much faster after inducing anesthesia than their non-pregnant counterparts. A very small amount of this is due to a 20% reduction in functional residual capacity and a corresponding decrease in oxygen store. The primary reason for rapid desaturation during apnea is greatly increased oxygen consumption from the fetus.

***Note from the Editors:** This charming arch is found in a quiet and serene public space that is nestled in the remains of the grounds Glasgow Royal Maternity Hospital (Fig. 166.1). The hospital was founded in the Victorian era in the 1860s. The hospital still exists and was relocated to another area of Glasgow. Most of the original building was finally demolished in the early 2000s, but it was decided to retain the arch and some of the foundations to make a quiet picnic spot as a tribute to the generations of babies who were born there.

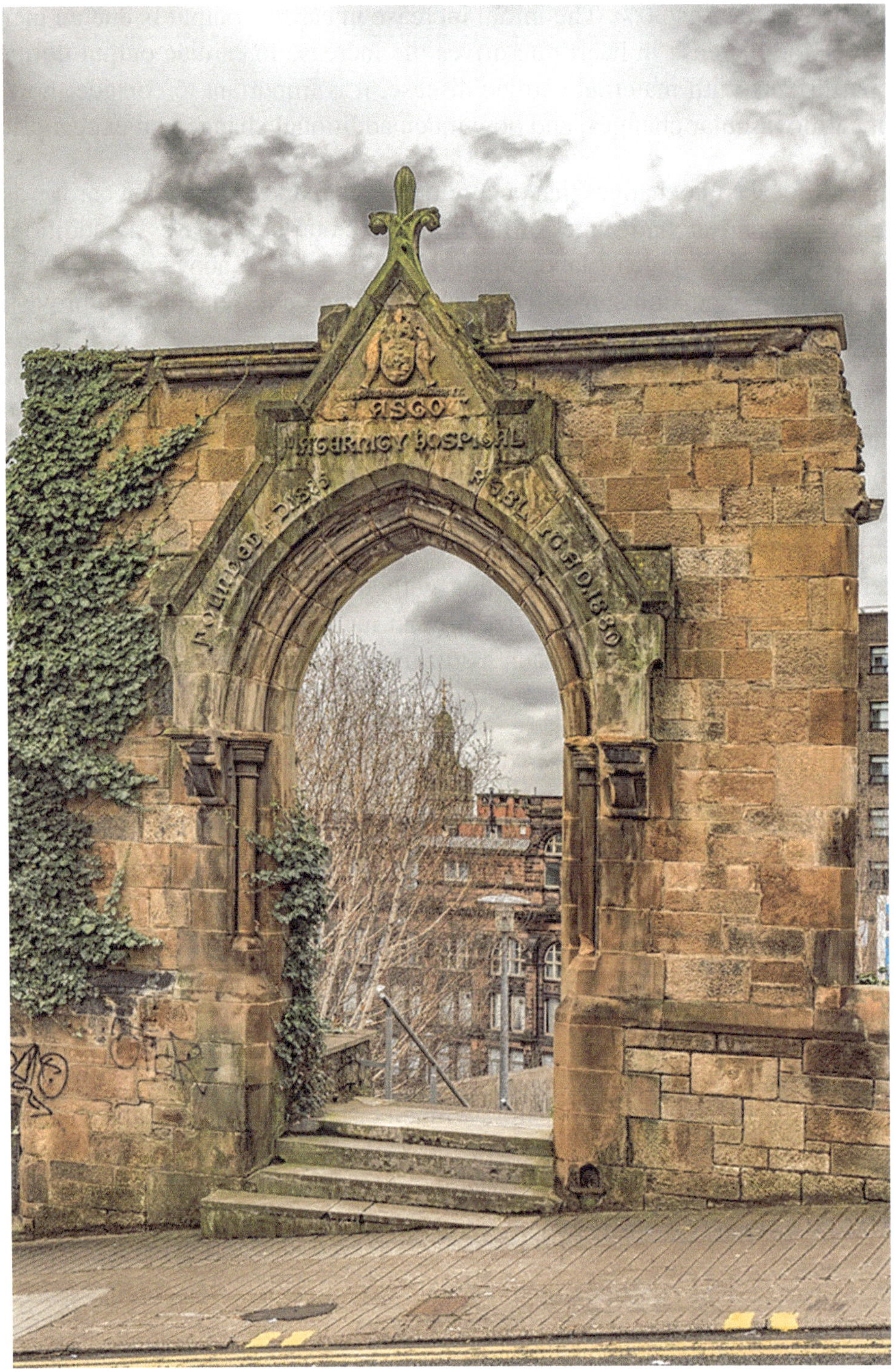

Fig. 166.1 A preserved arch on the former grounds of the Royal Glasgow Maternity Hospital. Photo: Image used under standard license from stock.adobe.com

On the Labor Deck

- Taking care of pregnant patients is the only place in all of anesthesiology and medicine where you are taking care of a group of people—especially if the mother has a multi-gestation pregnancy—in front of a group of people. You will be evaluating the patient and making therapeutic decisions and interventions in full view of the patient's partner and/or family members and the doula.—**Editors**

- OB anesthesia is kind of a special calling; we will admit it. But give it a really decent look before you decide that you want to create a practice without it. Those of us who have spent extended periods of time in the OB suite come to feel that it is one of the most elegant types of anesthesiology. It's just about the only area of anesthetic practice where the goal is to keep the patient safely awake rather than safely asleep. Think about it—the more awake you can keep the patient, the better. You are conducting a full anesthetic—for a major medical intervention—and it's better if you can get the patient through without needing benzodiazepines or opioids. You have to really know what you are doing to accomplish that.—**Editors**

- Labor patients with elaborate and lengthy birth plans frequently need to change course, either by choice or by the situation. Some of these patients have a sense of failure and guilt for not "sticking to the plan." The OB anesthesia team should approach these patients with compassion and understanding. Positive support and themes such as providing care for safe outcomes of mother and baby go a long way to gaining acceptance as part the "new" plan.—**DCM**

- In the last 10–20 years, there has been considerable thought given to NPO requirements before surgery and what actually constitutes a "full stomach." The draconian NPO requirements of 20 years ago have been revised and rightfully so. Do not think this means that the consideration of parturients and even non-term pregnant patients as full stomachs should be similarly relaxed. The "full stomach" mantra for OB patients is going away any time soon, we don't think, and rightfully so.—**Editors**

- I have never regretted replacing a labor epidural that was not working well. Every one of these patients may go for an urgent cesarean, and there are countless times I have noted that we prevented needing GETA because we replaced that labor epidural.—**DCM**

- Labor and delivery nurses are your biggest asset in providing optimal care to laboring women. They are your eyes and ears to provide the best possible intrapartum care. Establishing relationships with them is super important and makes the care team so much stronger.—**DCM**

- How your OB cases go depends not only on whether your epidural fails, it also depends on whether your IV access fails. I've never understood this practice of putting a 20 g or, heaven forbid, a 22 g IV in a laboring parturient in order to "improve the childbirth experience." Gracious, the necessity of inducing a stat general anesthetic with a 22 g IV is not improving the chances of a good experience for anybody! We are supposed to be pros at IV access, so use lidocaine and do yourself and your patient the favor of a decently running 18 g IV.—**CM**

- Anesthesiologists are very concerned about organ perfusion. Keep in mind that the fetal heart rate monitor is the most sensitive indicator of end-organ perfusion. Use this additional tool to craft a safe plan for the mother and her neonate.—**BMT**

- On the labor floor, regular assessment of the fetal heart rate tracing can mean the difference between an emergent surgery and one that can be predicted.—**BMT**

- The level of concern with a fetal heart rate tracing should directly correlate with the frequency of patient visits. Parturients *without* an epidural catheter require airway assessment and, at times, encouragement to receive a neuraxial technique. Parturients *with* an epidural catheter require confirmation that it is adequate to provide surgical anesthesia.—**BMT**

- And when you sign out the labor board at the end of your shift, make sure you've checked how that IV is running and sign that out as well. Don't make any assumptions. Parturients move around a lot. I once had a patient who pulled out three IVs in one shift.—**CM**

- What is the threshold platelet count required for safe neuraxial placement? No one really knows. We know that the complication of epidural hematoma occurs much less frequently in the obstetric, compared to the general surgical, population. In the obstetric population, it is now common to use a threshold of 70,000. Some providers will go even lower than 70,000 if neuraxial placement means avoiding a general anesthetic for cesarean delivery. It's a judgment call.—**BMT**

- And if you do a neuraxial technique with a lower-than-you'd-like platelet count, feel free to take every safety action pertaining to that neuraxial technique. Call the hematologists, check serial platelet counts, do neuro checks as often as you want, and put the actions in place for very close monitoring for epidural hematomas. Remember that patients suffer untoward complications from epidural hematomas if they are not promptly recognized, identified, and treated. If you have a difficult decision to make and you make it in favor of neuraxial analgesia/anesthesia, think about how you would defend that decision, because you might have to. Way back in the day, several of the *Bridges* editors were taught to leave the catheter in until the platelet count had normalized. We've seen post-partum patients go to the ICU for close surveillance and monitoring, including neuro checks.—**Editors**

- Every obstetrical anesthesiologist will spend time at parties talking to people about their labor epidurals. And talking to pregnant friends and the wives of friends late at night on the phone. Generally, we usually find a way to work this factoid into the conversation fairly early: anesthesiologists in labor always, always choose epidural analgesia for themselves. We're not aware of any pregnant anesthesiologist ever who chose "natural" labor and childbirth, are you?—**Editors**

- I am not sure what my coauthors would say, but I've also been asked if a home birth with a midwife is "just as safe." Meaning here in the United States. My answer has always been a single word—<u>NO</u>! Personally, I think it's insane. I've not done as much OB anesthesia as Brandon and David, but I've done enough to have seen *multiple* cases when there was a question whether the patient was going to live long enough to get her back to the OR, much less live long enough to get into a hospital from home. Not to mention the times the baby unexpectedly had to be intubated or go urgently to the NICU.—**CM**

***Note from the Editors:** The Firth of Forth Bridge is a UNESCO World Heritage site and is considered a national symbol of Scotland (Fig. 166.2). It is a cantilevered railway bridge that was opened in 1890. We think it looks a little bit like a tracing of labor contractions. ☺

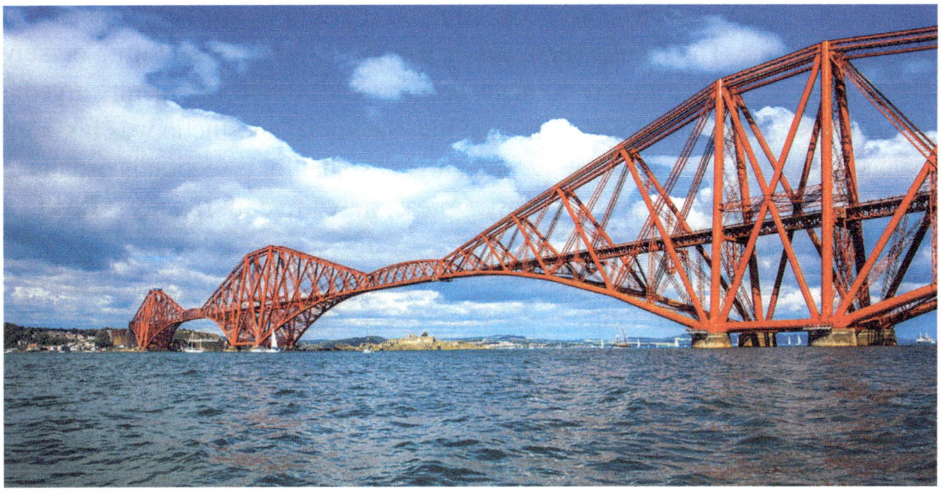

Fig. 166.2 The striking and famous Firth of Forth railway bridge in Scotland. Photo: Image used under standard license from iStock.com

In the Delivery Room

- In general, women come to the operating suite on magnesium for one of two reasons: (1) to prevent seizures in the setting of preeclampsia and (2) as a neuroprotective agent for fetuses at high risk for premature birth. Magnesium decreases uterine contractility and predisposes the uterus to atony. Thus, if a woman comes to the operating room on magnesium—ask why. If it is for preeclampsia, keep the infusion running and be prepared to treat atony. If it is for preterm infant neurological protection, you can stop it upon arrival to the operating room.—**BMT**

- Is left uterine displacement a useful tool to avoid hypotension or an outdated practice without evidence of benefit? Left uterine displacement is commonly performed in the operating room immediately after spinal placement. While it has not been shown to improve neonatal acid-base status, it does improve maternal hemodynamics. Furthermore, left uterine displacement is most helpful for the 8% of pregnant women that develop supine hypotensive syndrome. Since we have no pre-spinal method of determining who is at risk for supine hypotensive syndrome, I tilt all women after spinal placement. It is a cheap, simple procedure that is unlikely to cause harm.—**BMT**

- In Chap. 120, which discusses the lessons the anesthesia community can continue to learn from the aviation industry, **Mitch Robbins**, a commercial airline pilot describes the process of "chair flying." This is a technique of sitting in front of a poster of the cockpit and visualizing and even miming pilot techniques in a variety of situations. I was taught something very similar when I was a junior resident rotating through the OB suite. We were sitting at the conference table one day and the faculty said, "okay, people imagine you have to do a really urgent spinal for a surgical delivery. Not so urgent that you have to do an emergent induction, but urgent. The C-section itself might not be that fast, but the spinal has to go in quickly and reliably. What are you going to do? We are going to go over this and over this until you can visualize this in your sleep. What would you get a hold of out of the med cabinet as you go into the room—what are going to be your go-to techniques to get this spinal done? What local anesthetic are you going to use and how much?"—**CM**

- After some discussion of the questions above, we hit upon the simplest possible spinal anesthetic dose of 10 mg of 0.75% bupivacaine. The faculty then had us use that exact dose and time ourselves for the next twenty spinal anesthetics we did until we were really comfortable with it. The faculty urged us to become so proficient with our chosen "most reliable" technique that the spinal anesthetic was not appreciably slower than doing a general anesthetic. My go-to dose for an urgent spinal for c-section is usually 12 mg of 0.75% hyperbaric bupivacaine +15 mcg fentanyl + 100 mcg preservative-free morphine.—**BMT**

- Assisted deliveries—for spinal anesthesia to facilitate forceps delivery, I would give 5 mg of bupivacaine or 20–25 mg of 1% chloroprocaine.—**BMT**

- For a vacuum-assisted delivery I would give less a smaller dose, 2.5–3.75 mg of 0.25% bupivacaine.—**BMT**

- Take the opportunity to talk to senior and experienced OB anesthesiologists about their "spinal needle preferences and practices." What you are interested in hearing about is what needle they routinely use, what do they use for patients with high or very high body weights, and what they would use if the spinal has to go in urgently or emergently and they need to know for sure that they are in the CSF and that they can inject the local anesthetic quickly and definitely.—**Editors**

- If you are very new to the practice of anesthesiology or don't routinely do spinals, here is a quick pictorial review (Fig. 166.3). A lot of us trained at Hopkins, which stocked the Whitacre and Quincke needles.—**Editors**

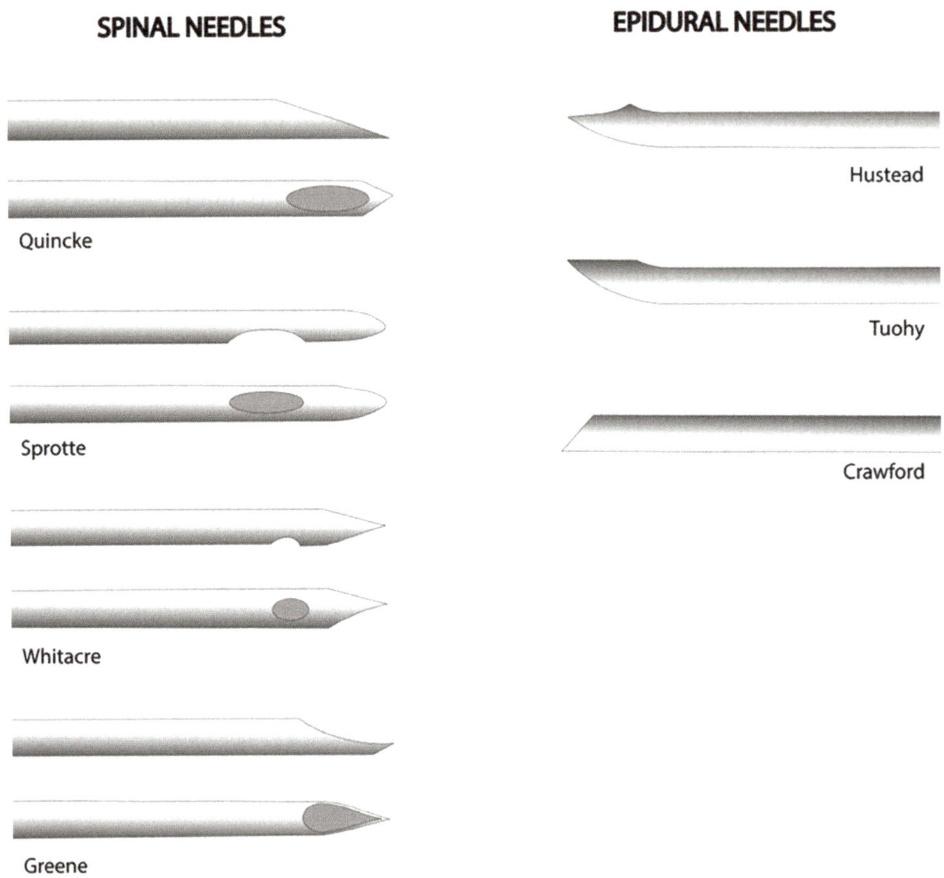

Fig. 166.3 The business ends of the common types of spinal and epidural needles. Only the Quincke is considered a cutting needle. Illustration: Image used under standard license from adobe.stock.com

- As we put this chapter together, we had a brisk discussion on spinal needle size for operative delivery for parturients, especially in high urgency or emergency cases. **Brandon Togioka**, who has done a huge amount of OB anesthesia, hasn't really ever used any spinal needle larger than a 22-g cutting needle and those weren't even in the OB suite, they were for hips or knees. He has searched his memory banks and doesn't recall using a larger diameter needle than a 25-g pencil point needle for an obstetric patient. In his expert opinion, the use of neuraxial ultrasound has reduced the need to use large diameter spinal needles.—**Editors**

- Should you use a cutting needle in an OB patient? Well, you technically can, but we don't *really recommend it for routine use*. If there is a complication with a PDPH, it would be too easy to find somebody in the expert witness category who will say that a pencil point needle should have been used instead.—**Editors**

- *Anesthesia Bridges* editor **Ray Graber** was kind enough to take the time to consult with the OB anesthesia team at Case Western about needle size and preference and the largest and "sharpest" needle they use—for their difficult and urgent cases would be a 22-g Quincke needle.—**RGG and Editors**

- I generally concur with Brandon's thinking and Ray's report of the practice at Case Western. However, my advice is to accept that sometimes a bigger needle is ultimately less risky overall. You always want the smallest needle that gets the spinal meds reliably into the intrathecal space on the fewest attempts, but the emphasis is on smallest, reliable, and fewest attempts, all at the same time. While minimizing the risk-benefit ratio for PDPH at all times. It's a tricky clinical problem, which is why we recommend that you think carefully about it.—**CM**

- Getting into the details—it's undeniably harder to feel the dural pop, appreciate the backflow of CSF, and inject local anesthetic with a 27-g than with a 22-g. It's also sometimes harder to redirect a 27-g needle because you really do have to withdraw the introducer an adequate distance. And it's harder to teach residents with a smaller needle, we will admit it. For these purposes, when Brian is teaching spinal-through-epidural needle techniques, he has his trainees use a 25-g spinal needle. I was taught to at least *consider* starting with a 22-g Whitacre if the patient is above a certain weight—as I recall, the threshold was about 100–110 kg—and the spinal needed to go in urgently or emergently.—**CM**

- Another option for patients with higher body weights is to start with a longer needle. We forget that spinal needles—both cutting and pencil point—come in a variety of lengths. I have seen the "standard" length spinal needle that is in the spinal kit fall short of the reaching the intrathecal space any number of times, even when the positioning and orientation of the needle were perfect.—**CM**

- Also remember that risks such as epidural hematoma are associated with number of needle passes and the amount of needle re-direction in the epidural space. The injection of the anesthetic is also more reliable through a larger needle.—**Editors**

- Supplemental oxygen is commonly administered in the operating room for cesarean delivery. The theory is that supplemental oxygen may improve oxygen delivery when hypotension occurs after spinal placement. The evidence to support this practice in healthy women undergoing scheduled cesarean delivery is poor. Supplemental oxygen does not appear to improve 1 or 5-minute Apgar scores, and the impact upon neonatal umbilical artery and vein oxygenation is minimal. Furthermore, supplemental oxygen may cause harm by increasing free radical activity—therefore the decision to use supplemental oxygen should be made on a case-by-case basis. All healthy women undergoing cesarean delivery do not require supplemental oxygenation.—**BMT**

- It has been hypothesized that difficult intubation is less of a concern in contemporary obstetric practice, due to a higher frequency of neuraxial placement and the availability of video laryngoscopes. This hypothesis is incorrect. The risk of difficult intubation in the obstetric population remains significantly above the general surgical population. Continue to have great respect for the obstetric airway.—**BMT**

- Remember that in a true emergency requiring general anesthesia, the obstetricians *can* start the section under local anesthesia if they have to until you can get the airway secured. I've seen it and I've done it. It's not pretty, nobody is very happy about it, but it's better than a lost airway.—**CM**

- Once as a resident on Cathy's first-ever OB call, she took over an operative delivery and the block just wasn't working very well. The obstetricians had a while to go. We did **not** want to have to do a general anesthetic in the middle of the case and couldn't give enough sedation. She called the faculty who said, "Chloroprocaine 2% or 3%! It's in the glass med cabinet. Have the OBs start pouring it right into the incision." She thought what the heck? And then asked how much they could administer into the wound. Her attending said, "As much as in the cabinet." Remember that chloroprocaine is an ester local anesthetic. It has relatively low potency, so you need a lot of it, but also has extremely low toxicity. It is rapidly metabolized by plasma cholinesterases, on the order of minutes. It can be used in spinal, epidural, and caudal blocks and in pudendal and paracervical blocks in OB.—**CM** and **BMT**

- Think about what you are going to give to an awake C-section patient for anxiety after the baby is out. A surprising number of patients need this. Where I practiced OB anesthesia, the go-to drug was ketamine—in small doses—with an also-small dose of benzodiazepines.—**CM**

- It's always a great idea to ask senior OB anesthesiologists what they have tightened up on and what they have loosened up on as they have gained experience in the OB suite. So, we did just that of David and Brandon. Their interesting answers are below and show the nuanced evolution of their clinical practice.—**Editors**

- From **David Mayer**—I have:

  - Tightened up on sterile field/prep/jewelry removal.

  - Tightened up on early and aggressive second line uterotonics.

  - Tightened up on putting in a second IV.

  - Loosened up on left-lateral tilt for most cases.

  - Loosened up on when OB Calls for a section and the patient has not fasted 6 or 8 hours. Always depends on the "why," though. Unless the patient refuses neuraxial anesthesia or has a contraindication to neuraxial, I am less concerned with aspiration and waiting compared to increased risks of chorio, fetal issues, and uterine atony and bleeding.

  - Loosened up on admission platelet count. I never withheld neuraxial analgesia for labs in the past, but now I hardly even care—provided history and physical exam and OB issues are non-contributory

- From **Brandon Togioka**:

  - I agree with David with regards to earlier second IV placement. I now request it for all patients with pre-eclampsia with severe features.

  - I also tightened up with regards to cordis placement for all patients with more than focally adherent placenta accreta spectrum disorder on ultrasound or MRI imaging. I have had two women experience myocardial damage due to rapid (> 1 liter/minute) blood loss.

  - I have also loosened up on left uterine displacement, though I still usually do it. I prioritize starting phenylephrine over left uterine displacement.

  - I have tightened up on early aggressive use of phenylephrine after spinal placement.

  - I no longer have the nurses give a fluid preload. It is often not helpful. Rather, we now administer a fluid co-load (fluid bolus with pressure bag once we enter the operating room).

  - I tightened up on labor epidural assessments. This is the best way to predict which epidurals may not provide adequate anesthesia for cesarean delivery.

  - I tightened up on administration of anti-emetics prior to prophylactic cephalosporin administration during cesarean delivery. Many patients get nauseated when the cephalosporin is administered.

Post-Dural Puncture Headaches

- Post-dural puncture headaches (PDPH) are much more than a simple headache. They are associated with significant morbidity including subdural hematoma, cranial nerve palsy, impaired early maternal-neonatal bonding, and they can be the inciting event that triggers future migraine attacks. PDPHs require regular follow-up. Severe headaches should be treated with a blood patch. Caffeine, fluid boluses, supine positioning, and bedrest are like band-aids, treating the symptoms. The blood patch is the only modality that addresses the underlying pathology.—**BMT**

- The "national average" for PDPH in OB suites is about 1–1.5% in hospitals that do more than 500 deliveries. If your personal or hospital numbers are higher than this, there needs to be of thorough evaluation of what's going on.—**Editors**

- Agree with the above! I noticed after only a short time that parturients were pretty philosophical about epidurals that didn't work, but really had a tremendously hard time with a severe PDPH. They "remembered" it long after the delivery and had a hard time getting over it. I have seen patients who have come in adamantly refusing every single intervention except general anesthesia for urgent or emergent operative delivery.—**CM**

- So just to review (for the board exams): conservative and supportive measures for PDPH include rehydration, acetaminophen, NSAIDs, opioids, and anti-emetics. Other therapeutic modalities that have been described include intravenous or oral caffeine, sumatriptan, desmopressin acetate, and adrenocorticotrophic hormone. But as Brandon says, blood patch is the current definitive treatment.—**Editors**

- Remember that you can do serial blood patches. If a patient is still having severe PDPH symptoms after a blood patch, you can repeat it several days or a week later. A blood patch should be immediately effective in relieving the headache pain and distress, but it is just a patch, it is not a repair of the dura, and it is possible that headache symptoms can recur.—**BMT and Editors**

- When completing a blood patch, how much blood should you administer and how quickly should you inject it? A blood volume of 20 ml appears to provide equal efficacy to a volume of 30 ml, while decreasing the frequency of side effects. Just remember that when you complete a blood patch, you are giving your patient an epidural hematoma. This hurts and can result in significantly lower back pressure. The pressure typically dissipates over time, but it can be more uncomfortable than the headache. If blood is administered too quickly, you can cause temporary paralysis. For this reason, always ask the patient to tell you if the pressure in their back is becoming so severe that they wish you to stop injecting. Monitoring pain is a great way to ensure that blood is not injected too quickly or in too large a quantity.—**BMT**

- We were taught that the person who does the epidural blood patch should be different if possible, than the person who inadvertently did the wet tap or did the neuraxial technique that was antecedent to the PDPH. We have seen patients inadvertently wet-tapped a second time by the same provider and this caused the patient to become enraged and threaten legal action if that provider "comes near me again."—**Editors**

- Epidural blood patches can be done in Jehovah's Witness patients with continuous tubing and three-way stopcocks. There are a number of case reports describing the various techniques in the literature.—**Editors**

- If you have a patient who refuses blood patch for religious reasons, you can *consider* saline infusion into the epidural space. It's being evaluated in anesthesia and oncology patient cohorts [2].—*Editors*

- At some point in your career, you will meet a patient with a PDPH that strongly desires to avoid a blood patch. For these situations, there are two less invasive options with some evidence of effectiveness. The sphenopalatine ganglion block has been used to treat migraine and postdural puncture headaches. It is performed by positioning the patient supine, placing cotton swabs soaked in local anesthetic through the nares until resistance is encountered, and resting the cotton end immediately superior to the middle nasal turbinate for five minutes. The sphenopalatine block is hypothesized to work by blocking parasympathetic-induced cerebral vasodilation, the proposed vascular mechanism for PDPH and migraines.—**BMT** and **RGG**

- Another less invasive option for treating PDPH is co-administration of neostigmine and atropine [3]. Please note that this approach has been associated with side effects such as abdominal cramping and bladder spasms. Neostigmine is hypothesized to work by causing direct cerebral vasoconstriction and increasing cerebrospinal fluid pressure. Atropine is hypothesized to inhibit cerebral vasodilation and increase cerebrospinal fluid secretion.—**BMT**

- There are also several recent fascinating case reports and retrospective case reviews that looked at acupuncture to treat severe PDPH [4, 5, 6, 7]. Also, a 2016 case report described immediate amelioration of PDPH pain with only two acupuncture treatments in a male patient who refused conservative therapies and epidural blood patch [8]. —**Editors**

- I really blush to think that, back in the olden days, we would tell patients that spinal headaches could be very uncomfortable, but they weren't that "dangerous." We also didn't routinely request a consult and management from the pain service for our PDPH patients. Gah! I wish I could go back in time and re-deliver that clinical care.—**CM**

- Our point is that perhaps the headache itself isn't dangerous, but it is *the prime symptom of a serious iatrogenic complication that does carry serious morbidity or danger*. If you recommend or place an epidural and inadvertent dural puncture occurs, you are obligated to work completely through the treatment algorithms to treat and resolve the complication. As we mention above, this should include a very low threshold for speedy consultation with the pain and complementary medicine services.—**Editors**

Preeclampsia

- Preeclampsia is not going anywhere as a public health issue. In fact, it's just the opposite. Preeclampsia and related hypertensive disorders of pregnancy affect up to 8% of all births (or more if there are multiple risk factors present). Unfortunately, the rate has increased about 25% in the 20 years. Preeclampsia/eclampsia are leading causes of infant and maternal mortality. They are really serious diseases and deserve the clinician's utmost attention.—**BMT**

- The precise cause of preeclampsia/eclampsia is not known. Risks factors include: first pregnancy, previous history of preeclampsia, multiple gestation, history of hypertension, diabetes, kidney disease, organ transplant, increased body-mass index, extremes of maternal age (over 35 years and under 20 years), family history of preeclampsia, polycystic ovarian syndrome, history of autoimmune disease, sickle cell disease, and African American race.—**Editors**

- Symptoms of preeclampsia can include headache, abdominal pain, shortness of breath, blurred vision, photophobia, visual auras, dizziness, and anxiety.—**BMT**

- Edema is no longer considered a diagnostic criterion for preeclampsia, in part because the incidence of edema is so high during normal pregnancy. However, it is the author's experience that patients with preeclampsia develop greater extremity swelling than non-preeclamptic patients. To this extent, place a second intravenous line as soon as preeclampsia with severe features is diagnosed. Intravenous line insertion will only get harder as labor progresses.—**BMT**

- Similarly, conduct a history and physical that includes an airway exam when induction of labor is initiated for preeclamptic patients. Remember that the airway will become more difficult as induction progresses: oxytocin administration is associated with fluid retention, airway edema will worsen, and the likelihood of bleeding with laryngoscopy manipulation will increase. —**BMT**

- In one study, 100% of patients who experienced a stroke in the peripartum period had severe uncontrolled hypertension (SBP > 155 mm Hg). Almost all these patients suffered permanent disability or death. Treat hypertension aggressively in preeclamptic patients on the labor floor.—**BMT**

- Remember that anti-hypertensive medications and magnesium only alleviate the symptoms and some of the risk factors. They are not "cures" for pre-eclampsia.—**Editors**

- Magnesium is really an interesting drug. Remember that although is it widely used as co-adjunctive therapy for preeclampsia, it is also a tocolytic agent. The molecular action includes competitive calcium blockade, which decreases the calcium conductance of presynaptic voltage-dependent calcium channels. It also limits the outflow of calcium from the sarcoplasmic reticulum. All together, these mechanisms result in decreased release of acetylcholine from the end plate of the presynaptic neuromuscular junction. This increases the patient's sensitivity to nondepolarizing muscle relaxants.—**Editors**

- Magnesium is also a non-competitive N-methyl-D-aspartate (NMDA) receptor antagonist, which may contribute to its role as a useful adjuvant pain medication. —**Editors**

- Keep in mind that magnesium, especially prolonged administration, may decrease requirements of intravenous anesthetics and opioid narcotics.—**Editors**

- The only definitive "cure" for preeclampsia is delivery of the infant and placenta. And this is a cure only for the baby, not for the mother. So, you can say that delivery is the beginning of the "cure." It is imperative that the health of the mother be monitored post-partum. The editors have worked in hospitals where severely pre-eclamptic patients went as a matter of policy, to the ICU step-down for monitoring post-partum.—**Editors**

- Don't hesitate to put an arterial line in a preeclamptic patient if you think you use it to guide therapy for an operative delivery. If you need it, you need it. This is no time for a gingerly approach to blood pressure management in a patient who may become critically ill at any point in time.—**Editors**

- One of the most common questions from our obstetric colleagues is, "how low can the platelet count be for my patient to receive an epidural?" The Society for Obstetric Anesthesia and Perinatology published a taskforce opinion that neuraxial anesthesia is likely safe in patients with a platelet count ≥70,000/microliter, in the absence of other bleeding risk factors. Generally, it is not recommended to perform a neuraxial technique when the platelet count is <50,000/microliter. The decision to perform a neuraxial technique when the platelet count is between 50,000 and 70,000/microliter depends upon the indication (labor pain relief or to facilitate surgery), obstetric and patient risk factors, the airway exam, and, as always, patient preference.—**BMT**

- Patients with rapidly declining platelet counts should be encouraged to receive neuraxial analgesia early, before severe thrombocytopenia develops, even if labor pain scores are low. Catheters can be infused with a very low hourly rate of local anesthetic solution to avoid hypotension and motor block. This allows the patient to obtain neuraxial labor analgesia when it is desired, and it provides a definitive method of anesthesia for possible cesarean delivery.—**BMT**

- It is common practice to co-load with crystalloid when placing a neuraxial catheter. Patients with preeclampsia are at greater risk for pulmonary edema due to greater hydrostatic pressure, lower oncotic pressure, and capillary leak. These patients typically receive intravenous fluid for hours-days in the form of oxytocin and magnesium. It is best to minimize fluid administration to these patients. The authors have found that a fluid load is often not necessary to prevent hypotension in these patients when they receive a low-concentration local anesthetic epidural solution. —**BMT**

- Patients with preeclampsia can be more sensitive to the effects of vasopressors. Start with smaller dosages when treating hypotension, for example, 50 mcg phenylephrine and 2.5 mg ephedrine.—**BMT**

- Patients with HELLP Syndrome (hemolysis, elevated liver enzymes, and low platelets) are higher risk for morbidity and mortality than patients with preeclampsia. Severe right upper quadrant pain should be quickly addressed and considered a serious finding. The authors have seen patients rapidly deteriorate multiple times after the complaint of right upper quadrant pain. Bedside ultrasound or CT should be performed to assess for liver rupture and hepatic bleeding.—**BMT**

- Patients with HELLP syndrome should have normal prothrombin (PT), partial thromboplastin (PTT), and fibrinogen concentrations. If PT/PTT are prolonged, or if fibrinogen is low, the patient likely has co-existent disseminated intravascular coagulation (DIC), which is much more common in the setting of HELLP syndrome.—**BMT**

***Note from the Editors:** Motherwell Bridge and Engineering, Inc. is a Scottish structural and bridge engineering firm that has been in business since 1898. We thought the name of the firm was perfect for this chapter. They work in heavy industry, but their work is also recognized for its aesthetic and even lyrical quality. They built this bridge over Argyle St in the Glasgow Central Station (Fig. 166.4).

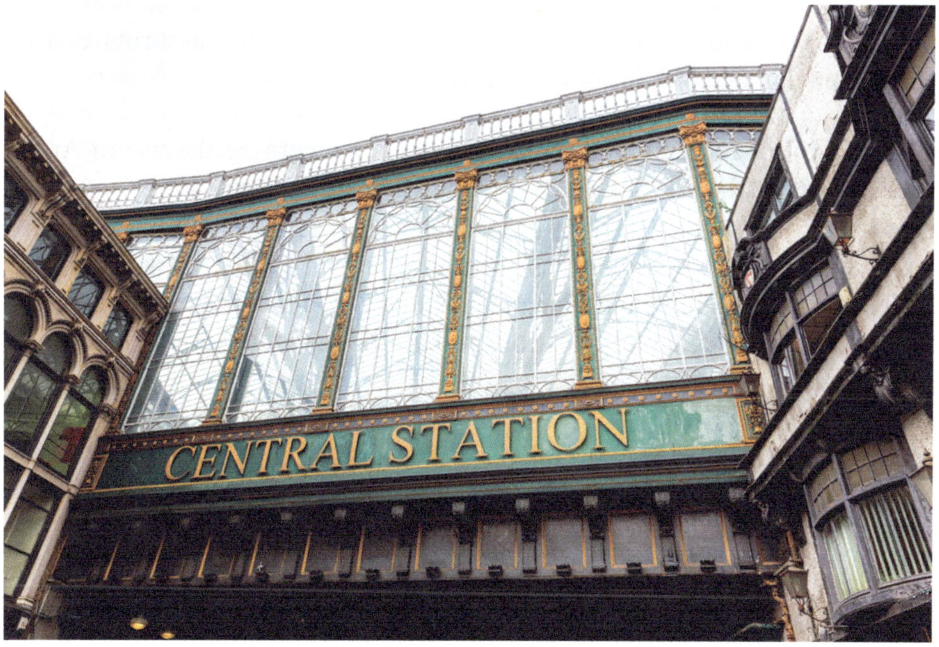

Fig. 166.4 The bridge over Argyle Street in Central Station is also known as "Hielan" Man's Umbrella. Photo: Image used under standard license from shutterstock.com

- Don't get behind on the care of a pre-eclamptic patient or *you* will be the one with the hypertension and headaches!—**CM**

Apgars

- Virginia Apgar was a surgeon turned obstetric anesthesiologist who invented the "APGAR" score for assessing newborns (see below). The Apgar score has remained relevant for 30+ years. "Apgar" has become an acronym, or more correctly, a backronym. It stands for *appearance, pulse, grimace, activity, and respiration*. Each category is scored 0, 1, or 2 at one minute after delivery and 5 minutes post-delivery.—**ECR** and **Editors**

- The basic form of the Apgar evaluation has remained fairly constant over the decades, but the understanding of the appropriate clinical meaning has evolved. The 1-minute Apgar score was originally used to determine if a distressed infant required resuscitation. However, it is now recognized that resuscitative efforts should be initiated immediately. Accordingly, the Apgar score may have more utility in determining when resuscitative efforts should be terminated.—**ECR** and **Editors**

- Recognized determinants of the Apgar scores include gestational age, birth weight, maternal medications, drug use or anesthesia, and congenital anomalies.—**ECR** and **Editors**

- Seventy years after the introduction of post-natal Apgar score, the predictive value of a low Apgar score is still incompletely understood. Low Apgar scores (0–3) at 1-minute have little predictive value. Low Apgar scores at later time points (5- and 10-minutes) are associated with cerebral palsy; however, most infants with low scores will not develop cerebral palsy. —**ECR** and **Editors**

- While we were putting this content together, an interesting discussion occurred between the authors as to whether Apgars of 4 and 7 could be considered a recognized harbinger of later neurologic sequelae (severe cerebral palsy). The answer is technically no, although the scores themselves are certainly lower than we like to see, and it seems a bit outside our normal thinking to call Apgars of 4 and 7 "normal." But remember that a score of 7–10 is considered reassuring that hypoxia has not caused neonatal brain damage.—**ECR** and **Editors**

- There is still quite a bit of research and debate going on concerning the use of Apgars. This ranges from inter-rater reliability, the use of the "extended" 10-minute Apgar score, and whether the *change* in Apgar scores from 1 minute to 5 minutes has any short or long-term predictive value. There are also those in the OB and pediatric communities who have suggested that it is time to retire the Apgar score. We don't see that happening any time soon. Rather, we think the ongoing debate is an interesting reflection that many fundamental questions remain open in the care of obstetrical and neonatal patients.—**Editors**

Other Special Topics

- Unfortunately, the OB suite carries its own special category of malpractice risk. We were taught that you have to accept this and be mindful of it, but not intimidated. And it's okay to practice a bit "defensively" if we may use that term. For example, we were advised that this is not the place to try out new drugs without a clear indication or drugs that are new to you. This is a place for the tried-and-true techniques. We've talked to clinicians who have been pressed hard in depositions about their drug choices and how familiar they were with drugs and how many times that had used a particular drug.

We know of at least one person who was antagonistically queried about every single drug on the anesthesia record.—**Editors**

- However, an exception to the above can be made if there is a clear indication for a new drug. I have never given intralipid to a patient in the OB suite but have used in the ICU where we were able to avoid intubation and cardiac arrest. I would not have hesitated to use it for a parturient—even when it was a brand-new drug, if the clinical indications were met, and to avoid emergency intubation and resuscitation. I asked Brian about this, and he concurred with my thinking.—**CM**

- If you do maintain proficiency in obstetrical anesthesia and find your way to a career where that patient cohort is not avoided, you may find that you will become and remain highly employable. An OB anesthesiologist once put it this way, "I don't look at it as avoiding jobs where *I have to do* OB cases. I look at it as where are the jobs where *I get to do* OB cases."—**Editors**

- Always remember that the OB suite is a place of high blood loss cases. The average blood loss for an uncomplicated vaginal delivery is around 500 ml and the average blood loss for an uncomplicated C-section is about 1000 ml. Would you start a case in the regular ORs with an expected liter of blood loss with a 22-g IV? Once again, we think not.—**Editors**

- Speaking of obstetrical bleeding, it is my (unofficial) opinion that it seems to come up on boards quite a bit. Disclaimer: I am not a boards examiner or question-writer. But, on my oral boards, I was asked, "You hear the words placental accreta mentioned. What does that mean to you and what would you do?" I know of at least two other people who essentially got the same question. I must know at least six people (at least) who have been asked obstetrical bleeding questions of some type on their board exams.—**CM**

- The answer to the above question is that you secure extra IV access, call for blood in the room, and prepare to volume resuscitate if necessary. —**CM**

- I agree with Cathy. *One more time*—never start a delivery for a patient with concern for accreta spectrum disorder without blood in the room.—**BMT**

- The bleeding emergencies in the OB suite—including placental abruption, placenta previa, and uterine atony—are scary and dangerous for everybody, but perhaps the worst of catastrophic events for the parturient is amniotic fluid embolism (AFE). This is a "non-bleeding" emergency but associated with extremely high maternal mortality—various studies range from 60–80%. I have seen one case and Brandon Togioka has also seen several cases and, tragically, all the patients we have seen with AFE died. If you are going to talk to experienced OB anesthesiologists about their practice experience, ask if they have seen AFE and talk to them about how they managed it.—**CM**

- The exact precipitating events for AFE are still not understood, but risk factors are thought to include advanced maternal age, multiple gestation, male fetus, and trauma.—**Editors**

- The cardiovascular and hemodynamic collapse associated with AFE can manifest as sudden cardiac arrest or acute onset of severe and progressive dyspnea, tachypnea, and hypotension. It can occur during delivery or in the postpartum period.—**Editors**

- As we stated above, this is a catastrophic complication. It is very rare, so there aren't large retrospective studies, but the literature does contain case reports. There is a new treatment for AFE called A-O-K, which stands for atropine, ondansetron, and ketorolac [9]. ECMO has also been used successfully [10].—**Editors**

- There doesn't seem to be a standard practice for anesthesia preparations for external cephalic version (ECV). It varies by institution and provider. We have seen versions done without so much as an IV (when we were students, not when we were attendings and had any say in the matter). The key to dealing with versions is that they can rarely be the cause for emergent surgical delivery. We have seen them associated with total loss of fetal heart tones. We've seen it. For early ECV (36–37 weeks), Brandon usually places a spinal to achieve a T4 level without Duramorph. For late ECV, he usually has a combined spinal-epidural, again without Duramorph. We've also seen OB anesthesiologists place an epidural and test it but not dose it as the obstetrician wished to know if the patient was feeling excessive discomfort or sharp pain during the procedure.—**BMT** and **Editors**

- Marijuana and other cannabis products are now legal in many states. But just because a substance is legal does not mean it is safe. Many pregnant women and parturients use it for a variety of reasons—to combat nausea or on the basis of small studies that state it *might* decrease the risk of pre-eclampsia. Evidently, non-medical personnel at marijuana dispensaries are known to recommend it to pregnant women for nausea. Studies have reported that up to 20% of pregnant women 24 years old and younger will test positive for marijuana, although self-reported rates are much lower. I am personally aware of a chronic recreational user smoking a huge amount of marijuana just before leaving for the hospital to give birth. Her statement was, "Gotta smoke enough to get me through the next 36 hours." This is both sad and scary!—**CM**

- Smoked marijuana has over 500 active compounds in it, and no amount of marijuana is considered "safe" in pregnancy. It is associated with a large number of complications and deleterious effects in pregnant women, including fetal growth restriction, increased risk of pre-term birth and stillbirth, low birth weight, and negative long-term brain development effects in the baby, including decrements in memory, learning, and behavior.—**Editors**

- Smoked marijuana has the same drug–drug interactions as smoked tobacco, including induction of CYP1A2. Habitual recreational use also effects the mother-to-be in unhealthy ways, including increasing the risk of accidents, especially traffic accidents. A good resource is below.—**Editors**

  https://www.samhsa.gov/marijuana/marijuana-pregnancy

Responsibility and Honor

- No one remembers the anesthesiologist that did their lap chole. But most patients do remember the anesthesiologist who took care of them during labor. Whether that is a positive one or negative one is completely in your hands.—**DCM**

- The privilege of being part of such a critical and personal time as a new human is born and a family grows, never gets old.—**DCM**

- Over time, I realized that we all have access to the same literature and techniques. I wondered what separates the average obstetric anesthesiologist from the truly great one. I have to come to realize, "Compassion and excellence are in the details."—**BMT**

Clinical Wisdom from *Avoiding Common Anesthesia Errors, 2nd Edition*

Bridges editor Brandon Togioka was instrumental in developing, writing, and editing the OB anesthesia content for *Avoiding Common Anesthesia Errors, 2nd Edition,* nicknamed "Green2." We recommend you take a look at that extensive compilation of clinical wisdom.

Green2 OB Anesthesia Chapter Titles We Recommend:

- Be Prepared for the Presence of a Doula in the Both the Labor and Delivery Room
- Guests on the Labor Deck and in the Delivery Room—How to Manage It and Keep Your Professional Demeanor
- Alternatives to Epidural Analgesia for Labor Pain—What to Consider, What You Might Be Asked
- Epidural Labor Analgesia: Does It Prolong Labor?
- We Were Taught Once a C-section, Always a C-section…What to Do When Your Hospital Now Wants to Provide Trial of Labor after Cesarean (TOLAC) Services
- Should We Place a Spinal for a Version? Anesthesia for External Cephalic Version
- Management of an Accidental Dural Puncture in the Laboring Patient—When the Hanging Drop Becomes a Flowing River
- "We Have an Urgent C-Section!" The Pitfalls of Intrapartum Monitoring of the Fetus
- Stat C-section—The 30-Minute Rule and Beyond
- Postpartum Hemorrhage: Don't Forget That Having a Baby is Major Surgery
- From Glad to Sad (Part 1): Pain Control after Cesarean Section
- From Glad to Sad (Part 2): Postpartum Neuropathy of the Lower Extremity
- Obstetric Anesthesia/Analgesia Can Work in a Small Hospital: The Key Principles Are Commitment, Flexibility, and Planning
- Resuscitation of the Pregnant Cardiopulmonary Arrest Patient: Not Just Standard ACLS
- The Pregnant Anesthesia Provider (Part 1)—Managing the Occupational Exposures
- The Pregnant Anesthesia Provider (and New Adoptive Parent)—Part 2

Avoiding Common Anesthesia Errors, 2nd Edition, is available on Amazon and all the major medical book websites.

Bonus Content! Virginia Apgar, MD—Emily C. Rhinehart, BS

Virginia Apgar, MD is one of the all-time great pioneers in anesthesiology and one of very first female academic leaders (Fig. 166.5).

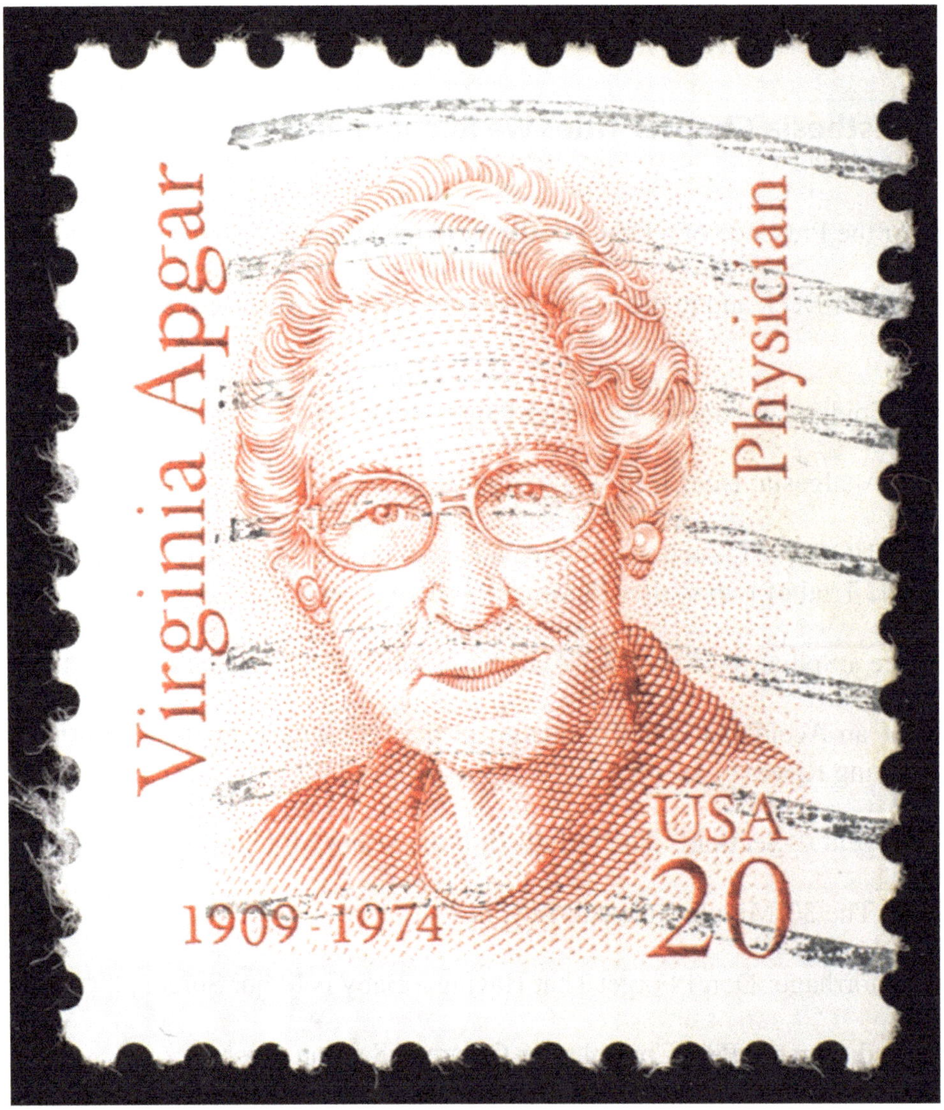

Fig. 166.5 Virginia Apgar MD was honored as a great physician and great American on a US postage stamp. Photo: Image used under standard license from shutterstock.com

She was born in Westfield, New Jersey in 1909. Even in her early years, she was sure she wanted to pursue a medical career. She attended Mount Holyoke College where she studied zoology and excelled in her academic studies. She not only supported herself with numerous part-time jobs but also played in the orchestra, worked on the college newspaper, participated in the dramatic arts, and was on seven different sports teams. In 1929, Virginia Apgar started at Columbia University's College of Physicians and Surgeons, where she was 1 of 9 women in the 90-person class.

In 1933, Virginia Apgar graduated from Columbia University's College of Physicians and Surgeons. She abstained from the traditional doctoral robes and instead elected to wear scrubs to show her dedication to medicine. She started in a surgical residency at Presbyterian Hospital; but was discouraged from continuing this pathway by her mentor Dr. Alan Whipple—evidently, women already had great difficulties in starting and maintaining careers in surgery and the Depression was exacerbating that unfortunate fact.

Dr. Whipple suggested she look into the upcoming specialty of anesthesiology, believing that she had the energy and curiosity to contribute greatly to this new field. He hoped that she would learn the specialty and come back to Presbyterian Hospital where they could work together. Surgery was advancing much faster than anesthesiology and much of anesthesiology was being performed by nurses who had little training in the field, which led to distressingly poor clinical situations. Whipple wasn't the first surgeon to recognize that having physicians trained in anesthesiology and who also had the drive and stamina to undertake significant advancements would be extremely helpful and create better surgical outcomes.

After finishing a year of surgical residency, Dr. Apgar began her difficult pursuit of anesthesiology training. She had few options since at that time there were only five anesthesiology residency programs in the country, three of them unpaid. With the two paid residencies full, she stayed at Presbyterian Hospital for another year, but instead of continuing with her surgical residency, she spent a year in a program with the nurses who performed the anesthesia at Presbyterian. Dr. Apgar then moved on, attending residency positions at the University of Wisconsin under Ralph Waters and Emery Rovenstine at Bellevue Hospital. In 1938 after completing this, training, she returned to Presbyterian as the director of the new division of anesthesiology, the first woman to head a division at Presbyterian. She worked to recruit medical students, teach, and expand the division. For the first 5 years of her tenure, this was incredibly challenging as the division was underfunded and consisted of only her.

After 11 years of building, the division was finally large and functional enough to become its own department. Dr. Apgar was passed over for the position of department chair, which was given to her male colleague Emanuel Papper. Dr. Apgar was no longer in charge of administrative duties and soon after became the first woman to be a full-time professor at the Columbia College of Physicians and Surgeons, where she was already a part-time professor who was beloved by her students.

With her "extra" time, she was able to focus on advancing the field of anesthesiology through research. She had noticed as more and more births were in hospitals instead of at home that greatly decreased the maternal mortality rates were greatly decreased, but the neonatal mortality rates had not changed. In 1952, Dr. Apgar developed the evaluation tool eventually known as the Apgar score, which evaluated the baby within minutes of birth in order to develop a quantitative measurement of how the baby was adjusting to life outside of the womb. This test focused on heart rate, respiration, movement, irritability, and color. One of her residents reworked the measured aspects to *appearance, pulse, grimace, activity, and respiration*—this made it so "Apgar" became a reverse acronym, which greatly amused Dr. Apgar. The Apgar scale and evaluation were first presented at an IARS meeting in 1952 and published in *Anesthesia & Analgesia* in 1953 [9]. She worked with many physicians to relate this score to maternal anesthesia practices, the development of the child, and the overall birthing process with the goal of improving all three.

In the late 1950s, she had witnessed over 17,000 births and been published over 60 times, revolutionizing obstetric anesthesia. With these 17,000 births, she had seen hundreds of birth defects, which began to intrigue her. With her research requiring more statistical analysis, she decided to enroll in an MPH program at Johns Hopkins so that she could master statistics and supplement her work. During her time at Johns Hopkins, she thought deeply about the birth defects she witnessed and how they could be treated or even prevented.

After receiving her MPH degree in 1959, she was offered a position as the head of the new Division of Congenital Malformations for the National Foundation for Infantile Paralysis (NFIP), now known as the March of Dimes. The NFIP was looking to expand after the creation of polio vaccines.

She was extremely successful at the NFIP—raising a significant amount of money for the organization as well as pioneering research on the subject of teratology, which is the study of birth defects. Also, caring about making medical information more accessible for people, especially mothers, she published a book called *Is My Baby All Right?* This book was an easy-to-understand guide to birth defects for mothers of children with birth defects. She eventually taught teratology at Cornell Weill Medical School. She died in 1974 after contributing a great deal to the new field of anesthesiology and the American medical community in general, and was remembered not only for her intelligence but for her warmth, energy, personability, and sense of humor.

References

1. Soma-Pillay P, Nelson-Piercy C, et al. Physiological changes in pregnancy. Cardiovasc J Afr. 2016;27(2):89–94.
2. Kiki I, Gundogdu M, et al. A simple, safe, and effective approach to prevent postdural puncture headache: epidural saline injection. Eurasian J Med. 2009;41(3):175–9.
3. Mahmoud AAA, Mansour AZ, et al. Anesth Analg. 2018;127(6):1434–39.
4. Dietzel J, Witstruck T, Adler S, Usichenko TI. Acupuncture for treatment of therapy-resistant postdural puncture headache: a retrospective case series. Br J Anaesth. 2013;111:847–9.
5. Sharma A, Cheam E. Acupuncture in the management of post-partum headache following neuraxial analgesia. Int J Obstet Anesth. 2009;18:417–9.
6. Sohn J. Preventing post-dural puncture headache in obstetric patients. SOAP annual Meeting Abstracts. 2020. Available from: https://www.soap.org/assets/docs/Abstracts2020/Sohn_Jackie.pdf
7. Acquah J, Chang A. Acupuncture and postdural puncture headache. Volpe Anesth Digest. 2019;5(1). Available from: https://uknowledge.uky.edu/vad/vol5/iss1/4/
8. Chang A, Acquah J, et al. Acupuncture for the management of postdural puncture headache: a case report. Glob Adv Health Med. 2016;5(1):103–6.
9. Apgar V. A proposal for a new method of evaluation of the newborn infant. Anesth Analg. 1953;32:250–9.
10. For the following online resources, Springer Basic style does not have a strict rule but you can adapt this way.

Authors

Brandon Togioka is an associate professor and vice chair of clinical research at Oregon Health and Science University. He trained at Hopkins for anesthesia residency and OB anesthesia fellowship. Among his many clinical and research interests is a focus on high-risk parturients healthcare disparities, especially in the Hispanic community. His article on eliminating disparities in labor pain management in Hispanic parturients was featured on the cover of the October 2019 issue of *Anesthesiology.* He has been recognized numerous times by Portland Monthly as a top doctor and anesthesiologist.

David Mayer has been a teaching clinician in the department of anesthesiology at the UNC School of Medicine for over 30 years. Although a native of Louisiana, he has adopted Tarheel sports teams over the years. In his free time, he enjoys playing tennis and attempting to play golf.

Emily Rhinehart grew up in the metropolitan Baltimore area. She is a pre-med student who graduated from the University of Southern California with a major in health promotion and disease prevention and a minor in health policy. She is interested in an eventual career in anesthesiology. In her spare time, she loves music, the guitar, and playing soccer. She exemplifies the bright young student who is our specialty's future.

Cathy Marcucci considers obstetrical anesthesia to be a favorite of hers, second only to vascular, thoracic, and transplant anesthesia. She is thankful for the solid teaching she received in OB anesthesia by the outstanding Hopkins faculty, including the opportunity to attend conferences with the late, great Dr. Robert Abraham.

Wisdom on Neuro-anesthesiology

167

Michael D. Altose, Brian T. Gierl, Robert E. Minahan,
Ziyad O. Knio, Allan Gottschalk, and Catherine Marcucci

Introduction

Neuroanesthesiology is a fascinating anesthesia subspecialty for several reasons. First and foremost is the complex physiology that underlies it. Second, it crosses disciplines with all the other areas of anesthesia practice, and neuro-anesthesiologists take care of a lot of different patient cohorts. That's why a classic oral boards question has always been a patient with (something big—take your pick) who needs a craniotomy. The "something big" could be a pregnant patient or somebody with severe coronary artery disease or liver failure.

Neuro-anesthesiology also has many levels of acuity—it encompasses urgent and emergent adult and pediatric cases, peripheral and central nervous system cases, trauma cases, routine sedation cases, care of the chronic pain patient, and its own subspecialty of critical care medicine. We were delighted to tap into the thoughts and teaching points of three experienced neuro-anesthesiologists—**Mike Altose**, **Brian Gierl**, and **Allan Gottschalk**—and neurologist **Rob Minahan**.

General

- Just because you take a job that is "no hearts, no heads" doesn't mean that you won't be working with neurosurgeons and doing neuro-anesthesia. One of the editors was trained at a location where carotid endarterectomies were routinely done by the neurosurgeons.—**Editors**

M. D. Altose
Department of Anesthesiology and Perioperative Medicine, University Hospitals Cleveland Medical Center, Cleveland, OH, USA
e-mail: Michael.Altose@UHhospitals.org

B. T. Gierl
Neuroanesthesiology and Neuroanesthesiology QI, University of Pittsburgh Medical Center Presbyterian, Pittsburgh, PA, USA

R. E. Minahan
Real Time Neuromonitoring Associates, Glen Burnie, MD, USA

Z. O. Knio
Department of Anesthesiology, University of Virginia, Charlottesville, VA, USA

A. Gottschalk
Department of Anesthesiology and Critical Care Medicine, Johns Hopkins University, Baltimore, MD, USA

C. Marcucci (✉)
Departments of Transfusion Medicine, Clinical Center, National Institutes of Health, Bethesda, MD, USA

S. Mohamed et al. (eds.), *Anesthesia Bridges*, https://doi.org/10.1007/978-3-032-08294-7_167

- Similarly, if you are training or practicing at a location with a neurosurgery practice, expect to see neurosurgery cases outside the "neuro rooms." At Hopkins, back in the day, it was not unusual to be posted in a room with a pediatric neurosurgeon doing rhizotomies in older adult patients.—**Editors**

- If you are considering employment in the VA Health Care System, remember that Level II VA hospitals do neurosurgery cases. What qualifies a VA hospital to do neurosurgery cases is having a neurosurgeon on staff, not neuro-anesthesiologists or a dedicated neuro-ICU. I did neurosurgery cases several times a week while on staff at a mid-sized VA hospital.—**CM**

- For some reason, still unknown to me, I was assigned to do my neuro-anesthesiology rotation in my second month as a CA-1. I did my preceptor month and then, boom, straight to the neuro rooms. I remember flailing around pretty badly, until somebody finally said to me, "Okay, just focus on these things—head over heart in terms of physiology (almost always) and quick, effective, safe turns with little wasted effort. And remember, whichever way you turn 'em to start the case, you gotta turn 'em back when the case is over." Pretty good advice even for experienced anesthesiologists.—**CM**

  Have you ever noticed that the neuro rooms are one place where the surgeons don't tend to blare music? We've been in rooms where the surgeon has specifically requested "no music." Wonder if there is any lesson there for the other surgeons?—**Editors**

- Show extra empathy to families of pediatric patients who require a middle-of-the-night ventriculoperitoneal (VP) shunt revision. It's our observation that these are some of the most stressed-out parents you will interact with, even if they have been through an urgent shunt revision before. Their child has most likely had a period of steadily worsening neurological status, right before their eyes, and they understand that the solution is in the operating room, and they must get their child there. It has to be excruciating. One of the few times I ever saw a set of parents really lose complete composure was many years ago when an urgent VP shunt revision was temporarily bumped for some sort of vascular rupture. The parents just went ballistic.—**CM** and **Editors**

Anatomy and Physiology

- Neuroanesthesiology is interesting and challenging to do because of the variation in pain receptors and pain physiology between the central and peripheral nervous systems. Remember that there are no somatic pain receptors in the brain itself. But the scalp is a different story, of course.—**Editors**

- And surgery for the peripheral nerve pathologies can often involve people who are experiencing terrific pain. Nerve pain and/or neuropathic pain can be excruciating. Trigeminal neuralgia is among the most painful syndromes in all of medicine. If you plan to make neuro-anesthesiology a part of your practice, make sure that you are comfortable caring for chronic pain patients.—**Editors**

- Cerebral blood flow autoregulation over a range of cerebral perfusion pressures, carbon dioxide responsiveness, and flow-metabolism coupling are the predominant determinants of cerebral blood flow in the healthy brain. Pathologies such as traumatic brain injury, subarachnoid hemorrhage, or meningitis can disrupt their ability to control blood flow and alter ICP.—**BTG**

- Head elevation always helps to drain venous blood and CSF, but hydrocephalus can blunt its impact. The ability of propofol to reduce $CMRO_2$ and provide direct cerebral vasoconstriction is almost always preserved.—**BTG**

- Paradoxically, increasing MAP to preserve CPP (~60–80 mmHg) will actually decrease ICP by causing arterial vasoconstriction.—**BTG**

- You almost always want your $PaCO_2$ to be less than 40 mmHg in a craniotomy case. Often the target is 25–30 mmHg. The subsequent respiratory alkalosis will cause hydrogen ions to shift into the bloodstream. When albumin loses hydronium ions, calcium binds to albumin, and the ionized calcium concentration is reduced. Cells exchange H+ for K+, and plasma potassium declines.—**BTG**

- Hyperventilation starts working almost immediately, and it only works for about 6–8 hours before the pH of the CSF returns to normal.—**MDA**

- After that, you will get rebound *HYPER*perfusion when you return to normal ventilation. Therefore, don't start hyperventilation until you need it (at/after incision) and stop it as soon as you can (as soon as the tumor is out). This gives time for the CSF pH to return to normal. It also allows brain tissue to fill in the "cavity" where the tumor was, and you'll get less air trapped under the dura after closure.—**MDA**

- We "get away" with a lot of hypotension in anesthesia, but neurosurgery might not be the place for it. Cerebral blood flow can be very low in some regions due to hyperventilation, surgical retraction, and other mechanisms of injury/ischemia. It's really a good idea to maintain normal blood pressure in most procedures unless the surgeon requires otherwise.—**MDA**

- Likewise, When I was training >15 years ago, I was taught that the goal in a typical craniotomy for tumor was "normotensive hyperosmotic euvolemia." That is how I have practiced ever since for cases where brain relaxation is needed, unless the surgeon is specifically requesting a negative fluid balance, usually in a last-ditch and probably-not-evidenced-based attempt to remedy a tight brain. I suspect that all organs, the brain included, will fare better when volume status is optimized, and vasopressors are used sparingly.—**MDA**

- One common hemodynamic goal in craniotomy for tumor is to lower cerebral blood flow to relax the brain and allow for optimal surgical conditions. This goal is often achieved with hyperventilation and IV anesthetic agents. But not all craniotomies are alike! For a neurovascular procedure, the surgeon may be relying on adequate collateral circulation, in which case volatile agents and normal ventilation may be more appropriate.—**MDA**

- We typically focus on the plasma sodium concentration as an indicator of plasma osmolarity. However, mannitol (similar to hyperglycemia) will induce a pseudohyponatremia that will not result in cerebral edema; it is osmolarity that determines brain hydration/edema.—**BTG**

- A patient with a neurologic deficit prior to a general anesthetic will often have a worsening of that deficit postoperatively until they clear their anesthetic because the healthy neurons surrounding the damaged area need to work that much harder to make up for the damaged neurons and are unable to do so with residual anesthetic present. This pertains to volatile anesthetics and the GABA agonists propofol and benzodiazepines. Dexmedetomidine and low dose opioids have less of an impact.—**BTG**

- A patient who had a deficit with a stroke—particularly one that required physical rehabilitation—will often experience a transient re-emergence or worsening of stroke symptoms postoperatively. That phenomenon is known as recrudescence and should be considered before treating the patient for an acute stroke. An experienced anesthesiologist or neurologist can be helpful.—**BTG**

- Patients for mechanical thrombectomy can be managed with or without an endotracheal tube, as long as the patient is induced and intubated expeditiously and CPP is maintained. A stroke patient for mechanical thrombectomy under general anesthesia needs a higher MAP and CBF to drive collateral blood flow and a normal to elevated P_aCO_2 so that cerebral vasoconstriction does not reduce CBF.—**BTG**

- Speaking of anatomy, the fixture of the head in an optimal 3-D spatial position is of great importance to the surgeons. The anesthesia team should be aware of this and work collaboratively with the surgeons to ensure the patient is safely positioned for the surgical procedure. It sounds trivial but remember that small changes in neck position with change the position of the patient's head and vice versa.—**Editors**

- The ideal position of the head is the position that provides optimal surgical approach to the target brain area and is based on two principles.—**Editors**

- An imaginary trajectory from the highest point at the skull surface to the area of interest in the brain should be the shortest distance between the two points.—**Editors**

- Whenever possible, the exposed surface of the skull and an imaginary perimeter of craniotomy should be parallel to the floor.—**Editors**

***Note from the Editors:** Neural regeneration strategies or the concept of "nerve bridges" are some of the most exciting areas in medical research. While work continues in the field facilitating nerve autografts, the bioengineers are working hard on developing off-the-shelf, readily available nerve allografts and nerve scaffolds. Of course, nerve regeneration is heavily dependent on initiating axonal bridges (Fig. 167.1).

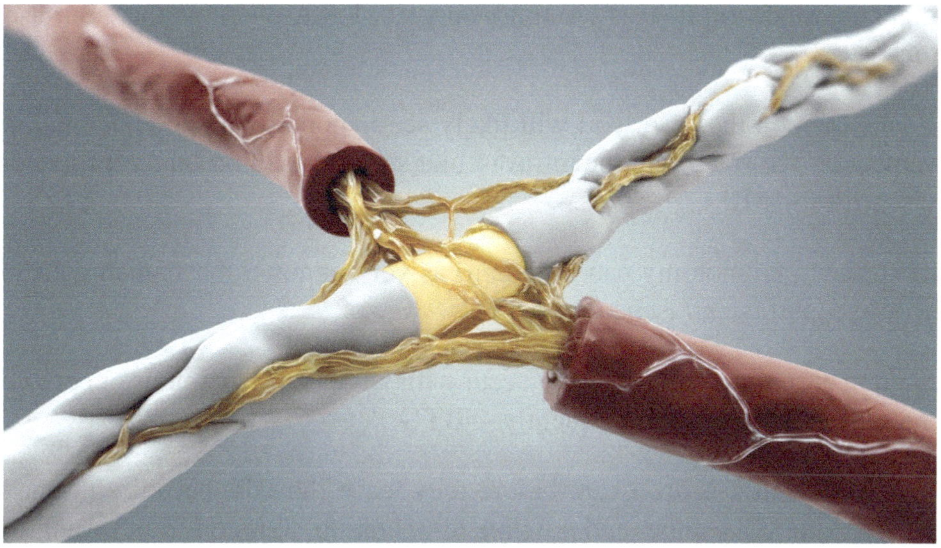

Fig. 167.1 An illustration of the development of a nerve bridge. On the microscopic level, vascular bridges form first, and then that vascular scaffolding is used by migrating nerve component cells. Illustration. Photo: Image used under standard license from stock.adobe.com

Clinical Assessment and Patient Monitoring

- There are number of ways that a radiologist can tell you that the patient's intracranial pressure is elevated or that will be elevated soon, other than a midline shift: enlarged ventricles (hydrocephalus), effaced of ventricles, empty or obliterated basal cisterns and other CSF spaces, herniation (of anything), loss or blunting of sulci, or loss of grey-white matter differentiation.—**BTG**

- The best way to test the integrity of neurological functions is your a physical examination. You should have a good baseline neurological exam before providing an anesthetic to anyone. If you don't routinely do neuro-anesthesia, leave time for the neuro exam in your general pre-op assessment.—**BTG**

- The baseline neurological exam should also include a Mini-Mental Status Exam (MMSE), especially in head cases. You should be able to do this in less than five minutes. Use the time you would have used to place an arterial line that you don't really need (see below). Make sure you report the MMSE results to the postoperative care team.—**Editors**

- If the patient has an intraventricular drain, you should monitor intraoperative intracranial pressure. There are a number of issues that can lead to an increase in ICP, including but not limited to: elevated $PaCO_2$, high doses of volatile anesthetics, metabolic acidosis, hypo-osmolarity, impaired venous drainage, or seizure, increasing $CMRO_2$. Elevated intracranial pressure for an entire case can lead to long-term complications.—**BTG**

- Remember that the arterial line must be at the level of the heart to give accurate readings! When the patient's head (and heart) are raised, up the transducer goes on the pole. And don't forget to lower it when the patient comes down. It's easy to think oh yeah, I already know that! But it happens all the time.—**Editors**

- If you check labs early in the case, you will likely see hyponatremia and anemia due to mannitol, causing movement of free water into the intravascular space. It will probably resolve on its own once urine output increases.—**MDA**

- Rising lactate during a craniotomy can be due to as yet unknown mechanisms. It doesn't indicate hypovolemia or hypoperfusion / ischemia.—**BTG**

- Rising urine output during a craniotomy can occur without diabetes insipidus or cerebral salt wasting. If it occurs, monitor plasma sodium frequently.—**BTG**

- Craniotomy patients need a neuro exam before they leave the OR, because an unexpected deficit might mean a trip to the CT scanner and possible re-operation. Surgeons don't want to find out about a deficit after the patient is in PACU, and if there's any question the surgeon needs to give the ok to leave the OR.—**MDA**

- Facilitate the exam by planning ahead—avoid benzodiazepines unless absolutely necessary, turn off propofol early whenever possible, and minimize opioids until after extubation—I give acetaminophen in pre-op and rarely have issues with post-op pain. Consider extubating before the neuro exam if that's what is best for the patient, such as to avoid coughing or hypertension. Then stay in the OR until the surgeon is satisfied with the neuro exam.—**MDA**

- If you check labs early in the case, you will likely see hyponatremia and anemia due to mannitol, causing movement of free water into the intravascular space. It will probably resolve on its own once urine output increases.—**MDA**

- Then there is the issue of arterial line placement. Leaving aside patient specific comorbidities, I typically do not place an arterial catheter for intracranial cases. We now have continuous capnography and pulse oximetry to guide ventilation and oxygenation.—**AG**

- Exceptions to the above are vascular cases, those where tumors are adjacent or attached to large vessels, and posterior fossa cases where the tumor is deep within the posterior fossa. Since I generally find little need for extensive use of laboratory studies, I find that a strategically placed IV will permit me access to all the blood samples I require. When we looked at this practice, one thing was very clear: an arterial line adds an *average* of 11 minutes per case without any measurable benefits. Of course, the time to place an arterial line may be less if placed by an experienced anesthesiologist, but is often longer if placed by a trainee.—**AG** and **Editors**

Airway

- Much is often made about tracheal intubation in association with cervical spine surgery. Even in the presence of significant myelopathy, I rarely feel compelled to perform other than standard direct laryngoscopy.—**AG**

- If the patient can flex and extend without symptoms, the lesion is not high (most flexion/extension is C0-C1 and C1-C2), and the anatomy is intact (no trauma), I am quite comfortable with direct laryngoscopy, but probably would move on if successful intubation would require extremes of extension. If one is uncomfortable with this concept, look at how the patients are positioned for surgery for an ACDF.—**AG**

- In a past era, patients with severe cervical and sometimes lower myelopathy would be intubated and positioned awake to ensure the integrity of the spinal cord. However, modern intraoperative monitoring with both SSEPs and MEPs supplants this and provides continuous assurance.—**AG**

- Along this line, the "wakeup test" is rarely used as a routine assessment. However, I have performed several just after positioning when intraoperative monitoring indicated a new deficit, where the subsequent exam confirmed a new loss of function which resolved with repositioning, sometimes with fluoroscopic guidance and at other times due to a revised surgical approach (posterior vs. anterior).—**AG**

***Note from the Editors:** Among Allan Gottschalk's favorite bridges is the Verrazano Narrows Bridge (Fig. 167.2).

> I am a big fan of the Verrazano Narrows Bridge. I enjoyed watching it go up when I was a small child. I was also fascinated by the fact that the curvature of the Earth had to be considered when determining the distance between towers. And I liked that it finally provided a shortcut alleviating the passage through midtown Manhattan on the way from Long Island to my mother's family in New Jersey—something very much appreciated during summer visits when air conditioning in in cars was not yet standard.

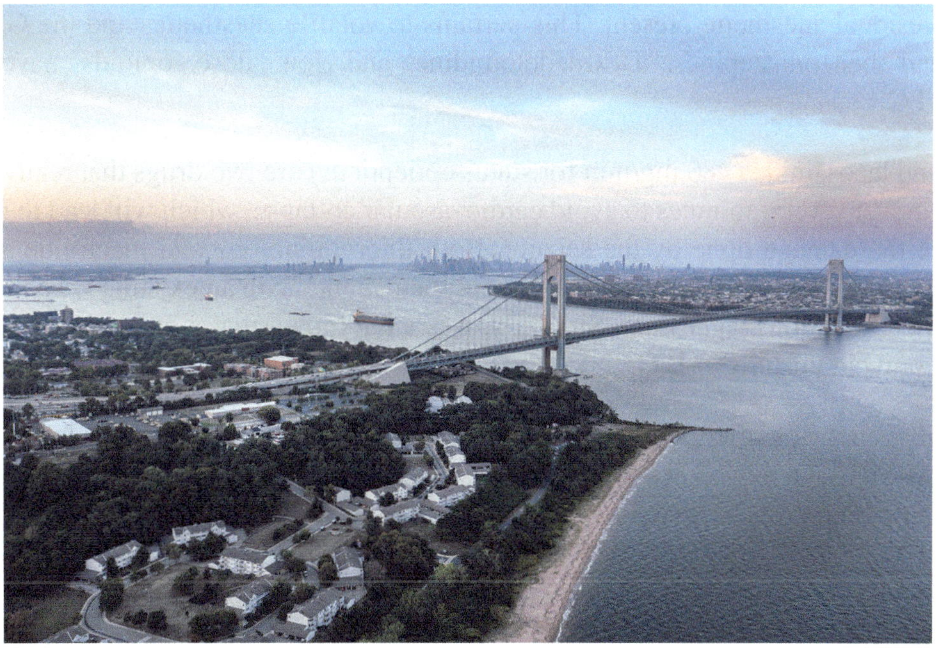

Fig. 167.2 The Verrazano Narrows Bridge opened in 1964 and at that time was the longest suspension bridge in the world. It connects Brooklyn and Staten Island and also acts as a major interstate connector between Long Island and the Mid-Atlantic states. The huge towers are 1.675 inches farther apart at the top than at the bottom to account for the earth's curvature. Seasonal expansion and contractions of the steel suspension cables cause the road surface to be 12 feet lower in the summer than in the winter. The photo above really gives a sense of how the bridge connects the boroughs of New York. Photo: Image used under standard license from iStock.com

Medications

- Neuro-anesthesia is the one subspecialty in which you may be routinely dealing with patients on chronic, high-dose steroids, with all the awful side effects those drugs entail.—**Editors**

- And what are those chronic steroid side effects? The most important ones for perioperative physicians are weight gain, which can change airway diameter and anatomy, leading to difficulty in intubating and sleep apnea, hypertension, and disruptions in blood sugar regulation.—**Editors**

- Also, remember that steroids are both CYP 3A4 substrates and equivocal inducers. But they are much more likely to be the "victims" in a drug-drug interaction (DDI) than cause increased metabolism of other meds. Perioperative physicians, including neuro-ICU docs, should scan the medication list for other CYP 3A4 substrates such as verapamil, diltiazem, azole antifungals, and ciprofloxacin, as these are all known to cause clinically relevant increased metabolism of steroids. The seizure syndromes may not be as well-controlled as thought.—**Editors**

- Gabapentin, tricyclic antidepressants, anti-convulsants (sodium valproate, carbamazepine, oxcarbazepine, lamotrigine) are all drugs commonly seen in the medication lists of neurosurgical patients. All have a somewhat complicated clinical pharmacology, including multiple pharmacodynamic and pharmacokinetic DDIs, so make sure you review them before starting a neuro-anesthesia rotation. And all these drugs are used as mood stabilizers for psychiatric patients. Might be a good idea to do a joint resident lecture on these crossover drugs?—**Editors**

- A patient with a neurologic deficit prior to a general anesthetic will often have a worsening of that deficit postoperatively until they clear their anesthetic because the healthy neurons surrounding the damaged area need to work that much harder to make up for the damaged neurons and are unable to do so with residual anesthetic present. This pertains to volatile anesthetics and the GABA agonists propofol and benzodiazepines. Dexmedetomidine and low dose opioids have less of an impact.—**BTG**

- Phenytoin and lacosamide (<80 mg/min for status epilepticus) are two drugs that really do need to be administered over several minutes to avoid cardiovascular collapse, which will lead to hypoperfusion and increase the damage done by the seizure. Both fluoroquinolone and macrolide antibiotics can trigger arrhythmias (torsade de pointes) in susceptible patients with an existing QTc prolongation, or low serum potassium or magnesium. Similarly, it is well known that a quick vancomycin dose can lead to vancomycin flushing.—**BTG**

- Emergence hypertension after craniotomy is very common. Plan by giving some labetalol toward the end of the case as soon as you see the blood pressure creeping up. Start with 5–10 mg IV and keep giving 5–20 mg boluses as needed. Esmolol is a good short-acting option, but labetalol is more effective at lowering blood pressure. Remember that hydralazine takes 15–20 minutes to have an effect.—**MDA**

- Once there's labetalol on board, hydralazine can be very potent! I usually limit myself to 5 mg at a time in that setting. Have a calcium channel blocker available such as clevidipine or nicardipine in case the blood pressure gets away from you.—**MDA**

- Run mannitol through an IV that you can see! Sometimes a small hole happens in the back wall of a vein during IV placement. The IV runs fine throughout the case. But mannitol can sneak out of that hole and bring fluid with it. Nobody wants to call an intraoperative (or worse, postoperative!) hand consult for a cold, swollen, mottled hand. And having a waveform on the pulse oximeter does NOT rule out compartment syndrome!—**MDA**

- On the issue of mannitol as a vesicant. I never run it on an infusion pump to avoid higher pressures (say when a proximal blood pressure cuff inflates, or a limb is repositioned) and to minimize the catastrophe with an unrecognized infiltrated IV. This last scenario (infiltrated IV with mannitol on infusion pump) is the only time I have known patients to have an injury from mannitol.—**AG**

- More on mannitol—when using mannitol, always keep in mind how it affects hemodynamics and laboratory values. Initially, in patients with healthy hearts, there may be an increase in blood pressure, which can be ridden out with a small increase in anesthetic concentration. Once diuresis begins in earnest, a "softer" blood pressure may result, one of the reasons for suggesting more reversible interventions acutely.—**AG**

- Similarly, at the beginning of the case, the use of mannitol will dilute laboratory values but concentrate them toward the end. Thus, the hemoglobin concentration tends to understate red cell mass early on and do just the opposite later on. I personally avoid checking labs in a stable situation to avoid related concerns, particularly by the surgeons.—**AG**

- Though its use is treated as anachronistic by some, nitrous oxide still continues to play a major role in my practice and that of some of the more senior faculty. For intracranial cases, our neurosurgeons always irrigate below the dura just before they close to check for hemostasis and eliminate any gas pockets. In combination, at 70%, with scalp blockade (see below) and a little fentanyl, the entire closure following that of the still-sensitive dura is possible without anything else (the 0.25% of isoflurane is discontinued upon dural closure). The patient can usually be extubated before the head wrapping is completed.—**AG**

- For procedures of the spine, I like to think of nitrous oxide as inhalational ketamine. Its NMDA antagonism is known to reduce chronic postsurgical pain months after surgery, and a modest exposure has a positive effect on pain-related behavior in animals with chronic pain.—**AG**

- Once closure begins, 70% nitrous oxide is generally sufficient if the amount of opioid is adequate. Only when opioid dose is inadequate, requiring high concentrations of volatile anesthetic, is there meaningful interference with intraoperative monitoring. Think about this carefully and try it.—**AG**

- At 70% NO2, there is a small but not overwhelming or unacceptable effect on SSEPs. Nitrous oxide may also improve affect analogous to ketamine's role in depression. Why deny this to our patients?—**AG**

- On use of vasopressors during spine surgery—most of the arrests in association with surgery of the spine that I have observed have been facilitated by use of vasopressor infusions. Once this starts, the only thing that saves the patient is that the surgeon completes the operation before an arrest occurs.—**AG**

- With a vasopressor reducing vascular volume, hemoglobin concentrations are falsely reassuring.—**AG**

- If I do not find a need for an infusion of vasopressor right after induction, one is never started. The most typical reason is a hypertensive patient whose post-induction blood pressure is now low due to ongoing use of antihypertensive medication in whom adequate perfusion pressures, particularly for the spine, are indicated. This does not preclude an occasional bolus of a vasopressor until one catches up with volume resuscitation due to hemorrhage.—**AG**

- When patients are opioid resistant, a common situation with spine surgery, it's not immediately clear what the opioid dose should be. Like with many things in anesthesiology, titration is the answer!—**AG**

- Following a suggestion in the literature, I titrate fentanyl until pain is at an acceptable level and/or the respiratory rate goes to 5-6 breaths per minute. I just watch for the initiation of a breath and start to count slowly. If I get to ten before the next one, it is time to complete the induction. From my perspective, fentanyl is best because it redistributes over 20 minutes, so even if you have overdone it, you did not really.—**AG**

- When starting out with large doses of fentanyl, get the muscle relaxant in quickly to avoid chest-wall rigidity. If you are doing a big case, a repeat dose of fentanyl right before incision, often 30–50% of original total, is generally indicated. This process also helps you decide if use of drugs like ketamine may be indicated and guides postoperative PCA dosing.—**AG**

Equipment

- Know how to properly operate a lumbar drain. If you aren't sure, just ask the surgeon. And make sure your resident also knows. Catastrophic things happen when lumbar drains are mismanaged.—**MDA**

- Some of the most important equipment considerations for neuro-anesthesiologists concern the placement of the head pins. This is a bit ironic since we often don't even touch them. There is some variation, but the Mayfield frame is a 3-pin device often used for fixation for craniotomies. For other brain and skull cases, such as a burr hole or a functional neurosurgery (like deep brain stimulator placement), a 4-pin device is used.—**Editors**

- Recognized complications of pin placement include scalp vessel damage and hematoma, epidural hematoma, pin site infection, air embolism, pneumocephalus, shunt tube damage, skull fracture, and brain parenchyma damage. In one case series, a catastrophic hematoma was reported in 5/766 (about 0.65%) of cases [1]. That is not that small of an occurrence, as adverse events in anesthesia go.—**Editors**

- Complications from the pins should be on the differential in the ICU or even in the OR whenever the patient seems to be having a rockier emergence or post-op course than would be expected.—**Editors**

- The *Anesthesia Bridges* editors asked the authors for their comments and wisdom and thoughts about pins and specific pin placement. They all answered back that they felt did not have the expertise to critically evaluate the literature. It's pretty fascinating reading, though. For example, one paper looks at the response of different cranial bones to pin placement [2]. The stated premise of the paper is below. What it says to us is that although pins and head fixation have been used for many decades (Frank Mayfield designed his skull clamp in the 1960s), the physiologic and anatomic effects are still not completely understood. We think it would be a great topic for an interdisciplinary lecture by the surgeons.—**Editors**

- Despite the daily use of the head-fixation device (HFD) in the operating room, there are no evidence-based guidelines for its use, especially for adequate pinning forces to avoid complications during its utilization. The goal of this research was to study the cranial responds to the HFD. It experimentally determined the response of the bone to the pin of the single-pin side of the HFD depending on three factors, the pin angle, applied force, and the different pin placing locations.—**Editors**

- This paper also makes the point that children are generally at greater risk than adults, due to thinner cranial bone thickness, the presence of fontanelles, and mobile anatomic structures and landmarks. There is more literature available on pediatric head fixation complications than adults, but there is probably under-reporting in both patient cohorts.—**Editors**

- One thing we can say is that it is critical not to let the patient cough or buck while in the pins. We were taught not to reverse the neuromuscular blockade until they were out of the head fixation device and to keep a syringe of propofol handy if you even see the patient swallowing. This is conservative, yes, but you don't want the patients inadvertently pulling themselves out of those pins!—**Editors**

Intraoperative Management

- I perform scalp blockade at the beginning of virtually every intracranial case I do. Since the volume is small, I use 0.75% bupivacaine (plain) because, in the literature, the blocks where decreased postoperative pain appears most measurable were with higher concentrations of local anesthetics.—**AG**

- The scalp blocks permit one to run with very light levels of general anesthesia for prompt emergence and leaves one confident and well-prepared for awake craniotomies.—**AG**

- When an image guidance system is used in conjunction with intracranial surgery, we typically place the scalp block after the image guidance system is calibrated against the previously placed markers on the patient's head in order to prevent a wheal underneath one of these markers from producing an offset error.—**AG**

- Pin sites outside of the field of the block are dealt with directly, with local anesthetic injected just caudal to the pin site. Consider injecting the pin sites for spine cases when head fixation is used.—**AG**

- Sometimes, particularly with vascular cases, image guidance is not used and a standardized anatomic approach is made so the block can be placed prior to head fixation, helping to blunt the related hemodynamic response. This requires a more extensive block, particularly to cover the pins placed in the occipital area. But it can be very effective.—**AG**

- When performing scalp blockade for midline approaches to the posterior fossa, do not neglect consideration of the third occipital nerve which passes through the fascia on either side of the midline at the level of the mastoid. Until I did this, my blocks for these surgeries were not as compelling.—**AG**

- Also, when blocking the auriculotemporal or great auricular nerve, in front or behind the ear, respectively, always direct the needle cephalad in order to avoid an inadvertent VIIth nerve block, which may confuse things if this nerve is being monitored intraoperatively.—**AG**

- When the brain is swelling, surgeons are having problems with exposure, and additional osmotherapy is being implemented, there are some quick moves that can be made. Certainly, the level of hypoventilation should be checked, and any PEEP turned off to reduce venous congestion—it is amazing how high some people will turn up the PEEP. A bolus of propofol to reduce brain metabolism and associated blood flow will work almost instantly. Eventually, additional mannitol and hypertonic saline with furosemide will get things under control.—**Authors**

- The eyes are such an important consideration in neuro-anesthesia. First, remember that the eyes are an extension of the brain. Second, all the turns can put the eyes at risk. Third, any time the head is above the heart, you must always keep the potential for visual loss at the front of your mind.—**Editors**

- The editors know many anesthesiologists who will categorically not place a patient at greater than 45 degrees, except in the case of the true sitting craniotomy.—**Editors**

- One of the senior neuro-anesthesiologists at Hopkins back in the day said to me once, "If the patient is seated, we are standing." His point is that you really have to keep your vigilance up in a seated craniotomy case. As he clarified, "This is not a case that's going to be a long day of charting and not much else."—**CM**

- Negotiate with the surgeons if they want to do a 180 degree turn in the supine position. You just don't want to be looking only at the bottom of the feet. Usually, a turn of 160 degrees or 170 degrees is acceptable, and they can get their personnel and tables positioned adequately.—**Editors**

- As you are turning prepping and draping and turning, plan and preserve a route of access to the patient. Can you get to the arterial line? Can you get to the pulse ox? Can you get to a hand, forearm, antecubital space, groin, or foot for a new IV or arterial line is necessary or to draw labs? —**Editors**

***Note from the Editors:** Rob Minahan is from Green Bay, Wisconsin. To show our appreciation for his help with this chapter, we thought it would be fun to feature the Leo Frigo Memorial Bridge (Fig. 167.3).

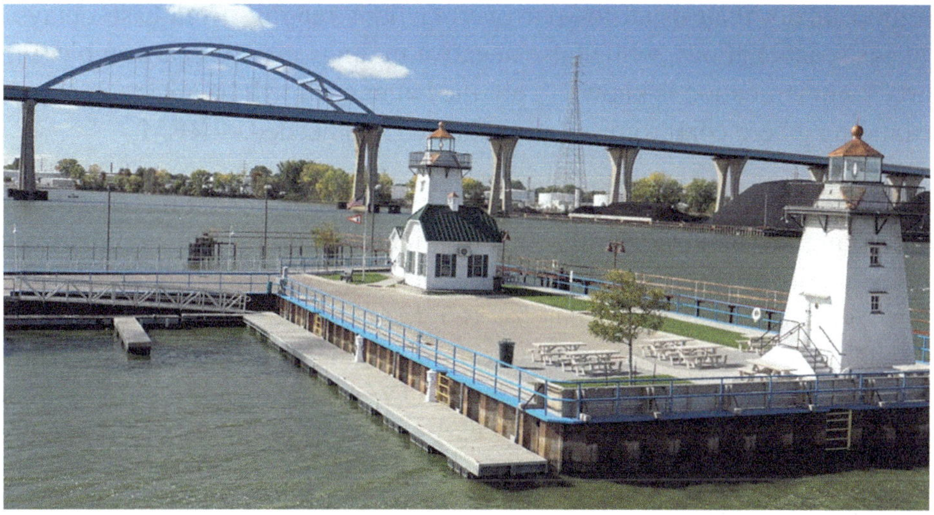

Fig. 167.3 The Leo Frigo Memorial Bridge, formerly known as the Tower Drive Bridge, spans the Fox River just south of the mouth of Green Bay. Leo Frigo was a civic and philanthropic leader in the city. Among his legacy projects was the creation of Paul's Pantry, one of the nation's largest food pantries. This view also shows the Grassy Island Range Lights in the foreground. Photo: Image used under standard license from stock.adobe.com

Evoked Potentials Monitoring

- Delivering an optimal anesthetic regimen for procedures utilizing intraoperative neuromonitoring (IONM) is complex but can be guided by some simple general principles. And this starts with the unfortunate fact that in many cases, the anesthesiologist's goals of comfortably deep anesthesia, analgesia, and amnesia work against the intraoperative neurological monitoring team's ability to measure neurologic function with clarity.—**REM**

- It's important for us to remember that we have a wide range of tools with which to deliver anesthesia. There are many ways to get the case done! Therefore, communication with the neuromonitoring team is important in order to weigh what they view as important for the greatest sensitivity and specificity of the IONM data. And that's a good question for the neurology team before every case.—**REM** and **Editors**

- It is in the patient's best interests that a balance be struck such that adequate anesthesia is delivered safely while at the same time maximally maintaining the neuromonitoring team's window into the patient's neurologic function. And this is important to emphasize. In general, there is usually good rapport between the anesthesia team and the IONM team but if there is a disagreement on the clinical plan, it doesn't come down to what the IONM wants or needs. It's a question of their expert assessment as to what's best for the patient.—**REM** and **Editors**

- In addition, the anesthesiologist's motivation to provide regimens that optimize neuromonitoring may be impacted by communication with the surgeons and their view of the importance of the IONM for each case. If the surgeons' concern for neurologic injury is heightened in a given case, this knowledge may sway the anesthesiologist's balance more toward IONM because false positive findings in this scenario are more likely than usual to spur overreactions ranging from case delays to incomplete procedures to case cancellations, while false negative findings may be catastrophic. Finally, the more this three-party communication is known to all, the better each will be able to accomplish their goals while understanding where compromises are indicated and needed.—**REM**

- Once a plan for anesthesia is made, flexibility is key as well as open lines of communication! For example, in a young and neurologically intact patient with idiopathic scoliosis, one would normally expect to acquire adequate transcranial motor evoked potentials with low-level potent inhalational agent. As such, an initial plan for 0.5 MAC of gas could be made. Unfortunately, occasionally such patients can only generate trans-cranial motor evoked potentials (TcMEPs) with propofol-based total intravenous anesthetic (TIVA). Understanding that one is dealing with an exceptional case and conversion to TIVA early enough in the case to allow baseline signals before critical surgical steps may be the only way to allow for ongoing assessment of motor function and avoidance of a wake-up test at the end of the case. And remember that nobody really wants a wake-up test.—**REM**

- There is no one best anesthesia regimen for neuromonitoring with the preferences for a given case dependent upon the tests to be monitored. For example, TIVA yields best monitoring results for TcMEPs. However, TIVA frequently negatively impacts EEG monitoring so cases where EEG is primary for the monitoring, for example carotid endarterectomy, are often best monitored purely with inhalational agents.—**REM**

- Use intraoperative neuromonitoring (IONM) to your advantage. Think about this—rarely do we have such ease of access to quantitative twitch monitoring, or to EEG assessment of anesthetic depth.—**ZOK**

- Not only are motor-evoked potentials (MEPs) more sensitive than somato-sensory evoked potentials (SSEPs) to the effects of anesthesia, but they are also inherently more sensitive to anterior spinal cord ischemia. SSEPs only monitor dorsal column function. This is particularly relevant during major vascular cases.—**ZOK**

- Brainstem auditory evoked potentials (BAEPs) are the least sensitive EPs to the effects of anesthetic medications. Intraoperative recall is most commonly described as *hearing* operating room conversations. Coincidence?—**ZOK**

- Diminished signals may also be secondary to blood loss—both overt, such as on the surgical field, and occult, such as an accumulating subdural hematoma.—**ZOK**

- If volatile (versus true TIVA) is desired, use the start of the case to determine an upper limit of end-tidal volatile concentration (%).—**ZOK**

- Ketamine is your friend, in many situations, but especially during IONM as it increases the amplitude of evoked potentials.—**ZOK**

- Of the routinely used testing modalities, most would probably agree that TcMEPs are the most challenging potentials to monitor. At the same time, when employed they are typically the signals of greatest interest and the signals most likely to alter the surgical course.—**REM**

- Let's caution this one more time—use of a propofol-based total intravenous anesthetic (TIVA) is ideal from the neuromonitoring perspective when TcMEPs are used. In the unfortunate case of a postoperative neuro deficit, we all want to be able to say that we optimized the acquisition and maintenance of IONM to the best of our knowledge and ability.—**REM**

- And here's why—TIVA yields the highest amplitude signals, produces signals in the greatest number of muscles assessed, shows the greatest stability of responses over time, allows acquisition of signals in difficult patients, and may allow monitoring in cases that otherwise would not have useful TcMEP signals and as a result of these factors is expected to give the highest sensitivity and sensitivity.—**REM**

- Ketamine, etomidate, and narcotics may be added with little or no negative impact on the TcMEP monitoring protocols.—**REM**

- Balanced anesthesia using potent inhalational agents (typically ≤0.5 MAC) with propofol may be desirable in some patients for reasons unrelated to the neuromonitoring (for example, reducing the risk of recall). This can be tolerated in patients with good signals.—**REM**

- When signals are lost (or weak at baseline), have a differential—traumatic disruption of pathway, generalized ischemia, drug effects. Give an honest workup to each potential explanation. The most unusual culprit I've encountered was an mis-programmed infusion pump (200 mL/hr propofol, versus 200 mcg/kg/min). The overdose was enough to diminish signals, but surprisingly not enough to cause any hemodynamic compromise.—**ZOK**

- *Remember!* Varying degrees of patient sensitivity to anesthetics does not allow preoperative prediction of the impact for individual patients.—**REM**

- An initial plan for balanced anesthesia might be employed but when safe, the inhalational agent portion may need to be eliminated or reduced to allow monitorable TcMEP signals.—**REM**

- More frequent testing of the TcMEP should be employed to allow identification of a gradual anesthetic-related fade over time.—**REM**

- Challenges in TcMEP monitoring are more likely to be problematic in patients with preexisting neurologic deficits, such as myelopathy.—**REM**

- Dexmedetomidine is at times added to TIVA regimens and may improve the delivery of anesthesia unrelated to the neuromonitoring. Unfortunately, when dexmedetomidine is used at infusion rates of ≥0.3 μg/kg/hr, TcMEP signals are impaired relative to propofol alone. —**REM**

- When possible, avoid relying on neuromonitoring-attenuating agents for blood pressure control. In patients with frequent swings in blood pressure, bolus-dosing or rapid adjustments of inhalational agents cause analogous swings in monitored signals. When poorly timed, these swings can disable the neuromonitoring—for example, a bolus of propofol at the time of clamping for carotid endarterectomy is likely to suppress EEG at that critical time. Less dramatically, with frequent dosing signals rarely completely return to their baseline state. This can significantly dull the precision of neuromonitoring.—**REM**

- The *Bridges* editors asked me to comment specifically on drugs that are commonly given in EP cases that shouldn't be. There is not straightforward answer to this. The anesthesiologist must manage a range of bodily functions while weighing the impact of possible anesthetic regimens against its impact on the neuromonitoring. Learning what this impact is and how to more comfortably manage neuromonitoring-friendly regimens is a skill that allows effective monitoring to proceed. Gaining this skill is a worthy goal but it is probably not appropriate to say any drug "shouldn't be given" in a contextless setting.—**REM**

- That being said, from a narrow neuromonitoring perspective, nitrous oxide is particularly unpopular. For somatosensory and motor evoked potentials, nitrous oxide likely has a similar effect to potent inhalational agents in terms of "inhibition/MAC." When used in combination with potent agents, nitrous oxide may be synergistic in its suppression of evoked potentials.—**REM**

- Finally, nitrous oxide has the added disadvantage that lung concentrations may be rapidly increased or decreased, which translates to a relatively rapid impact on neuromonitoring signals that more closely mimic changes related to surgical injury.—**REM**

- Given these factors and the typical availability less impactful alternative anesthetic agents, nitrous oxide should be avoided, when possible, all other things being equal and with due respect to the senior anesthesiology authors.—**REM**

- Any anesthesiologist who is interested in doing neurosurgery cases is more than welcome to learn the EP business from the neurology side of the electrode. What the anesthesia probably doesn't know is that neurology residents don't do IONM in a serious way during residency training. Fellows when starting out tend to get one of several introductory texts. One that is pretty good is *A Practical Approach to Neurophysiologic Intraoperative Monitoring* by AM Husain, Demos Medical Publishing, 2014. The neurologists are also happy to do joint conferences and educational exchanges.—**REM**

***Note from the Editors:** Doesn't this bridge look like it could represent a nerve and axon? It looks huge but is actually quite a small bridge across the entrance to a bay in Canada (Fig. 167.4).

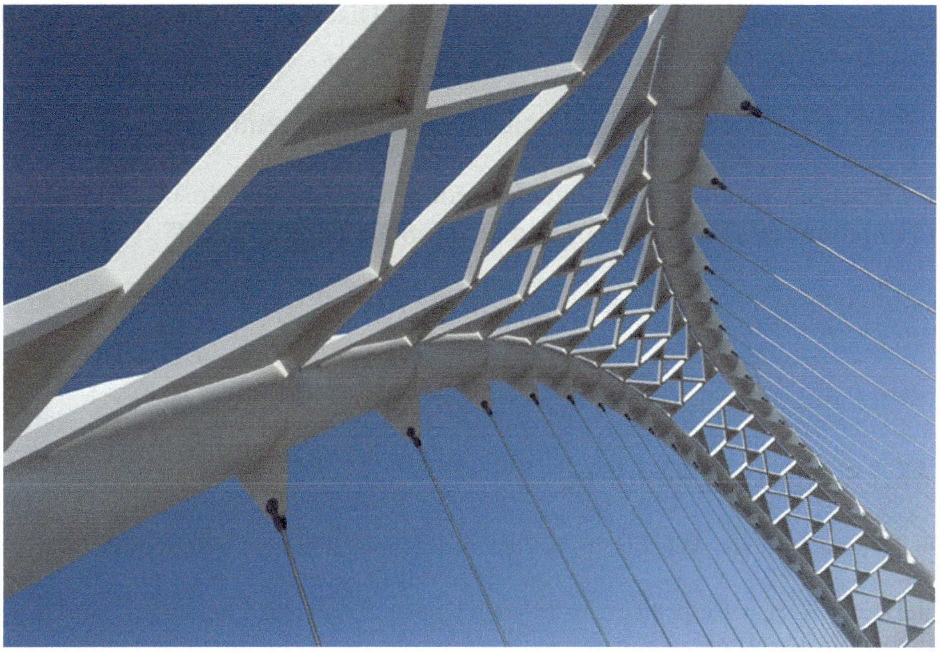

Fig. 167.4 The Humber Bay Arch Bridge near Toronto, CA. Photo: Image used under standard license from stock-adobe.com

More Wisdom from *Avoiding Common Anesthesia Errors, 2nd Edition*

There is a wealth of additional tips, teaching tidbits, and overall wisdom on doctor-patient relations in our previous book, which is nicknamed "Green2." Please check out this information and remember that every single penny of royalties goes to FAER in perpetuity!

Green2 Chapters with More Wisdom on Neuro-Anesthesiology:

- The Neurophysiology You Learned in Medical School Is Always Relevant—Get a Grip on It and Don't Let Go
- Cerebral Aneurysm Versus "Routine" Craniotomy—the Anesthetic Goals Are Not the Same
- Perioperative Visual Loss Is One of the Most Feared and Devastating Complications of Spine Surgery
- Being Maximally Prepared for Minimally Invasive Pituitary Surgery
- Evoked Potentials: Don't Approach the Surgeon for Neurophysiologist Until You Know These Principles
- Awake Craniotomy

- Anesthesia for the Pregnant Patient with Neurosurgical Disorder: These Cases Actually Do Happen in Real Life….and on the Oral Boards
- Don't Forget There's No Such Thing as a Brain Transplant: Preventing Perioperative Stroke
- Anesthesia for Emergent Neurointeventional Procedures: "Neurology Just Called, They Have a Stroke Patient for Thrombectomy Down in Neuroradiology, Start Time Is 2 AM"
- Encephalopathy and Intracranial Hypertension in the Acute Liver Failure Patient Are Not the Same Thing!

References and Suggested Readings

1. Rozet I, Vavilala M. Risks and benefits of patient positioning during neurosurgical care. Anesthesiol Clin. 2007;25(3):631–x.
2. Visentin A, van Dooren K, et al. Respond of the different human cranial bones to pin-type head fixation device. Acta Neurochir (Wien). 2021;163(4):885–93.
3. Holt F, Strantzas S, Zaarour C, Chamlati R, Vreugdenhil I, Luginbuehl I, Karsli C, Faraoni D. The effect of dexmedetomidine on motor-evoked potentials during pediatric posterior spinal fusion surgery: a retrospective case-control study. Can J Anaesth. 2020;67(10):1341–8.
4. Mahmoud M, Sadhasivam S, Salisbury S, Nick TG, Schnell B, Sestokas AK, Wiggins C, Samuels P, Kabalin T, McAuliffe J. Susceptibility of transcranial electric motor-evoked potentials to varying targeted blood levels of dexmedetomidine during spine surgery. Anesthesiology. 2010;112(6):1364–73.
5. Sloan T, Sloan H, Rogers J. Nitrous oxide and isoflurane are synergistic with respect to amplitude and latency effects on sensory evoked potentials. J Clin Monit Comput. 2010;24(2):113–23.

Authors

Mike Altose grew up in the Cleveland, Ohio area. After four years away from home studying chemistry at Brandeis University, he returned to his hometown, where he joined the MD-PhD program at Case Western Reserve University, followed by residency in anesthesiology at University Hospitals of Cleveland, where he is now on faculty and serves as the section head for neurosurgical anesthesia. He is thrilled to be fulfilling his lifelong interest in teaching: he teaches both pharmacology and physiology to the anesthesiology assistant students at CWRU, coordinates the orientation boot camp for anesthesia interns, runs the department simulation center, serves as chair of the Program Evaluation Committee, and teaches residents regularly in the classroom and clinical setting. He especially credits Helmut Cascorbi MD, Howard Nearman MD, and Murray Altose MD for their support and mentorship in guiding him toward a career in education and academic medicine.

Brian Gierl is from the Pittsburgh area originally. He holds a BS in chemical engineering from Cornell University and is now a neuro-anesthesiologist in the UPMC system as well as the director of the neuro-anesthesia fellowship. He has a wide variety of clinical and academic interests and was a lead editor for *Avoiding Common Anesthesia Errors, 2nd Edition*. In his spare time, Brian is an avid cyclist and international traveler.

Rob Minahan grew up as an avid Packer fan in Green Bay, WI. He graduated from Yale University in 1987 with a degree in mathematics and then obtained his MD degree from Duke University. While a resident and fellow at Johns Hopkins University he developed an interest in clinical neurophysiology and has focused his clinical activity on intraoperative neuromonitoring ever since. Rob initially remained at Johns Hopkins as Director of the Intraoperative Neuromonitoring service for 6 years and then moved to Georgetown University as Professor as Neurology and Director of intraoperative neuromonitoring for the next two decades. Rob is also a former President of the American Society of

Neurophysiological Monitoring and currently works for Real Time Neuromonitoring Associates. Together with his wife, Lara Diamond Minahan DDS, he is the proud parent of two young adult daughters.

Ziyad Knio grew up in Baltimore County, Maryland. He received his bachelor's degree in biometry and statistics from Cornell University and his medical degree from Wake Forest School of Medicine. He did his anesthesiology training at the University of Virginia, where he was chief resident. He began a critical care fellowship at Columbia University in 2024. His academic interests include perioperative outcomes research and critical care medicine. He lives with his partner, Margo, and their cat Ewok.

Allan Gottschalk is a second-generation anesthesiologist raised on Long Island who graduated from Boston University in 1978 with a degree in biomedical engineering. He then matriculated at the University of Pennsylvania where he ultimately obtained his MD, PhD, and MS degrees in both systems engineering and biomedical engineering. While a resident and research fellow in the Department of Anesthesiology at the University of Pennsylvania, his interests in sensory biology naturally led to an interest in perioperative pain. After serving on the faculty in the Department of Anesthesiology at Penn, Dr. Gottschalk joined the faculty at Johns Hopkins in 2000, where he is now a professor of anesthesiology and critical care medicine with a joint appointment in the Department of Neurosurgery. Dr. Gottschalk sails a high-performance multihull on the Chesapeake whenever possible and when off the water, he is an avid woodworker. His wife Barbara and their three adult daughters are all in healthcare.

Cathy Marcucci is a senior academic anesthesiologist and inveterate anesthesiology educator. She is also fellowship-trained in transfusion medicine. She survived that early rotation in the neuro rooms, as did her patients, and has always been grateful for the superb training she received there from outstanding anesthesiologist including Jeff Kirsch, Laurel Moore, and Mark Mirski.

Wisdom on Cardiac Anesthesia

168

Raymond G. Graber, Christopher A. Troianos, Mark Nelson, Edwin G. Avery IV, Louise Y. Sun, and Ronald S. Bank

Contributors:

Edwin G. Avery IV, MD (EGA)

Brian P. Barrick, MD (BPB)

Catherine Marcucci, MD (CM)

Ziyan Song, MD (ZS)

Introduction

Taking care of patients undergoing cardiac surgery is a rewarding experience, but it can be challenging. There is a lot of cardiac and coagulation pathophysiology and pharmacology you need to learn. There are a lot of line placements and other technical skills you will have to master. You have to invest time in learning how to perform and interpret transesophageal echocardiography. However, this foundation will make you a more skilled anesthesiologist and prepare you to tackle the daily challenges in your noncardiac rooms, too. In this chapter, we present some tips and aphorisms that hopefully will help the reader in their practice of cardiac anesthesia.

R. G. Graber · E. G. Avery IV
Department of Anesthesiology and Perioperative Medicine, University Hospitals Cleveland Medical Center, Cleveland, OH, USA
e-mail: Raymond.graber@uhhospitals.org

C. A. Troianos (✉)
Anesthesiology Institute, Cleveland Clinic, Cleveland, OH, USA
e-mail: TROIANC@ccf.org

M. Nelson
Department of Anesthesiology, Virginia Commonwealth University, Richmond, VA, USA

L. Y. Sun
Department of Anesthesiology, Perioperative, and Pain Medicine, Stanford University, Palo Alto, CA, USA

R. S. Bank
Department of Anesthesiology, INOVA Fairfax Hospital, UVA School of Medicine, INOVA Campus, Falls Church, VA, USA

S. Mohamed et al. (eds.), *Anesthesia Bridges*, https://doi.org/10.1007/978-3-032-08294-7_168

Basics

- For those who are starting their independent practice in cardiac anesthesia, be confident in your skills, but never shy away from asking for a second opinion when you are not 100% sure. In my early days, I quickly realized that figuring out what I didn't know was just as important as demonstrating what I knew well.—**LYS**

- Cardiovascular physiology is analogous to pipes and circuits: capacitance, resistance, conduction, flow, and effective circulating volume. Solid understanding of physics and engineering concepts is an asset to a cardiac anesthesiologist.—**LYS**

- Or put more simply, cardiac anesthesia is simply making blood go round and round by manipulating preload, contractility, and afterload.—**ZS**

- Study and understand the physiology and management of patients with right heart failure and pulmonary hypertension. You will avoid a great deal of morbidity and mortality over the course of your career by doing so.—**RSB**

- I love the right ventricle (RV). RV function is key to the success of a heart and/or lung transplant, and any complex cardiac case.—**LYS**

- Don't let the pulmonary artery (PA) pressures get higher than the arterial pressure. If it does, *fix it.*—**CAT**

- Don't let the potassium get higher than the hemoglobin. *Fix that, too.*—**CAT**

- One of the fastest and most easily titratable ways to control blood pressure is via bed position—Trendelenburg and reverse Trendelenburg. This is especially useful in cardiac cases when blood pressure management is critical. This helps to precisely titrate blood pressure at critical times without overshooting in either direction.—**RSB**

- Don't assume the cardiac rooms are done until the cardiac catheterization lab is closed for the day! You need to stay ready—personnel and room—for an emergency case.—**Editors**

- The practice of cardiac anesthesiology is filled with acronyms and abbreviations, which are second nature to veteran cardiac anesthesiologists. Make sure the beginners and students, and everybody else, are clear about what means what. I once sat in on a QA review where the term "Echo" was repeatedly used instead of "ECMO." Not joking.—**CM**

Communication

- I think there is more intraoperative communication and teamwork with surgeons during cardiac surgical cases than in any other surgical specialty. It starts with a discussion prior to the case about things like radial artery harvesting and cannulation strategy—this will affect where you put your lines. Communicate your transesophageal echocardiogram (TEE) findings to the surgeon pre- and post-cardiopulmonary bypass (CPB). They frequently ask for TEE confirmation of wires when doing a femoral cannulation. Let them know what your plans are for inotropic strategy prior to separation from bypass. Is ongoing bleeding surgical or coagulopathy? The more complicated the case, the more issues there will be to discuss! So put your courtesy hat on and be ready to collaborate.—**RGG**

- Get to know your perfusionists and what they are doing. During the pump run, there's a lot going on. At the time of the huddle, there should be group discussion about temperature and blood pressure goals, acceptable hemoglobin levels, cardioplegia delivery, and so forth. During the pump run, check in regularly with them to see what kind of issues they are dealing with.—**RGG**

- It is also important to have good communication with your ICU team post-op. If you don't have it, get together with the cardiac anesthesiologists and the intensivists, and develop a report sheet that details all the important aspects of care—lines, airway, fluids, drips, TEE findings, and intraoperative problems.—**RGG**

- Work to develop protocols in your cardiac anesthesia group. This helps ensure consistency and quality of care and makes it easier for the residents you are training. This is especially important for cases like heart and lung transplantation, which are both complicated and lower in volume. When you are doing a case only several times a year, it is helpful to have protocols and guidelines to review ahead of time. Make sure the surgeons are generally onboard with your group's practice paradigms and guidelines.—**RGG**

Cardiac Bridges

- Speaking of communication, bridges are about connecting one point in time and space to what's on the other side. Understanding the cardiac bridges in this anesthesiology subspecialty is critical to practicing in the cardiac surgery rooms. Ray Graber put together a great summary for us.—**Editors**

  - *Myocardial bridge*: This is a condition in which there is a band ("bridge") of myocardium overlying a segment of coronary artery. When the muscle contracts, blood flow through that artery can be impaired, leading to angina symptoms. This is usually treated medically, but in some situations, surgery is necessary.— **RGG**

  - *Bridge to transplant*: A therapy used to support a patient's physiology until they can make it to organ transplant. For example, a left ventricular assist device (LVAD) may be implanted to serve as a bridge to heart transplantation.— **RGG**

  - *Bridge to recovery*: A therapy used to support a patient's physiology until they can recover from a reversible event. Examples include extracorporeal membrane oxygenation (ECMO), Impella catheter insertion, and LVAD placement.— **RGG**

  - *Bridge to nowhere*: The unfortunate situation where a patient is placed on support such as ECMO, but the underlying disease proves not to be reversible, or the patient becomes not eligible for transplant. *Editor's Note*: We found a number of "bridge to nowhere" photos on the internet. The one below is the most striking (Fig. 168.1).—**RGG**

  - *Anticoagulation bridge*: Temporary anticoagulation, typically with heparin, used during the preoperative period when a patient's regular long-term anticoagulant therapy, for example, warfarin, is suspended. The goal is to still provide anticoagulation, but in a manner that can be rapidly terminated, or reversed if needed, when the patient is ready to undergo surgery.—**RGG**

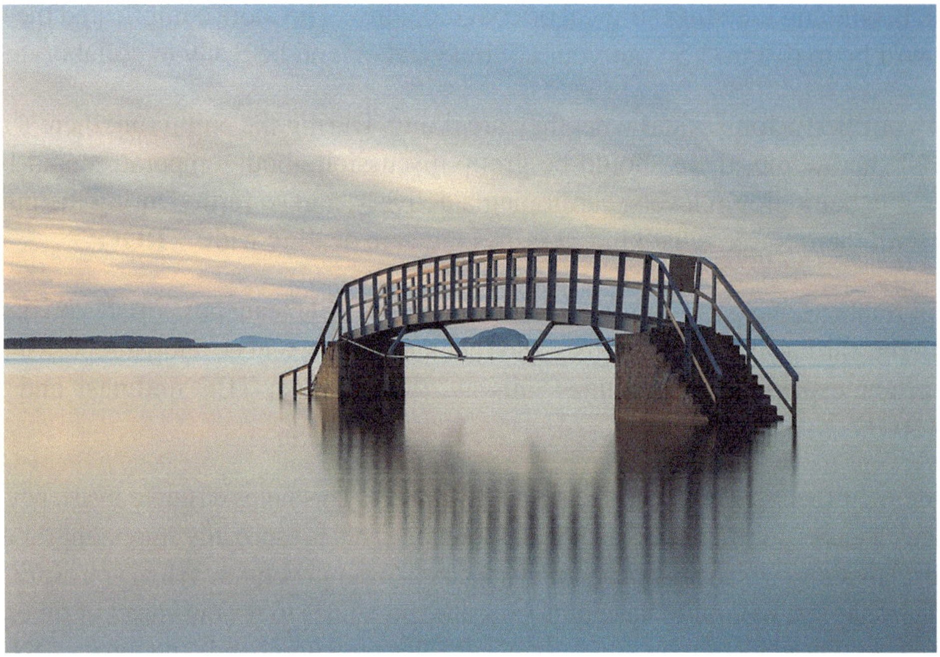

Fig. 168.1 The Belhaven Bridge crosses the Biel Water near the coast of Scotland. When the North Sea high tide comes in, it becomes a "bridge to nowhere." Photo: Simon Wootton used with permission

Line Placement

- Beards are a hindrance to sterile technique during central line insertion. Before surgery, I will discuss this with patients, and most are then willing to let their beards get trimmed back. I have been known to get an electric shaver, throw a sheet around the patient's neck, and shave the patient's beard in pre-op hold, much to the delight of their friends and family. My goal is to shave hair up to the jaw line, and I usually do both sides so that it looks good. If you have a patient who has a religious reason for not wanting their beard trimmed (for example, we have a large Amish community near us), I will try to do a minimal shave near the insertion site, and then use wide tape or strategically placed surgical mask to keep hair out of the way.—**RGG**

- Before prepping the neck for a central line insertion, I always take a quick look with the ultrasound to check out the anatomy. I like to see that the vessel is reasonably-sized, and also get an idea of the carotid location. This is especially important in patients who have had previous central lines. I have seen many patients with completely thrombosed right internal jugular veins (IJs). I have had at least one patient who had both IJs completely thrombosed. By taking a quick scan, you choose an appropriate site before you prep and drape.—**RGG**

- Always, always, always use ultrasound for central venous cannulation. There is nothing to prove and nothing to be gained by "trying first" to see what happens! Yes, the success rate with a landmark guided technique is over 90%, but you don't want to be that one anesthesiologist who places an introducer in the carotid, a pulmonary catheter in the spinal canal, or causes a life-threatening hemothorax. These complications have all occurred and are reported in the literature.—**CAT**

- Ultrasound is readily available these days, and so easy to use, but must be used in real-time to observe the needle tip inside the vessel. There should be no excuse for not using it. Some have stated that we need to know the anatomy in case we don't have it available, but I would argue that I have learned more about anatomy using ultrasound routinely than I would have going in "blind." There is no compromise of sterility when standard techniques are employed.—**CAT**

- Here is something I learned from Chris Troianos. When positioning for IJ placement, try to limit the head rotation of the patient. The more you rotate the head, the more you rotate the carotid under the IJ. Similarly, when you are scanning with ultrasound, try to position your probe more perpendicular to the floor rather than perpendicular to the neck. This will help give you a view with the carotid less likely to be posterior to the IJ [1].—**RGG**

- For an excellent summary of the evidence supporting ultrasound-guided cannulation of both venous and arterial sites, and also technique recommendations, read the 2012 paper by Chris Troianos and colleagues titled "Guidelines for performing ultrasound guided vascular cannulation: Recommendations of the American Society of Echocardiography and the Society of Cardiovascular Anesthesiologists." [2] It's a worthwhile read.—**RGG**

- A "fool-proof" confirmation of venous (versus arterial) placement of a central venous catheter is imaging the guide wire in the superior vena cava (SVC) with TEE. This should be done before inserting a large-bore catheter over the wire. People have been fooled by using dark color of blood and even by pressure measurement of the cannulating needle to confirm venous placement, but there is no way that imaging a wire in the SVC with TEE can be anything other than a venous cannulation. Therefore, my typical practice is to induce general anesthesia and place the TEE probe before central venous cannulation in the absence of any contraindications.—**CAT**

- When you place female patients in Trendelenburg position for line placement, sometimes breast tissue can be pulled by gravity towards your insertion point and be a hindrance to line placement. I frequently will get some wide tape and tape the breast towards the foot of the bed to help open up that space. I'll do this on guys, too!—**RGG**

- Don't use the entire length of a #11 scalpel for a skin nick when you are placing a 7 or 8 Fr central line, as it will ooze the entire case and ultimately require a stitch or two at the end of the case to stop the bleeding. The skin nick should match the diameter of the catheter you are placing.—**EGA** and **RGG**

- Always check the ECG to make sure that your patient does not have a left bundle branch block before placing a PA catheter. A right bundle may be induced during or after PA catheter placement, which would leave the patient with complete heart block, which is not how you want to start your case. It is best to either not use a PA catheter, or to pass it once the epicardium is exposed during a cardiac surgical case. This allows placement of epicardial pacing leads with the occurrence of complete heart block.—**CAT**

- When I float a PA catheter in a ventilated patient, I typically try to time my advancement to the ventilatory cycle. At end expiration, venous return should be improved, so I try to take advantage of this and advance the catheter a few centimeters with each expiratory phase.—**RGG**

- In some patients, getting the PA catheter past the tricuspid valve can be difficult. Patients with severe tricuspid regurgitation or large right atriums can be a challenge. In the cardiac rooms, if after several attempts I am not able to float past the tricuspid valve, I will place my TEE probe and obtain a modified bicaval view—which shows me both the superior vena cava and the tricuspid valve. Using this view for guidance, with the balloon up, I will pull back the PA catheter to remove any loops in the catheter, then try to advance the catheter to an appropriate depth so that the balloon is above the valve. You can also rotate the catheter within its sheath to better position the balloon above the valve. Once you are positioned above the valve, you can attempt to advance through it.—**RGG**

- When floating a PA catheter, if you're having trouble getting from the RV to the pulmonary artery, remember the Valsalva technique. Once in the RV, hold a breath at an inspiratory pressure of around 30, and as soon as you let the bag go, advance the catheter. This technique works surprisingly well.—**RSB**

- Always watch the EKG when advancing a central line guidewire, central line catheter, and floating a PA catheter. Some patients won't tolerate well the dysrhythmias, which can result. If you're not watching the EKG and don't pull that guidewire/line back quickly, the situation can deteriorate very rapidly, leading to otherwise easily preventable morbidity or even mortality.—**RSB**

- If your patient is not tolerating the advancement of a PA catheter, stop trying. Pull it back to the CVP position and leave it there. This way, you still have at least a CVP, and you don't have patient who arrested from repeated attempts at floating the Swan-Ganz (S-G) catheter. When you do so remember to change the PA tracing to CVP, if it's a S-G with an infusion port remember that this port is no longer in the patient and connect the infusions elsewhere and be sure to turn the CVP transducer stopcock off towards the transducer so that the saline from the pressure bag does not fill the cover of the S-G catheter with saline.—**RSB**

  When attempting to float a PA catheter through a left IJ, sometimes you will meet some resistance at the end of the introducer. Anatomically, the left IJ meets the left subclavian vein to form the left brachiocephalic vein. The PA catheter has to make a right turn at the end of the IJ to enter the brachiocephalic. If the introducer tip is too close to the wall of the brachiocephalic, it will have trouble making the turn and advancing. The solution is to pull the introducer back a few centimeters, then try advancing the PA catheter again.—**RGG**

  Once the PA catheter has been advanced into the heart, you can advance the introducer back over the PA and stitch it in place. Some clinicians choose not to sew the left IJ introducer into place on a routine basis until after they have successfully placed the PA catheter. On another note, be very careful how far you advance a dilator in the left IJ since it is possible to perforate the brachiocephalic at the IJ junction.—**RGG**

- Everybody seems to agree about the brachial artery line in the cardiac rooms:

  - Consider going straight for a brachial arterial line for complex cases. These will give you less dampening and more reliable MAP measurements after prolonged bypass runs, enabling precise titration of vasoactive meds and minimizing vasoconstrictor doses.—**LYS**

- We commonly place brachial arterial lines for many of our hearts, since the waveform tends to be more reliable throughout the duration of the case, especially when separating from cardiopulmonary bypass. We always place these with ultrasound. This minimizes the number of attempts at placement, but also helps protect the median nerve, which typically lies just medial to the artery.—**RGG**

- Don't be afraid of brachial arterial lines for cardiac surgery! We published our study of over 21,000 patients at the Cleveland Clinic in 2017, showing that brachial artery cannulation for hemodynamic monitoring during cardiac surgery rarely causes complications (0.19% incidence) [3].—**CAT**

Monitors

- I have delved deeply into the matter and advise not to sell short the use of intraoperative cerebral oximetry monitoring for any cardiac case, as this underused technology has the ability to provide a first alert indication of many common and one-off negative physiologic changes and is also ultimately highly useful to assess if there is adequate oxygenation to the brain.—**EGA**

- **Editor's Note:** Ed Avery is an educational consultant to Medtronic on the subject of cerebral oximetry and has received research funding from Medtronic support for *investigator-initiated* protocols evaluating the use of cerebral oximetry in thoracic surgery. This doesn't mean his advice above is not worthwhile—we totally agree with him that the principles of cerebral oximetry monitoring are something you should be learning about.

- The use of goal-directed fluid therapy devices—for example, arterial pulse contour analysis, echocardiography, thermodilution cardiac index, bioimpedance of chest and lower torso, pulse pressure variation—to optimize intravascular volume status in surgical procedures with large fluid shifts is supported by hundreds of studies worldwide-so use these adjuncts religiously.—**EGA**

- If possible, employ the use of thromboelastography (TEG) routinely in cardiac cases. This is especially important if the patient is bleeding, and you are trying to decipher what products may help reverse a coagulopathy. Unnecessary administration of intravenous factor concentrates, for example, prothrombin complex concentrates or fibrinogen concentrate, has both a significant pharmacy cost and may also increase the risk of thromboembolic events.—**EGA** and **RGG**

- When using pressure transducers, always be sure that the trace is indeed the one that you and the rest of the room think that it is. When flushing or zeroing, be sure that the color matches what it's supposed to be. Otherwise, incorrect decisions can be made.—**RSB**

- For example, if the surgeon thinks that the retrograde cardioplegia pressure is being read off of the central venous pressure (CVP) transducer stopcock and it's instead connected to the PA stopcock, they can think that the coronary sinus (CS) cannula is not correctly in place when in fact it is. This can lead to the CS while continuing to try to place the CS cannula. This is just one of many bad things that can happen with such a mix-up.—**RSB**

Induction of Anesthesia

- Induce patients with just the right amount of anesthetics and wait just long enough to achieve anesthetic goals without causing hypotension.—**LYS**

- How you induce anesthesia in the cardiac rooms is more important than what you induce with. Over the years, many induction paradigms have been used. Induction isn't usually what makes or breaks the success of a case, except in the situations of stenotic valves and delayed awakenings.—**Editors**

- When inducing a patient for coronary artery bypass grafting (CABG), don't be fooled by how good a patient with a high-grade proximal left main lesion and a normal EF can look. While these patients can look robust, it's critical to induce very carefully! Avoid hypotension on induction, as they can crash fast and hard and be very difficult to get back. Do a very careful induction with small, incremental doses of your induction agent. Often, it works well to give a small dose of phenylephrine up front. Have esmolol immediately available to treat tachycardia.—**RSB**

- Respect critical aortic stenosis, critical mitral stenosis, severe pulmonary hypertension, and right heart failure patients! These patients can crash fast and hard on induction. These conditions are very unforgiving, so show them some love and the anesthesiologists who take care of them (Fig. 168.2). Consider starting an inotrope up front prior to induction, do a very careful, measured induction, stay ahead of, and aggressively treat hypotension and don't let the latter patients get hypercarbic.—**RSB**

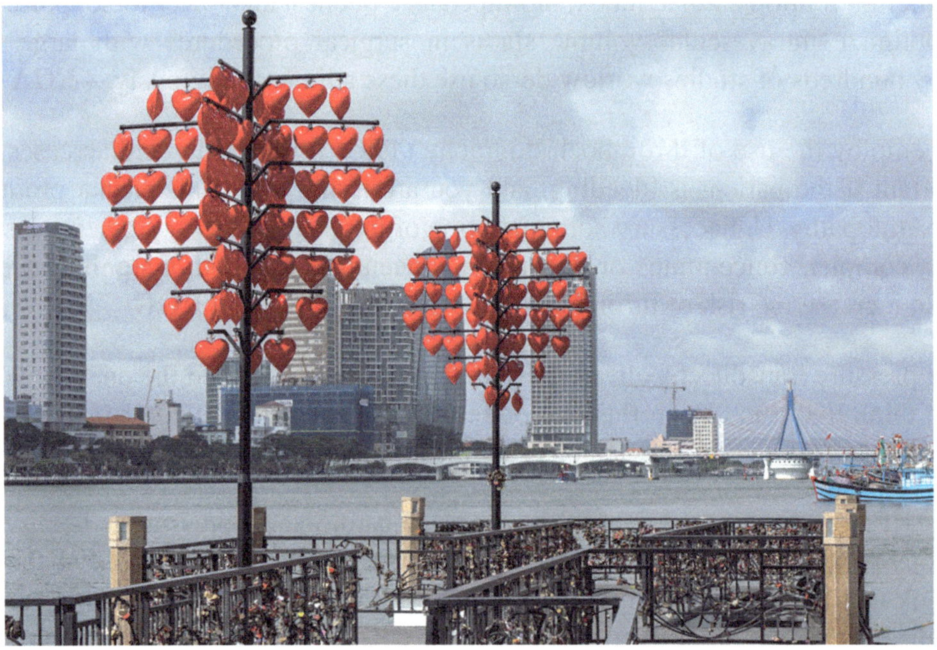

Fig. 168.2 Always make sure there is plenty of love to around! We love this "heartful" pier with a cable-stayed bridge way in the background. Photo: Image used under standard license from stock.adobe.com

Case Management

- Here are some generic goals that I teach my residents: Maintain glucose <180 mg/dL, keep potassium between 4 and 6 meq/L, avoid respiratory acidosis—and frequently mild hyperventilation is better when you have pulmonary hypertension or right heart issues—keep MAPS 70–90 mmHg, keep HR <90 bpm, and keep Hb >8.0 g/dL.—**RGG**

- The way to make off-pump CABGs smooth is to move with the surgical team. Anticipate and get ahead of their every move. Know the grafting sequence ahead of time. Recognize the signs of acute myocardial ischemia and communicate promptly. And keep the patient warm!—**LYS**

- Epinephrine is not the solution to everything. Lay eyes on the patient, evaluate their acid-base status, and assess their disease on echo. These will reveal whether inotropy is necessary.—**LYS**

- Be in tune with the surgeon: know when vasoactive boluses are necessary and when they'll make us end up chasing our tails with numerous boluses of uppers and downers. Every drug comes with side effects, as does hemodynamic lability. You want a smooth ride, not on the rollercoaster!—**LYS**

- Always check the field before treating the pressure!—**RSB**

- Have someone double-check any vasoactive drips that you hang. Do the same for your colleagues.—**RSB**

- Go light on fixed and long-acting hemodynamic depressive agents in the cardiac rooms. They are not easily reversible, and you may end up chasing your tail, round and around.—**RSB**

- One of my mentors (John Ammon) told me: "A good cardiac anesthesiologist, under-reacts, aggressively!" implying to not "overtreat" to produce large swings in blood pressure with pressors, and vasodilating drugs.—**CAT**

- When I was starting out, I did not have an appreciation for the metabolic side effects of beta agonists. Specifically, that serum glucose will rise, and serum potassium will fall. This is frequently seen in the extreme in cardiac transplantation because the high dose steroids in combination with beta agonists administered to these patients will cause an "upregulation" of these side effects. High glucose levels will require treatment with increasing doses of insulin, which will further drive the potassium down. It is not uncommon for a patient to require 80 meq or more of potassium supplementation during a cardiac transplant, especially if they are a diabetic.—**RGG**

- Lactic acidosis (LA) is very common post cardiac transplantation—is seen in greater than 90% of patients. It starts near the time of initiation of inotropes, peaks at 4–8 hours later, and lasts 12–24 hours. It has been hypothesized that the LA commonly seen is due to a Type B mechanism (aerobic)—specifically as a result of beta-2 stimulation of glycolysis in skeletal muscles by the commonly used inotropes such as epinephrine.—**RGG**

- Lactic acidosis after heart transplant seems to occur despite good cardiac index and oxygen delivery and is correlated with onset and dose of inotropes. An additional factor may be the use of high dose steroids. Steroids are known to increase beta-2 receptor numbers and function—so thus may exacerbate the effect of the administered beta-2 agonists. Decreases in hepatic or renal function will also slow clearance of lactate. Bottom line—don't panic when you see increasing LA post cardiac transplant, it is a normal phenomenon. Treat by hyperventilation, weaning beta-2 agonists as appropriate, and deploying judicious sodium bicarbonate treatment as needed.—**RGG**

- Leave the use of activated factor VII as a last resort if the use of allogeneic blood components, prothrombin complex concentrates, and fibrinogen concentrates have not resulted in correction of severe coagulopathy.—**EGA**

Favorite and Not-So-Favorite Cases

We asked our authors to tell us a bit about their favorite and not-so-favorite cases, and they didn't have any trouble knowing what they think.

From Chris Troianos:

- My favorite cardiac case without question is a mitral valve repair because of the comprehensive discussion and interaction required between the cardiac anesthesiologist and the cardiac surgeon. The cardiac anesthesiologist performs and interprets the intraoperative TEE, gains an appreciation of the effects of changing hemodynamics on the degree of regurgitation, relates the anatomical issues causing the mitral regurgitation to the surgeon, and often suggests a potential surgical correction, such as resecting flail, redundant mitral leaflet tissue, or adding artificial chordae tendineae.

- The cardiac anesthesiologist also manages the separation from CPB and evaluates the success of the surgical repair and potential complications that might be associated with the repair. This might include systolic anterior motion of the mitral valve, causing outflow tract obstruction. Less than perfect repairs prompt further discussion between the surgeon and anesthesiologist as to the risk of another bypass run versus the consequences of the existing repair. The condition of the patient and the capabilities of the surgeon must always be factored into the discussion. This requires considerable experience, emotional intelligence, and great communication skills.

- A close second favorite case is septal myectomy for hypertrophic obstructive cardiomyopathy, particularly those cases that require careful differentiation between mitral valve pathology causing mitral regurgitation, and mitral regurgitation from left ventricular outflow tract obstruction. Again, a thorough and comprehensive review and understanding of the pathophysiology, and discussion between the anesthesiologist and the surgeon are paramount.

- My least favorite case is one in which, thankfully, we are not doing as much anymore. Automatic internal cardiac defibrillator (AICD) implantation in the past involved a thoracotomy with placement of epicardial patches, in patients with recurrent arrhythmias or dilated cardiomyopathy. It was a big operation (thoracotomy incision) without immediate patient benefit, for prophylactic prevention of a sustained malignant arrhythmia. I am thankful that these are now done with sedation for intravascular lead placement, similar to placement of a transvenous pacemaker.

From Louise Sun:

- My favorite type of case is LVAD implantation, and a close second favorite is heart transplant. I find these cases satisfying because they encompass the fundamentals of managing patients with severe LV or biventricular failure at induction, and team-based approach to RV failure management after bypass and in the CVICU.

- Amongst my least favorites are the robotic cases, mainly because of their duration and monotonic nature.

From Ron Bank:

- I have a lot of cases that I like for different reasons. One of my favorites is repair of an ascending dissection. I like that they are interesting, challenging cases in which you're outright saving someone's life. I don't like their emergent and unscheduled nature—frequently in off hours, but I like the case itself.

- My least favorite was lung transplants when we used to do them with double lumen tubes (DLETTs); we now do them with single lumen endotracheal tubes. DLETTs, especially in cases with a lot of blood in the lungs and the ETT, are very hard to manage and to troubleshoot due to difficult visualization from the blood and secretions. This, combined with how sick these patients are and how difficult it sometimes is to manage them on one lung (the ones that we didn't do on bypass), made these among my least favorite.

From Ray Graber:

- It is hard to pick a favorite case. Different cases have appeal to the various parts of my personality.

- The adrenaline junkie side of my persona really likes doing ascending aortic dissections *and heart* and lung transplants. There is much at stake with these patients, a lot of things that can go wrong, a lot of potential problems I have to work my way through. These cases are a ton of work and frequently in the middle of the night—and are the medical equivalent of going into battle. These are the cases that are bonding experiences for me and my residents. These are the cases that, afterwards as I start my drive home, I feel like I have really accomplished something, but then as the adrenaline comes down, I just hope to get home and not fall asleep and crash my car.

- The calmer side of my persona enjoys doing aortic valve replacement surgery for aortic stenosis. Yes, you have to maintain perfusion pressure and avoid crashing on induction, but most of these patients who are presenting electively seem to have good LV function, and these hearts really like coming off pump with their new valve and lower afterload.

- My intellectual side enjoys doing mitral valve repairs for regurgitation. It is fun to perform the echo, interpret the results, and help guide the surgeons as they do their valve repairs. These cases are like puzzles we are trying to solve.

- As for least favorite cases, I would probably vote for descending thoracic aneurysms. These are also very detailed cases with a lot of tasks, a lot of risk, and can be long and bloody. If you have ever spent all day working on such a case, feel like you have done good work, and then wind up with a paraplegic patient, you know how I feel.

From Ed Avery:

- In the favorite case scenario, we are probably working with a very skilled and friendly cardiac surgeon who supports our opinion on a particular patient being an ideal early extubation candidate in a cardiac surgery case involving CPB. I experience a great feeling of accomplishment when I plan an "ERAS HEAVY" approach for a CPB case that allows for an expeditious extubation at the end of the case. This always entails more work for the anesthesia team, but it is worth it.

- "ERAS HEAVY" entails setting up extra IV drips in addition to the standard fare. Depending on one's approach, this may mean a small bolus of ketamine with a low-dose drip along with a magnesium drip and a lidocaine bolus and drip. It is also important to pretreat these patients with at least two antiemetics and run them on a propofol drip after separating from bypass, so the wakeup is quicker.

- Finally, I find the bilateral serratus anterior plane chest wall nerve blocks with catheters/pump or pain ball are a great adjunct, which allows for up to 3 days of pain relief, and don't forget the IV acetaminophen, if you can get your hands on some, along with a dose of ketorolac. It is shocking how awake and comfortable these patients are compared to a more standard cardiac anesthetic.

- As far a least favorite case, I think most will agree it is really a huge bummer when one is just going on or coming off CPB and you pick up an iatrogenic or spontaneous aortic dissection. It means more pump time, almost certainly more bleeding to deal with, and probably a somewhat crippled heart. Not to mention that you for sure will be getting out much later than one may have planned.

***Note from the Editors:** We think that this is the perfect bridge for this chapter (Fig. 168.3).

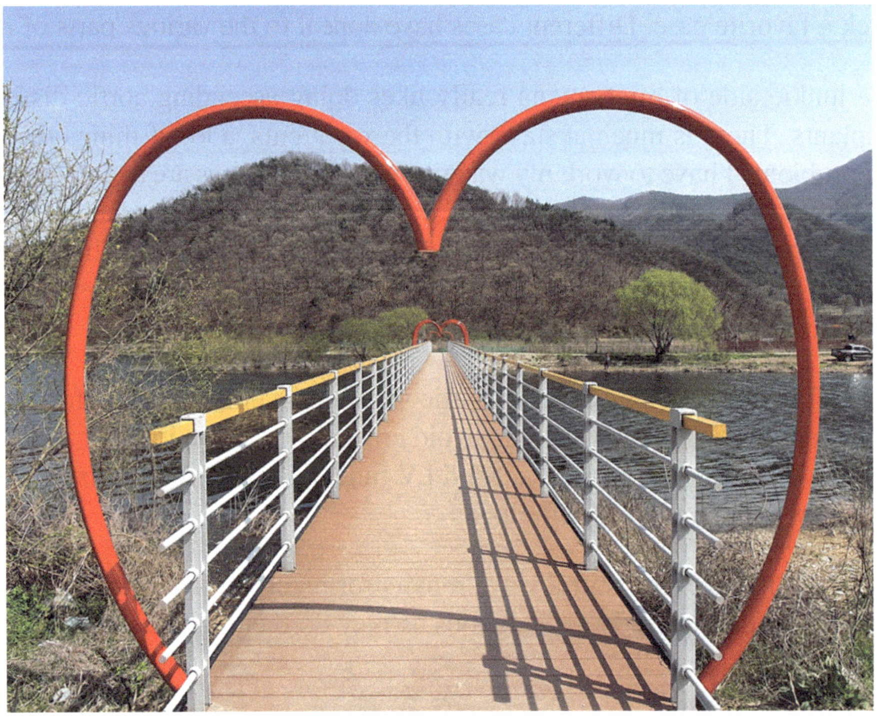

Fig. 168.3 Heart-shaped bridge portal in Gui Reservoir in Wanju-gun, South Korea. Photo: Image used under standard license from iStock.com, credit to Yeongsik Im

Transesophageal Echocardiography

- When placing a TEE probe, make sure you have adequate lubrication in the mouth and on the probe. *Never force the probe*—it is possible to cause a pharyngeal or soft palate injury. If you are having trouble placing a TEE probe, try using laryngoscope to lift the larynx out of the way. If at the end of the case, there appears to be ongoing bleeding coming from the oropharynx, suspect an injury, and have an ENT surgeon come and evaluate the patient before you leave the room. I have seen several cases where ENT either cauterized bleeding or had to put a few stitches in. Better to deal with this problem early.—**RGG**

- In patients in whom TEE probe placement is difficult—especially small, elderly patients—consider using a pediatric TEE probe to minimize the chance of morbidity from the probe.—**RSB**

- If you're going to use a TEE in a case, be sure to put the TEE in prior to placing the line. Despite using ultrasound to place a central line, the guidewire can perforate distal to where you are imaging. Seeing the guidewire in the RA provides a great measure of safety as it confirms that the guidewire has made it to the heart. Having the TEE in prior to line placement can also assist with floating the PA catheter.—**RSB**

- TEE probes are expensive. It's good practice to always use a TEE bite block—to protect both the probe and the patient. The exceptions are if the patient has limited mouth opening, or do not have teeth to keep the bite block in place. In these situations, use cotton gauze between the probe and teeth and wrap around over the lip surface, and tape in place. I have seen a patient with an injury similar to a rope burn from the probe being maneuvered in and out against an unprotected lip. Nobody was very happy about this.—**RGG**

- The machine doesn't make the sonographer. Become expert so that you can answer clinical questions with varying machine quality.—**MTN**

- What is the most common missed finding on TEE? The second finding. Do not focus solely on the first or major finding. Always finish the complete exam and have a systematic way of doing it so nothing is missed.—**MTN**

- When in doubt, assume the patient has the disease and get on with the case! In other words, sometimes we are verifying disease seen in pre-op echos, but don't get good imaging. In that case, move on. You can't spend countless time doing follow-up echos when you have other tasks to do.—**LYS and RGG**

- TEE is just transthoracic echocardiograph upside down. We know this, of course, but remember to make this point when you are teaching echo skills to students, who are used to looking at and thinking about the heart in an anterior view. It takes a bit of thought and concentration to reorient the heart in your mental and visual perception.—**ZS and Editors**

- Utilize sector width and depth whenever possible. It will only sharpen the image and make you look like an expert. It can't hurt.—**MTN**

- Always check color gain and scale when using color Doppler. It is easy to assume they are appropriately set and give faulty information to the surgeon.—**MTN**

- Use TEE to personalize hemodynamic goals. In the setting of multiple cardiac lesions that carry conflicting hemodynamic requirements, determine the chronicity of each lesion, and identify the primary lesion. Treatment is most effective when tailored to the primary lesion.—**LYS**

- Try to avoid quantifying regurgitant lesions while under general anesthesia. Regurgitant lesions are almost always affected by the hemodynamic changes associated with GA. When asked "how much mitral regurgitation is there?" while under GA, simply open the awake study and evaluate the images.—**MTN**

- Don't just evaluate RV function on TEE; also look over the drape. RV is the most anterior chamber and can be clearly visualized in the surgical field.—**ZS**

- Organized pericardial effusions can be difficult to see. Be suspicious and search diligently for pericardial boundaries.—**MTN**

- Dilated atria are always bad. Atrial dilatation is always the result of elevated LA pressures. Be suspicious to call a heart normal with atrial dilatation regardless of whether there are no other findings.—**MTN**

- Aortitis can be mistaken for intramural hematoma. If the IM is too symmetrical without significant atheromatous disease, consider the diagnosis of aortitis.—**MTN**

- Acute pulmonary embolism with hypotension will always have a leftward septal shift and right ventricular dilatation. Search for another cause of hypotension in the absence of these findings.—**MTN**

- Laminated thrombus in the LV apex is difficult to rule out on TEE. Echo contrast agents can be helpful if apical thrombus is suspected.—**MTN**

- The TEE has been termed to be "The Great Distractor"—don't let it be that in your OR! Always pay attention to the patient.—**RSB**

  The TEE can be helpful, neutral, or an enemy of the patient. Be certain of the findings you report. Always consider pretest probability. TEE findings are like a lab test, the likelihood of their validity is directly proportional to the pretest probability.—**MTN**

  TEE is not just about patient anatomy, pathology, and physiology. It is also a helpful procedural guide. It is used to help float PA catheters, to check that surgeon placed arterial and venous wires are where they are supposed to be, to check that femoral venous cannulas are in the correct position in the heart, to see that coronary sinus catheters are placed to an adequate depth, to check position of intra-aortic balloon pumps, to check position of Impella catheters and LVAD apical cannulas, to check that the left heart is adequately de-aired before coming off pump—and I am sure this list will continue to grow.—**RGG**

  I use a worksheet to write a draft of my TEE report after I record my images. The American Society of Echocardiography has established normal values and grading systems for valve lesions and chamber sizes. I built a worksheet that includes all these values. This serves as a guideline that I can use as I interpret my images and record the results (Fig. 168.4).—**RGG**

Lt. Ventricle: Diameter (cm): Men ☐ Normal (4.2-5.8) Dilation: ☐ Mild (5.9-6.3) ☐ Mod (6.4-6.8) ☐ Sev (>6.8)
Women ☐ Normal (3.8-5.2) Dilation: ☐ Mild (5.3-5.6) ☐ Mod (5.7-6.1) ☐ Sev (>6.1)

Wall Thickness (mm): Men ☐ Normal (6-10) Hypertrophy: ☐ Mild (11-13) ☐ Mod (14-16) ☐ Sev (>16) WMAs:
Women ☐ Normal (6-9) Hypertrophy: ☐ Mild (10-12) ☐ Mod (13-15) ☐ Sev (>15)

Function: EF%: ______ Men ☐ Normal (52-72) Dysfcn: ☐ Mild (41-51) ☐ Mod (30-40) ☐ Sev (<30) Diastology:
Women ☐ Normal (54-74) Dysfcn: ☐ Mild (41-53) ☐ Mod (30-40) ☐ Sev (<30)

Lt. Atrium: Diameter (cm): Men ☐ Normal (3.0-4.0) Dilation: ☐ Mild (4.1-4.6) ☐ Mod (4.7-5.2) ☐ Sev (>5.2)
LA Appendage clot: Y N Women ☐ Normal (2.7-3.8) Dilation: ☐ Mild (3.9-4.2) ☐ Mod (4.3-4.6) ☐ Sev (>4.6)
LA Appendage velocity (cm/sec): ☐ Normal (>40) ☐ Mildly reduced (20-40) ☐ Reduced (<20)

Right Ventricle: Enlargement: ☐ None (≈ 2/3 LV size) ☐ Trivial/mild (2/3-LVsize) ☐ Mod/Sev (≥ LV size)
Basal Diameter (cm): ☐ Normal (2.5-4.1) Dilation: ☐ (>4.1) TAPSE (cm): ☐ Normal > 1.7
Mid-RV diameter (cm): ☐ Normal (1.9-3.5) Dilation: ☐ (>3.5)
Wall Thickness (mm): ☐ Normal (1-5) ☐ Hypertrophy (>5)
Function: ☐ Normal Dysfcn: ☐ Mild ☐ Moderate ☐ Severe Comments:

Rt.Atrium: Diameter (cm): ☐ Normal (<4.6) Dilation: ☐ Mild (4.6-4.9) ☐ Mod (5.0-5.4) ☐ Sev (>5.4)

Atrial Septrum: ☐ Nl ☐ Aneurysm (>15 mm from midline) ☐ Lipomatous Hypertrophy ☐ ASD Type __________ Shunt: r→l l→r)

Aortic Valve: Structure: ☐ Trileaflet ☐ Bileaflet ☐ Bio Prosthesis ☐ Mechanical Prosthesis
AVA (cm²): Stenosis: ☐ None ☐ Mild (>1.5) ☐ Mod (1.0-1.5) ☐ Sev (<1.0)
Mean PG (mm Hg): Stenosis: ☐ None ☐ Mild (<20) ☐ Mod (20-40) ☐ Sev (>40)

$$(CSA_{AV}) = \frac{CSA_{LVOT} \times VTI_{LVOT}}{VTI_{AV}}$$

Regurg: ☐ None ☐ Trace ☐ Mild ☐ Moderate ☐ Severe Comments:

PHT (msec):	>500	200-500	<200
Jet Ht Ratio %:	<25%	25-64	≥65
VC (cm):	<3	.3-.6	>.6

Holodiastolic flow reversal? Y N

Mitral Valve: ☐ Normal ☐ Ring ☐ Bio prosthesis ☐ Mechanical Prosthesis
MVA (cm²): Stenosis: ☐ None ☐ Mild (<1.5) ☐ Mod (1.0-1.5) ☐ Sev (>1.0)
Mean PG (mm. Hg): Stenosis: ☐ None ☐ Mild (<5) ☐ Mod (5-10) ☐ Sev (>10)
Regurg: ☐ None ☐ Trace ☐ Mild ☐ Mod ☐ Sev Jet Directions:

VC (cm):	<.3	.3-.69	≥.7
Jet area (cm²):	2-4	4-10	>10
EROA (cm²):	<.20	.20-.40	≥.40

Comments:

Annulus (mm)(LAX in diastole): ☐ Normal (≤35) ☐ Dilated (>35) ☐ Sev Dil (>39) ☐ Calcified

SAM Predictors:
Basal septum > 15mm
C-sept < 25 mm (systole onset)
AL/PL ≤ 1.3 (systole)
PL > 15 mm (diastole)
Aorto-mitral angle <120°

Tricuspid Valve: ☐ Normal ☐ Ring ☐ Bio prosthesis ☐ Mechanical Prosthesis
Mean PG (mm Hg): Stenosis: ☐ None ☐ Significant (≥ 5 mm Hg)
Annulus (mm)(4Ch in diastole): ☐ Normal (≤35) ☐ Dilated (>35) ☐ Sev Dil (>39)
Regurg: ☐ None ☐ Trace ☐ Mild ☐ Moderate ☐ Severe Comments:
Abnormal Leaflet Morphology/Motion Comments:

Pulmonic Valve: Comments:

Ascending Aorta (cm): ☐ Dilated (♂ > 3.8; ♀ >3.7) Annulus (cm): Sinus (cm): ST Jcn (cm): ☐ Dissection
Descending Aorta: ☐ Dissection Plaque (mm): ☐ Normal (<1) ☐ II/Intimal thick (<3) ☐ III/Atheroma <5 ☐ IV/Atheroma ≥5 ☐ V/Mobile
Flow Patterns: Hepatic Veins/IVC: Pulmonary Veins:
Pericardial Effusion: ☐ No ☐ Small (< 1 cm) ☐ Mod (1-2 cm) ☐ Large (> 2 cm) ☐ Tamponade

Fig. 168.4 Example of the pertinent information for a TEE report form. (Illustration: Content used courtesy of Ray Graber)

- Most hospitals will have some sort of echo database to which your studies will be uploaded, and these databases may also be where you write your echo report and do billing. The cardiologists have very complex templates they use to write their reports. We were able to work with our cardiology IT people to develop a short template for anesthesia use, which makes our reports much easier to write.—**RGG**

- Try to do your TEE reports on the same day you performed the exam. I fill out a paper report sheet in the OR, then transcribe this to our hospitals cardiology department electronic echo database. Ideally, I will try to write my pre-pump report during cardiopulmonary bypass, and then only have to do my post pump report when the case is done.—**RGG**

Cardiopulmonary Bypass (CPB)

- Check with your perfusionist on regular basis during the pump run because if they are having a problem, then it usually means that you have a problem.—**EGA**

- Stay in constant communication with your perfusionist. If the pressure is down, is it because of lower pump flows or is it vasodilation? If they are giving multiple boluses of phenylephrine to support pressure when flow is adequate, you may need to assist them by starting a norepinephrine drip. If they have had to add multiple units of blood to the pump to maintain hemoglobin, you are more likely to have a dilutional coagulopathy and need clotting factors post-pump.—**RGG**

- Patients who have been on heparin drips may become heparin-resistant and may benefit from administration of antithrombin III. Potassium elevations secondary to cardioplegia will need to be treated with insulin prior to separation from CPB. Dextrose may or may not be needed depending on what the current glucose level is.—**RGG**

- Always check to see if there is a color change between blood in the arterial cannula and venous cannula.—**ZS**

  Your first attempt at bypass weaning is always your best attempt. Communicate well with the perfusionist and the surgeon, and make the most of it. Here's the hemodynamic mantra that's stuck with me and it works: *rate, rhythm, contractility, afterload*.—**LYS**

- When coming off cardiopulmonary bypass during a cardiac surgery, one of my attendings had a rhyming "paragraph" that helped you make sure you addressed everything.—**BPB**

  Rhythm, rate, ventilate. Check the labs and get them straight. Warm the patient, cut your flow. Come off the pump and then do the echo.

- The little saying above sounds simplistic, like a nursery rhyme, but it actually applies to every CPB case. Try it.—**BPB**

- There are multiple reasons why patients become coagulopathic after CPB. Values for fibrinogen, platelets, and other factors drop by 25–50% due to hemodilution when a patient is put on pump. CPB causes inactivation of platelets. Blood salvaged off the surgical field or residual pump blood gets processed through a cell salvage device, which washes out platelets and other clotting factors. You can sometimes make an educated guess about what products you need based on pre-op values that are low, normal, or off. Also, use TEG results to help guide you. Understanding the coagulation issues—including following the literature is part of being an expert in the cardiac rooms.—**RGG**

- Remember that plasmapheresis can be done via the CPB circuit. Read up on this before there is a request, so you are not flummoxed when it arises in clinical (often transplant) situations. The plasmapheresis part of the combined circuit is overseen by the transfusion medicine staff. They will be happy to give you a lecture on the subject.—**CM**

Closing Time

- I usually will take a last look at LV and RV function once the chest is closed. Similarly, if I have a PA catheter, I will obtain a cardiac output measurement at that time. Bad things occasionally happen when the chest is closed—chambers get compressed, grafts can become compressed or kinked. I once diagnosed a kinked left internal mammary artery to left anterior descending artery graft, once the chest was closed, the anterior wall became severely hypokinetic.—**RGG**

- Once the chest is closed, make sure the chest tube blood levels are marked with a time. Periodically check the chest tube output during closure and prior to taking the drapes down. Excessive chest tube output can either be coagulopathy or surgical bleeding. A seemingly dry patient can start bleeding when a sternal wire nicks an artery. If there is significant chest tube output, discuss with surgeons. If heparin is adequately reversed by ACT, and TEG parameters are normal, then surgical bleeding is a possibility, and the patient may need to be opened back up. Otherwise, consider giving an additional small dose of protamine (25–50 mg) and start getting clotting factors and platelets ready.—**RGG**

- If a patient does have excessive chest tube output, stay in the OR until the issue can be resolved. Ask the surgical team to leave the drapes up and the surgical field sterile. One of two things will happen—either the bleeding will get better with clotting factors, or the surgeon will have to reopen. Either way, better to address the problem prior to transporting to the ICU.—**RGG**

- Don't be afraid to extubate a cardiac surgical patient at the very end of the case if they are ready for it—that is, if the patient has appropriate respiratory function, is warm, on minimal vasoactive support, hemodynamically stable, dry chest tubes, appropriate analgesic/antiemetic regimens, no significant volume requirement.—**EGA**

- The ability to get patients extubated within a reasonable length of time (<6 h postop) at least partially depends on how we set them up for it in the OR. Early in my career we were in the era of high-dose narcotics, and it was not unusual to administer 100 mcg/kg of fentanyl for a cardiac case (along with significant midazolam doses). Elderly patients sometimes took days to wake up. We are thankfully past that era, but we still have to control our intraoperative narcotic dose to allow adequate wake-up times.—**RGG**

- Cardiac anesthesiologists are nowadays employing a variety of strategies to try to improve analgesia as the patient emerges, such as regional blocks (erector spinae, serratus anterior plane, pectoral-intercostal facial plane blocks), dexmedetomidine infusions, and preoperative methadone. Follow this research closely; you don't want to get left behind the curve on these techniques.—**RGG**

- OK, now it is time to get out of the room. There are a lot of tasks that may need to be accomplished. Doing postop blocks, removing the TEE probe, replacing IJ neck dressings that have been messed up by the surgical prep, taking off old monitors and transitioning to transport monitoring, placing an oral gastric tube, gathering medications for transport, gathering paperwork, including your report sheet for the ICU. The key is to not wait to the last minute—have your supplies organized and ready to go. As soon as the sternum is closed, and the patient is stable, you can start simplifying and preparing.—**RGG**

- Once you get the patient out of the operating room, you have to get them out of the ICU and then out of the hospital. Do every single thing that is recommended by your cardiac rehab team. And there is also plenty of room for complementary medicine techniques, as well. These ideas are not new—we found an article dating back to the 1970s and the use of acupuncture to decrease the amount of anesthesia needed for cardiac surgery patients [4].—**Editors**

- Remember that integrative medicine techniques often start even before the patient gets to the OR. Several studies have suggested that even a few preoperative acupuncture treatments will help improve outcomes, including getting patients off CPB more easily or mitigating the effects of CPB on the lungs [5, 6].—**Editors**

- It has been known for some time that acupuncture has efficacy for both general postoperative symptoms such as nausea and arrhythmias, but just as this chapter was going to press, a really fascinating study was published in JTCVS Open, the peer-reviewed open access platform of the American Association of Thoracic Surgeons [7].— **Editors**

- This study is named the Results from the Acupuncture After Heart Surgery Study. The mean number of postoperative acupuncture treatments was 3.8 over 4–5 days. Acupuncture was associated with a reduction in pain, nausea, stress, and anxiety after each session and patients receiving acupuncture had reduced postoperative stress and anxiety across admission compared with standard care. What was interesting is that acupuncture was associated with reduced postoperative atrial fibrillation incidence, fewer discharges on amiodarone, and fewer hours in the intensive care unit. There were no reported adverse events from the acupuncture treatments.—**Editors**

- There are also similar studies that found efficacy with complementary techniques such as massage and visualization. The point is to keep seeking better outcomes and keep an open mind!—**Editors**

*__Note from the Editors:__ Is a drawbridge doing its job when it is up or down? (Fig. 168.5) It's an interesting metaphysical question to ponder over a beverage. Similarly, is a cardiac anesthesiologist doing her true job when she gets the patient safely *on* or *off* bypass? This photo was selected to remind our readers that the real goal of a cardiac anesthetic is get the patient *out of the room*. Plan every second of your case with that aim and goal in mind.

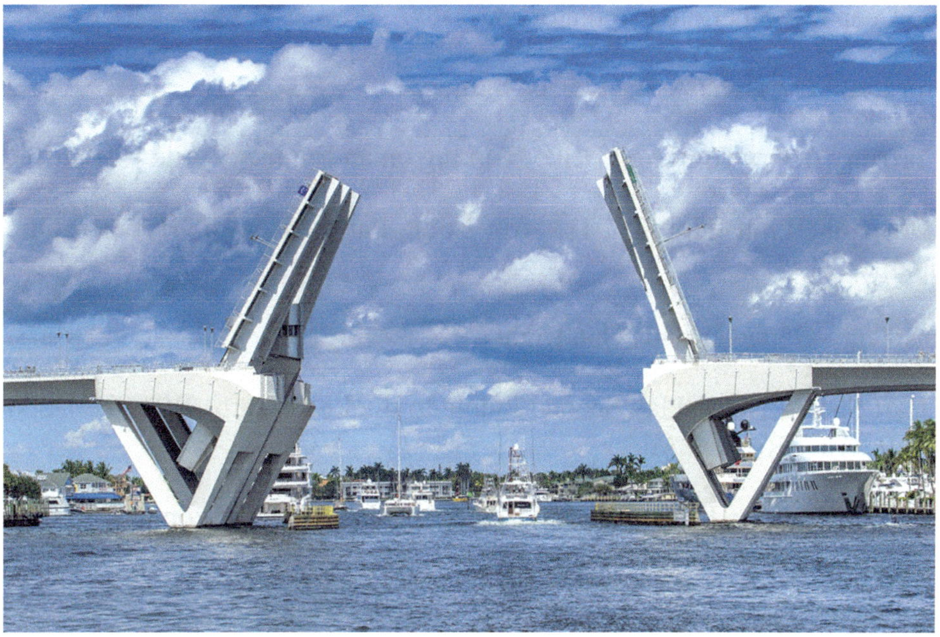

Fig. 168.5 A drawbridge in action—no way to tell if it's opening or closing, but one follows the other, always. *Photo: Image used under standard license from* stock.adobe.com

Clinical Wisdom from *Avoiding Common Anesthesia Errors, 2nd Edition*

The *Anesthesia Bridges* editors thank Ray Graber (the first author of this chapter) for being a great academic cardiac anesthesiologist and a great colleague. He was the associate editor for *Avoiding Common Anesthesia Errors, 2nd Edition,* nicknamed "Green2," and wrote and/or edited the following short chapters in that book that are each packed with additional clinical advice, tips, and wisdom. Many of the titles are teaching points in and of themselves. We highly recommend you check them out!

Green2 Cardiac Anesthesia Titles

- Cardiac Surgical Coagulopathy—You'll Need the Blood Bank and a Genie in a Bottle
- A Is for Aortic, C Is for Cannulation, B Is for…..Be Careful!
- Transesophageal Echocardiography in the Cardiac Surgery Suite—Strategies to Stay Out of Trouble
- Myocardial Protection Strategies During Cardiopulmonary Bypass—Do Everything You Can but Realize That Some Ischemic Damage Is Inevitable
- The Heartbreak of Left-Sided Valvular Dysfunction
- Anesthesia for the Descending Thoracic Aorta—Initiate Damage Control Measures
- Buckle Your Seat Belt: Taking Care of the Patient with Ascending Aortic Dissection

- Rolling in the Deep Hypothermic Circulatory Arrest
- Anesthesia for Left Ventricular Assist Device Surgery
- Off-Pump Coronary Artery Grafting Is Like Working on an Engine (While It Is Still Running)
- What To Do and What Not To Do for Your Patients with Hypertrophic Obstructive Cardiomyopathy
- Cardiac Transplant—Gotta Get This One Right
- The Right Heart Should Never Play Second Fiddle to the Left Heart—What To Do When the Right Heart Just Really Ain't Right at All

Avoiding Common Anesthesia Errors, 2nd Edition, is available on Amazon and all the major medical book websites.

Final Thoughts on Cardiac Anesthesiology

- More than any other specialty, you have to keep all the details locked down tight to make these cases go well (Fig. 168.6). Every aspect of your plan must be worked out and buttoned up because these are cases when there can be competent surgical and anesthetic techniques, and the patient still does not get out of the room alive. And then, you just have to set aside the fact that you are working on somebody's heart and just execute your plan to get everybody to the other side (Fig. 168.7).

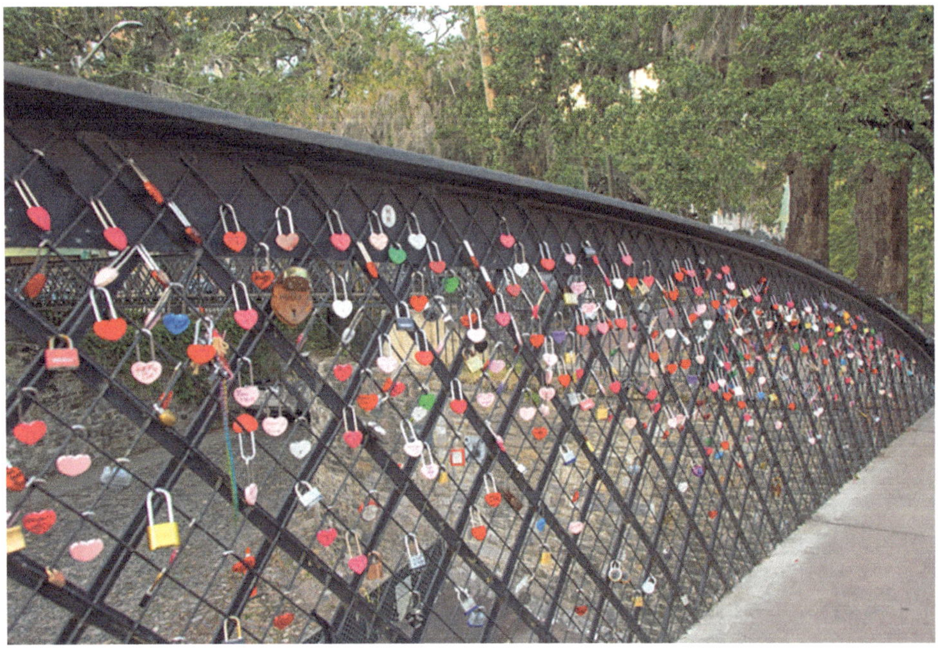

Fig. 168.6 Love Lock Bridge in Savannah, GA. Photo: William Reagan, used under standard license from iStock.com

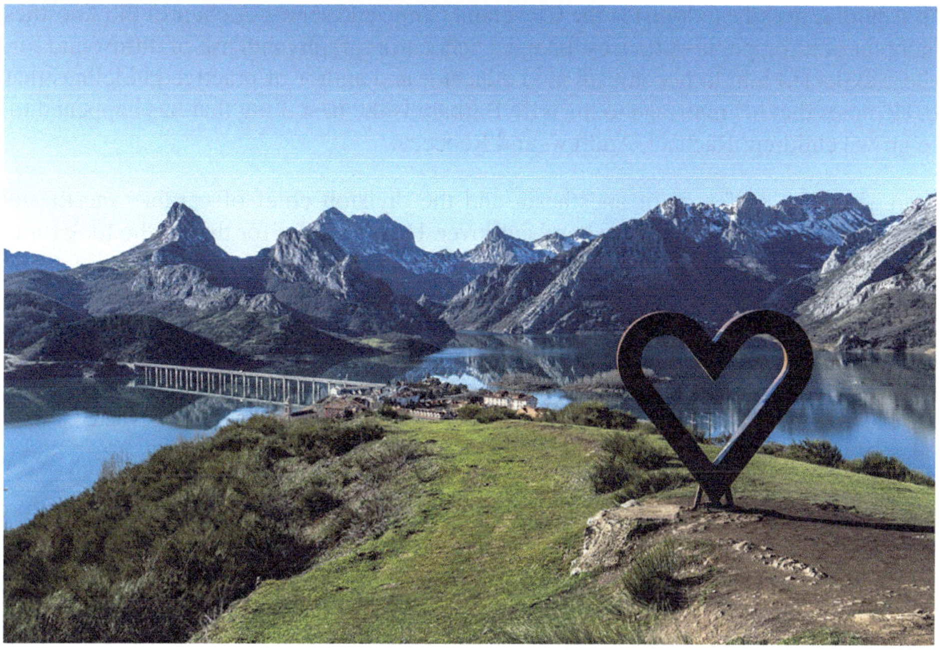

Fig. 168.7 Heart sculpture at entrance to mountain bridge. Photo: J. J. Farquitectos, used under standard license from iStock.com

References

1. Troianos CA, Kuwik RJ, Pasqual JR, et al. Internal jugular vein and carotid artery anatomic relation as determined by ultrasonography. Anesthesiology. 1996;85(1):43–8.
2. Troianos CA, Hartman GS, Glas KE, et al. Special articles: guidelines for performing ultrasound guided vascular cannulation: recommendations of the American Society of Echocardiography and the Society of Cardiovascular Anesthesiologists. Anesth Analg. 2012;114(1):46–72.
3. Singh A, Bahadorani B, Wakefield BJ, et al. Brachial arterial pressure monitoring during cardiac surgery rarely causes complications. Anesthesiology. 2017;126(6):1065–76.
4. Hollinger I, Richter JA. Acupuncture anesthesia for open heart surgery: a report of 800 cases. Am J Chin Med. 1979;7(1):77–90.
5. Dhar E, Zhang L, et al. Electroacupuncture ameliorates cardiopulmonary bypass induced apoptosis in lung via ROS/Nrf2/NLRP3 inflammasome pathway. Life Sci. 2019;238:117058.
6. Acupuncture strikes happy nerve with heart patients | 2000-11-01 |... [Internet]. Clinician.com. 2025 [cited 2025 Jul 27]. Available from: https://www.reliasmedia.com/articles/47277-acupuncture-strikes-happy-nerve-with-heart-patients
7. Feingold KL, Moskowitz JT, et al. Acupuncture after valve surgery is feasible and shows promise in reducing post-operative atrial fibrillation: The ACU-Heart pilot trial. JTCVS Open. 2023;3(16):321–32.

Authors

Ray Graber serves as the anesthesia departmental vice chair for quality at University Hospitals Cleveland Medical. He has dual interests in cardiac and orthopedic anesthesia. During his 30+ year career, he has focused on process improvement, reduction of errors, and improving patient outcomes. He is enjoying the opportunity to pass on some of what he has learned during his time in the cardiac arena.

Chris Troianos is a cardiac anesthesiologist at the Cleveland Clinic and serves as chair of the Anesthesiology Institute. He was an early adopter of intraoperative transesophageal echocardiography and use of ultrasound for vascular access. His passion for these skills led him to become an avid educator and author of practice guidelines that supported their daily clinical use. He notes that his marriage to his wife Barbara is the best thing that has happened to him, along with raising their three grown children, Rachael, Andrew, and Rebecca.

Mark Nelson is an associate professor of anesthesia and the division chief of cardiac anesthesiology at Virginia Commonwealth University. He is also an animal and car lover. He is grateful for those who took time to be mentors—mentors in medicine and mentors in life. Mentorship is one of the most important traits of any successful organization, institution, or culture. He is proud to be an American.

Ed Avery is a New Englander who trained and worked at the MGH for over a decade before moving to Cleveland. He is a cardiac anesthesiologist with multiple areas of interest—including blood pressure control, the coagulation system, and improving patient outcomes—and has participated in numerous clinical trials. In his spare time, he enjoys a good glass of wine, and working on his cars, usually not at the same time!

Louise Sun is a professor of anesthesiology and the chief of cardiothoracic anesthesiology at Stanford Medicine. She is grateful to her parents, and the beautiful people of her hometown (Guelph, Ontario), for always believing in her and motivating her to aim higher. She is proud of her decisiveness in the operating room but regrets that she is often indecisive about lunch.

Ron Bank is a senior cardiac anesthesiologist at INOVA Fairfax Hospital. He teaches at all levels in the University of Virginia academic medical system and mentors pre-med students. Ron believes and teaches his trainees that half of the success in a complicated cardiac case is due to the thought you put into it before the patient ever reaches the door of the operating room. Besides his family, patients, and community, Ron is devoted to outdoors sports activities, especially those in or under the water.

Wisdom for the ICU

169

Bradford D. Winters, Brant M. Wagener, Andrew B. Barker,
Rajen V. Nathwani, and Catherine Marcucci

Contributors:

Meena Bhatia, MD (MB)

Carol F. Bodenheimer, MD (CFB)

Edward J. Damrose, MD (EJD)

Vincent L. Hoellerich, MD (VLH)

Alexander S. Kuo, MD (ASK)

Michael A. Ramsay, MD (MAR)

Amy J. Robbins, MD (AJR)

Neil B. Sandson, MD (NBS)

Troy G. Seelhammer, MD (TGS)

Kenneth T. Shelton, MD (KTS)

Megan E. Terek, MD (MET)

B. D. Winters
Department of Anesthesiology and Critical Care Medicine, Johns Hopkins University, Baltimore, MD, USA

B. M. Wagener
Division of Critical Care Medicine, Division of Molecular and Translational Biomedicine, Birmingham, AL, USA

Department of Anesthesiology and Perioperative Medicine, Heersink School of Medicine, The University of at Birmingham, Birmingham, AL, USA

A. B. Barker
Department of Anesthesiology and Perioperative Medicine, Heersink School of Medicine, University of Alabama at Birmingham, Birmingham, AL, USA

R. V. Nathwani
Department of Anesthesiology and Pain Medicine, University of Washington School of Medicine, Harborview Medical Center, Seattle, WA, USA

C. Marcucci (✉)
Department of Transfusion Medicine, Clinical Center, National Institutes of Health, Bethesda, MD, USA

S. Mohamed et al. (eds.), *Anesthesia Bridges*, https://doi.org/10.1007/978-3-032-08294-7_169

Brandon M. Togioka, MD (BMT)

Kamila Vagnerova, MD (KV)

Introduction

The key to providing great ICU care is to first do no harm, try to remove as much of the pathophysiology as possible, and then stand by so that the patient can heal. Remember, everything that can happen in the OR can and does happen in the ICU, including drug errors, airway mishaps, and procedural mistakes. ICU care is like a 24-hours OR case, but one that you do every day and over and over. You must have constant vigilance, use common sense, and be an effective communicator and care team member. And please get the patient out of bed as soon as possible!

Dao of ICU Care

- Patients don't become suddenly critically ill; they are only recognized as such.—**BDW**

- Conflict is inevitable. Always be the poised consultant and handle conflict with tact and grace.—**BDW**

- As important as critical care is to help save a life, it is equally important to help usher that life out in a peaceful and dignified manner when critical care has failed. Take the time to do it right and think carefully about your approach to the issues. Empathize and communicate with significant others or loved ones of your patient.—**MET**

- It is important to have a realistic understanding of death. Modern medicine is amazing, and we can do so much with so little. We can fully support every organ system, and it is important to know what that looks like and how much work that can be. It is also important to know that often, we still will not keep someone from dying.—**ABB**

- We do *not* heal patients. Patient's bodies heal themselves. We only temporize pathophysiology and put the patient in the best position possible to heal.—**BMW**

- None of your patients read the book. They have their own different problems due to the life they have lived and the co-morbidities they have obtained. Do your best to return them to their personal physiology and let them do the rest.—**BMW**

- My career advice for critical care medicine—the ICU is a place to interface with the hospital at large. You work with all kinds of consultants and care teams. Foster these relationships, learn from everyone, and collaborate clinically and academically.—**ABB**

- To deliver the best critical care medicine to a patient in the ICU, one needs to develop and maintain the culture in the unit. It must be appreciated that each ICU has a different culture for many reasons. Changing culture is challenging and takes time.—**ABB**

- The intensive care unit is just a place. As an ICU doctor, you can provide intensive care wherever a patient needs it.—**ASK**

- The hospital and the ICU can be a very dehumanizing place for patients and their families. Sometimes just the normal human behavior of sitting down, addressing people by their name, and asking them how they are feeling can make all the difference.—**ASK**

***Note from the Editors:** Speaking of Dao, many bridges are harmonious and beautiful. But not every bridge has to be a work of art; sometimes it just has to get the job done (Fig. 169.1).

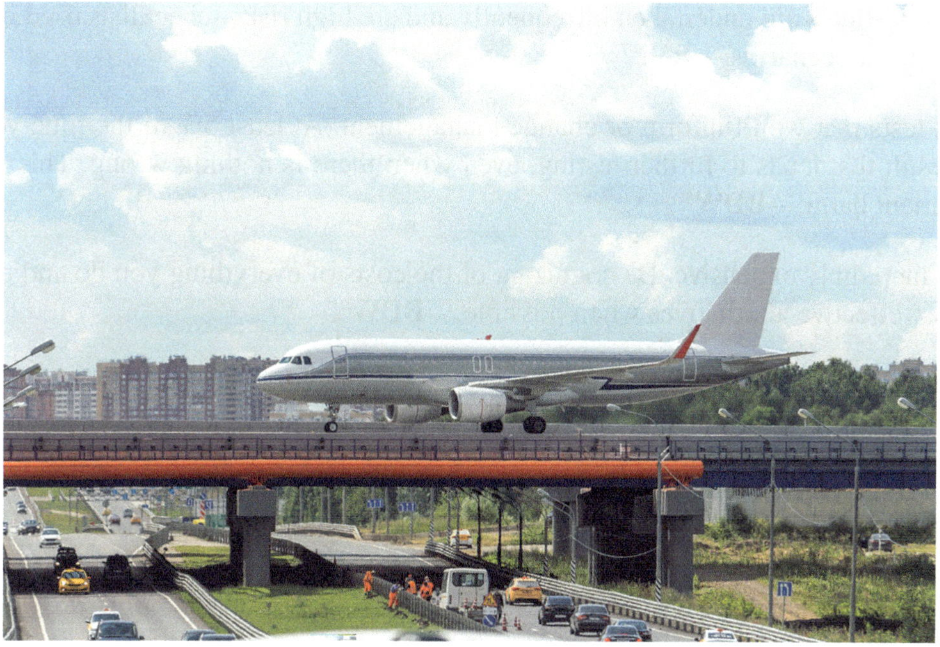

Fig. 169.1 A taxiway bridge over a busy highway. There are at least 40 airplane bridges in the world. They present unique civil engineering and design challenges, especially as airplanes continue to get larger and heavier. Not only must they withstand the weight of the largest airplanes, but they must also be designed for the substantial forces exerted by aircraft braking, thus affecting the lateral load in substructure design. Photo: Image used under standard license from iStock.com

General Principles of ICU Care

- Care in the intensive care unit is by definition intense, but it is always, always predicated on doing the basics well. The fanciest new modality or most expensive new drug isn't going to help you or your patient if you neglect the basics.—**RVN and Editors**

- Physics was the most important course you ever took. If you don't remember it, go back and review it. An intrinsic knowledge of physics is essential to the practice of critical care medicine. You don't need to be able to do differential equations; it is the principles that matter in everyday application.—**BDW**

- Be wary of "eminence-based" medicine. Embrace evidence-based medicine.—**BDW**

- Despite all of the technology and monitors, it is still good to put a hand or a stethoscope on the patient; it gives you time to think if nothing else.—**BDW**

- When we were training, we had ICU attendings who made a practice of standing in the doorway of the ICU bay for a few moments, either right before or right after rounds, just to observe the patient and what was going on in the room. When asked about this, our attendings told us that it was to see how much the patient was moving on his own, how the nurses were interacting with the patient, and especially how the family was interacting with the patient. Families can pick up on non-verbal clues that the ICU staff sometimes misses. It's not a bad practice to ask the families every day about their impression of how the patient seems to them. Especially the patient's mother, if she is available.—**Editors**

- Checklists are very useful to avoid cognitive overload and make sure crucial steps are not missed. Many ICU procedures are undertaken infrequently and are high risk—checklists used in real time are excellent for these scenarios.—**RVN**

- Don't order tests that won't inform or change management. At least 5% of the time you will get an abnormal result that leads to further testing, even when there is nothing wrong. This wastes money and risks patient harm.—**BDW**

- ICU care is incredibly expensive. Be cognizant of the costs of everything you do and order and look for more cost-effective alternatives when possible.—**BDW**

- Despite being in the ICU and usually incredibly sick, patients often remember substantial portions of their time in the ICU. Make sure anything they could hear, see, or remember is as positive and professional as possible.—**BDW**

- Just because you can doesn't mean you should. Consider each procedure or intervention carefully. Risks may be minimal or minimized, but never zero. Does this procedure or intervention contribute meaningfully to the patient's management? Try to think of every reason *not* to do something; if the benefits outweigh, then proceed.—**MET**

- Don't just do something, stand there. Assess the situation and stop to think before you act or give orders. Give time for interventions to take effect before doing more or changing tack.—**MET**

- You know ACLS—but your goal is not to use it. Subtle changes in vitals or lab trends might portend trouble ahead. Anticipate clinical decompensation and do what you can to avoid it. Stay at least two steps ahead of your patient.—**MET**

- You must think about and evaluate the patient every time you make a decision, even briefly. What you evaluated at rounds may no longer be true. Also, that previous evaluation was just a snapshot or picture. The physiologic picture may have changed.—**BMW**

- Everything that you do or order (fluids, meds, procedures, out of bed to chair) has benefits and drawbacks. Treat every decision as such. The wrong fluids can hurt a patient just as badly as a tension pneumothorax secondary to a CVL misadventure.—**BMW**

- A good question to ask yourself every day with every patient: Is everything in the right place? Line and tube placement seem to be the big ones. Endotracheal tube in wrong spot, vascular access in wrong spot, nasogastric or Dobhoff tube in wrong spot. But there can also be other things out of place. Have the drips been set up correctly? Are the drains where they are supposed to be? Is the patient's ID band where it is supposed to be? Are they properly covered? Is there anything in the bed that is not supposed to be there?—**BMW and Editors**

- We once saw a patient get a moderately bad pressure sore from a roll of tape that somehow got under him. And we have seen patients burned by warming devices and lights. It's kind of an entropy thing—things will migrate out of place and to a state of disorder if there is not constant vigilance. This is true even in the ICU, where there is supposed to be intensive monitoring and surveillance at all times.—**BMW and Editors**

- The pleural of "anecdote" in critical care is not "data," we should strive to use rigorous clinical trials to guide life-and-death decisions.—**KTS**

- Critical care provides an opportunity to use the collective wisdom of a multidisciplinary and cross-specialty ICU team to drive medical care.—**KTS**

- In the SICU, patients have poor nutritional status. Generating a white count or fever requires lean muscle mass that they may not have. A small increase in WBC (even if not abnormal) along with other signs of end-organ dysfunction, such as coagulopathy or hyperglycemia, should make you consider pneumonia or some other infection that is brewing.—**BMW**

- When a patient becomes quiet—that is not a good thing. It is more likely a sign of hypoactive delirium or some other bad omen.—**BMW**

- Remember to treat your nurses well. They have been at the bedside longer than you if you are in training. They did not go to medical school, but they may have common sense and have seen something before that worries them. They can help you think of problems and make you look good to your attending.—**BMW**

- When you do a procedure, leave the room cleaner than you found it.—**BMW**

- Patient's illnesses typically have a predictable time course. The medical issues will resolve over a certain period and complications during that time are usually predictable. It is important to understand this timeline and the pattern to illness in order to provide the most effective supportive care, medical management, and to anticipate complications.—**ABB**

- Patients need to show daily progress. If they are not moving forward and responding, or they are clinically the same from day to day, then they are moving backwards.—**ABB**

- In the ICU if the patient does not show clinical progress in response to treatment within a reasonable timeframe, there may be an issue in the effectiveness of the treatment. One must stop and reconsider the underlying issues and make sure you aren't missing anything. Think of another organ system to involve in your differential, consider antibiotic resistance, or stop and do something different.—**ABB**

- There is no substitute for an astute and experienced bedside nurse in the ICU. They are our eyes and ears. So much of a patient's clinical course depends on the bedside nurse.—**ABB**

- There is no substitute for a clinician making effective and timely decisions at the bedside.**—ABB**

- Medical therapeutic interventions need to be clear and concise. You are treating one problem with one intervention with close surveillance of efficacy. The minute you use a treatment's side effect as a primary outcome, you have lost control of the big picture and treatment plan. For example, using a sedation medication as an antihypertensive.—**ABB**

- Clinical courses are dynamic in the critically ill, and it is always better to choose a single therapy for a single problem to keep the physiologic picture clearer. For example, use metoprolol for heart rate and amlodipine for blood pressure management rather than carvedilol. When less acute and more static clinical course, then tailor management carvedilol for easier outpatient compliance.—**ABB**

- To be effective in care delivery, the ICU care team needs to be informed and empowered. Every team member needs a clearly defined role and responsibility to function efficiently and effectively. The team management style is not always a top-down dictatorship. There are many moving parts to a team, and everyone needs to be empowered to bring their experience and opinion to the discussion for the patients benefit.—**ABB**

- The continuous renal replacement machine must be understood. If nothing else, understand the basic prescription and how much work the machine is doing and can do. If you have a prescription for high solute clearance, using a zero-potassium bath, and your patient with ischemic bowel or limbs has hyperkalemia, something is wrong.—**ABB**

- Find a way to have a private word with the anesthesiology attending for every bigger case coming to the ICU. Transport and sign-out of a big case can be hectic—the surgeons are there, the residents and fellows are there, the nurses are trying to start their own care of the patient. Even if you place a quick private phone call, attending to attending, before the patient leaves the OR, you want to hear from the anesthesiologist of record how the airway, lines, and resuscitation went and how the junior anesthesia staff and surgeons did.—**Editors**

- ICU training that has teams composed of both surgeons and anesthesiologists seems to be efficacious in building career-long professional relationships. Take every opportunity to get to know the surgeons you are working with in the ICU.—**Editors**

- Make your documentation matter. So often with today's electronic health records (EHRs), clinicians' notes are nearly useless, the result of endless "cut and paste." At the very least, make your impression and plan unique to the patient for that day's events. This is so helpful to others caring for ICU patients with you, but always meaningful when doing retrospective chart reviews to best assess the course of the patient and medical decision-making.—**VLH**

- Constipation in the ICU is common and miserable for the patient—treat it early. Develop a protocol with your pharmacy and have "bowel management" as part of the daily ICU rounds. Acupuncture helps. The link below discusses two recent meta-analyses and gives a bit of background on Traditional Chinese Medicine.—**RVN and Editors**

  https://www.medicalnewstoday.com/articles/acupuncture-for-constipation

- Keep an ear open for the OR. At Hopkins, available ICU docs would respond to emergency calls in the OR. I had only two truly emergency re-intubations in the eight years I was there—airway obstructed by a mucus plug and post-carotid endarterectomy bleeding in the neck—and both times **Brad Winters** heard the call and came over from the ICU, which was just across the hall in those days, to help me re-intubate. I still remember those cases, and that it was Brad who came over to help me.—**CM**

- *ALWAYS* take seriously a family member who says the patient is worse and work up the complaint *they describe*. On more than one occasion, I have had families complaining of change in facial appearance or slight slurring of a few words, a full hour before the nurses or doctors could appreciate the change.—**CFB**

- The ICU is a place of frequent palliative medicine consults and support. A large portion of my palliative practice was for critically ill patients in the ICU. The palliative team can support the patient, family, and care team in the face of life-threatening illness. The palliative team rides alongside the patient and family when the clinical course may improve and assures a level of continuity beyond the ICU to step down units, the med-surg floor, and even into rehab and the outpatient setting. If the patient should worsen or approach end of life that same team can provide direction and options both in and out of the ICU. Think about consulting palliative medicine early and often!—**AJR**

***Note from the Editors:** We asked Brad Winters for his favorite bridge and why and he sent back two words: "Tappan Zee." We weren't sure if he meant the new or old bridge. He was in the ICU that week and we didn't wish to bother him, so here are both (Figs. 169.2 and 169.3).

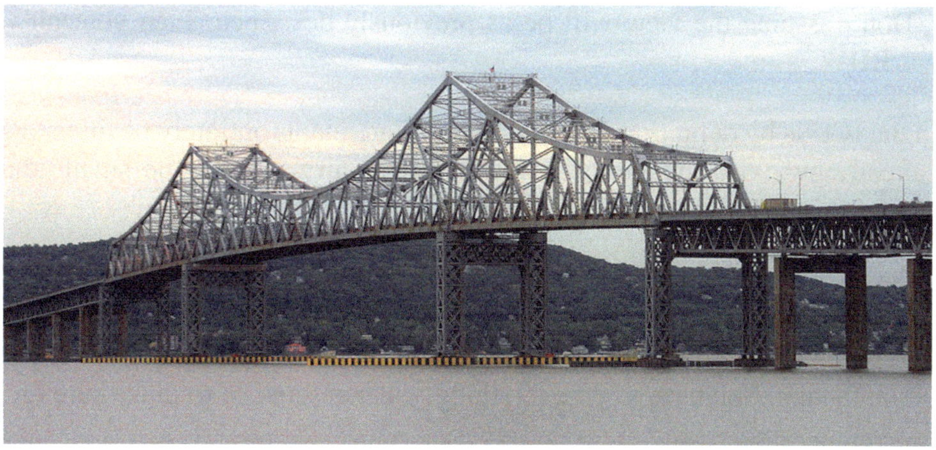

Fig. 169.2 The Tappan Zee Bridge (1955–2017). Located about 25 miles north of Manhattan, the bridge's name is derived from the name of the Colonial-era river crossing at that location, which derived from the Tappan Native American tribe that inhabited the area and the Dutch word for "sea." It was built from 1952 to 1955 on a budget of $81 million. Due to a gigantic political dispute, it was located just outside the boundaries of the New York Port Authority and so crossed the Hudson at one of its widest points. Construction of the bridge was considerably enabled by World War 2 technology. Photo: Image used under standard license from iStock.com

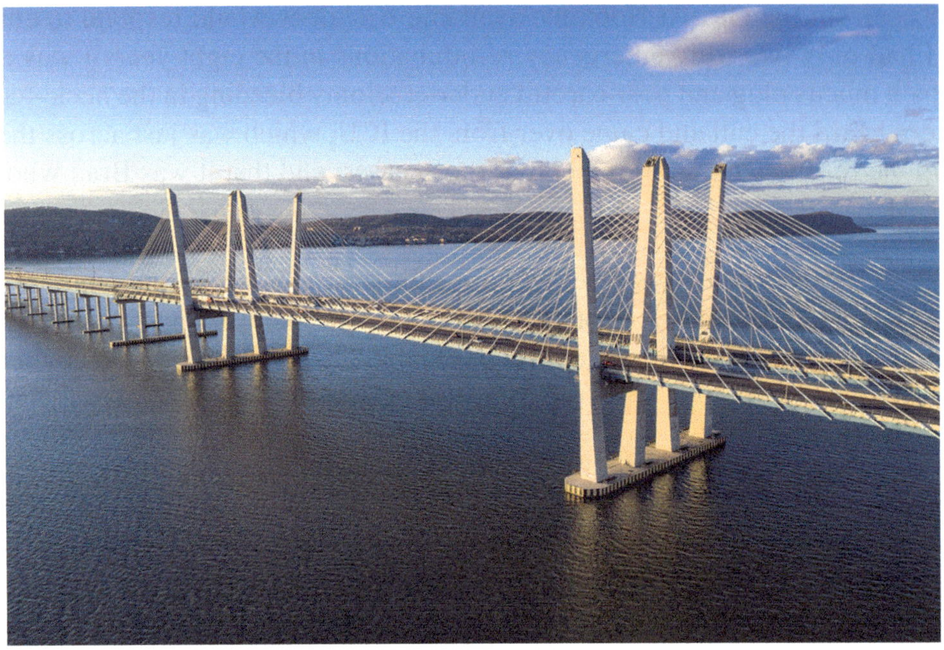

Fig. 169.3 The new Tappan Zee, which is officially named for former New York Governor Mario Cuomo, opened in 2017. It is a twin, cable-stayed bridge over the Hudson River, located just to the north of the original bridge. The project cost over $3 billion and was plagued by controversy. Photo: Image used under standard license from stock.adobe.com

Airway and Ventilator Management

- In the ICU, even a previously easy airway can become a disaster especially after a prolonged time on a ventilator. Don't assume the view will be as previously described. Plan your airway maneuvers accordingly.—**BDW**

- Intubation in the ICU is by definition difficult, patients are inappropriately positioned/slumped in the bed, likely already hypoxic, and the only available oral airways may be small adult or pediatric size.—**KV**

- I agree with the above contributors! Every intubation in the ICU is a potentially difficult intubation. *Aim for first pass success.* Optimize position before you start, use a checklist, and make sure the best intubator is present—either doing the intubation or supervising. Don't just hope it goes okay with a junior person intubating. You have to do everything you can think of to make sure of it.—**RVN and Editors**

- Remember that the Difficult Airway Algorithm is not just for the OR.—**Editors**

- ICU nurses are clinically astute and often have advanced training, but they do not train in anesthesiology or the OR. Therefore, do not assume or expect ICU nurses to be helpful with difficult intubation. They are not CRNAs, they don't have formal airway training. If you really need help with a difficult airway, get another anesthesiologist or anesthesia-trained person.—**KV and Editors**

- Similarly, there are hospitals where respiratory therapists have intubating privileges. We were taught to assume that their experience and skill levels in advanced airway management is about the same as staff in the emergency room.—**Editors**

- Endotracheal tubes can get soft when in place for several days. They can rise above the vocal cords as they soften. When repositioning the ETT, in this case, it is best to use a flexible bronchoscope, as using a more rigid bougie or tube exchange catheter can run the risk of straightening the ETT and dislodging the tube from the airway even further.—**ABB**

- Ventilators are our tools we use to help people. It is our job to understand everything about how they work and how to implement them for each patient. We need to understand physiology and our patient's pathophysiology and apply our tool effectively. So, start with the patient and what they need and apply the ventilator settings accordingly to achieve the clinical goals of support without causing harm. That may mean using a different mode, flow pattern, or I:E ratio than what is normative, and that is ok.—**ABB**

- When you are first starting in providing ICU or need to refresh, start with studying and learning assist control/volume control and assist control/pressure control for lung transplant patients.—**KTS and Editors**

- Re-intubations are never a good thing and should generally not be part of the planned airway management. Most experienced ICU physicians do not do a "trial of extubation, we can always reintubate." For one thing, it incurs risk. A failed extubation is no less serious in the ICU than in the OR. It stresses the patient physiologically, including any period of hypoxemia or hypercarbia. As noted above, it can be technically difficult. It's also emotionally deleterious to the patient and the family to have such a setback in the clinical course. Plan your care so that you have a very low re-intubation rate.—**Editors**

- And reintubation rates should be tracked and discussed in QA meetings.—**Editors**

- A tracheostomy is like a handshake—if you think about doing it, you should strongly consider carrying through with it.—**BMW**

- Do not extubate anyone that needs a tracheostomy. Patients do not have to prove they will fail extubation to require a trach.—**ABB**

- When a patient needs a tracheostomy, it does not reflect on your skill to liberate the patient from the ventilator. Tracheostomies allow you to move quickly forward with the clinical process.—**ABB**

- I don't worry particularly about vent settings *per se* or try to fit patients to a specific vent management protocol if they show me that they can't do it. I set PEEP to best compliance (wherever that is), set the tidal volume to 4-6cc/kg, dial down FiO2 to SpO2 of 90ish, and let the patient over-breathe the vent by 1-2 breathes—that way they get rest, but also control ventilation and therefore acid-base balance. They know what they need physiologically and what they can handle. Then wean to PSV and extubation as they get better.—**BMW**

Medication Management

- Have a pharmacist join you on your ICU ward rounds to help minimize iatrogenic injury.—**RVN**
- We give a lot of drugs in ICU—anaphylaxis and drug toxicity should be on the differential for nearly every situation.—**RVN**
- Medications that are titrated need clear physiologic parameters to target. Whether it is systolic blood pressure, mean arterial pressure, cardiac output, Richmond Agitation and Sedation Scale, or train-of-4, it must be clearly written and communicated. This makes sure the clinical goals are planned and achievable, and that the bedside nurse's license is protected. Try and have one medication for one parameter.—**ABB**
- I don't worry about weaning pressors. Mainly because it is the *reason* for the pressors that matters and is what I worry about. The more a patient can control their own physiology and the faster they can do it, the better off I think they are. For example, if a patient is on two pressors and it is due to acute blood loss anemia, I would expect the pressors to wean quickly with adequate resuscitation. Similarly, for sepsis, once antibiotics and source control are achieved, or are being achieved, most people come off drugs pretty quickly.—**BMW**
- At MGH (now MGB), we wean pressors quickly and have a quite low threshold to start oral midodrine. However, inotropes, not as fast.—**KTS**
- I prefer to stay away from benzodiazepines if possible as they can cause delirium in sepsis. I do use them for ARDS to help with vent synchrony. I usually prefer propofol/fentanyl or another narcotic. The same principles apply in the ICU as in the OR—treat pain as well as providing sedation/amnestic. Dexmedetomidine is great if the patient tolerates (not usually) or you are working towards extubation in the next few hours.—**BMW**
- We also do not utilize benzos heavily for sedation of intubated patients. Our typical sedatives are either propofol or precedex—we are using precedex much more lately.—**KTS**
- Remember that haloperidol does not treat delirium! It is a sedative, nothing more. It is advantageous for the ICU because it has several routes of administration, is not appreciably anti-cholinergic, and does not cause appreciable drug-drug interactions, but it does not treat the delirious state *per se*. The only treat to "treat" delirium is to treat the underlying cause.—**NBS**
- ICU delirium is very multi-factorial—inherent disease states, drugs or drug withdrawal, electrolyte imbalances, and more. When seeking an etiology for delirium, *suspect everything* until each possibility is definitely ruled out.—**Editors**
- The ICU setting is a set up for the occurrence of drug-drug interactions (DDIs). For one, medication panels in the ICU are fluid and dynamic. When making additions to the med regimen, always consider that the risk of pharmacodynamic interactions is increased.—**NBS and CM**

- Pharmacokinetic DDIs can occur when meds are either stopped or started. This can represent either the introduction or removal of an inducer or inhibitor.—**NBS and CM**

- ICU patients are also at risk of DDIs because of the ever-present risk of fungal infections. The azole antifungals are prime instigators for inhibition of **CYP3A4**, which metabolizes a huge number of exogenous compounds. It is imperative that you review the patient's med list for possible interactions any time you are starting an azole antifungal. Substrates of **CYP3A4** include some of the statins, calcium channel blockers, some antipsychotics, steroids, and carbamazepine, to name several.—**NBS and CM**

- The presence or development of acute kidney injury (AKI) in the ICU patient should prompt review of every single medication on the list. Since up to 40–50% of critically ill patients will develop AKI at some point in their clinical course, make up your mind that this will be necessary. Of course, your ICU pharmacy staff will help you, but as the physician, you are responsible for getting this right. Have a good go-to summary and refresher on the topic and review it frequently. There are many available, but one we like, because it's short and to the point, is below.—**Editors**

  Drug dosing in critically ill patients with acute kidney injury and on renal replacement. Saran S, Rao SS, and Azim A. Indian J Crit Care Med. 2020 Apr; 24(Suppl3): S129–S134.

- Many IV infusions, for example, nicardipine, will provide a large volume of fluid to the patient, so be mindful of this.—**RVN**

- Chloroprocaine is a great drug for ICU dressing changes, which can be incredibly painful. As we note elsewhere, there is extremely low toxicity for this drug and rapid onset. The technique could not be simpler—simply open the vials in a sterile fashion, pour the local anesthetic on the dressings until they are saturated, and also pour it on the wound edges. Wait 5–10 minutes or so and then do the dressing changes. One of the *Bridges* contributors requested this before dressing changes when she was in the ICU for necrotizing fasciitis, as the team taking care of her was entirely made up of surgeons and they had never heard of this technique. It greatly decreased the amount of pain medication needed for the procedures.—**Editors**

- Pay attention to your local antimicrobial bio gram and change antibiotic regimens as resistance patterns change.—**RVN**

***Note from the Editors:** We put out a request to our authors to tell us about an intensivist who had made a big impact on their career and Mike Ramsay sent us the wonderful obituary piece he had written for Roy Simpson, aka Dr. Bernard Roy Jerome Simpson, who was the esteemed chair at Baylor for many years (Fig. 169.4).

> Dr. Simpson was born in Wales in 1922, got his medical degree from London University, and trained in anesthesia at the Radcliffe Infirmary under Robert Macintosh. He was also a veteran, serving as a physician in the Canadian Royal Air Force. Dr. Simpson was involved in many of the leading developments itn the practice of anesthesiology of his day, including publishing early influential data on the efficacy of pain control for postoperative respiratory function and recovery, describing monitoring of cerebral function under anesthesia, initiating the training of anesthesia technicians, and researching the causes of post-anesthesia hepatitis.

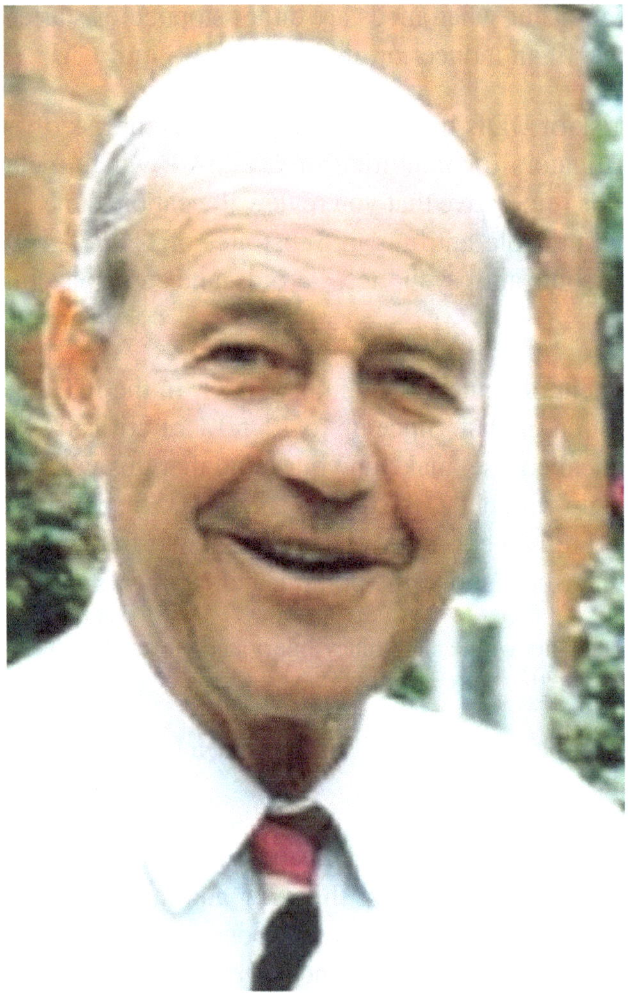

Fig. 169.4 The late and very esteemed Roy Simpson (1922–2012). His forceful and forthright personality made a big impact on both his people and his hospital system. Photo: Image used with permission from the Simpson family

- Roy Simpson was the mentor who had the greatest impact on my professional career. He insisted on the acronym ITU (intensive therapy unit) instead of ICU (intensive care unit) because, he said, "We treat patients as well as care for them." I was working as a resident in his unit when I developed the sedation control scale that later became known by my name. Professor Simpson was a remarkable man who loved life as much as he loved the practice of anesthesiology.—**MAR**

Bleeding and Fluid Management

- What goes in must come out. Classify fluid therapy as an intervention and be both judicious and intentional with its use as you would with any other medication or procedure.—**TGS**

- Resuscitate or do not, there is no slow code. In an emergency, it is your role to rapidly assess, evaluate, and intervene without delay.—**TGS**

- When should you have a high suspicion for bleeding—retroperitoneal or otherwise? It depends. I work in a surgical ICU, so if it is pancreatitis or there was a pancreatic resection, it can be a lot of vessels that bleed. Or a femoral artery graft can pop (has happened!), or GI bleeding if on anticoagulation. The important point is *to transfuse* if you think bleeding is contributing to the patient's sudden instability, rather than waiting for labs. Or get imaging. Or go to interventional radiology or the OR. It really depends on the specific clinical situation—but don't sit around and just watch it happen. Investigate and do something.—**BMW**

- The *Bridges* editors specifically asked me to include some wisdom on when you can't trust your drain outputs. Again, the answer is when the clinical situation does not make sense. Sometimes we have to upsize drains. If everything slows, but the patient is not better clinically, time to be suspicious.—**BMW**

- Always carefully consider bleeding risks in the surgical ICU when starting therapeutic anticoagulation. Monitor anticoagulation carefully. Use more than one monitoring parameter if able, such as anti-Xa and aPTT together. We affect one part of the clotting cascade with heparin; sepsis affects many different parts.—**ABB**

Longitudinal Care and Rehabilitation of ICU Patients

- Post-ICU syndrome is a real thing. Do what you can to prevent it; avoid and treat delirium, use spontaneous breathing trial and spontaneous awakening trials to expedite liberation from the ventilator, avoid paralytics, if possible, encourage early mobility, prevent hospital acquired infection, and adhere to prophylactic guidelines, such as for venous thromboembolism, when indicated.—**BDW**

- Many ancient texts describe the poor effects of bedrest and inactivity. In his *Treatise of Hygiene*, Maimonides said in 1199, "Anyone who lives a sedentary life and does not exercise…all his days will be painful ones and his strength shall wane." It is absolutely nuts to physiatrists that during the nineteenth and twentieth centuries that bedrest was prescribed as a *cure*. Finally, at the end of the twentieth century and beginning of the twenty-first century, our understanding of the consequences of disuse increased. Much of our current data on bedrest is from the space program.—**CFB**

- The average ICU stay in the US is 3.3 days (2018 data). The average patient spends 1.5 *additional* days in a non-ICU bed. A single ICU stay increases the time spent in the hospital by 50%. Every day in ICU on bedrest decreases muscle strength by 3–11%.—**CFB**

- Remember that each day in the ICU requires *one week* of rehab time. Consider very early physiatry consults for all of your ICU patients, especially if they are going to be there for more than 24–48 hours. Ask them if there would be efficacy in formal PT and/OT sessions to prevent loss of muscle memory. We have seen OT therapy sessions have great efficacy for TBI patients, even if the OT staff has to put the dice in the patient's hand, close their fingers, shake their hand, and then roll the dice for them.—**CFB**

- ICU patients should be out of bed to a chair or in bed in "chair position" *twice a day.*—**CFB**

- One thing that is now well-known in the rehab of critically ill patients is establishing daytime and nighttime. The best way to do this is by controlling lighting.—**CFB**

- There isn't a lot of prospective data at present, but whatever you can do that establishes periods of alertness during the day is probably helpful on some level. If somebody asked me for my unofficial but expert opinion, I would say that daytime engagement and conversation is good, even if your patient is intubated and sedated. Anything that promotes daytime alertness and engagement will be helpful. The nurses do this, but the physician staff can do it as well, a bit more than I think they currently do.—**CFB**

- Tell your patient what is going on around them and talk them through their day. Don't forget to ask them questions and ask them to interact with you. But don't stand in the door and yell questions in a sing song voice, either. Try to use as normal a conversational tone as possible. Tell them who is in the room. Tell them who you are. Tell them jokes and ask them who their favorite comedian is. Tell them who won the game and what's in the sports page, and ask if they have ever been to Lambeau Field themselves. Tell them what day it is, what the weather is. Show them pictures of their families. Tell them the daffodils are up. Tell them how long they have been in the ICU and when you are hoping they will be transferred out.—**CFB**

- I agree with the above! I once had a patient who was in the ICU for months, early one spring. An organ transplant and then a redo organ transplant. Heavily sedated, drips, pressors, dialysis, everything. Finally, the patient got better in mid-April. The very first thing he said to his family when he finally swam up to the surface and could talk was, "Did anybody file the taxes?" Not, "Where am I and what happened?" Somehow, despite not appearing to have alertness or awareness for weeks or even months, at some deep-brain level, the patient's sense of time had remained intact. So, interact with your ICU patient exactly as you would with a patient in the regular PACU or on a regular floor.—**CM**

- Somebody told me once that, besides embryogenesis and fetal development, wound healing is just about the most complex process the body has, perhaps second only to digestion, but in reverse. The healing cascade is packed with multiple interdependent pathophysiological and immunological mediators. It's not just the initial scar formation—scar formation is just the start of wound healing. What the body is trying to accomplish is the repair and restoration of cellular integrity where there is just space and the absence of tissue.—**CM**

- The line between an acute wound and a chronic wound is blurry. It's been said that even the most chronic wound becomes acute every time the dressing is changed.—**Editors**

- Vacuum-healing devices need separate pain and anxiety management considerations. They are painful, but in a weird and hard-to-describe way, and they itch like crazy. They are also a tad bit difficult psychologically, and they disrupt sleep. Ask me how I know.—**CM**

- Want to read some interesting literature on wound healing? Look at the papers on *medical grade honey* healing both chronic and acute wounds [1]. Turns out that honey has all kinds of desirable properties for wound healing. First of all, it's topical. Second, it's strongly anti-microbial. Its active compounds include phenolic acid, flavonoids, enzymes, organic acids, and vitamins. It has applications as both primary and rescue therapy in a wide range of clinical situations, including burns, malignancies, leg ulcers, amputation, ruptured abdominal wounds, and septic and other surgical wounds. The biomedical engineers are busy developing tissue-engineered scaffolding for drug delivery, of course.—**Editors**

ECMO

- ECMO is a therapeutic modality in transition. In the old days, it was considered as a bridge therapy only—for example, until another heart could be found. It wasn't a definitive modality. Was it the recent pandemic that has changed this? It seems as if it has now thought of like dialysis—invasive, unfortunate, lifesaving, and... indefinite, especially by families. We once heard a patient's mother inquire about arranging for "home ECMO."—**Editors**

- If you are debating and struggling with whether to put a patient on ECMO or not, they should probably be on it.—**MB**

- Truth be told, even prior to COVID, ECMO had matured into a longer-term bridge technology with typical runs exceeding 7–14 days. COVID runs were much longer, and outcomes even better, but longer runs have become much more commonplace.—**TGS**

- ECMO does *not* treat the underlying pathophysiologic state. Rather it offers physiologic support to buy time for other interventions and natural recovery processes to manifest meaningful improvements.—**TGS**

- The central concept in ECMO hinges around the importance of restoration of adequate oxygen delivery to vital organs. All indications, adjunct therapies, and exit strategies are contingent upon this same underlying principle.—**TGS**

- ECMO represents an exceptional model of contact phase activation that involves the sequential and concurrent activation of the primary and secondary hemostatic cascades. Advances in materials and circuitry have improved the tolerance of blood to the foreign material surface necessitated by ECMO, but to date have not mitigated these challenges entirely.—**TGS**

- The most common complication associated with ECMO continue to be hemorrhagic and thrombotic in nature. Broadly, 10–30% of all ECMO patients will suffer major complications in this realm.—**TGS**

- Much about ECMO remains to be elucidated, including indications, duration of support for various clinical states, cannulation configuration, anticoagulant type and intensity, and assay utilized, and how to leverage mixed technologies to optimize outcomes, for example, Impella + ECMO, intra-aortic balloon pump + ECMO, and bi-ventricular assist device +/- oxygenator.—**TGS and Editors**

- Every patient on bridging therapies should have a poster of a beautiful bridge in a beautiful garden posted within eyesight (Fig. 169.5). Data are accumulating on the outcomes and benefits of such a simple intervention.—**Editors**

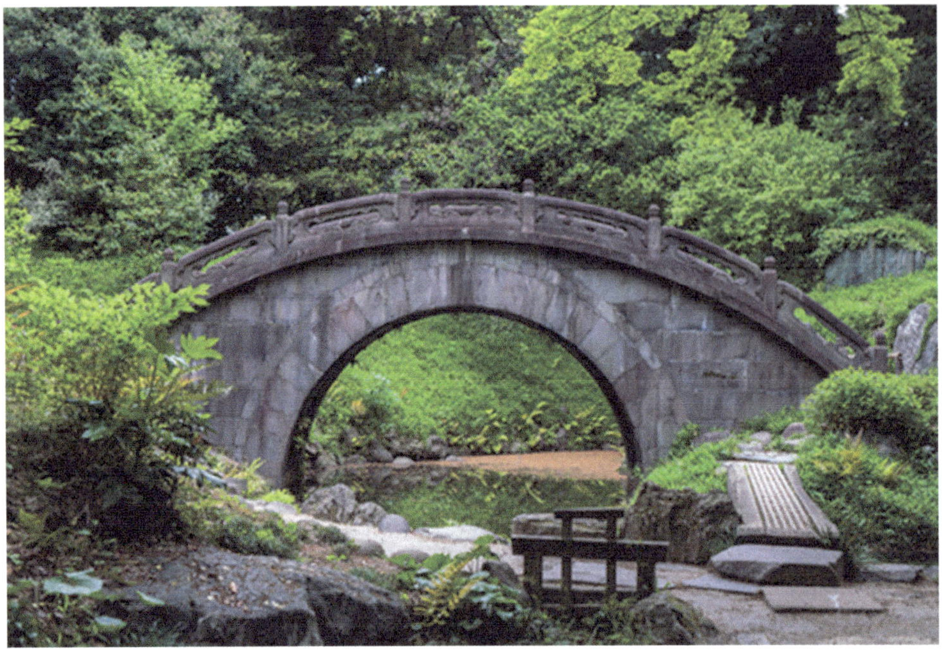

Fig. 169.5 A lovely old stone bridge in a beautiful botanical garden. Photo: Image used under standard license from shutterstock.com

Pregnant Women in the ICU

- Procedures go best when they are performed in locations with experienced personnel and standard equipment. It is easy to recommend that a high-risk parturient delivery in the ICU, instead of on labor and delivery. However, in my experience complications involving the baby, such as fetal bradycardia, occur at much higher frequency than maternal complications. Further, most complications involving high-risk parturient occur after delivery, not during the labor process. In this manner, I have become less likely to recommend that high-risk parturients labor in the ICU over time.—**BMT**

- The fetal heart rate is a much more sensitive indicator of global tissue perfusion than serum lactate, central venous oxygen saturation or urine output.—**BMT**

- Keep the mother as the priority. Generally speaking, the fetus will die if the mother does not survive. Thus, while it is important to consider drug effects on the fetus, a general rule of thumb is to select the drug that is best for maternal physiology. Most drugs including opioids, sedatives, and neuromuscular blocking agents, are safe. There are only a few drugs that should generally be avoided: warfarin, nonsteroidal anti-inflammatory drugs in the third trimester, angiotensin-converting enzyme inhibitors, valproic acid, and methotrexate.—**BMT**

- Most radiographic studies expose the fetus to a low and safe level of radiation, especially if there is lead shielding of the fetus. Accordingly, if you believe a radiographic study is indicated for maternal reasons, you should generally pursue it.—**BMT**

- Remember that pregnant women will come to the ICU after delivery as well—especially for severe pre-eclampsia and eclampsia (monitoring and continuation of therapy such as magnesium for up to 24 hours) or if there was a bleeding complication in the OR. Don't argue the matter, if the OB suite calls you for an admission, they need one. Remember that you no longer have the gravid uterus, but the physiological changes of pregnancy essentially continue through the immediate post-partum period. You should be current and comfortable with post-partum care and patient-centered medicine as you must remember that you have a new mother in your midst, assuming the baby has done okay. Utilize every resource to maximize time with the parturient's time with the newborn and the family and support group.—**Editors**

- Back in the day, when I was training, we tended to send all pregnant women to a monitored bed for 24 hours postoperatively or post-procedure for fetal monitoring and tocolysis, if necessary. Find out what your department's policies are or develop them and lean to the conservative side of the issues.—**CM**

- <u>The single most difficult case</u> I ever did during the eight years I was at Hopkins—and in my entire career—was a pregnant trauma case who came to the OR one night as a helicopter transport from a major nearby highway with severe blunt trauma from a motor vehicle accident. I remarked to the charge nurse that I was sure the patient would go to Shock Trauma. "Nope," said the nurse, "They're on flyby. The patient's coming here." She was very young—like 22 years old—but she had chest trauma (hemothorax, pneumothorax), abdominal trauma, extremity bony and soft tissue trauma, and a broken pelvis. And she was pregnant—about 20–21 weeks' gestation—just under viability for that era.—**CM**

- <u>Most difficult case, part 2:</u> I was a fairly new attending at the time, and I remember calling down to the OB suite to ask them to send a nurse up to do fetal monitoring. They initially declined—nonviable fetus by dates and what seemed like an impossible barrier to the monitoring itself, given the amount of trauma—but changed their minds and sent a nurse up when I offered to pay somebody coming off shift out of my own pocket to do it (the nurse that came up refused to let me pay her separately but said the offer told them how desperate I was for fetal monitoring). The very experienced OB nurse did manage to establish a fetal trace and did a fantastic job throughout the case, which was about 10 hours long. We didn't compromise trauma care of the mother, but I evaluated and considered the fetal hemodynamics with every clinical decision we made. I just remembered thinking, "I hope the baby is getting some of this oxygen."—**CM**

- <u>Most difficult case, conclusion:</u> I still don't know how we kept that mother and fetus alive during that massive transfusion protocol, which went on and on as different surgical teams rotated through, and we gave her about 90 units of blood. I think it was because the higher powers intervened on our side, I truly do, and the fact that she was very young. I remember that **Pete Pronovost** was the ICU attending covering that night and talking to him several times during the case, and that he came in from home around 4 AM to receive the patient in the ICU. She did go into labor about 24 hours later, which was successfully terminated with tocolysis. This was the single most technically challenging case I ever did. As I recall, she went on to deliver a healthy infant.—**CM**

The Burn ICU

- Burn injuries are absolutely devastating. Not only are they incredibly painful but they are also psychologically and emotionally difficult for the patients and families. It is the only type of traumatic injury that has a dedicated ICU location.—**Editors**

- Large burns are terrible, of course, but patients also can have life-long sequelae and emotional distress from burns suffered on the face, hands, and genitals, even if the burned surface is relatively small. The depth of the burn is also very important.—**CFB**

- For inhalation injury or suspected inhalation injury, intubate at the first sign that criteria are met, for example, stridor or increased work of breathing, before the airway closes. *Don't wait.*—**BDW**

- Carboxyhemoglobin levels do not correlate with risk of mortality though >30% COHb is considered severe carbon monoxide (CO) poisoning.—**BDW**

- The pulse ox is unreliable in face of CO poisoning. Get frequent blood gases preferably with a co-oximeter that can differentiate OxyHb and COHb.—**BDW**

- Burn patients seem to be on the forefront of microbial resistance. They get infected with the worse organisms; *Mucor species, Candida auris*, multi-drug resistant *Acinetobacter*, multi-drug resistant *Pseudomonas species*, and so forth. Be aggressive with infection control and treatment while still trying to be a good steward of antibiotics. It's a tough balance.—**BDW**

- Separating systemic immune response syndrome from the burns and the special dressings and grafts like allograft, from infection can be difficult. Once infection sets in, though, it can be a disaster.—**BDW**

- Despite best efforts in the OR, the burn patient almost always comes out of the OR under-resuscitated or if they are adequately resuscitated, they get behind quickly once back in the unit. Be generous with the fluid and blood. This is, of course, after the initial first 24-hour resuscitation, which follows one of the standard formulas like the modified Parkland formula.—**BDW**

  https://www.uab.edu/medicine/anesthesiology/faculty

- Ketamine is a great agent for helping with pain management in addition to narcotics and gabapentin.—**BDW**

- Burn rehab can be very, very challenging. Please feel free to consult and confer with your rehab team frequently. Some burn units have the rehab staff round on patients several times a week.—**CFB**

- Positioning patients properly, using splints, and at times, even a rigid cast that gets bi-valved can be critical.—**CFB**

- Shoulder range of motion and finger range of motion are particularly challenging in burn patients. Plan positioning and line placement so that these can be optimized.—**CFB**

A Surgeon's Perspective

- As a surgeon, getting my patient out of the ICU as quickly as possible so rehab can begin is very important to me. Extubation as soon as reasonably safe facilitates this. It can be a source of frustration waiting for medications to be weaned so that the patient is conscious enough to safely extubate, and even more frustrating when disinhibition necessitates sedating the patient again. Those precious days slipping by can increase the odds of iatrogenic complications—ventilator-associated pneumonia, hospital-acquired pressure injuries, urinary tract infections and the like. As much as I appreciate the care my patients receive in the ICU, I do appreciate the patient leaving the ICU as soon as possible.—**EJD**

- It is important to me that I am on the same page as the intensivist. Any decisions about the de-escalation of treatment should be handled jointly. It is sometimes surprising how perceptions and points of view differ—what looks hopeless to one provider may be routine and par for the course to another. Getting the message straight before approaching the patient and their family is critical, as is a mutually agreeable joint plan of action.—**EJD**

- If the patient was a difficult intubation to begin with, there is nothing in the ICU environment that will make this easier should the patient require reintubation. Consider extubation in the OR—it is a controlled environment where the surgeon and anesthesiologist may have more light, tools, and help at their disposal to manage a situation should it deteriorate.—**EJD**

- Note: The *Anesthesia Bridges* authors and editors agree with Ed Damrose's concerns in the above wisdom, but perhaps not his conclusions for *every case*. Because the one thing the ICU offers that the OR doesn't is time.—**Editors**

- Elective tracheostomy in these situations may be preferable to uncertain extubation as reestablishment of mechanical ventilation may be made simpler. When in doubt, do the tracheostomy.—**EJD**

- Sometimes colleagues insist on carrying on treatment even when the situation is futile. Consider an ethics consult if you feel you are being forced to provide treatment that is inappropriate. Sometimes the viewpoints and input of other members of the care team is necessary to facilitate the decision to deescalate. The same situation applies if family members are unrealistic and insist on futile life-sustaining measures.—**EJD**

- If the drain output is low, but the patient is not responding clinically the way you expect, trust your judgment. The drain may be malfunctioning and not doing what you think it's doing. It may need to be replaced.—**EJD**

Are Regional Anesthesia and Complementary Medicine Techniques Underutilized in the ICU?

- The most common regional anesthesia techniques seen in the ICUs are probably epidural catheters and femoral catheters. This isn't likely to change any time soon but be careful with your ICU epidural catheters. First of all, *they do migrate!* The very first time I gave intralipid was in the little ICU at the

Philadelphia VA and an epidural catheter had been dosed. Evidently, the whole dose went intravascular, and the patient arrested. The intralipid worked like a charm, as I recall. Fifteen minutes later the patient was sitting up in bed, talking to us and said, "Did a bunch of people rush in here for some reason?"—**CM**

- Second, we can't tell you the number of times that ICU epidurals get dosed, and then the team is dealing with a confusing clinical situation in trying to figure out why the patient is hypotensive. Especially if they also spike a fever. Or if the patient has to go urgently to the OR. Or if you are trying to make a clinical assessment about the volume status. They can be really effective in pain management but make sure you have control of the epidural and not the other way around.—**Editors**

- There's a good article on the NYSORA website that makes the point that, right now, there are no large randomized, controlled trials or large prospective trials looking at continuous upper extremity blocks in critically ill patients [2]. This is a shame as upper extremity trauma is very common in a number of injury situations, such as falls and blunt chest trauma, and there are a number of approaches and blocks that can be used such continuous interscalene and continuous cervical paravertebral blocks.—**Editors**

- In terms of integrative medicine techniques, we think they are also underutilized. As we were talking about this amongst ourselves and looking at the literature on the use of integrative medicine, we were surprised how little of it was in the anesthesiology and critical care journals. It's not a competition between specialties (including nursing), but let's change who is leading this area of clinical research?—**Editors**

- The integrative medicine interventions to improve sleep quality and quantity, especially meditation and acupuncture, seem to be fairly effective and easy to do.—**Editors**

- But the range of integrative techniques that have been tried is pretty big—guided imagery, biofeedback, aromatherapy, massage, healing touch, music therapy, mind-body sessions, and (get this) garlic tablets.—**Editors**

- But we think the coolest complimentary technique is, hands down, pet therapy. And, yes, it can be done in the ICU. The medical critical care and rehab medicine departments at Hopkins got together and published a review and editorial in 2018 in *Critical Care* in which they called animal-assisted interventions the "exemplars" of non-pharmacologic modalities to reduce suffering and encourage recovery behavior [3]. Honestly, it seems as if there are pretty much no clinical issues that a dog isn't going to help, ranging from "I can't breathe, I'm dying" to "I am worthless and a burden." It appears that the trick is to put the dog right in the bed with the patient (Fig. 169.6).—**Editors**

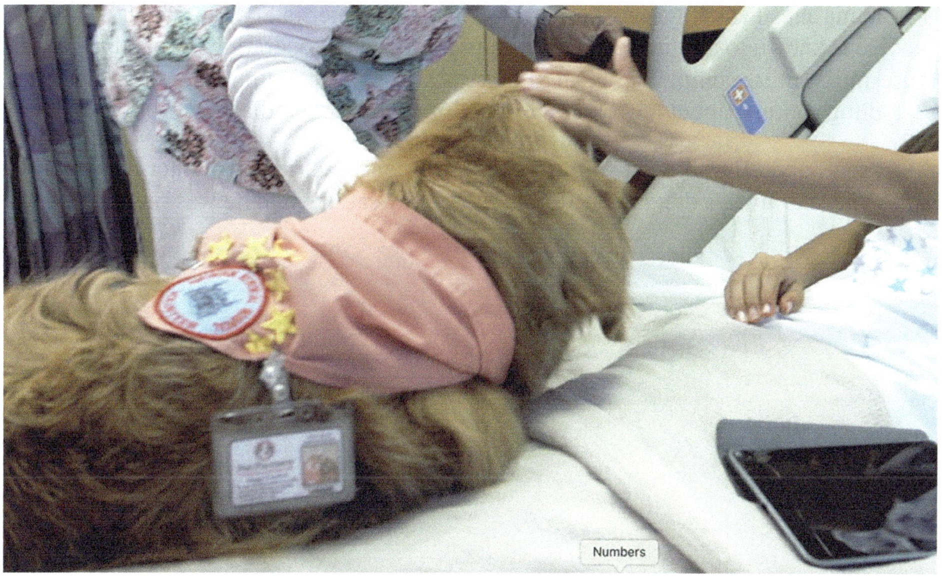

Fig. 169.6 A good boy suited up and getting ready to work his magic. Notice the patient has put her tablet down to interact with the dog! Photo: Image used under standard license from iStock.com

References

1. Tashkandi H. Honey in wound healing: an updated review. Open Life Sci. 2021 Oct 6. Published online.
2. Operater. Regional Analgesia in the Critically ill Patient—NYSORA [Internet]. NYSORA. 2018 [cited 2025 Jul 27]. Available from: https://www.nysora.com/topics/sub-specialties/comorbidities/regional-analgesia-critically-ill/#toc_PERIPHERAL-NERVE-BLOCKS-FOR-THE-UPPER-EXTREMITIES.
3. Hosey MM, Jaskulski J, Wegener ST, et al. Animal-assisted intervention in the ICU: a tool for humanization. Crit Care. 2018;22(1):22.

Authors

Brad Winters is an intensivist, long-distance cyclist, kayaker, model train geek, and *former* mountain and ice climber—because when you hit 60 years old, you slow down a bit. Despite his protests, his daughter has gone into medicine, and he is immensely proud of her. His son is studying to be a pastry chef, and Dr. Winters has had to increase his cycling to deal with the side effects of his son's excellent career. His lovely wife of over 30 years is a good sport about his hobbies and said he can buy a motorcycle when he retires since he gave up mountain climbing.

Brant Wagener is an intensivist, anesthesiologist, and scientist at the University of Alabama at Birmingham. He tries to provide four things at his job every day—dad jokes, movie/book quotes, song lyrics, and common sense. He and his wife Jennifer are the parents of three great kids that want to rule the world and one obnoxious Labrador dog that wants to eat it. He reads eclectically and as much as he can, always makes time to play with kids, doesn't travel as much as he wants, and would love to run a marathon, but cannot find the time.

Andrew Barker is an anesthesiologist and intensivist at University of Alabama at Birmingham where he is the associate medical director of the SICU and program director of the critical care Medicine fellowship. At work Dr. Barker is a fun guy and never met a fungal infection he didn't want to do battle with. Outside of work, Andrew holds the position of household chief entertainment officer, where he spends his time managing entropy and herding cats.

Raj Nathwani is a trauma anesthesiologist at Harborview Medical Center in Seattle, which is part of the University of Washington system. He is known to be a careful and calm presence in the operating room, and especially enjoys delivering anesthesia care in the most complex clinical situations. Besides spending time with his wife and busy young family, Raj enjoys cycling and just about any other activity done outdoors in the beautiful Northwest.

Cathy Marcucci is a senior anesthesiologist who trained in residency with Brad Winters and then was junior faculty with him at Hopkins. She was always delighted to sign out her OR cases when he was on service.

Part IX

Personal Stories

The Chesapeake Bay Bridge—Annapolis, MD

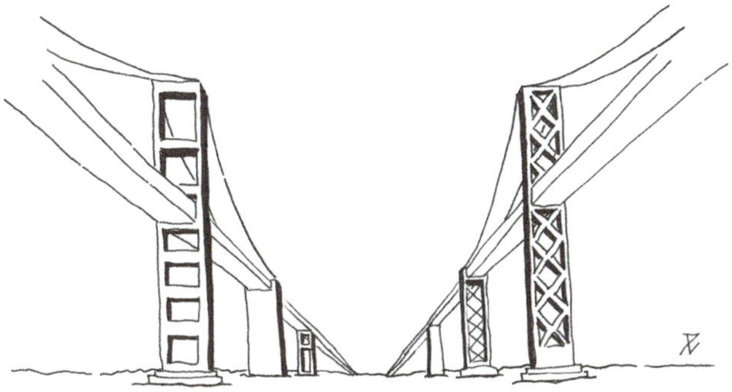

The Chesapeake Bay Bridge, which is officially named the Gov. William Preston Lane Jr. Memorial Bridge, is a dual-span bridge that spans the Chesapeake Bay in Maryland. It was selected as a favorite bridge by editor **Ron Bank** and author **Allan Gottschalk**.

It connects the capital city of Annapolis on the west side of the bridge to Stevensville, Maryland on Kent Island on the east side. The original span opened in 1952 and had a length of 4.3 miles. It was the world's longest continuous over-water steel structure. The parallel bridge was constructed and completed in 1973. Because of its height, the narrowness of the spans, the lack of hard shoulders, the low guardrails, and the frequency of high winds, it is often cited as one of the scariest bridges in the United States. However, for many Marylanders, it is a sentimental favorite as it is the literal and emotional gateway to a lifetime of summers spent at the Maryland and southern Delaware beaches. It is also a beautiful gargantuan sky sculpture for the people who sail back and forth under it on the Chesapeake Bay.

Ron, Allan, and the editors of *Anesthesia Bridges* thank **Daniel Nemec** of The Architectural Team in Boston, MA, for this stunning perspective drawing of the bridge.

170 Introduction

Catherine Marcucci

It's so important to remember that anesthesiology is a living, not a life. My mother once wondered if anesthesia is something that people had a lot of fun with in their spare time and advised that it was perhaps a good idea to keep up my outside interests and activities. Since most things in life benefit from a balancing test, we asked our authors and editors to tell us about their own backgrounds and life journeys and how they combined anesthesiology with the priorities in their lives outside the OR and hospital. We were delighted when the essays and personal photos started arriving with words of wisdom on how our colleagues managed their family and home lives and outside interests at various stages of their careers. For instance, we were intrigued that **Nee Dalal** negotiated a planned move for her family by telling her husband, "I'm open to considering any location, as long as it has at least a million people."

We extend our deepest thanks to the Dalal-Taylor, Gottschalk, and Peterson families and Drs. Zvara, Cattaneo, and Axley for searching their files and taking the time to send us their collective experiences, advice, and wisdom. Always remember, though, that families come in all shapes, sizes, and configurations, and not every life is about raising children. What's most important is that your personal story be centered around you—your own priorities and experiences—whomever and whatever that may involve. And that you support your team and the people that depend on you (Fig. 170.1).

C. Marcucci (✉)
Department of Transfusion Medicine, Clinical Center, National Institutes of Health, Bethesda, MD, USA

S. Mohamed et al. (eds.), *Anesthesia Bridges*, https://doi.org/10.1007/978-3-032-08294-7_170

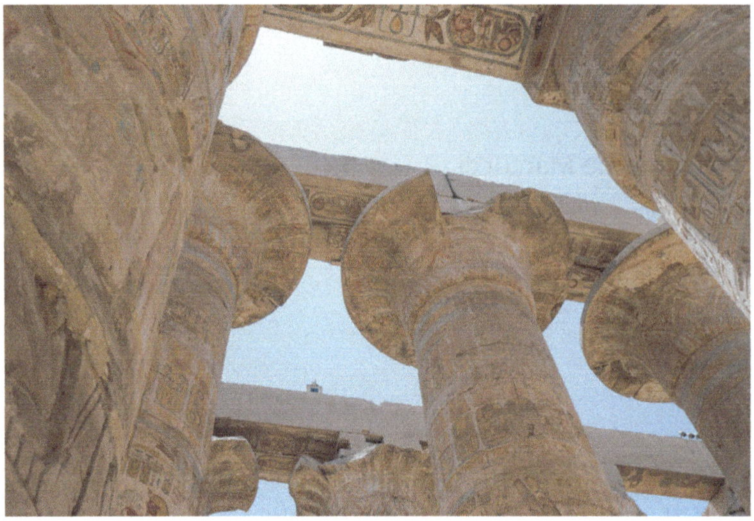

Fig. 170.1 Beautiful columns supporting beams in an ancient temple structure in Egypt. Photo: Juan Marcos, image used under standard license from iStock.com

Author

Cathy Marcucci is a senior academic anesthesiologist and inveterate anesthesiology educator. She is also fellowship-trained in transfusion medicine. When not taking care of patients and/or putting the latest book together, she dedicates her time to mentoring junior colleagues, writing copy for animal rescues, and travel.

Med School, Marriage, and a Medical Family

171

Niloofer F. Dalal, Nicholas B. Taylor, Zachary R. Taylor, and Catherine Marcucci

Contributor:

Catherine Marcucci, MD

Introduction

Niloofer "Nee" Dalal and **Grant Taylor** were members of the Temple University School of Medicine Class of 1991. Nee stayed at Temple to train in anesthesiology and has had a busy life as full-time clinician, spouse, and mother. She practices in the larger Emory health care system. Grant is a general surgeon in a small practice in Douglasville, Georgia. Nick Taylor is a surgical resident at Jefferson Abdingdon Hospital. Zachary Taylor is a chemist by training who is transitioning into an IT career. Here is their advice.

Early Days

I was born in India and came to the US as a toddler, while my dad did his Fulbright scholarship at Penn. My parents relocated to Philadelphia permanently when I was seven years old. I attended a suburban public high school, then went on to Swarthmore College, followed by a master's degree at Temple, before moving to Penn. Eventually, I decided that research was not for me. My mentor advised me to attend medical school, and I was accepted to several places, but I ended up at Temple, where my father was teaching and where I had free tuition. Grant and I came from two ends of the medical school spectrum

N. F. Dalal
Emory Clinic, School of Medicine Faculty, Emory Health Care, Atlanta, GA, USA

N. B. Taylor
General Surgery Residency Program, Jefferson Abingdon Hospital, Abingdon, PA, USA

Z. R. Taylor
Philadelphia, PA, USA

C. Marcucci (✉)
Department of Transfusion Medicine, Clinical Center, National Institutes of Health, Bethesda, MD, USA

S. Mohamed et al. (eds.), *Anesthesia Bridges*, https://doi.org/10.1007/978-3-032-08294-7_171

when we met. Grant had always wanted to be a doctor and came to medical school straight from college. He was from a small town in western PA, the first in his family to go to college, let alone medical school.

Courtship and Wedding

Our first sustained contact was when he was invited, simply because he had a station wagon, on a sailing trip to the Keys just after our neuroanatomy exam in January 1988. The rest of us on the trip were older and somehow connected to Swarthmore.

We became roommates with others the next few years, and I found it comforting to have someone to go out to dinner with or on a bike ride when I hit a wall studying. It allowed us to stay grounded and not isolated during stressful times. We lived together for two years, but there was always an extra bedroom on the premises to appease my mother's "sensibilities." After we decided to get married, she gave up, and we lived in my old bedroom at home to save money.

We were engaged at the Taj Mahal when we went for a family wedding. The trip was the first time Grant had left the US (a whole other story). My parents were British-educated in India, and very Westernized, but still had Eastern values to some extent. Grant and my mother pretty much decided on our wedding details. I had grown up being the kitchen help for my mother's large parties so I knew she would do a great job organizing everything for our civil ceremony. I wore my mother's wedding sari (easier than shopping for a dress), my cousins in the party wore their wedding saris, and all the men wore suits. My parents' attitude was they had brought me to this country and therefore accepted my decision to marry outside our religion, which meant that I would no longer be considered a Zoroastrian.

Doing Residencies with Two Babies!

We did the couples match—but not with a lot of thought. We ended up in Philadelphia, which was not what we expected. Grant matched at Hahnemann for categorical surgery, and I stayed at Temple. Residency was a trying time. I found out I was pregnant during my CA1 year while we were in Japan for an endoscopy rotation that Grant was doing.

I delivered Nick in November of my CA-1 year and went back after 4 weeks. We tried daycare, but then realized that we needed a nanny. Marie was a single Italian lady who had just retired from AT&T. She ran the house and me, but truly loved Nick as her own. I didn't breastfeed because I was on my CT rotation and never thought of asking to pump. I somehow became chief resident and allowed everyone else to pick their electives, so I ended up with mostly NICU/Peds and ICU rotations. In fact, as an attending, I had to teach myself blocks, without ultrasound, since I only did 1 month of pain.

I took Nick to visit my grandmother in India and found out I was pregnant again with Zack. Needless to say, I never left the US for a long time after! I took my written boards 6 months pregnant, and the orals were just postpartum. It never occurred to me that I should defer for a year.

When Nick was born, Grant had decided to do two years of research at CHOP after his second year of general surgery residency. So, I knew that I would have to get a job in Philly for a few years until Grant finished. I decided not to stay at Temple but to go into private practice—which paid more.

I was hired by Allegheny Health Network when it owned Hahnemann and Medical College of Pennsylvania, but I worked at their small community hospitals. It was a transition from university anesthesia with lots of support to an old-school captain of the ship OR mentality. My mentor, Alan Jay Schwartz, taught me by example how to advocate for patients during discussions with questionable surgeons. I have never felt the need to back down or compromise clinical care. I have often been told I have a surgical temperament, in the sense of gaining their respect. I think being around the best and brightest during my formative years at Swarthmore has a lot to do with who I am today.

We had Zack while we were still in Philly and realized I would have to compartmentalize my work from my home life. Though I had really enjoyed research, I knew I would have to "just" be a staff anesthesiologist. It has not always been the easiest fit—for example, many of my recent bosses find me intolerant and abrasive, but I get very positive feedback from the clinical staff. I've been told they can trust what I say because I am blunt and do not play games.

Pennsylvania and Georgia

I followed Grant to his small town in Western PA after he finished, and tried my best to fit in. But seven years later, I told him that we had to move for the kids, and he could pick any city with more than a million people. We have been in Atlanta since 2005. It has worked well professionally—Grant works in a small rural hospital with two partners that he enjoys working with and I am part of the Emory system.

When I joined Emory Anesthesia, we were just forming an outpatient community service that was separate from the main university. We were a money maker and therefore had autonomy. But when we had to close down surgical centers (17 or so) for COVID they had to support us. They are now in the process of trying to merge us into their university fold—with all the bureaucracy that goes with it.

Family First!

Family life has always been of primary importance to us. When we moved to Atlanta, Grant was fixated on the boys going to public school, so we looked up the relevant ACT and SAT scores and moved to East Cobb, Georgia. We have since downsized and moved to Vinings, which is closer to the city for the airport, restaurants, and theater.

Vacations have always been our family's favorite way for the four of us to connect. The boys learned to ski in Stowe, Vermont, when they were four and seven years old. They took weeks of lessons, and by the time we took them out west to Colorado or Utah, they were on double black trails, and Grant and I were cruising blue runs. They still go on trips together when they can. We have also taken several backroad biking trips, since they are tailored to different skill levels.

We started taking the kids abroad early, and they have been to most of Europe (Fig. 171.1). We have also been farther from home—to India for two weeks and to Australia to SCUBA for two weeks. Our last big trip was over the Christmas/New Year's holiday in 2019–2020. We traveled and biked through Korea, Singapore, Vietnam, Cambodia, and Thailand. We were on 15 flights and all got COVID, although we did not know what it was at the time, of course. Luckily, we were all well enough to travel home.

I tried to direct both our boys away from medicine in college since they did not have the drive at that stage to excel in medicine. Both Emory and Wake Forrest have great business schools and great STEM programs. Nick decided to go into medicine, and Zack is a natural science/engineering/tech guy and said thanks, but no thanks to medicine. They each seem to have chosen their career directions for good reasons—intellectual curiosity and the right fit for their personalities. They are well prepared because of their multigenerational/ethnic upbringing and watching us through the years. Nick got engaged to Sarah whom he met at Emory, and she went to Drexel Med, graduating in 2023. She decided on a career in anesthesiology, go figure. All three of these young adults are really great people!

***Note from the Editors:** Nee loves the Ponte Vecchio in Florence (Figs. 171.1 and 171.2). She tells us: "My favorite Italian city is Florence for its art and history. Many family vacations have included this city since I never tire of visiting it."

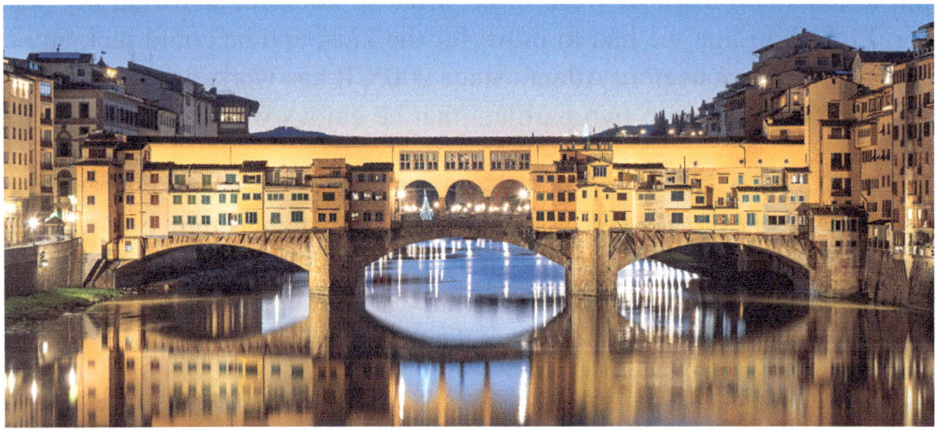

Fig. 171.1 The Ponte Vecchio Bridge in Florence. This famous bridge, whose name means "Old Bridge" in Italian, was constructed as a close-spandrel segmental arch bridge over the Arno River in Italy. It is built on the site of a Roman bridge at the narrowest point of the river. It is first referenced in history in 996, but has been swept away and rebuilt several times. It has always hosted shops and merchants, which at one point were all butcher shops, vegetable stalls, and tanners. Today, only jewelers, art dealers, and souvenir shops are allowed. It was the only bridge in Florence that was not purposely destroyed in WW2. Photo: Image used under standard license from shutterstock.com

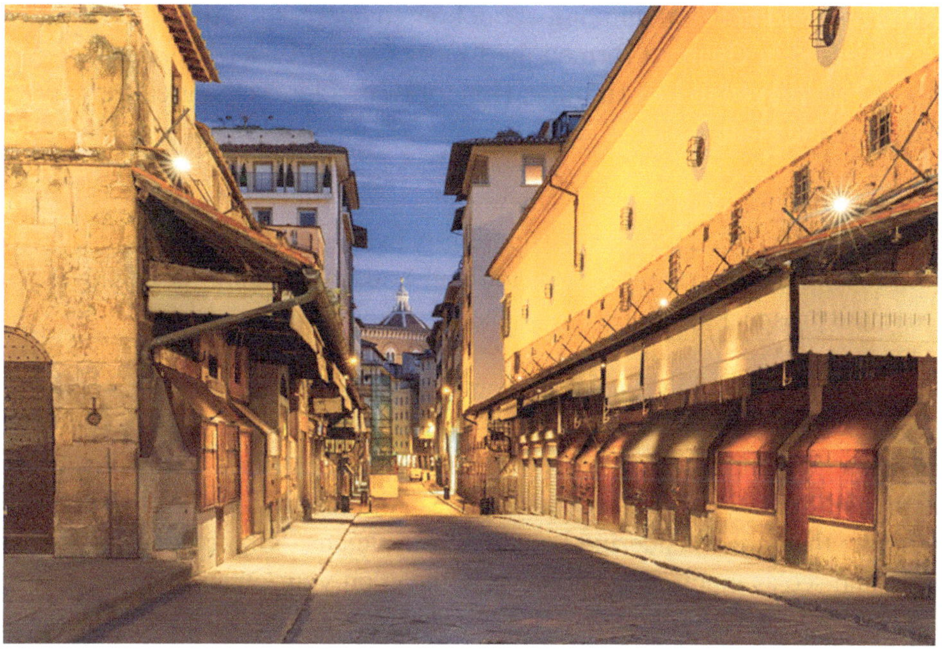

Fig. 171.2. A stunning view looking down the Ponte Vecchio. Photo: Image used under standard license from shutterstock.com

From Nick Taylor

I was raised by physicians, and this caused some humorous moments when I still lived at home—for instance, I remember well my friend James' mouth hanging open as he sat motionless at my family's dinner table. He looked a little ill but also intrigued. We listened as my dad spoke in detail about managing a perforated bowel on the OR table, while my mom chimed in about profound hypotension and used the words, "trying to die on rocket fuel." We continued our animated conversation, but James was too stunned to eat. That was the first time it struck me that our normal household dinner conversation might not be so commonplace.

I entered college at Emory University with a love of high school science and thoughts of applying to medical school, but was strongly advised by both family and mentors to avoid the tunnel vision of many college freshmen. So, I took classes I never imagined I would enjoy—who knew that a course centered around the question "Why are we?" would have made me think I could be a lawyer or professor of philosophy. To heed the advice of those I admired, I enrolled in a variety of classes and participated in activities such as backpacking, club tennis, and volunteering in my community.

My desire to go into medicine remained, however. But I was determined to experience medicine on my own terms, and this led me to join Emory's Global Medical Brigades. In Ghana, I saw hospitals that were wall-less huts, disposable medical supplies were often reused, and people were suffering life-threatening complications from diseases that could easily be treated with a $2 prescription at home. There, I realized that the scope of medicine was much bigger than a dinner table conversation or summer break days spent shadowing friends of my parents.

When I came home, I could not stop thinking about how to address the root causes of the public health problems that I witnessed in Ghana. I formed the Emory Global Water Brigades under the auspices of Global Brigades. We journeyed to Los Hatillos, Honduras, to address the greatest public health need in that community: access to clean water.

After returning from Honduras, I discovered a new enthusiasm for science, fueled by the hope to impact public and global health. I pursued a research opportunity in a neuroscience laboratory where we focused on the effects of anesthesia on cognitive function and how to mitigate its negative outcomes, which opened my eyes to the prospect of a career in academic medicine.

Having a family in medicine helped me to get an intimate glimpse into the world of healthcare, of course. But I feel very grateful that my parents, at every step, encouraged me to develop wide general interests and increasing personal ownership of my medical career. They were beyond supportive of my efforts to work on public health projects outside the US. And that is my advice to the younger members of medical families if they are considering becoming physicians—branch out from what you've heard at the dinner table and see as much of medicine as you can on your own.

From Zachary Taylor

Growing up with parents who are physicians, I often tuned out the dinner conversation which centered around caring for patients because it wasn't hugely interesting to me. I was also encouraged to explore many different disciplines while in college at Wake Forest. I was a chemistry major and took both liberal arts courses and science courses, including elective courses on medicinal chemistry and biochemistry. I became interested in the central role proteins played in the human body, so I wrote a grant to study mutations in a bacterial protein originally found in cystic fibrosis patients. Because I wasn't in the pre-med grind, I had the chance to really delve deeply into my protein research. I also spent a lot of time in the lab working on my honors chemistry thesis.

I also founded, chartered, and launched a club called Wake for Warriors, which was deeply meaningful but took a lot of time that I might not have had if I had been preparing to apply to medical schools.

The *Anesthesia Bridges* editors asked me for my specific advice for medical families with kids considering, or not considering, medical school. I would say that my parents got it right by insisting that I not consider a career in medicine to be a foregone conclusion. They were always supportive and asked that I take a variety of courses and pursue other activities that didn't necessarily lead to medical school. I am very grateful for my degree in chemistry and the time I spent in career-enriching and life-enriching activities that weren't about pursuing a medical career. These days, I am working on my coding skills and considering additional coursework to add IT credentials to my CV. My parents are totally fine with me not being a physician—they aren't the types to insist on something that I am not strongly called to do.

Lessons Learned (From Nee Dalal)

- I make a point of telling fresh grads the few things that I have learned along the way. It's important to share what's worked for you.

- I was only one of two women when I joined the specialty arm of Emory. We are now over 50% women with two in leadership positions. To get to where we are today, we needed broad shoulders and had to keep pushing for what was right.

- Your clinical skills and judgment are your saving grace. Stay on the call schedule for 5–10 years. That is where you learn to be independent.

- We have come a long way with accepting childbearing in our specialty, but juggling small children and work will be your greatest challenge. Ask for help, but be aware of the strain it may cause the group and try to compensate.

- We had a medical household, and my children grew up listening to medical conversations at the dinner table. But of course, they were raised by parents who were medical school classmates! One son is a physician, and our other son is a tech guy. We insisted that their college experiences be as well-rounded as possible in terms of coursework, clubs, and travel and that they develop their own approaches to their careers, determining for themselves what is right for them.

- Figure out what you want your family's methods of connecting and enjoying each other to be and don't be afraid to invest in them. *Always remember that your kids are your legacy!* (Fig. 171.3)

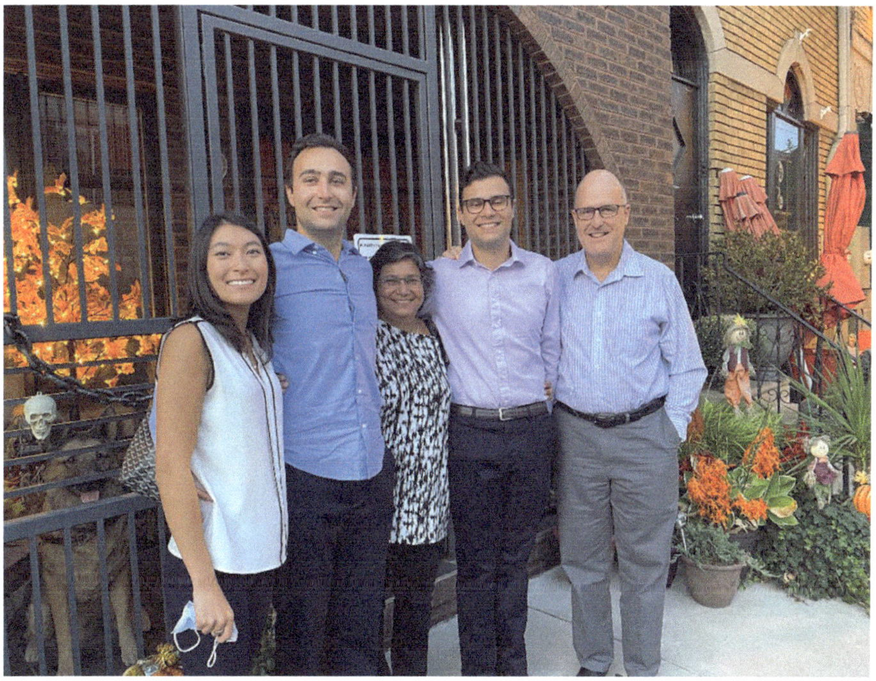

Fig. 171.3 The wonderful Dalal-Taylor group on a recent family outing. From left to right: Sarah Lee, MD, Nicholas Taylor, MD, Niloofer Dalal, MD, Zachary Taylor, and Grant Taylor, MD. Sarah graduated from Drexel in 2023 and is starting her career as an anesthesiologist. Photo: Collection of the Dalal-Taylor family

Authors

Nee Dalal found fun and family time during long weekends in Sarasota, Florida after buying a house there during the first year of the COVID epidemic. She and Grant get there as often as they can. Their Sarasota dream house is under construction.

Nick Taylor is a busy general surgery resident but still finds time to enjoy Philadelphian culture with Sarah Lee, whom he is helping to learn to ski. Local hills, however, do not compare with Vermont or out West, so major ski trips are always in the works.

Zack Taylor is a chemist by training who lives in Philadelphia. He has totally embraced the Philly sports teams, including the 76ers and, of course, the Phillies. His Bernese Mountain Dog and brother Gus remain at home in Atlanta with good old Mom and Dad, so Zack is now the proud papa to his own 100-pound baby, Berner Winston.

Cathy Marcucci is a senior academic anesthesiologist and inveterate anesthesiology educator. She is also fellowship-trained in transfusion medicine. When she is not taking care of patients and/or putting the latest book together, she dedicates her time to mentoring junior colleagues, writing copy for animal rescues, and travelling.

Grant Taylor On Life with His Favorite Anesthesiologist

172

Grant Taylor and Catherine Marcucci

Contributor:

Catherine Marcucci, MD

Introduction

Grant Taylor and **Nee Dalal** were one of the four couples from the Temple University School of Medicine Class of 1991 to marry. He took time from his busy life and practice to fill us in on some additional parts of their story.

Early Life

I grew up in a very small town in western Pennsylvania with a population of only 5000 people. My family was lower middle class. My father worked in a steel mill, and my mother worked in the catalog department at JCPenney's. My parents did the best they could to provide a good life for us. I always idolized the physicians in town and at a very early age decided to pursue a career in medicine.

Med School at Temple

I worked hard in high school and college and was fortunate to be accepted to medical school at Temple University. I certainly experienced culture shock going from such a small town to a major metropolitan city. Since I knew nothing about Philadelphia, I chose to live in the East Falls section of the city. I did not know anyone at medical school and so lived alone. It was difficult, but I soon made friends with my anatomy group.

G. Taylor
Wellstar General Surgery, Douglasville, GA, USA

C. Marcucci (✉)
Department of Transfusion Medicine, Clinical Center, National Institutes of Health, Bethesda, MD, USA

S. Mohamed et al. (eds.), *Anesthesia Bridges*, https://doi.org/10.1007/978-3-032-08294-7_172

One of my partners in anatomy planned a trip to Florida after the neuroanatomy exam that we took in January 1988. During his planning, he did not consider transportation. I owned an older station wagon, and when one of the guests dropped out, I was invited to go, most likely for my transportation. The car was an old Dodge station wagon with red vinyl seats that I bought for $1000 before coming to medical school. Certainly not a luxury ride.

Meeting Nee Dalal

I had noticed Niloofer during our anatomy dissection classes. I thought it was very cute that she required a small stepladder to be able to see the dissections. During this trip we connected, and we became friends and started dating. Our first date was in February 1988 after we returned from our trip. We went to see *Good Morning Vietnam*, starring Robin Williams. Niloofer still distinctly remembers our first date, since I had to borrow money to pay for the movie. I stayed in Philadelphia for the summer to work, and our relationship blossomed. We decided to live together starting in the second year. For the second and third year, we shared large apartments with roommates. During our fourth year, we lived in Niloofer's parents' house to save money.

I must admit that it had been very lonely just studying and eating during my first year. Since I was new to the city, I was very shy about traveling outside of my apartment. Niloofer expanded my horizons as she introduced me to big city life. It was very comforting to have somebody going through the same process, as she was able to understand the stress involved with medical school. No matter how many times we explained it to our parents and hometown friends, our situation was beyond their comprehension. In fact, even today, I feel our parents still don't understand what we have experienced.

Our Early Life Together

I thoroughly enjoyed my time with Niloofer, as she became the love of my life and my best friend. Her parents planned a trip to India for her cousin's wedding during our third year, and I was invited to go. I decided to ask her to marry me while we were visiting the Taj Mahal during the visit—and we set a date for the week after we graduated from medical school. This was a very busy time for us and somewhat overwhelming. We did the couples match and actually matched in Philadelphia, which made our transition from med school a little easier.

Our residencies were both very demanding, and it was comforting to have a spouse who was experiencing the same type of schedule. During residency, I decided I wanted to do pediatric surgery. To enhance my CV, I decided to do research at the Children's Hospital of Philadelphia. During this time, we had our first child, Nicholas. To this day, I'm still not sure how Niloofer was able to handle our family life, anesthesia residency, and having our first son. Our second son, Zachary, was born when Niloofer was a first year attending. I had returned to my general surgery residency and was no help with the children. Again, I'm not sure how we made it through this time, but I give Nee the credit for managing to keep us going forward (Fig. 172.1).

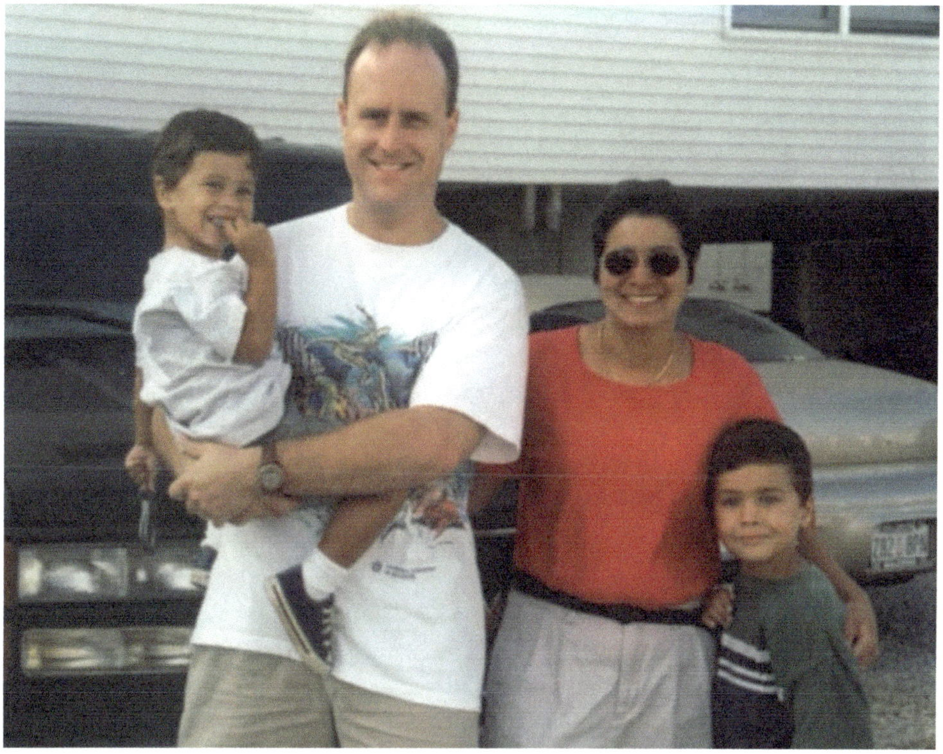

Fig. 172.1 Nee and Grant, in the early days in Hermitage, PA, with their adorable boys, making it look easy. Zack is in his father's arms, and Nick is next to Nee. Photo: Collection of the Dalal-Taylor family

Real Life

When I finished general surgery residency, I had decided that I did not want to do two more years of training or a pediatric surgery fellowship. I therefore took a job in general surgery. The best job for me at the time was in the area where I had grown up. It was now time for Niloofer to experience culture shock. I moved her from her large metropolitan area to my very small town. After 7 years, she decided it was time to return to a large city. At the time of our move to Atlanta, our children were 11 and 8. We both started new jobs and hired an *au pair* to help with the children. We enjoyed having Lina to help care for our children, but she decided to return to Germany. Fortunately, Niloofer's parents moved in with us. They were a great help while we were getting our careers started (Fig. 172.2).

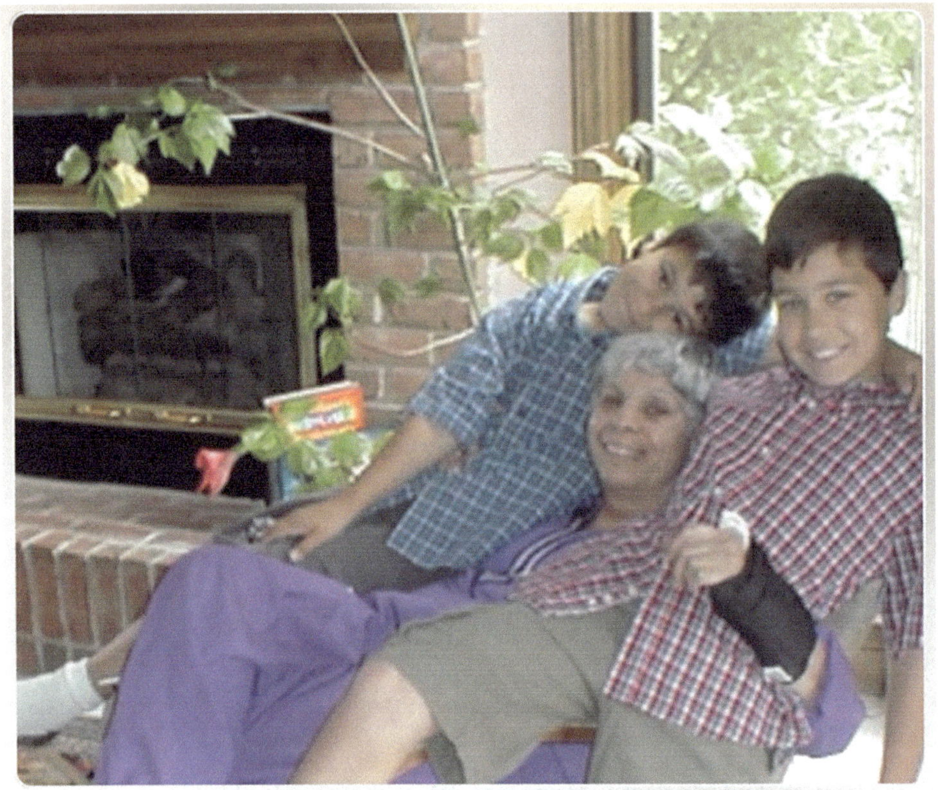

Fig. 172.2 The boys with Jeroo Dalal, their beloved Nana and Nee's beautiful Mom, around 2004. Photo: Collection of the Dalal-Taylor family

The Kids

One of our sons has decided to pursue a career in medicine, the other is a chemist, although his mother and I think he would also be an excellent engineer. Even though they had many disappointments at our missing childhood plays or concerts, as they grew older, they understood our dilemmas. Niloofer and I would frequently talk about our experiences in medicine around the children. I am sure these discussions helped the children decide on their careers in and out of medicine, since they saw up close what we did—both the good and the bad.

Our older son, Nicholas, graduated from Temple Medical School. Nick is now a general surgery resident at Abington Jefferson Hospital. Our younger son, Zachary, graduated with a degree in chemistry. He still has not decided on his ultimate career; however, he is leaning towards additional coursework in IT and/or computer science. We have completely paid for our children's educations. Since I financed my education completely on loans, we felt that it was important to give our children a head start, finishing their schooling with zero debt.

Advice

As I reflect on my career, I'm not sure I could have done it married to somebody outside of medicine. Our experiences are very unique to medicine. I'm not sure anyone outside of medicine fully understands the process. I have enjoyed being married to an anesthesiologist. Since there's always a difference of opinion between surgery and anesthesia concerning work–life balance and the urgency of a case, it was easier for me to see their side of the story.

We are currently planning on retiring when I turn 62 and have already purchased our retirement home in Sarasota, Florida.

Lessons Learned

- To the editors, it seems very clear that this couple has always derived comfort and companionship in their dual medical careers, even from their student days. It's interesting that Grant's anesthesia-like perspectives arise from his relationship with Nee, but that she feels that her direct and no-nonsense surgeon-like approach originates from her (pre-Grant) college days. That's Swarthmore for you? ☺
- Our younger readers should please take note of how often Nee and Grant undertook major efforts of cooperation, flexibility, and compromise—for example, the couple's match, Grant's choice to detour into 2 years of research, Nee's relocation to Grant's hometown for a period of 7 years, and then Grant's relocation back to a larger metropolitan area.
- Nee and Grant also used several different arrangements and accepted available family support for help with their kids. It's important to keep working out solutions to the challenges.
- "Living lean" when a young couple and then prioritizing the kids' educations when their resources were greater is a great set of choices. Although they both had full-time careers, they found their own way to do family first.
- As Wendye Robbins said her in interview elsewhere in this book, *marry the right person!*

Authors

Grant Taylor has practiced in a variety of settings and continues to be entirely happy in his current general surgery practice. He remains a devoted family man and was proud to have the family together in Philadelphia at the time of Nick's graduation from Temple, even though they were not able to be at the ceremony itself due to COVID restrictions.

Cathy Marcucci is a senior academic anesthesiologist and inveterate anesthesiology educator. She is also fellowship-trained in transfusion medicine. When she is not taking care of patients and/or putting the latest book together, she dedicates her time to mentoring junior colleagues, writing copy for animal rescues, and travelling.

Our Inspiration: Sally (Sabina) Sikorski Gottschalk, RN BSN and Carl Gottschalk, MD

173

Allan Gottschalk, Chelsea L. Gottschalk, Laura M. Gottschalk, and Catherine Marcucci

Introduction

Allan Gottschalk is a neuro-anesthesiologist at Hopkins. His wife, Barbara N. Gottschalk BSN MSN, is a nurse practitioner in neurotology, also at Hopkins. They live in the Baltimore metropolitan area and are the proud parents of three adult children, Chelsea, Lindsey, and Laura. Chelsea is a physician. Lindsey and Laura are public health professionals (Fig. 173.1).

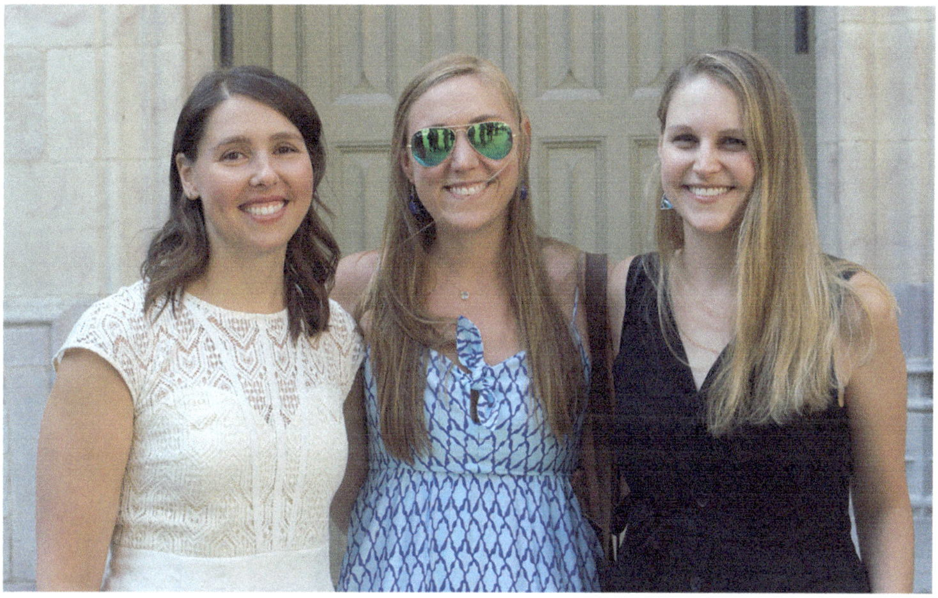

Fig. 173.1 Lindsey, Laura, and Chelsea from left to right in Dijon, France, at the civil ceremony for Lindsey's marriage to Henri Guenancia, a French mathematician she met when he was on a fellowship in the US. Photo: Collection of the Gottschalk family

A. Gottschalk (✉)
Department of Anesthesiology and Critical Care Medicine, Department of Neurosurgery, Johns Hopkins University, Baltimore, MD, USA
e-mail: agottschalk@jhmi.edu

C. L. Gottschalk
Lexington Eye Associates, Lexington, MA, USA

L. M. Gottschalk
National Specialist, Health Promotions, American Lung Association, Chicago, IL, USA

C. Marcucci
Department of Transfusion Medicine, Clinical Center, National Institutes of Health, Bethesda, MD, USA

S. Mohamed et al. (eds.), *Anesthesia Bridges*, https://doi.org/10.1007/978-3-032-08294-7_173

From Allan

As a second-generation anesthesiologist in an academic setting, now briefly reflecting on how I got here as well as some other facets of my life, my current situation can in retrospect appear so preordained, though little was actively pursued—it sorta just happened.

My Father

Carl Gottschalk, MD, grew up in Germany, the son of an American businessman married to a German woman (Fig. 173.2). In 1938, the family returned to the United States for what should be obvious reasons and took up residence in the Washington Heights area of New York City. He enrolled in college as a chemistry major but midway, joined the army when the US entered the war. There, he was a member of the Army Air Core, serving as a meteorologist, achieving the rank of Master Sergeant upon discharge.

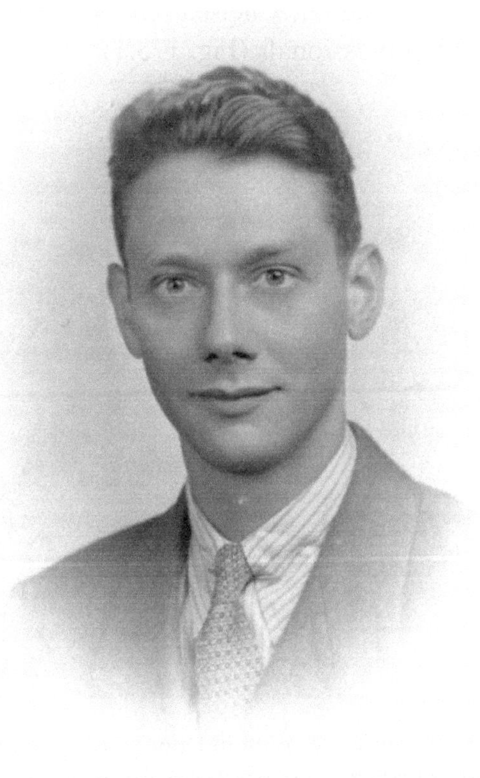

Fig. 173.2 Carl Gottschalk, MD, Allan's father, as a young man in an undated passport photo. Photo: Collection of the Gottschalk family

My father then returned to college, completed his degree, and entered medical school. He was attracted to the emerging specialty of anesthesiology and trained under Rovenstine—there is even a Gottschalk and Rovenstine paper! [1]. While at Bellevue Hospital, he met my mother, Sally, who was then the head nurse on the labor floor. Not too long after that, he accepted an opportunity to work at a hospital on the South Shore of Long Island as the first anesthesiologist to practice there. He bought a house on the water adjacent to Great South Bay and soon convinced my mother to marry him. They had five children, of whom I am the oldest (Fig. 173.3). We enjoyed regular opportunities to go boating, fishing, and visit the beach.

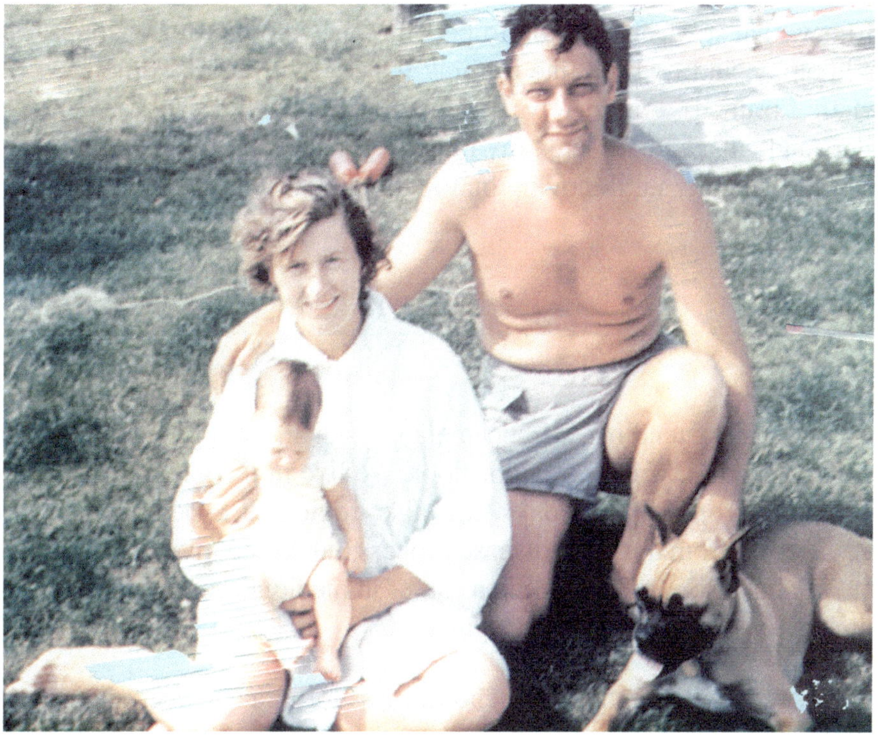

Fig. 173.3 Carl, Sally, and Allan with Cleo in the beginning 1956. Photo: Collection of the Gottschalk family

My Role Models

As I grew up, I saw my anesthesiologist father as a valued member of the local community of physicians who were our family's friends and his colleagues. After dinner, my father typically returned to the hospital to make rounds. If he could, he snagged a kid or two for company, and we would hang out in the hospital lobby while he saw patients, conferred with other physicians, and performed all of the usual pre- and post-operative stuff. Unfortunately, one evening when I was thirteen, he suffered a massive subarachnoid hemorrhage and died the next morning. My mother went back to nursing full-time, first on the labor floor and, later, as nursing director of a rehabilitation hospital. She then became my connection to medicine and taught me what caring, whether for patients, family, or others, was all about.

With my mother's encouragement and advice from her circle of medical friends, I went off to college with a career in medicine as my goal, but with very few specifics. At Boston University, I studied biomedical engineering and was ultimately accepted to the University of Pennsylvania School of Medicine. While rotating in obstetrics, I met Barbara, then a new nurse on the labor floor, and we would move in together and marry in short order.

University of Pennsylvania

While at Penn, I also pursued a doctorate focusing on the neurosciences (then there was no Neuroscience Department, so all of this was in the Department of Anatomy), applying engineering principles to information processing by the visual system. It seemed natural to consider a career in ophthalmology. However, on the first morning of the first day of the week-long medical student specialty rotation in ophthalmology, I knew that it was not in me to become one (though my youngest has completed her training in ophthalmology, and I would like to think that as a little girl, some seed was planted while visiting the lab where I trained). Fortunately, Penn had an outstanding Department of Anesthesiology, and I came to understand what had attracted my father. I subsequently trained there, did research there, and was a member of the faculty until moving on to Hopkins, where most of my time is devoted to the care of neurosurgical patients.

Today

So, without ever consciously intending it, I became a physician, even going into the same specialty as my father. I also married a nurse from the labor floor. We live in the Chesapeake Bay area, so we can continue the boating habit from my early days. It is also ironic that I spend a huge amount of my time caring for patients suffering from the same disease process that killed my father. But here I am. Through my parents, I got to see how rich and rewarding a career in medicine could be and also understood what one's responsibilities were if such a career was pursued.

As for the specifics, like my father in medical school, I was fortunate to encounter anesthesiology being practiced in its best form, he with Rovenstine, and me at Penn. In making my decision about specialty, I was also encouraged by the example of my father, recognizing that a scientifically oriented person with some similar personality traits could enjoy the practice of anesthesiology to the extent that he did. In elucidating the impact of my father's early death on my career, I think it was best summarized by one of our vascular neurosurgeons who, upon hearing my history, pointed out how important it was that I viscerally understood the many ways that neurovascular disease could affect patients and the people around them and, therefore, acted accordingly. I still have no specific insight about marrying a woman from the labor floor, but it was a good choice and, like my career in anesthesiology, we are having an amazing run together with our three girls, the one in ophthalmology and two in public health.

From Chelsea Gottschalk

As a child growing up in a medical family, it took a little more than the garden variety bump and bruise to elicit a sympathetic response from my parents. We knew that we could milk any illness a little longer with my mother, and unless there was an arterial bleed, we were unlikely to get more than a raised eyebrow from my father. Not that growing up this way did not have its perks. We (my two older sisters and I) would often play around in our parents' offices on school holidays and sick days, drawing on the whiteboards with medical posters and pamphlets surrounding us in the background. On family vacations, we had two built-in first responders for any mishaps. I also accompanied my father on field trips around the OR in middle school on Take-Your-Daughter-to-Work Day, which encouraged my early interest in medicine—although looking back, these types of visits from adolescents are probably now strictly prohibited.

The details of my grandfather's career in medicine were not something I knew much about growing up, mostly due to my lack of questioning on my part. I had not realized how much his career had molded my father's, but I saw through my father that medicine could be an intellectually challenging and rewarding career path. After my acceptance into medical school, my dad handed down my grandfather's black doctor's bag, and it really shed light on the significance of becoming a third-generation physician (see Chap. 195). I am now starting out my career, and while I chose ophthalmology over anesthesia, and private practice over academia, I can say that I am very proud to be another Dr. Gottschalk (Fig. 173.4).

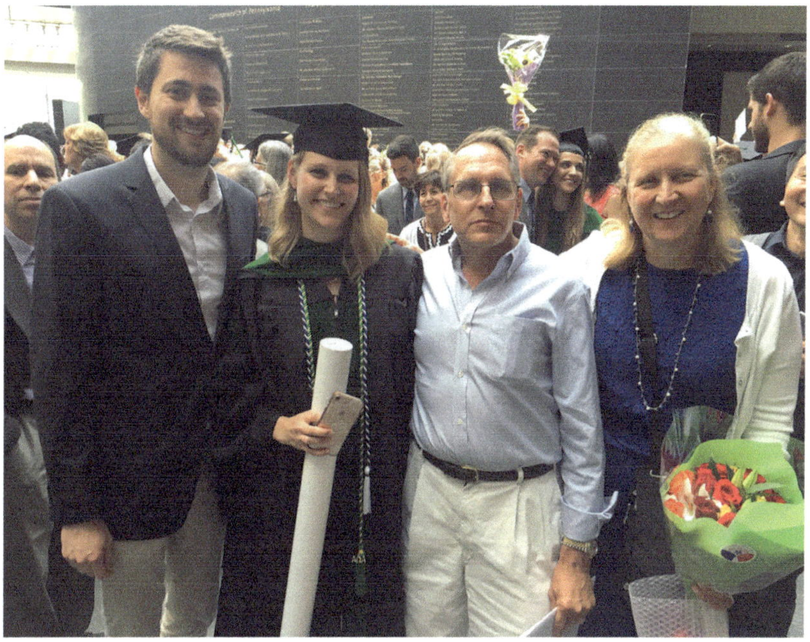

Fig. 173.4 Chelsea Gottschalk MD, graduating from the Sidney Kimmel Medical College at Thomas Jefferson University in 2018, with her husband Dillon Shook and parents. Photo: Collection of the Gottschalk family

From Laura Gottschalk

While I was in grad school, I accompanied one of my friends to an ER visit for moral support. My friend sat in the exam room with a blank expression and nodded, feigning understanding, as the nurse explained what they thought was going on and why. I stepped in on her behalf and asked a list of questions that I thought were important. The nurse asked, completely seriously, "Are you in medicine?" I quickly said no and labeled myself as just a concerned friend, but it has been through experiences like these where I see how my parents have shaped me. I have learned from them how to be an advocate for both myself and others in my orbit, while not being intimidated in a medical space.

I have never been mathematically or scientifically inclined and therefore felt that the field of healthcare was a no-fly zone for me. However, I became fascinated with human behavior and the field of psychology and found myself in an MSW program years later. In one of my classes, we participated in a regular exercise family therapists use called a genogram. This entails reviewing generations of family and highlighting common themes. When I did mine, various themes arose, but one of the most prominent ones was that the majority of family members had worked or are working in a field that helps people.

While I may have thought time after time that I was so different from my parents, the above genogram exercise helped to highlight how my grandparents passed down those same values to my parents that they have then passed to my sisters and me. This drive to help and the natural curiosity my parents stoked later led me to pursue an MPH—in Australia! (Fig. 173.5). While I will never be the one diagnosing or drawing blood, I have felt at home working in the field of public health and working to make healthcare accessible and equitable in my own community.

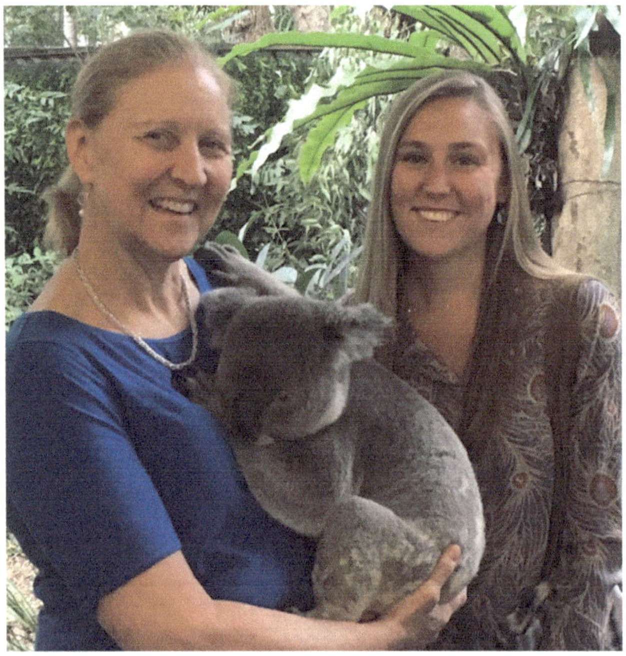

Fig. 173.5 Laura and Barbara with a furry friend in Australia while Laura was working on her MPH. Photo: Collection of Gottschalk family

Lessons Learned: Thoughts from Allan Gottschalk

- Consistency between what you say and do—kids are smart and will spot when things don't match up.
- With regard to gender roles, what you pattern at home is what they will expect in life. I was always very conscious of avoiding certain stereotypes at home. For example, my wife Barbara handles all the money, often drives the family, and can pursue her career as she sees fit.
- Encourage education, independence, and new experiences by example and supporting these activities.
- Our children have told us they greatly appreciate that they were always spoken to as equals, and they strive to extend the same courtesy to others in their lives.

Reference

1. Gottschalk C, Orkin LR, Rovenstine EA. Nisentil: a preliminary screening study of its clinical applicability. NY State J Med. 1955;55(1):90–4.

Authors

Allan Gottschalk was born and raised on Long Island. He went to Boston University for a BS in biomedical engineering and got both his MD and PhD in anatomy (neuroscience) at the University of Pennsylvania. He stayed at Penn for his residency in anesthesiology, a two-year research fellowship, and as a faculty member in the Department of Anesthesiology. He moved to Johns Hopkins in 2000, where he is a professor of anesthesiology and critical care medicine with a joint appointment in neurosurgery. He and his wife Barbara live in the Baltimore area and have three adult daughters—one an ophthalmologist and two in public health. They regularly sail their trimaran Triple Threat on the Chesapeake Bay, and, in the winter, Allan is an avid woodworker with a particular affinity for box forms, such as jewelry boxes and turned boxes. The family gets together to sail, ski, and scuba dive as often as they can.

Chelsea Gottschalk graduated from Tufts/New UK Eye Center ophthalmology residency in June 2022 and started her career as a comprehensive ophthalmologist in private practice in the greater Boston area. She lives in Woburn, MA, with her husband, Dillon, and enjoys taking hikes with their rescue dog, Nali.

Laura Gottschalk is working in public health with a focus on health promotion and disease prevention as part of the American Lung Association's national team. She lives with her boyfriend, Dylan LaPlante, and their bloodhound, Mabel, in the Black Hills of South Dakota. She is an avid traveler and enjoys all things outdoors.

Cathy Marcucci is a senior academic anesthesiologist and inveterate anesthesiology educator. She is also fellowship-trained in transfusion medicine. When she is not taking care of patients and/or putting the latest book together, she dedicates her time to mentoring junior colleagues, writing copy for animal rescues, and travelling.

My Journey

174

David A. Zvara

Introduction

Anesthesia Bridges editor **David Zvara** is a cardiothoracic anesthesiologist at the University of North Carolina at Chapel Hill. He trained at Ohio State and rose through the academic ranks becoming a professor of anesthesiology at Wake Forest, and then went back to Ohio State to be chairman before landing at UNC-Chapel Hill as professor, chair, chief executive officer for UNC faculty physicians as well as UNC Hospitals' chief medical officer, and now professor emeritus. David is also a veteran and deployed as an Air Force physician anesthesiologist during Operation Desert Storm. He and his wife Bharathi live in Chapel Hill and are the proud parents of four daughters and five grandchildren (Fig. 174.1).

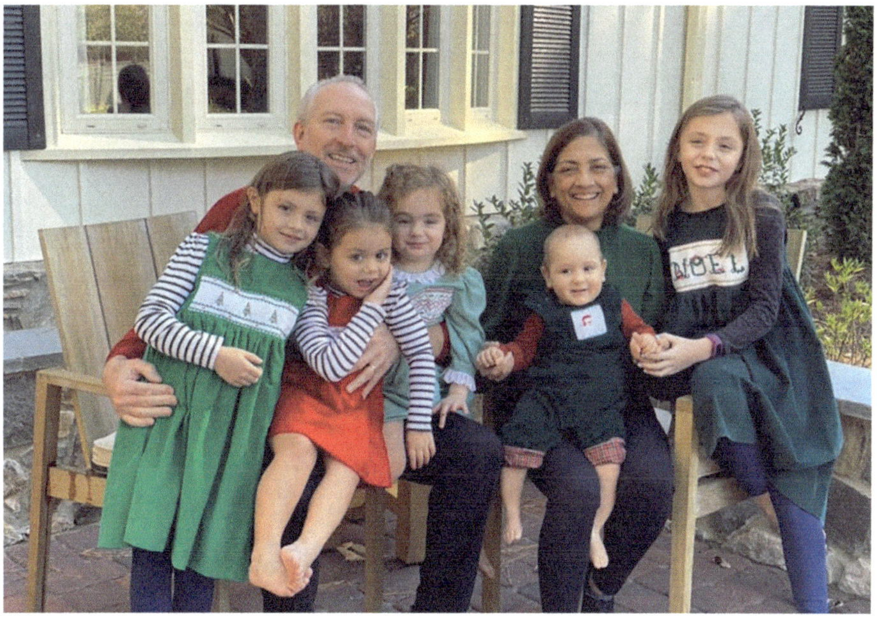

Fig. 174.1 David and Bharathi Zvara and their five beautiful grandchildren, at home in Chapel Hill, North Carolina, November 25, 2021. Photo: Collection of the Zvara family

D. A. Zvara (✉)
(Emeritus) Department of Anesthesiology, The University of North Carolina at Chapel Hill School of Medicine, Chapel Hill, NC, USA
e-mail: David_zvara@med.unc.edu

S. Mohamed et al. (eds.), *Anesthesia Bridges*, https://doi.org/10.1007/978-3-032-08294-7_174

Beginnings

I needed a job. That much was clear, and when opportunity came to me as a junior in high school to either flip burgers or work as a transporter in physical therapy at the community hospital, I took the one that paid a dime more an hour. No kidding, physical therapy here I come. I had no idea about medicine, nurses, doctors, or what pain and suffering looked like. But I found that I loved working with people. I had that job, weekends, summers, and breaks all the way from high school until I signed a commission with the United States Air Force that paid my tuition in medical school at (yes) *The* Ohio State University.

Meeting and Marrying Bharathi Jayranthi

I loved medicine, I loved the hospital, and three-fourths the way through medical school, I found a love for anesthesiology. But my real story, the improbable one, centers around, then a girl, and now my wife, of 40+ years (Fig. 174.2). I met Bharathi as a second-year undergraduate and asked her to marry me before we hit our first dating anniversary. To her great credit, she said no. Persistence pays, and four years later, as a second-year medical student, we tied the knot. Four jobs, three states, four daughters, five grandchildren, four decades, and here we are.

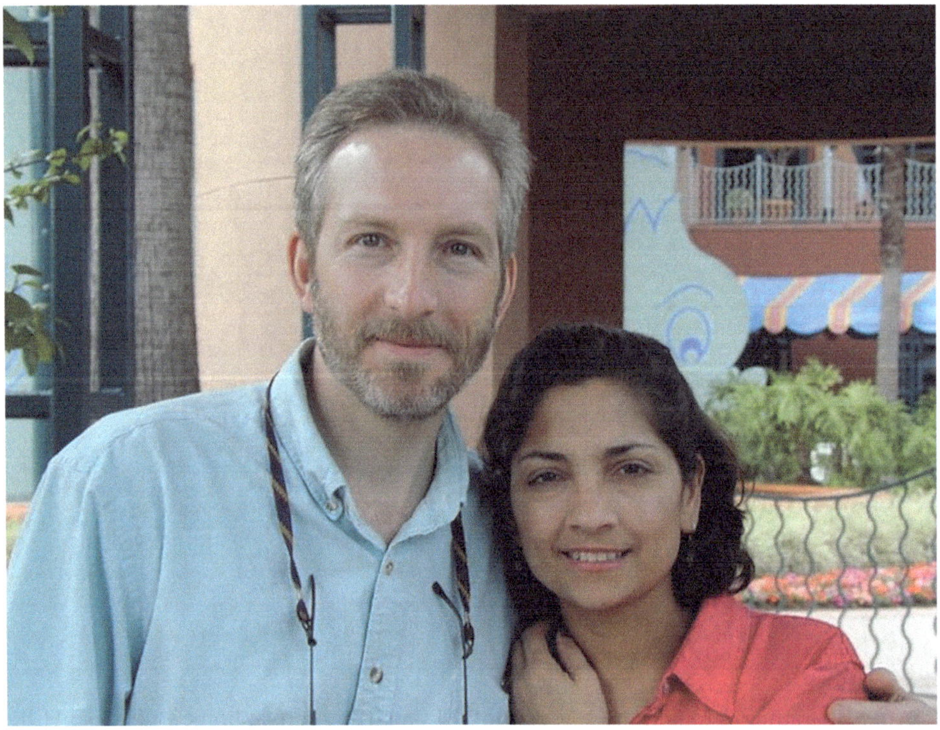

Fig. 174.2 David Zvara and Bharathi Jayanthi Zvara in 2003. Photo: Collection of the Zvara family

Building Our Life Together

The crazy part is that Bharathi, born in Andhra Pradesh, came from generations of farmers in rural India, and we visit India to this day (Fig. 174.3). Her father, a mathematics prodigy, discovered as a youth, earned a chance to complete his Ph.D. in Berkeley, California, a million miles away from home and anything anyone in his family had ever known before. Me? My father immigrated from a tiny, one schoolhouse, one church, one graveyard town about 100 kilometers outside of Budapest (Fig. 174.4). My mom's family came from Enna, Sicily. Somehow, within a generation, Bharathi and I met, in chemistry class, navigated all the family and cultural differences, and became one. At any step along this immigrant journey, the outcomes could have taken a turn. I guess that's true for all of us, but sometimes, we wonder at it all.

None of the achievements, our family, my professional success, Bharathi's PhD, and research could have happened without this happenstance of good fortune. From modest means, our families came to this country, and from their roots, our plenty.

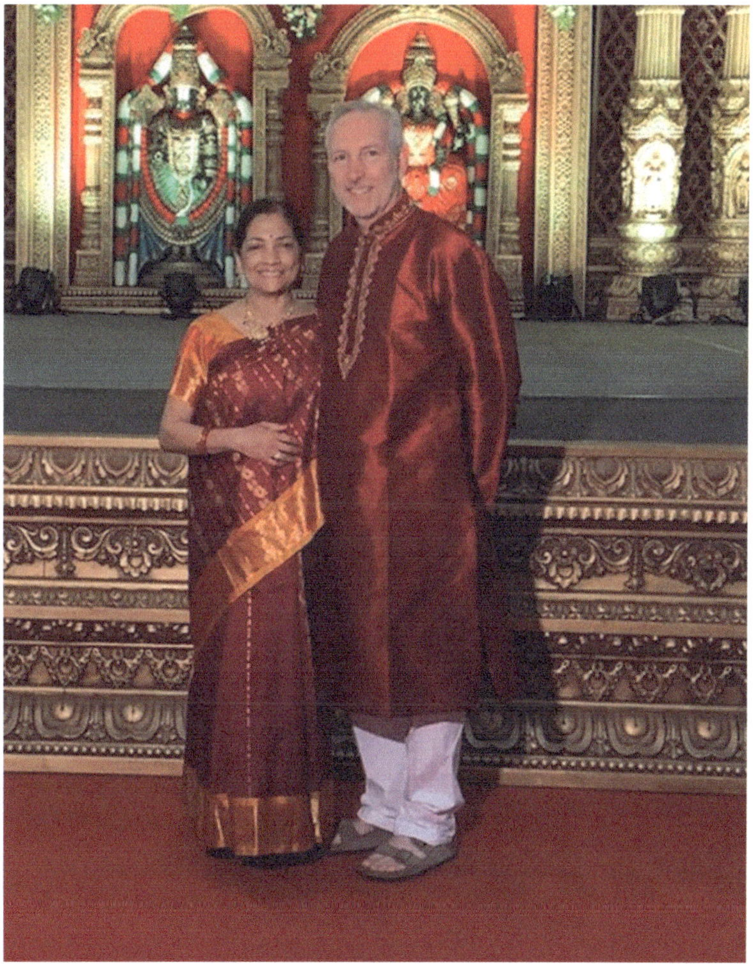

Fig. 174.3 David and Bharathi in Hyderabad, India in 2019. Photo: Collection of the Zvara family

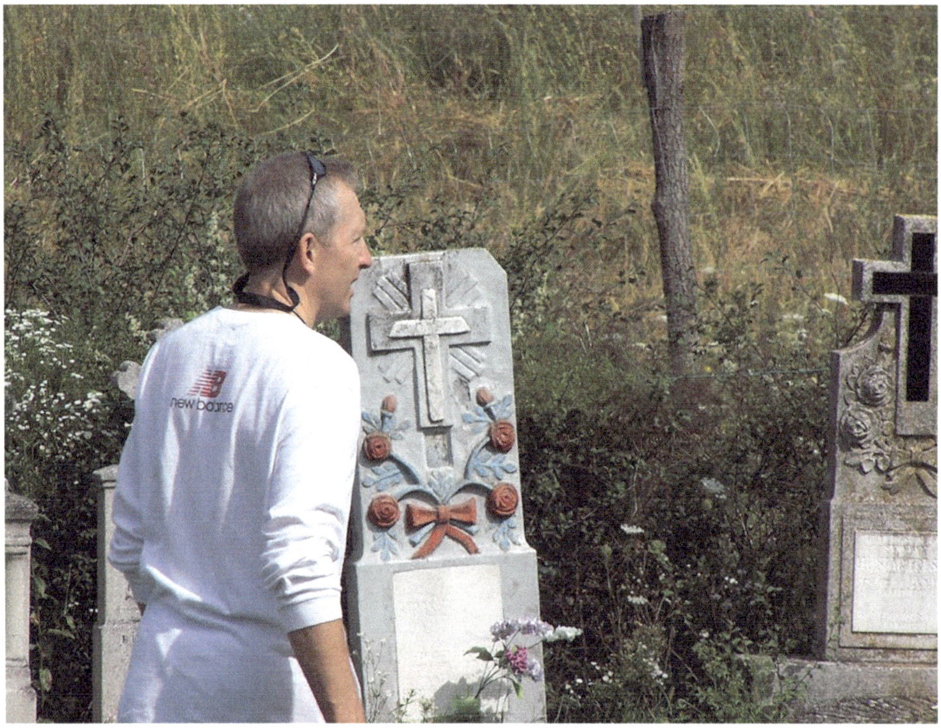

Fig. 174.4 David walking the ancestral graveyard in Terpes, Hungary in August 2006. Photo: Collection of the Zvara family

Lumps, Bumps, and Three-Fifty Will Get You a Cup of Coffee

Reflections are great, and advice comes easily with a little scotch and the passage of time. Still, there are lessons I've learned, I've tried to live by, and I'd love to share in an essay like this. So, here we go…

Jump in and get wet—Commitment matters. At the start of any endeavor, you simply need to decide are you in, or are you not? I remember so vividly the reaction my family and friends had when I declared I was directing all my efforts and studies to getting into medical school. It seemed an impossible reach. I remember walking home from the library after a fourteen-hour day of classroom lectures and study, and thinking, *I can do this.* I remember taking the oath of the United States of America when I received my military commission. I remember my wedding vows, holding our first-born, taking that job. So, what's the point? If you do something, go all in. You want to swim? You've got to get wet. Jump in with both feet.

Fencing thoroughbreds—Leaders manage teams, and I truly believe that teams succeed over individual success. And still, on every team, there is a driver, a catalyst, a motivator, an organizer, the heart or soul, the workhorse. It could be different people fulfilling different roles. Nonetheless, recognizing the individual talent and harnessing that talent for the group's success is the leader's talent. Making this point, sometimes I like to say: *You know what you do when you have a thoroughbred? You let him run.*

Standing in a canoe—Teaching anesthesiology and the pharmacologic management of brittle vasculopathic patients in the heart room, I'd often ask that question. *Can you stand up in a canoe?* The answer is, of course, you can, but you'd better do it slow and steady. No quick moves. Stay in balance. Same thing holds in managing the extremely ill. Slow, steady, directed care, and you won't find yourself overboard in the water of your own making.

Don't step on their neck—This one's not an original. Sheryl Hudspeth is one of the first heart surgeons I ever worked with at Wake Forest. He's an old-school, crusty surgeon with no time for nonsense. He was brilliant and fearless in the operating room. Not reckless nor foolish. Whenever a team member (read anesthesiologist, intensivist, consultant, or whomever) might express doubt about a patient, he'd sum it up like this: *If you don't step on their neck, they'll do alright.*

What'd he mean by that? Basically, if given half a chance, the body and spirit will find a way. Healing is sometimes beyond our intervention, so the "best" care, sometimes, is to not *do* too much. Let 'em be. Don't gum the works with some fancy clinical trick. Simple is usually better than complicated. Don't worry so much, and above all, don't step on their neck.

Pouring from an empty cup—It's cliché these days, and sometimes counterintuitive. I urge our folks to think bigger, give more, and *do* more. I don't preach "work-life balance," rather, I preach "productivity matters!" Am I out of step? Insensitive? Olympic champions don't practice 24 hours a day; rather, they blend practice with purposeful rest, mental relief, and directed nutrition. When it comes time to perform, their body, mind, and soul are at their peak. Purposeful replenishment maintains a full cup. Here's one small bit of advice in that vein: no emails after 7 pm. Don't look, as you will be sucked in if you do. I practiced this at home nearly all the years I was chair, and you know what? The place is still standing.

Haste, grace, and knowing what to ignore—Seventeen years as a chair, 40+ years as a husband, 1046 cumulative years as a parent of four daughters, and now acting as the executive for an entire medical staff provides me with some perspective on keeping my nose out of trouble. Don't judge others too fast; there are always two sides to every story. Be forgiving. No one is perfect people make mistakes all the time. And lastly, not everything is a crisis. Time and temperance give people the opportunity to find their way. Let them.

Final Thoughts

I am grateful for all the professional opportunities that came my way. While in the service, I was deployed in Operation Desert Storm; I came to Wake Forest University and established a nascent research team and educational platform. Mid-career, I returned to Ohio State as chair, and I was lucky enough to be selected first chair, then chief executive of the faculty physicians at the University of North Carolina at Chapel Hill. A place our family calls home. All of it blows my mind when I think about that first job, and the difference a dime an hour has made in my life.

Lessons Learned

- The editors had fun reading David's essay on his family's personal story. First, it is the quintessential American saga. The Zvara daughters were blessed with a really interesting set of grandparents—South Asian, Hungarian, and Sicilian. We bet that all the women in the older generations (on both sides!) were happy to see their offspring pull up to the table and fill their plates. And probably some of the senior men in the family were happy to see everybody eat, too.
- We ask our readers to notice how strongly the thread of home and family runs through David's journey, as well as his sense of good fortune and even luck.
- There is also an overall lesson here not to take yourself too seriously. *Anesthesia Bridges* author Neil Sandson (a psychiatrist) chuckled at how David was willing to poke fun at himself when relating that the lady of his affections had the good sense to turn down his first marriage proposal. Neil remarked, "Well, you gotta be pretty chill to tell that kind of story on yourself."
- We thank David for sharing his journey with us!

Author

David Zvara has had many professional appointments, responsibilities, and achievements in addition to being a professor and the immediate past chair of his department. These include serving as the chief operating officer of UNC Faculty Physicians and the director of the medical center's ambulatory COVID response team. He has been named as a fellow by the American Heart Association and has also been recognized in Best Doctors in America, Inc. Dr. Zvara is a fellow of the American Society of Anesthesiologists and has given back to the national professional community by donating his time to be a senior examiner for the American Board of Anesthesiology.

Making It Work

175

Linda M. Peterson, Kailey L. Peterson, Kelsey Peterson Ostergren, and Catherine Marcucci

Contributor:

William P. Peterson, MD

Introduction

Linda Peterson is a psychiatrist and the chief medical officer of McLaren Greater Lansing Hospital in Lansing, Michigan. **Bill Peterson** is a cardiac anesthesiologist at E.W. Sparrow Hospital and heads the cardiac anesthesia group. Together they raised two beautiful daughters, Kelsey and Kailey, while balancing priorities and negotiating the challenges of a two-physician marriage and household.

Starting the Journey

Our journey started in the first weeks of medical school. Dating through those intense and formative years provided a platform for understanding what it took, the costs emotionally and financially, and the rewards unique to the amazing profession of medicine. We were married in 1987 (Fig. 175.1). We continued in our training, retaining that same awareness of the need for understanding and support. At each step, this base of understanding, acceptance, communication, and respect has served us well.

L. M. Peterson
McLaren Greater Lansing Hospital, Lansing, MI, USA

K. L. Peterson
Kohler Company, Kohler, WI, USA

K. P. Ostergren
Michigan Health & Hospital Association, Okemos, MI, USA

C. Marcucci (✉)
Department of Transfusion Medicine, Clinical Center, National Institutes of Health, Bethesda, MD, USA

S. Mohamed et al. (eds.), *Anesthesia Bridges*, https://doi.org/10.1007/978-3-032-08294-7_175

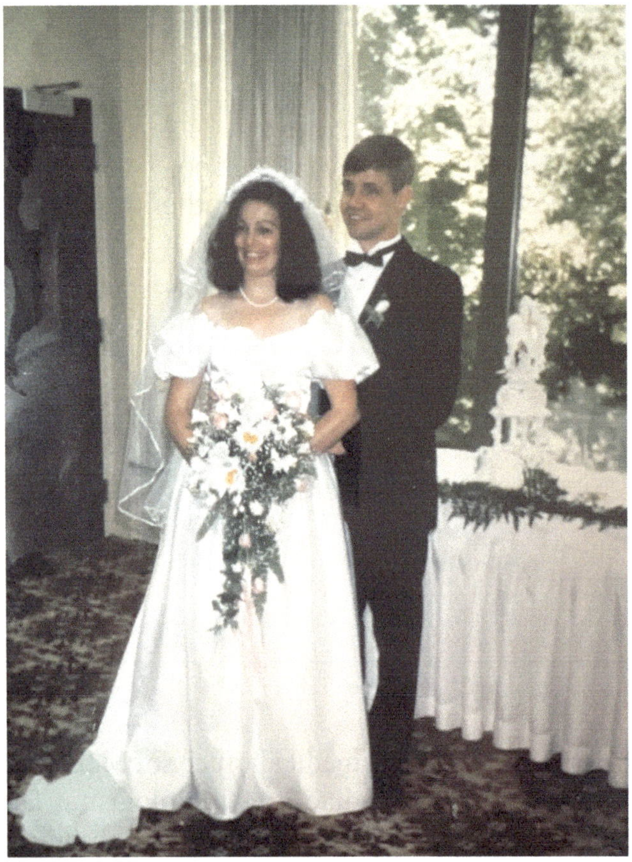

Fig. 175.1 Linda and Bill Peterson on their wedding day—June 12, 1987. Photo: Collection of the Peterson family

What's the Secret to Making a Medical Marriage Work?

No secret! Ultimately, it is about respect, commitment, and communication. It is navigating the myriad challenges and curve balls of life by listening and seeking to understand before speaking and trying to be understood. To nurture the relationship, we made it a rule that every year we would take a vacation by ourselves. No kids, no family, no friends, just us. What started as kind of a fun excuse to get away has proved to be a cherished time of reconnecting and strengthening our relationship even after nearly 40 years together.

Our Family

Children add their own unique joys and needs, of course. Only by leaning hard on that awareness and understanding were we able to navigate the challenges. There was no "this is your job" response to anything. Each hurdle or curve ball was met with a conversation of how to handle it, who could do it, and how it could be done best. We were fortunate to have grandparents present locally in the lives of our children, and they were a blessing in managing some of those inevitable moments when life hands out more than you thought you could handle in the moment.

Kailey Peterson on Her Childhood

From a very early age, I can remember my father telling me that I could do anything I set my mind to. Now in my mid-twenties, I can reflect on those formative years and how instrumental my father's occupation was in creating my worldview and aspirations. The profound impact of watching my father spend hours caring for others, being a relentless patient advocate, and always striving to be better than he was the day before, has shaped me in more ways than I could express. Not only did he have a successful career, but he was also an incredible father and husband while doing so. Being a physician, let alone an anesthesiologist, can be a demanding profession, but my Dad has shown me that you truly can achieve anything you set your mind to.

Kelsey Peterson on Growing Up with Her Dad

As a young child, I did not have a good understanding of what my Dad did—all I knew was that he worked really long days, missed a lot of weeknight dinners, and stayed up really late working on his computer. This routine was normal for our family, so while some of my friends had a family dinner every night at 6 PM, that was not our life. That said, it never occurred to me that I was "missing out" on anything because I felt like a priority to him when he *was* home.

While many movies depict a "hard working, always absent father," this was not how my Dad operated, as my sister and I have always been (and continue to be) a priority for him. He gave 100% at work, but when he was home, he was passionate and fully invested in raising his daughters. Whether this meant proofreading essays, helping with trigonometry homework, or designing a project for the school science fair, he made every effort to develop us as students, young women, and engaged members of our community—even if that meant doing so over another cup of coffee at 9 PM, on the heels of a 14-hour day in the OR.

The time, energy, investment, and love my Dad pours into my sister and me are something I will forever be grateful for. While he worked a lot (and still continues to), he set an example of what it looks like to follow your passion, showing us the value of hard work, dedication, persistence, and the power of simply "showing up."

As a professional in my mid-30s, with my first baby on the way, I have spent a lot of time reflecting on my own childhood and how I was raised. I can wholeheartedly say that balancing a fulfilling professional life alongside a rich family life is possible, and my Dad showed me what that can look like. No family is perfect, but we all do the best we can to juggle the things that are most important to us, and I have come to appreciate this more than ever before, as I know I was one of the things that were most important to him.

The Best Advice That Bill Peterson Ever Got or Gave

Approach your work and your marriage with a mind set to do more than "your share." If you and your spouse each endeavor to do 70% of what needs doing, you will be wildly successful. Same in your practice. Do your best, prioritize your faith, family, and friends—life will reward you richly. And family is everything! (Fig. 175.2).

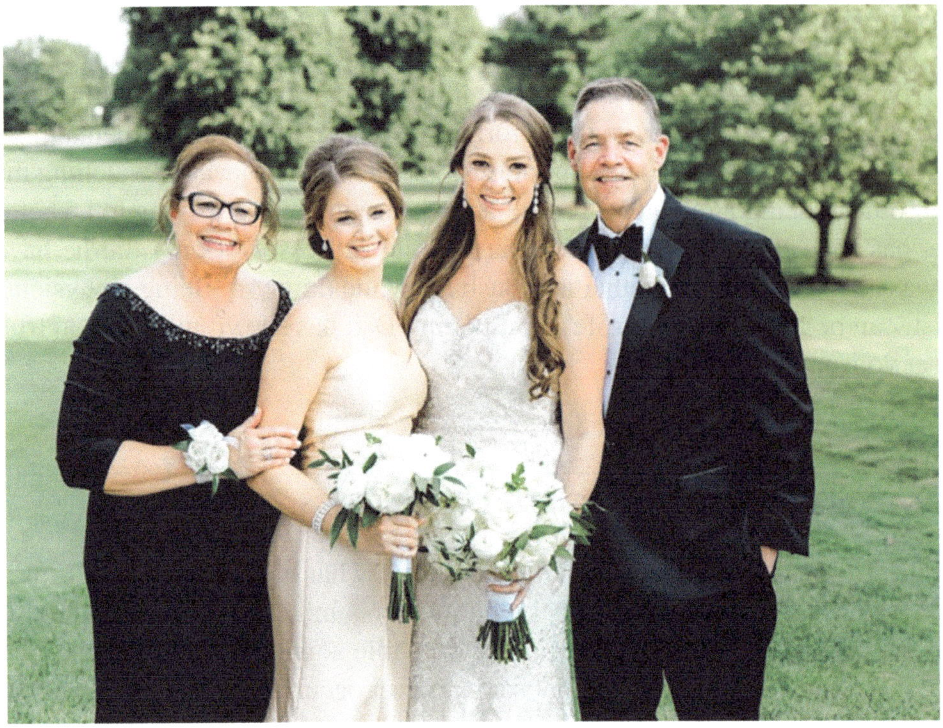

Fig. 175.2 The wonderful and devoted Peterson family—Linda, Kailey, older sister and bride Kelsey, and Bill. Photo: Collection of the Peterson family

Gratitude (From Kelsey Peterson Ostergren)

- I am grateful that my father's career allowed him to follow his passions and have a fulfilling professional life.
- I am grateful that his anesthesiology career afforded my sister and me enriching opportunities that many other kids didn't have.
- I am grateful that his career provided us with the resources to travel extensively together as a family.
- I am grateful that my Dad's love of learning was something he passed on to his daughters.
- I am grateful that my Dad showed up day after day for his girls and always made us a priority.

Lessons Learned

- It is very clear that the Peterson parents worked together to build a family life that prioritized their children—but at the same time, carved out that time for just the two of them. No kids, no other family, no friends, no exceptions.

- Please notice that these kids do not appear to have suffered serious damage to their young psyches because their folks worked long hours, and there wasn't the traditional family dinner hour. Kids will generally feel very positive about their parents' devotion to them, no matter what form it takes—as long as it does not cross over into being overcontrolling, which can breed resentment and rebellion.
- The trick for parents is to accept that the day's work is not done when you come through the door at home after a shift in the hospital. Your real life's work is just beginning. That's why Bill was sometimes drinking coffee at 9 PM.
- Congratulations to Linda and Bill for raising such a beautiful family!

Authors

Linda Peterson is a psychiatrist and chief medical officer in Lansing, Michigan, where she lives with her husband Bill. In her spare time, she loves anything to do with the outdoors, especially golf, pickleball, and kayaking. She also enjoys travel and dinners with friends but most of all, time with family.

Kailey Peterson works as a global buyer for raw materials for the Kohler company. Her responsibilities also include leading the company's carbon strategy and contributing to the overall corporate sustainability goals. She currently lives in Littleton, Colorado, and enjoys hiking, yoga, cooking, and all the great activities Colorado has to offer.

Kelsey Peterson Ostergren currently serves as the director of health policy initiatives at the Michigan Health & Hospital Association, where she helps inform changes to healthcare delivery models for hospitals and healthcare facilities across the state. She currently lives in Kalamazoo, Michigan, with her husband Brand and dog Charles and looks forward to expanding their family in the very near future. In her free time, Kelsey is an avid crafter, an outdoor enthusiast, and loves trying new vegan recipes.

Cathy Marcucci first met Bill and Linda Peterson in the 1990s. Bill was a young cardiac anesthesiologist at her training program and Linda was her husband's chief resident. Cathy and Neil remember meeting Bill and Linda and (baby) Kelsey for dinner at a Chinese restaurant and Bill carried Kelsey in one arm and an even bigger purple Barney in the other.

Devotion and Diligence

176

Christine Garcia Cattaneo and Catherine Marcucci

Contributor:

Catherine Marcucci, MD

Introduction

Christine Garcia and **Stephen Cattaneo** met while training and in med school at Hopkins. Christine is an anesthesiologist at Anne Arundel Medical Center, and Stephen is a cardiothoracic surgeon there. They have four beautiful children—twins Sophia and Isabella, and sons Stephen and Matthew. They live in suburban Maryland.

We Are Partners and Friends!

I met my husband, Stephen, in May during my Osler medicine internship at Johns Hopkins Hospital. It was his first clinical rotation in medical school, and he was assigned to my team. He and I spent a few nights on call together, got along immediately, and began dating a few months into my anesthesia residency at Hopkins. Stephen finished his medical school and matched/started at Hopkins for a 9-year residency program in general and cardiac surgery, while I finished my residency, completed my fellowship in cardiac anesthesia, and took a job in private practice in Annapolis, MD.

By the time Stephen finished his residency and fellowship, I had been a partner in my practice, worked full-time, and had four kids under four years of age. Stephen eventually took a job at the hospital where I work, and we have both worked there for 20+ years (me) and 15+ years (him).

C. G. Cattaneo
Anne Arundel Medical Center, Annapolis, MD, USA

TeamHealth, Inc., Knoxville, TN, USA

C. Marcucci (✉)
Department of Transfusion Medicine, Clinical Center, National Institutes of Health, Bethesda, MD, USA

S. Mohamed et al. (eds.), *Anesthesia Bridges*, https://doi.org/10.1007/978-3-032-08294-7_176

Over the years, working at our hospital, we have spent time together serving on the medical executive committee. We decided NOT to do any clinical cases together. We tried to have nightly family dinners with the kids, and they would often complain that we talked about work too much.

Managing a Medical Marriage

I have found that we have had a better understanding of each other since we are both physicians who frequently work long hours or overnight. We have a deeper understanding and empathy for each other, given our common situations, and rarely have any conflicts over time spent at the hospital or taking calls on the weekends. In fact, my husband was very supportive of my sharing a job, which has allowed me to decrease the number of days I work each week, as well as the concentration of my late nights and overnight calls. This has given me the best of both worlds—working as a physician as well as having time to be a mom to our kids.

We have both worked collaboratively to raise our kids the way we feel is best, make the most of their sporting and academic events, help them through the college application period, and work through other stressful life events. Of our four kids, three feel they will pursue careers in medicine, I take that as a positive reflection of our work and family lives.

Our Domestic Details

I have generally worked 30–40 hours clinically per week, depending on my call schedule. I was president of our practice for 10 years and probably worked another 10–15 hours per week administratively, often at home. Stephen works probably 55–70 hours per week. He is now the medical staff president which adds a lot of evening meetings.

We have had *au pairs* since our twins were toddlers. In fact, at the time I wrote this essay, we were on our 20th au pair, who helped with driving our youngest (no license yet!) to school and swim practice, and also made the kids dinner and did a lot of the shopping. The kids attended private schools in Baltimore, and our kids are now in college. We prioritized college savings for the kids from the time each was born.

We started taking big vacations when the kids were 5–9 years old. We do have a big house, and we need it with seven people living there! We have a pool in the backyard, as the kids are big swimmers. We have rarely done date nights—we prefer to spend time with the kids.

Our Final Wisdom

I would suggest that medical couples allow themselves to connect by sharing medical stories and events, but not too much. We have both benefited from our shared understanding of the medical lifestyle and the ability to discuss issues with each other. We have been able to comfort and support each other in challenging times. Medicine is a way we are connected, and administrative positions have kept us close and aligned with each other. However, we have many other interests in common outside of medicine and have spent time doing things together—watching football, attending kids' sporting events, traveling, and working out. We were delighted to celebrate our 25th wedding anniversary and continue to look forward with anticipation and excitement.

Lessons Learned

- Our readers should note that Christine and Stephen invested in the help they needed to get done what they wanted to get done for the kids—whether that was school elsewhere in the metropolitan Baltimore region or a home-cooked dinner every night. As we have mentioned elsewhere in the book, invest in what's important to you, and don't feel guilty about it.

- We have found that having a physician spouse is a great comfort, as it has been for the Cattaneos. We don't know of any two-physician couples where this hasn't been the case. But notice that they made the sensible decision not to do cases together, and they have lots of other shared interests outside of medicine.

- We thank Christine for taking the time from her full-time career, full-time personal life, and graduate school studies to share the details of how she and Steve are guiding their family through these hectic years. This is a great family, by all accounts, and it's not hard to understand why—these parents have given the issue of balancing their careers and children much thought and careful planning.

***Note from the Editors:** Christine, Stephen, and the kids love Ohio and attending Ohio State football games as often as possible. For her favorite bridge, Christine suggested, "Any beautiful Ohio bridge would be great!" We thought this natural rock bridge in Hocking Hills State Park fit the bill (Fig. 176.1).

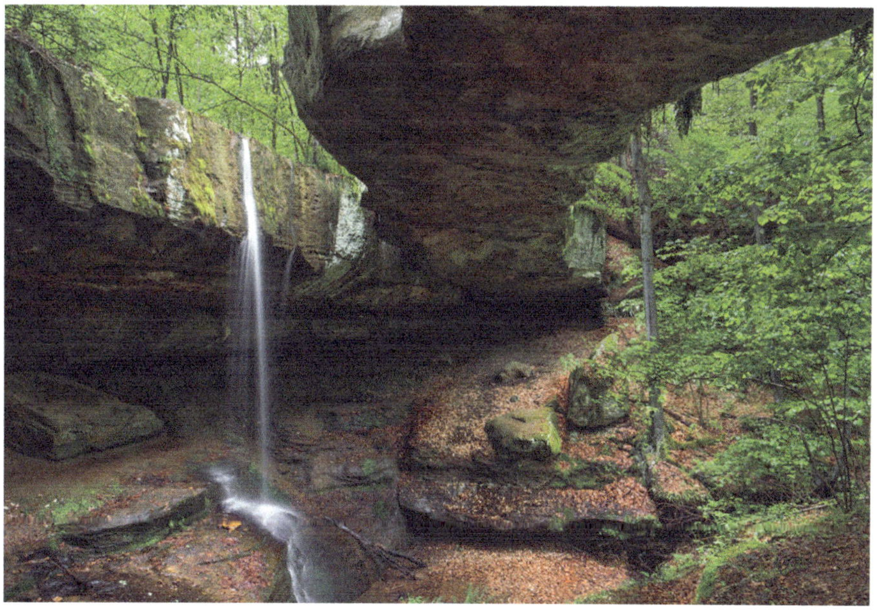

Fig. 176.1 The natural rock bridge in Hocking Hills State Park in Logan, Ohio, is in southeast Ohio. The bridge is over 100 feet long and 10–12 feet wide. It arches gracefully above a ravine with a small creek and a waterfall. The Black Hand sandstone sedimentary rock of the bridge formed millions of years ago when Ohio was under a warm inland sea. The sea drained about the time the Appalachian Mountains formed, exposing the rock to erosion. Ohio has at least 12 natural rock bridges, but we think this one is the most striking. Photo: Image used under standard license from stock.adobe.com

Authors

Christine Garcia Cattaneo is an anesthesiologist in Annapolis, Maryland. She also held a variety of management positions with her practice group. In addition to being the wife of a busy surgeon and chief medical officer *and* the mother of a large family, she somehow recently found time to get an MBA and accept a position as an anesthesiology executive with a large privately-owned healthcare company. In her very rare spare time, she loves travelling and celebrating holidays with her group.

Cathy Marcucci is a senior academic anesthesiologist and inveterate anesthesiology educator. She is also fellowship-trained in transfusion medicine. When she is not taking care of patients and/or putting the latest book together, she dedicates her time to duplicate bridge, swimming, writing copy for animal rescues, and travelling.

To My Younger Self

177

Michael S. Axley and Catherine Marcucci

Contributor:

Catherine Marcucci, MD

To My Younger Self

Looking back on it all from my vantage point now, if I had it to say to myself 20+ years ago, I'd say this: the journey you are about to embark upon has the potential to be immensely satisfying, and you will see, experience, and learn things that are not possible to encounter in any other setting or profession. On the other hand, you may have underestimated, substantially, two important things:

- The amount of real difficulty and complexity inherent in this particular field of study.
- The sheer duration of time involved. If you want to have a classic family life that includes children's sports on the weekends, honestly, this may not be the field for you. If it is going to bother you that your friends who went to business school are at the beach while you are at the hospital, this may not be the field for you.

Healing

With those caveats, I think there are a lot of different ways to be a good, or even great, doctor, and that's fine. I have found that physicians are often engaged in some sort of internal healing process as well as striving to heal others. Since injury knows no boundaries, it's appropriate that we should come from all walks of life. I would suppose that if I have regrets regarding medicine, they mainly fall into the cate-

M. S. Axley
Oregon Anesthesiology Group, Portland, OR, USA

C. Marcucci (✉)
Department of Transfusion Medicine, Clinical Center, National Institutes of Health, Bethesda, MD, USA

S. Mohamed et al. (eds.), *Anesthesia Bridges*, https://doi.org/10.1007/978-3-032-08294-7_177

gory of "I wish I had found anesthesia earlier." It did take me several years of specialty shopping, including an internal medicine residency, to locate my final specialty, and that process involved a lot of unnecessary stress.

Final Thoughts

I guess for me, medicine is not one of those professions where you can reasonably think you're going to leave it as the same person who entered. You're going to have to wrestle with your own demons throughout the process, and the person who emerges is not going to be the same. It is to be hoped that it's someone we can all live with and enjoy, a person who is kind and caring to their spouse, children, partners, patients, and ultimately, themselves.

Lessons Learned

- There is much to think about in Mike's frank and heartfelt essay. We agree that there is an aura of uniqueness and exclusivity that attaches to the practice of anesthesiology. There are only a few other professions where saving lives is so manifestly apparent and so routine. This integral aspect of anesthesia practice can lend comfort on otherwise difficult and discouraging days.

- Are we all wounded healers? Or most of us anyway? It's an interesting existential thought experiment and difficult to know for sure. Because who among us has the complete measure of another's journey?

- Mike is right about the necessity of not caring that much about what the "money guys" are doing or buying. That kind of comparison, if you care about it at all, can make you dejected and/or disillusioned about your choices. If you are ever troubled by a whiff of this, reread the last two essays in this book—the letter that a grateful patient wrote to editor Ron Bank and the heroic story of Brandon Togioka's grandfather Noboru Togioka. This closing essay will inspire you and refresh your thinking about where the true rewards lie. They are not to be found in the monthly banking statements.

***Note from the Editors:** We asked Mike to choose his favorite bridge, and he sent us this wonderful little essay on the Sellwood Bridge and his love of the Northwest. (Figs. 177.1 and 177.2):

> My favorite bridge is the Sellwood Bridge in Portland. It spans the Willamette River to the south of Portland's City Center and provides access to the lovely little neighborhood of Sellwood-Moreland. This neighborhood is right next to a partner neighborhood, Eastmoreland, that hosts the campus where I happily attended school--Reed College.
>
> The Sellwood Bridge is one of the newest bridges in Portland, which has more than a few, and the construction seemed like it took forever. Fun fact, there are 12 bridges in the Portland city limits. In the summer, I'd often take my three kids and wife on a boat, and we'd glide under it along the water and take in all the details of the construction. It serves as a multi-use pathway, with corridors for pedestrians, bicycles, and cars, and has a clean, modern aesthetic that I associate with the best new architecture in the Portland area. It's also a sort of shortcut and back way into the east side and all of the food and adventures to be found there.

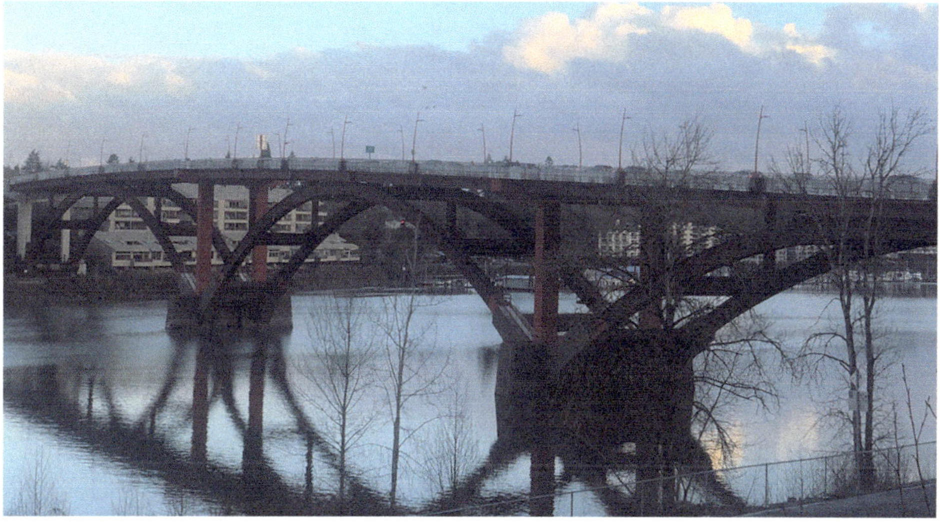

Fig. 177.1 The beautiful Sellwood Bridge reflected in the Willamette River in Portland, Oregon. Photo: Mike Axley

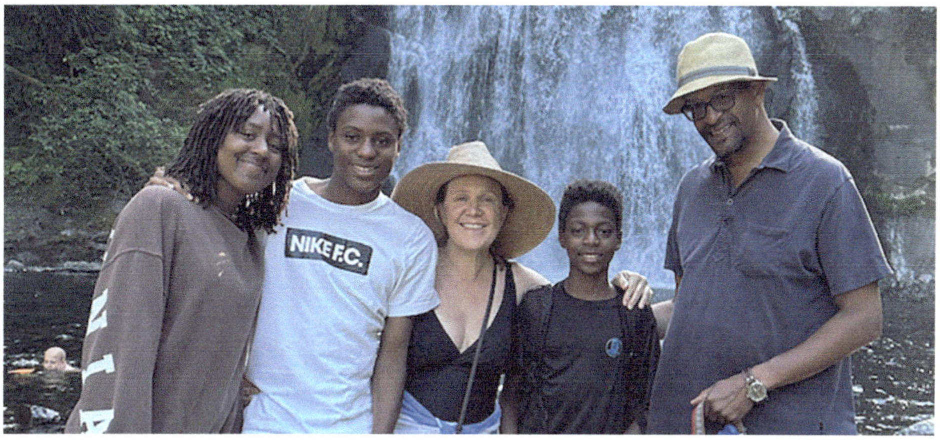

Fig. 177.2 Mike and Kim with their gorgeous kids, outdoors somewhere in the stunning nature of the Northwest. Photo: Collection of the Axley family

Authors

Mike Axley is a senior anesthesiologist in Oregon. Besides being devoted to his family and an outstanding clinician, he is a gifted journalist, writer, and editor. He tells us a bit more about his personal and family background in Chap. 201. We were delighted when he sent us this photo of his beautiful group (Fig. 177.2).

Cathy Marcucci is a senior academic anesthesiologist and inveterate anesthesiology educator. She is also fellowship-trained in transfusion medicine. When she is not taking care of patients and/or putting the latest book together, she dedicates her time to hunting for beautiful waterfalls and bridges.

Part X

Life Stories

Leonard P. Zakim Bunker Hill Memorial Bridge—Boston, MA

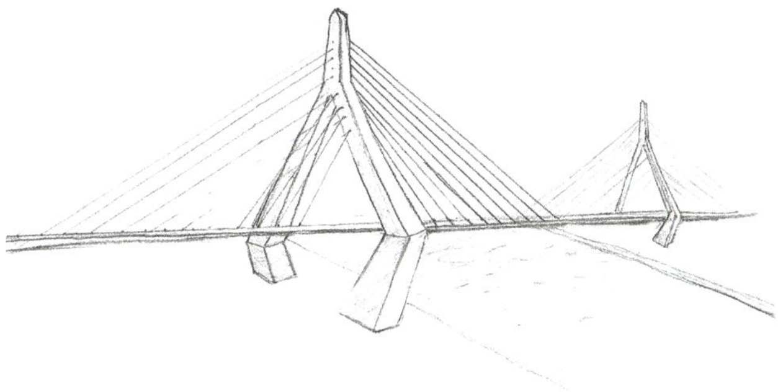

"The Zakim" was selected as a favorite by *Anesthesia Bridges* editor **Jake Seagull** and author **Jeanine Wiener-Kronish**. The bridge was named in honor of Lenny Zakim, who was a Jewish-American lawyer and influential religious and civil rights leader based in Boston. It is a cable-stayed bridge across the Charles River in Boston, MA.

It is one of the newest among our selected bridges and was completed in 2003, replacing the old Charleston High Bridge. The Zakim's harp configuration with cradles carrying each strand through pylons quickly become an icon for Boston and is often featured in Boston print media, on tourist souvenirs, and as landscape backdrops for news channels. Construction of the bridge required alteration of the Charles River Shoreline, and the designers and engineers took advantage of this to create a public landscape and art installation under the bridge. Dr. Wiener-Kronish wrote to us that the bridge is sentimental to her as it is adjacent to the arena where the Celtics play and brings light to short winter days and long winter nights.

Jake, Jeanine, and the *Anesthesia Bridges* editors thank **Kelsey O'Connor** of The Architectural Team in Boston, MA, for her pencil drawing that perfectly captures the exquisite and graceful geometry of the bridge.

178 Introduction

Edwin G. Avery IV

This section of *Anesthesia Bridges* is yet another mind opening collection of invaluable lessons from senior anesthesiologists. While the various topics in this section may initially seem somewhat unrelated, we hope our readers come away with the realization that these collected essays offer deep insights into our professional and personal lives from some of the best minds in the business.

Many of these chapters revolve around the difficult issue of trying to accomplish work–life balance. Our authors remind us of the value of getting involved with charity or other social action work as part of the "life" side of the equation. Other writers relate their stories of how they switched up their careers, including getting involved in international medicine. We also include one person's harrowing story of a life unraveling, his battle with drug addiction, and his ongoing recovery. He reminds us of the need for us to "monitor our own pulses," as anesthesiology can be a very stressful occupation, even for experienced and skilled clinicians.

Author

Ed Avery is a New Englander who trained and worked at the MGH for over a decade before being recruited to Cleveland. He is a cardiac anesthesiologist with multiple areas of interest—including blood pressure control, the coagulation system, and improving patient outcomes. He has served as chief of cardiac anesthesia, vice chair for research, and chair of the transfusion committee during his time at University Hospitals Cleveland Medical Center.

E. G. Avery IV (✉)
Department of Anesthesiology and Perioperative Medicine, University Hospitals Cleveland Medical Center, Cleveland, OH, USA

S. Mohamed et al. (eds.), *Anesthesia Bridges*, https://doi.org/10.1007/978-3-032-08294-7_178

179 Simple Truths

David A. Zvara

Introduction

In my many years in academic and clinical medicine, I've learned many lessons, some the hard way through mistakes, and some through the musings of my teachers and peers. The best lessons are those that can be distilled down to simple truths and captured in as few words as possible. Here you go.

Canoes and Care

Imagine anesthesia care like a gliding canoe through still water; effortless, quiet, and determined. Point A to point B. The best anesthesiology care is just like this: Unassuming, beautiful, and purposeful. Extending the metaphor, during those times of rough water or hemodynamic instability, one should strive to return to the effortlessness of the canoe. I often ask, "Can you stand up in a canoe?" Sure you can. Slowly, one can rise, without falling in the water, if one does so with deliberation, purpose, and balance. *That* is the art of anesthesia.

The X-Games of Medicine

Anesthesiology is the X-Games of Medicine. Think about it. A non-anesthesiologist worries at the bedside about the patient who is hemodynamically unstable, in critical, and precarious condition. *How will this person make it through the day, even with my best care?* An anesthesiologist assumes care of this same person, removes them from the safety of the ICU, induces a coma, controls and disturbs every physiologic function in the body, blunts an assault like none other (incision, organ removal, blood loss, cardiopulmonary bypass), and returns the person back to the ICU. *Intact!* All this in a day's work. Truly, anesthesiology is the X-games of Medicine.

D. A. Zvara (✉)
(Emeritus) Department of Anesthesiology, The University of North Carolina at Chapel Hill School of Medicine, Chapel Hill, NC, USA
e-mail: David_Zvara@med.unc.edu

S. Mohamed et al. (eds.), *Anesthesia Bridges*, https://doi.org/10.1007/978-3-032-08294-7_179

"Yes, Okay, and I Will..."

Here's some good advice for your first job: in the first six months to a year, what your partners would like to hear from you when asked to perform a task is "Yes, okay, and I will." Of course, one should never agree to something that is immoral, unethical, or illegal, but in the course of your usual work, this is the best response. Your value to the practice will shine in time. In the first 6 to 12 months, keep your opinions to yourself, offer little advice, and when asked to do something, respond, "yes, okay, and I will."

Be a Good Doctor

I give this advice to every new physician in our practice regardless of how many years of experience they may have: "*You have only one job in your first year here: be a good doctor*." So many times, I've seen physicians enter into our academic practice and wish to set the world on fire in research, education, or administrative service, only to fall flat. Before you can establish yourself as a researcher, educator, or practice administrative leader, you must gain the trust of the surgeons and your anesthesiologist colleagues. Without this respect for you as a clinical physician, none of the other secondary achievements are possible. I feel so strongly about this, I prohibit all new physicians fresh from training from participating in any committees in their first year. "When the surgeon looks up and asks a question about the patient," I advise, "I want you to be in the operating room to answer it." Gain clinical trust and the rest swiftly follows.

Finding a Project Partner

"I can find a hundred people who can start a project; I'm looking for the three who can finish it." Dr. John Butterworth, IV, former chair at Virginia Commonwealth University, passed this advice down to me when I was an assistant professor at Wake Forest. The best partners are those who stick with the work well beyond the initial euphoria of the inception and deliver on time. When picking people to help you with a project, find the three who deliver, and avoid the 97 looking for a ride.

MBA Versus OJT

What does it take to be a successful chairperson of a department? Sure, an MBA or other business education and experience are great, but a simple medical degree and a little "on the job training" (OJT) are fine, too. Here are the essential elements of being a chair: Be honest, be considerate, be fair, be consistent, paint an inspirational vision of the future, provide the resources necessary to achieve this envisioned future, and never deviate from the rules of simple arithmetic. Budgets and forecasting are little more than an exercise in addition and subtraction. Keep it simple, follow the principles outlined above, and your OJT degree will suffice.

Listen, Listen, Listen

You can self-analyze and seek 360 evaluations until you spin in circles. The single greatest advice I've received, and I've received it repeatedly throughout my career, is *listen*. To succeed as a leader, one must listen to those around them. Active, engaged listening, with interest and empathy, is the greatest talent of a leader.

Speak Less and Say More

Nothing further to add.

One Thing About Something

The most common error inexperienced presenters make is the idea that they must include every bit of information ever known or published on their selected topic. The listener is treated to a superficial review of an ocean of information rather than a focused review of the most important. Depth does not exist. The talk is like scanning the table of contents of a text, and never once opening the book. Limit your topic. Go deep. When you think you've cut enough and it is as bare bones as can be; cut more! I beg of you, when we come to the end of your lecture, please let me learn at least one thing about something, rather than nothing about everything.

About Competition

In our free market economy, no one cares that your faculty are smart. No one cares that your department carries the cost of educating residents. No one cares that your department sponsors unfunded research. What your payers care about is your cost (quality is assumed!). They care about your competitiveness in the market. An academic chair does carry the burden of education and research, but when negotiating in the open market, there is no quarter for these missions. Compete for outside work on the terms of the market, not on ivy tower views of how the world *should be*. A successful academic program, like a well-balanced retirement portfolio, will balance education, research, administrative contributions, and entrepreneurial clinical care contracts, matching, toe-to-toe with the best private practice in town.

The Rule of 85/15

Dale Carnegie, in his great book *How to Win Friends and Influence People,* speaks of the balance between building relationships and content knowledge. Essentially, he rhetorically argues that 85% of your success is based on your ability to develop meaningful relationships, and 15% of your success is based on your expertise in the area. It's true. Everyone expects an anesthesiologist to know how to deliver exceptional, safe anesthesiology care; those who move ahead in leadership are those who can nurture, develop, and create meaningful relationships with colleagues, peers, administrators, patients, and others around them.

***Note from the Editors:** Speaking of Dale Carnegie, he was born and spent his youth in Maryville, Missouri. We went looking for cool bridges therein and found this little gem—the "Kissing Bridge" on the campus of Northwest Missouri State University (Fig. 179.1).

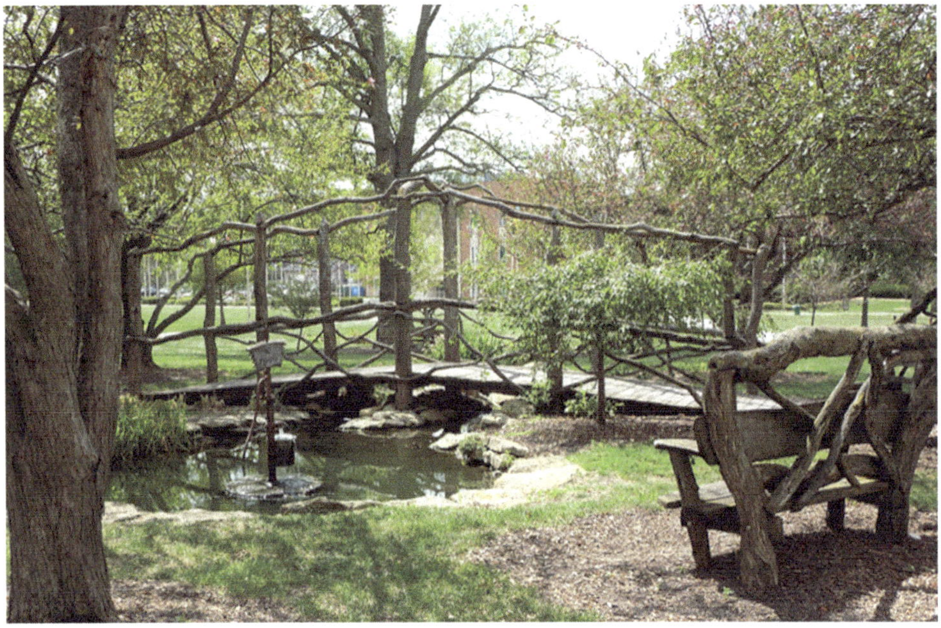

Fig. 179.1 From the university: A small rustic bridge, known as the "Kissing Bridge," is located on the campus of Northwest Missouri State University in Maryville, Missouri. According to Northwest lore, a freshman is not considered a bona fide coed if they are not kissed on the bridge before the first snowfall. Throughout its history, the bridge has become a destination for first dates, engagement proposals, and weddings. Photo: Image used with permission of Northwest Missouri State University

Care for Your People

Always care for your team. Always. If people believe in you, they will sacrifice for you. In an environment of trust, no task is too great for the team. But trust always starts with you. Folks may disagree with your decisions, but if they trust you as a caring leader, they will follow. Care for your people. Develop trust. *Then,* tackle your problems.

A Hundred Problems

As chair, I was often asked by applicants "What are the major problems in the Department? What am I most worried about?" I responded, "You want problems? We got a hundred of them. We have 100 today, we'll have 100 tomorrow, and we'll have 100 five years from now. I just hope they aren't the same ones!" Here's the point: there is no perfect. Each day brings a new challenge. Successful teams navigate, manage, and solve problems. Every place, every job, has a hundred problems… every day. Don't worry about that part of it. Ask, rather, "How does your group solve problems? How does your group deal with conflict?" And, then, listen closely to the answer.

Crisis Management

Sometimes in anesthesiology, one must simply push forward. There are no good alternatives, the outcome appears bleak, and the task is *hard*. In these times, my best advice is to "plant both feet firmly on the ground, hug the one you love, and do your job." Said another way, grounding yourself in the knowledge of your ability, understanding that there is a support team behind you, and focus on delivering care in the moment. Act.

"Anesthesiology Is Hard…

…So, let's not make it any harder." Avoid unnecessary conflicts. Avoid the bait of gossip. Avoid pettiness. Value sincerity. Value integrity. Value work. Value relationships. Value each other. The practice of anesthesiology is hard enough all on its own, let's not make it any harder.

Role Modeling

People judge you on your appearance. People judge you on what you do. People judge you on what you say. This is to be human. If you wish to be treated like a professional, then you must model professionalism. Look professional. Act professionally. Speak professionally. You set the example and tone for how others will treat you. You set the example for those around you. An exemplary team has exemplary role models. Choose to be a role model.

Lessons Learned

- In the first six months to a year in a new job, what your partners would like to hear from you when asked to perform a task is "Yes, okay, and I will."
- You have one main job in your first year of practice—to be a good doctor.
- The best partners are those who stick with the work well beyond the initial euphoria of the inception and deliver on time. Be a "finisher," not just a "starter."
- *Listen. Care for your people. Nurture relationships.*

Author

David Zvara fell into health care at age 16 when taking his first hospital job as a transporter for a physical therapy department. Struck by the generosity of a senior surgeon allowing this naïve high school student a look into the mystery of the OR, Dr. Zvara set his sights on entering this world. The joy of personal connection, the joy of mentorship, and the joy of scholarship motivate him. "Leadership is less about coaching, and more about being a good water boy: Check your ego, and make sure the team has what it needs to succeed. Now, get going."

180 Monitor Your Own Pulse

Mark J. Baskerville

Introduction

Many years ago, I remember sitting in the hospital auditorium listening to the annual compulsory lecture on blood-borne pathogens, proper hand washing, and of course, substance abuse. The program director had recently sent a fellow resident to a treatment center after discovering him to be diverting fentanyl from the operating rooms.

The Talk

We were taught that addiction was a disease, and as an at-risk specialty, we were encouraged to remain vigilant for signs of this occupational hazard among our colleagues. Addiction was not a choice nor a moral failing.

I didn't buy it. To me, this fellow resident was a "bad apple" that needed to be weeded out of our profession. It was one thing to become an alcoholic but to steal drugs from the hospital?

I convinced myself that this talk was not meant for me. It was unfathomable that I would ever succumb to drug addiction, let alone to the tools of my chosen trade. This lecture was not meant for me, or so I thought...

Many years later, I became the poster child for the impaired physician. A destructive combination of arrogance, a reckless disregard for boundaries, an inability to ask for help, a genetic predisposition for addiction, unrecognized depression, and grief all led me to do the unthinkable.

Today, I have evolved into a role model for personal and professional recovery. I have not only survived my circumstances but have thrived. Moreover, I am delighted to share that my fellow resident, whom I once ignorantly characterized as a bad apple, has flourished beyond anyone's expectations. He was not a bad doctor but a sick doctor.

M. J. Baskerville (✉)
Department of Anesthesiology and Critical Care, Oregon Health and Science University, Portland, OR, USA
e-mail: baskervi@ohsu.edu

S. Mohamed et al. (eds.), *Anesthesia Bridges*, https://doi.org/10.1007/978-3-032-08294-7_180

I would like to share my addiction history, professional sanctions, and successful recovery. I hope to communicate who I am, what happened, and my subsequent journey into recovery. Hopefully, in the end, you'll realize that I, too, was not a bad doctor, but a sick doctor—a sickness that can infect any anesthesiologist given the right circumstances.

The Start of My Story

After graduating college, I attended medical school and subsequently completed two residencies in emergency medicine and anesthesiology. After five rigorous years of training, I took a welcome break—working and teaching as a part-time attending in the operating rooms. This reprieve afforded me the opportunity to complete my specialty board certification exams, travel, and get married.

Eventually, we decided to move to the West Coast to raise a family. Although I worked primarily as a cardiac anesthesiologist in a community hospital, I remained on the staff at my former training institution as a part-time clinical associate. I would fly back several times per year to work in the operating rooms and tutor residents. I incredibly enjoyed these teaching experiences—a stark contrast with my private practice world, which progressively grew more unsatisfying.

Ultimately, my professional disillusionment and personal discontent reached a peak. A series of life stressors—in the face of an unrecognized clinical depression—breached my ability to cope. A series of bad decisions and clouded judgments resulted in my crossing boundaries that were never meant to be violated. For two months, I found myself in a lethal struggle with a fentanyl addiction. I lost my job, my license, and my dignity. But in sobriety, I found humility, gratitude, and integrity.

***Note from the Editors:** Mark Baskerville's choice for a meaningful bridge in his life is the St. John's Bridge in the Portland, OR metro area (Fig. 180.1a and b). When we asked Mark what prompted his choice of this bridge, he sent back a remarkable answer:

> Actually, my choice of this bridge merges well with my chapter. I pulled a person I am monitoring for the state bar off the edge early one morning during a suicide attempt. When the *Anesthesia Bridges* editors asked me for my favorite internet picture of the bridge, I said I could do much better than that! My colleague Laura Chess lives in the area of the bridge, and this is the view from her house—lucky person! From her house, the spires frame a view of Mt. Hood.

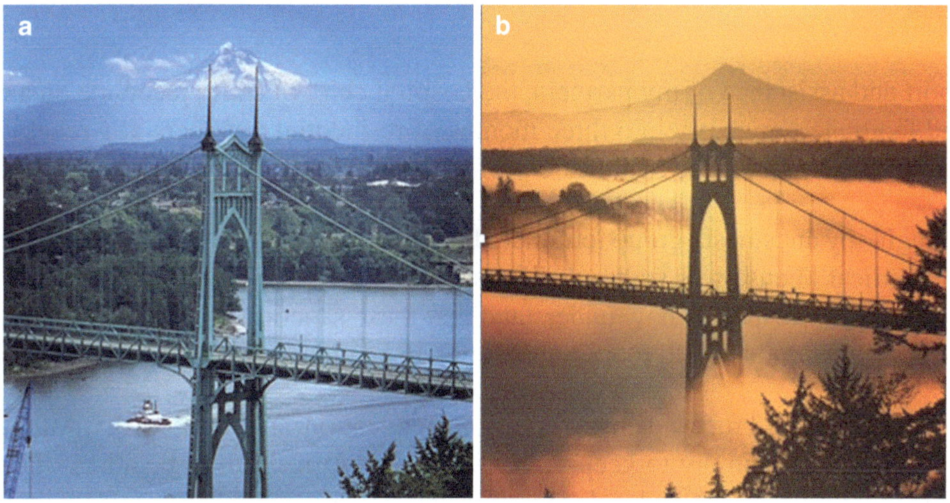

Figs. 180.1 (**a** and **b**) The St. John's Bridge in Multnomah County, OR. This steel suspension bridge crosses the Willamette River and connects the Cathedral Park neighborhood of North Portland with the neighborhoods of Northwest Portland. It was dedicated in 1931 and held many construction records at the time. It is associated with quite a bit of renown and notoriety. Municipal officials waited until St. Patrick's Day in 1931 to announce that the bridge would be painted green. In bright sunlight, it is the color of lima beans, but we also love it when the marine surroundings make it blue and when it is shrouded in fog. Photos: Laura Chess

Acute Illness

One morning, I suffered a grand mal seizure in the operating room, triggered by the progressive accumulation of drug metabolites within my system. By the grace of God, this patient, as well as many others, was not harmed. I had turned into a liar and a thief, as I actively hid my addiction and falsified my wastage of drugs on controlled substance logs. Although most ascribe my dishonesty to my disease, I now realize it was much more than that—it was an inevitable consequence of the progressive erosion of my character that began years before I ever picked up a syringe.

I acted in reckless disregard for the safety of my patients. The hallmark of addiction is denial and minimization—neither of which I wish to ascribe to my conduct. I violated the trust of my colleagues, the hospital, and most importantly, my patients. I was deeply sorry that I had disappointed so many. I always thought it "could never happen to me." But it did. I never realized the power of an addiction to take over your life and to force you to act in ways that you never thought possible. But it does…

Boundaries weren't for me. It was a slippery slope of prescribing antibiotics for a family member, to bringing syringes home for my wife's fertility injections, and ultimately diverting wasted fentanyl for my dying dog. I hate that word—"diverted." Let's call it what it was: **theft.**

As my life was unravelling, I did a poor job of monitoring my own psychological and emotional pulse. I thought I could control the uncontrollable. Why did I not ask for help? I feared that I would lose my job and my license. Ironically, that is exactly what happened. Yet, I was one of the lucky ones who did not lose their life.

Recovery

With the support and assistance of my partners, the hospital chief of staff placed me on a medical leave of absence and facilitated my entry into three months of residential treatment at a rehabilitation center that specialized in treating addicted healthcare professionals.

Ultimately, though, my anesthesia group terminated my employment and reported me to the state medical board. My medical license was suspended for several years, despite my participation in the state's diversion program. In retrospect, I now understand that these sanctions were the exact accountability I needed to atone for my conduct, and more importantly, to keep me sober and to protect the public.

During this mandated break, I focused on my family, my education, and my recovery. Although I enrolled in business and law school simply to keep my brain busy, it turned out to be a blessing in disguise. I enjoyed being back in a classroom and truly learning again. I will always be grateful for this opportunity to hit the proverbial "reset button" mid-career. It put everything into perspective and gave me the necessary clarity to understand who I was, why I failed, what I wanted, and how to get it back.

I realized that the traditional practice of anesthesiology was not an option. Going back to the operating room would be akin to making an alcoholic become a bartender. However, intensive care units and emergency departments were a particularly fitting clinical environment in which I could leverage my skills and experience to care for patients, while at the same time, providing the necessary safeguards to mitigate any risk of relapse.

However, before I could embark down this new clinical path, I had to convince the state medical board that I was worthy of a license. Without a doubt, the primary role of the medical board was to protect the welfare of the public. Obviously, an opioid-addicted physician would pose a great threat to the public. Before granting me an active license, the medical board needed to be convinced that I had been successfully rehabilitated: Had I embraced recovery? Was my addiction in sustained remission? Had I accepted full responsibility and been held accountable for my conduct? Was the likelihood of this ever happening again vanishingly remote? Could I be trusted to care for a close friend or family member? Thankfully, they said yes...

Gratitude and Growth

I would be remiss to suggest that I made a successful comeback on my own. Many had to put blind faith in me and to provide opportunities I did not deserve. Most critically, my former program director—the same person who showed compassion for that resident when I failed to do so—stood unwaveringly by my side and selflessly advocated for my return to medicine. Without his support, I would never have been able to salvage my career.

Opioid addiction is a chronic disease that, like any other incurable condition, requires diligent management and uncompromising self-discipline to always prioritize my recovery. In medicine, I had made the deliberate decision to never put myself or my patients at risk again. I did not return to anesthesiology, where it is inherent to the job to have unfettered, unsupervised access to potent opioids. Fortunately, critical care and emergency medicine have allowed me to use my clinical skills and medical knowledge under the direct supervision of a close-knit team, while at the same time, shielding me from access and direct exposure to opioids.

Today...

Now well into my 20th year of recovery, I have tested my sobriety and have performed well despite the rigorous workload and the high-stress environment of a busy ICU. I participate in a comprehensive recovery program, including strict monitoring, psychiatric care, toxicology screens, cognitive behavioral therapy, fellowship groups, and continual interaction with the addiction community. I am monitored rigorously by the state's physician health program, while my individual care is managed by an addiction psychiatrist. My abstinence is confirmed with daily phone calls randomizing my mandatory observed drug tests. Transparency remains the key to my success with day-to-day accountability to my colleagues, as well as a no-cause drug testing policy.

I am not the same person I was 20+ years ago. I am no longer that arrogant, controlling person who had no respect for boundaries and refused to ask for help. Time has allowed my brain to rewire and recovery has taught me how to live life on life's terms. I have accepted complete and full responsibility for my conduct. I do not blame anyone or anything, except my disease and my arrogance. Even though the safe-harbor provisions afforded by the prior diversion program broke down in my situation, the added accountability had only strengthened my recovery, taught me the importance of humility, and made me a better person, and ultimately, a better doctor.

Although the opioid epidemic respects no boundaries, I hope to mitigate its effect by making the impaired practitioner a "never event." My experience—successes and failures—provides a rich background and a valuable perspective to counsel other physicians on how to care for others, while caring for themselves.

I accept this duty. I no longer view the publicity of my addiction and my sanctions as a stigma, but as an opportunity to be a role model. I volunteer my professional skills and personal experiences on both a local and national level, where I internally and externally champion the use of more proactive, preventive measures to help protect our healthcare practitioners, and most importantly, our patients.

I remain deeply indebted to all who have afforded me a chance to rehabilitate my career. Without fail, I will continually prove my worthiness to practice medicine, while never taking for granted the privilege of being a physician. In the end, if the purpose of my life was to serve as a warning to others, then I have succeeded. Please do not make the sentinel error I had made—that is, telling yourself, "that could never happen to me."

Lessons Learned

- **Monitor your own** pulse! Anesthesiology can be a very stressful occupation, even for experienced and skilled clinicians.

- Mounting work-related stress, along with unrecognized depression, and a disposition for addictive behaviors has the potential to permit almost anyone to develop a lethal (to both self and others) addiction to alcohol or opioids.

- Leave control in the OR, it's **both okay and necessary** to take a break from what we do clinically.

- Respect boundaries, the rules are **not** just for everyone else.
- Learn to ask for help, it could save your life.
- Embrace humility.

Author

Mark Baskerville practices as an intensivist, an attorney, and an ethicist. He has a passion for medical education with a particular interest in leveraging high-fidelity simulation to improve patient care and team performance across the perioperative arena. When not treating patients in the ICU, he can be found in a courtroom defending the rights of prisoners. He devotes any remaining free time to travel with his wife and three children.

Manipulation: Is It a Good Thing or Bad Thing?

181

Neil B. Sandson, Catherine Marcucci,
and Raymond G. Graber

Introduction

The usual definition of manipulation is to "control or influence (a person or situation) cleverly, unfairly, or unscrupulously." We agree with clever influence; we don't agree with unfair or unscrupulous influence. We, therefore, explore the nuances of this definition below.

To start with, from Neil Sandson: **Get it out of your mind that manipulation is necessarily a bad thing.**

> The term "manipulation" generally has a negative connotation, and some explicitly define it as attempting to influence others to one's own advantage. However, as a psychiatrist, I see benevolently directed manipulation as a critical skill set. I've gone so far as to tell trainees that they are being taught to be effective manipulators of others' acute and chronic emotional states, for their patients' benefit rather than their own, and that the sooner they become comfortable with that concept, the more effective they will be in learning those important skills.
>
> Some may wish to avoid this language, instead couching therapeutic manipulations as "persuasion" and "guidance." Certainly, persuasion, guidance, supportiveness, collaboration, and myriad other concepts are also part of the therapeutic armamentarium. Effective therapists need to be deliberately and skillfully titrating interventions, based on what they believe would be more effective, best tolerated, most appropriate, and the like. This requires the therapist/provider to be fundamentally in control of more dimensions of the interaction than would be healthy in a reciprocal relationship.

N. B. Sandson
Department of Psychiatry, VA Maryland Health Care System, Baltimore, MD, USA

University of Maryland, Baltimore, MD, USA

C. Marcucci (✉)
Department of Transfusion Medicine, Clinical Center, National Institutes of Health, Bethesda, MD, USA

R. G. Graber
Department of Anesthesiology and Perioperative Medicine, University Hospitals Cleveland Medical Center, Cleveland, OH, USA

S. Mohamed et al. (eds.), *Anesthesia Bridges*, https://doi.org/10.1007/978-3-032-08294-7_181

I Include Myself

We can try to use language to sanitize this communication paradigm and cater to our sensibilities, but what is being described is, at heart, a kind of manipulation. So long as it's not fundamentally selfish, when I'm able to discern others attempting to manipulate me, I regard it as a compliment; they care enough about how I feel to try to exert some influence over that. But of course, I will keep my own counsel on if and how I allow myself to be affected.

Manners, consideration, solicitude: these things can arise from altruistic places, but to the extent that they also represent socially learned behaviors, they are manipulations that we are all too happy to invite and accept. I don't think this is Machiavellian reductionism. Rather, I think it is a worldview that acknowledges the realities of our internal and external emotional landscapes and provides a map with actual landmarks and features, instead of an array of comforting mirages.

***Note from the Editors:** Speaking of manipulation and gaming, Neil Sandson's favorite "bridge" is **duplicate bridge**, hands down (Fig. 181.1). He tells us why:

> Bridge is intellectual combat! And you fight with a partner on the battlefield, which is often disguised as a card table in a church basement.

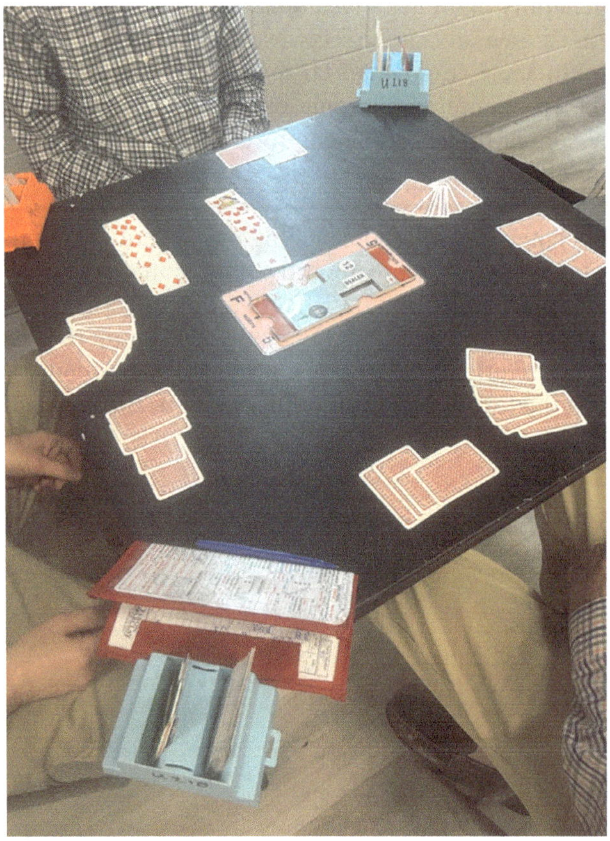

Fig. 181.1 A typical duplicate bridge hand. Unlike chess, bridge is a game that is unlikely ever to be solved, as only half the cards are revealed to the player at the start of the hand. It is Neil Sandson's favorite game to play. He is a Ruby Life Master. Photo: Cathy Marcucci

From Ray Graber: **But unfortunately, we have all seen the dark side of manipulation**

On the other hand, be aware of manipulation that is not altruistic and is self-serving. Most of us have stories about surgeons who will try to manipulate the OR schedule to get their cases in at a time that works for them. It is an inconvenient reality that cases added onto surgical schedules must wait for an available spot, and surgeons will plead their case.

I like to tell the story of a urologist who called me on a Sunday morning early in my career to book a newborn for repair of bladder exstrophy and insisted that it had to bump all other cases. After cases and staff were rearranged to accommodate this request, the surgeon called back to say he had to delay the case because the newborn was more premature than he had realized. When asked how long he was going to delay the case, he responded "about 4 weeks." That surgeon lost all credibility with the staff that day.

So, how do you deal with the scenario where a surgeon wants to bump other cases? First, there are some cases that just have to go ASAP—for example, patients who are actively hemorrhaging. But more often, there is a safe window of time for most surgeries. On weekends and evenings, most surgeries proceed in the order in which they were booked. One method experienced OR staff use is to have the surgeon who wants to jump the line call the surgeon he/she wants to bump to discuss which case should go first. Our colleagues believe that a surgeon is less likely to try to "put one over" on another surgical colleague. If the two surgeons are within the same department, the department chair can help resolve the issue of who has priority. Some hospitals also have a surgeon on call (a "surgical safety officer") to deal with disputes such as this in the OR.

On another note, long surgical wait times due to inadequate staffing can only lead to exacerbation of the above issue. Ideally, hospital leadership should endeavor to have adequate staff to match the caseload of the operating room suite. This is perhaps something you can inquire about when looking at a job. If operating rooms are constrained by the availability of nursing teams, that manpower and scheduling tension may be reflected onto and born by the anesthesia and surgical teams and result in manipulation and jockeying in the schedule.

From Neil Sandson and Cathy Marcucci

Sociopathic, heavy-handed powerplays, as Ray described above, do represent an extreme pole of toxic manipulation, for sure. Just as it is more challenging to mobilize subtle and benevolent manipulations on behalf of patients, it is also more challenging to recognize and thwart subtle and clever malevolently intended manipulations in the workplace.

Skilled and effective leaders have the knowledge of the rules and power dynamics to address the former situations, and they have developed the pattern recognition to recognize the later. But what do you do if you are junior faculty and you don't yet have tons of the experience or institutional authority, but your manipulation Spidey-sense is tingling?

- **First**, don't be mad that it is happening. If you are going to work in the operating room, then you must recognize that this is the only place where care is shared with two independent providers. This unique situation inevitably leads to conflict, which in turn can lead to attempts to inappropriately manipulate. People who see a shortcut to what they want, or what personally serves their interests, will try to take it. There may be name-calling, aspersions cast upon your clinical skills and acumen, and all sorts of other underhanded ad hominem attacks. **Don't take the bait.**

- **Second**, don't hesitate to first consult your own conscience as to how much support you would receive from your senior folks in trying to ward off any level of ill-intended manipulation. When Cathy was working for Denny Bourke at the Baltimore VA, she made it a practice to let him know what conflicts she was involved in as she was inappropriately pressured to do things or not do things. She didn't ask him to walk over to the OR to fight off the manipulations or even involve him in any group conversations. But she would find a way to quickly let him know what the issues were, what the ECHO showed, what she was being asked to do, what she was going to do, and what she was not going to do. He mentioned several times that this information was very helpful when, occasionally, somebody stomped over to the anesthesiology office suite to make a fuss.

- **Third**, unless it is a clear matter of patient safety or clearly an anesthesia clinical decision, don't rush to get in front of any trains. Don't let anybody dictate your care plan to you, but there is no need for you to get flattened.

- **Fourth**, we wish we could give you detailed replies to malevolent manipulation, but of course responses need to be tailored to the specific situation and attempted malfeasance. However, we **will** recommend that you develop a couple of bland and innocuous delaying and defusing statements that nobody could ever criticize, even in the most hostile management review. These are not definitive ways to end toxic manipulation, rather these are space and time fillers to slow down the tempo of the interaction to give you time to think. We have touched on several of these elsewhere in this book, but they merit a second consideration. We've highlighted the one-liners.

Responses that cannot be impeached:

That doesn't seem quite cricket from an anesthesia viewpoint.

It's best care not to skip these steps.

A repeat EKG is indicated in this situation and would be very helpful. We will be giving the patient the benefit of this reasonable standard of care.

We are going to start the case when the proper and necessary preop eval is completed and we've reviewed. We won't start the case before that. We will let you know the minute the patient is ready to go.

We need to make all parts of the case match each other.

Can we all just slow down and think about what's best for the patient?

I do think it's best if the anesthesia decisions are made by the anesthesia team. Wouldn't you agree?

That feels a bit ad hominem.

This seems to be taking on the dimensions of a personal attack rather than a patient-centered discussion of care.

I understand that we have the same goal of patient care, maybe different approaches, though. Whether or not it's intentional, I believe that what you are asking me to do is not strongly indicated.

Yes, I agree. My decision is indeed moderately conservative, but I think that level of caution is warranted here. This is not the patient that we want to have to reintubate in the PACU.

We're just trying to be careful.

Lessons Learned

- Positive manipulation is done to add to safety, security, and increased standard and quality of care. It should decrease interpersonal tension and lead to positive feelings and outcome. Negative manipulation is generally about persuading people to do something they shouldn't do. It leads to regret, bitterness, and anger.
- With respect to the positive manipulation skills that mental health providers are taught—perhaps there is also a lesson here to be learned for anesthesia providers? We know that the anesthesiologist's personal qualities and communication styles—calm, knowledgeable, confident—has great effect on a patient's anxiety level, sense of comfort, and even resulting pain levels. What is this but a degree of altruistic manipulation? Every single one of the descriptors noted above in "titrating interventions" can be applied to selecting an anesthesia technique, determining an overall anesthetic management plan, and presenting it to the patient with the appropriate discussion of risks and benefits.
- Speaking of calmness, it is a highly valuable personality trait when seeking to deploy benevolent manipulation and defending against the malevolent version.
- Emotionally balanced persuasion is also a very necessary skill when dealing with trainees, surgeons, nurses, ancillary clinical staff, and the wider clinical care setting. Especially when you are trying to convince people that they need to decide to care. Remember, you can't really make people deliver superlative care—you have to instead make them want to.
- Unfortunately, sometimes people will use manipulation as a control game or power play. Deflect this with the most minimal and oblique defense that gets you and the patient out of harm's way of the manipulation. No need to create open conflict. We repeat, no need to step in front of a speeding train and get flattened. If the priority levels of surgical cases are set by the hospital, don't overcall them. If a surgeon wants to post a Level 1 case and bump a Level 2 case, that is not something to get in the middle of.
- Use the deflecting statements above only if they work for you. If they don't, think carefully about one that would work for you and have them ready in your mind for deployment.

Authors

Neil Sandson is a psychiatrist in Baltimore, MD. He has worked his benevolent powers of persuasion in many situations ranging from the Baltimore City jail to his patients in four different hospitals to his children. There is no dissuading the dog, though—she pretty much sleeps where she wants including on the upholstered furniture and under the covers of whichever bed looks good to her that night.

Cathy Marcucci is an anesthesiologist and transfusion medicine physician. She plans to review this chapter at regular intervals, being herself something of a black-or-white person and always looking for ways to better finesse the situation. She doesn't mind being (kindly) manipulated but intensely dislikes being lied to.

Ray Graber is a senior anesthesiologist at Case Western. He is known for his calm and diplomatic demeanor, regardless of the situation. His colleagues have suggested that he could give lessons in this.

Learning from the Greats

182

Ronald H. Wender

Introduction

Why do we choose to teach? We teach because we take out a tremendous amount from the profession and we need to put something back. The "put back" is training those who come after you. It is also a way of saying thank you to those who spent the time, effort, and expertise on our education. What advice would I give to a much younger version of myself? Say thank you to your mentors both in and out of medicine for their help and commitment.

Margaret Mead and Isidor Rabi

First is Margaret Mead, the matriarch of modern anthropology. She was my advisor and teacher during my year of independent research at the Museum of Natural History in New York. Working one-on-one with a legend in anthropology taught me to never be afraid to leave my comfort zone, which opened entire new worlds of knowledge. I learned to never be afraid to ask a question, even if it demonstrates lack of knowledge. Doing research for a 135-page paper by spending days in the bowels of the Columbia University library taught me perseverance and the challenge of pursuing new information.

Contrast that with today's ability to get instant gratification via the computer and PubMed. Taking graduate courses at Columbia allowed me to interact one-on-one with Dr. Isidor Rabi, who won the Nobel Prize in Physics for discovering nuclear magnetic resonance. Dr. Rabi clearly demonstrated the importance of humility and dignity in the face of ultimate achievement. Dr. Rabi's ability to talk to students on a level they could easily understand without talking down to them has been a guiding principle in my 45+ years as an educator.

R. H. Wender (✉)
Department of Anesthesiology, Cedars-Sinai Medical Center, Los Angeles, CA, USA

S. Mohamed et al. (eds.), *Anesthesia Bridges*, https://doi.org/10.1007/978-3-032-08294-7_182

The Reverend Dr. King

Fate, time, and circumstance can often shape a career unexpectedly. That certainly was evident in my career. Unexpectedly, I was able to get a job doing radio, including news, sports, weather, and interviews, for the only African American-owned radio station in the United States. This was during the heart of the Civil Rights movement in Atlanta. Being the token Caucasian working for a radio station with only African American staff and talent taught me what it is like to be a minority. My office was in the Southern Christian Leadership Conference, a two-story building, and my office was right above that of the Reverend Dr. Martin Luther King, Jr. This time left an indelible mark on my psyche, about understanding and helping to improve the plight of others.

When Dr. King would return to his office, he would take a broom and bang on the ceiling, which was the floor of my office. I would run downstairs to interview him. I spent many hours of one-on-one time with the giants of the civil rights movement, including Dr. King, and was the only white reporter allowed in the Student Nonviolent Coordinating Committee headquarters during the Rap Brown/Stokely Carmichael era. To have one-on-one time with a man who shaped history and to "pick his brain" was truly a blessing and an opportunity very few people have.

Dr. King knew longevity was not in his future. Yet, it did not deter him from his message in life. He showed me what real dedication means. I am thankful for the time we had together. After spending this personal time with Dr. King, the lesson learned was, "No matter how you are treated, no matter what your circumstances, you are always responsible for your actions."

***Note from the Editors:** A view from the east side of the bridge where Dr. King attempted to lead 2000 civil rights marchers towards Montgomery AL on March 7, 1965 (Fig. 182.1). They eventually reached the capital on March 21.

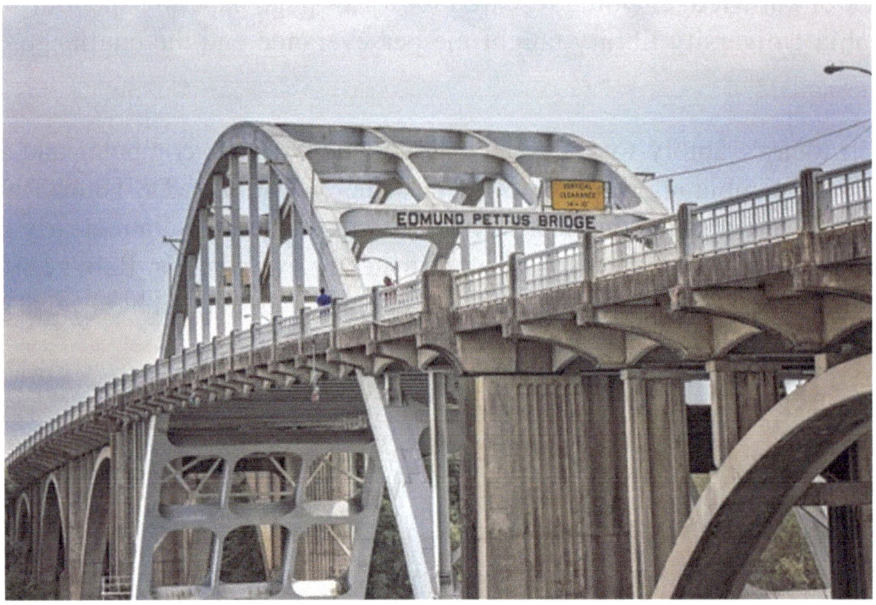

Fig. 182.1 The Edmund Pettus bridge was built in 1940 and is a through steel bridge. It spans the Alabama River in Selma, AL. It is now a National Historic Landmark. Photo: Image used under standard license from stock.adobe.com

Cedars-Sinai

Arriving at Cedars-Sinai in 1976, I had the honor and opportunity of working with two giants in cardiology—Jeremy Swan and William Ganz. These two brilliant physicians demonstrated ingenuity, humility, and grace. "Don't be afraid to push the envelope" was the motivating paradigm. Unfortunately, in many areas of medicine, there is resistance to change. I was very fortunate to learn from two pioneers in medicine who opened many doors for me.

This really taught me the meaning and value of mentoring. It showed me what it means if you are lucky enough to be mentored. This allowed me to take on an anesthesia chairmanship at age 29, knowing well that I would have to literally grow up in the job, which I would have for 42 years. I have had many mentors in the anesthesiology community, such as Stan Schneider and James Schauble, who taught me how to navigate the operating rooms but also to develop an empathetic and humanistic approach to patients. I have always loved saying "smart people surround themselves with smarter people and you will always look good." I have tried to live by that advice.

Lessons Learned

- Do not be afraid to leave your comfort zone.
- Humility in the face of achievement is enviable.
- "You are responsible for your actions."
- Being a mentor is an honor.
- "Better to be board certified than certified bored."

Author

Ron Wender was born and raised in Atlanta, Georgia. He met his wife of 50+ years, Fern, at Columbia University in New York. They became the only married undergraduates at Columbia. Fern has been a Beverly Hills divorce lawyer for 30+ years. Most importantly, she gave Ron a kidney. Ron has been at Cedars-Sinai since it opened in 1976.

183 Pay Attention to the Interface Because That's Where All the Innovation Will Happen

Raymond G. Graber, John Matthew Hess, Charles H. Sandson, and Catherine Marcucci

Introduction

We are convinced that the statement in the title is one of the most important pieces of advice that we can give our colleagues but also possibly one of the more difficult topics for anesthesiologists, of all ages, to turn and face. We cannot say it too bluntly: Do not let yourself get behind the technology curve! And if you are a bit behind, start making plans now to catch up. Here are some recommendations.

Pay Close Attention to the Interface

And just what is the "interface?" In the business John Hess is in (component and connector design), it's precisely defined in computer hardware lingo, but a general definition for anesthesiology could be the shared boundary where two systems meet and information is shared. The exchange of information can be between software, hardware, peripheral devices, humans, and any combination of these. In our daily work, maybe the most important interface is between us and the patient. Other important interfaces are those between the patient and our monitoring equipment, our monitors and us, and our data with the wider data systems of the hospital. Be aware that all these interfaces are continually evolving, and accept that you must stay up to date with these developments.

Patient–clinician interface: A good example is the adoption and implementation of ultrasound-guided techniques for blocks and line placement. The same old anatomy exists for the internal jugular vein and peripheral nerves. The Seldinger technique and delivery of local anesthetic through a hollow needle are essentially the same as 50 years ago.

R. G. Graber
Department of Anesthesiology and Perioperative Medicine, University Hospitals Cleveland Medical Center, Cleveland, OH, USA
e-mail: raymond.graber@uhhospitals.org

J. M. Hess
Tessco Technologies, Inc., Hunt Valley, MD, USA

C. H. Sandson
ZS Associates, Washington, DC, USA

C. Marcucci (✉)
Department of Transfusion Medicine, Clinical Center, National Institutes of Health, Bethesda, MD, USA

S. Mohamed et al. (eds.), *Anesthesia Bridges*, https://doi.org/10.1007/978-3-032-08294-7_183

But the interface is no longer just the anatomical landmarks and the anesthesiologist's eyes and fingers. If you were initially reluctant to adopt the use of ultrasound, you were immediately off the curve. Another good example is the development and increasing use of video laryngoscopy. This technology has literally given us the ability to see around corners and made what were previously difficult intubations routine walks in the park. We are also using increasingly advanced transesophageal echocardiography equipment with 3D imaging to guide both our cardiac surgeons in the OR and our cardiology interventionalists in the catheterization labs.

Patient-monitor interface: Our monitors are getting more and more sophisticated and are giving us new ways to look at our patient's physiology. It's not just about measuring blood pressure and heart rate anymore.

New types of cardiac output monitoring systems give us the ability to deliver goal-directed fluid therapy. We have devices to measure depth of anesthesia, neuromuscular transmission, and cerebral blood flow. Point-of-care laboratory devices such as new-generation thromboelastograms (TEGs) are giving us more detailed information about the clotting system. Most of these devices are linked by wires and cables to our main anesthesia monitor system—generating at best clutter, and at worst hazardous trip-inducing working conditions. In the future, we'll see the more frequent use of technology such as Bluetooth to link our equipment together.

Clinician-monitor interface: As the amount of potential physiologic data increases, our equipment manufacturers will continue to work towards finding effective and meaningful ways to display all this information. For example, depth of anesthesia devices typically displays a number based on an algorithmic interpretation of a patient's EEG.

What about recording all this data? During the course of our careers, we have seen anesthesia record keeping move from charting on paper to the development of Anesthesia Information Management Systems (AIMS). These allow the automatic collection, storage, and presentation of patient data, along with giving us access to entering drug data and the rest of the typical perioperative documentation that we do. Our access to AIMS was initially by using computers mounted to or adjacent to our anesthesia machines but has moved to tablet devices in some systems. The integration of clinical decision support tools is another ongoing area of development. Built-in artificial intelligence applications will warn us of dangerous trends or remind us of antibiotic redosing—maybe by pinging our wearable smart devices (watches, headsets and glasses).

Data, Data, and More Data!

The decisions we make in the operating room do not exist in a vacuum. Each time we make a choice or complete an action, we are also affecting the wider system we exist within. We are constantly creating data.

There are multiple types of data generated, stored, and hence available for analysis. There are patient **physiologic** and **outcomes** data that have been collected in our electronic anesthesia records and can be used for process improvement and for quality assurance activities. There are **financial** data, for example, automated anesthesia billing and pharmacy charges abstracted from anesthesia records. And then there are OR **management** and **efficiency data**. Do cases start on time? How long do they last? How long does room turnover take? To sum, be aware that <u>your</u> data are being collected and analyzed.

If You Are Reluctant to Consider and Accept Innovations at the Interface, You Will Eventually Be Replaced

This is because innovations at the anesthesia interface will be focused on making things safer for patients and less costly for both patients and the health care system. These pressures will continue to be overwhelming and immutable, although they won't result in unanimous positive results in every instance—some of the failures of mandated electronic patient records come to mind. But overall, to refuse to accept interface innovations will be, in essence, to obstruct patient-care progress that must and will happen, either with you or without you.

Don't Take It Personally!

It is part of human nature to resist change. And this problem happens in every industry, including the tech sector. John tells us of a situation that occurred in his first professional engineering job, back in the day. There were engineering designers still working on drafting tables, and the boss was trying to convert the office to workstations and computer-aided design. John and a couple of other people were already onboard.

By the end of the week, about half of the rest of the group agreed to convert somewhat reluctantly, and the remaining people were gone. As in, escorted out of the building with their final paychecks. And these shown-the-door people were youngish engineers who had been specifically hired to be designers, inventors, and innovators. They were most definitely not old-timers.

Usually, though, tech is not your enemy! Charlie Sandson tells us that the vast majority of the new technology we will see coming into our hospitals in the next decade is going to be specifically designed to make it possible for doctors to do their jobs faster and more safely. A common complaint of physicians is along the lines of "My unit is already doing the best job it can, and only other physicians know how to make the little tweaks we might need."

In a sense, they are actually right! Qualitatively, we have made modern medicine about as efficient as it can get. We've picked off all the easy changes through doctors doing anecdotal analyses of their own units. The only way to continue to improve is through data-driven analyses, and while change can be disruptive and resistance is natural, these are the steps needed to continue to improve the efficiency of our ORs.

Start Looking Around

Work to recognize effective innovation ideas and don't be a "patent hoarder."

Here again, we feel the anesthesia community has much to learn from innovation in the technology business. John Hess received 11 patents in 16 years with a previous company. The patents are clustered around seven big ideas. Only one patent is held just by him—some are held by a whole team of people.

Why is this important? Because those 11 patents "sold" for about $2,000,000,000 in business. Of course, meaningful innovation in the anesthesia business isn't just measured in dollars, but the point is to look for and develop ideas that are understandable, effective, and able to be implemented—or in other words that will "sell."

And there is no need to be stingy with your efforts and ideas. "Patent hoarders" out in the tech sector are those people who are over-claiming and attempting to hoard credit and ownership of ideas and innovation. In our medical situation, we feel this would be a mistake. There is plenty of creative work to be done—there is room for everyone to have a robust role in innovation and to do well by doing good, both for ourselves and our patients.

***Note from the Editors:** We are grateful to coauthor John Hess for sharing his time and expertise with the anesthesia community. Since John is originally from Lancaster County, PA we wanted to feature a beautiful Lancaster covered bridge in his honor, but we couldn't decide on which was the coolest. We ended up choosing the Weaver's Mill Covered Bridge (Fig. 183.1). The bridge's single span crosses the Conestoga River and was built in 1878. It has wooden double Burr arch trusses with additional steel rods. As is tradition with Lancaster Country bridges, it is painted red inside and out and the approaches are painted white.

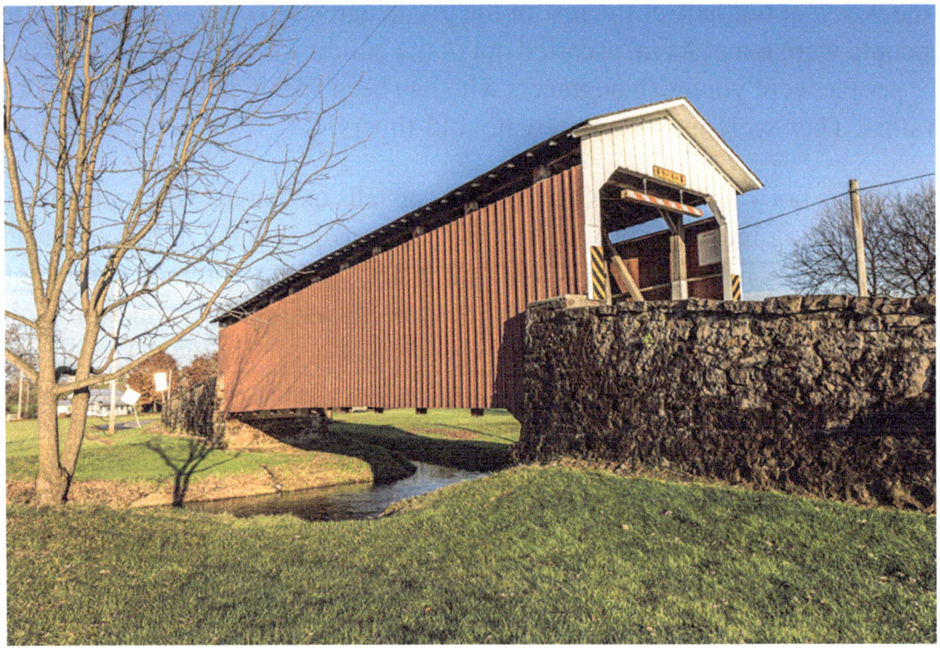

Fig. 183.1 The Weaver's Mill Bridge over Conestoga Creek in Lancaster County, PA. John is married to Josie Weaver Hess, but there is no relation. Apparently, there are hundreds of Weaver families in Lancaster County. Photo: Image used under standard license from adobestock.com

Keep Your Eyes Trained on Society!

If you can't see areas for innovation by looking closely at our working environments, refocus your gaze on what's going on in society.

The anesthesia business has been the leader in some areas of patient care and safety, and other medical specialties and businesses have adapted and adopted our research and innovations. In other areas, we are perhaps a bit behind on the innovation curve. Here are three areas that are actively emerging:

Artificial intelligence (AI): This is most simply a system's ability to correctly interpret external data, to learn from such data, and to use those learnings to achieve specific goals and tasks through flexible adaptation, thus simulating human intelligence. It is already here, but not yet fully deployed, of course. Many experts believe it is the most important and powerful development in the technology and innovation sector.

We recommend that you attend every lecture and do every online learning module that you can find on how AI will impact medicine, especially the practice of anesthesiology. Most applications of artificial intelligence for anesthesiology are still in research and development, and the focus is not on replacing clinician judgment or skills but on investigating ways to augment them. In the future, we may see automated delivery of anesthetics and automated responses to hemodynamic instability as machine learning concepts and applications get increasingly sophisticated.

Nanotechnology: This is science, engineering, and technology at the level of the atom (or about 10^{-9} meters). The concept was first suggested by legendary Richard Feynman in 1959. There are dozens of medical technology companies already focused on nanomedicine applications such as imaging and diagnosis. Probably the most promising work involves methods to target specific cells and tissues for delivery of drugs or therapeutics by building "molecular machines." What's next after nanotechnology? Pico technology and even femto technology. These involve the manipulation of matter on the scale of 10^{-12} and 10^{-15} meters, or at the level of protons!

Sustainability: The U.S. health care sector has been estimated to contribute up to 10% of the nation's greenhouse gas emissions. In order to reduce health care waste and pollution in the operating room, it is now understood that we need to go way, way beyond just scavenging waste anesthetic agents. The operating room also generates a ton of waste from disposables used during the course of surgery. A wealth of articles in the medical literature and lay press already exists. If you haven't read them, please do so at the soonest possible opportunity. And don't resist this movement—it's here, it will continue to be here, and it's necessary and important.

Finally, Find the Knowers and Doers

If you are an anesthesiologist without a STEM degree and without an outsize interest in technology and innovations, start hanging around those people who are and do.

There are always at least a couple of people in every department who are the go-to equipment and tech folks. Ask them what seminars they attended at the last meeting or what they thought of the most recent tech-y journal articles. If you are an anesthesiologist with a science, STEM, or engineering degree—a not inconsiderable number of us—keep up your networking with engineering and tech people in other businesses and sectors, particularly the mechanical, industrial, materials science, and computer engineers.

Lessons Learned

- Our business is the delivery of anesthetics and perioperative care. We would do well to borrow freely and shamelessly from the folks whose business it is to write the code, develop the machines and materials, and move the personnel and materials. Hijack and apply whatever engineering principles will benefit your patients!
- Think often and carefully about the interface—this is where the innovation will happen. Focus on how the interface is characterized, understood, managed, and even manipulated.
- **Don't resist the tech advances!** If you do, they will sweep past you. And you will be swept out the door in the currents.
- Start reading and learning about artificial intelligence, nanotechnology, and sustainability. These are several of the current cutting-edge topics.
- **Do not be afraid.** There will always be room for humanism and the human touch in patient-centered medicine.

Authors

Ray Graber holds a BS in biomedical engineering from Rensselaer Polytechnic Institute. He feels the problem-solving skills he learned as an engineer are invaluable to him during his daily work as an anesthesiologist. His son, Colin, holds a PhD in artificial intelligence and machine learning at University of Illinois, and serves as a resource for his Dad.

John Matthew Hess holds a BS in mechanical engineering from the Pennsylvania State University and an MBA from the Pennsylvania State University. He and his wife Josie, are the proud parents of two boys, both of whom enjoy keeping them busy. John worked as a new product design engineer, product manager, and, most recently, senior product manager in the electrical components and telecommunications industry. He managed a $150-million-dollar annual revenue business and is most proud of his patent: "Electrical isolation device capable of limiting magnetic saturation even upon receipt of high power direct-current bias and method for making the same and connector for incorporating the same." He is particularly interested in the emerging sustainability and reuse community as it pertains to local environmental conservation.

Charlie Sandson holds a BS in industrial and management engineering from Rensselaer Polytechnic Institute. He is based in Washington DC and works as an analytics associate for an international management consulting firm specializing in the pharmaceutical and healthcare industries. He especially enjoys market research, negotiation of strategic business partnerships, salesforce sizing, and supply chain operations. He has been a supporter and fan of the anesthesia community for many years. His most recent anesthesia publication was "What's in a Name?" in *Avoiding Common Anesthesia Errors, Second Edition.*

Cathy Marcucci holds a BS in chemical engineering from Cornell University. Before going to medical school, she worked in organic chemicals research, production design, and production engineering for several large chemical and energy corporations, including Dow Chemical, Northern Petrochemicals, and several Enron subsidiaries. She remains proud of an analysis she did for filling and maintaining a large liquid natural gas tank facility in Ventura, Iowa, as this work involved the use of novel (at the time) software for the prediction of the pertinent gas phase equilibria.

You Can Have Whatever You Want, You Just Have to Pay for It

184

Dawn Dillman

Introduction

This piece of advice in this title is one that my father has given me many times in my life, for many different purposes. It's true when considering buying a house or a car, but it's also true for broader life as well. There is a common thread of wisdom that you should always say yes to an opportunity. While that attitude and approach will open new doors for you, it is important to be aware of the costs when taking on new projects or roles. Sometimes the cost will be obvious, sometimes less so but all the costs and resources below that deserve special attention.

Monetary Costs Are Usually the Most Obvious

This could be the direct cost of tuition for an academic program like a master's degree or development meeting, such as a teaching workshop. These will help you build skills and may be of considerable interest to you. You may need to accept the upfront or ongoing costs like membership dues or maintenance of equipment. The harder thing to assess is what the opportunity costs? For example, will taking a program director position mean you are less productive clinically and will you make less because of that?

Time Is Finite and Should Also Be Considered a Cost

Does the committee you are going to join have meetings at 5 pm on Tuesday afternoons? That may mean the cost is not being able to attend your child's soccer practice. Time can be particularly relevant for maintaining relationships outside of the workplace. It can be helpful to have explicit discussions with intimate family or friends in this regard. This is closely related to the saying "You can have it all, just not at the same time." If you spend time on one thing, you are by definition not spending it doing something else. It is worth noting, though, that time spent doing work may also be considered time spent as a role model in some circumstances. For example, my mother was an anesthesiologist, not a stay-at-home mom, and her love of her career had a positive influence on me choosing my career.

D. Dillman (✉)
Department of Anesthesia, University of Iowa, Iowa City, IA, USA
e-mail: dawn-dillman@uiowa.edu

S. Mohamed et al. (eds.), *Anesthesia Bridges*, https://doi.org/10.1007/978-3-032-08294-7_184

Social Capital

Social capital, meaning the influence you have on others, may be relevant in your decision-making.

If your chair is asking you to be involved in a project, is there a possibility that turning it down may close the doors to them offering you a different project? If you don't spend time communicating to your group, is the cost that they trust you less as a leader? Social capital can and should be spent at times to get things done, but it helps to be cognizant of when you are using up that finite resource.

Social Stature and Its Perception by Self (Aka Ego) May Also Be a Cost

Choosing to focus solely on being as clinically active as possible to minimize economic costs may lead to the cost of not being recognized for promotion, and a loss of sense of efficacy at a job. Perhaps there is a person that you cannot imagine yourself working for—the cost to ego would be too high to consider that role or job. Another facet of this is the perception of self-impact on the world. The cost of taking a teaching role may mean the cost of not being able to spend as much time directly taking care of patients, but a greater perceived impact on patient care overall by teaching others how to take care of patients.

Ultimately, only you can judge the balance of the costs versus the benefits for yourself. The more explicit you can be with yourself about what you are choosing and what you are ready to give up, the more likely you will be to both advocate for what you want and be happy with the ultimate outcome of your decisions.

Lessons Learned

- Almost every opportunity has a cost.
- The dimensions that we barter with in life/career decisions can be viewed as monetary, time spent, social capital, or ego.
- To remain satisfied with your life/career decisions, be explicit with yourself about what you really want and what you are willing to give up.

Bonus Content!

For my own life, this has played out differently at times or with varying opportunities. For example, I was on the medical student progress committee at our college for 6 years, and the committee met at least monthly from 5 PM to 6:30 PM. I enjoyed the work and made some very helpful professional connections through that committee. My significant other at that time, however, later told me he felt marginalized by my choosing to do extra work in the evening instead of spending time with him. I had my first child as my term on the committee was ending, and when I was eligible to reapply, I had to weigh whether the benefit I would get out of working with that group again would outweigh me missing time with my young daughter. At that point, I decided not to apply for the committee again.

I didn't always choose time with my family, though. I chose to continue to be an oral board examiner because I felt the connections I was making at a national level were important enough to balance the week away from my children. The choices are not always easy, and you do the best you can with the information you have at the time and give yourself grace if it turns out differently than you expected.

***Note from the Editors:** Dawn chose the High Trestle Trail Bridge as her favorite bridge, and it is a fantastic structure (Figs. 184.1 and 184.2).

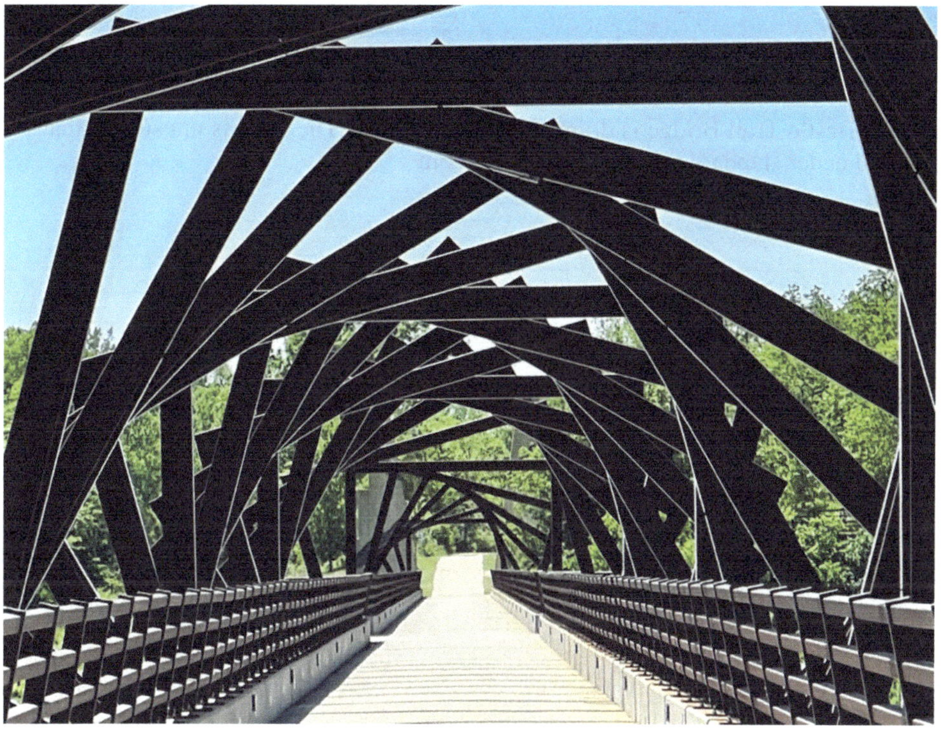

Fig. 184.1 The High Trestle Trail Bridge outside of Madrid, IA. The bike and walking High Trestle Trail winds 25 miles through five Iowa towns and is part of the national Rails-to-Trails movement. The stunning design of the bridge, which crosses the Des Moines River Valley and is 13 stories above the river, is intended to convey the feeling of descending into a mine shaft, a nod to the area's coal-mining heritage. Photo: Image used under standard license from stock.adobe.com

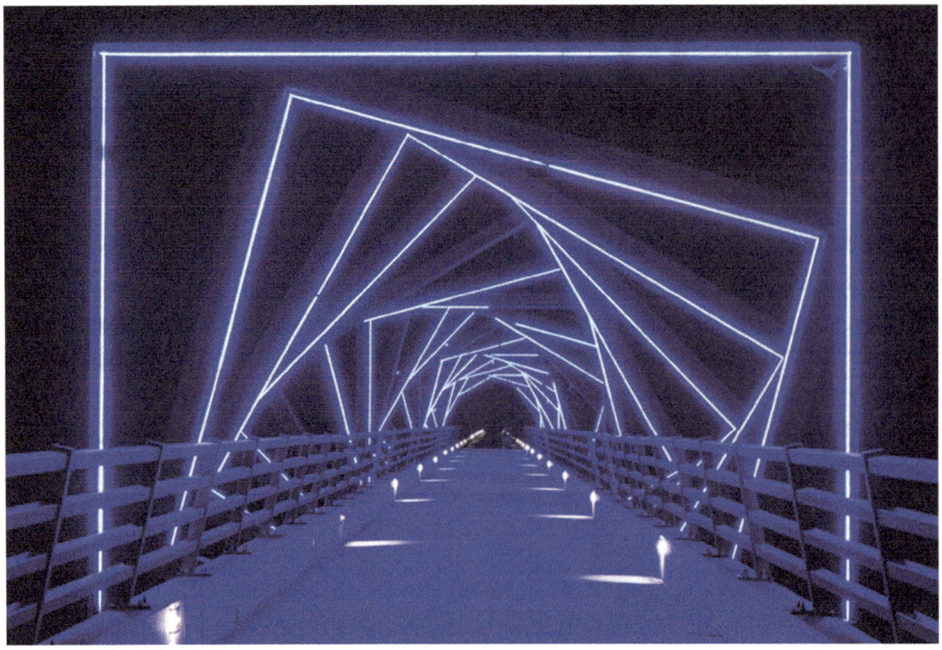

Fig. 184.2 The High Trestle Trail Bridge is dramatically lit at night. The Trail is unusual in that it is open 24 h per day. Photo: Image used under standard license from iStock.com

Author

Dawn Dillman grew up in Iowa, and thought she was escaping to residency in Maryland and then an academic practice in Texas. She *then* thought she was really and truly settled when she spent 18 years in Oregon, but it turned out that home was still Iowa. She's dedicated to her children Dahlia and David and to teaching and mentoring at all levels.

Does Life–Work Balance Exist?

185

Mojica Remskar

Introduction

It was my first night on call. In fact, it was my first day at work in the American medical system as an intern in surgery.

The Beginning of the Beginning

As soon as everyone else left the hospital, the pages started: "I need pain medicine orders…sleeping medication orders…anti-nausea medication orders…TPN orders…a veteran closed himself into the closet and presumably has a gun." For that last one, I asked politely if perhaps security should be contacted as well. At about 2 AM, the pager went off and an order for relief of constipation was requested for a patient who I knew had chronic constipation.

And so, it continued until the morning…and many of the nights I was on call. I am sure this sounds very familiar to anyone who has ever been a resident. The rest of my internship I spent in a somewhat dazed state of constant tiredness, sleepiness, and fear of missing something important related to one of my many patients. Night calls were frequent, sleep deprivation was real, and I kept trying to remind myself why I decided to pursue medicine as a profession.

The End of the Beginning

In spite of sometimes feeling as if the residency would never end, it suddenly did, and before I knew it, I was done with my fellowship as well and started down the path of attending-hood. I anticipated having an amazing amount of time—and money—for all sorts of things I like to do—hiking, reading, playing tennis, skiing, traveling, and mission trips. All the things that were supposed to fill me back up with the energy I once had before medical school, residency, and fellowship.

M. Remskar (✉)
Department of Anesthesiology, University of Minnesota, Minneapolis, MN, USA
e-mail: mremskar@umn.edu

S. Mohamed et al. (eds.), *Anesthesia Bridges*, https://doi.org/10.1007/978-3-032-08294-7_185

Surprised and Sad

To my surprise, commitments of all sorts and pressures on my time increased rather than decreased with the transition into the "adult world" of attending-hood. Clinical demands, call demands, academic productivity, departmental needs, and resident education needs. I must admit that I was well on the way to becoming someone I promised myself never to become: a disgruntled cynical physician who is tired and upset all the time, has a pale face from infrequent exposure to daylight, and the expression of someone who has aged prematurely under external demands and the inability to balance work and home life.

I looked for sources of my dissatisfaction outside of myself. All the people and everything in my environment were blamed for my unsatisfying predicament: the leadership of the department and the hospital, the operating room disorganization, old equipment, call schedules, and an unreasonable scheduling office. Everything but me and my complete absence of planning for my own professional direction.

I was adding to my own stress by committing to too many things: a committee here, a lecture there, a book chapter. As the frustration inside of me was building, I of course, as any typical Type A person would, used multi-tasking as a way to get things done. In fact, I felt quite productive, except that at the end of the day, I had very little to show of anything that would propel me forward towards my goals—and I was just keeping my head above water. And, like many women, I was doing an awful lot of what I later learned has a name: office housework.

Thinking It Through

Looking back, I also know that I failed to think through my professional goals in any organized manner. Of course, I knew I wanted to progress academically and clinically, but I had not really carefully considered what that "progress" would ideally look like, and what it would take to get to where I wanted to go.

In parallel to increasing tensions at work, tensions and pressures at home were also increasing—due to long work hours. I was coming home at 6 or 7 PM, sometimes later, always very tired, unable or unwilling to participate in home activities. Every weekend, I brought home many projects I did not complete during the workweek. I thought I would have more time to concentrate at home, but it was all at the expense of my family time. If I am honest, I know I was inefficient at work. I spent a lot of time chatting with people in the office and in the operating rooms, instead of finishing a few things here and there while at work. This led to an inability to relax at home and really disassociate from work, which was a big dissatisfaction for everyone around me.

Scrimping on Self

Unfortunately, self-care activities were the first thing I cut out of my day. I claimed I had no time, but I know I spent significant amounts of it blankly staring at the TV screen with an empty head. Time passed, and hours of sleep were taken away by unproductive activity that did nothing to help me feel better and remain healthy. In the meantime, I was reading and listening to a variety of discussions on the topic of the importance of work–life balance. I wondered who the superhumans were who were able to achieve this elusive ideal, which seemed to be completely unattainable for me personally.

As far as planning my academic path, the only thing I did pursue intentionally early on was education. I became Teacher of the Year several times, so when the position of a program director presented itself, I gladly took it on. I also got involved in education with simulation and eventually became the medical director at our school's simulation center. Several years into my attending-hood and very early on in my program directorship, an opportunity to pursue a master's program in healthcare education presented itself. I took it.

Mastering the Graduate Degree and Life

As a young program director, I understood I had to gain some theoretical knowledge in education to be effective in the role I was taking on. At the same time, I questioned the sanity of my decision to pursue yet another thing which would negatively impact my work–life balance.

Amazingly, the opposite happened. The master's program was not only good for my official educational roles in the department but also for my personal and professional growth. My mentors taught me valuable lessons in how to manage and control my time at work and at home, and how to be in charge of my career. I'd always felt in control of things I did in my life, but I failed to approach the initial years of being an attending in a systematic way involving a plan and outlining the specific steps I would take. As opposed to letting external influences be the main factor in pushing me in various directions (write a book chapter, join this or that committee…), I started to become the guide of my own academic path. I engaged in every activity after first asking myself a question: Will this activity contribute to my development towards my stated career goals?

More Controlled but Greater Freedom

The resulting feeling of control was liberating, allowing me space to breathe. It may have been easier to blame everyone else for all my misery, but thoughtfully examining my career like it was a patient that needed my attention and outlining what I really wanted to do and who I wanted to become as a physician and educator was the most invigorating thing I have done since graduating from residency and fellowship. One of the most important lessons that came out of the master's program was the homework that asked me to outline the things I needed to do to get to where I want to be. This forced me to focus my attention on and choose the activities that would be most productive and satisfying for me on any given day.

***Note from the Editors:** Mojca is from Slovenia, and we think the Dragon Bridge is one of the coolest bridges in this beautiful European country (Fig. 185.1).

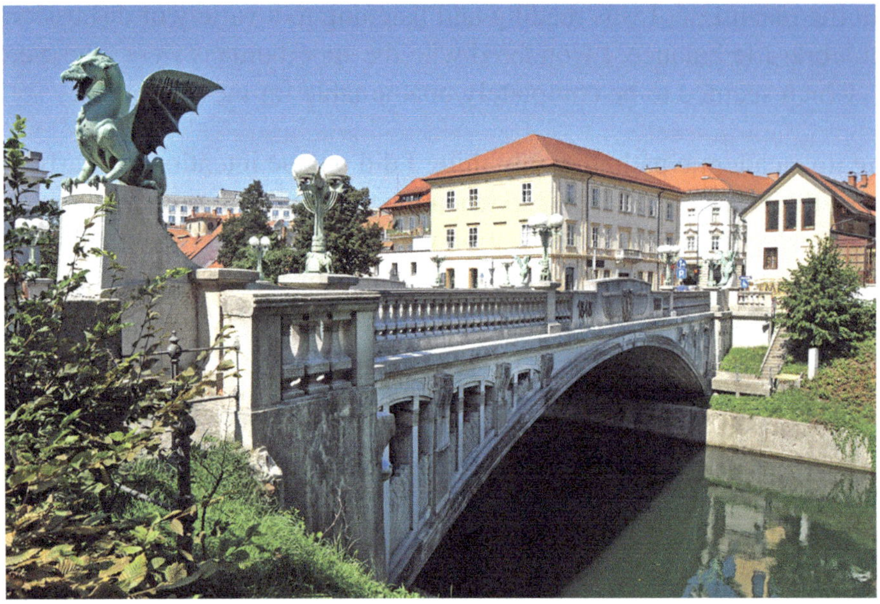

Fig. 185.1 The Dragon Bridge spans the Ljubljana River in Ljubljana, Slovenia. It was built in the early 1900s and replaced an older oak bridge. It is considered one of the most beautiful bridges produced under the Vienna Secession, an art movement that is closely linked to the Art Nouveau movement. It was extensively rehabbed and reinforced with concrete in the 1980s. Photo: Image used under standard license from shutterstock.com

Is Work–Life Balance Real?

Surprisingly, even though I took on additional work, I suddenly had more time for myself, my family, my workouts, and other things I like to do. At work, I pursued something I was really passionate about in a structured way, which filled me up with positive emotions and made it fun to go to work. As I was learning how to manage my time, how to filter through requests for committees and other departmental functions, how to be deliberate and know when to say no, I was finally taking full responsibility for my choices and my work–life balance. Rather than blaming that lack of balance on external factors over which I have little to no control, I learned to focus on the daily choices and lack of planning that are in my control.

As I was redefining my path, I read an article that argued that work–life balance is a false concept—that it does not exist. So many of our waking hours are spent at work that unless we find something inspiring and fulfilling in that work, we will keep chasing the illusory idea of work–life balance, like one chases the treasure beneath the rainbow. I now firmly believe that the author was correct. Too much of our day is spent at work for us to be able to achieve fulfillment with the short time we have outside of work.

Perspectives

As physicians, the work we have chosen is a critical, life-enhancing profession, not just for others but for ourselves, which inherently carries a commitment to what we do…and that often goes beyond the 9–5 schedule of a mere job. Inevitably, our mind remains preoccupied with things that happened at work—decisions we had to make with apparent confidence, often quickly and with limited information, to ensure patient safety. The work we do is incredibly creative if we choose to practice it that way.

Think about what we anesthesiologists do on a daily basis: Meet the patient, often for the first time; somehow gain their trust in the initial 5–10 minutes we spend with them while they are conscious; safely get them through surgery in spite of surgical procedures constantly challenging physiologic homeostasis; help with pain management; and sometimes literally save peoples' lives. It is a very beautiful profession. There is so much in it that can be inspiring and fulfilling, but we need to **choose** to see it that way. If we do, every day at work becomes time spent creatively, doing something very meaningful.

Looking back at those earlier phases of my career, I see that I perceived all the reasons for my stress to be external to me. I perceived all the reasons were out of my immediate control. It took a few more years of personal growth to recognize that I do have the ability to take control of my own professional career. I learned that I need to change the only thing that is in my control: myself and my own approach to how I lead my professional life. Through that, I can find a balance, but I'm not sure I would call it "work-life balance," as if those are separated by a clear line. I think I would prefer to call it personal and professional contentment.

Lessons Learned

- Looking back at my career, I know I have achieved a lot in a relatively short time. But it took someone wiser than I to tell me that I can and **should** be in control of my professional faith—of my belief that what I do really matters, even when it is a struggle.
- I could have avoided several years of frustration with the people and systems around me if I'd understood that **I am in control of my path, if not always the woods that surround it**. I had to learn several lessons to become a confident, satisfied physician, one who enjoys and believes in what I do.
- Ask yourself pointed questions about what it is that you want professionally and then lay out the specific actions it will take for you to get there.
- Find inspiration in something you do at work—an activity so meaningful or fun that it does not feel like work, but like **purpose**. We all need a creative outlet that fills and refreshes our soul. I found that in pursuing education in healthcare is my academic career path.
- Maintain your personal health and emotional balance by consciously making time for whatever you do to remain healthy. I suggest some form of physical activity and some form of mindfulness activity, in whatever form that allows you to calm and focus your mind and body.
- Structure your day intentionally: Literally, make a plan for each and every day. Spend only as much time on the activity as you have intended for it. If you were going to spend 30 minutes a day writing, only spend 30 minutes at it.
- Consciously dedicate time to home life without interruptions. You can do this, no matter how busy, if you structure your day. Always have time dedicated to activities that relax you and keep you healthy.

- Finally, remind yourself constantly that very few humans in the world are as fortunate as we physicians are, to have a profession where you spend your days keeping patients safe through some of the biggest challenges they will encounter in life, participate in development of the next generation of physicians, and create new knowledge. These are the reasons most of us decided to pursue what we knew would be an arduous path. Don't let whatever is going on in the woods cause you to stray from that path when it is within your power to keep moving forward.

Author

Mojca Remskar is a native of Slovenia but feels at home in Minnesota. She loves to take care of adult and pediatric cardiac patients at UMN and the Minneapolis VA. She loves her family, which consists of wife Elisha, daughter Remi, the dog, and Brki, the cat. She is passionate about the protection of pollinators.

You Can Do Everything, But Not All at the Same Time

186

Lisa Leffert

Introduction

During my 25+ year career as an academic physician anesthesiologist, I have heard a lot of people speak. These people have included formal lecturers, interdisciplinary colleagues, patients, friends, and family members. Many of the sentiments expressed were context-specific and failed to stay with me after the encounter was over. However, some of them contained pearls of wisdom. These "life mantras," as I will call them, have helped to guide me in my subsequent professional and personal encounters. Not infrequently, I share them with colleagues, in the form of advice, counsel, or comfort, and hear their stories about how these mantras have been helpful to them. Now I will share them with you.

"You Can Do Everything, But Not All at the Same Time"

This was said to me by my mother. These were high-impact words coming from her. By age 35, she had graduated from the Wharton Business Program at the University of Pennsylvania in the first class to include women, worked as a Wall Street stockbroker, married a surgeon, raised two children, and enrolled in law school (Fig. 186.1). These accomplishments were notable for a woman born in 1938. My mother's path had also included a 9-year hiatus between the end of her Wall Street career and the start of her career as a litigator, during which she focused on child-rearing and other pursuits.

"You can do everything, but not all at the same time," she told me as I considered how to balance becoming a physician, having a family, and actively maintaining other interests. She was not suggesting that parents should not or could not simultaneously have a family and build their careers. Rather, she was highlighting that there are many stages to one's life and career, and that some facets might be more feasible at some stages more than at others.

For me, this advice was actualized in the following manner. As an academic physician, I aspired to be a master clinician, administrative leader, and researcher. My husband was an academic physician

L. Leffert (✉)
Department of Anesthesiology, Yale School of Medicine, New Haven, CT, USA
e-mail: Lisa.leffert@yale.edu

S. Mohamed et al. (eds.), *Anesthesia Bridges*, https://doi.org/10.1007/978-3-032-08294-7_186

with similar career aspirations, and we both wanted to have children. Whereas the idea of "taking turns" satisfying our major career goals seemed ideal in theory, the reality was that both of us wanted to finish training in a timely fashion, both wanted to take advantage of the invitation to be chief resident, and so on.

What ultimately worked for us was to pace both of our careers in a series of stages. I decided to focus on two of three of my career missions (clinical work and leadership opportunities) at the outset. I knew that having a scholarly component to my career was important to academic advancement and to my intellectual nourishment, but I simply could not do it all "at the same time."

I had one son during medical school and a second in my first year as faculty and took the slower road to professorship. If I reflect and could speak to my 30-year-old-self, I would probably recommend some revisions—first, taking the time to attain tools in statistics and experimental design. And second, reallocating some of my administrative work to an earlier investment in scholarly activity. However, the overall approach would have been the same. As I continue to grow and learn in my wonderful career, it's joyful to see our sons find their paths—one into medicine and the other into education.

***Note from the Editors:** Lisa Leffert with her gorgeous and inspirational mother, Linda Leffert (Fig. 186.1).

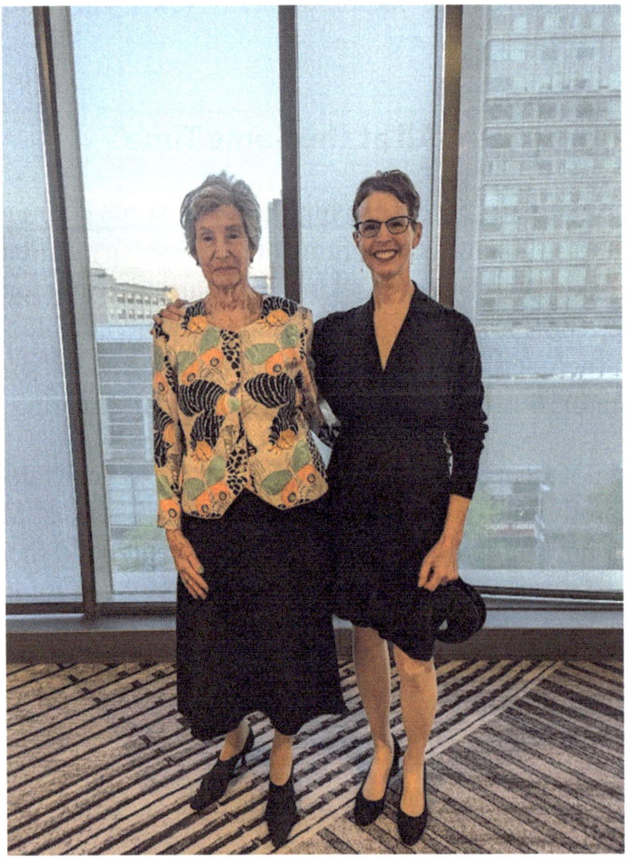

Fig. 186.1 Linda Leffert is originally from New York City and now calls Boston home. She attended the University of Pennsylvania and Northeastern Law School. Lisa credits Linda's wise advice and outstanding example as a great help in helping organize her own priorities and career. Photo: Collection of the Leffert family

"The Best Revenge Is Living Well"

My husband credits this mantra as the phrase that linked our fates. We were in the Harvard Medical School Quad when I approached him soon after the failure of his serious romantic relationship. Although we were not close friends at the time, I was motivated to offer him support. I had been struck by the difficult way in which the relationship had ended, and the discretion that he had displayed in his response. He remembers my having said, "the best revenge is living well" to highlight how he controlled his narrative and focused his energy on his positive path going forward, rather than on dwelling on the past.

Our professional and personal lives are full of challenges. We may experience being passed over for a promotion, being the recipient of disrespectful comments, or not being seen or heard. To be clear, unprofessional, or discriminatory behavior requires swift corrective action, not just a positive attitude. Structural change is required to bring about true diversity, equity, and inclusion. That said, maintaining ownership of your narrative as you face adversity and work to right what is wrong and hold on to your positive path will greatly help to facilitate "living well."

"Don't Narrate"

These words are attributed to a female supervising surgeon. They were said to a female surgery resident who was articulating each step of an ongoing surgical procedure, pausing to seek reassurance. The intent of "don't narrate" was to highlight that empowered professionals do not repeatedly ask permission. Nor do they preface public comments with qualifying (or disqualifying) phrases such as: "sorry, but I just wanted to say….", or "it may just be my opinion but…."

This is not to discount the importance of seeking education and guidance from one's peers and supervisors. Nor is it to blur the line between fact and opinion. Rather, it is to highlight that if you want others to have confidence in your ideas or actions, then it is important to portray that you have confidence in them. Understanding and presenting the potential pitfalls of your thoughts and actions is also desirable at the appropriate time and plan. Balancing these behaviors is a critical aspect of one's professional development.

"If One Person Is Bothering You Today, Then It's Probably Them. If It's Two People, Then It's Probably You"

This mantra was shared in a lecture delivered by an erudite senior female scientist.

Each of us has colleagues with whom it is challenging to work. Similarly, each of us has bad days. Distinguishing between the two can be important, as the paths forward are often quite different. The former requires an analysis of what about the interaction makes it challenging, and what you can do to try to foster a productive relationship. If there is a disagreement about a particular position, then taking a step back to find the common ground—for example, you are both committed to excellent patient outcomes—can often make the discussion less personal and more productive [1].

If the disagreement is about core values or fundamental differences in beliefs, then the conversation can be more difficult. This is where the hard work lies. Assuming the other individual's stance doesn't compromise key institutional missions and basic principles of respect, then I remind myself that the ultimate sign of professionalism is being able to converse with those with whom you fundamentally differ. Minimizing emotion improves ones' equipoise and helps to facilitate subsequent conversations.

Alternatively, if on a given day everyone is irritating you, then it is reasonable to think about whether you are not at your best. In these cases, self-care may be the remedy. For this, we need tools to nurture ourselves when we are depleted, irritated, or even clinically depressed. Just as we build an armamentarium of tools with which we care for patients (clinical content knowledge/evidence base, technical skills, use of technology), we need to assemble a personal survival toolkit. This toolkit might include important non-work-related passions—such as physical activity, cooking, meditation—and mental and physical health resources and social connections.

In summary, you will hear many people speak over the course of your career. In these pages, I have shared with you some of the life mantras that have guided me.

Lessons Learned

- Your career will be long. You will undoubtedly have to prioritize some things over others at any given time, but you will find a time and a place for your key missions.
- Focus your energy on a positive path going forward rather than on dwelling on the past.
- Be humble but speak with confidence. Do not apologize for your thoughts and questions.
- When you are in conflict with a colleague, taking a step back to find common ground will often make discussions less personal and more productive.
- Recognize that there are times when self-care is needed.

Reference

1. Fisher R, Ury W, Patton B. Getting to yes: negotiating agreement without giving in. Penquin Books; 2011.

Author

Lisa Leffert spent the first 30 years of her career in Boston, at Harvard, and thought she would never leave. There, she focused on obstetric anesthesiology, faculty development, neurologic disease in pregnancy, and administration. She and her husband, Lee, raised two wonderful sons. Life took a totally unexpected, but wonderful turn, when she became chair at Yale. It just goes to show—keep an open mind and go with your gut feel.

187 Feeling a Bit Disappointed and Discouraged with Medicine? Consider the Farmers!

Randy G. Jensen, Matthew L. Rorie, Ruth A. Jensen, and Catherine Marcucci

Introduction

If you are suffering significant depression, demoralization, and burnout, seek help, at the professional level if necessary. *But* if you are just somewhat mad and grumpy—if you are mildly disgusted and disappointed in the practice of anesthesiology specifically or medicine in general—perhaps thinking about the career and business pressures faced by today's farmers might put things into perspective and help to cheer you up a bit.

RJ Acres is a 700-acre farm outside of Blair, Nebraska that is farmed by partners **Randy Jensen** and **Matt Rorie** (Figs. 187.1 and 187.2). The farm is a historic, beautiful, and well-managed property that has been in the Jensen family for several generations. Randy's grandfather, Frederick Jensen, first moved to the farm in 1920 and Randy's father, Kenneth Jensen, started farming it with Fred in the years right after WW2.

Randy joined the farm operation full-time after graduating from college in the mid-1970s when they primarily raised hogs as Porker Valley, Inc. Ruth Jensen arrived at the farm in 1977 when she married Randy but also always had a full-time career as a chemical engineer. She is the treasurer of the farm corporation, which now concentrates mainly on crop farming. Matt joined RJ Acres as a partner in 2016. Ruth, Randy, and Matt all took time out of their busy summer schedules to tell us what their challenges and rewards are and how they deal with the unique stresses of farming.

***Note from the Editors:** RJ Acres farmers Randy Jensen and Matt Rorie (Figs. 187.1 and 187.2).

R. G. Jensen · M. L. Rorie · R. A. Jensen (✉)
RJ Acres, Blair, NE, USA

C. Marcucci
Department of Transfusion Medicine, Clinical Center, National Institutes of Health, Bethesda, MD, USA

S. Mohamed et al. (eds.), *Anesthesia Bridges*, https://doi.org/10.1007/978-3-032-08294-7_187

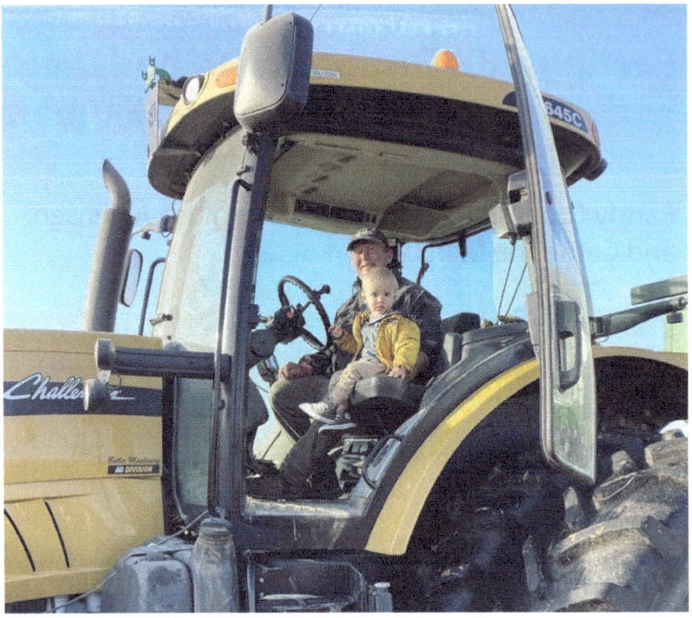

Fig. 187.1 Randy Jensen with grandson Gavin in the big tractor

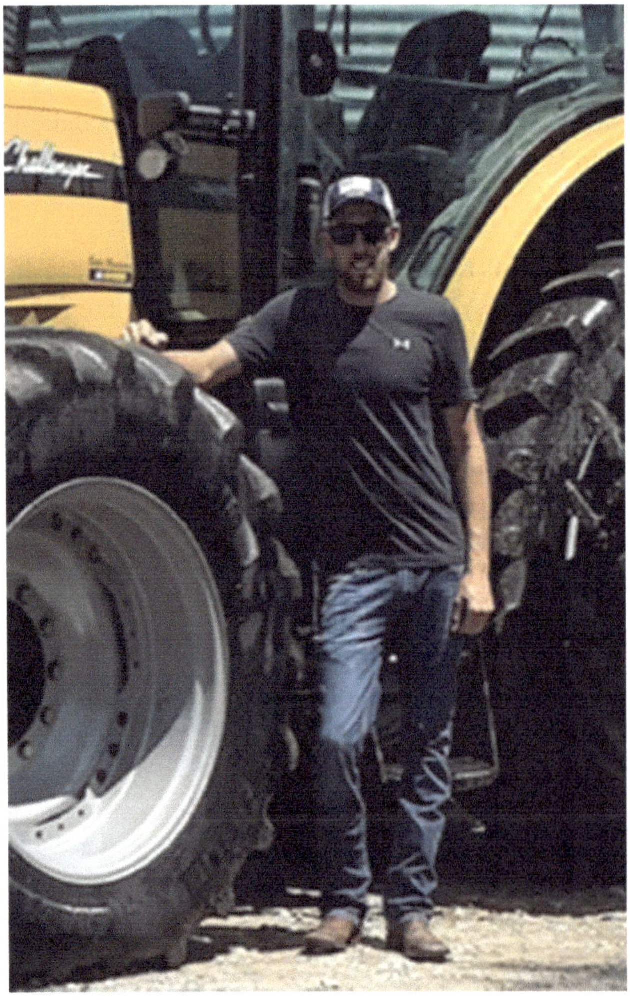

Fig. 187.2 Matt Rorie in front of the big tractor, with a grain bin behind him. Photos: Courtesy of Matt Rorie and the Jensen family

From the Interviews: Lessons from the Farmers

- First of all, farmers work hard. They work as hard as we do or maybe harder. And not just long hours—farming is extremely labor-intensive, especially livestock farming. My various practice locations have drawn patients from farming communities in Maryland, West Virginia, and Pennsylvania. I am not in the habit of proceeding with cases if the patients have missed their pre-op cardiac workups, but I will make an exception if the patient is actively farming, especially if they have a large animal operation. I once waved a West Virginia farmer through to the OR with no workup, as he had never smoked, had normal blood pressure, and managed 70 head of cattle with only his elderly father for help.

- They work seven days a week, particularly if they have animals as part of their operation. When I asked Randy if they worked constantly, he demurred a bit, "Well, not constantly. For instance, we only work a partial day on Saturdays and Sundays. We would rarely work until dark on the weekends. But the animals have to eat every day, of course." There are periods in the winter when crop farmers aren't working in the fields, but they are still working on their equipment and other farm administrative tasks. They have a bit more free time in the deep winter months, and this is when they like to get their volunteer work done. Randy can often be found in town during the winter season, discharging his civic duties. They also use these months to concentrate on church and family activities, watch sports, and catch up on their journals and continuing education.

- During planting and harvest, they do nothing but that. They do not even stop to eat. I asked Randy if he takes time every day to check the farm news such as grain prices and he said, "Not during planting." Planting or harvesting is like doing an intense OR case that lasts a week or more.

- However, farmers do have one advantage over us—they don't work in the dark, which for them means they don't work at night. They are up early—usually not later than 6 AM—so they can start working when it gets light, but they don't work in the fields after it gets dark. It's too dangerous.

- Think our loan payback pressures are terrible? A farmer's payback period until he is in the black is around 50 years—at a minimum. Somebody starting in farming today would hope to have his operation in the clear for the second generation of his descendants—at the earliest. The buy-in for a farming career is as if we had to buy our own anesthesia machines, fiberoptic scopes, and cardiopulmonary bypass machines. Randy estimates that there is about $750,000 dollars of equipment sitting in his barn (five different tractors and associated other equipment like a grain cart and sprayer), and he works and plans hard to keep equipment purchases to a minimum (Figs. 187.3 and 187.4). The big tractor shown above would be about $300,000 to replace.

***Note from the Editors:** The RJ Acres barn is full of farm equipment. Imagine if you had to figure out a way to support yourself and pay off your student loans, pay off the million-dollar mortgage on your land, and still find the money to buy these vehicles (Figs. 187.3 and 187.4).

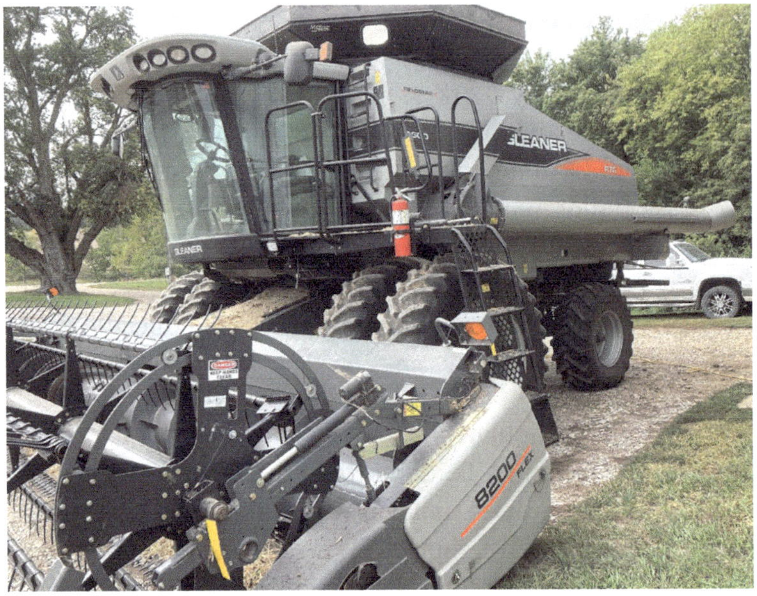

Fig. 187.3 This monstrosity is a combine with a soybean head. Photo: Courtesy of Randy Jensen

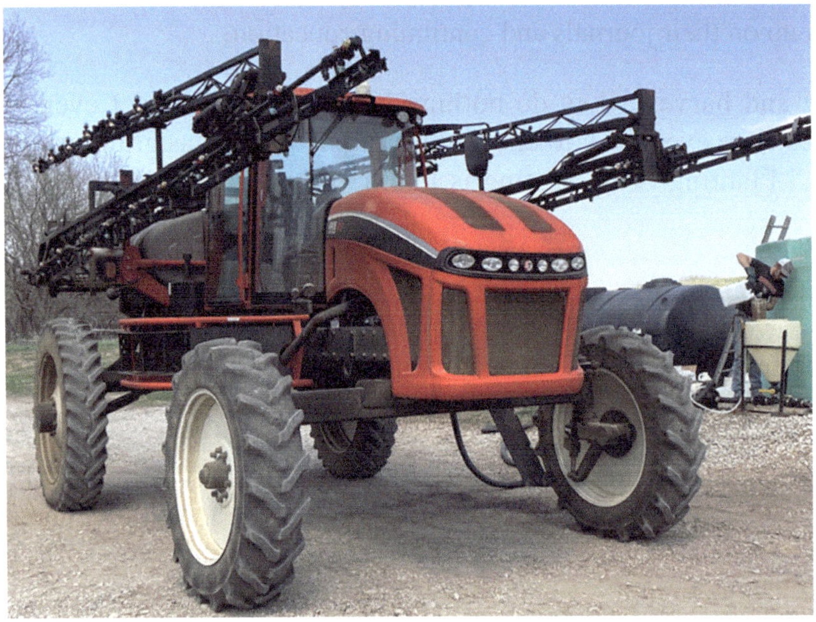

Fig. 187.4 This is the sprayer—the cost was about $110,000. Matt is looking at a laser retrofit to greatly minimize the use of chemicals. Photo: Courtesy of Randy Jensen

- This doesn't include the cost of the land—a general estimate for farmland is about $10,000 an acre, although there is some variation in the price of farmland in Nebraska, as it is not as flat as Iowa. Let's say you are 50 years old, and your land is paid off, but a nice 100-acre parcel of bottom land adjacent to yours comes on the market or your brother wants to sell some land that your dad farmed. It's going to cost you a mortgage of a million dollars or more to buy it.

***Note from the Editors:** RJ Acres is a magical place. I asked Ruth for a picture of the creek, and she sent me this beautiful picture looking down the driveway towards the creek in the distance with a double rainbow bridge up to the sky (Fig. 187.5).

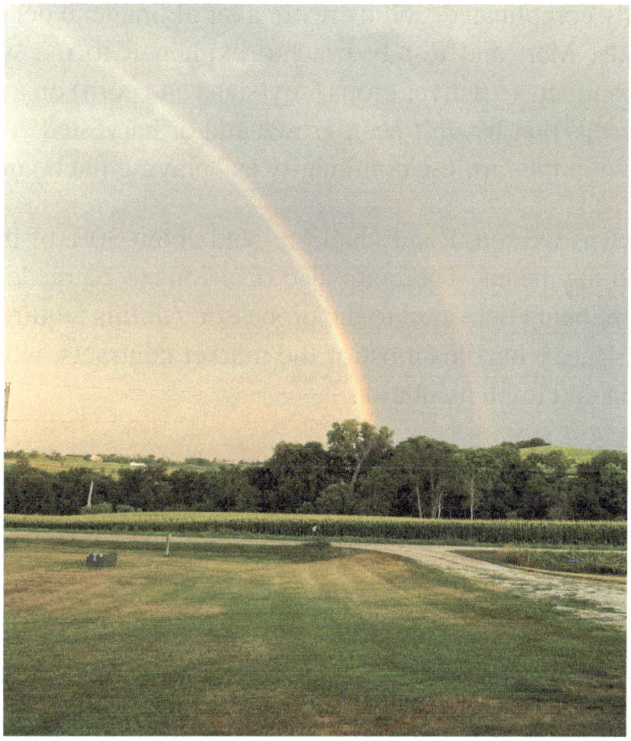

Fig. 187.5 The view from the house, looking over RJ Acres corn towards the creek. Photo: Ruth Jensen

- Today's farmers are educated. Randy estimates that at least half of all American farmers have college degrees. His degree is in animal science, and Matt's degree is in agricultural economics, both from the University of Nebraska, Lincoln. Farmers don't usually get graduate degrees unless they plan to teach.

- They seek continuing education on a regular basis. Randy and Matt read *Nebraska Farmer*, *Farm Journal*, and *AgPhD*. They also attend courses, seminars, and workshops on a regular and as-needed basis to follow the advancements in farming technology.

- Farmers employ a lot of cutting-edge technology, as much as we do or perhaps more. They really don't have the option not to if they want to stay competitive. For example, RJ Acres has GPS on two of the tractors, which feeds "drive data" to a satellite, which beams it back down to a monitor in the tractor to map each field. This allows Matt and Randy to keep track of what's been plowed, what hasn't been plowed, and what's been planted, so that there isn't an overlap. GPS access is purchased through a commercial farm technology vendor and is generally available for intervals of 3, 6, or 12 months.

- They also have auto-steer on their tractors, which will drive the tractor on whatever course they plot on the monitor. Newer autosteer systems will even turn the tractor around for the farmer. Matt is just in the process of pricing laser-based sprayers, which can analyze plants in the ground for the presence or absence of weeds and will automatically turn the sprayer on and off. He also tells me that they are not one bit afraid of the AI technology that is on the horizon—anything that will help them with farm management and increase the per acre yield is something that they will look at and lean into.

- Farm economics are really complicated, and there are a lot of financial decisions that have to continually be made and remade. Matt and Randy tried to explain it to me without enormous success. Essentially, they set up contracts to deliver crops (soybeans and corn) on a monthly basis for a certain price. This can involve crops that haven't been grown and/or harvested yet, so it's a high-priced and risky game and it's known in the farming community as "playing the board."

- At the time this chapter was written, Randy had pre-sold about 30% of his corn while it was in the field but had not yet sold any beans. There are also decisions to be made on how and how long the crops will be stored before being delivered to the processor. All this requires a lot of experience so, as the more senior partner, Randy handles most of the market contracts, while Matt generally handles the technology evaluation and implementation.

- A general goal for farm profits in the region that RJ Acres is in is to generate profits of $100 per acre. Randy stressed that this is just an average across a number of years. There might be a good year with profits of $300 per acre or more, but then a string of three years when there really isn't much of a profit at all. Imagine if we spent three years in a row working day in and day out doing anesthesia cases, covering all the costs, with the knowledge that it might not be until the fourth year when our practices generated a positive balance sheet.

- Operating costs are considerable in farming. A bag of seed corn costs $300 and seeds about 2.5 acres. So, if the guys have 250 acres in corn (and I think it is usually more than that), that is about $30,000 per year, just for the seed for just the corn. This does not include the soybeans. This would be as if we had to buy our own anesthesia drugs as well as all of our own equipment. Are you getting the picture that there is an enormous and continual drain on the finances of a farmer above and beyond the investments of time and labor?

- The margins in farming are paper-thin. Grain prices vary daily, and I gather that a fluctuation of 10 cents in the price of a bushel of corn can make a fairly sizable difference one way or the other. And speaking of margins, Matt remarked to me in our interview, "It is certainly possibly to go bankrupt in one year."

- Farming is physically demanding and even dangerous. As Randy says, "Sometimes the only way to get a 500-pound sow to move is to move her yourself." We get carpal tunnel syndrome and are exposed to radiation in the OR. Farmers put tremendous stress on their shoulders, hips, and knees and many, many farmers need joint replacements in middle age. Matt recently sustained a dislocated shoulder when he was kicked by a calf he was vaccinating. They are also exposed to radiation—only their exposure is from ambient sunlight all day, every day, in the fields. They work with hugely dangerous equipment and can be exposed to dangerous chemicals, even if every effort is made to farm with a low-chemical footprint.

- Our work location is climate-controlled. Theirs is not. They are at the mercy of the weather. And all kinds of weather—too hot, too cold, too wet, and too dry.

- We visit RJ Acres as often as we can and, on the last trip out, my son Charlie Sandson was invited to the early AM (like 6 AM) coffee group at a local diner. He came back saying, "It's true what they say about farmers and rain. I have never heard such in-depth discussion about yesterday's weather as I heard today." Harry Truman, who grew up on a farm outside of Independence, Missouri and farmed it as a young man, retained an intense interest in the weather until the very end of his life.

- Farmers are generally courteous to each other but not universally collegial. We were surprised to hear that there is sometimes even a bit of competition. Both Randy and Matt described it this way, "Not every guy wants to let you know how he is doing and what is going on over at his property." Of course, as you might imagine, the farmers who participate in formal farming groups and informal social groups have the advantage in large and small ways. But the loners still persist in their lonely ways.

- They don't make gigantic amounts of money. Even established, successful farmers make much less than we do because a high percentage of the profits is plowed right back into the farm (get it, plowed ☺). Randy gave me permission to quote his and Matt's salaries, which we will not do in the interest of discretion but think five figures, which is pretty typical for their Nebraska farming community.

- The RJ Acres partners draw a bit less from their farm corporation than average, as they are planning on buying additional land. Matt tells us that there are farmers who draw bigger salaries, but this is usually if they are at the end of their careers and are planning on cashing out their operation or selling their land, sometimes to developers. If you are a working farmer who plans to stay in business and pass your farm down in your estate, your salary is going to be approximately what a mid-career public school teacher makes for your entire career. There is just no way to draw a bigger salary and still make the necessary investments in equipment and technology and pay your notes. So, think about this—we sometimes feel mad and sad, and that most everything going on in the anesthesia world is bad. And rightfully so, our frustrations and concerns are very real. But we must keep in mind that the lowest paid working anesthesiologist is still making about five times what the highest paid working farmer is making.

- Farmers usually, although not always, live on their farms, so there is some break there for them. But living in a house that's on the property doesn't send your kids to Spain for their senior trips, or put them through college, or buy a top-notch comprehensive health insurance policy that includes vision and dental.

- Farmers work long years. They retire even a bit later than we do. I once asked Randy if his dad Kenny was still farming—I mean really farming, like loading hogs and such—and Randy said, "Oh sure, he's only 77." The senior Mr. Jensen was still out and about on the property into his nineties—mowing and turning over the garden at the house and hitching up the snow blade on the small tractor to plow the lane (Fig. 187.6).

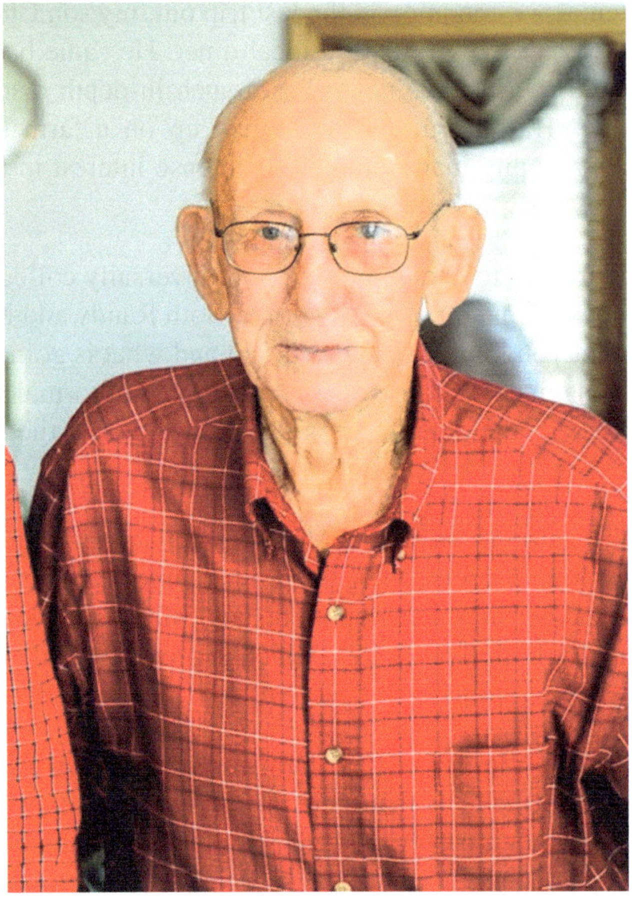

Fig. 187.6 Randy's dad, Kenneth F. Jensen (1922–2015), in his later years. It was Kenny, really, who was the bridge from his family's Depression-era farming before the war to the more modern farming era, sending Randy off to college to get a degree in agricultural sciences. Photo: Collection of the Jensen family

- Kenny was also a WW2 veteran, of course, enlisting in 1942. He was a tank mechanic and driver who saw action with the 11th Armored Division in Europe, including intense combat in the Battle of the Bulge, where the 11th was charged with defending the highway to Bastogne against fierce assault. He was a quiet man who always maintained that he had done nothing special in the war and deserved no medals, but he lived and worked the rest of his life, climbing on and off his tractors, and died 70 years after WW2 with German shrapnel still in his leg. He was yet another hero of the Greatest Generation, in spite of his denials, and was much loved by his family and esteemed by his community.

- Just in case you thought that perhaps we are kidding about farmers working forever, we aren't (Fig. 187.7). *Anesthesia Bridges* editor Brandon Togioka's grandfather was Noboru Togioka, and his dramatic and inspiring story is told in Chap. 208. When Brandon reviewed this chapter, he remarked that his grandpa also farmed well into his eighties.

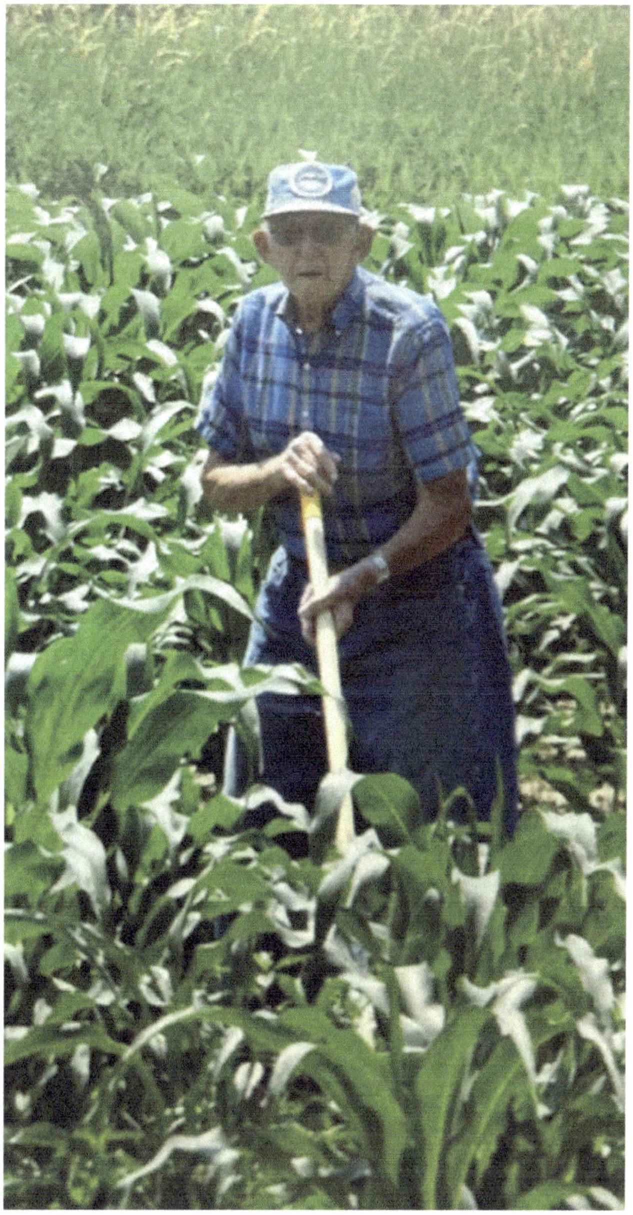

Fig. 187.7 The senior Mr. Jensen caught hoeing the sweet corn patch at the age of 90. He was supposed to be taking it easy that day but did not feel that Randy was keeping the weeds under control to the proper standard. Look at Kenny's strong arms and hands—the result of many decades of intense physical work. Photo: Collection of the Jensen family

Lessons Learned: How Do Farmers Cope and What Wisdom Can We Gain?

- I asked the three RJ Acres partners how they cope with farm life. Their unanimous answer was that they don't "cope"—they could not imagine any other career or way of life. Randy Jensen and Matt Rorie are educated, hardworking, and tech savvy—it seems that they surely could have set their sights on law school, med school, or business careers (which in a way they did—farm business—but I am talking about Wall Street careers or consulting for Deloitte). Ruth had a very successful career as a senior engineer but also always embraced the farm as the way of life for her family, although they did live in town when the kids were younger. They don't really even consider the issue of work-life balance. To farmers, their work is their life. They even live at their place of work—imagine if we lived in the hospital. Elsewhere in this book, our authors have suggested the same thing—that work–life balance is actually a false dilemma. The take-home message and lesson is to arrange our professional careers to minimize the need for that boundary. This might not be entirely possible, but it is something to work towards.

- They also could not imagine having somebody else be their boss. They can't change the weather, and they can't change grain prices, but they view everything else as potentially amenable to change. Apart from the immutable circumstances, what happens on their farm is what they make happen and they wouldn't have it any other way. They don't spend a lot of time complaining about what they can't change, and they also don't spend time complaining about what they can change, because they just do it. Randy one time asked me why physicians stop trying to optimize our practice conditions if we don't like them, and there are still things that can be changed.

- It's all about the land. They care about it tremendously. As Randy said to me once, "It's not the tractor that grows the corn." His point is that people see a tractor and think that's the farm. The RJ Acres farm equipment is carefully considered and well-maintained but to Randy and Matt, it's just the means to the end, and they are careful not to over-invest in it. What they really care about is the land and land management issues. They work tremendously hard at all aspects of farm operations but really like most to be out in the fields. And just like in the movies, they do walk up and down the rows in the early morning and evenings, just checking out what's going on with their crops from the viewpoint on the ground. The analogy for us is that we should not focus on any one anesthetic technique or latest gadget, they're just the equipment in our barn. What's important is cultivating and staying grounded in the overall landscape of patient management.

***Note from the Editors:** RJ Acres is actually two parcels of land. This is the older historic land that has been farmed for four generations (Fig. 187.8). A separate parcel of bottom land is about two miles away.

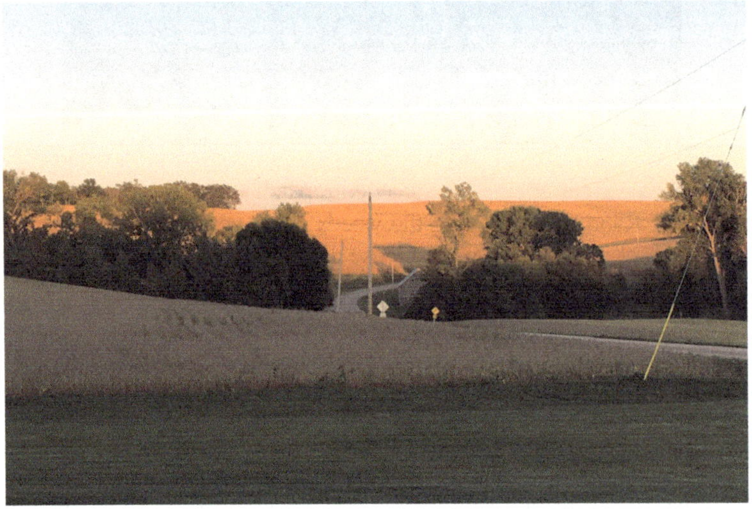

Fig. 187.8 The view from the house, looking over corn that is ready to harvest. Ruth and Randy and Matt all live on the property; Matt's house is just on the other side of the tree line. You can catch a glimpse of the old wooden barn in the center of the picture, between the road signs. This structure, which is over 100 years old, could be in a picture book or on a calendar and is Ruth's favorite place on the farm. The Jensen family now uses it for get-togethers and parties—daughter Taryn Jensen LaFlamme had her wedding rehearsal dinner and party there. Photo: Ruth Jensen

- They have a really strong and organized lobby - stronger than ours perhaps and more united in striving to represent farmers. Although farmers usually work in small teams (often but not always family members) on any one farm, there is an entire network of professionals who support the working farmer, from the government level on down.

- There are not really paraprofessionals in commercial farming. You are either farming or you're not. It's too expensive and dangerous to do it half-way. There are farm workers, who do farm work but don't own the equipment or land, and they have their own unions and political lobby. Their issues are important—they are rightfully looking for fair wages and safe working conditions—but those lobbies are not attempting to redistribute "ownership" or tell farm owners how they can practice farming in terms of land management or who owns what part of the contracts. Randy is somewhat bemused at how fractured the practice landscape is for today's physician, from the government level on down. His question to me once was, "How did the doctors let control of medicine get taken away from them?" I had no good answer for him. The lesson for us today is to redouble our support for the organizations that are working on the issues that are most critical to physicians in general and anesthesiologists in particular.

- All of their professional help is specialized in dealing with the farming community. The lawyers, accountants, and tax and estate planning people they consult are all hyper-experienced in the specific issues that farmers face and the structure of farm corporations. Even the physicians they go to know what's involved in farming and the correct farm lingo. Randy recently had hip surgery and the orthopedic surgeon at the university hospital in Omaha said to him, "Okay, you got to wait at least four weeks until you climb up on a grain cart." This highlights our advice elsewhere in this book—hire consultants who are experienced in dealing with the specific issues facing physicians and anesthesiologists, just as our farming friends do.

- They never lose sight of their mission. Like us, farmers consider themselves the invisible and unsung heroes of America. Randy said to me years ago, "Well, I guess you could consider that our clients are anybody who wants to eat." In their minds, there is a vast societal need for food, which, of course, there is, and they are the ones who are going to fill it. This unshakeable faith in the critical nature and manifest importance of what they do helps to prevent disillusionment and burnout. There's a lot for us to think about here. Perhaps the foremost question to unpack is: Why are we letting certain forces promulgate the position that **physicians** are not really needed that much in medicine today? How did we get to where we are with these issues, and where are we going?

Bonus Content! More Insider Information from the Farmers

Because I am an old and dear friend of RJ Acres, I asked Randy and Matt a few more questions about what it's really like to be them.

- They both told me that farmers are fully aware that they are subject to a degree of stereotyping and clichés in the media and popular opinion that is as bad as ours, or worse. They don't particularly care about this—they truly don't—although Randy did once remark to me, "Well, I guess some people might say we are hicks, but I don't think it's true that we're dumb hicks. You can't farm if you are dumb, or at least you won't be farming for long." Conversely, I asked Matt if farmers sit out on their farms and **laugh at us** for being dumb for jamming ourselves into cities. And he hesitated just the tiniest second and said, “No, not really”—while laughing, of course.

- They don’t care about being flyover country. In fact, they quite like it that way. Their view is, “Okay, why don’t you be where you want to be, and we’ll be where we want to be.” And this isn’t said spitefully. All three of the Jensen kids chose careers that weren’t in farming—two live on the East Coast in metropolitan areas—and their parents are perfectly fine with that. And by the way, the U.S. state with the most flyovers isn’t even Nebraska or any other state in the Midwest. It’s Virginia [1].

- Their political positions and recreational and civic interests are as individual as ours are. They are knowledgeable and regular voters, but not monolithically—there are both registered Democrats and Republicans and lots of independents in their community, as in ours. They vote the issues and their consciences, just as physicians do, and perhaps as physicians should do a bit more. They are knowledgeable and concerned about worldwide humanitarian issues, especially food issues. For example, Ruth and Randy’s church cares a lot about what’s going on in Africa and has several outreach programs, which the Jensen’s actively support.

- They travel. Their horizons do not end at the edge of their properties. Farmers cover for each other so they can travel regionally, nationally, and internationally. They go to the Caribbean and Hawaii and meet their adult kids for Thanksgiving weekend at lake houses and resorts, just like everybody else.

- They are very civically minded. Towns in farming communities are often small enough that there aren’t the municipal programs that larger suburban or metropolitan regions have. So, if their town is too small to have a municipal recycling effort, they just get together and organize and run the program themselves. The Sandson kids know that if they are visiting RJ Acres over a weekend, they are heading into town with Randy on Saturday to sort recyclables. Farmers are also often quite active with local 4H clubs and Grange Hall programs. An award for 50 continuous years of membership in the National Grange Association is kind of a big deal and will be mentioned in your obituary.

- They are not gun crazy. Every farmer has a shotgun, of course. There is no way of telling when a rabid animal will get on the property, or some sort of poisonous snake will come crawling out of the woods and decline to turn around and go back in without any trouble. And remember that bears and bobcats are making a comeback in some parts of the country, and there are often calves and lambs on farms. The first time my daughter Lisa asked Randy if he had a gun, he said yes, he had a shotgun, but he would have to look around to find it, he thought maybe it was in the basement. Then he would have to look around to find the shells, they were maybe in the basement too, but a different part of the basement. But, if she would give him 20 minutes or so, he would see if he could get everything together that he needed to fire the gun. Lisa looked at Randy with a shocked expression on her face. She ended up writing a well-received college application essay partly about this very conversation as she realized that her pre-conceived notions were not correct.

- They were hit hard by the Missouri River floods in 2011 (Fig. 187.9). It was really tough on the land and on them in terms of the labor required to recover. The RJ Acres bottom land was completely underwater, and an entire house had even washed down the river and was in the center of the acreage. They managed to be ready to plant the next year, but it wasn't easy getting that done. Randy and Matt had farmed responsibly and done everything by the book, but it had happened anyway. It's just a risk of farming bottom land. They were insured, and there was nothing they could do about it but go forward and keep farming, so that's what they did. Sort of like getting hit with a major malpractice suit when you didn't do anything wrong in the case? Something to think about.

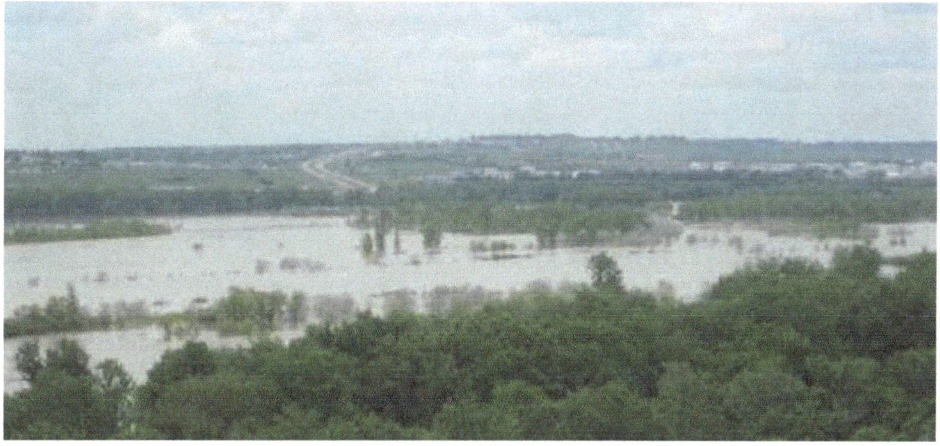

Fig. 187.9 The Missouri River Flood in 2011, looking east into Iowa. The roadway that is visible is I-680, a major spur of I-80. The roadbed of the bridge across the river and the cloverleaf exchange with I-29 were completely underwater, as the river crested at almost 37 feet. The RJ Acres river parcel is not shown but is north off to the left of this photo and was completely underwater. Recovery was done in 1 year, but it was an enormous amount of work and required specialized equipment. Photo: USGS.gov, public domain

- But to finish up on a lighter note—farmers do have one big advantage over us—they don't have to hire people to get their kids back and forth to school! Farm states such as Nebraska, Iowa, Kansas, North Dakota, and South Dakota will grant driving permits to farm kids at the age of 14 for the purposes of driving themselves to school and home, if they live more than five miles outside town. And they can drive younger siblings to school as well (with restrictions). Matt grew up on a Nebraska farm and drove himself to school at 14, and the Jensen kids also started driving at 14 after they moved out to the farm.

More Scenes from a Farm Life

Isn't it interesting and informative to peek into other professionals' lives and see what their challenges and daily realities are (Figs. 187.10, 187.11, and 187.12)? It puts what we do into all kinds of perspective (Figs. 187.13 and 187.14).

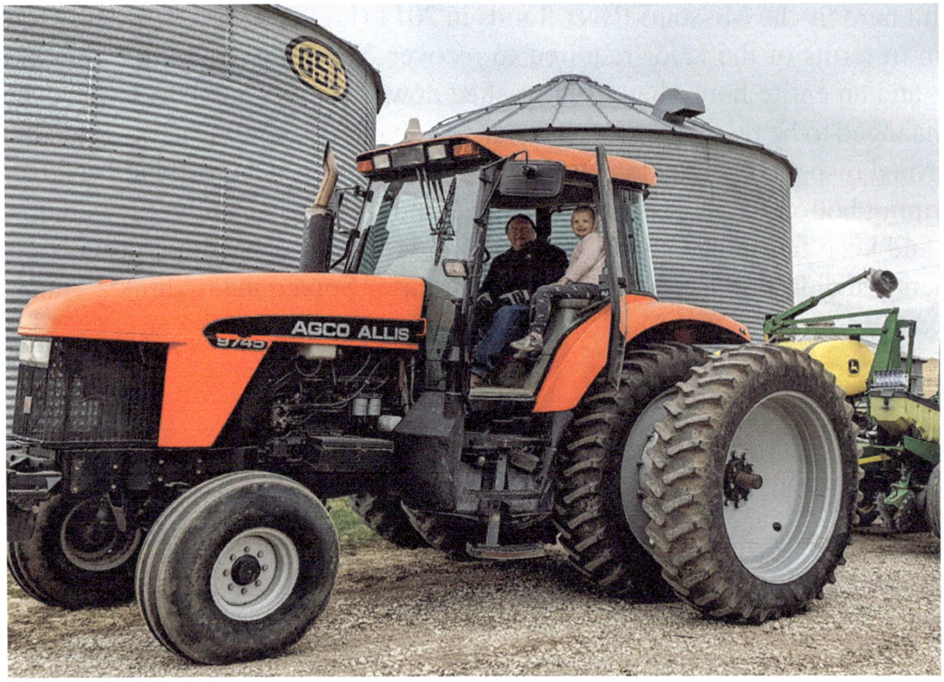

Fig. 187.10 Randy and granddaughter Claire are in one of the little tractors with the planter hooked on the back and grain bins behind. Photo: Ruth Jensen

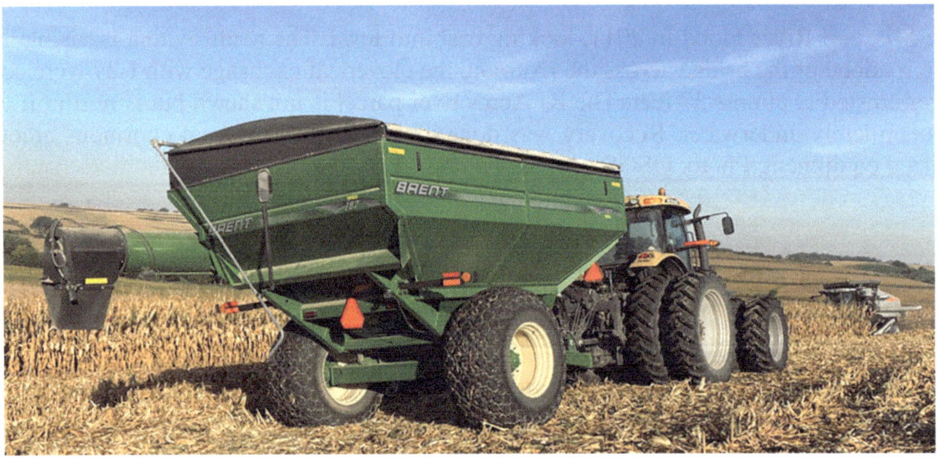

Fig. 187.11 Getting the corn harvested on a lovely Nebraska fall day. It really is a beautiful state, in case you haven't noticed. Photo: Randy Jensen

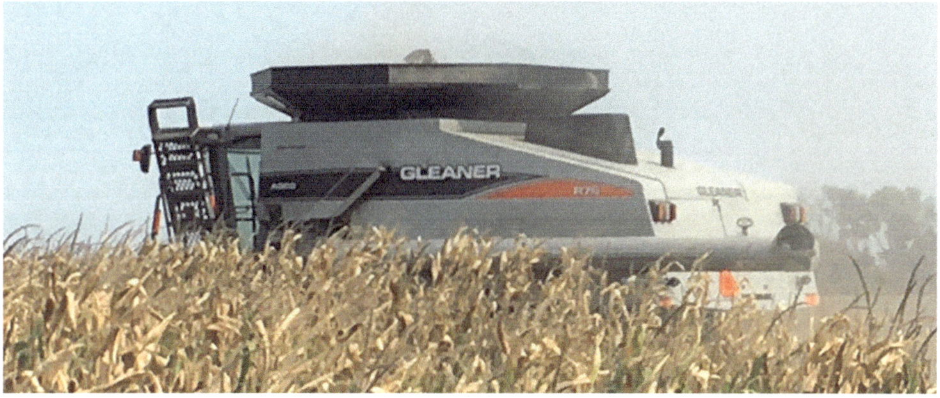

Fig. 187.12 They could never in a million years get somebody intubated and extubated, nor could we ever in a million years get the corn into the ground, out of the field, and into the grain bin. Photo: Randy Jensen

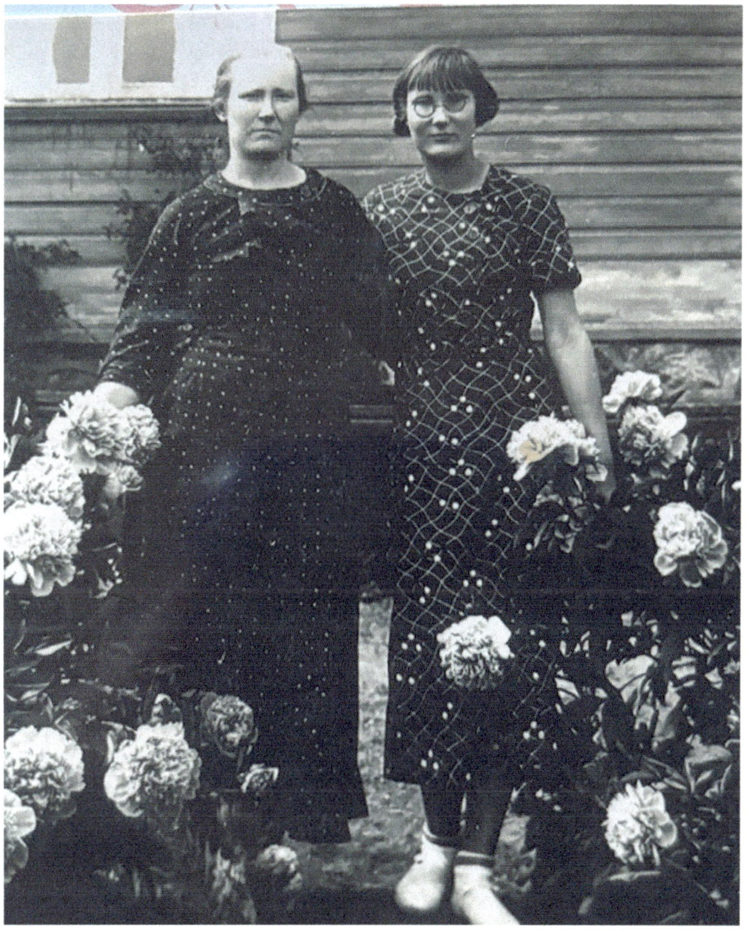

Fig. 187.13 Ruth's mother, Erna Muzikants Auers and grandmother, Martha Antonia Muzikants, in Latvia in the late 1930s. Ahead of them was the awful task of getting out of Nazi-occupied Latvia as the Soviets were advancing in 1944. They eventually made it to a displaced persons camp but imagine if the safest place you could get to was actually to flee *inside* the German borders at the end of the Second World War. They finally got to the US in the late 1940s or early 1950s. These women had to summon more strength and bravery and face more danger in those wartime years than many of us will have to in our lifetimes, and it is important that we put our professional trials and tribulations in perspective. We must remember that in the end, it's just a job, not the literal life-or-death situation these women faced. Photo: Collection of the Auers family

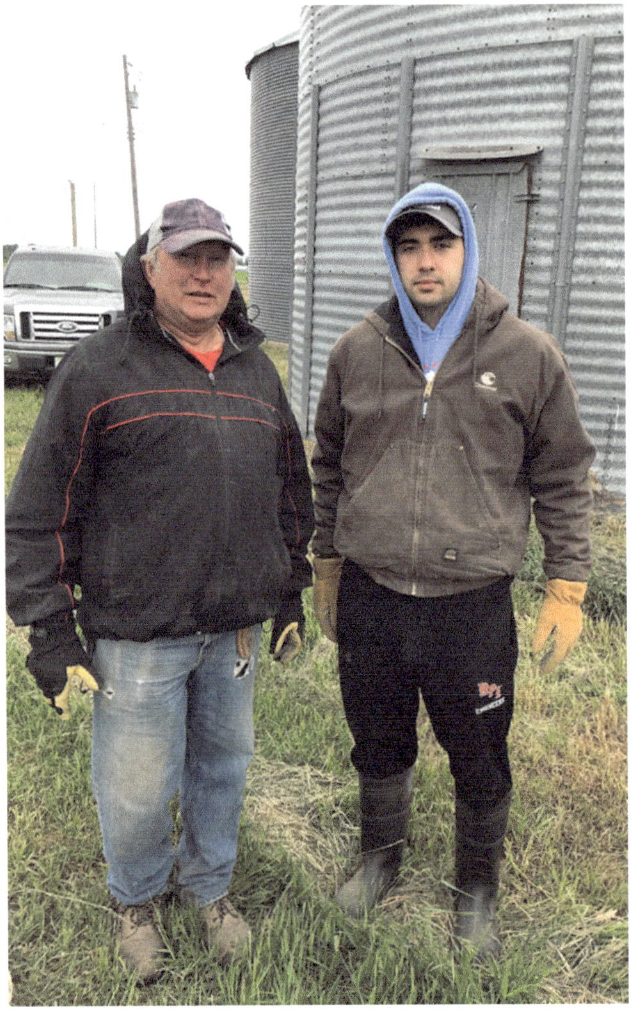

Fig. 187.14 Randy Jensen and graduating RPI senior Charlie Sandson in 2021, out at the all-important grain bins, getting ready to load the truck for the trip to Cargill. Photo: Cathy Marcucci

Reference

1. Munore R. Which state is actually flown over the most? What if? Serious scientific answers to absurd hypothetical questions. Houghton Mifflin Harcourt; 2014. p. 147–9.

Authors

Matt Rorie is from Elmwood, Nebraska, where he grew up on his family's farm. He began farming with Randy shortly after college and became a partner in 2016. In his spare time, he enjoys boating, fishing, antique tractor pulls, and tinkering around with vintage farm equipment. He is Gavin's and Margot's uncle.

Ruth Auers Jensen grew up in Lincoln, Nebraska with her own fascinating family history. Her incredibly brave and hard-working parents were born in Latvia and were caught up in the terrible events of WW2, eventually prevailing over and evading the Nazis, the German Reich, *and* the Red Army (Fig. 187.13). They immigrated to the United States where they built a life and raised four successful children. As a child, Ruth spoke fluent Latvian, one of the most complex and difficult-to-learn languages in the world. She holds a BS in chemical engineering as well as a Professional Engineer license and held numerous senior positions in several large gas pipeline companies before retiring several years ago. Even during her own busy professional career and while raising three children, she was intimately knowledgeable and supportive of all aspects of the farm operation and holds the title of treasurer of RJ Acres. Besides sharing Randy's devotion to their children and grandchildren, travel, and the Nebraska Cornhuskers, Ruth is a superb cook, is very active in her church, and collects beautiful antique jewelry.

Randy Jensen grew up on the RJ Acres property. He attended the University of Nebraska-Lincoln where he met Ruth Auers—and a party that he took Ruth to while they were dating has gone down in family history as the reason Ruth graduated with a 3.99 GPA and not a perfect 4.0. Randy is first and foremost a family man and is beyond proud of his three adult children and four beautiful grandchildren—Henry and Claire LaFlamme and Gavin and Margot Rorie. In spite of the labor-intensive nature of farming, he and Ruth have found time to visit every U.S. state (except Alabama and Delaware) and 60 foreign countries. He also loves to garden and anything to do with the Nebraska Cornhuskers.

Cathy Marcucci met Ruth Jensen in 1982 when they were both young chemical engineers working for InterNorth (which later became Enron). She soon became Randy's friend as well and has been a big fan of RJ Acres and Porker Valley (the farm's previous incorporation), since her first visit in the early 1980s. She now gets to Blair, NE as often as she can, with her kids in tow, if possible. Her son Charlie Sandson once got the unofficial prize for most interesting summer vacation as there was not one other kid in the incoming class of September new hires at his first permanent job—not one single kid—who had made a trip to Cargill to deliver grain (Fig. 187.14). Matt Rorie was driving the truck on that grain delivery day if memory serves correctly.

Put Down That Hard Cider and Pick Up a Fishing Pole!

188

Amberly Hall Brown, Austin Brown, F. Jacob Seagull, and Catherine Marcucci

Introduction

In addition to their successful music industry careers, **Amberly Hall** and **Austin Brown** are avid outdoors people. First among their favorite activities is fishing. They are so passionate about it that they have launched a YouTube channel at *The Beauty and The Bass* to concentrate on fishing content. At one point in our interview about music, we were discussing the similar stresses of their profession and ours—arduous schedules, constant and necessary contact with people (audiences and fans for them, patients and families for us), nights away from home, performance pressures, and how to stay focused, healthy, and grounded. The subject of fishing came up, and Austin and Amberly were curious as to whether fishing was a popular leisure activity for anesthesiologists and physicians in general. We didn't think so but got on email with Jake Seagull, who insisted that there are **lots** of anesthesiologists who fish (no, really Jake, don't think so). The collective response was okay then—any anesthesiologists who don't fish should most definitely start!

What followed was an exchange of pictures of proud people holding up huge bass (Jake also flyfishes) and two Zoom meetings in which Amberly, Austin, and Jake made a compelling case for this time-honored sport and hobby.

The Conversations

- **First of all, fishing is an extremely easy way to be in nature.** Which is so good for everybody! Just like golf is considered to be "a good walk spoiled" flyfishing is a good excuse to stand knee deep in a river without looking crazy. And from a human factors standpoint, it is well understood that being in a location with wide horizons (large-scale visual range and lots of three-dimensional features)

A. H. Brown · A. Brown
The Beauty and The Bass, Nashville, TN, USA

F. J. Seagull
Center for Bioethics and Social Science in Medicine, University of Michigan Medical School, Ann Arbor, MI, USA

C. Marcucci (✉)
Department of Transfusion Medicine, Clinical Center, National Institutes of Health, Bethesda, MD, USA

S. Mohamed et al. (eds.), *Anesthesia Bridges*, https://doi.org/10.1007/978-3-032-08294-7_188

leads to feelings of euphoria, especially in contrast to the inside of a hospital operating room or intensive care unit.

- **It is almost always geographically available.** Okay, granted, nothing is going to do it for deep-sea fishermen except being 30 miles out on the ocean. But apart from those people, a vast amount of fishing is done in local lakes, ponds, streams, and rivers, regardless of population density. Drive to the reservoir for any metropolitan area or across a bridge in any size town, and you'll see people fishing from the banks and the roadway.

- **It is financially accessible.** Amberly spent her young life fishing with a cane pole but eventually decided to advance to the rod and reel level of the sport. When I inquired if you could do an equipment buy-in for something around $500 dollars, she burst out laughing. Her advice? "Go get yourself a Zebco 33 for $30 and that's it, you're equipped to go out there and get started on a new way of life." Apparently, this is the rod and reel that the whole world starts fishing with—who knew? Seems like an absolute pittance, especially when you think of the money we spend on take-out food after a call shift. It is entirely possible to fish for a lifetime without spending more than the cost of a yearly fishing license. Very different than the accrued costs for court and golf club fees and lift tickets, especially if you are paying off med school loans or paying private school tuitions.

- **It puts the "Z" in Zen!** You must understand—you cannot rush fishing! There are certain techniques, of course, and various types of flies and lures, but there really is no guaranteed way to make that fish get on your line any faster than it's going to. Fishing is mentally engaging but not mentally stressful. It is all about being one with the process but detached from the outcome. Remember, they call it "fishing", not "catching." And remember that the presence of water (both running and still) has been considered to be healing in every culture throughout history.

- **It is enjoyable as a solo or group activity.** All three of these fishing fans will grab some fishing time both by themselves and in social groups. Amberly often will take a break and fish a bit at lunch. They sometimes listen to music while fishing and sometimes not. It really depends on what sort of boat they are in. Metal boats will reflect the sound into the water and scare the fish.

- **It is accessible to people in a wide variety of health states and doesn't cause much wear and tear.** In today's more inclusive society, there is something nice about going in seriously for an activity that has such low participation barriers and such a level playing field. You can fish standing or sitting in a wheelchair while exhausted or in ill health. Because, honestly, the fish won't take much notice. Similarly, it doesn't matter how great you look, how your last show went, how many likes you get on a video, or how many lives you have saved—the fish won't be that impressed.

- **It is generally pretty safe.** Fishing safety is generally about boating safety and avoiding intoxicating substances. Amberly remembers that she did once get hurt coming down her asphalt driveway on her way to fish and fell on a slick spot and scraped her knee. Although she cautions that you **do** have to be careful of your hands when you are baiting your hook. Amberly and Austin are very conservative about wearing life jackets if they are on water with a current or undertow or if they do not know the water. They also do not fish in boats without a buddy.

- **It is an ethical way to be a sportsman.** This one is really important. Here is not the place to make any statements about blood sports. Properly licensed and responsible hunting is still the choice of millions of people. It's legal. But it is just not everybody's thing. A lot of people who fish practice catch-and-release fishing, which helps to mitigate these concerns. Austin and Amberly do eat the very occasional fish they've caught, but a great number of their fishy friends go right back in.

- **Don't just do catch and release, do best practices catch and release.** There is a lot of information readily available on the internet on this. The first realization is that catch and release done poorly or roughly can cause the fish to die even if released. To summarize, the goal is to minimize the stress to the fish. First, minimize the time the fish is out of the water. It should always be less than a minute at the most. Try to keep it to seconds, if possible. Study baiting techniques so that the fish is not deeply hooked or hooked through the gills. If you are going to take a quick picture before release, **always** hold the fish securely and horizontally by the middle, never by the mouth, and not by or over the gills. If possible, place the fish gently back in the water and hold it there a second before releasing. Kudos to coauthors Amberly Hall Brown and Austin Brown for using correct holding techniques in the photo illustrations (Figs. 188.1, 188.2, and 188.3). Austin also mentioned to Cathy that they are now limiting fishing in their own pond as repeated catch-and-release fishing can cause overfishing stress to the animals and will increase mortality.

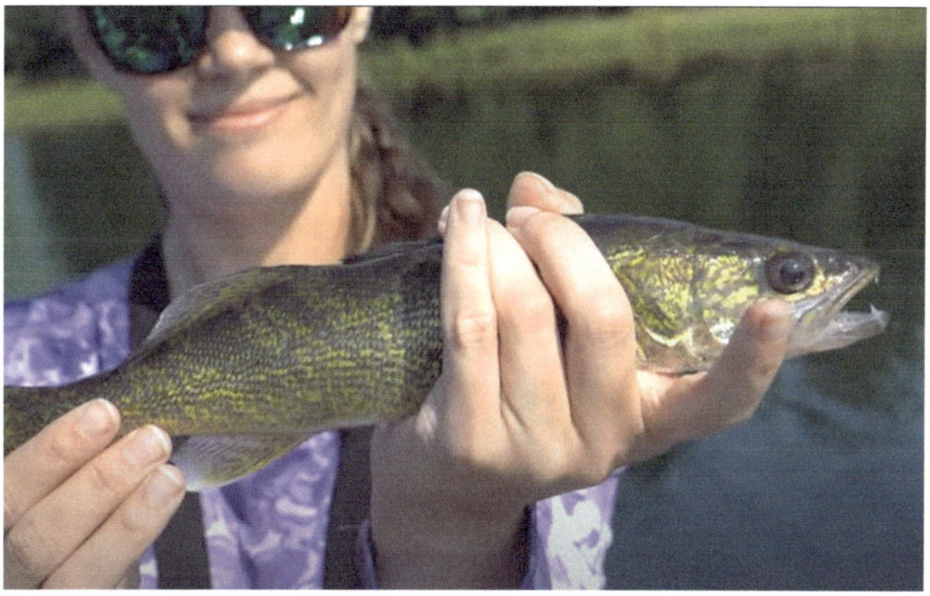

Fig. 188.1 Amberly Hall Brown demonstrates the correct way to hold a catch-and-release fish. Photo: Austin Brown

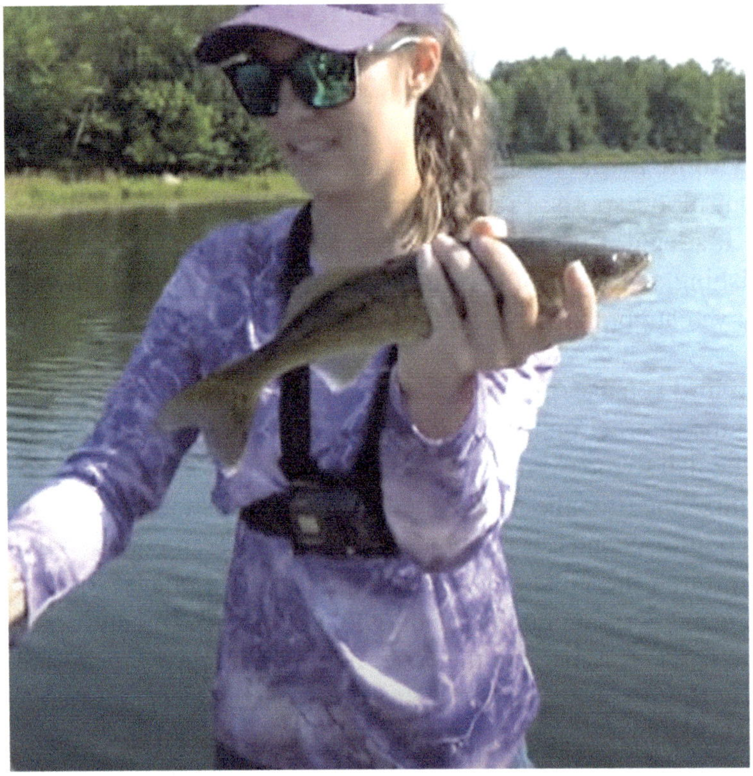

Fig. 188.2 Notice that Amberly does not have any part of her hand over the gills. Photo: Austin Brown

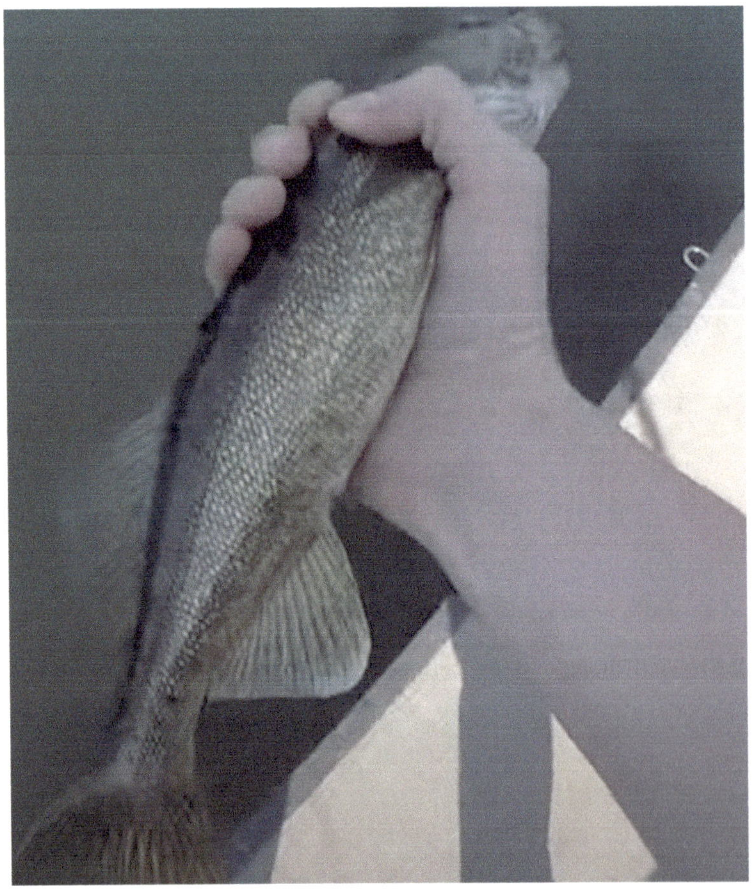

Fig. 188.3 Coauthor Austin Brown holding a catch-and-release fish securely by the middle before leaning over and placing the fish in the water. Photo: Amberly Hall Brown

- **It's a fantastic way to relate to patients**. Elsewhere in this book, Steve Frank makes the point of really talking to our patients, even though our time with them is limited. It's important to establish that human contact—to take just a few moments in the stress of the perioperative period to find out what matters to them. Cathy tends to ask people if they play bridge. This is completely ridiculous because in 33 years as an anesthesiologist she has never found a single patient who did. But Amberly, Austin, and Jake advise that just a bit of fishing knowledge and experience will allow us to quickly establish rapport with a huge range of people—young, old, rural, urban, and suburban. Apparently, it's as easy as saying, "Tell me, Mr. Washington, do you fish?" The proper response then being, "Hey, me too! What do you go for?"

- **It's a readily available vacation and travel activity.** But you don't have to pack a trailer of gear to do it. There's a You Tube video of Amberly and Austin leaving a concert venue after a show to head to Wisconsin for a 48-hours fishing vacation for walleye and perch. This was in the middle of an extended tour schedule, so their truck was packed pretty full of luggage and other tour gear. But in the back, compartment was still room for no less than nine fishing rods! Imagine trying to go on vacation with nine pairs of skis or nine bags of golf clubs or nine touring bicycles. Of course, if you do want to pull out all the stops, there's no end of "destination" fishing locations. On Amberly's and Austin's bucket list is a week-long guided bass fishing trip to Lake Okeechobee in southeast Florida. Evidently, this is one of the premier bass fishing locations, and many tournaments for the fishing pros are held there due to the size, energy, and attitude of the fish. But it is accessible to even beginning fishermen due to the abundant shoreline and calm waters.

- **What's a good lifelong fishing program?** First, anything that gets you started. You can spend your whole fishing career using an inexpensive rod and reel and fishing from a bank or a dock. But small flat-bottomed Jon boats can be had for just a couple of hundred bucks. Austin got his for his 14th birthday, and he is still using it decades later. With a little outboard motor, you can then fish for a lifetime on lakes and ponds. Everybody who fishes eventually fishes for bass, but the trout fishermen are out there as well. They're a fun fishing community and very devoted to their segment of the sport. The best overall advice that Amberly and Austin have is to base your fishing itinerary on where you want to be and where you want to go. There is fishing everywhere!

Lessons Learned

- The practice of anesthesiology is rewarding but can be oh-so-hard on its practitioners. Fishing might be just what the doctor ordered.

- The affordability and easy accessibility are two of its most attractive aspects. If you want to fish at a higher price point, that's readily available too.

- It's an engaging, stimulating, yet relaxing activity that doesn't depend on speed, performance, or physical fitness.

- Remember, fishing safety largely means paying attention to boating safety. And a bit of caution about your hands.

- You can be every bit the fisherman at 90 that you were at 30.
- The fishing community straddles every demographic. This makes it hugely advantageous when seeking to connect with patients (and everybody else in the world).

Authors

Amberly Hall Brown lives in Nashville, where she is busy developing her fishing and outdoor channel *The Beauty and the Bass*. She is hoping to take up fly fishing in the very near future in the northern USA and Canada. In the meantime, she fishes as often as she can in her local waters.

Austin Brown lives in Nashville, where his favorite place to fish is his own pond. His dream fishing indulgence—in the future—would be a fully equipped high-end bass boat. He describes himself as the original catch-and-release guy.

Jake Seagull loves to fish for bass all over the north-central part of the US and Colorado. He is also an avid fly fisherman. As a human factors expert, he especially appreciates the Zen aspect of fishing (of course). He heartily endorses Amberly's and Austin's fishing ethics.

Cathy Marcucci remembers fishing for large catfish called "channel cats" while spending summers in Georgia with her extended family. Her Eagle Scout son and Boston-based daughter both already like to fish, and they are all working on Neil for some family fishing time in the near future. In the meantime, she is still casting about for bridge players.

189 Continuous Professional Development: Necessary for the Pursuit of Mastery

Cynthia A. Lien

Introduction

It's easy to get comfortable with your current job, location, and responsibilities. However, if you really want to pursue career development, consider periodically reinventing yourself. While a move from a major metropolitan city on the East Coast to the Midwest may not be for everyone, it allowed me to re-explore goals, learn new skills, discover new talents, and meet new challenges with the benefit of at least some added wisdom. Whatever career path you have chosen or will choose, it will be work—with all of its challenges, so genuine commitment is necessary to continue to move forward.

My Personal Path

Writing about one's own path is an interesting undertaking. It was much more difficult than I had anticipated—and much more personal. As I often do, I reached out to my daughters for their advice (Fig. 189.1). They suggested that it would be best to share a sense of vulnerability. As a woman in medicine, even one who has had her share of accomplishments, I am not yet sure that I am convinced of that. So much professional energy has been devoted to building bridges, disagreeing pleasantly, and sublimating critical thoughts that it is refreshing to see a growing presence of women in the leadership of anesthesiology, education, and medicine—many of whom are less guarded than I am.

My desire to succeed and make a difference was fueled by an education system that should have been cheering me on but frequently was not supportive. If I may reminisce for a moment, in middle school "home economics" was not my area of interest—and to this day I don't sew—so I lobbied the school administration to allow girls to take "shop" instead. I continued to play trombone and worked to hold the seat of first trombone in the high school band because our music teacher said that I played like a girl—whatever that meant. I thank my guidance counselor, whose name I cannot remember, for motivating my choice of college and my drive, as he said that I would never be accepted to an Ivy League college. This perseverance is a characteristic that has contributed to my resilience and enabled me to push through the more challenging times.

C. A. Lien (✉)
Department of Anesthesiology, Medical College of Wisconsin/Froedtert Hospital, Milwaukee, WI, USA
e-mail: clien@mcw.edu

S. Mohamed et al. (eds.), *Anesthesia Bridges*, https://doi.org/10.1007/978-3-032-08294-7_189

***Note from the Editors:** Cindy Lien's wonderful family (Fig. 189.1).

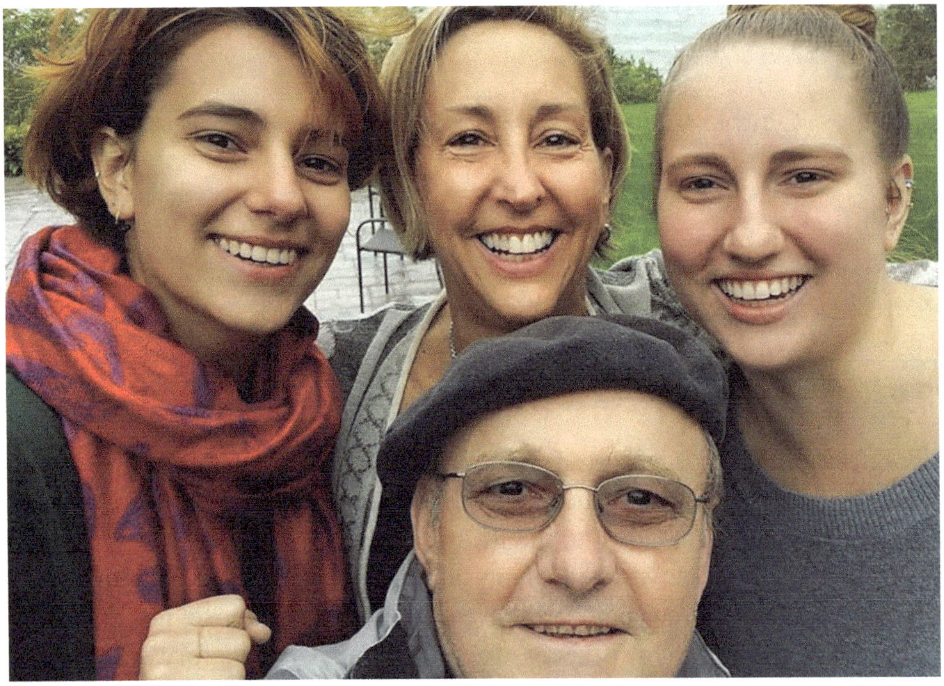

Fig. 189.1 Cindy Lien's group. Husband Dan Brinzac, looking very dashing in a beret (it's not every man that can pull off that look), with daughter Christina on the upper left and daughter Erika on the upper right. Photo: Collection of the Lien-Brinzac family

Starting My Journey

I spent my first year after college working in a tissue typing lab and considering pursuing a PhD. After several months of plating trays to look at compatibility between kidney donors and potential recipients, I knew that I wanted to be involved more in the translational and application pieces of science; I wanted to impact patient outcomes. So, I applied to medical school. While I truly did enjoy every rotation in medical school, I ultimately decided to pursue a residency in anesthesiology, which, to my less experienced self, seemed like an interesting specialty where someone could develop an academic career without having to rely on the sponsorship of others.

Now, many years later, I have come to appreciate that I could not have been more wrong about the ability to accomplish much without the input of others. Success, regardless of your specialty of practice, requires teamwork and active collaboration. Medicine, especially anesthesiology, is truly a team sport—whether we are considering the anesthesia care team, research collaborators, or our collection of colleagues and mentors—each of whom brings something unique to the specialty and the delivery of patient care. Moving the specialty forward and improving patient care, whether through research, education, or managing a patient's perioperative experience, requires discussion and consideration of diverse points of view and teamwork.

Building a team has been the subject of so many books and is dependent on too many different factors to list. What I have found to be important is to never forget why you chose a specialty and to never lose sight of yourself as you move toward your ever-evolving goals. It is important to surround yourself with people who challenge you and propel you toward your goals, while they pursue theirs.

Feedback Is Fundamental

While I am pleased by the path my career has taken, it would have never been possible had I not stood "on the shoulders of others." In addition to the many mentors and sponsors, what stands out is the feedback I have received from so many individuals along the way. Feedback is so important as we critically appraise our performance—it helps us look for ways to improve and also allows us to reflect on what we do well.

Our successes, however small, provide grounding for the work of refining our performance. Historically, underrepresented individuals don't recognize either their successes or the importance of those successes, so positive feedback is crucial for development. Similarly, while we should be able to recognize our own areas for development, that process is facilitated by the honest appraisal of our shortcomings by others.

Full mastery of anything is an illusion, and when I entered medicine, I committed to continuously learning and increasing my skills as a clinician and an educator. While we would all likely prefer that all our feedback come in polished, neat, and easily digestible little packages, the reality of our hectic days is that is rarely the case. Working through initial defensiveness to actually hear what is being said is essential to processing the information and enhancing our skills. Honest and raw feedback may take us back for a moment (or longer!) and diminish our sense of accomplishment, but, with time, it allows us to reframe goals and our approaches to achieve them and permits us to become our better selves.

Gratitude

So, I end this essay with much gratitude. Thank you to all of those who have given and continue to give me feedback during my career: my patients, my mentors, my colleagues, my students, those who chose their words carefully, and those who did not, those who responded to a request for feedback, and those who spoke their mind at unexpected times. All have been an essential piece of my ongoing and relatively lengthy career, and will continue to be so moving forward, none of which would have been possible without them.

Lessons Learned

- One way to pursue career development is to periodically reinvent yourself.
- Having perseverance and resilience enables one to work through the more challenging times in life.
- Success requires teamwork and active collaboration.
- Really listening to honest and raw feedback allows us to become our better selves.

Author

Cynthia Lien completed her residency at Columbia University Medical Center and then remained in Manhattan to practice at New York-Presbyterian Hospital. After raising two daughters in New York City, she and her husband, Dan became Midwesterners; the girls stayed in New York. When not at the hospital and advocating for the highest standards of medical care, she can be found on the tennis court or walking the dunes of Lake Michigan with her husband.

Don't Neglect Your Social Action Efforts: Kirk Lalwani Shares His Thoughts

190

Kirk Lalwani and Catherine Marcucci

Introduction

We more than understand the life, work, and financial pressures faced by junior anesthesiologists. Practice parameters are changing on an ongoing basis, and often not for the better, it seems. Raising children becomes ever more hectic and complicated in multiple and sometimes weird ways. And nobody's student loans and mortgages are magically vanishing. In the midst of all this life stuff, we truly implore you not to neglect your social action efforts. Kirk was kind enough to give us his personal philosophy and approach to social action below.

From Kirk

Giving back to your community is what defines each of us as a members of the community. We all feel passionately about different causes, but the common denominator is that every social action effort affects your community in a positive way. It may be that you do your job well, or volunteer after work, or serve as a leader of a charitable organization, or donate cash or kind to charities. Choosing a charity that serves a cause close to your heart is often the easiest. Sometimes, specific life events like illness motivate us to donate to a cause. Others respond to a call for action, such as when natural disasters strike or local blood shortages are announced.

Ensuring that your chosen charity uses donated funds wisely and without excessive waste or administrative expense is crucial when choosing a charity to donate to. An excellent website that rates charities on their financial transparency and accountability, and in some cases, their impact as well, is Charity Navigator (www.charitynavigator.org), where a four-star rating is the highest. GuideStar (www.guidestar.org) is another website offering detailed analysis of nonprofits but requires a paid subscription for some features.

K. Lalwani
Department of Anesthesiology, Oregon Health & Science University, Portland, OR, USA

C. Marcucci (✉)
Department of Transfusion Medicine, Clinical Center, National Institutes of Health, Bethesda, MD, USA

S. Mohamed et al. (eds.), *Anesthesia Bridges*, https://doi.org/10.1007/978-3-032-08294-7_190

I have worked with children's charities like Save the Children, domestic violence nonprofits like The National Coalition Against Domestic Violence and LifeWire, and food security organizations like Feeding America. These charities have inspired me over the years because they are apolitical and help foster basic human rights, dignity, safety, and the end of food insecurity.

In the following chapters, we describe several additional social action efforts that have had great meaning for us. Similar to the causes listed above, these causes have intrigued and motivated us for many years.

Lessons Learned

- It is in the very nature of being a physician to care deeply and get involved. Why fight against this nature when it comes to social action?
- Follow your heart!
- But there's room for a cool and level head as well. The charity rating websites can provide efficient and thorough evaluations and analysis of a wide range of charities.

***Note from the Editors:** Speaking of social action and social awareness, the Tilikum Crossing in Portland, Oregon is one of Kirk's favorite bridges (Fig. 190.1). This stunning structure permits only light rail traffic, buses, bicyclists, and pedestrians—it is the only fully operational roadway bridge in the country that is not open to cars. However, emergency vehicles are permitted.

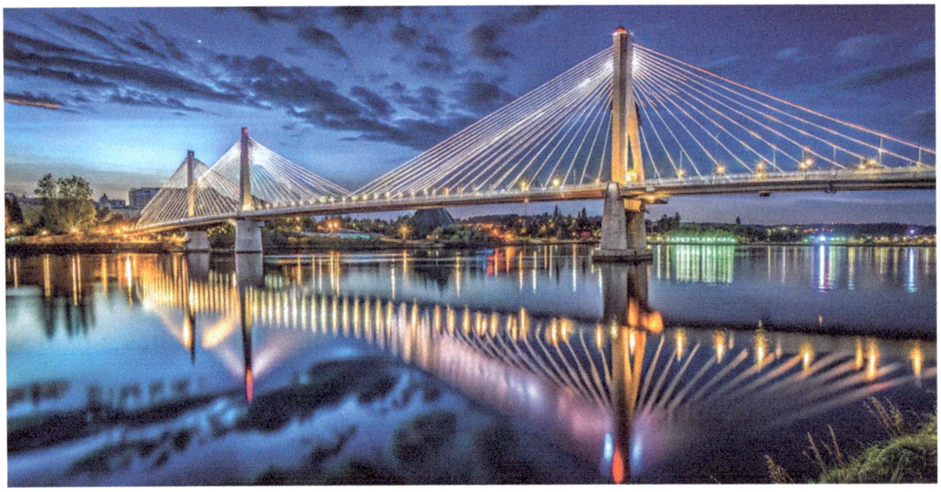

Fig. 190.1 Tilikum Crossing, or the Bridge of the People, is a cable-stayed bridge over the Willamette River. *Tilikum* is a Chinook jargon word meaning people, tribe, or family and the name is intended to honor the Multnomah, Cascade, Clackamas, and other Chinookan peoples who had inhabited the area for around 14,000 years. The bridge is dramatically lit at night in different colors based on input from monitors that record the river's current speed, water height, and temperature. Photo: Image used under standard license from stock.adobe.com

Authors

Kirk Lalwani is a pediatric anesthesiologist and professor of anesthesiology at Oregon Health and Science University. His earliest social action recollection as a child is helping his family prepare and distribute meals to children at a community orphanage. He has instilled the value of community service in his children through shifts at the food bank and other volunteer activities.

Cathy Marcucci has participated in a number of charity efforts, both for the anesthesia community and in her private life. Recently, she did a short chapter for Kirk's new benefit book published by Oxford University Press entitled *Professional, Ethical, Legal and Educational Lessons in Medicine: A Problem-Based Learning Approach* for the charity **Feeding America**. This is a really great compilation of information on important topics, go pick up a copy.

191 You Cannot Miss with Animal Rescue: We Started with Rabbits

Catherine Marcucci

Contributing author:

Susan Wong, BS

Introduction

On our last big wedding anniversary, my husband Neil Sandson and I were doing some of the life review that often happens around the notable milestones, and he remarked to me, "Well, you know, we've rescued six animals, that's gotta be up there on our list of successes." And so, it is.

We started with four rabbits. We had badly wanted a dog and the kids did too, but we couldn't do the middle of the day care and didn't have the budget at the time for a really good doggy day care—private dog sitters and walkers being out of the question at that time. So, we did the full complement of goldfish—Speedy, Goldie, Ultrafast, and Finn populated the goldfish bowl at various times. This worked when Charlie and Lisa were little but didn't cut it when they got to school age. My sister-in-law was a dialysis nurse and had to set out in the wee hours to get to her shift starting at 6 AM. She had hit upon the solution of house rabbits and recommended it to us.

The Rabbits Arrive

And so, Cardigan, Zeus, Shemp, and Jake joined the family. And it turned out that house rabbits were the perfect pets for our medical household! By "house rabbit" I mean rabbits that are 100% indoor pets—there should be no wire hutch in a corner of the backyard in the modern day. Other than committing to living inside with your animals, and understanding that rabbits will be rabbits, for us personally, there were almost no downsides to owning house rabbits as pets.

First of all, there is an active rabbit rescue community, both nationally and internationally. There are many, many, *many* abandoned and needy rabbits in search of a good home—third only behind dogs and cats. The people working in rabbit rescue are as dedicated as any. We worked with Friends of Rabbits

C. Marcucci (✉)
Department of Transfusion Medicine, Clinical Center, National Institutes of Health, Bethesda, MD, USA

S. Mohamed et al. (eds.), *Anesthesia Bridges*, https://doi.org/10.1007/978-3-032-08294-7_191

(FofR), a 501(c)(3) nonprofit, that is incorporated in Virginia, and places rabbits in the metropolitan Washington DC/Baltimore area.

The people at FofR were totally supportive and available every single day of the year for questions, advice, and support. They also guaranteed that they would rehome the rabbit in the rare event that a placement situation didn't work out—for instance, every once in a while, an adoptive family finds that somebody is allergic to rabbits or the hay that is used for their bedding. Also, most rescue rabbits are mixed breed, so there is a range of phenotypes in the rescue population. We did not have pre-conceived ideas about size and color but generally rescues can work with adopters to find a match on physical characteristics.

Rabbit Feeding and Care

We also found the care of house rabbits to be remarkably easy. We set a kiddie pool up with a folding gate as the walls. We knew that we might not have a lot of time on any given day to interact and play with the rabbits, so we opted for a bonded pair and then a second bonded pair. Because their pen was of sufficient size, if we were not able for a day to take them out and interact with them, they were fine snuggled up together, and we made up the exercise time on the next day.

Also, rabbits love music that is soothing and melodic. All we had to do for morning care was make sure they had clean water, food in their food dish, and then tune the radio into a classical music station with the volume on low. No early morning walks in the ice and slush and dark. Of course, rabbits should never be left for long periods of time without care and fresh water and food. In most areas, the costs for rabbit sitting are generally in line with those for cat sitting as it requires about the same level of involvement.

That said, we did make every effort to interact with our animals daily. But keep in mind that "play with the rabbits" is not a terrible evening chore for a school age kid. When house rabbits are allowed the free run of a room, they will do the bunny kicks and hops and zoomies that delight kids. They love to be petted but do not like to be extensively handled, off the ground, or on the furniture. Two of our rabbits essentially thought they were dogs—they were extremely affectionate and affiliative and had a small vocabulary of about 10 words. In contrast, our black and white Dutch girl was very independent and was the boss of all the boys.

Rabbits will litter train themselves if given a regular cat litter pan. They do require their litter box to be changed every couple of days and the hay in their pool to be changed every week. They do not require bathing at all and other grooming needs, such as keeping their fur maintained, depend on their breed mix. We chose rabbits with short coats who did not shed a lot. A long-haired rabbit will shed and require regular professional grooming—remember that angora sweaters are made from combed rabbit fur. Rabbits also do not carry a lot of communicable disease if they remain house rabbits. So, although they should have a yearly routine checkup, there is less expense for shots and so forth than with dogs. Rabbits are considered exotic pets, but most decent-sized veterinary practices will have a rabbit person, although you will want to do your due diligence on this and just not assume. Rabbit rescues are located throughout the country and your rescue will be able to direct you to an acceptable caregiver for your animal. If you move, just contact a local rescue in your new location and they will be glad to tell you where their rabbits are seen.

A well-cared for house rabbit will live about eight years, although all of ours lived past 10. But it is imperative that potential adopters understand that a rabbit is always going to do its rabbit thing. They are inveterate chewing machines, and their teeth never stop growing. If they are not supervised when out of their pool, they will find your lamp cords and baseboards and may try to "rearrange" your couch cushions. So, there is this caveat—rabbits *DO* require an ongoing and infinite supply of toys and boxes to eat. We used to clean yard sales out of wicker baskets, priced at a dollar or less. A large wicker basket or even cardboard box (take off all the tape!) will do the trick for almost a week, depending on how many rabbits you have. We lost a lamp or two over the years to those chomping bunny teeth, but we have to say that both of our dogs have proved to be more destructive and worse chewers than any of our four rabbits. This is the nature of pet ownership.

Although most rabbits can exist in a household with most cats, greater consideration should be given if you wish to include a dog in your household as well. Friends of Rabbits have done multiple placements with adopters who have dogs. On the other hand, sometimes a dog's innate prey drive will just be too strong, and rabbits have been known to suffer fatal heart attacks and strokes even when taken into situations where certain breeds of large or hunting dogs are present in the room. As with all cross-species households, it just depends on the specific animals.

Finally, there is a group of rescue rabbits that is especially needy—the ones with the pink eyes. Sadly, these rabbits are often considered to be less desirable by adopters—sort of the "black dog syndrome" that is seen by dog rescuers. We decided to look past this and adopt a former laboratory rabbit—the late great Jake—and came to love his pink eyes that exactly matched his pink ears.

***Note from the Editors:** This isn't Jake, but he looked just like this (Fig. 191.1).

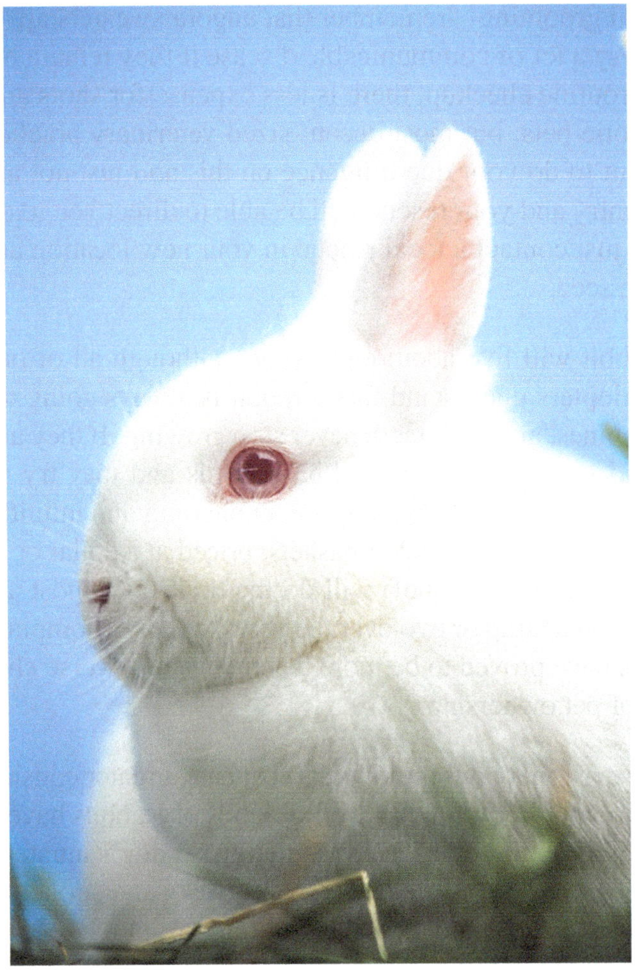

Fig. 191.1 Pink-eyed white rescue rabbits are the hardest to place and rescue pros now call them "ruby eyes" to try to counteract the stigma. If you would like to add a rabbit to your family, please consider opening your hearts to a bunny like this. (Photo: Image used under standard license from shutterstock.com)

Lessons Learned

- Animal welfare/rescue is one of the most important social action efforts you can make. If you can't adopt an animal, there are many ways to contribute. You can volunteer to care for or foster animals or help at adoption events.

- **The Friends of Rabbits website is www.friendsofrabbits.org** (Fig. 191.2). Contributions are always welcome, and no amount is too small. Donating money comes with the knowledge and satisfaction that you will make an immediate impact—guaranteed.

- House rabbits were great pets for our medical family. We found our rabbits to be wonderful and tolerated the frustrations and quirks of owning rabbits easily. The set-up is relatively inexpensive and straightforward. They do not need middle-of- the-day care, do not require regular bathing (but may require regular grooming) and do not carry communicable diseases. Remember to consider allergies to bunny fur and/or hay, though. Ruby-eyed bunnies are often most in need of a loving home.

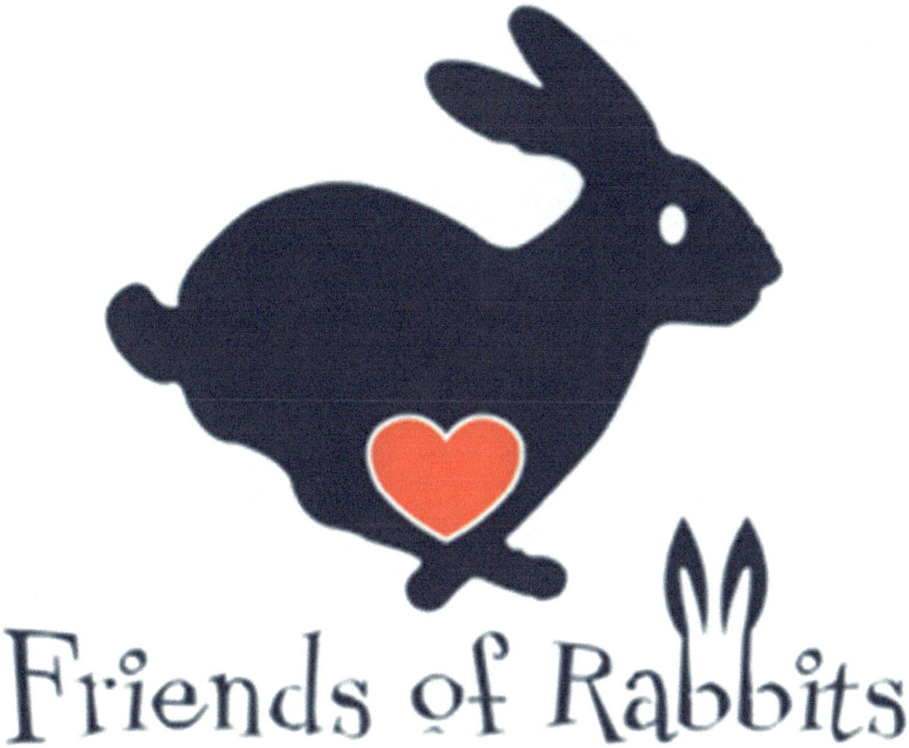

Fig. 191.2 The logo of the wonderful rescue where we got our bunnies. We had a great experience with this group and our rabbits. Illustration: Image used with permission of Friends of Rabbits

Author

Cathy Marcucci was raised with animals and couldn't imagine raising her own children without the pleasure of a household pet. After the bunnies arrived, one of her online avatars became "Zmanmom." Someone once asked her, "Mother of a boy named Zach, I presume?" and there was a bit of surprised look when she said, "No, mother of a rabbit named Zeus." She is hopeful that at least one reader of this book will consider adopting a rescue rabbit for their own family.

Man's Best Friend!

192

C. J. Barilleaux-Badger and Catherine Marcucci

Introduction

The Marcucci-Sandson family are dog people—first, last, and always.

From Cathy

Our love of dogs is something inborn, we think. Sheltering four rabbits worked and we loved them, but eventually we decided to take the plunge, rearrange schedules, expand the budget, and get a family dog. For us, there was no other solution than to rescue a dog. Although we would have adopted ten needy dogs if we could, our little pittie-mix is probably best as an only dog. She's not aggressive, but she's not interested in sharing the love with another animal. We take the best possible care of her that we can, but we still have doggie love left over!

So, we decided to find several dog rescues that we could contribute to and develop a relationship with, the only pre-condition being that it had to be a nonprofit organization and really needy. We started out by contributing to a popular online site that collects for hundreds of dog rescues and one day I clicked on a feature story described as "dogs who need the most help."

There, at the top of the feature, was a picture of a medium size mixed-breed dog with crooked ears named Whitney (Fig. 192.1) with the tagline, "Just another kill-shelter dog." And that was it—I was hooked on helping individual dog rescues save as many dogs as I reasonably could within the boundaries of financial probity. I didn't adopt Whitney, but I did sponsor her care, which was hugely rewarding. She is safe and being well-cared for but is still waiting for her forever home.

C. J. Barilleaux-Badger
Barking Mad Animal Refuge, Ltd, Hemphill, TX, USA

C. Marcucci (✉)
Department of Transfusion Medicine, Clinical Center, National Institutes of Health, Bethesda, MD, USA

S. Mohamed et al. (eds.), *Anesthesia Bridges*, https://doi.org/10.1007/978-3-032-08294-7_192

***Note from the Editors:** This is Whitney (Fig. 192.1).

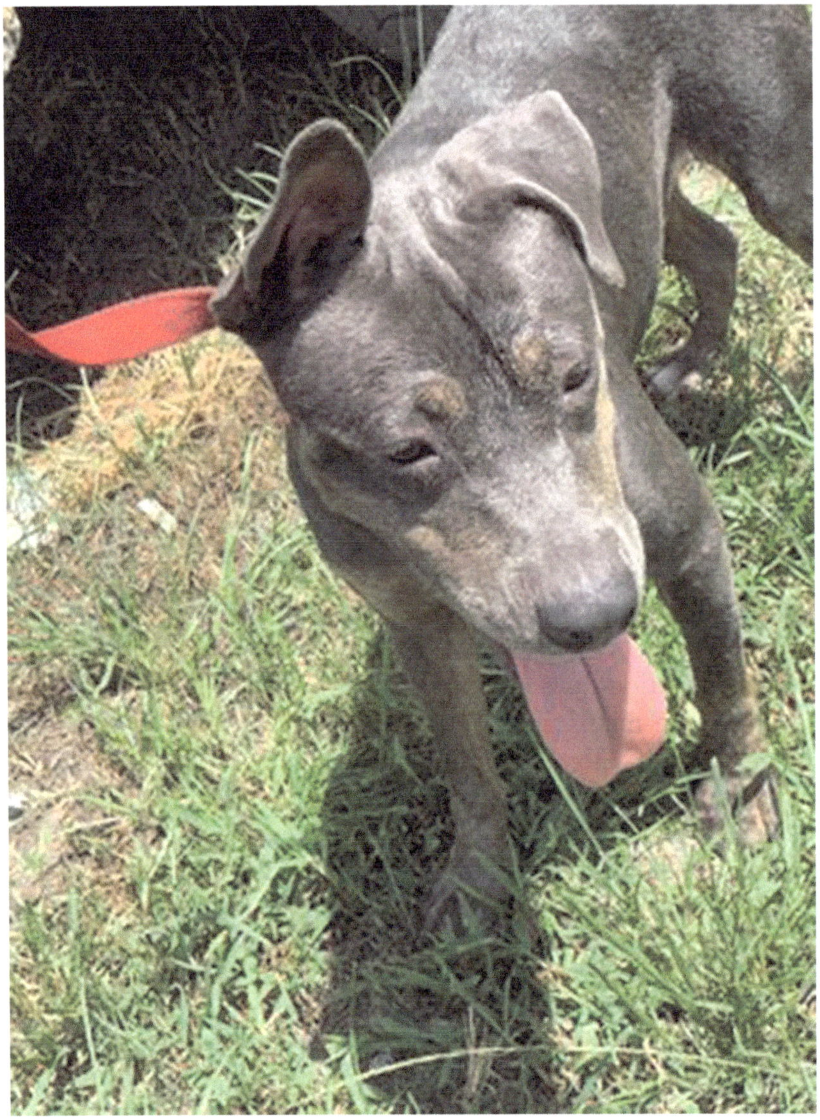

Fig. 192.1 This beautiful girl is dog-friendly and people-friendly and still at BMAR waiting for her forever home. We continue to love those wonky ears. Photo: CJ Barilleaux-Badger

Dog rescues work well as social action for physicians because *so many* of the dogs in shelters and rescues need medical attention. For instance, we try to help at least a tiny bit with every rescue dog that we can find who is suffering from burns. We have also contributed larger amounts to particular dogs who are facing surgery or intensive heart worm or parvo treatments but some months we will just donate $100 worth of flea treatments or a couple of bags of dog food. The point is that you can make an enormous impact for a cash-strapped rescue with even a small donation or gift of goods.

When our monthly dog rescue budget is tapped out, we work a bit on our current project—Doctors for Dogs. This involves developing physician donor groups for certain types of medical problems—trying to find orthopedic surgeons who will donate for dogs with fractures or who were struck by cars or ophthalmologists to donate to dogs with eye problems. If we can get that up and going, we're next going to use our grant-writing skills and volunteer to help rescues apply for grants.

We also look for dog rescues that work in underserved areas. I started watching the dogs who were posted for donations by the rescue who saved Whitney and found Barking Mad Animal Rescue/Barking Mad Animal Refuge (BMAR). They are a registered 501(c)(3) no-kill rescue in Hemphill, Texas. They run a large operation for dog rescue, rehabilitation, and placement, in a three-county area in rural east Texas where there are *NO* municipal funds or facilities for abandoned, injured, or unwanted dogs (Fig. 192.2).

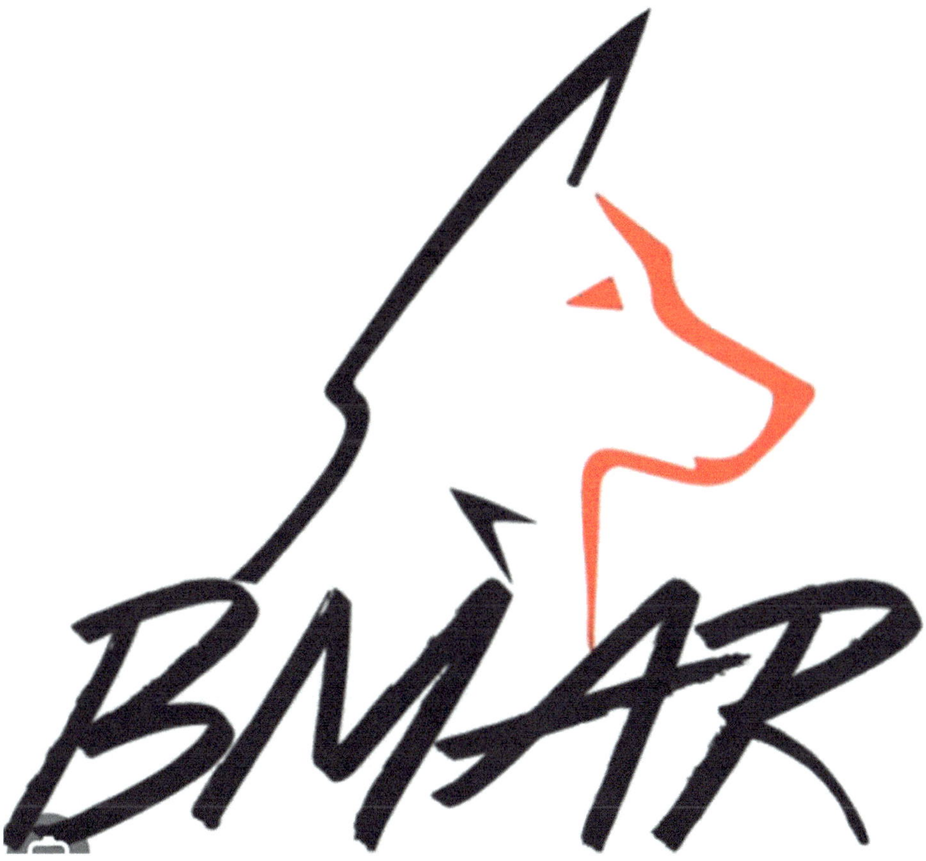

Fig. 192.2 The logo of Barking Mad Animal Refuge. There are thousands of deserving animal rescue operations, but this one is especially needy and deserving. Every single dog that crosses their gate would have otherwise perished. Please consider donating if you are able. Their email is barkingmadanimalrescue@gmail.com. They get hundreds of emails weekly from people looking to surrender dogs, so it is best to identify yourself in the subject line as a potential donor. Illustration: used with permission of CJ Barrilleaux-Badger for Barking Mad Animal Refuge

They also function as a sanctuary for dogs who cannot be placed for various reasons and as a hospice for end-of-life care and this is the Barking Mad Animal Refuge part of their operation. They are a 100% percent volunteer operation that raises all of its funds through private donations. The people who run the rescue use a lot of their own money as well. They have a calling and mission as great or greater than we do, since they are willing to pretty much go broke helping their patients. They do not have the advantage of operating in a wealthy area and choose to put all available funds into the dogs, taking dogs that no one else will take. I asked CJ Barilleaux-Badger, the founder and director of BMAR, to tell us in her own words about the lives she has saved and why she does what she does.

From CJ Barilleaux-Badger

Barking Mad Animal Refuge is truly a mission of love offering help to animals and any person who asks, who reaches out. We are believers in second chances for our four-legged friends and the humans whose lives need companions.

Our dogs are the best friend of a disabled vet, a companion so that elderly lady living by herself is not lonely, that hermit gentleman who doesn't interact with anyone…except a rescue dog that managed to win his heart and give him something to live for. The antics of rescue dogs are the givers of smiles to the sick, the homebound, the mentally ill. They can break the ice and give someone a reason to reach out, to ask for help, to get a visit that will change a life….for a dog or a human.

We change lives for these dogs and the people who love them. Rescues bring people together, educate the willing, and make the world a better place for people and animals to coexist. Our supporters are worldwide, and many countries are involved with our efforts to give these dogs a will to live, freedom from abuse, proper care and best of all, placement in a loving home…a family of their own. We can be their whole world. We can help you do your job and make the world a better place.

Conclusions

Need we say anything more?

Lessons Learned

- If you are a dog person, there is no better social action than dog rescue.
- My family likes that we can make an impact on the medical status of a lot of dogs with a relatively small amount of money. For instance, I talked CJ into starting a regular donor drive called Medicine Mondays, which has helped keep her rescue stocked with the non-prescription medical supplies that an animal rescue with 400 dogs boarding at any time needs on a constant basis.
- We chose a rescue in an underserved, rural area to develop a relationship with but it's a great thing to donate to make a local impact for the dogs in your own area. Need doesn't really have boundaries.

BMAR almost went under and was hours away from closing during the pandemic, staying open only by deploying desperation measures. But they reorganized, got straight with their paperwork, renewed their nonprofit status and have vowed to stay open if humanly possible. They are constantly in need, as are most dog and animal rescues.

- CJ's motto, when deciding how best to help BMAR's dogs, is "we love differences." Being less than picture perfect or having medical needs shouldn't disqualify a dog from obtaining sanctuary, rehabilitation, and a home.
- Barking Mad Animal Rescue/Barking Mad Animal Refuge is on Facebook, TikTok, and Instagram. Their website is at barkingmadanimalrescue.com and has their nonprofit and tax information.

Authors

CJ Barilleaux-Badger's life in animal rescue began as a young girl when she saved a litter of puppies that she found abandoned in a grocery store sack. She was a successful businesswoman in Houston before relocating with her family to a small farm in Sabine County, Texas in 2005. She operated Barking Mad Animal Rescue as a private family enterprise until 2014, when she registered as a 501(c)(3) nonprofit due to the overwhelming needs of the homeless dogs in that area. In 2022, she formed the in-house Barking Mad Animal Refuge, also as a 501(c)(3), to emphasize Barking Mad's sanctuary mission. She and her dedicated volunteer staff, including her husband Myron Badger and son Justin Barilleaux, work 365 days per year, caring for the dogs. She estimates that she has taken in and saved the lives of over 10,000 animals.

Cathy Marcucci's favorite dog breed is the American rescue dog. She is the proud mother of Cocoa, a chihuahua-pit bull mix who was rescued from Puerto Rico in 2017 on the last Jet Blue flight out before Hurricane Maria. Her beloved girlhood dog Posy came to the Marcucci family in 1973 from a listing in the paper advertising a litter of puppies "free to a good home."

Please Consider Donating Blood!

193

Tsung-Lin Tsai, Leonard N. Chen, Harvey J. Alter, and Catherine Marcucci

In life, we often talk about giving something of ourselves to others, but this is typically just a thought or a concept to be achieved at a later time. When donating blood, one actually and physically gives something of themselves to selflessly benefit the health of another, often anonymous, recipient. To do so, creates a wonderful feeling of satisfaction and fulfillment. Try it..........you'll like it.

- **Harvey J. Alter, MD**
  Distinguished NIH Clinical Investigator
  2020 Laureate, Nobel Prize in Medicine or Physiology

The Pressing Need for Blood Donations

This is a straightforward plea—if you are eligible, please consider donating blood or blood components. The reasons are so compelling! First, the simple math—around 10 million units of red blood cells and 2 million units of platelets are transfused each year in the USA, and one patient is transfused in the USA about every two seconds. This means that it takes around 40,000 blood donors per day to fulfill the nation's need for blood products. The relatively short shelf-life of these living drugs also demands periodic replenishment of the entire national inventory, from weekly (such as platelets) to annually (plasma).

Second, donating blood is one of the most direct ways to help patients but the supply chain is shockingly fragile. Only about 38% of the adult population in the US is eligible to give blood at any one time. And the fraction of those who can give that do give is surprisingly small—all of the blood supply in the USA comes from around only 5% of the eligible population. Even within the cohort of donors, the demographics are skewed—almost half of all donated blood comes from donors over the age of 50.

In recent years, the U.S. allogeneic nondirected donor pool has shrunk precipitously, from 9.2 million donors in 2011 to 6.8 million donors in 2015. The decreased number of donors was partially offset by a similar decline of blood transfusions (30% decrease in last decade), the wide adoption of patient blood management (PBM), minimally invasive surgical technologies, and improved pharmaceutical agents that spare marrow. However, the aging donor pool is of great concern—sophisticated models have shown that the supply of blood will soon be outrun by the demand.

T.-L. Tsai · L. N. Chen · H. J. Alter · C. Marcucci (✉)
Department of Transfusion Medicine, Clinical Center, National Institutes of Health, Bethesda, MD, USA

S. Mohamed et al. (eds.), *Anesthesia Bridges*, https://doi.org/10.1007/978-3-032-08294-7_193

Despite of decades of research and promising work by the engineers, we still do not have FDA-approved, factory-manufactured replacements for human blood components, including red cells, platelets, plasma, and granulocytes. So, for the foreseeable future, we will continue to depend on the selfless donors that give not only the blood but their time, again and again, to fulfill patients' needs.

***Note from the Editors:** Lin Tsai and Len Chen are from Taiwan. To thank them for helping us with this chapter, we are including the Sanxiantai Dragon Bridge in Taitung, Taiwan (Fig. 193.1).

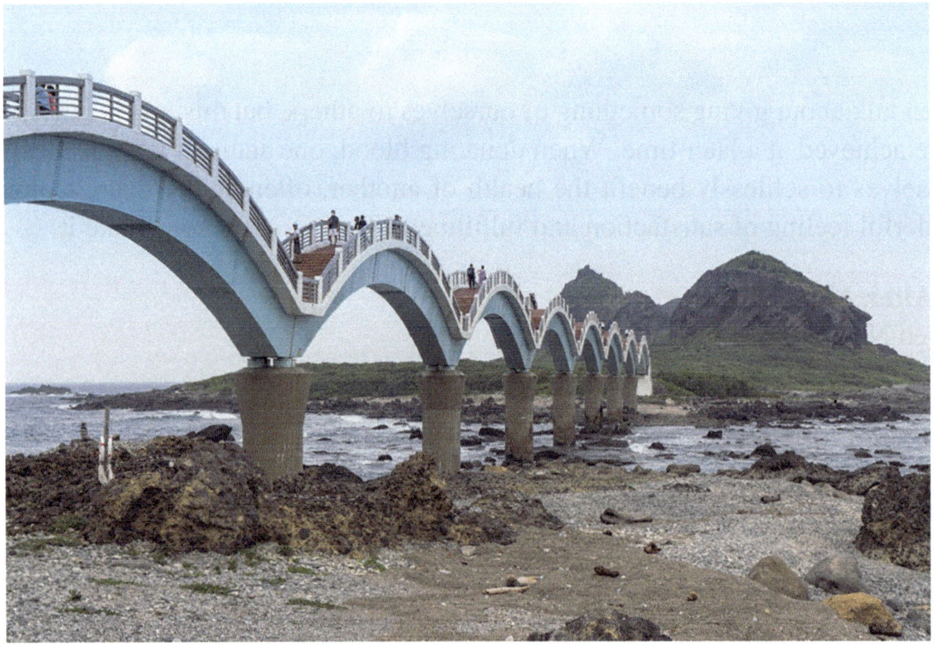

Fig. 193.1 The Sanxiantai Dragon Bridge in Taitung, Taiwan. We think it looks like a beautiful Asian sculpture. Photo: Imaged used under standard license from shutterstock.com

Donor Benefits

The benefits of blood donation for the donor are considerable. Blood donation decreases the body's stores of iron, which can have a direct therapeutic effect for donors with hereditary hemochromatosis. There has also been a suggestion that regular blood donation decreases cardiovascular risks, especially for donors aged 43–61 years, possibly due to changes in blood viscosity and improvement in free radical scavenging.

Blood donation may also slightly decrease the risk of liver, colon, throat, and lung cancer. And although blood centers do not advocate this as the prime motivation to give, the pre-donation and post-donation vital signs and infectious disease screenings are highly accurate and can provide valuable and regular health information to the donor. In addition to these physical benefits, blood donation may also help the mental state. Such a volunteering action has a positive effect on happiness and may reduce the risk of depression.

People donate blood for various reasons. Psychologists have looked into various generations of repeat donors to try to understand what is the biggest driver for these donors; who undertake the inconvenience of taking time off work to roll up their sleeves again and again. The reasons exceed simple altruism. The abstract idea of "saving life" can only motivate a potential donor so far. This vague and general altruistic urge may be sufficient for a potential donor to resolve to donate in the future but may not be enough to get over the hurdle of deciding to and taking action to donate. As Dr. Alter notes above, it's the self-identity and sense of immediacy as a "blood donor" that serves to get people in the door and eventually cements the behavior of a repeat donor.

Pandemic Donors

Many brand-new donors came forward during the early pandemic, willing to donate convalescent plasma "so other people will not suffer what I had gone through after getting infected by COVID-19." Unfortunately, only a small fraction of those donors continued to donate either whole blood or platelets once the demand of convalescent plasma waned. But the great people who stayed in our donor pool have proudly assumed their new role and identity as regular blood donors. No matter what drove the donor into a collection center the very first time, be it a pandemic, a significant life event or to help loved ones, we hope the experience of donating will be mentally fulfilling and emotionally satisfying to ensure a repeat donation in the future.

Lessons Learned

- A small percentage of U.S. adults donate the entirety of the blood supply. And the supply chain is in jeopardy as the donor population ages.
- There is no synthetic blood component on the development horizon. For the near future, the ability to transfuse blood will depend on donors rolling up their sleeves.
- Regular blood donation has several health benefits and can decrease cardiovascular and cancer risk.
- We believe, however, that the greatest benefits are emotional and psychological—an inimitable sense of belonging to a special cohort of citizens as well as increasing a sense of well-being.
- Year in and year out, anesthesiologists administer about half of all the blood transfused in the country, so it is the ultimate social action for our community. Like us, blood donors play a largely unseen but critical role in keeping the delivery of clinical care possible.

Authors

Lin Tsai is originally from Taiwan and lived for the last 14 years in Madison, Wisconsin and Irvine, California. He relocated to Bethesda, Maryland in 2021 to do a transfusion medicine fellowship at the National Institutes of Health. As part of his fellowship training, he also explored the possibilities of cellular engineering as an enormously impactful modality in the future of medicine. He then relocated to the Seattle area to start his professional career in transfusion medicine, including teaching, clinical work, and research. He and his wife are the proud parents of two boys.

Len Chen was born and raised in Taiwan, but has lived in Washington, DC since graduate school. He considers himself a Washingtonian. He thought he was leaving medicine for bench research when he embarked on immunogenetics research at Georgetown University. He is glad that being a physician in transfusion medicine at NIH allows him to enjoy both clinical practice and research. He and his wife Marcy have two sons, and they enjoy cooking, gardening, and camping as a family.

Harvey Alter has been designated a Distinguished NIH Investigator, only one of 23 NIH scientists to hold that honor. In his long career in clinical research, Dr. Alter has played a key role in the discovery of two hepatitis viruses, namely hepatitis B virus (HBV) and the non-A, non-B virus, later designated the hepatitis C virus (HCV). In long-term prospective studies, Harvey helped define the natural history of NANB/HCV infection and proved its frequent progression to chronic hepatitis and its evolution to cirrhosis and liver related mortality and documented the progressive decline of transfusion-associated hepatitis incidence from 33% in the 1960s to near zero in 1997. For his cumulative research accomplishments, he was elected to fellowship in the American Association of Physicians and received the prestigious Clinical Lasker Award and the Canada Gairdner International Award. Harvey was elected to both the National Academy of Sciences and National Academy of Medicine and achieved Master status in the ACP. In 2020, Dr. Alter was awarded the Nobel Prize in Physiology or Medicine.

Cathy Marcucci's first fellowship was in vascular, thoracic, and transplant anesthesiology. The nature of her clinical caseload resulted in a lifelong interest in transfusion medicine. She estimates that she has given at least 30,000 units of blood products in the OR and ICU and hopes that she eventually gains the understanding and depth of knowledge that her coauthors possess in this fascinating branch of medicine. On behalf of the *Anesthesia Bridges* editors, Cathy thanks Drs. Tsai, Chen, and Alter for their generosity to the anesthesia community and for taking an interest in this project.

A Career in International Anesthesiology

194

K. A. Kelly McQueen

Introduction

I always planned to have an international career. By "planned" I mean that I grew up with wanderer parents, was intrigued by the faraway and the unknown, and ultimately felt called to serve those less fortunate. But as I headed to medical school, I really had no idea on how to follow through on these ideas.

Early Career Initiatives

Early in medical school, with many thanks to the engagement of a local pediatric psychologist with an interest in health education for children, I learned about an emerging (it was the mid-1980s) health crisis, that I could contribute to at home and abroad—HIV/AIDS. This early interest in public health and his encouragement to join the effort to educate children about important health topics offered me the opportunity to begin writing children's books and to work locally to educate children. Together we published two children's books. *What's A Virus Anyway* explains the essentials of HIV/AIDS and *Let's Talk Trash* is a book on recycling for children. Both books were illustrated by Vermont children. This unexpected experience provided a steppingstone toward an eventual career in global public health.

Later, during my clinical rotations, one of my pediatric professors who knew of my international aspirations gave me the opportunity to complete a month of pediatrics in the Dominican Republic. I spent a month living in a community along the southern coast of the island with five nuns and a priest who ran the local hospital and a school. It was a pivotal month for me. I spent my days traveling up into the Compos with a cooler of vaccines to vaccinate young children whose families rarely left the hills, and teaching health education with the nuns at the school.

I witnessed for the first time a truly resource-constrained system and was further inspired to serve the underserved. When I returned to the University of Vermont to complete my medical studies, my profes-

K. A. K. McQueen (✉)
Department of Anesthesiology, University of Wisconsin School of Medicine, Madison, WI, USA
e-mail: kelly.mcqueen@wisc.edu

S. Mohamed et al. (eds.), *Anesthesia Bridges*, https://doi.org/10.1007/978-3-032-08294-7_194

sor asked, "Did you get that out of your system so you can focus on your medical education?" When I confessed that in fact it was not "out of my system," but rather affirmed as my aspiration, he recommended "Well, I hope you're prepared to dig toilets." Indeed, I could do that too.

Anesthesiology Rotations Abroad

Choosing anesthesiology as my specialty seemed to many to be a confounder for my international career. After all, global surgery was not yet on the radar—not for public health and certainly not for anesthesiologists in the USA. Naïve as I was, choosing anesthesiology didn't seem like a barrier to serving in low-income countries. From my perspective, my plan was intact, but the journey remained unknown, as it would be for some time.

Residency offered several opportunities to better understand underserved areas of anesthesiology, and when I had the opportunity to participate in a People-to-People overseas service trip focusing on obstetrics and OB anesthesia in my second year of residency, I jumped at the chance. Just a year after the dissolution of the USSR, in early spring, I accompanied a team of physicians to Russia, Latvia, and Lithuania to evaluate the OB/GYN and OB Anesthesia medical specialties. This experience contributed significantly to future choices of service and eventually additional education.

Early in the 1990s, the countries previously known as the Union of Socialist Soviet Republics (USSR) were reeling from a long history of integration and were struggling to create a future of independence. Most of these countries were ranked as middle-income countries at the time, but the syphoning of resources during communistic rule had created a dichotomy in health care. Eager to impress and compete with the United States (US) and Europe, the USSR had invested in high-end health care programs such as large-scale cardiac and transplant programs. These programs, while productive and valuable in treating the growing burden of chronic disease, meant that the health care system neglected other populations, namely women and children for basic health care—including OB care.

I experienced a difficult-to-describe and side-by-side, comparison—resources and operating rooms that looked like the USA, adjacent to poorly resourced birthing suites and operating rooms that, I would come to learn, looked like the lowest-resourced countries in Africa. And the outcomes matched the investment. The cardiac and transplant programs touted outcomes similar to the USA and Europe, whereas the maternal mortality and neonatal mortality rate were sky high, similar to Sub-Saharan Africa. I was shocked by the disparity and struggled to make sense of a way forward for these countries.

The People-to-People team of physicians met with Russian, Latvian, and Lithuanian physicians and discussed approaches to OB care in the USA. I presented lectures on modern OB anesthesia and shared reasons to move away from general anesthesia for Cesarean section and taught options for neuraxial anesthesia for both labor and delivery. At that time, women in these three countries were not offered analgesia for labor.

When I asked why—after all local anesthesia is cheap and epidural techniques were common the world over, they shared stories of paralyzing spinals and catastrophic epidural infections. The hospitals were reusing spinal and epidural needles (as unusual in the 1990s as it is now) and they shared how they had tried to compensate for poor sterility by injecting antibiotics into the epidural space along with the local anesthetic. Not surprising, the subsequent epidural scarring left women with lasting impairments and future fears of neuraxial anesthesia. I witnessed many preventable tragedies while in Russia, Latvia, and Lithuania, and these experiences shaped my commitment to a future of education and training in low and middle-income countries (LMICs).

***Note from the Editors:** Kelly McQueen did a global health rotation in Latvia during training that had an enormous impact on her future academic and public health career. In addition, *Anesthesia Bridges* author Ruth Jensen's parents were WW2 immigrants from Latvia and Ruth grew up speaking Latvian and going to Latvian school on the weekends. To honor this, we choose two stunning bridges in Riga—the Railway Bridge and the Shroud Bridge (Figs. 194.1 and 194.2).

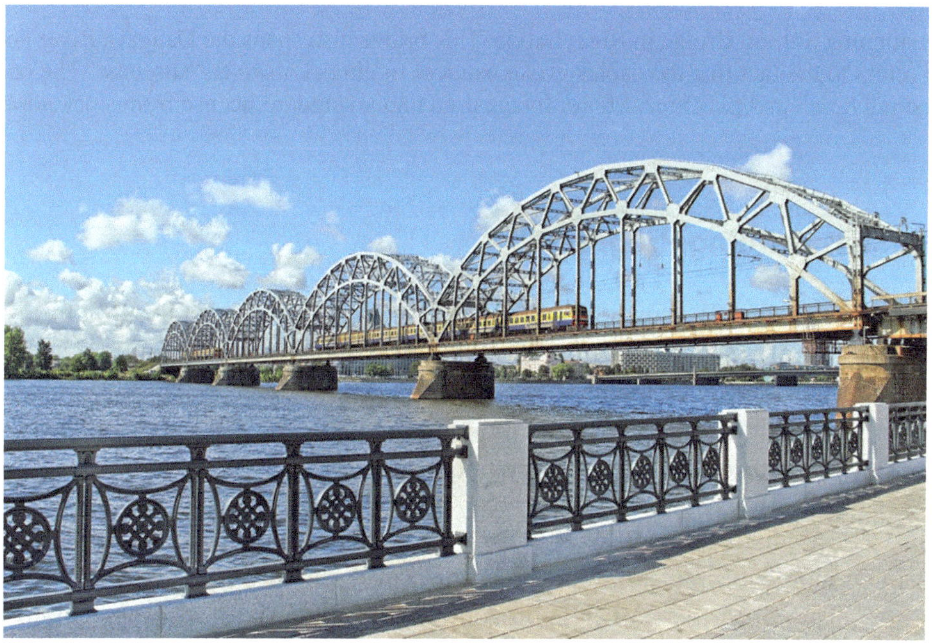

Fig. 194.1 The Railway Bridge in Riga, Latvia. The iron bridge spans the Daugava River and was inaugurated in 1914, replacing an older iron bridge that was built in 1871. The Railway Bridge was unfortunately shelled to the point of destruction in both WW1 and WW2 but was rebuilt after each war. Photo: Image used under standard license from stock.adobe.com

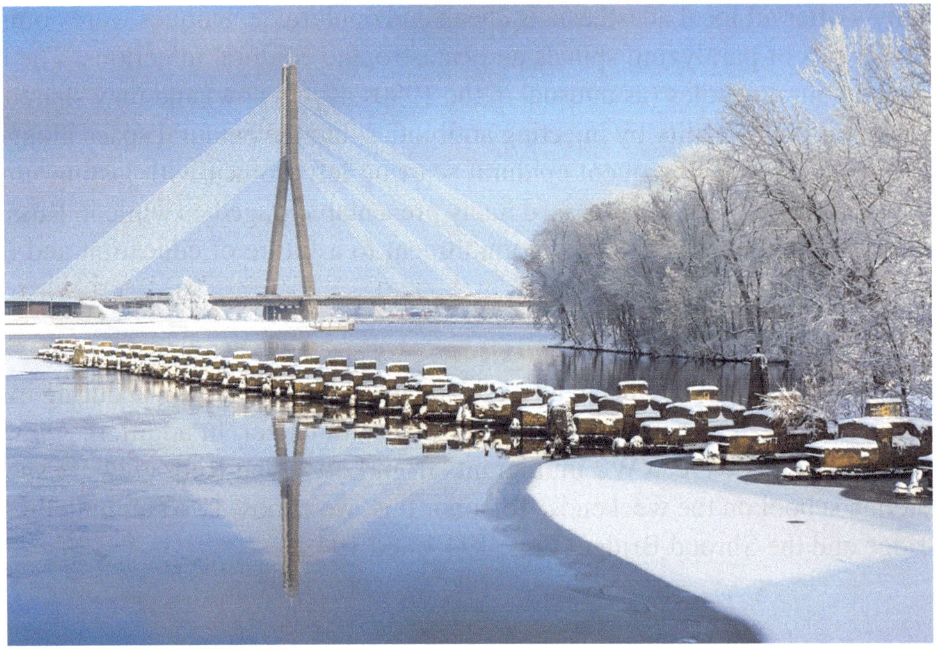

Fig. 194.2 The stunning Shroud Bridge in Riga, Latvia. This bridge also spans the Daugava River and was opened in 1981. The name refers to the fact that the cables evoke nautical riggings known as "shrouds." The park at the base of the bridge has a small beach and play area. Photo: Image used under standard license from stock.adobe.com

The ASA Overseas Training Program

Following my fellowship in OB anesthesia at the Mayo Clinic, I was finally able to test my plan and begin the journey to a career in global health. Shortly after completing my training, I had the opportunity to teach and provide service for the American Society of Anesthesiologists (ASA) Overseas Teaching Program (OTP) in Tanzania. This was a pivotal moment in my career where I came to value the essential role that the non-physician provider plays in low-income countries.

The ASA OTP was established by Dr. Nicholas Greene. Over many years, Dr. Greene convinced the ASA to invest in training non-physician providers in Sub-Saharan Africa where physician providers were critically low. This train-the-trainer approach taught hundreds of non-physicians to give a safe anesthetic, primarily spinal anesthesia and ketamine. Even today, this approach contributes significantly to meeting the global anesthesia crisis in low-income countries.

Combining Private Practice and Global Health

I joined a large private practice in Phoenix, Arizona following completion of my training. My contract with the group allowed for nine months of clinical service, and three months "off" at a reduced salary, and year-round benefits. This allowed me to work overseas three months a year, continuing my journey toward an international career. I worked for short-term surgical mission organizations— Operation Smile and Interplast, and for international organizations such as Medicine Sans Frontiers—Doctors without Borders. It was during a longer assignment with this organization in Sri Lanka that I realized that providing anesthesia for one patient at a time, would not lead to improving the circumstances I had experienced in Russia, Lithuania, and Latvia, nor those working for the ASA OTP in Sub-Saharan Africa. When I returned from Sri Lanka, I enrolled in a Master of Public Health (MPH) degree program at Harvard. My journey had changed course.

Global Health Research and Policy Development

I completed an MPH in 2002 with a focus in international health and wrote my thesis on the importance of surgery and anesthesia to international health. My professors acknowledged the role of anesthesia and surgery in disaster relief and humanitarian crises but questioned its value to public health. It would be another decade before the case for the latter would be made, but my journey continued. Leaving Harvard, I spent a year in Washington, DC as a fellow for the American Association for the Advancement of Science where I served in the Office of Naval Research, supporting infectious disease surveillance for the Navy field offices.

In 2003, I returned to private practice, working nine months a year, and now leveraging my relationships at Harvard to begin conducting anesthesia and surgery infrastructure research in low-income countries in Africa. Within five years, my research and publications intersected with the work of other internationally focused surgeons and anesthesiologists, and by 2008 we began gathering to discuss collaborating and advocating for the role of anesthesia and surgery in global public health. In the same time frame, I was asked to lead the ASA Committee on Global Humanitarian Outreach, and I founded a global workgroup which eventually became an Integrated Society of the International Society of Surgeons, the Alliance for Surgery and Anesthesia Presence (ASAP)—a multi-disciplinary society committed to advocacy for surgery and safe anesthesia in LMICs.

In 2015, this work culminated in three pivotal events—a World Bank Publication focusing on essential surgery and anesthesia, the Lancet Commission on Global Surgery, and the World Health Assembly Resolution supporting emergency and essential surgery and safe anesthesia. Anesthesia, surgery, and global public health had finally intersected, and my personal journey was established, but not complete. In 2012, I was recruited away from private practice to Vanderbilt University Medical Center to direct the Department of Anesthesiology Global Health and Development. In this role, the research I started in 2003 became central to my academic work, and my career as a global anesthesiologist was official.

Lessons Learned

- Follow your passions and work hard to make them a reality.
- Be creative in pursuit of what matters most to you.
- Take the risks necessary to move ahead.

Do the work that's in front of you because it all matters. When I could help only one patient at a time, that's what I did. Later I was in a position to develop policy and design programs, and this larger platform has been enormously rewarding. But it doesn't make the individual care I gave any less meaningful.

Author

Kelly McQueen spent the first 23 years of her career as an anesthesiologist and public health expert serving providers and patients in low-income countries through her commitment to building infrastructure and providing education and training. She has worked clinically both in private practice and in academic departments and has led global programs and global initiatives throughout her career. She did not always aspire to lead a department of anesthesiology, but when the University of Wisconsin gave her the opportunity to apply her global leadership skills as the chair of the oldest academic department in the country, it was a career-changing decision for which she is grateful. Kelly lives in Madison, Wisconsin with her two dogs.

From North Philadelphia to East Africa: My Life and Career Journey

195

Rodger E. Barnette

Introduction

Several years back, we got a message from **Rodger Barnette** apologizing for a delayed email. It went something along the lines of, "*So sorry for the extra time to respond, internet has been very slow in East Africa lately.*" This was intriguing news, since Rodger had last corresponded from Philadelphia where he was chairing the Department of Anesthesiology at Temple. We knew we had to hear more about this, and we only had to ask one question of Rodger to get the fascinating story. Here it is: Why would a tenured professor of anesthesiology and medicine, who for 12 years had been chairman of an academic anesthesiology department, leave those positions to teach and practice anesthesiology and ICU medicine in rural East Africa?

A Story of Africa Brought Us Together

My wife and I share a long-standing interest in medical missions. That was the reason we met; I was the student who had spent three months at a hospital in Nyankunde, Zaire during the fourth year of medical school, and my wife Ginny was the ER nurse who wanted to hear the story.

Early in our marriage we considered full-time overseas work, but a number of circumstances prevented that from happening. We did intermittently travel to remote areas of the world to serve short-term for anywhere from a few weeks to a few months, and we believed that would be the extent of our involvement. Then in 2008 my wife accepted a position at Serge Global, Inc., a non-denominational mission agency, as a recruiter for teachers, pastors, and medical personnel willing to work in East Africa. While in that role she met Mark and Sue Newton, who were based in Kijabe, Kenya.

R. E. Barnette (Retired) (✉)
AIC Kijabe Hospital, Kijabe, Kenya

S. Mohamed et al. (eds.), *Anesthesia Bridges*, https://doi.org/10.1007/978-3-032-08294-7_195

Committing to Kijabe

In the fall of 2012, we volunteered for a month at Kijabe hospital. And in January of 2013 we followed up that visit with a video call to Mark and Sue Newton. Mark at the time was the only anesthesiologist at Kijabe hospital, and he challenged us to consider returning to Kijabe on a full-time basis. He said, "You two love Africa and love the people—and Rodger, you're a seasoned academician so you know how to teach, and you're not frightened by old technology or old medications." In the weeks after that call Ginny and I spent hours praying and discussing Mark's invitation. We talked it over with many friends and family members and ultimately decided to accept the challenge and move to East Africa.

My wife and I are Christians; we believe Jesus is the Son of God. That he suffered and died on a Roman cross for our sins, was buried, and rose from the dead. Christianity states it is not possible to earn forgiveness by doing good works. Instead, through faith, we believe and accept Jesus as our Savior and Lord, and we are made right in relationship to God because of Christ's sacrifice. Any good works come after we are believers—they are a result of our relationship with God, not the cause. These good works are "faith working through love" (Galatians 5:6). We could never serve and love others without a relationship with Jesus, because faith in the work of Christ provides the foundation and motivation for our love and service.

We applied to Serge and went through the process of being evaluated and accepted into that organization. This provided us with an incredible group of people who were not only supportive of the work we were preparing to engage in at Kijabe but prayed for us and helped financially, as we received no salary from Kijabe hospital. We lived in a small apartment that was about a two-minute walk from the hospital.

The Kijabe Care Model

We left the USA in July of 2015 having made a commitment to spend 5 years in rural East Africa, teaching and practicing at Kijabe hospital. For a significant portion of that time, I was the only anesthesiologist and was responsible for 8–9 operating rooms and one procedure room. The model in many ways was like a small ICU in the USA. There was a KRNA (Kenyan Registered Nurse Anesthetist) and one or two students in each room. Mark and/or I were the consultants available to teach, help, and intervene as the need arose. There were no billing or government regulations that constrained our practice structure.

Mark Newton had started the first nurse anesthetist school in East Africa, and one of my major responsibilities was to teach and evaluate the NA students. Though nurse anesthetists filled a huge need, it was apparent that physician anesthesiologists were desperately needed. And so, Mark and I, with Drs. Liz Drum, Greg Sund, Matt Kynes, Jeff Lane, and a number of other anesthesiologists, began the process of creating an anesthesiology residency at Kijabe hospital under the authority and guidance of the leadership of the Pan African Academy of Christian Surgeons (PAACS).

Practicing medicine in a low- or middle income-country has many challenges. Resources are often limited or absent. UpToDate is a great resource, and I used it often, but what I missed most was being able to easily consult with colleagues from a variety of specialties. This lack of availability of colleagues forced a greater sense of collaborative dependence among the Kijabe physicians. I met and practiced with physicians from Australia, the UK, the USA, Kenya, Uganda, Tanzania, and other areas of the world. I did not meet any who were there for fame, glory, academic advancement, or materialistic reasons. Holistic patient care was a shared focus, as was training and mentoring our trainees.

***Note from the Editors:** The Kilifi Bridge in Kenya is an example of the modern infrastructure in the more developed areas of the country (Figs. 195.1 and 195.2).

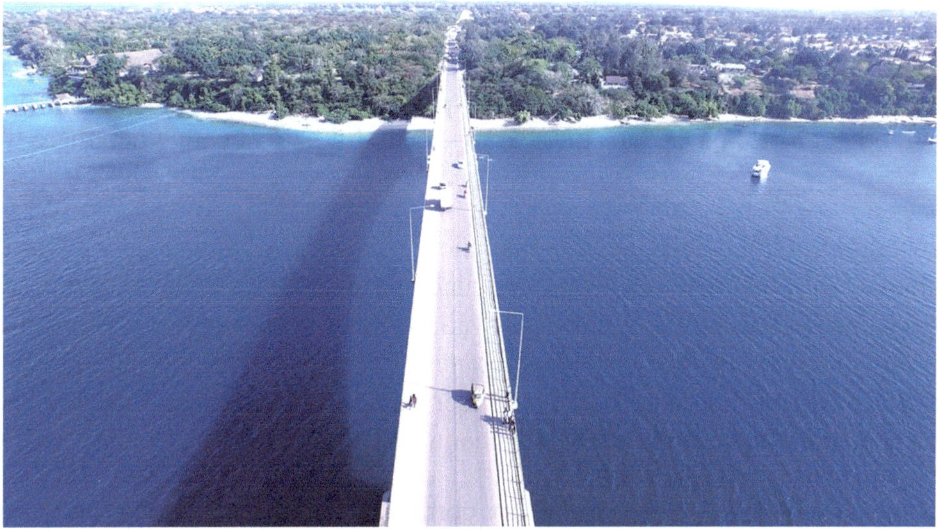

Fig. 195.1 The Kilifi Bridge is the longest bridge in Kenya. It was completed in 1991. Kenya must be very beautiful—look at the sand and blue water. Photo: Image use purchased from iStock.com

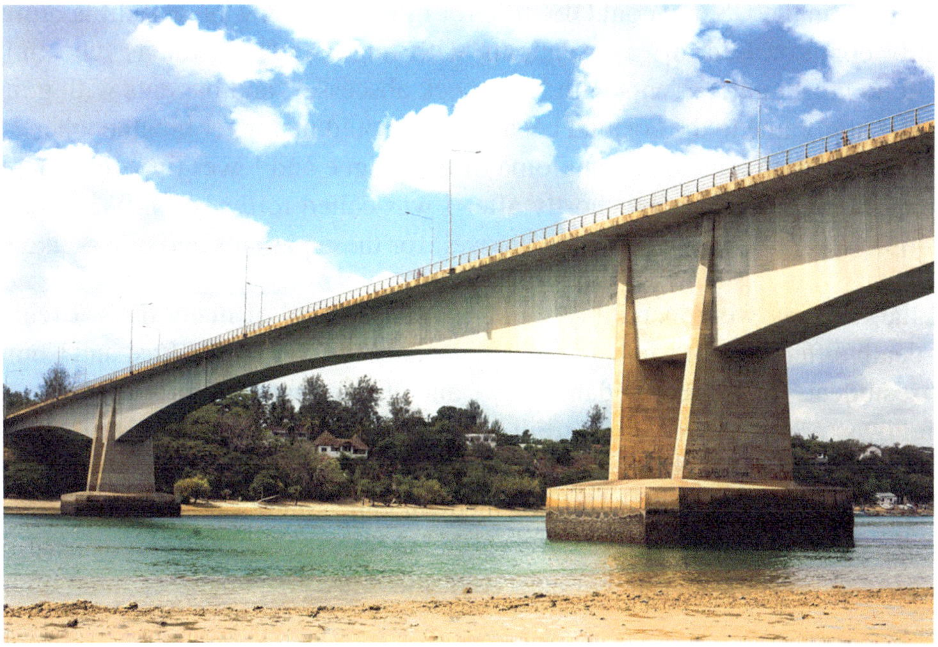

Fig. 195.2 The Kilifi Bridge. The superstructure is a prestressed continuous box girder. The bridge is narrow compared to bridges in the USA and has only two lanes. Photo: Image used under standard license from stock.adobe.com

Teaching, Learning, and Providing Care

I learned a huge amount during the five years we lived in rural East Africa; I discovered there was value to having trained with older technologies, older medications, and older ACLS algorithms, because many of the newer medical discoveries were not available in that part of the world. I found I could not only do quite well with just a history and physical exam—but as I learned decades ago—the history and physical were absolutely paramount. It helped that I had 30+ years of clinical experience and also held board-certification in critical care medicine and internal medicine. But many times, it was a process of problem-solving with other on-site physicians that led to successful patient care when there was no obvious path forward.

If a surgical procedure could be done under spinal anesthesia—then that was how it was done. We used 0.5% bupivacaine for all spinals. An old ultrasound machine allowed for upper extremity nerve blocks—again 0.5% bupivacaine was used. Halothane was available to us via a supplier in India—so we used that agent or isoflurane (though in the last year sevoflurane became available). For anesthesia machines, we primarily used older Drager Narkomed 2B or Drager Fabius GS machines that had been donated or purchased for a very modest price after they had been rehabbed.

Blood bank resources were also very rudimentary compared to the US. We had no fractionated blood products at all—only whole blood. The hospital blood bank was not part of a national or regional blood bank system; we were on our own. If we needed blood, we would ask families to donate and we would often put out messages for urgent needs on a KJ hospital staff WhatsApp group.

I have many stories of caring successfully for unstable patients with serious diseases; and sadly, patients I could have cared for in the US, but could do little for in Kenya. I saw an incredible number of patients with significantly compromised airways. Patients with huge ameloblastomas who only sought care when they could no longer eat, patients with large neck abscesses, and patients with goiters the size of melons, many of whom came to the hospital because they could no longer breathe when lying flat. I will never forget the patient with a large hemangioma of the tongue and lower lip who progressed to a cannot-ventilate–cannot-intubate situation shortly after I was called to the room. With the help of physicians from multiple specialties, I was able to care well for these patients and others like them.

The work and the teaching were incredibly satisfying. At the end of many days, I realized that I had made a life-or-death difference for a patient. Teaching eager residents from East and Central Africa, and nurse anesthetist students from South Sudan, Kenya, and other countries was a privilege. Anesthesiology residents and fellows (primarily from Vanderbilt University and Temple University) came out to Kijabe on 1-month overseas rotations. For the majority of those U.S. trainees, practicing at Kijabe was a dramatic taste of engaging in a very basic form of medical care. Many said it felt like traveling decades back in time to an era of medicine they had read about but never expected to experience. It was exciting to work with them and demonstrate how much could be done for patients in such a resource-limited environment.

Africa

In the midst of all of this, there was time to visit with and get to know Kenyans, Tanzanians, and folks from South Sudan and Somaliland. We now count many from that part of the world as dear friends. And, of course, we took time to travel to game parks, the elephant orphanage in Nairobi, rhino conservatories, beautiful national parks, the Indian Ocean coast, and Zanzibar. East Africa is an incredibly rich and beautiful part of the world.

My wife and I are now back in the US, our full-time commitment completed. But we are staying involved. Our plan became spending half of each year in East Africa—and continuing to teach and care for patients in Kijabe before "retiring" to Tennesee. Our current schedule is to alternate throughout the year three months in the USA with 3 months in Kenya. Until very recently, I still practiced part-time at Temple University in Philadelphia during our time in the US.

Lessons Learned

- Don't be afraid to move out in faith when presented with a new challenge.
- In spite of the impressive technology available to practicing physicians, a good history and a careful and complete physical exam are key to excellent patient care.
- By practicing medicine in low- and middle-income countries (short-term or long-term), you will gain more than you give. You will also find that working with limited resources *expands* your knowledge and skills.
- A great deal of good patient care can be provided in a setting of limited resources.
- As an interesting aside, many Kenyans speak English, which is the official language, but not everyone speaks it. Almost everyone speaks Swahili, and everyone speaks their tribal language. I spent three months in Swahili language study in 2015, with six weeks in Zanzibar and six weeks in Kenya, and then had a weekly tutor for several years. I get by using Swahili with patients.

Author

Rodger Barnette spent a significant portion of his career at Temple University in anesthesiology, critical care medicine, education, and a variety of leadership roles. He and his wife Ginny, moved to rural East Africa in 2015 where for 5 years they worked at a faith-based hospital. Rodger taught and practiced anesthesiology and ICU medicine and was also actively involved in starting an anesthesiology residency while Ginny worked in infection control. They were both involved in mentoring. After alternating three months in Africa with three months in the USA, Rodger retired from Temple, and they now reside just south of Nashville when they are in the States. They have an adult son and daughter and two lovely granddaughters.

Everybody's Journey Is Different

196

Michael Lin, Lynn Knox, and Catherine Marcucci

Contributor:

Catherine Marcucci, MD

Introduction

In this chapter, **Lynn Knox** was interviewed by **Michael Lin**, who was a senior medical student at the time.

Interview

Michael Lin: Hi Dr. Knox, thank you for agreeing to meet with me today. I would like to start off the interview with a brief introduction about your anesthesia background.

Lynn Knox: Of course, Michael, I am currently the vice chair for education at UTMB and have recently stepped down from my position as the anesthesiology residency program director for the past 20 years. However, I continue to be very much involved with resident education. As far as my anesthesia background, I actually came through a very different pathway than most, starting with nursing school. I had a neighbor, who was an OR nurse and who motivated me to pursue a career in nurse anesthesia. I completed nursing school in Tennessee.

M. Lin
University of Texas Medical Branch School of Medicine, The University of Texas Medical Branch at Galveston, Galveston, TX, USA

L. Knox
Department of Anesthesiology, The University of Texas Medical Branch, Galveston, TX, USA

C. Marcucci (✉)
Department of Transfusion Medicine, Clinical Center, National Institutes of Health, Bethesda, MD, USA

S. Mohamed et al. (eds.), *Anesthesia Bridges*, https://doi.org/10.1007/978-3-032-08294-7_196

However, in order to get into a CRNA (nurse anesthesia) program, I required ICU experience. I was able to obtain an ICU position at Baptist Hospital in Nashville. I thought I would be there for at least a year before I could apply for anesthesia school. As things often happen, luck intervenes. I ran into a lot of student nurse anesthetists on the IV start team and discovered an unexpected opening for anesthesia school. At the time, training for nurse anesthesia was completed through a certificate program. These days, nurse anesthetists get their master's, some even their doctorates in nursing practice.

Career Transition

Michael: Can you describe your career transition?

Lynn: I had two years of training as a nurse anesthetist, worked for some time in Nashville and ended up moving to Texas. In Dallas, I was the chief nurse anesthetist at Baylor and became invested in advancing my education and clinical practice. I thought about pursuing a nursing master program but ultimately decided to apply to medical school.

By the time I got around to attending Southwestern medical school in Dallas, I was about 35 years old. Yes, you can still go to medical school at age 35, because it is really never too late. It worked out great for me. I matched to UTMB for my anesthesia residency. I was really happy to match at UTMB. I found I liked the academic atmosphere and stayed on as faculty. So that is how I've been faculty here at UTMB since 1998, seeing a lot of changes and growth, really enjoying it, and never regretting it.

Michael: Did your prior nursing background compliment your anesthesia residency training?

Lynn: Yes, having given anesthesia as a nurse made my residency easier when I started learning the basics in the first years. I was very quickly able to go into more complex cases, and it was great. Medical school was a humbling experience because I found out about how much I really didn't know. Likewise, in anesthesia residency, I discovered that there is always something new to learn, despite giving anesthesia for 10 years as a nurse anesthetist.

Challenges and Lessons Learned

Michael: What are some of the most difficult challenges that you have faced throughout the years? What did you learn from these experiences?

Lynn: One big challenge was just realizing that I could become an anesthesiologist, then working towards that goal. Prior to medical school, I took a lot of premed courses at night and worked full-time as a nurse anesthetist during the day. All of which I think was good preparation for medical school, where I had to study and work. When I moved on to residency, I was used to organizing my studies around a full-time job. I think that made the transition much easier. Over the years, I have learned that this transition to residency from being a full-time student can be challenging for many residents. Everything changes. Not only are you studying, but you are also an employee and part of the staff with clinical duties and patient responsibilities.

Michael: With the added responsibilities, what is your secret to achieving a work-life balance?

Lynn: Right, work-life balance is difficult. Throughout the years, there have been a lot of production pressures within anesthesiology and the ORs. In some cases, it seems autonomy is being taken away from physicians by administrators. I believe this is where some of the pressures that cause burnout come from. I think being aware of this and remembering why you are there in the operating room—what got you started into anesthesia and taking care of patients in the first place—can help a lot. Sometimes, you feel like a cog in a wheel, and you must remind yourself of these things. Using your free time for something you really enjoy, spending time with family and friends, having these things to look forward to—I think really helps as well.

Michael: What are some of your most important qualities or attributes that have made you successful?

Lynn: I think part of that is perseverance. It is a long road when you have already been working, and have to give up salary, and have eight years ahead of you. It is a big decision. Once I did it, I never looked back, I just went forward. For the younger people that I get to mentor, I often remind them to have a goal. Every day can seem long. However, at the end of the year, you are like, "oh my goodness, I'm already going onto my next thing." Senior resident anesthesiologists come and tell me they can hardly believe they are done. Personally, perseverance to me means finishing what I started.

Flexibility is also very important. I have worked with a lot of different surgeons, colleagues, and nurses. I try to be receptive to all these different ways of doing things, even though I may have done it in a different way before I came to UTMB. I believe this helped me to be successful as a resident and continues to be key. It's just good to be flexible and realize you can do things safely, but without rigid adherence to only one solution, if you are to have an armamentarium to deal with unexpected clinical challenges. And indeed, flexibility allows constant improvement and is key to developing a successful resident education program as well.

Our Specialty

Michael: How has anesthesiology changed throughout the years? What are your thoughts on the future of anesthesiology?

Lynn: I think the anesthesia care over the years has become much more complex, allowing surgeons to do increasingly complex cases. When I started as a nurse anesthetist, it was not rare to hear that patients would never make it through surgery, and that they were inoperable. Now, these high acuity patients come into surgery every day. There used to be a sort of cut-off age to get a CABG. Now, our patients are candidates for CABG, PCTA, and stents into their 90s. Patients used to be admitted to the hospital for a week for a cholecystectomy; this is often a same-day surgery now.

As a result, the expectations of perioperative anesthesia care are also much higher from patients and surgeons. They want the patient to be street-ready. Our drugs and technology have improved over the years. Anesthesiology is a very challenging specialty now, but I believe it allows miraculous things to happen in the whole surgical world.

Michael: How do you make the tough and difficult decisions? How do you cope with failure and celebrate success?

Lynn: Failure is the hardest. A failure for us could mean a patient was harmed. I think what really becomes important for coping is your environment, colleagues, and having a support system at work and at home. There could be a lot of guilt involved with any kind of failure having to do with a patient. It is tough. You become very confident over the years that you can handle anything. When you finally find the one airway you actually can't intubate or have a poor patient outcome, it is very tough. I think one important thing is having the humility to ask for help. That's why it is important to find a place you fit in well and can depend on the support system of your colleagues. You do have help, and you feel like you can ask for it. It is not taking away from you; it is just adding to good patient care.

Michael: What are some life lessons that you would like to pass onto the next generation of aspiring anesthesiologists?

Lynn: It comes back to the golden rule. You want to treat others as you want to be treated. This is so true to becoming a success. When you get out of a residency program, you are able to give anesthesia. However, whether you are successful within your group depends a lot on your communication skills, interpersonal skills, really how well you are a supportive person and patient advocate. As a successful physician, you want to be seen as that person who people can go to with a problem and get help without feeling like a failure.

As far as a clinical pearl that never changes, remember the old "KISS" principle: "Keep it simple, stupid." Don't get your anesthesia technique so complicated that it gets too confusing. I still believe in that. The simplest thing I tell residents from day one is you can always give more of any anesthetic, any medication, but you can't always take it back, so *titrate everything*—because every single patient is different.

Michael: Thank you so much, Dr. Knox, for your time and for sharing your life experience with all of us. In closing, do you have any last words?

Lynn: Anesthesiology has been a really fulfilling career for me. Every day is different. The complexity and perioperative responsibilities of the specialty continue to grow, so I am optimistic that physician led anesthesiology is going to be a rewarding field for a long time.

Lessons Learned

- To be successful, you must have perseverance. It's a long road to get through school and training—*don't look back* and keep your goals in mind.
- Success depends a lot on your communication skills, interpersonal skills, and how well you can be a supportive person and patient advocate.

Authors

Michael Lin is a first-generation American who completed his undergraduate degree in human nutrition and foods at the University of Houston and received his medical school training at UTMB Galveston. He enjoys cruises and tennis. He is currently working towards improving his proficiency and hand-eye coordination in table tennis.

Lynn Knox credits her path as a "non-traditional" student with igniting an interest in adult education and life-long learning. After medical school at UT Southwestern, she completed an anesthesiology residency at UTMB, Galveston and never left. Her greatest privilege has been shepherding over 400 residents through the rigors of anesthesiology training. She and her husband Steve are avid travelers, having visited all seven continents.

Cathy Marcucci is a senior academic anesthesiologist and inveterate anesthesiology educator. She was also a non-traditional medical student, starting at Temple Med at the age of 30.

I Wish I Had Figured Out a Better Post-Call Routine

197

F. Jacob Seagull and Catherine Marcucci

Introduction

Life is busy and complicated for all of us, nobody what career stage we are in. And when you add in working all night in high-pressure, high-stakes situations, you have a recipe for fatigue and inefficiency to follow.

From Cathy

To be honest, I never really solved the post-call routine problem. You might think that I would have because I certainly did my share of in-house calls through the years. My first big mistake was that I didn't really have much of a *pre-call* routine. My second mistake was to wait to see how tired I would be. My third mistake was to consider the post-call day as a wide-open day with limitless potential, like a weekend or vacation day.

Of course, the three big decisions for any post-call person are deciding when and how much to sleep, when and how much to exercise, and how much to advance the household agenda (even if the household has only one person). If I had it to do over again, I would standardize everything, and at a very, very simple level. And I do mean everything—what time I left the hospital, what I ate, what my family ate. I would make exceptions only for big, important stuff like urgent medical appointments or car repairs or the really big programs at school or if the kids had other pressing needs, which wouldn't include running to Michael's for poster board[1].

[1] *Who am I kidding? Of course, it would have included running to Michael's for poster board! But maybe I could have limited that to once a month.*

F. J. Seagull
Center for Bioethics and Social Science in Medicine, University of Michigan Medical School, Ann Arbor, MI, USA

C. Marcucci (✉)
Department of Transfusion Medicine, Clinical Center, National Institutes of Health, Bethesda, MD, USA

S. Mohamed et al. (eds.), *Anesthesia Bridges*, https://doi.org/10.1007/978-3-032-08294-7_197

Regrets

When I took in-house call, my call nights were almost always preceded by a full day in the OR and frequently almost sleepless, so I am not sure why I just didn't come to expect it. I am a true morning person, so it is difficult for me to sleep during the day, when I want to be up. I would head home and try to get to sleep at ten in the morning—it rarely happened; I was always too jazzed up. And the sleep was supposed to be so that I could do a full workout later in the day—and that rarely happened either. I usually didn't manage to exercise at all post-call. I also tried to do extra cooking, cleaning, and childcare (as if it was a weekend day that I wasn't working), which in hindsight was ridiculous. It was nuts to try to make gains in the household program when what I should have done was just minimized and corrected the sleep deficits.

Looking back, all that attempted overachieving on post-call days was so not worth it. I remember one evening I was seriously exhausted after a tough night and it was the first year we had decided to put up a really big Christmas tree for the kids. My great-but-Jewish husband was doing his best trying to get a tree into a stand—and that tree was 10 feet tall if it was an inch. I was so tired and so strung out that I just couldn't even tell him how to do it. By the time we abandoned the tree for the night—on its side on the floor in the dining room—the kids were crying, I was crying, and Neil was wondering if we should maybe just cancel Christmas altogether that year.

Routines

In hindsight, the first thing I would do is figure out a better pre-call routine. In this day and age, you will often be off during the day before taking an overnight call. If you have this advantage, I advise that you try to sleep a bit later, even if that means sleeping in the bedroom in the basement. Hopefully, your partner will not mind getting the household going. And the other important pre-call thing I would do is to bring more fruit and healthy snacks with me to call—I ate way too much pizza and other delivery food on call. Sleep-deprived people generally do eat more junk.

The second thing I would do is figure out a non-sleep wind-down once I got home from the hospital. For me, it would be a warm, not hot, shower and a half-hour of yoga. I'd eat a calorie-dense protein meal—maybe some complex carbohydrates like oatmeal but NO doughnuts. Or a Western omelet might do the trick, as well. Then, I'd maybe rest a bit and watch the morning gardening or cooking shows for an hour. I'd stay up if I could manage until my husband got home or just after dinner, whichever was later. It was a mistake for me to spend the morning trying to sleep, then getting to sleep at noon and getting up at dinnertime. That meant a second almost sleepless night because it was too soon to go back to sleep 4 hours later. But delaying sleep would mean no driving or cooking. So, after unwinding, then maybe some light household stuff. And I do mean light. A couple of loads of laundry or straighten the kids' rooms or change the water in the goldfish bowl or do some online banking. And then the rest of the day, dare I say it, something relaxing or fun.

Anesthesia practice is getting busier and busier—it's not the easiest way to make a living. If you've had a double dose or overnight dose of it, there is nothing wrong with a bit of mitigation. But I made that mistake over and over again. I had the means to have the kids picked up from daycare on post-call days and to order food, but I rarely did. I had this idea that I had to be the one to be in the pickup lane at school because I hadn't seen them the night before. A total miscalculation.

When the kids were older, they didn't care that they hadn't seen me—if you don't believe this, wait and see. When they were younger, I should have created a fun routine when the babysitter brought them home from daycare or school, such as everybody was going to have dinner in their pajamas before Mom went to bed. Dinner would have been something really, really simple and sort of picnic-y and fun. But the same thing or the same couple of things. So, whoever went to the grocery store the previous weekend would automatically know to get the sliced turkey breast and pimento cream cheese for the turkey roll-ups, the baby carrots, corn chips and ice cream, or the eggs and English muffins for breakfast-for-dinner.

Although the pressures to be productive can be strong, I would also try not to do any "academic" work on post-call days unless I had had a decent amount of sleep. Trying to deal with your research and data on no sleep can make you resent it a little bit, even if you otherwise are engaged and passionate about your work. Who needs that extra stress? And you're not going to be that efficient or productive anyway.

***Note from the Editors:** Speaking of rest, Korean traffic designers and architects often build futuristic-looking rest stop bridges over roads and highways to expand services for travelers but minimize the construction footprint and land use. Larger rest stops sometimes include capsule hotels for long-distance travelers (Fig. 197.1).

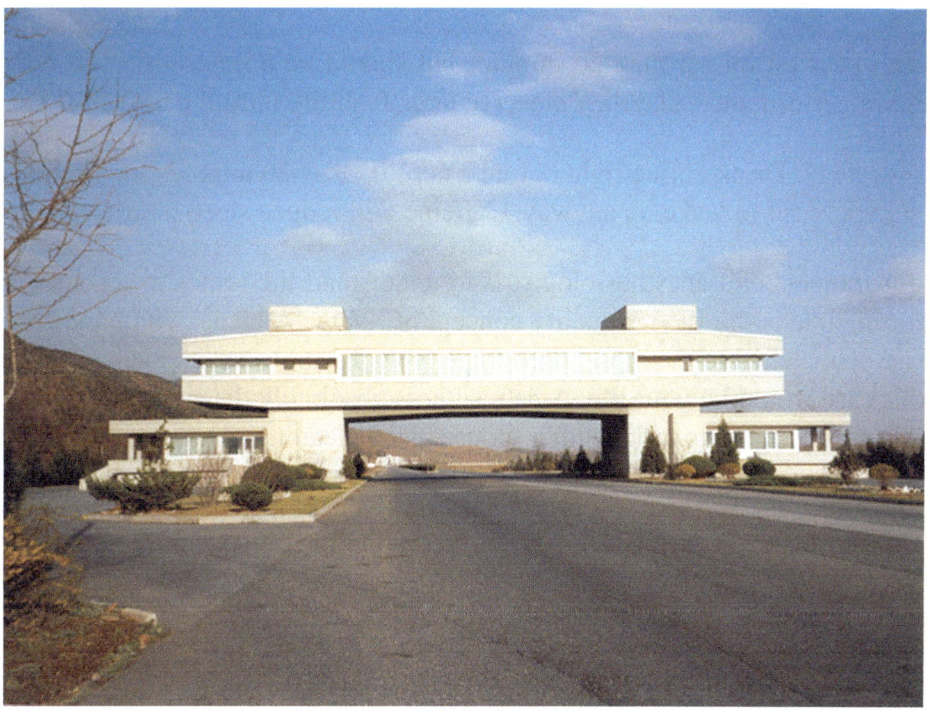

Fig. 197.1 A modern-looking highway rest stop in Korea. The central windows belong to the capsule hotel. Photo: Image purchased under standard license from iStock.com

From Jake

A lot of what Cathy arrived at intuitively is backed up by science and human studies principles, with several caveats. I agree that the most important thing is to understand the issues that go with sleep deprivation. Whole books have been written on the subject, of course. And I would also recommend that every anesthesiologist review the following papers. These were written specifically about people training in anesthesia, which makes them especially informative and important:

- Wong et al. [3]

- Williams et al. [4]

If you are just too busy (or too tired!) to read those papers, here are some common-sense sleep tips that might be helpful:

- Most sleep and human factors experts would not agree with trying to go completely without sleep until the next night. The key is "short napping" (see below).

- You <u>should</u> act like a baby: Develop routines to get yourself to bed.

- There are gateways to sleep, so don't miss your sleep window. And honor those sleep gateways. These are the parts of the circadian rhythm when you can sleep easily. So, when you start feeling sleepy, sleep for 20 minutes.

- Your body is light sensitive, so manage light to help shift circadian rhythms. Use bright/blue light when working and when you first get off call, then a dark room to sleep.

- Micro naps can be a bit longer than 20 minutes but should be no more than 60 minutes. They are known to restore performance, and they preserve mental ability until the next full sleep opportunity.

- One napping strategy: Drink coffee right before a nap! It takes 20 minutes for the caffeine to kick in, which is when you want to wake up anyway. Caffeine will reduce sleep inertia, which is good.

The next task for the post-call anesthesiologist is to understand the issues of resource allocation. The most important principle is the LEAN/quality concept of "Value Added," which indicates that the type of activity should be matched to the most appropriate type of worker to "add value" to the overall product, which in this case would be your life. A babysitter is absolutely the right resource to deploy for an exhausted anesthesiologist. Swap tasks with a spouse, get a cleaning service, and order in.

Remember, you yourself are a scarce resource during residency. *Place a large value on your time*. A bit of good time with "rested you" is better than a lot of crappy time with grumpy, exhausted you, for both socializing and for getting stuff done. Cooking, cleaning, and household stuff is not only extending your fatigue, it is also being done by an exhausted person. Not a great way to add value.

Closely related is the principle of productivity. An exhausted you is an inefficient you—a dull axe. And a dull axe is more dangerous than a sharp one. I also agree with Cathy's advice about taking a day off the practice of anesthesiology if possible post-call. Taking a mental break will result in higher productivity when work resumes.

The topic of work-life balance has become a giant field of research, and the research clearly shows that having a balance leads to more productivity as well as less burnout, less depression, and less anxiety. Burnout enormously affects the ability to perform as a physician, get through residency, and overall health. There are countless studies showing stress-health-burnout is detrimental, and that balance, including breaks and time off, results in higher productivity. It is always much, much better to prevent burnout than to try to heal, remediate, or resolve it.

And, finally, I am a strong advocate for sensible call schedules optimized with the help of software. The complicated process of satisfying every individual's special requests, ideal schedules, and work hour constraints is time-consuming and difficult for people to calculate, while relatively trivial computationally for a software program. Software can save time and headaches. If I may be permitted, here is a paper on the topic [5].

Lessons Learned

- Take the time to figure out your post-call routine, but first address your pre-call routine! Try to go into call as rested as possible, not over-exercised, and stocked up with healthy food.

- Cathy was always a full-time working Mom when her kids were at home and Neil always worked full-time, as well. If your partner works full-time maintaining the home front, you have the flexibility of tweaking the call routines a bit. But we still advise making the routines. You want to have the healthy habits become as automatic as possible.

- Research exists that shows that high quality sleep time is positively correlated with eating cereal/pasta and negatively correlated with eating meat. Sleep quality seems to be negatively correlated with eating beans and positively with eating oil. So, for better sleep, eat pasta Bolognese with olive oil but no meat.

- Please, please take our advice and do not try to do too much. It's not worth it, and you will look back, wonder why you tried to do it, and even regret it.

Further Readings

1. Haghighatdoost F, Karimi G, Esmaillzadeh A, Azadbakht L. Sleep deprivation is associated with lower diet quality indices and higher rate of general and central obesity among young female students in Iran. Nutrition. 2012;28(11–12):1146–50.
2. Mota MC, De-Souza DA, Rossato LT, Silva CM, Araújo MBJ, Tufik S, de Mello MT, Crispim CA. Dietary patterns, metabolic markers and subjective sleep measures in resident physicians. Chronobiol Int. 2013;30(8):1032–41.
3. Wong LR, Flynn-Evans E, Ruskin KJ. Fatigue Risk Management: the impact of anesthesiology residents' work schedules on job performance and a review of potential countermeasures. Anesth Analg. 2018;126(4).1340–8.
4. Williams GW, Shankar B, Klier EM, Chuang AZ, El Marjiya-Villarreal S, Nwokolo OO, Sharma A, Sereno AB. Sensorimotor and executive function slowing in anesthesiology residents after overnight shifts. J Clin Anesth. 2017;40:110–6.
5. Ballard TN, Grenda TR, Cohn AM, Daskin MS, Seagull FJ, Reddy RM. Innovative scheduling solutions for graduate medical education. J Grad Med Educ. 2015;7(2):169–70.

Authors

Jake Seagull holds a PhD in human factors and is currently a lead research specialist at Michigan Medicine's Center for Bioethics and Social Science in Medicine. He and Judy Smith are currently parenting a young adult son who needs much more sleep than he gets, and share custody of a rescue dog, who sleeps much more than she needs. He builds his personal schedule around the facts that he is a true night owl and a lifelong fan of micro-naps, way before they were a thing.

Cathy Marcucci figures that she has taken about 1000 nights of call (at least). These days, with her empty nest, her post-call routine is yoga, reading, and little else. The ever-steady Neil remains more than willing to fetch the gyoza or Caesar salads, and his grateful wife is now smart enough to simply say thank you.

Music as Metaphor

198

Amberly Hall Brown, Austin Brown, F. Jacob Seagull, and Catherine Marcucci

Introduction

We knew right away when we got the contract for this book that we wanted to do a piece on music. It's such an interesting metaphor for anesthesiology—the most salient point being the parallel between any live music and working in the OR. Everyone has their roles, but nobody has a specific script—much like a performing group or band, with each instrument having a role, and an idea about the blueprint of the song. But improvisation is the key to making good music.

Fundamentals

Everyone knows when their solo is. Everyone hears the drummer tracking the bars and the transitions. Everyone knows the chord changes. No one knows exactly what is going to happen when everyone plays. To succeed at music or anesthesia, you have to be good at your role, flexible in your responses, and a good communicator, so people know what you are doing.

For this chapter, we also had the fun opportunity to speak with country music professionals **Amberly Hall Brown** and **Austin Brown**. Together they run Austin Brown Music, LLC—Austin is the eponymous performing partner and Amberly is the talented businesswoman and managing partner who makes it go (Fig. 198.1). Austin also sang lead/high tenor with the successful vocal band Home Free, and that was a huge part of his professional life for many years. Amberly and Austin were kind enough to take time out of their busy performing and recording schedules to hear about the issues and problems of our specialty and talk about theirs.

A. H. Brown · A. Brown
Austin Brown Music, Nashville, TN, USA

F. J. Seagull
Center for Bioethics and Social Sciences in Medicine, Michigan Medicine, Ann Arbor, MI, USA

C. Marcucci (✉)
Department of Transfusion Medicine, Clinical Center, National Institutes of Health, Bethesda, MD, USA

S. Mohamed et al. (eds.), *Anesthesia Bridges*, https://doi.org/10.1007/978-3-032-08294-7_198

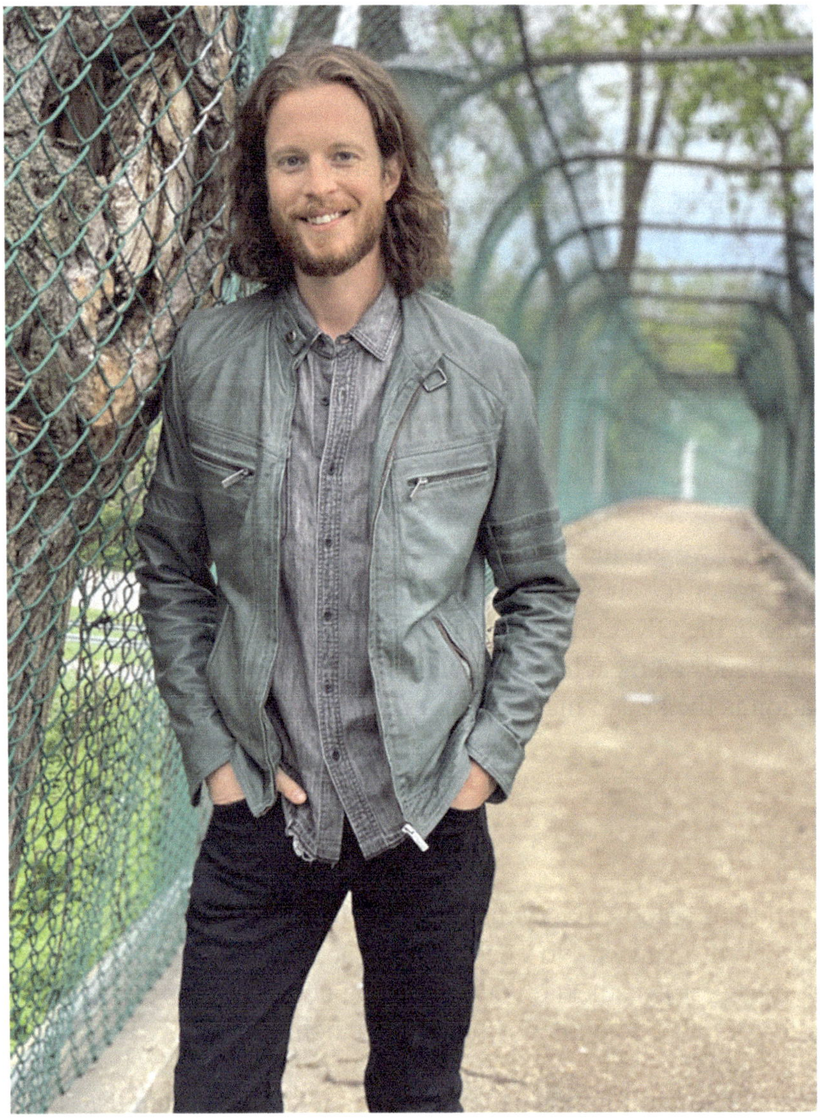

Fig. 198.1 Austin Brown, performing partner for *Austin Brown Music* and former lead tenor for *Home Free and Sweet and Low Music Co.* Photo: Amberly Hall Brown

Cathy is a novice listener of country music but has figured out that its themes of transition and renewal are energizing for her. She asked Austin, "would you say that hip hop is too edgy and negative to replenish the spirits of busy, tired physicians?" His reply was, "I would never say that nor would most music pros that I know." Apparently, the roots of hip hop are quite similar to those of country music and many songs are actually quite upbeat and positive. What generally distinguishes country music from other music styles is the enormous emphasis on storytelling and the rural roots. Hip hop music often has equal storytelling values, just with more urban roots.

Keep Your Ears Open!

We also assumed we would be talking *only* about country music and that Amberly and Austin wouldn't have much time or interest for other music genres. Nothing could have been further from the truth. They listen to other musicians and other types of music constantly. And they are quite egalitarian—they will jump on TikTok to see what's new; they listen to classical music when cooking and cleaning and even get on You Tube and listen to meditation videos and music. We thought they might diss Broadway show tunes—too trippy, too pop—but no, they love this type of music and laughed their heads off at The Book of Mormon, just like the rest of us. Apparently, this how music pros work—they are constantly going outside their own music spaces to see what's going on elsewhere.

We feel there's a lesson for us here—we don't do this enough! When Cathy was in her early and mid-career years, she didn't think or read about anything in the entire field of medicine that wasn't anesthesiology. She rarely even got outside her subspecialty training in vascular, transplant, and thoracic anesthesia—and she didn't consider going to a SOAP meeting after a certain point. She needed to produce clinical and research results in her own little corner of anesthesiology, and it felt like there was just no time for anything else. Professional musicians also have constant production and performing pressures, but they find a way. There's an enormous amount of anesthesia content online these days—why not put on a YouTube video or podcast and just let it play?

Collaborating and the Community

Musicians are also always looking for professional collaborations. Talent, personality, and charisma, even in spades, aren't going to be enough. They need an extensive network to make it and keep making it. They also need to evolve and grow their catalogue constantly. If you watch a number of AustinBrownMusic.com videos online, which Cathy did to prepare for the interview, you will see the various rotating combinations of musicians (and friends) that get together for different songs and video releases and how they all networked during the SARS-CoV-2 pandemic.

They also don't have the option of not having an online presence, which Amberly initiated and managed for AustinBrownMusic.com in a disciplined way. It's business, yes, but somehow it still seems to be about the relationships. This is advice that senior anesthesiologists have often given to junior anesthesiologists that has not always been received with credulity. When you are getting into a tense situation with a surgeon or colleague, how often are you thinking, you know, maybe this isn't the right approach—maybe I need to start thinking about what publications and research we can do?

A number of years ago, Austin and his vocal band Home Free had the opportunity to have a long meeting with the late, great Kenny Rogers. He had invited them to appear with him on *The Tonight Show* with Jimmy Fallon. The appearance didn't happen due to cancelled airline flights, but they still had the chance to see him in New York and have an extended conversation. They came away with two lasting impressions. First, Austin related that after the appearance Rogers took the time to personally talk with and thank each member of the show's crew. Valuable advice that we can borrow, for sure. When was the last time you actually spoke to and thanked each person in the OR, including the cleaning people who turned your room over for you?

Second, Kenny also advised Austin and "the boys" to build their careers steadily and carefully with solid, quality work that they felt genuinely good about, as this would make the decline of their careers gentler and more tolerable. This is really fascinating advice. When Cathy was a junior anesthesiologist, she had a lot of valuable mentoring, but it was always about the next step or the next two steps. Thirty years ago, nobody was advising her about the end of her career. But Jake Seagull, human factors guy extraordinaire, also advises the people he is mentoring to look as far into the future as possible, and this is one reason why. Evidently, the music and entertainment people know and understand from their salad days that the waning of their popularity and careers is inevitable. And so, the senior people advise the junior people how to mitigate this, even on the way up.

Confidence and Competence

Music professionals are all about confidence and making it look cool and fun and easy but that belies their education, training, focus, and discipline. Austin might be singing, "I heard the rooster crow" in a country music song, but scratch one millimeter below that and two seconds later, he's in a conversation about music theory or Shakespeare or how to conduct an orchestra. Honestly? It was somewhat comforting to be reminded that we are not the only people who have the public-facing vs. professional-facing dichotomy. We're not on a stage performing every day, of course, but we're in the pre-op area consenting patients and talking to families. And it is certainly equally incumbent on us to project confidence and knowledge and mastery of anesthesia—to make our highly specialized training and skills look effortless and to communicate with our patients at the educational and information levels where they live.

Personal Playlist

Finally, we asked Amberly and Austin for their thoughts about how to develop and expand a really energizing personal playlist. Their advice was a bit surprising—just find music in any genre that reflects back to you the best of who you were, who you are, and where you want to go. They just aren't willing to use private or professional time listening to music that doesn't reflect their personal values. They work in the country music space because, even more than love or loss, country music is about coming home, and they truly value their families and personal histories. They also understand the impact and power of subliminal messaging and advise that music listeners look carefully at the lyrics of a song before playlisting it—what you hear over and over again will eventually seep into your soul, which is pretty good general life advice. I also asked if it's best to start at the beginning of an artist's catalogue and work forward or start with the most recent releases and work backwards. Their answer was "just jump in!"

Amberly's and Austin's (current) playlist:

- Ben Rector—especially his most current work
- Joe Jonas

- anything by Alabama
- Randy Travis
- Garth Brooks
- Maren Morris
- Dear Evan Hansen—especially the last aria
- the great Dolly Parton—of course!

Lessons Learned

- It's a blast to spend an hour talking to a professional in a different field about their life and professional rewards and challenges. Do this at every opportunity, and you will come away with ideas and insight.
- Music is a fun metaphor for anesthesia—it's all about making the song happen, regardless of what happens unexpectedly or what your teammates do. *As long as the patient is okay*, you just have to keep perspective about it. If you ever need a chuckle, search You Tube for "Austin Brown forgets the words" and watch his Home Free bandmates, especially lead tenor Rob Lundquist, trying not to laugh.
- Country music just strips everything down to the bone. Cathy was watching a Willie Nelson interview, and he said, "Country music is three chords and the truth." She ran this quote by Austin who said, "Well, sure, of course. That's one of the most common sayings in the business. That's our truth about singing the truth."
- Is there a parallel in anesthesia? And not that tired old trope about boredom and terror, that is annoying as all get out, as we say elsewhere. So how about, "Anesthesia is three principles of physiology and making them match" or something along those lines? Anyway, the point is to think deeply enough about our practice to develop your own "truths." Ours are sprinkled liberally throughout this book but here are a couple more:
  - Anesthesia is physiology, pharmacology, and anatomy and maintaining their harmony, even in the most challenging of circumstances.
  - Critical care medicine is knowing when to act, how to act, and the best way to evaluate the action you just took.
  - Hospice medicine meets three needs the patient has: for peace, resolution, and not getting in the way.

  - Palliative medicine is three holistic ways to support your patient and helping them live better and happier with a serious illness.
  - Regional anesthesia is where the needle is, where the needle isn't, and what's in the syringe.
  - OB anesthesia is about making sure the mother, the baby, and the obstetrician are happy, comfortable, and stable when the procedure or delivery is over.

- It's also fun to talk to a trained voice professional—their knowledge of airway anatomy is every bit as good as ours.
- A carefully thought-out social media presence is imperative in today's world. The online space has really been crowded since the pandemic started, but Amberly was able to begin to build AustinBrownMusic.com with several well-placed videos, especially Austin's cover of *Unchained Melody*, accompanied by his good friend Steven Martinez. This classic song has been covered dozens of times, but Austin's rendition has over 18,000,000 views—go watch it, you'll be impressed. Anesthesia content isn't going to get that type of exposure, of course, but medical content can still do okay—for instance, the Blood Bank Guy (www.bbguy.org) does pretty well. Don't think the space is already full—it's never full if it's the right new material.
- Music professionals are constantly looking outside of their own music spheres. Those of us who work exclusively in an anesthesia subspecialty should borrow this strategy. Why not spend an hour seeing what was new at the latest ambulatory anesthesia conference? Or maybe look completely outside anesthesiology. How about attending a cardiology conference or dropping into the cardiac surgery meetings to learn about advances in revascularization?
- They also collaborate and network constantly. Kenny Rogers wanted to meet and work with new people right up to the very end of his career. We should always be on the lookout for the next joint publication or research team.
- The country music space has some fun advantages for the listener. First, it's been around a while, so there's a lot of it. Most of the best country music songs have been covered and recovered, so you can always find your own favorite version of a song. It's also very accessible and affordable if you are interested in listening to live music—most towns, even small towns, will have at least one or two country music groups performing live in bars or other small venues. And a lot of country music has crossover appeal, so it's a subject that you can use to establish contact with colleagues and patients.
- Try to build the most robust "catalogue" (aka CV) that you can as you go up. It will provide support and comfort on your way down.

Authors

Amberly Hall Brown hails from Chattanooga, Tennessee. After 12 years in the restaurant business, she is now an experienced country music professional and the managing partner of Austin Brown Music. Her loves include travelling, collecting crystals, fishing, anything involving being outdoors, and animals. She is currently in the process of starting her own animal sanctuary/rehabilitation facility and looks forward to living her dream of working with animals. She is the proud mother of two dogs, two cats, three Bass, three Bluegill, and a Redear Sunfish that she shares with her loving partner, Austin Brown.

Austin Brown was born and raised in Tifton, Georgia. After obtaining a degree in musical theater at Oklahoma City University, he spent time performing in regional theaters, amusement parks, and on cruise ships. In 2012, he met Home Free on a cruise ship and joined the band full-time as the high tenor in January of 2013. During 2020, when the world locked down, Austin followed his entrepreneurial instincts and began a solo career with his business partner and love of his life, Amberly Hall. When he wasn't touring with Home Free, performing with Sweet and Low Music Co., or working on solo music, Austin has always enjoyed working in the yard, fishing, going to gem/mineral shows, and giving back to his community at AustinBrownMusic.com.

Jake Seagull holds a PhD in psychology and has published widely in many areas of human factors research. As somebody who is finely attuned to the human condition, he feels that music is perhaps *THE* universal language. He enjoys listening to a wide variety of music, with jazz being the first among favorites.

Cathy Marcucci grew up listening to 1970s rock and little else. She once attended a spring prom where "Stairway to Heaven" was played in its entirety—more than once. She is now a big fan of both Home Free and Austin Brown Music and is working her way through their entire catalogues. Her current favorites are 'Good Ol' Boy Good Time' and 'Earn It,' which she listens to both on the way to work and on the way home.

Physician Burnout: Prevent the Creeping Dread

199

Neil B. Sandson and Catherine Marcucci

Introduction

Most physicians embark on a career in medicine because, at least in large part, they are drawn toward a life of service. Granted that they will generally be financially well-rewarded for their labors, but folks do not gravitate toward medicine unless they are attracted to the prospect of helping others. Fueled by their idealism, theirs' and others' expectations, and appealing fantasies of what their lives will be like after their training, tens of thousands of trainees each year progress through medical schools and residency programs in order to reach their promised lands.

Real Life!

Then the reality arrives. For many, the reality matches their expectations, and they pursue fulfilling careers in their desired branch of medicine. For many others, however, the disillusionments and frustrations hit either soon after training or even in the midst of training. The excitement and anticipation have gone away; the work does not feel fun, interesting, or gratifying anymore, producing indifference and even antipathy toward their work.

Some try to make the best of it, staying in their profession despite their demoralization and lack of engagement/investment, tolerating the ever-increasing sense of inevitability and hopelessness. If and when other parts of their lives also descend into dysfunction, the synergistic misery can even culminate in suicide. Career change is often a superior option, but the almost unparalleled amount of time and sunk cost of a medical career keep unhappy doctors in their unsatisfying jobs. This is what burnout looks like.

N. B. Sandson
Department of Psychiatry, VA Maryland Health Care System, Baltimore, MD, USA

University of Maryland, Baltimore, MD, USA

C. Marcucci (✉)
Department of Transfusion Medicine, Clinical Center, National Institutes of Health, Bethesda, MD, USA

S. Mohamed et al. (eds.), *Anesthesia Bridges*, https://doi.org/10.1007/978-3-032-08294-7_199

Burnout: What and Why

Most physicians intuitively understand what is meant by the term "burnout." It can be characterized by apathy, cynicism, detachment, emotional exhaustion, and despair. Burnout can result in higher physician turnover, wastage, errors, addiction, and malpractice episodes. The causes can be both systemic and highly individualized.

On a systemic level, changes in the practice of medicine have been heavily implicated. Physicians now spend less time with patients, are expected to do more, and have to engage in ever-increasing labor to address documentation requirements, insurance company requirements, etc. The demands of regulators and insurance companies can come to feel both burdensome and intrusive, leading physicians to feel frustrated and overwhelmed.

Physicians are also often required to learn and relearn the quirks and operational specifics of electronic medical record systems, which can become tiresome at best and debilitating at worst. The "business of medicine" has produced a consumer-based and monetarily driven ethos that is often at odds with the idealized notions that brought folks into medicine in the first place, as opposed to, say, investment banking. Additionally, despite seniority, many physicians continue to have to work punishing schedules, comparable to residents.

The prevalence of physician burnout is striking. Rates run at approximately 50%. In one 2021 survey of 13,000 physicians across 29 specialties, the specialties most likely to produce burnout are emergency medicine (60%), critical care medicine (56%), and obstetrics and gynecology (53%). Anesthesiology was ranked ninth at 47%.

Clearly, physician burnout is not some occasional aberration of what is otherwise a system that fosters adaptive, gratifying occupational longevity. If "our" goal is to have burnout be the exception rather than the rule, then it seems obvious that many basic, core elements of how the practice of medicine is structured are fundamentally ill-conceived. The entire system needs an overhaul, and it will take many years and a coordinated multi-level set of processes to even begin to comprehensively address this issue.

Seeking Solutions

However, some reasonably helpful measures have been undertaken to address burnout, on the scale of individuals and specific health systems. Mental health referrals are never a bad idea for identified individuals who are suffering from burnout. Since underlying, unrecognized, and thus undertreated depressive and anxiety disorders can predispose vulnerable individuals to develop burnout, addressing these issues through readily available and effective treatment can be very helpful.

Many systems are investing time and effort into supporting "wellness programs." However, these programs seldom involve deconstructing or otherwise restructuring destructive aspects of programs; rather, they seek to provide some sort of distraction and/or mitigation, but they unfortunately leave the inciting influences intact. At the level of the individual, solutions to burnout need to involve some sort of change, whether that person changes aspects of their job that are under their control, leaves that specific job entirely, or is fortunate enough to be the beneficiary of systemic changes enacted by enlightened leadership.

Burnout Never Resolves on Its Own

However, one can never "outlast" burnout. It can be endured and tolerated, but if the person and their circumstances never change for the better, then neither will the enduring state of burnout. It is only starting to be understood that an overzealous commitment to efficiency is rendering many workplaces unsustainable in the long term. However, most workplaces are generally *not* committed to the happiness and self-actualization of their employees, and in order to maximize productivity (and not incidentally profits), high employee turnover is tolerated as the price of this maximal efficiency model. Sadly, on a systemic level, we are *very* far from addressing this pernicious phenomenon in the manner that our profession deserves. Prevention and treatment of burnout are mostly happening on an individual rather than a systemic level.

***Note from the Editors:** Neil Sandson loves Japan and Japanese culture. We asked him for a favorite bridge in Japan, and he chose the Kin Tai Bridge in the Yamaguchi Prefecture (Fig. 199.1). This incredibly beautiful wood pedestrian bridge was built in 1673 and spans the Nishiki River. There are five arches that rest on stone piers. It was built without nails and remained intact for 273 years but fell into disrepair during WW2 and was washed away by a typhoon in 1950. It has since been rebuilt and refurbished and is currently under regular maintenance. For flood protection, the bridge is built so that the wooden planks "float" on a mesh substructure, and flood waters will wash the walkway away but leave the underlying structure intact.

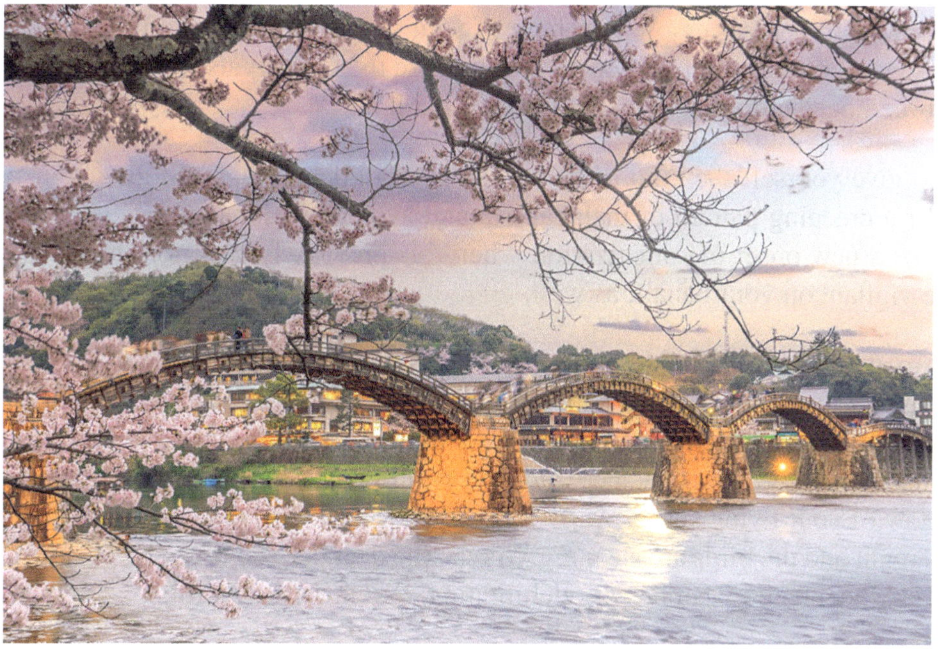

Fig. 199.1 The Kin Tai or Kintaikyo bridge was declared a Japanese national treasure in 1922. It is surrounded by cherry trees and lit every evening. Photo: Image used under standard license from Shutterstock.com

From Neil Sandson

If a young physician approached me, having seen a senior colleague struggling with significant burnout, and requested information on developing proactive safeguards against burnout, I would give the following advice:

1. Make time and space for what is most important to you and the people who depend on you, outside of work—and to the extent that you have control over it, within your work as well.

2. Try to maintain variety within your workday or week. Having a mix of different kinds of tasks and subroutines can keep the work fresher and more stimulating.

3. Collaborate with leadership to pursue goals for professional growth and development. If this is a living, breathing part of your career trajectory, then it will be much more difficult to experience the stuck, dead-end position that can lead to burnout.

4. For these first three pieces of advice, leadership can be an invaluable resource in helping to convert good ideas into tangible realities. So long as it does not entail obvious wastage, supervisors generally recognize that happy employees are more productive employees, and they will often work with you to help accomplish this.

5. Cultivate the habit of quiet, radical honesty – to yourself, most of all, and with those you love. People can create enormous stress for themselves by driving towards goals they do not really want. You might find yourself in a less enjoyable phase of your work or career, and it is okay to admit that, at least to those you trust, and actively work to minimize those intervals. If you think to yourself, "Am I getting burned out?" you probably are. Call it what it is.

6. Continue to give yourself the kind of compassionate vigilance that you give your patients. Watch carefully for a creeping pattern of maladaptive and avoidant behaviors or a sudden inability to get out of bed or a new onset of somatization when this previously was not an issue. Ask your inner circle to be vigilant on your behalf, as well.

7. Keep your experiences varied at home, even if all you can manage are microvariations. If you feel that you must have certainly worn a path on your carpet or ruts in your wood floors due to the soul-crushing tedium and restricted patterns of your daily routine, make sure that you go into every room of your house every day. Tiptoe in and watch your children sleeping for a few moments. Look out at every window of your living space. Walk out onto your back deck and see what the birds are doing, even if it is night and the birds are sleeping. Maybe the deer and the foxes will be out and about. That hamster-in-a-wheel feeling can be very debilitating. Watch for it carefully.

8. Do not try to "force" yourself to do too many difficult things. Sometimes you have to buckle down and be disciplined about something at work. Nobody can learn the new regional technique for you but you, or do your CMEs. But you do not have to force yourself to do the taxes, or declutter the garage, or count your reps at the gym. There are people you can hire to do that. Do not try to be an automaton, not even for one second.

9. Find one thing that can be experienced in 5 minutes or less that works for you. Pictures of gardens, all things Japanese, a blog devoted to puppies, or a sports team. "Go" there at least twice a day.

10. Do not fear change. If one allows fear of the unknown to keep one in a static, unchanging, and unfulfilling position, then burnout awaits. Of course, one must be practical. Incremental change is preferable to impulsively gambling one's life savings on a shaky business deal.

11. It is generally not helpful to think in terms of sunk cost/time. Even if one has invested a great deal of time and money in the pursuit of a career, if it has become clear that the career is no longer fulfilling, then the sunk cost and time should not oblige one to stay in that career. A fresh start is often the right answer. This is easier if you have set your arrangements up so that you have at least some degree of situational and financial flexibility.

12. Do not be afraid to seek help, whether it is a therapist, psychiatrist, or even a life coach. Even cognitive behavior therapy has been shown to be of some help in warding off the initial stages of burnout. Even the act of seeking the help can be a catalyst to achieving the change that helps improve matters.

Lessons Learned

- All the editors concur with all of the above points!

- Remember, burnout is not just depression or anxiety. It is demoralization. And it does not just arrive when you find yourself in a highly regulated or rigidly structured, repetitive work environment. Pilots work in these conditions and suffer much less burnout than physicians because they could not imagine doing any other job and so find tolerating these aspects of their jobs worthwhile because of their love of flying. The same with the farmers, who work constantly in stressful conditions, and make a tiny fraction of what we make. Burnout happens when you work in these conditions and feel there is no way out.

- The wellness programs are sometimes helpful for people, but do not get down on yourself if the various workplace wellness programs do not seem to be working for you. Truthfully, Neil Sandson finds most of them trivial if not downright laughable. Distracting yourself from the problem *versus* facing and solving the problem are very different things. Receiving an email at work urging you to journal for 20 minutes a day is not really going to be a universal solution to the pressures that physicians face. If you feel burnout creeping up on you, give them a try, but if it does not click, keep moving until you find a solution.

- *Vigilance always*. It is much better to be on the lookout for burnout on the horizon than to realize it is already upon you. Also, keep a strong lookout for compassion fatigue.

- If you realize that you are in a battle with burnout, deploy every offense and defense that you can access. Do not try to tough it out. Employ the short-term and mitigating strategies that are offered to you—they probably would not hurt—but recognize that true burnout cannot be willed away. *Resolution will involve change*.

- In addition, do not feel ashamed. You are not weak, lazy, or incapable. Understand that people who are sensitive and intelligent are at increased risk.

Authors

Neil Sandson is a psychiatrist with appointments at the University of Maryland and the VA Maryland Health Care System. His areas of clinical expertise and research interests include the treatment of PTSD, major depression, and anxiety disorders. He enjoys playing squash and bridge and spending time with his family.

Cathy Marcucci is an anesthesiologist who has always found major vascular and large blood loss cases to be particularly interesting and challenging in a good way. She also refreshes her soul with plants, reading, games, and puzzles of all sorts, including duplicate bridge, the color blue, attending minor league baseball games, and writing anesthesia textbooks for charity.

If You Have Inherited a Gladstone Bag, Pass It On!

200

Olivia Liao, Raymond G. Graber, Allan Gottschalk, and Catherine Marcucci

Introduction

"Gladstone bag" is the actual name of the iconic black leather doctor's bag that is so well-known in literature, the movies, and in real life, especially if one of your family's elders was a physician.

Background

William Gladstone was the English Prime Minister four separate times between 1868 and 1894 and became known for walking among Parliament buildings with a small, lightweight leather bag with a wide top opening that made the contents easily accessible. The Gladstone bag was adopted by the medical profession in the late Victorian era and was in ubiquitous use until about the 1960s. Neurologists still use them to this day to carry their reflex hammers and tuning forks.

If your father or grandfather was a physician, he surely had a black doctor's bag at some point in his career. Sadly, although we searched, we were unable to find anyone who has a Gladstone bag that belonged to their grandmother or great-grandmother. This is perhaps because the percentage of physicians who were women actually declined from 10% in 1900 to less than 4% in 1940. Rest assured that we were both sad and mad when we discovered that infuriating fact.

O. Liao
Carnegie Mellon University, Pittsburgh, PA, USA

R. G. Graber
Department of Anesthesiology and Perioperative Medicine, University Hospitals Cleveland Medical Center, Cleveland, OH, USA

A. Gottschalk
Department of Anesthesiology and Critical Care Medicine. Department of Neurosurgery, Johns Hopkins University, Baltimore, MD, USA

C. Marcucci (✉)
Department of Transfusion Medicine, Clinical Center, National Institutes of Health, Bethesda, MD, USA

S. Mohamed et al. (eds.), *Anesthesia Bridges*, https://doi.org/10.1007/978-3-032-08294-7_200

But anyway, although the "modern" form of the doctor's bag might date from 1870 or so, physicians have always carried their supplies around with them. There are multiple references in antiquity to physicians' kits—including Greek texts from around 350 BC describing small, fitted cases with supplies and Egyptian hieroglyphics from about 100 BC showing a set of surgical instruments in a case.

The Gottschalk Family Bag

The patina of this great little leather bag shows that it has seen some serious service (Fig. 200.1). It has become a cherished heirloom in the Gottschalk family. The senior Dr. Gottschalk's story is told in Chapter 173, *Our Inspiration: Sally (Sabina) Sikorski, RN BSN, and Carl Gottschalk, MD,* in the Personal Stories section.

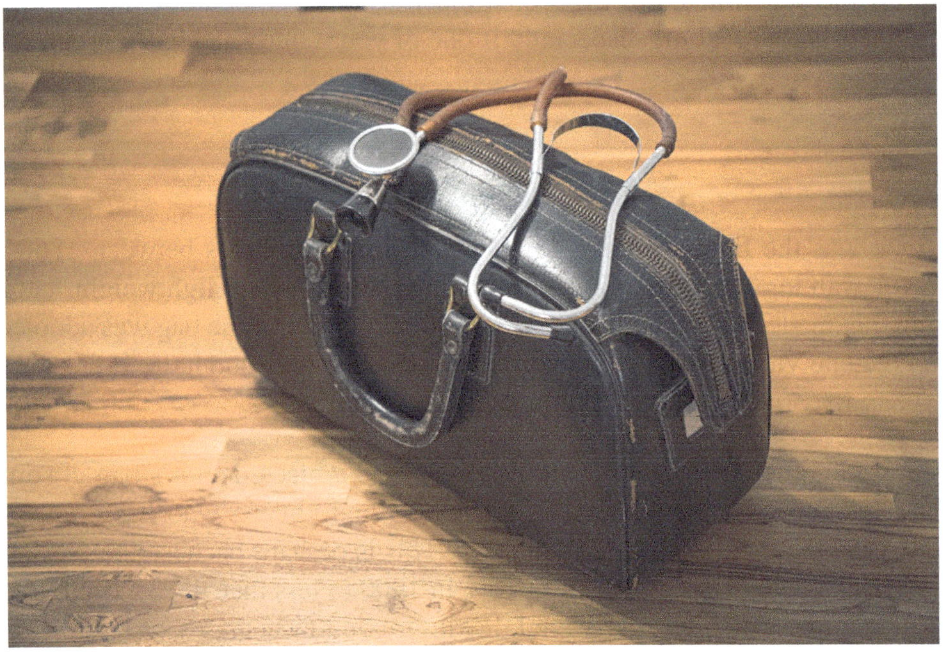

Fig. 200.1 The Gottschalk bag. This bag and stethoscope were owned and used by the late Carl Gottschalk MD, as he started his medical and anesthesiology career in the 1950s. They were presented to his granddaughter, Chelsea L. Gottschalk MD, upon her graduation from medical school in 2018. Photo: Dillon Shook

The Graber Family Bag

Ray Graber was delighted to receive his father's Gladstone bag (Fig. 200.2). A bit more of the senior Dr. Graber's story is told in Chapter 98, "Why You Should Talk to Your Patients" in the Doctor-Patient Relations section of this book.

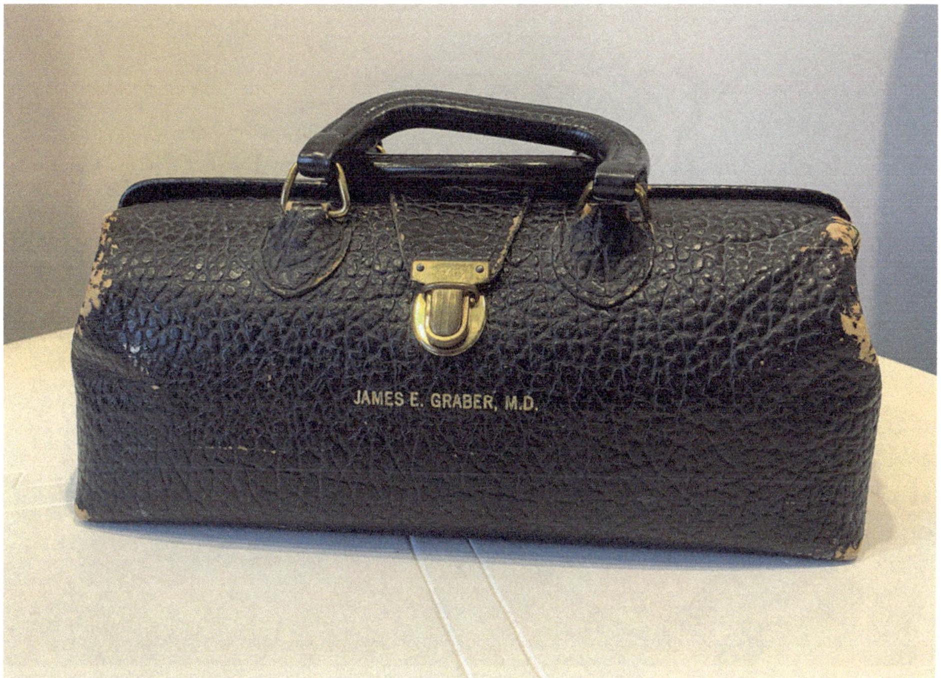

Fig. 200.2 The Graber bag. This bag was owned by the late James Graber, MD, Ray Graber's dad. Jim Graber was a highly respected clinician, led the anesthesiology department at St. Peter's Hospital in Albany, NY for many years, and was the past president of the New York State Society of Anesthesiology. It is so nice and so fitting that his Gladstone bag was passed down to Ray. Photo: Raymond Graber, MD

The Liao Family Bag

The late Schue-Yuan Liao, MD, was the father and grandfather of *Anesthesia Bridges* authors Albert Liao and Olivia Liao, respectively. The Liao family has their doctor's bag and we were delighted when they sent us a picture of the bag and its contents (Fig. 200.3). Dr. Liao received his Gladstone bag in 1960 when he graduated from the first class of Kaohsiung Medical College, now Kaoshiung Medical University, a prestigious private tertiary care and research institution in southern Taiwan.

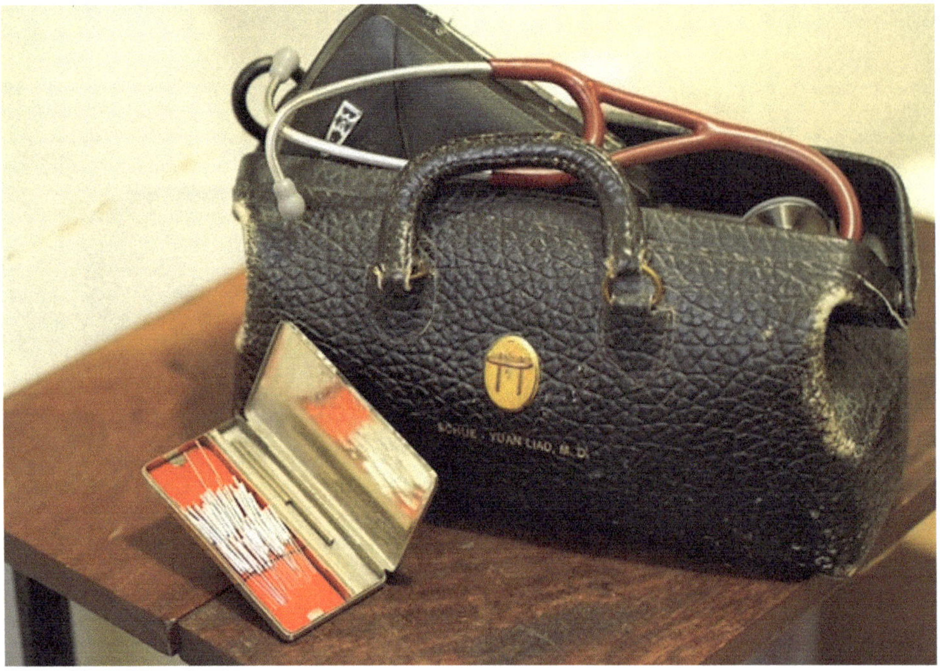

Fig. 200.3 The Liao bag. This Gladstone bag was owned by the late Schue-Yuan Liao, MD. Dr. Liao received his doctoral degree in 1960 when he graduated from the first class of Kaohsiung Medical College in Taiwan, now Kaohsiung Medical University. Then, as now, the medical school taught a modern medical curriculum in English, which is why the name of the new medical graduate is embossed in English letters and not in Mandarin Chinese. Dr. Liao's Gladstone bag supplies included a stethoscope, blood pressure cuff, reflex hammer, tuning fork, prescription pad, alcohol swabs, and acupuncture needles. Photo: John Liao

He arrived in the United States five years later with nothing but an apple and twenty dollars in his pocket. In the following years, he moved all over the country to obtain board certification in neurology and start his US medical career. He finally settled in Maryland in the early 1970s and opened his own neurology practice, adding acupuncture as a method of pain management. By the time he retired in 2016, acupuncture was his primary treatment method.

The Sandson Family Bag

The Sandson family (*Anesthesia Bridges* authors Neil, Charlie, and Lisa Sandson) is the proud owner of the Gladstone bag used in an internship in 1960 by Gerald B. Sandson, MD—Neil's dad, and still a practicing psychiatrist at the age of 88. It was presented to Neil by his parents when he graduated from Temple University School of Medicine in 1991. We wanted to photograph it for this essay, but could not find it—it's not totally lost, but seems to be lost somewhere in the house. Neither of the Sandson kids is bound for a medical career, but both have indicated interest in inheriting the bag in the fullness of time. As Lisa said, "I'll definitely take Grandpa's doctor's bag if it's up for grabs! I can line it with satin and use it for jewelry boxes or even carry it as a handbag. But can I pass on Grandma's dishes?"

The Doctor's Bag Then and Now

The doctor's bag is still in use today, although chloroform in a dropper bottle is no longer a regular staple. In Australia, the Royal Australian College of General Practitioners Standards 5th edition requires that all practitioners have ready access to a well-stocked doctor's bag, although bags may be shared among physicians in a practice [1].

Many standard and/or required items for the bag have not changed in the last hundred years—hand cleanser, stethoscope, sphygmomanometer, thermometer, ophthalmoscope, and auriscope. A sharps container, mask, and gloves are now mandated, of course. What's interesting to us is the array of drugs that are permitted in the bags of general practitioners in Australia. You would expect the epinephrine, nitrates, naloxone, penicillin, and glucose/glucagon. More surprising is that Australian general practitioners are also permitted to carry clonazepam, diazepam, midazolam, morphine, tramadol, and—get this—ampules of methoxyflurane for self-administered inhalation in trauma situations. Needless to say, the standards mandate careful and secure maintenance and storage of the bag.

Lessons Learned

- The traditional doctor's black leather bag with a top opening is also known as a Gladstone bag.
- Every anesthesiologist alive has carried a bag, of course, at least during training or on call, but somehow these nylon tackle or camera bags don't have quite the same panache. They get a bit of blood on them, and you dump them in the trash and order the next one from Eddie Bauer. And we don't think we've ever seen a surgeon or even a surgical resident walk around the hospital with a bag of gear and supplies, have you?
- We have noticed that families that have a Gladstone bag proudly pass it down, especially if the younger generation has somebody graduating from med school. Better yet, if the name of the original owner is embossed in gold letters.
- No generation of young people really wants their parents' and grandparents' fancy, fragile, and outdated stuff, we are learning. But a Gladstone bag might get some takers. It can be repurposed to hold jewelry and small belongings, and maybe even has a whiff of steampunk style about it. But no matter what, it beats a bunch of teacups and saucers.

Reference

1. RACGP – Criterion GP5.3 – Doctor's bag [Internet]. Racgp.org.au. 2018. Available from: https://www.racgp.org.au/running-a-practice/practice-standards/standards-5th-edition/standards-for-general-practices-5th-ed/general-practice-standards/gp-standard-5/criterion-gp5-3-doctor-s-bag.

Authors

Olivia Liao, Allan Gottschalk, and **Ray Graber,** in their respective careers, are proud to honor the legacy of hard-working physicians who gave the best of themselves to their patients and passed their competency and strength onto their families. **Cathy Marcucci** is not from a medical family; instead, she hopes to provide such an example to her own children.

201 Dr. Axley's Microscope

Michael S. Axley and Catherine Marcucci

Introduction

We just happened to send a draft of the previous chapter to *Anesthesia Bridges* author and editor Mike Axley, who wrote back:

> Turns out that I also have a Gladstone bag! But I also inherited the microscope my great grandfather used to go to medical school with back in the early part of the last century. He passed it on to his son, my grandfather, who was also a physician. My grandmother gave it to me when I went off to medical school. Up to that point, I hadn't known it existed. It still has the original test slide intact.

When we got this from Mike, we asked if he could send us a picture of the scope. Even though he was busy negotiating contracts or some such pressing business, he found the time to send us a photo of this beautiful piece of antique medical equipment (Fig. 201.1).

M. S. Axley
Oregon Anesthesiology Group, Portland, OR, USA

C. Marcucci (✉)
Department of Transfusion Medicine, Clinical Center, National Institutes of Health, Bethesda, MD, USA

S. Mohamed et al. (eds.), *Anesthesia Bridges*, https://doi.org/10.1007/978-3-032-08294-7_201

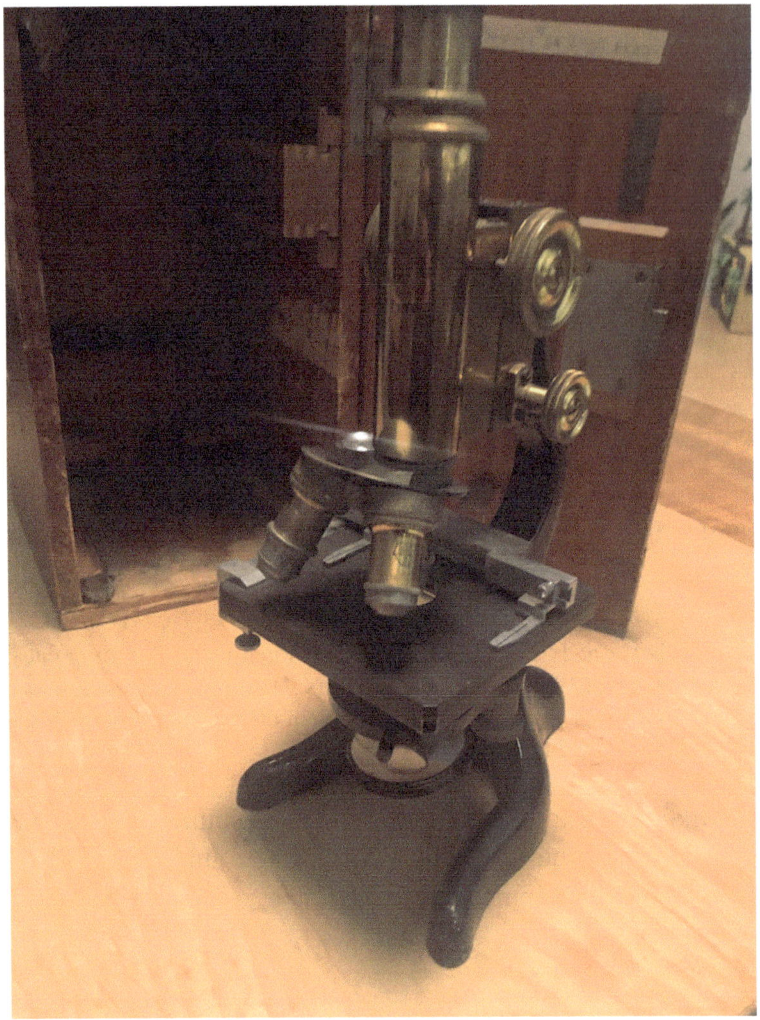

Fig. 201.1 The microscope owned and used by Albert Wilson Axley, MD and Albert Walter Axley, MD when they attended medical school at the University of Wisconsin. It is now the property of their great-grandson and grandson, Mike Axley. Photo: Mike Axley

From Mike

My maternal great-grandfather was a generalist who had a clinic outside of Madison, Wisconsin. As I understand it, he did the whole thing, from minor surgeries to birthing babies. Part of the wave of emigration from Germany in the nineteenth century, he was probably born in the United States but was the son of an emigrant household. There are stories in our families of how he would take a sleigh around in the winter to make house calls on the cranberry farmers. My microscope would be from this era, and he almost certainly used it himself in medical school at the University of Wisconsin.

My grandfather's name was Walter Axley (Fig. 201.2). He followed his father to medical school at the University of Wisconsin; this would have been in the early 1940s. If I remember correctly, he met his wife while he was in medical school, and they initially settled in the Midwest outside of Chicago. I believe that he did a residency in that city as well. They later moved to one of the most rural places in the country—Havre, Montana. Havre is a town in northern Montana that sits on a passage called the Hi-Line, a stretch of highway and railroad cutting across the plains of Montana close to the Canadian border.

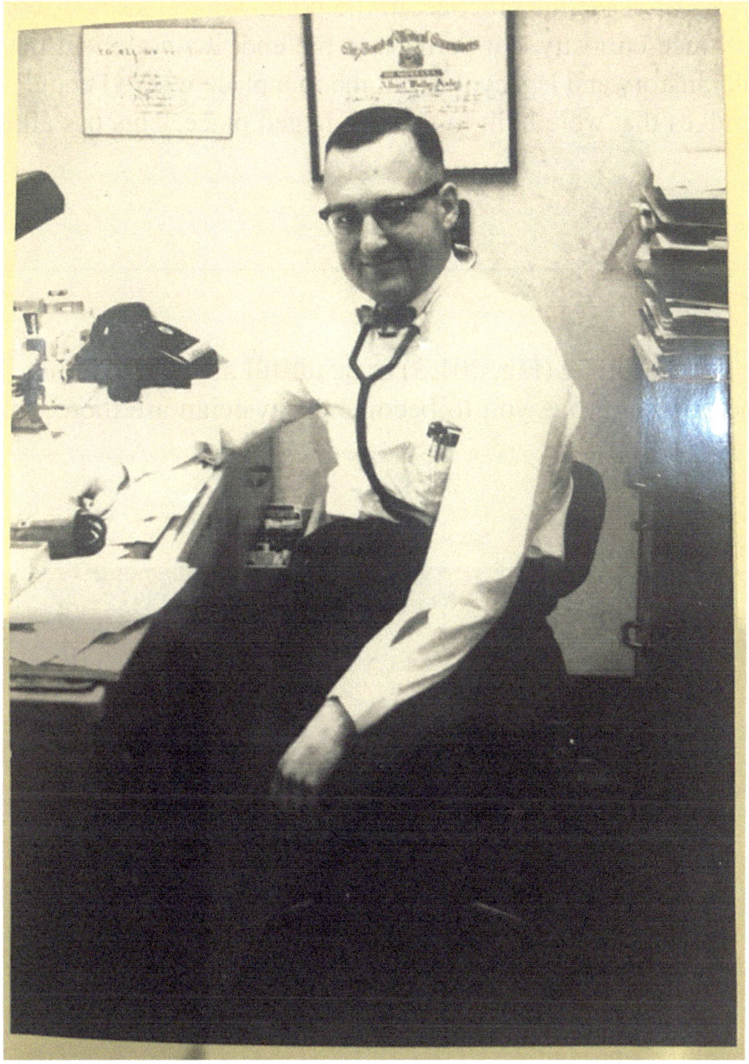

Fig. 201.2 Walter Axley, MD, in his medical office, probably in the 1950s. Photo: Collection of the Axley family

My grandfather loved fishing. This was good because there is not a lot to do in this part of Montana besides fishing and hunting. He liked fishing on lakes, and the family spent a lot of time at the summer cabins you could find back then on Lake Flathead. But what he really loved was fly fishing. In addition to his microscope, my grandmother preserved a number of his bamboo poles, reels, and flies. I then spent the early part of my twenties breaking many of those poles and losing many of those flies in the trees around Portland. I still have the bulk of the fly libraries, however.

As a physician, he too was a generalist, and I think widely respected in the area around Havre. I've had at least a few people tell me how he treated someone in their family. He spent his whole career there and worked until he passed away at the age of 52. I would have been around two years old at that time. Right around 25 years later, I started medical school at Cornell.

I always thought that I wanted to be a doctor. It was a very motivating aspect of my childhood. I did not really know my grandfather, since he died when I was a baby, but I wanted to be like him in some way and perhaps act in the role that he had played. This drive had enough power to propel me through a number of pretty difficult times. It had enough power, in fact, to put me through medical school, two residencies, and 10 years of academic practice, to the point where I sit now, contemplating my microscope. And it is a very nice curiosity, but perhaps in the end, it's not about the hardware. To put it in context, I have a family history and legacy that put me in a place where I could aspire to be a doctor—I am grateful for the bridges that were built to this privileged place. This has allowed me to become the person I am today.

Lessons Learned

- You may not have a doctor's bag (Fig. 201.3) or beautiful medical antiques, but your own personal history and the factors that drove you to become a physician are there. Just open your eyes and look around.

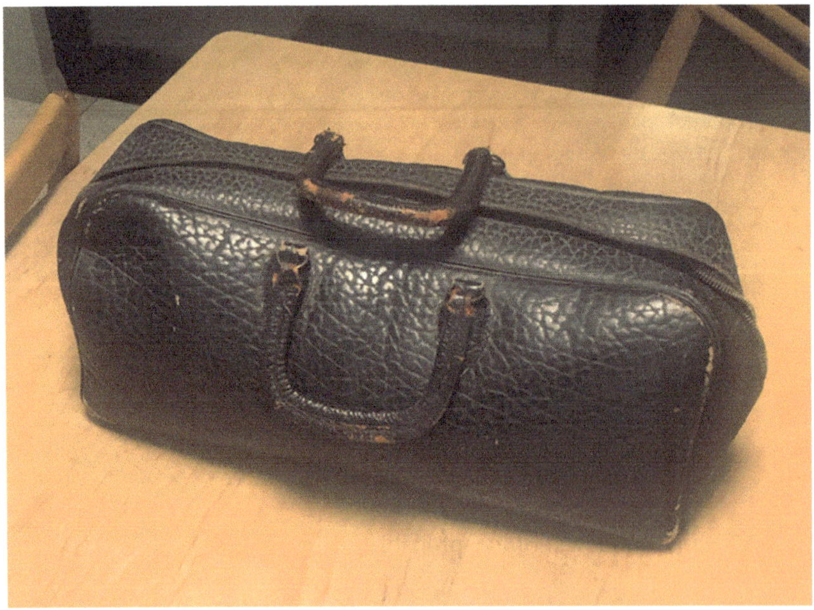

Fig. 201.3 The Gladstone bag owned originally by Dr. Walter Axley. We bet he used it every day. Photo: Mike Axley

- Doesn't the senior Dr. Axley look like he had some really great stories to tell? (Fig. 201.4)

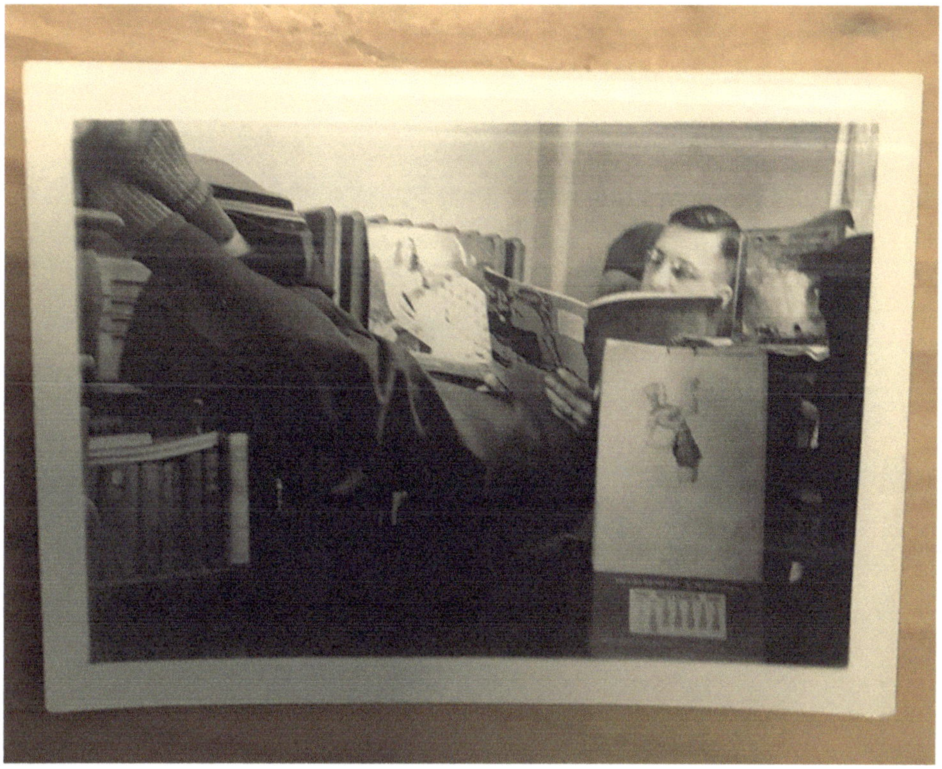

Fig. 201.4 Walter Axley, MD relaxing at home, sometime in the 1940s or 1950s. Photo: Collection of the Axley family

Authors

Mike Axley is an anesthesiologist in Portland, OR. He has many interests besides his family and anesthesiology and has been a lifelong writer, reader, and editor.

Cathy Marcucci is a senior academic anesthesiologist. Unlike Mike's medical family, her grandparents and great grandparents made their living as a piece-work garment worker, carpenter and bricklayer, and peasants in the hilltop area of Abruzzi, Italy.

Words of Wisdom: Quotes on Money and Wealth

202

Catherine Marcucci, F. Jacob Seagull, and Neil B. Sandson

Contributor:

Austin Brown

Introduction

We thought it would be fun to include some thoughts about money vs. wealth for our readers. Physicians often are not extremely expert at money matters—by definition, the practice of medicine means we place others' interests above our own. This doesn't have to carry over to the financial and business realms, but unfortunately frequently does.

We wrote several drafts of this chapter before deciding to start with the basics and collect some classic quotes by the great thinkers and other notable figures.

Money Versus Wealth

When we started researching, the first thing that was impressed upon us is that **money** and **wealth** are not the same thing. Additionally, that a lot of the published money wisdom out there is just trite, clichéd nonsense. For instance, it is *not true* that everybody has the exact same potential for wealth because everybody has exactly the same number of minutes in a day. That's only true for people born into identical social circumstances and with identical states of health. But we did find a number of quotable quotes

C. Marcucci (✉)
Department of Transfusion Medicine, Clinical Center, National Institutes of Health, Bethesda, MD, USA

F. J. Seagull
Center for Bioethics and Social Science in Medicine, University of Michigan Medical School, Ann Arbor, MI, USA

N. B. Sandson
Department of Psychiatry, VA Maryland Health Care System, Baltimore, MD, USA

University of Maryland, Baltimore, MD, USA

S. Mohamed et al. (eds.), *Anesthesia Bridges*, https://doi.org/10.1007/978-3-032-08294-7_202

that seem both relevant and helpful. Of course, as they are direct historical quotes spanning many centuries and translated from other languages, there is much non-inclusive language. Please recognize that we assert gender-neutrality in our intention. So, in no particular order:

- A wise person should have money in their head, but not in their heart.—**Jonathan Swift**
- Who is rich? The one who appreciates what they have.—**Pirkei Avot 4**
- Are you rich or do you just have money? —**Frank Sonnenberg**
- The price of anything is the amount of life you exchange for it.—**Henry David Thoreau**
- A love that does not make you feel rich is poor in heart.—**P.S. Jagadeesh Kumar**
- Opportunity is missed by most people because it is dressed in overalls and looks like work.—**Thomas Edison**
- The quote is a good one! Just substitute “scrubs” for overalls and that’s us.—**Editors**
- Many people take no care of their money till they come nearly to the end of it, and others do just the same with their time.—**Johann Wolfgang von Goethe**
- I agree with Balzac and nineteenth-century writers…who say, “I write for money.” Yes, I think everybody should be paid handsomely; I insist on it, and I pay people who work for me, or with me, handsomely.—**Maya Angelou**
- It’s better to be remembered for what you said, not what you earned.—**Carla H. Krueger**
- Money is only a tool. It will take you wherever you wish, but it will not replace you as the driver.—**Ayn Rand**
- The only thing money really buys?—Space. A bigger house, a bigger car, a larger hotel room. First-class plane tickets. But it doesn’t even buy comfort. No one complains more than the rich and entitled. Comfort, security, ease. None of them come with money.—**Louise Penny**
- We are not sure about the quote above but included it to stimulate consideration. Personally, we think space often is comfort, security, and ease. Money may not bring a bigger car but often does bring a better car, meaning a safer car.—**Editors**
- Remember that the basic circular model of wealth has really never been discounted. It seems so simple, but the circle theory of the economy is that major economic exchanges are represented by continuous and circular flows between income, goods, and services. Work hard to keep your circle balanced and flowing smoothly.—**Editors**

***Note from the Editors:** This beautiful circle bridge is a great metaphor for the circle economic models (Fig. 202.1).

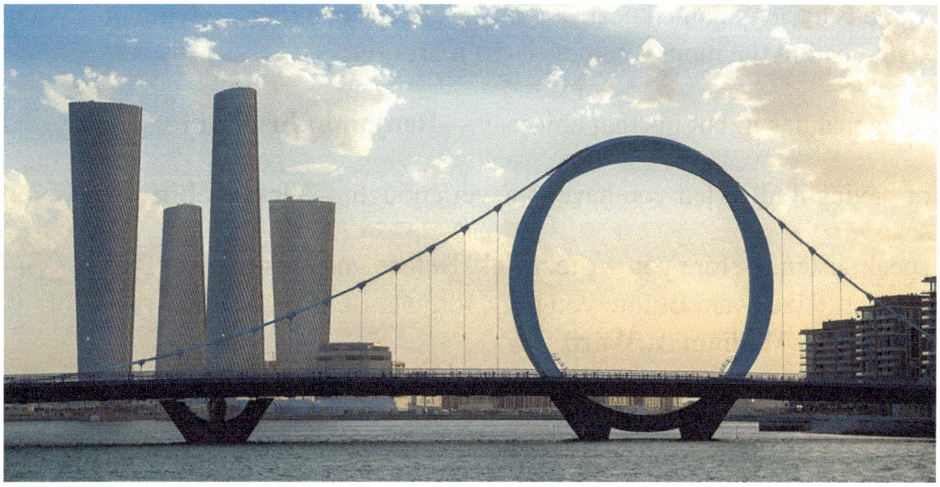

Fig. 202.1 A dramatic bridge in Qatar. It has a twin about 800 meters away. Photo: Image used for editorial use (non-fiction book) from shutterstock.com

- He who loses money, loses much; He who loses a friend, loses much more; He who loses faith, loses all.—**Eleanor Roosevelt**
- Do not save what is left after spending but spend what is left after saving.—**Warren Buffet**
- Happiness is not in the mere possession of money; it lies in the joy of achievement, in the thrill of creative effort.—**Franklin Roosevelt**
- It's good to have money and the things that money can buy, but it's good, too, to check up once in a while, and make sure that you haven't lost the things that money can't buy.—**George Lorimer**
- Money is a terrible master but an excellent servant.—**P.T. Barnum**
- We were very much a reading family, but we were a borrow-a-book-from-the-library family more than a bookshelves-full-of-books family. My parents valued books, but they grew up in the Depression, aware of the quicksilver nature of money, and they learned the hard way that you shouldn't buy what you could borrow. Because of that frugality, or perhaps independent of it, they also believed that you read a book for the experience of reading it.—**Susan Orlean**
- Wealth is the ability to fully experience life.—**Henry David Thoreau**
- You must gain control over your money or the lack of it will forever control you.—**Dave Ramsey**
- What if I told you that money is a game? How well do you play now? Would you consider yourself to be winning? Winning is not how well you do financially. It is how good you feel about playing.—**Ken Honda**

- The money game is a tricky game because the rules keep changing…My mentor Wahei Takeda once said, "There is no end in the money game." —**Ken Honda**
- Wealth is not his that has it, but his that enjoys it.—**Benjamin Franklin**
- If you live for having it all, what you have is never enough.—**Vicki Robin**
- Before you speak, listen. Before you write, think. Before you spend, earn. Before you invest, investigate. Before you criticize, wait. Before you pray, forgive. Before you quit, try. Before you retire, save. Before you die, give.—**William A. Ward**
- A budget is telling your money where to go instead of wondering where it went.—**John C. Maxwell**
- A man who both spends and saves money is the happiest man, because he has both enjoyments.—**Samuel Johnson**
- Not everything that can be counted counts, and not everything that counts can be counted.—**Albert Einstein**
- Boasting of wealth is an open invitation to others to divest you of it.—**Stewart Stafford**
- Those with many ideas are potentially rich people.—**Eraldo Banovac**
- (Our kids) just want to know what we stand for; our spending choices is one way that we articulate this.—**Ron Lieber**
- He who cannot economize will have to agonize.—**Confucius**
- Save money on the big, boring stuff so that you have something left over for life's little pleasures.—**Elizabeth Leamy**
- Money may not buy happiness, but I'd rather cry in a Jaguar than on a bus.
- (About money)—It is better to be roughly right than precisely wrong.—**John Maynard Keynes**
- The most important quality for an investor is temperament, not intellect.—**Warren Buffett**
- Enough is better than too much.—**Dutch Proverb**
- He who buys what he does not need, steals from himself.—**Swedish Proverb**

***Note from the Editors:** The Skeppsholm Bridge in Stockholm features a pair of gilt crowns that honor the Swedish royal family (Fig. 202.2).

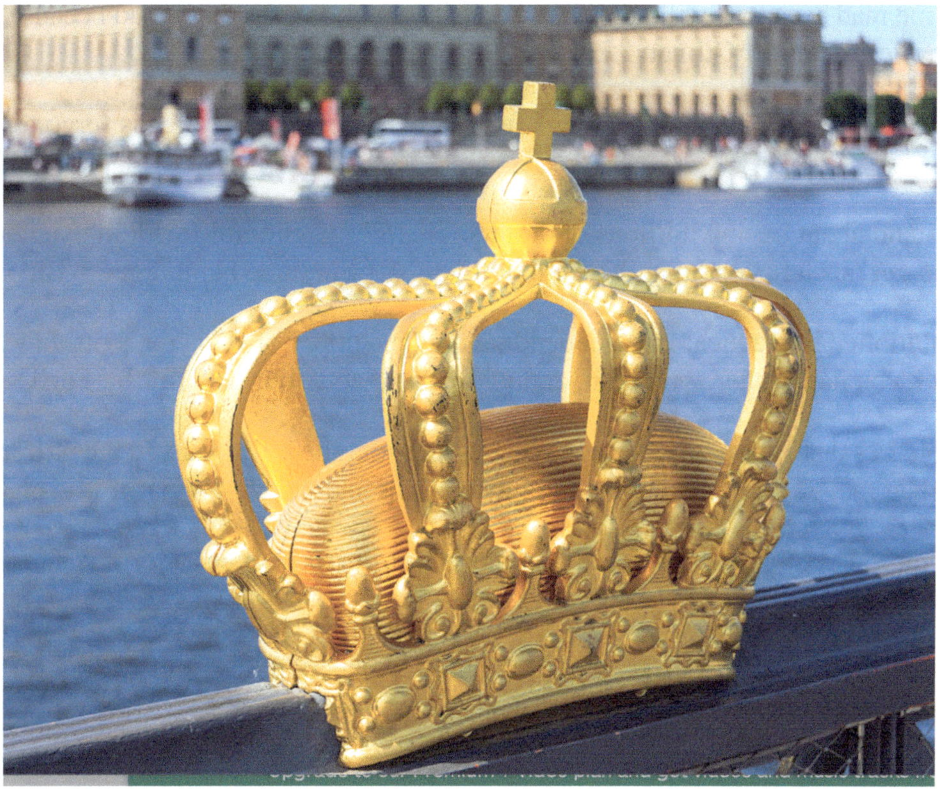

Fig. 202.2 The famous gilt crowns on the Skeppsholm bridge sit atop the iron railing. Photo: Image used under standard license from stock.adobe.com

- If you have trouble imagining a 20% loss in the stock market, you shouldn't be in stocks.—**John Bogle**
- Rich people stay rich by living like they're broke. Broke people stay broke by living like they're rich.—**Anonymous**
- The four most dangerous words in investing are, it's different this time.—**Sir John Templeton**
- Answer me this, if your TV wasn't broken in the first place then why do you need a new one? If your clothes still fit and aren't rags falling off you, why do you need more clothes? If your phone still does what it does, why do you need the newest brand out there? I could go on with these examples, but you get the gist. If it isn't broken, then why fix it? —**Harkin Headers**
- It is health that is real wealth and not pieces of gold and silver.—**Mahatma Gandhi**
- Money is like muck—not good unless it be spread.—**Francis Bacon**
- Frugality, I've learned, has its own cost, one that sometimes lasts forever.—**Nicholas Sparks**
- We're thrifty. We can live off our interest, save the principal, and let the kids go off and have a hoot.—**Keith Jackson**
- Know what you own and know why you own it.—**Peter Lynch**

- They deem me mad because I will not sell my days for gold, I deem them mad because they think my days have a price.—**Kahlil Gibran**
- The bitterness of poor quality remains long after the sweetness of low price is forgotten.—**Benjamin Franklin**
- I can understand about having millions of dollars. There's meaningful freedom that comes with that, but once you get much beyond that, I have to tell you, it's the same hamburger.—**Bill Gates**
- Money is multiplied in practical value depending on the number of W's you control in your life: what you do, when you do it, where you do it, and with whom you do it.—**Timothy Ferliss**
- Of the billionaires that I have known, money just brings out the basic traits in them. If they were jerks before they had money, they are simply jerks with a billion dollars.—**Warren Buffet**
- To acquire money requires valor, to keep money requires prudence, and to spend money well is an art.—**Berthold Auerbach**
- It's not how much money you make, but how much you keep, how hard it works for you, and how many generations you keep it for.—**Robert Kiyosaki**

Conclusions

To us, having money, or at least *enough* money, is just the beginning of wealth. We do not especially agree that you can be "wealthy" with little actual money—this maxim is a bit tired and from a different era. For one thing, we believe it is less likely that people can take the proactive steps to be healthy without sufficient funds.

In addition, it is also much harder to level out personal and professional crises or urgent situations without cold, hard cash—regardless of how rich you are in spirit. Sometimes a situation is simply easier to deal with by taking a ride-share home, even if it's a hundred miles, or staying in a hotel for 2 weeks. Conversely, wealth helps make money work to the most propitious level—and by this we mean emotional and psychological wealth as well as wealth of situation.

Lessons Learned

- Another favorite work hard/do well quote is from a country music song and is a great one for anesthesiologists:

  Pitter patter, let's get at her,

  Heard the rooster crow.

  If you ain't woke, it don't matter,

Cause it's time to go.

A hard day's work,

Getting in early.

—Austin Brown, "Earn It"

- Because that's what we do, we get up early, and we get to work. We've always liked getting to the hospital early and going into a dark OR to set it up for the day's cases. It kind of felt like opening the store and getting it ready for the day's customers, except that the commerce was the provision of anesthesia care. An added bonus was that our friends were often in the next room, setting up for their cases.

- Money and wealth are not the same thing! They are codependent variables.

- It seems like there is a book from the Japanese simplicity and serenity universe on everything. Each of the Sandson kids is getting a copy of Ken Honda's *Happy Money* as a holiday present this year. Some of it is just basics, but there are some good thoughts on the links between money and emotions. The author makes a clear distinction between money IQ and money EQ that we could all probably stand to review.

- The quotes above are just some of the editors' favorites on money, wealth, and success. If they don't resonate with you, there are many others out there. Find a couple to live with.

Authors

Jake Seagull holds a PhD in human factors psychology. Money has never been the main motivation for any of his life's choices. He doesn't claim to be an expert in finance, accounting, or economics, but has had a lifelong personal and professional interest in how and why people do what they do.

Neil Sandson and **Cathy Marcucci** have shared investment accounts and expense books since 1992. They count themselves beyond fortunate to have never had a serious disagreement about either, even when Cathy gave way, way too money to dog rescues.

Commonsense Considerations About Money and Wealth

203

Cobin Soelberg, Harriet W. Hopf, Amy J. Robbins,
Amr E. Abouleish, Richard G. Sheffield,
and Catherine Marcucci

Contributors:

Edwin G. Avery IV, MD

Ronald S. Bank, MD

Christine A. Doyle, MD

Raymond G. Graber, MD

Vincent L. Hoellerich, MD*

Introduction

There was some discussion between the editors over whether we should do a chapter with specific practical money and wealth topics. The point was made that we aren't able to give actual financial advice. And we're not! Even though one of us *is* a financial planner, the content herein is not intended to be specific financial advice but rather some of the valuable information that we received in our own

C. Soelberg (✉)
Bend Anesthesiology Group, Principal Advisor – Greeley Wealth Management, Bend, OR, USA

H. W. Hopf
Departments of Anesthesiology and Biomedical Engineering, University of Utah, Salt Lake City, UT, USA

A. J. Robbins
Stanson Health, a Premier Inc. Company, Charlotte, NC, USA

Atrium Health, Carolinas Palliative Care and Hospice Group, Charlotte, NC, USA

A. E. Abouleish
Department of Anesthesiology, The University of Texas Medical Branch, Galveston, TX, USA

R. G. Sheffield
Author – Medium Platform, Managing Editor UPS.com (retired), Atlanta, GA, USA

C. Marcucci
Department of Transfusion Medicine, Clinical Center, National Institutes of Health, Bethesda, MD, USA

S. Mohamed et al. (eds.), *Anesthesia Bridges*, https://doi.org/10.1007/978-3-032-08294-7_203

salad days. There are a hundred ways to put together a personal and family financial plan, and legions of certified professionals to help you do that. We are not those people—we wish to make that abundantly clear.

However, there are three reasons that we decided to go ahead and pull together a checklist:

First, every conversation Cathy Marcucci had with her mentors or spouse concerning a significant career change started or ended with the question, "Can you (we) afford to do it?" **Wendye Robbins** made the same point when asked how to prepare for a major career jump—get your financial house in order and keep it that way. We think financial planning and topics are just a continuation of career development and planning. A great financial plan should plan for many contingencies, of course. But at the end of the day, what you are doing when you make this plan is creating better options for your future.

Second, a draft copy of this chapter was pounced on by a group of young professionals in a different field and circulated as an informal worksheet.

Third, one of the editors commented, "I wish there had been something like this tucked away at the back of the anesthesia books I was reading way back when. It would have reminded me regularly to at least consider these topics."

Fourth, building financial security and learning about these topics is a process! You don't need to do all of this at once. Some of these issues will resonate with you, and others will not. Think about building your financial foundation over the course of many years. Building habits takes time.

So, here goes, and remember this is what we were advised and found useful. The information below doesn't replace the detailed and ongoing discussions you will need to have with your life and financial partners and your advisors, but hopefully will serve as something of an outline:

- Wanting to be financially successful in your anesthesia career is a reasonable aim. But what does that mean? We work hard in somewhat hazardous conditions and don't have an infinitely long career span. Having a big pot of money is not the end goal. It's what that money allows you to do that really matters!

- As you progress in your career and life, you'll find that dollars aren't the most important currency we have; time is. The older you get, the more precious time becomes.

- You will be asked about your priorities when meeting with your financial planner. Although when meeting with clients, **Cobin Soelberg** prefers to ask them about their values—not always the same thing as priorities. Starting as a young anesthesiologist, you might think, well, my priority is to do and have it all. First off, everything cannot be a priority! But life doesn't tend to work out that way. Every single one of us has made trade-offs. The most significant decisions tend to be about housing, schooling, who will be employed away from home, and how much. Some of us chose private schools or to have a spouse cover the home front full-time.

- While you get to make the decisions, you don't also get to control the consequences. Having one partner stay home might mean a smaller house and shorter or less frequent vacations. Some of us chose to live near excellent public schools and then had the funds for bigger houses or more home renovations and more elaborate (and expensive) recreational options, and vacations. But everybody eventually starts prioritizing in some way, especially when the kids arrive. Your life will feel richer and fuller if you live consistently with your values.

- Regardless of what priorities you decide for your family, accept that you may always wonder if you should have done it another way. Once, Cathy Marcucci was sitting outside the OR talking to the surgeon while waiting for the nurses to come in for a call case. She was wrestling with private school decisions and asked her surgical colleague what he had done and whether he had regrets. He replied that he didn't have regrets but still had doubts years later.

- His exact quote was, "You may never know for sure if it's the right thing. You have to accept that sometimes you won't know before, during, or after if this was the best use of your money. You decide the best you can on what you think is true at the time. And then, if you need to change the decision a year later, you remake it." His point is to try to know your children's strengths and needs as intimately as possible and then use your money and the options you have to foster those strengths and address any areas that might be helped.

- We structured this chapter in the ways we thought most critical to address, hence why protecting your income came first, then how to save, then covering what you might want to spend all your hard-earned cash on. Regardless of our individual decisions, we never regretted for an instant trying to do what was best for our families. Our families are always our overarching and main priority!

- Ultimately, what we are trying to accomplish by addressing all these financial topics is to give our future selves better options, whether it is saving money for our kids' college education, our own retirement, or a long sabbatical.

- Think back to who you were when you decided to be a physician. Could that version of you have imagined what you want and need 10 or 20 years later in life? Do you think you'll be any better at predicting what your future self will want?

- We guarantee one thing—your future self will appreciate better choices—better health, strong social ties, and a nest egg that allows you to live the way you want. And most importantly, time to spend with the people you love.

- We believe that wealth is the ability to spend your *time* doing what you love with the people you love for as long as your heart desires. What does this look like for you? If you take away nothing else from this advice, get clear in your mind that "wealth" is a nuanced and multi-layered concept. Our idea of what constitutes wealth is below. Each type requires investment and pays dividends.

Types of Wealth

- We often think of **financial wealth** first. It's easy to measure and compare. And while important, it is far from enough.
- **Physical and mental wealth** is arguably the most important state of wealth you can be in. Anything you do and any decision you make should not sacrifice your family's wealth in these areas. If you make the decision to short your own physical and mental wealth, make sure that the payoff is great indeed and the decrements to your health and well-being are ultra-short. You cannot burn through this wealth category and expect to "win" the long-term wealth game. It can't be done.
- **Social wealth** is what this entire book is about. As we say elsewhere, we are all on the same train. Your professional and personal relationships will make or break your life, way more than the dollars in your account.
- **Intellectual wealth** requires consistent commitment, energy, and persistence. In the medical field, you are what you know and what you know how to do. Don't let your acquisition of intellectual wealth slip too badly, no matter what else is going on in your life.
- **Time wealth is an incredibly important wealth concept.** What if you flipped the concept of time as desperately limited and viewed it as an incredibly valuable commodity to be utilized, resourced, and respected rather than feared? More on this below and in Chap. 207.

So, you've worked hard and thought deeply, and acquired wealth that is meaningful to you. How do you go about keeping what you've earned? Some thoughts on asset protection below.

Asset Protection

First, let's get this established—your unrestricted medical license may not be your most important asset, but it's way up there. Please do not do anything that will jeopardize it. One of us recently got a call from a family member with an extremely painful kidney stone—could they have a script for a week of narcotics or borrow some oxycodone left over from recent dental surgery? Sorry, but not able to help. Many doctors also get into trouble with Medicare or insurance fraud. No amount of money is worth losing your license!

Protecting Your Most Valuable Asset

What is your absolutely most valuable asset? Our answer is always your time and attention. But after that, your most significant asset is your future earnings. With this in mind, purchasing an individual, own-occupation disability policy is one of your most critical decisions. These policies tend to be less expensive the younger the age you buy them. The best disability policies cost about 3–4% of your income. And you win if you never have to use it! But if you are ever disabled and unable to work, an individual disability policy will be a financial lifeline.

- *Protect your hands!* Hire a lawyer as soon as you realize you need to use your short- or long-term disability, especially if you plan to continue working in a non-anesthesia context (e.g., an academic role or pre-op clinic). In Harriet's experience, disability insurance companies will ignore the own-occupation component and deny your claim because "you are still working full time." One letter from a lawyer and all that can change. Human resources can likely recommend an experienced lawyer.

- In many ways, a solid disability insurance policy is more important than a life insurance policy. Also, the lawyer in Cobin Soelberg will tell you that words (and definitions) matter! Read this policy. Have your financial planner read your policy. Aim to ensure 50–60% of your income—remember, this is a post-tax benefit.

- Owning an individual disability policy hits incredibly close to home for this author. Cobin's best friend from medical school, and a brilliant anesthesiologist, died from a Grade III astrocytoma in his forties. After the brain tumor was diagnosed, he never worked again for almost two years before he passed. His family would have been financially devastated had he not had solid disability insurance. Most importantly, he spent the last two years of his life with the people he loved, skiing, and mountain biking. What else can you ask for?

- Ok, time for just a few critical specifics—purchasing an own-occupation rider is a must. This rider means your policy will pay out if you cannot perform your duties as an anesthesiologist. A rider is an additional "piece" of coverage or protection you are purchasing. Kind of like a buffet for your insurance policy.

- Non-cancellable and guaranteed renewal is another mandatory rider. Otherwise, the insurance company could raise your rates or cancel your policy at any time.

- A few other riders worth considering:

  - *Partial disability*—this allows you to return to work less than full-time and still maintain your income

  - *Cost-of-Living adjustment*—the value of your benefit increases over time, *but only* kicks in once you become disabled

  - *Future benefit increase*—allows you to buy additional coverage. As you'd imagine, your income will grow as you get later in your career. This rider allows you to increase your benefit as well.

- Both the financial and legal professionals for the Sandsons strongly advised an umbrella liability policy as well. They felt this was really important to protect the assets of physicians, who are very easy to research online.

***Note from the Editors:** We asked Cobin Soelberg to tell us about his favorite bridge and he immediately sent us his short and succinct vote (Fig. 203.1):

> I was kind of thinking I would give a shout-out to the Ben Franklin in Philadelphia. It isn't pretty at all, but it's ALL Philly!

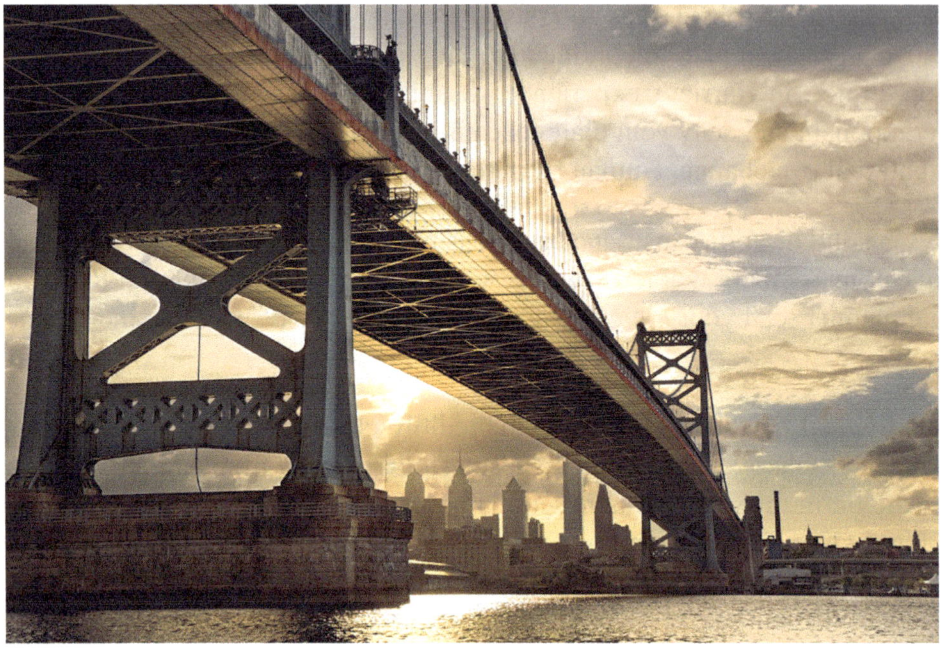

Fig. 203.1 The Benjamin Franklin Bridge, known to locals as "the Ben Franklin." It connects Philadelphia on the west to Camden, New Jersey, on the east, and is owned and operated by the Delaware River Port Authority. It was dedicated as part of the 1926 Sesquicentennial Exposition and was the longest suspension bridge in the world until 1926. The bridge carries pedestrian/cyclist, vehicular, and rail traffic. Photo: Image used under standard license from shutterstock.com

Life Insurance and Last Will *or* the Bets You Don't Want to Win—From Amr Abouleish*

Although applicable to others, I will focus on those readers who are married and have children. You need life insurance and a will. But God willing, you won't need either for many years. And Cobin feels strongly that you also need life insurance if anyone else, such as your partner or parents, depends on you for income.

Life Insurance

There are two major types of life insurance: term and whole life. Term life is when your premium just covers life insurance—if I stop paying, the insurance plan has no residual value. Whole life is term life, plus you pay an extra premium, like long-term savings. If you reach an age and are still alive, then there is value in the policy. I chose a term life policy since any excess income was used for college savings, paying off debt, or other investments.

How much life insurance you need is the next major question. If you have small children, consider the awful situation that you die tomorrow. What financial support do you want to give your surviving spouse and children? For example, let's say you want to (1) pay off the mortgage of your home, (2) fully fund a college fund for each child (at least $250,000 each), and (3) provide income for 10 years so your spouse can focus on the children as needed. You add this up for yourself… it won't be small. Finally, try to get term life insurance for an extended period, such as 20 years, with level premiums so your payment won't change.

- Watch out for people trying to sell you expensive whole-life policies—term life is much cheaper, and you can use the difference to pay down loans or invest the rest. The insurance agents make a bundle by selling you a whole life policy. These rarely make financial sense for physician households.

Last Will

In this case, you should be worried about the awful situation where both you and your spouse die at the same time, for example, in a car accident. You want to have legal documents that spell out who will care for your children, who will control their finances, and finally, a way so that your children don't inherit all the money at age 18 (create a trust fund), and the funds will be there in their twenties and thirties. Some experts recommend that young adult children not gain complete control of their inheritances until they are in their late twenties at the earliest.

Although everyone tends to want to ask the named guardian if they would be willing to be the guardian in this awful situation, I recommend that you don't for several reasons. Let's say you choose one set of grandparents. Then the other grandparents find out and get upset. Or you choose one of your siblings, but the other siblings find out. Further, what if circumstances change? The designated guardian gets divorced, gets older, or even dies. It's simpler to decide who you want to be the guardian. Change it over time if you need it to. Don't tell anyone other than your attorney. God willing, it will never come up, and you don't have to deal with drama.

We recommend that you invest in a good estate planning attorney to create your will and revocable trust—they will think of things you wouldn't. For example, if you have pets, you'll also want to make arrangements for their care. They are your dependents as much as your children. One estate planning attorney we know recommends that the family pets be endowed with a small amount from the estate to pay lifelong expenses—approximately $3000/year for a dog's remaining years of life expectancy, much more for a horse.

Estate Planning

I strongly recommend a revocable trust. A will still goes through probate. Probate takes time, is expensive, and is a public record because it goes through the courts. Having a revocable trust means determining what happens with your money and who cares for your loved ones when you pass, but avoids the public probate process. It is well worth the $5000–$10,000 you will spend to create a trust.

Finally, although this isn't strictly a wealth matter, make sure you have a living will and advance directives, even for young physicians who feel invincible. As mentioned elsewhere, the editors know a number of people who died young or suddenly!

***Note from the Editors:** The Galveston Causeway is a sentimental favorite of Amr Abouleish's (Fig. 203.2). He admits that it isn't a particularly beautiful bridge, but it is special to him because of the many times he drove back and forth over it to visit family and loved ones. We sent Amr several Causeway photos to choose from and he chose the one below because, in the upper right of the image, it also shows the pyramids of Moody Gardens. The Gardens were created by the Moody Foundation and are a public non-profit attraction that features the Aquarium Pyramid, the Rainforest Pyramid, and the Discovery Pyramid.

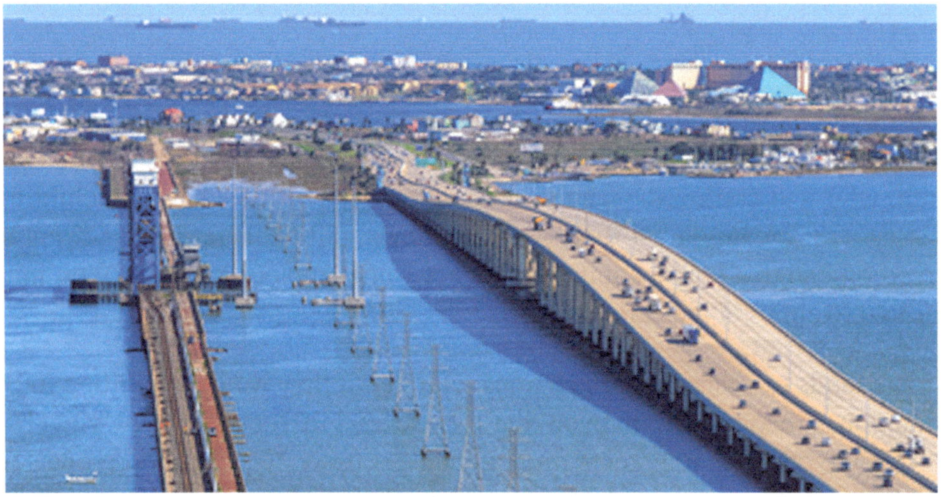

Fig. 203.2 The official name of the "Galveston Causeway" is the George and Cynthia Mitchell Memorial Causeway. It is actually a set of causeways that connect Galveston Island to "mainland" Texas. The original causeway was built in 1912 and carried both rail and auto traffic. Two causeways were built to the west of the original structure and opened starting in 1939. They carry the southbound and northbound traffic of Interstate 45. The original causeway now carries only rail traffic. This original route was listed on the National Register of Historic Places in 1976. The roadways were extensively rebuilt from 2003 to 2008, partially as a result of damage from Hurricane Ike. Photo: Image purchased and used under standard license from iStock.com

Saving

- Start by paying yourself first. Figure out a plan to repay your student loans and save for retirement. The best advice is to make this automatic. So that you do not even see the money coming out or need to think about it, then live off the rest. As others have said, spend time thinking about *your* priorities. Not the docs you work with or in your community. Not how your parents expect a doctor's life to look. Just yours alone.

- As a young attending, you'll have lots to save for—repaying your student loans, saving for retirement, and the first mortgage. Then there are all the ordinary expenses—saving for cars, a new furnace or roof, or a big vacation. These savings accounts are called vanishing funds—you save up for the expense, knowing you will drain the account at some point.

- It's also worth saving, just to save. Having cash on hand buys you time. It allows you to make decisions in your life that align with your values. You don't have to rush to a decision because you need to take a job that pays a higher salary or stay in a location your family dislikes. You won't have to sell assets when they have lost value. In short, having a cash cushion buys you peace of mind. Save a little bit each month. Start putting $1000 away each month as soon as you can.

- Don't get behind with the IRS or state taxing authority. Also, don't get too cute with your tax bill. It's one thing to have to pay a fine. It's another thing entirely to be looking at jail time.

- If you're not working hard enough in the hospital (ha!) and you don't mind working at home on the weekends and evenings, consider the following:

  1. Biomedical consulting can yield some impressive honoraria checks, and if you can become part of a speaker's bureau, the stream of both live and virtual lectures can help put a big dent in your expenses (for example, college tuition savings, 529 s, a new roof, a big vacation, or a vacation home).

  2. Additionally, if you are interested and willing to do medicolegal expert witness consulting, that pays very well and only requires a minimal amount of live travel. There are law firm listservs that you can sign up to be on and create a profile for your special interests or subspecialty, and lawyers will contact you.

  3. With both biomedical consulting and medicolegal expert witness work, you will be paid by 1099 (miscellaneous) income. Remember that 1099 income is taxed at about 50%, so keep at least half of what you earn to pay the taxes. Also, there are ways to lower your taxable income through thoughtful use of deductions, which your accountant can assist you with. Some individuals set up private companies or LLCs and give themselves a salary to avoid the 1099 tax rates but check with an expert first to see what is possible. You can also set up a solo 401(k) and save more money in a pre-tax manner.

From **Harriet Hopf:** When I first met Leo, I was a medical student, and he was a business student. He was appalled at my lack of knowledge of finance and demanded I read Andrew Tobias' *The Only Investment Guide You'll Ever Need.* It's still my go-to—it's useful and clear, echoing much of the above, and gets revised every few years. My favorite savings advice: buy tuna, or whatever your staples are, in bulk when it is on sale. Dependent, of course, on having the cash available to do so—going into debt on your credit card would wipe out the savings pretty quickly.

Retirement Accounts

- Saving in pre-tax retirement accounts is one of the few ways physicians have to save significantly on income taxes. It is worth maxing out these accounts whenever possible.

- Max out 401(k) or 403(b) or SEP-IRA early and always, if you can, and get the match, if offered. It's free money. Compound interest is amazing (Warren Buffet says it's the eighth wonder of the world!) if you start as a resident and look at how it's grown when you become 65.

- You'll have different options if you are in private practice, such as 401(k) and Cash Balance Plans vs. academics or government, such as 401(a), 403(b), or 457(b). While there are some critical differences, these are places to save pre-tax. Utilize as many as you can.

- Even as a high-income physician, you can make Roth IRA contributions—check out a backdoor Roth conversion. Having tax-free money in retirement is a huge win.

- If you have the extra funds, saving more in brokerage accounts gives you even more flexibility. You can access these funds at any time, tax-loss harvest, and use those capital losses directly against any capital gains.

- Dual incomes accelerate the ability to save and invest. If you have thought long and hard about both parents working and decided to go for it, the money helps cushion the emotions—it really does.

- The robo-investors are good these days for smaller amounts. Our kids used them for birthday and graduation cash from their grandparents.

But When Do I Get to Spend Some Money?

Housing

- From **Cobin Soelberg:** I strongly advise my early-career physician clients to consider renting, at least temporarily, for their first job. Many of you will leave your first job after several years. You won't know everything important to you about your career until you get into private practice or academics. You may find that flexibility is what's most important—or having a close-knit group of partners. When you are in a rental, changing jobs and cities is relatively painless.

- Buying a house is an expensive and often frustrating process. I am still amazed at the fees and expenses that get swept in under "closing costs." Additionally, when you own, you are responsible for taking care of the upkeep of your home. Even if that means calling a contractor, plumber, or repairman, someone must have the time to do this. Just in this past week, I've had partners need emergency repairs to their heater, and I had to take time off work to make these repairs happen.

  – From **Harriet Hopf:** When we bought our first house (at age 35), we found a general contractor (aka handyman) we loved. We trusted him enough to outsource repairs—if he couldn't do it himself, he'd hire someone to do it and oversee their work. When we moved to Utah, we did the same thing. In fact, he's here in our house, overseeing the installation of a new water heater as I write this! Costs a bit, but probably less than taking a day off the OR to do it yourself. And he is better at quality control than we would be.

- Cobin Soelberg and his spouse happily rented for the first few years. This gave them the resources to pay off over $400,000 in student loans and save for a down payment. They never bought into the old trope that renting is throwing money away.

- What you are getting when you rent is flexibility. If you need to move, you can. You can take the extra funds you save from paying a mortgage and invest or pay off debt.

- Another piece to remember about buying a house: it's not just the closing costs, repairs, and upkeep that add to your monthly expenses. You'll be furnishing and redecorating as well. None of this is to say purchasing a house is the wrong decision.

- Other considerations have to do with schools—public vs. private. We'll discuss those later. Think about what trade-offs you are willing to make in terms of size and location. Don't forget about your commute, either. Time in the car is time you will never get back. As a side note, look at your callback requirement for the hospital. If you live further away, you may be spending call nights in the hospital.

- That said, housing can be a great investment and way to build wealth. But you kind of have to know what you are doing. **Amy Robbins** bought her first house the year she was a CA-1 and has been able to add to her net worth with every house purchase and sale since then. She's not a commercial flipper but always took the time to study the real estate market deeply and has done well with every one of her primary family residences. Cobin adds the following, "Real estate can be a fantastic way to build wealth. If you want a second or third job." Amy does not disagree with this assessment of the time she invested in her family's real estate portfolio.

***Note from the Editors:** Are there bridges that are also houses? Of course there are. Here is one of our favorites (Fig. 203.3).

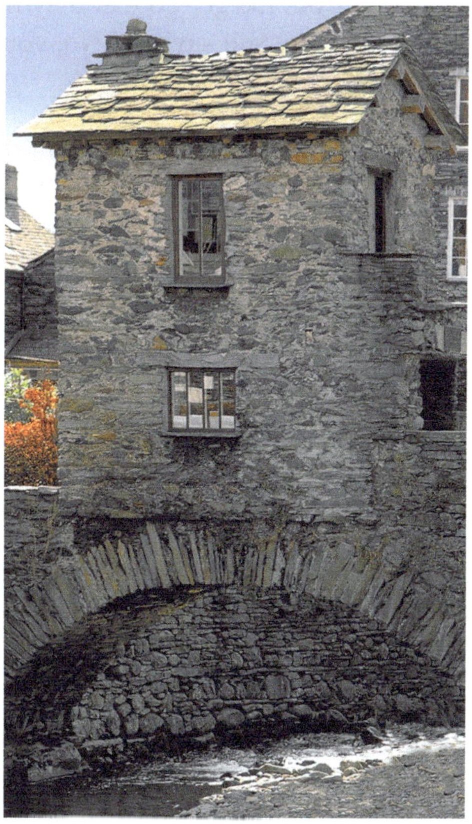

Fig. 203.3 The Bridge House in Ambleside dates back to the seventeenth century. It was originally built to store apples from the orchards on both sides of Stock Beck. It has also served as a counting house for a nearby mill, a tea room, a weaver's shop, a cobbler's, a chairmaker's, and a residential dwelling for a family of eight. It was restored in the 1920s and is a favorite building in the area and a popular attraction. Photo: Image used under standard license from stock.adobe.com

Cars

- The authors generally have not felt the need to put much money into cars. One quick way to burn money is to lease or buy a new car every 3–4 years.

- At one point, the Sandsons had two Honda Odyssey minivans—both green—named by the kids as "Big Green" and "Little Green." Cathy did not drive a "luxury car" until 2017 when she inherited her late mother-in-law's 2004 Lexus, which she drove until 2023. That car was 19 years old! She then gave it to her favorite neighborhood teenager—*Anesthesia Bridges* photographer Gavin Hess—who used it to go back and forth to school, work, and practice. But it has curtain airbags, doesn't burn a drop of oil, and has only 75,000 miles. Plus, it was thoroughly checked for safety by *Anesthesia Bridges* author **Bob Adolph**. So why not? Today, Cathy drives a 2013 Lexus. Neil went wild and crazy and bought himself a 2015 Honda CRV—in 2019, mind you.

- Ray Graber's wife drives a 2013 Audi, and he has driven a series of mid-value cars. One of Ray's partners, **Pete Matgouranis**, gave him a great tip—if you have kids, buy a cheaper safe vehicle (like a small SUV) about 4 years before your kid starts driving. Drive it for four years, then pass it down, which most of us in the editorial group have done in some way. However, a good policy is to retain ownership of the car—that way, the kids can use the vehicle, but you can control when and how that privilege is deployed. Stress to the kids from the get-go that they have the use of a car but not a car itself. Trust us, at least once you will hear yourself saying, "No, you can't drive there. You don't own the car, Mom and I own it, and the answer is no."

- For those who live in the mountains, a dependable AWD or 4WD vehicle is necessary. But so are winter tires. They are relatively cheap and worth their weight in gold! Never scrimp on tires or brakes!

- **Ed Avery** is the exception in our editorial group—he's a car guy. We thought for the longest time that he must be originally from Detroit, but he's not; he's from Rhode Island. You would think he'd maybe be into boats instead of automobiles. He has a sizable luxury and sports car inventory; however, he works very hard to earn "extra" money to support his car program so that it doesn't siphon money away from his other goals.

Vacations

- Here's where there was some variability among us. A bonding family summer vacation program was prioritized by some families, less so by others. Everybody gets so busy, and getting the gang together away from someplace inspiring is wonderful. The Grabers took family trips to Hawaii and a cruise from Barcelona to Rome and back. The Banks also made a big Hawaii trip recently with many bucket-list activities, but Ron commented that it was the first time he had ever taken a full two-week vacation. The Sandsons had a lot of money going out for two private school tuitions on their federal salaries, and so tended to hang out at the pool during the summer with just a tiny bit of family vacation time at the Delaware beaches. Good old Mom and Dad did manage to squeeze in a few short, focused-interest trips with the kids separately—for example, a sailing trip for Lisa and Neil in the Virgin Islands and the early rounds of March Madness and minor league baseball road trips for Charlie and

Cathy (sports Mom). The kids also went to cool places to see family friends and on Scout trips, but these were very cost-conscious.

- These are all great examples of how our families had different values and different priorities. At the end of the day, you will be most satisfied if you are living a life aligned with *your* values. In medicine, comparing outward signs of wealth is very easy. Teddy Roosevelt said, *"Comparison is the thief of joy."* And it's also a losing game. There will always be a family earning more, spending more, and having more toys. Don't get on this treadmill.

- Be oh-so-careful about acquiring extra stuff. It's so easy to get into this situation when you are younger. You work hard, and it's natural to want nice things. But then you get to the age when you have to clean out your parents' house, and it's a big eye-opener. All that stuff going out to the consignment shops and flea markets, and Goodwill. That your parents paid their hard-earned money for. It's sobering. And then you start looking around uneasily at your own house and all the stuff you have to store and heat and cool and insure and maintain and keep up. It's not simply the original cost, it's also the time you spend buying it and taking care of it. And if you have a big house on a large, manicured lot, all that green grass is really nothing more than a reflection of the money you've poured into it in mowing, watering, and fertilizing costs. If that's what's important to you, great, go for it. But those lawns that look like the putting greens at country clubs take a lot of dough, is all we're saying.

- *"The idea that material things can't bring happiness is only true if you buy the wrong stuff."* —Raval Navikant

- A corollary to the above is that it is not always true that experiences matter more than material things. Sometimes, the idea of what to do is just not enough to kick off the escapade or the adventure. Sometimes you just have to invest in the gear. And better gear often means a better experience.

Kids, Private Schools, and College Education

- Kids and money—the ever-important issue of the kids! It was so interesting and educational for us to compare notes. At first, it seemed like the only similarity was that we all gave our kids plenty of advantages. But as we discussed it amongst ourselves, it became apparent that each of the editors has been happy to support our kids, but those gifts came with an emphasis on productivity and achievement. Not one of us has just turned the money spigot on full blast.

- The school question—public vs. private. All of us prioritized education and invested heavily therein, tempered with expectations and common sense.

- A fair number of our kids went to private schools, K-12 through college, but were expected to treat that with respect and make the most of that opportunity.

- Of course, the kids who went to public schools did exactly the same. And the advantage of a mid-sized or larger public school is that they often have expanded opportunities for activities like marching bands and greater diversity of all sorts, always a good thing. Participation in a marching band requires discipline and commitment during the school year—and this often carries over to the summer season with "summer band practice."

- Virtually all our kids did a lot of volunteer work and social action as teenagers, which was prioritized by all of us. The list of the kids' volunteer work is long and, dare we say, quite impressive, given that these kids were also playing sports and instruments and studying.

- But even with busy sports and study schedules, the kids still found time for assisting in Sunday school at church, helping with youth sports, tutoring, advocating for diversity/equity/inclusion at school, Habitat for Humanity, and donating blood as older teens. Or a vast range of Scout projects, book drives, food drives, cooking at home for food kitchens, ecology projects, and volunteering hundreds of hours as hospital patient transport staff.

- One of our motivated teens even collected luggage and then decorated and filled suitcases with toiletries and other items for kids in foster care who were constantly moving from place to place and only had plastic bags to store their clothes and a few belongings. Social action efforts also seem to be prioritized by the colleges. We know a young person who landed his college spot (and scholarship!) when a recruiter called the high school, specifically looking for a kid with a specific minimum ACT score and a lot of social action.

- Many of our kids held part-time jobs in high school. And not do-nothing, fluff jobs, either—actual teenage jobs like we had back in the day. Collectively, they drove the pie cart and worked the deli counter at the grocery store, rented bikes and golf carts at the beach (**Vince Hoellerich's** kids), did maintenance work on school grounds, staffed YMCA daycare rooms, waited tables at a pizzeria, worked at bakeries, raked leaves, managed ice cream shops, did private babysitting, worked at summer camps, refereed youth soccer, did yard work, worked horse shows, shoveled snow, walked dogs, and lifeguarded. And the list goes on. Your kids have watched you work hard and impressions sink in.

- We parents of working kids saw to it that Roth IRAs were funded partially with the kids' earnings, but then parents tended to match contributions. We cannot overstate what a powerful gift this is! Teaching your kids about the value of saving and indirectly giving them an enormous leg up with the power of compounding. The Sandson kids were required to deposit half of all earnings into their Roth accounts, but then had leeway in what they did with the other half. But some of us did not feel so strongly about the kids working—if the academics were going well, that was enough. You will know your children best.

***Note from the Editors:** Vince Hoellerich's favorite bridge is the Bixby Canyon Bridge in California (Fig. 203.4):

> This bridge is a favorite of mine because it's framed by the spectacular beauty of Big Sur and the Pacific Ocean. It has incredible architecture and engineering and was completed during the height of the Depression for…..$200,000!

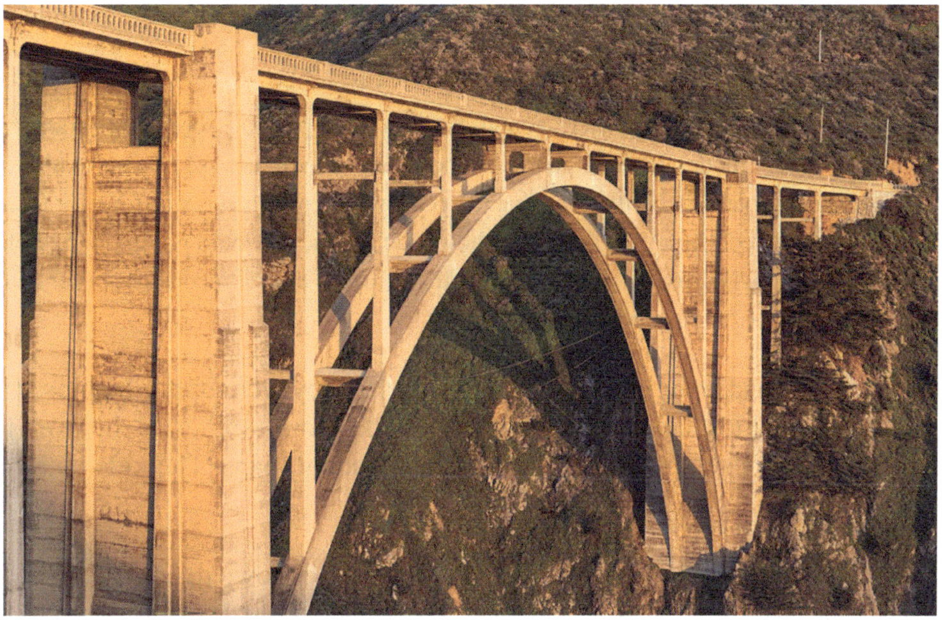

Fig. 203.4 The Bixby Canyon (Creek) Bridge is a reinforced concrete, open-spandrel arch bridge located about 120 miles south of San Francisco on State Highway 1. It is a treasured and much-photographed California landmark due to its aesthetic design and graceful architecture. It underwent a $20 million seismic refit in 1996. However, it still does not meet modern earthquake standards due to its narrow width. Photo: Image used under standard license from shutterstock.com

Financing College

- Start a 529 account for each kid as soon as they are born and max them out to your ability. Your state may give you a tax break; if so, it's worth considering. Otherwise, you can open a 529 run by any state—look for diverse investing options and low fees. Remember that anybody can contribute to a 529—grandparents qualify as donors. You can also change the beneficiary—so if one child doesn't use all their funds, it can be transferred. And you are allowed to take matching 529 money out penalty-free and tax-free if your kids get scholarships.

- One of us was able to put in only $200 for each kid per month. Still, with the stock market appreciation and the power of time and compounding, the 529 s covered seven semesters of private college tuition when the time came. During a phone call, the bursar's office even remarked, "Good thing you did this; otherwise, you would have been screwed when this tuition bill had to be paid." And this was the bursar's office saying this! Merit scholarships covered the rest.

- And with the passage of the SECURE Act 2.0, parents can transfer a lifetime maximum of 35,000 dollars from a 529 to a Roth IRA for the named beneficiary. This may not make sense for every family. But for those families with extra savings in a child's 529, this is a remarkable way for parents to jump-start savings for their children!

- But there are many ways to handle the college question. The Grabers decided to finance three college educations, and here was Ray's approach:

  Thinking like an engineer—when the kids were young, I set up three possible scenarios—state school (cheap), out-of-state public university (moderate), and private schools (expensive). I looked up current tuition and room and board, and tried to extrapolate with inflation what the costs would be when it was time for them to apply for college. I chose the moderate cost option to determine how much money I would put in our 529 plans each year to keep us on track for that goal. Reassess progress annually. If, in the end, someone gets a scholarship, great—the money can always be detoured to another kid.

- The Marcucci/Sandsons had a slightly different approach. They were up for helping with private colleges/universities, but the kids had to have some skin in the game—either do the work to get a significant amount of merit scholarship or expect to take out student loans. The kids both hustled and got the scholarship money.

- Let us repeat this—consider state colleges! It's now widely acknowledged that's where a lot of educational value is, and you have subsidized part of it already in taxes. Some are excellent schools, especially in the STEM fields. There isn't a major public or land grant university that doesn't have an *excellent* engineering college, and they are very competitive and prestigious. Georgia Tech, Virginia Tech, the University of Illinois, Purdue, Iowa State, NC State, and the University of Michigan come immediately to mind. Traditionally, the number one school in the country for chemical engineering is…the University of Minnesota. Tied for number one is the University of Wisconsin's department of chemical and biological engineering, which was chaired by *Anesthesia Bridges* author Mike Graham.

- If your child is applying to a field that requires a portfolio, don't forget to check to see if you can be considered for a portfolio scholarship or award. This can be a sizable five-figure sum—Lisa Sandson's portfolio prize covered an entire year's tuition costs. One of the Graber kids was also awarded a sizable portfolio scholarship.

- *Grad school:* We found that we tended to be very willing to help finance college, but that the kids were on their own for grad school or if they needed extra years due to changing majors. Have this discussion and set these expectations early with the kids.

What About Paying Off My Own Student Debt?

- Education of all types and at all stages of life is worth investing in. First, your own, and then those of the ones you love. Lately, so much has been written about crushing medical school debt. But the truth is that it can be dealt with if you take the problem on directly. It might require close and careful consideration of your daily budget, what job you take after training, where or what kind of house you buy, and where your kids go to school. So be it.

- For example, when they were first starting, Harriet Hopf and her husband made the disciplined decision to live on just half of his salary to knock out *all* of the student loans (over $150,000 in 1986 dollars, which is equivalent to $350,000 in 2019 dollars) and get the money together for a house down payment. They also saved enough in this very busy seven-year interval for a year of international travel. And *then* continued to live on this budget for a time, even after Harriet became an attending, to jumpstart the investment portfolio.

- There are many options for refinancing, both public and private student loans. One of your best returns on time will be understanding which program makes the most sense for your situation. You will save tens of thousands of dollars in interest by refinancing.

- Private loans should *absolutely* be refinanced to a lower rate. If you are not qualifying for Public Service Loan Forgiveness, refinancing your federal loans is likely a solid option as well.

Expert Help

- Professional help—get what you need! Be honest with yourself, and do not feel guilty about it. Trust us, it is fine to hire top-notch child-care, animal care, lawn care, cleaning help, legal support, meal services, or whatever is required so that you can focus on what is most important and valuable to you. Figure out what's making you anxious and stressed, and buy your way out as much as is reasonable and possible. *And do not feel guilty.*

- In the business realm, your team may include a financial planner, an accountant (CPA), and an attorney. Finding a CPA who helps with tax planning rather than just filing your taxes is a big help.

- Use a financial planner for physicians! Doctors can't automatically be expert investors, too! For one thing, they probably don't have the time. The best financial planners focus on your values and purpose. Money is a tool to help you and your family live your values.

- Get employment contracts reviewed with the best legal help you can find and afford.

- It should go without saying, but *read* your offer letter. What are the expectations of your role? What resources will you have to support your success? If you decide to negotiate (highly recommended), remember that salary is not the only component of compensation. Salary may be standardized; consider negotiating for protected time, start-up resources, or loan repayment. Negotiation shouldn't be about competition; the best negotiation is a collaboration with your chair (or other boss) to ensure you have the resources you need to succeed at what you are being hired to do. Consider reading Fisher and Ury's *Getting to Yes* before you start.

- Also, make sure that your employment attorney is experienced with restrictive covenants for local re-employment and can advise on this. These restriction clauses can greatly bedevil a career.

- You'll need a trust and estates lawyer to draft your will and revocable trust. Ideally, work with someone referred by someone you trust. We found ours by asking a colleague in the law school for recommendations.

- Consider hiring legal help for any other large contract you are dealing with. When you are a physician, sometimes you aren't offered great terms, as the other party has looked you up on the internet and decided that you should cover the difference for the major screw up on the swimming pool or the new slate roof. But your lawyers won't have trouble saying, "My client will need better terms," or "No."

- Speaking of large contracts, there is the question of pre-nuptial and post-nuptial agreements. Our advice is.....some people have them, and some don't. It's a personal decision, and what is right will not be the same for every couple. Individual and marital financial situations evolve over time. Harriet Hopf and Leo McKinley had a pre-nuptial agreement covering their student loan issues, but made a bonfire of it once the loans were paid off.

- A prenup is worth considering for those coming into the marriage with significant individual debt or assets. Likewise, for those of you in second or third marriages, coming into these relationships with substantial financial resources, discussing a prenup is helpful.

- Both the financial and legal professionals for the Sandsons strongly advised an umbrella liability policy as well. They felt this was really important to protect the assets of physicians, who are very easy to research online. Litigious people will sometimes go where they think the assets are.

Teaching the Kids About Money

- Federal salaries are all public information and online, down to the yearly bonuses. So, Neil Sandson decided to use this transparency to start his children's financial education early. To be clear, the kids did not have the passwords to the retirement accounts. Still, each sat in on some meetings with the financial planners and the tax preparers in their late teenage years so that they understood that the parental money pie could only be divided so many ways and that taxes must be paid. And the kids had to do the rough drafts of their own tax forms. These were only 1040EZ forms, but it was a start. They were also required to be prepared to discuss their banking and investment statements every couple of months with their parents.

- Six of the Sandson kids' eight great-grandparents were impoverished Italian or Jewish immigrants who found work as grocers, clothiers, piece-work garment workers, carpenters, and bricklayers, so the children were made aware that there would be no enormous generational wealth transfer. The facts are the facts; best not to let anybody have any illusions, especially if they are at school with the big-money kids, which they were.

Charitable Giving

- Don't neglect or forget to pay your resources forward with charitable giving of your time and/or money. We've included some thoughts on this elsewhere in the book, but it bears reiterating—do some good with what you've got. There are so many needy groups and worthy causes, and fun ways to give.

- You can donate to the places where your kids are participating or volunteering. You can give back to the schools that helped you with scholarships, like Harriet. You can develop charitable giving to a huge slate of local, regional, and professional non-profits, like Harriet again. Or you can focus your giving on a small, supremely worthy, and needy charity, like Cathy and Neil and Barking Mad Animal Rescue. Don't give more than you should, but do give what you can.

- Give back to the anesthesia community! It doesn't have to be a check—remember, time is money.

Oh, Wow, We Made It—Now What?!

- If there is one thing that physicians know how to do, it's work hard and hang in there. We wanted to end this chapter for young people by asking them to think *now* about what happens when everything they've thought about and planned for has been successfully accomplished. The kids are launched, the house is paid for, the retirement accounts are doing what they are supposed to be doing, and you've done something meaningful in philanthropy. How do you negotiate the big payoffs and payouts after a lifetime and career of careful planning?

- The basic questions revolve around deciding on the balance between generational wealth transfer (and when to transfer it) and retirement spending. There are certainly worse problems in the world.

- **We believe that wealth transfer is important to most anesthesiologists.** It certainly is to the 30 or so people we informally surveyed on the subject. For one thing, a professional career is often how people with refugee and immigrant backgrounds—or who came from families with nothing—make their way in the world and climb the economic ladder. It's one thing to take a position of eschewing generational wealth transfer and adopting the whole "die broke" paradigm if your grandfather was in the class of 1959 at Princeton and your grandmother went to Wellesley. But perhaps your choice will be different, and you will say no way to that uber-expensive cruise around New Zealand and decide to help the kids with a down payment for a house instead (Figs. 203.5). It's perfectly fine to make the choice to build generational wealth and get your family out of poverty.

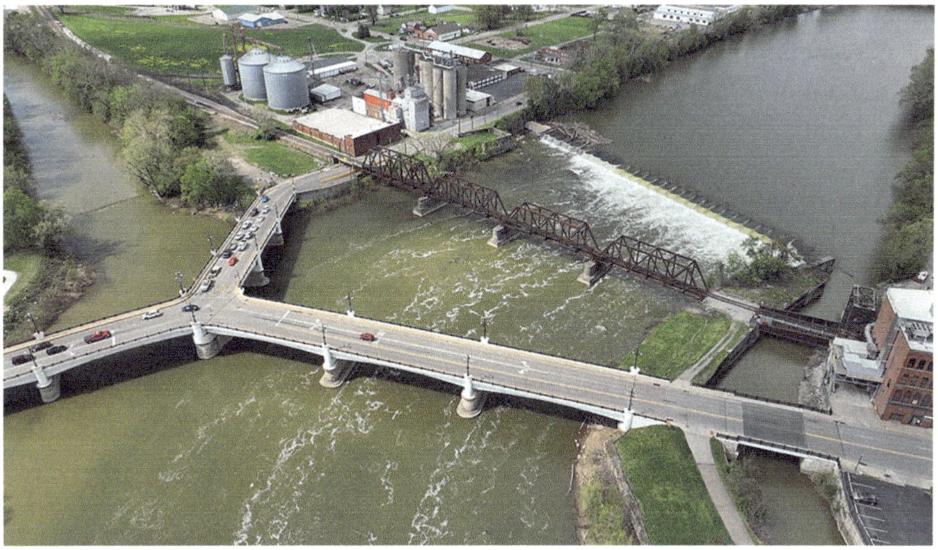

Fig. 203.5 The famous Y-shaped bridge in Zanesville, Ohio. Life is about choices and using what you have to get what you want. What is money but one of the most important tools life hands us? Go in the direction that meets your overall goals. Photo: Image used under license from stock.adobe.com

- **Because poverty does not make you strong—all it does is make you stoic in the moment**. The attendant damage, discouragement, or desperation usually has to be dealt with later. We could name at least six *Bridges* authors/editors who were the beneficiaries of family estates worth less than $5000, and we are not joking. This includes someone we know whose inheritance from her grandparents was one of the two spoons smuggled out of what is now Romania in the lining of a jacket. So, we remain firm in our advice that it is both prudent and rewarding to build generational wealth. **Everybody** wants to see their kids do better than they did—never met a parent yet who didn't.

- **But we also believe that you will want to spend some of that retirement money on yourself and that's a good thing, too**. Your personal interests and goals are as worthy as anybody else's, and it's your money. *Anesthesia Bridges* author **Richard Sheffield**, who is trained in industrial management as well as being an editor, blogger, and author, sent us the valuable thoughts and advice below. Keep them in mind as you travel your path. His wisdom is all about thinking clearly and constantly about what the destination is going to look like. He can be found online on Medium at *Spend Your Retirement Money!*

- **You saved for freedom—but don't be surprised if you have trouble flipping the switch from saver to spender.** Back in 2008, authors Michael Hurd and Susann Rohwedder described *The Retirement Consumption Puzzle*. They reported that over 30% of retirees expressed regret about not spending enough in retirement, even when they had the money. It's a real problem, and the sooner you admit to having it, the fewer years you'll waste being overly cautious.

- **Don't confuse getting older with getting less capable.** Society may want to start treating you like a child, but don't buy it. You're retired, not in kindergarten. You don't need to be coddled; you need fun, adventure, and stimulation of all the senses.

- **We'd rather look poor than indulgent**. Because luxury spending doesn't just cost money—it threatens identity. And identity? That's sacred ground. We don't fear running out of money as much as we fear looking indulgent. We can be addicted to modesty and afraid of looking or acting rich. But spending is something you do, not something you are. You built this wealth with hard work. Spending it is not a moral failure. You don't want to end up healthy, wealthy, and afraid to book a really nice hotel room.

- **In retirement, you're actually a time billionaire**. The term was coined by investor Graham Duncan, co-founder of East Rock Capital, during a 2019 episode of *The Tim Ferriss Show*. He pointed out that a billion seconds is about **31.7 years**—which means if you're in your fifties or sixties, you might have a *billion seconds* left to live. That makes you rich beyond measure… but only if you realize it.

- **Too much focus on wealth, and not enough on lifestyle**—We often end up sacrificing the thing we wanted (a rich, full life) for the thing that was supposed to get us there (money). If your net worth keeps growing and your joy doesn't, you're not thriving—you're hoarding.

- **Speaking of health, it's the best financial plan you never considered.** Physically active older adults spend up to 26% less on healthcare. That's not pocket change. That's a trip to Patagonia. Or at least a fancy massage chair. Every dumbbell you lift now might be a copay you dodge later.

- **There is no better version of you who is going to get things next week**. Psychologists have a name for this delusion: Future Time Slack—the idea that our future is somehow more spacious than the present. Every time you tell yourself you'll do something later, you're banking on a version of you that somehow has more energy, more motivation, and fewer distractions than you do right now. But the truth is, unless you change how you use your time now, next week will look exactly like this week… with slightly worse knees.

- **All retirement planning should start with one question**. **A:** Do I want my life to be very much like my life before retirement, just tweaked a bit to be more fun—or **B:** Do I want a life that is totally different from my life before retirement? Answering this question will let you confidently start moving, knowing that you're heading in the right direction, without all the pressure of having to figure out where you will eventually wind up.

- **Make space in your retirement for things you haven't thought of yet**. In the 1840s, the French called a new breed of idle ramblers "flâneurs." They were professional strollers—not the baby kind, the philosophical kind. They slowly walked through the city streets, just taking in the scene with no purpose or intent. The flâneur isn't lazy—he's just allergic to hustle culture. You need unfilled time and space to figure out how *who you want to become* is different from *who you are*.

- **No matter what happens with markets or politics—you are still getting older.** Political winds blow left and right, markets fluctuate up and down, but time only goes in one direction. The financial industry is always going to sell you on fear. That's how they get you to keep your money invested where they want it. Whatever happens to the Dow, this year is still happening to you. You can't time the market, you can't just wait it out, but you can absolutely waste your precious life trying.

Lessons Learned

- Please use the information above as a conversation starter with your partner or spouse, and your legal and financial advisors.

- Families and primary partner relationships come in all sizes, shapes, and variations. There are certain existing legal provisions pertaining to assets, wealth, and benefits if your family has a married couple and legally recognized children. If your situation does not, then you have increased needs for the best professional help you can find and afford, so do not scrimp on setting up your affairs completely to the best possible advantage. And remember that a family of one or two people is still a family and deserves as much thought and care, and careful planning as any. And pets are family members, too.

- Time is your most precious commodity—the years go by so quickly, and your family grows up and/or transitions through life stages before you know it. Remember that time is not a savings account, it's a melting popsicle.

- School decisions are big ones, and sometimes it seems like you have to "re-decide" them every year. Take comfort, you are not alone—a lot of us have been through this. Going in a different direction on the school's question doesn't mean that you aren't parenting well or that your initial decision was a bad one.

- Review the big issues and major decisions with a professional team—this might include your overall financial plans and goals, specific investments, important contracts, including employment contracts, life insurance, and wills.

- Give a bit to those who have worthy causes and financial needs. There are many groups for whom even $10 is a help. Such as every animal rescue non-profit in the country!
- Stay married if you can be happy and grow; don't get divorced unless you must—it can break you financially.
- Don't confuse what's truly valuable with what's merely expensive. And be really careful and thoughtful about acquiring too much stuff—nobody is judging you on the quality of your forks. Aim for the minimum amount of good quality possessions that allow you and your dependents to be comfortable.
- There will always be somebody who has figured out a way to make more money in their anesthesia career than you are making in yours. Don't spend too much time worrying or thinking about this—instead, wish them well, and concentrate on doing what's right for you.
- Work hard. Plan carefully. Enjoy the journey. When you get to a place of financial security, spend your money meaningfully and without guilt. And if you see a beautiful bridge, park yourself at a cafe and enjoy the view! (Fig. 203.6)

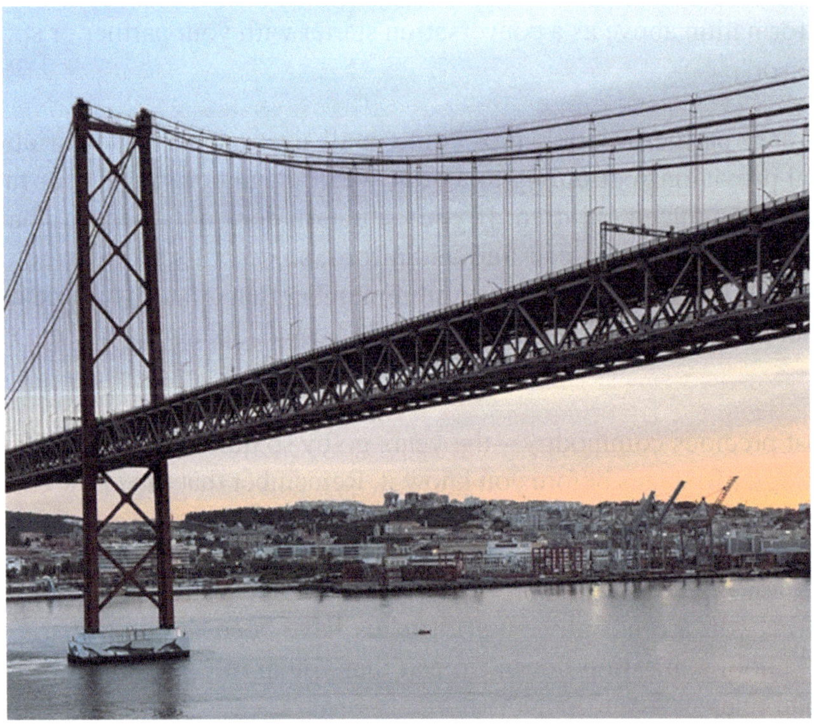

Fig. 203.6 The 25 de Abril Bridge in Lisbon, Portugal. The bridge was completed in 1966 and is often compared to the Golden Gate Bridge in San Francisco. Photo: Richard Sheffield

Authors

Cobin Soelberg is a private practice anesthesiologist and financial planner living in Bend, Oregon, with his young family and their sweet Rhodesian Ridgeback. He has always enjoyed learning and education, even if it meant a longer journey. And so, he took a leave of absence during medical school and earned a law degree. As a new academic attending, Cobin noticed the lack of financial knowledge and understanding from the residents and med students. After years of teaching and educating on financial topics, a close friend encouraged him to earn his Certified Financial Planner credentials and help other physicians earn financial freedom.

Harriet Hopf, Amr Abouleish, **Amy Robbins**, and **Cathy Marcucci** and the contributors to this chapter are all mostly through and on the other side of many of these issues. No one reports that they spent an enormous amount of time on car deliberations (except maybe Ed Avery?), but everybody agrees that a lot of time and thought was rightfully devoted to making the big decisions involving their families—and nobody regrets a second of time or a single penny invested in their loved ones. We reiterate that the information above is for educational and discussion purposes only. Your financial decisions should be made with the consultation and advice of your own qualified experts.

Richard Sheffield is a retired technologist and a successful writer and author. After graduating from Georgia Tech, he learned that understanding the latest wave of high-tech *and* being able to credibly write about it was a rare and valuable skill. He used this skill to surf the high-tech fields, jumping from solid state electronics, to microprocessors, to PCs and software, to the internet where he worked as the managing editor for the main website of UPS. He now finds himself neck deep in AI, still trying to not get left behind. When not traveling, he splits time between the heat of Atlanta and the more heat of Miami, where he loves spending time with his plastic surgeon girlfriend and avoiding the clinically horrifying procedure pics on her phone.

204 Anesthesia Paychecks—They Don't Exactly Come in the Same Shapes and Sizes

Edwin G. Avery IV

Introduction

It is well established that when we, as anesthesiologists, contract to provide anesthesia services for our employers, we will get paid for the work that we do. In this short essay, I want to share some of my recently obtained knowledge that was helpful in optimizing my salary in a manner specific for my own needs at a new anesthesia job.

In the interest of full disclosure, I am not offering financial advice, and I am certainly not a financial advisor. Rather, I am sharing some of my own research and my experiences in the hope that some of my anesthesia colleagues may see the topic of our anesthesia paycheck from a slightly different perspective.

Background

For the last 25 years as a practicing anesthesiologist, I derived the majority of my salary through a paycheck from my employer in the form of W-2 income. As a refresher, W-2 income means that the federal government is going to take a percentage of your wages for federal, state, local taxes, and Social Security (also known as a federal retirement benefit) from each paycheck. The rate that one is taxed at depends heavily on how much annual W-2-based income you receive from your employer.

There is a fairly short list of how an individual may be able to reduce their taxable income when one is paid through W-2 income. One way is to allocate a portion of your paycheck to a retirement savings account, such as a 401(k) or 403(b) account, in a tax-deferred manner, but you will have to pay those delayed taxes when you are retired and are withdrawing money from that account. In effect, by putting money into a retirement account, this temporarily shelters the money from being counted as part of your taxable income, and it grows tax-free during this period, if the markets are reasonably stable.

E. G. Avery IV (✉)
Department of Anesthesiology and Perioperative Medicine, University Hospitals Cleveland Medical Center, Cleveland, OH, USA

S. Mohamed et al. (eds.), *Anesthesia Bridges*, https://doi.org/10.1007/978-3-032-08294-7_204

One can also allocate pre-tax dollars to a college savings account, called a 529 fund. I have started tapping into the 529 fund that I set up for my daughter 17+ years ago, who is in college and is now using that money. As an incentive to promote education, the government allows these funds to remain untaxed if they are used for education-associated expenses—such as college or private grade/high school tuition, room and board, textbooks, a laptop for school, or food. Basically, these 529 funds are for qualified higher educational expenses (QHEE). Money that is withdrawn from a 529 account that is not deemed a QHEE is taxed at a standardized rate, and a 10% penalty is applied to the withdrawn funds.

My Personal Experience

To the best of my knowledge, these are two of the main ways by which we may reduce our taxable income when paid through the W-2 route.

Almost all of what I have just discussed is known by most of us and is the most common way anesthesiologists are paid. A second way that some anesthesiologists are paid is through a 1099 route, as opposed to a W-2. 1099 income is how independent contractors/business owners are paid. However, not all anesthesiologists who have 1099 income have a corporation or Limited Liability Company (LLC). For example, up until this year, I have always had 1099 consulting income from medical industry consulting and from medical expert witness work, but I never started a formal company. Instead, I kept all the 1099 income separate and filed both a W-2 and a 1099 (Schedule C) for my taxes. To be safe, I kept at least 50% of my 1099 income for taxes.

1099 income is taxed at a fixed rate, no matter whether the business is making a lot of money or is failing. The tax rate is dependent on the state you live in. Note that just because one is an independent contractor does not mean that they cannot have a three-or-four-year contract to provide services. Ultimately, the independent contractor negotiates with their employer, and a contract is set up that both parties agree to as far as benefits, salary, and duration of the employment.

***Note from the Editors:** Money should never be the sole endpoint, but it *can be* useful to get you over (some of) the crevices and cracks of life (Fig. 204.1).

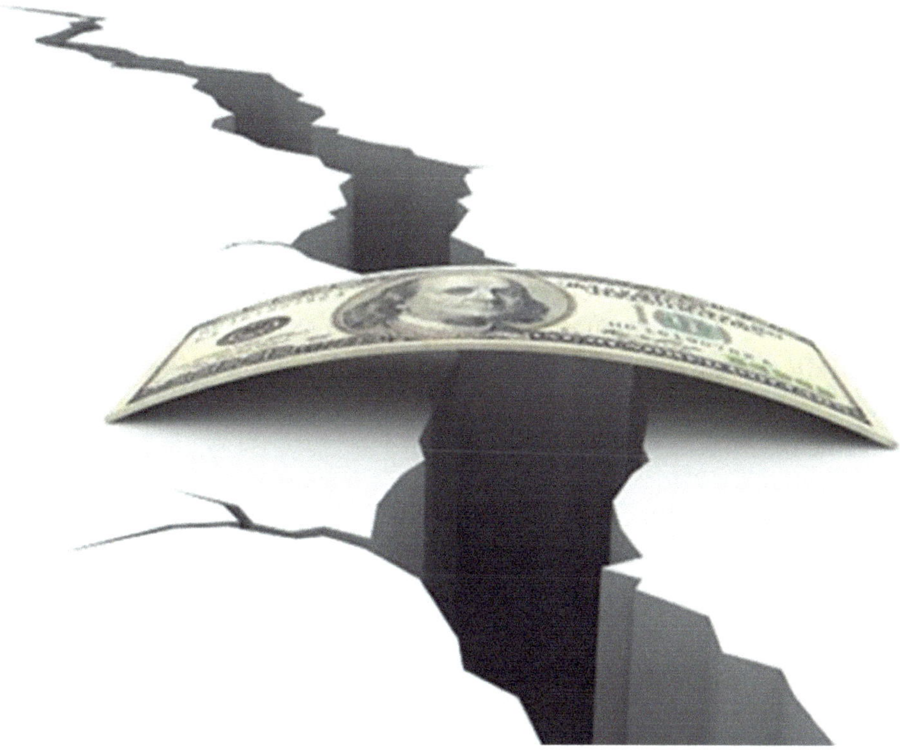

Fig. 204.1 A bridge built of Benjamins. Illustration: Image used under standard license from iStock.com

My Personal Research

In a deeper dive into the subject of how 1099 is different than W-2, let's consider that there are two major differences between 1099 and W-2 income. The first big difference is that when going the 1099 route, one's monthly salary does not have all of the standard withholdings and taxes taken out of the paycheck. This means that an individual has to plan to pay their federal, state, and local taxes on an ongoing quarterly basis or can pay all at once at the end of the year with a penalty. The second **huge** difference is that many business-related expenses that one accumulates as an independent contractor can be deemed deductible from one's taxable income.

As an example, if you purchase a vehicle with certain properties—such as a heavy-duty vehicle weighing greater than 6000 pounds, like a big SUV that is exclusively used for your business, a large amount of the cost of that vehicle can be considered a one-time tax-deductible expense. Similarly, the cost of gas and vehicle maintenance qualifies for a 58.5 cents/mile deduction. Other business expenses such as meals, travel, internet costs, computer, cell phones, and their usage fees, are fully tax-deductible.

As I previously stated, I think it is very important to understand that 1099 income is taxed at a set rate depending on what state one lives in, and could ultimately be a higher tax rate than the maximum that may be for a W-2 paid individual. However, the previously discussed business-related deductions serve to significantly reduce one's taxable income, and for that reason, the average tax rate for a 1099 individual is generally less than that of a W-2 paid employee.

An additional consideration is that 401(k) contributions are treated differently in each scenario. For the W-2 employee, the amount of retirement savings that can be contributed into a 401(k) is limited by two factors—a maximum annual contribution based on age, and how much money one makes—if your living expenses are too high, you may not be able to contribute the maximum amount for your age. On the other hand, an independent contractor can contribute an annual amount that is significantly higher—25% of annual compensation for specialized retirement accounts. As examples, a W-2 employee 50+ years of age can currently contribute a maximum of $27,000 annually to their 401(k), while in contrast, a 1099 employee with a SEP IRA (simplified employee pension individual retirement account) with an annual salary of $300,000 can contribute a maximum of $61,000. This is more than double what the W-2 employee can contribute.

One last consideration—as a health care provider with 1099 income and a LLC, one qualifies for the Safe Harbor 20% pass-through deduction, which permits married individuals to deduct an additional 20% of qualified business income if one's salary is below $315,000.

In summary, I have reviewed the very basic differences between how anesthesiologists are paid as a W-2 employee versus as an independent contractor/1099 employee. In my own transition from a mixed W-2/1099 employee to an isolated 1099 employee with a three-year contract, I am planning to contribute more for retirement and more to my children's educational accounts, because my tax rate will be lower and my salary higher.

I hope this information has opened the door for some readers to think a little differently about how we as anesthesiologists are paid. Lastly, there are two caveats. First, your employer must be willing to offer compensation on a 1099 basis; many employers do not extend this option to their employees. Second, there are a number of steps one must take to set up an LLC to leverage the possibilities of 1099 employment, and I strongly recommend consulting a professional financial advisor and/or legal team to accomplish this.

Lessons Learned

- Although most of us will probably start out our careers working as a salaried employee for a group or hospital, there may be some potential advantages to being an independent contractor if that form of employment compensation is available.
- The information above is the individual experience of the author and does not constitute financial advice. If you choose to explore the independent contractor route, make sure you have good legal and financial advisors to guide you on the legal and financial issues you will have to navigate.

Author

Ed Avery did both his residency and cardiac anesthesia fellowship at the Massachusetts General Hospital in Boston, where he stayed for almost 13 years before being recruited to Case Western Reserve University School of Medicine-University Hospitals, Cleveland Medical Center. He is a physician-scientist, having participated in over 20 clinical trials, and has authored dozens of book chapters and peer-reviewed manuscripts. He is an inveterate member of the hospital transfusion committee and is a great proponent for enhanced surgical recovery techniques. At home, he is the husband of his wife Lauren and father to his two young adult children, Sophia and Edwin. He is an avid exercise fanatic, and he relaxes by doing home projects and detailing the family cars.

Nine Hard-Won Pearls for Success in Academic Medicine (and Everything Else!)

205

Meghan B. Lane-Fall

Introduction

After years spent training and hungrily seeking knowledge about how to improve and succeed, I find myself now being asked for guidance on these same issues. Metaphorically, it is as if I am on an uphill hike toward the pinnacle of my career and have reached a clearing. There is clearly more ahead of me, but I've notched valuable experience under my belt and have a vantage point that offers a useful perspective. It has been an interesting and sometimes frustrating journey, made all the more difficult by navigating this challenge as a Black woman and first-generation scholar. As I reflect on what I have learned what I would have liked to know and what might be useful for others. I've distilled these lessons into nine key points:

1. **Practice gratitude**. It is so easy to get caught up in the quest for success (whatever that means to us) that our accomplishments and good fortune fade from view. Almost unconsciously, I practice gratitude daily. Sometimes it's taking a moment to enjoy a sunrise, a sunset, a warm day, pristine snow, a good meal, or my children's laughter. I am reminded of how many people cannot take these things for granted, which blunts the sometimes-daily annoyances, indignities, or frustrations that professional life can bring.

2. **Ask a lot of questions**. "Why?" is one of the most powerful questions we can ask. Indeed, one of my favorite techniques from quality improvement is "5 Whys," in which a clinical problem is stripped down to its root causes by asking this question five times. I find that many unspoken assumptions undergird our daily lives at work and home. These unspoken assumptions can keep us locked in unproductive patterns of behavior. They also reinforce systems that have led to inequality in care and outcomes and under-representation of marginalized groups in the hallways of power. Asking why, and then doing something about it, is one way to get closer to equity, improved performance, and better patient outcomes.

3. **Work smarter when possible**. When I started as a faculty member, I was a lab of one. I had to figure out scheduling, research logistics, graphic design, and more. As my lab and my research program grew, I just worked longer hours, still trying to do everything. It took me a few years to realize that just

M. B. Lane-Fall (✉)
Department of Anesthesiology and Critical Care, Vagelos College of Physicians and Surgeons, Columbia University, New York, NY, USA
e-mail: ml5302@cumc.columbia.edu

S. Mohamed et al. (eds.), *Anesthesia Bridges*, https://doi.org/10.1007/978-3-032-08294-7_205

because I could do something didn't mean I should. I learned how to delegate little things at first, like scheduling. As my team became more capable, I delegated more, also marshalling technology to help. By offloading some of my work, I realized that there were two major benefits. First, my time was freed to take care of work that only I could do, like writing grants. Second, the people to whom I delegated work learned new skills and sometimes surprised me and themselves with how capable they were.

***Note from the Editors:** Meghan Lane-Fall is at Columbia, which is in the Morningside Heights section of Manhattan, of course. The lovely and historic High Bridge is nearby (Fig. 205.1).

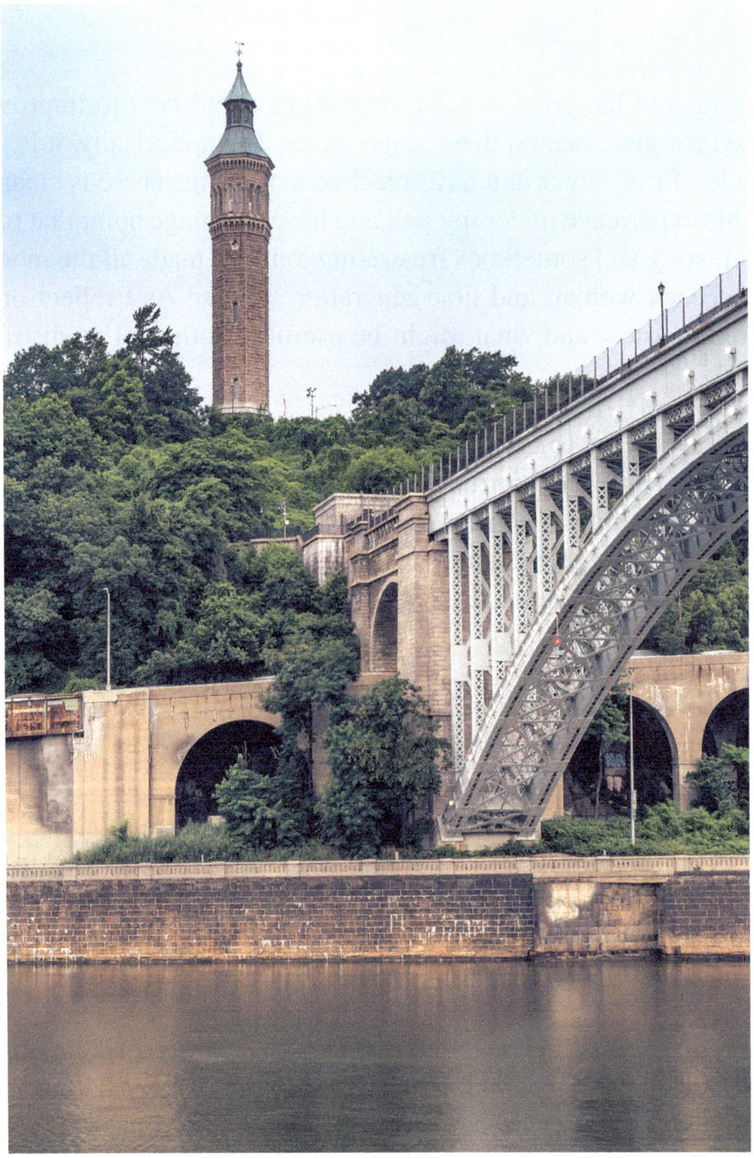

Fig. 205.1 The High Bridge in New York City spans the Harlem River between Manhattan and the Bronx. It is the oldest standing bridge in the city. It opened in 1828 as part of the Croton Aqueduct. It originally had 16 stone arches but underwent restoration in 1928, with five arches replaced with a single steel span. It underwent a second large restoration starting in 2009 and has been reopened to pedestrian and bicycle traffic. Photo: Image used under standard license from stock.adobe.com

4. **Give and ask for grace**. We all play multiple roles at home and work. While love is unlimited, time and energy are not, and sometimes we disappoint ourselves or others. To me, "giving grace" is the concept of extending understanding and forgiveness, even in the face of disappointment. I've found that assuming positive intent and extending grace, more often than not, results in better outcomes than becoming upset or disgruntled. Sometimes, I'm on the other end, having missed a deadline or disappointed someone. In these cases. I ask for grace—sometimes from myself—try to learn from the episode and keep moving forward.

5. **Network. A lot**. Although we tend to glorify individual industriousness, none of us is successful without help from many other people. Professionally, this includes mentors and sponsors, but it also includes countless other people with whom we interact over the course of time. I have found it useful to get to know (and, it should go without saying, be nice to) administrators, managers, non-physician clinicians, and support staff. In academic medicine, this principle extends to people in other departments and schools. You often will not know who you need to know before you need them, so better to have a long list of contacts.

6. **Say no**. When I was first getting started, I was acutely aware of my position in the hierarchy of academic medicine—that is, at the bottom. I did not feel empowered to say no to the multiple service requests that came my way to serve on committees, give ad hoc lectures, or advise medical students. These commitments squeezed out time for the activities that I was explicitly hired to do and that would determine whether I could be promoted—research, publishing, and cultivating a reputation outside my home institution. Developing the ability to say no, or perhaps "not now", while maintaining professional relationships is an essential skill that must be mastered to survive in academic medicine.

7. **Say yes**. While saying no is important, it's just as important to realize that saying "yes" to selected opportunities is just as critical to career progression. The key distinction for me is why I'm tempted to decline an opportunity. If it's because I truly don't have time or it's an obligation that is not aligned with my goals and objectives, then the answer should be no. On the other hand, if I'm worried that I'm underqualified or not ready, I have to reconsider. I ask myself whether the impostor phenomenon is at play, and I reach out to senior mentors for advice. Saying yes to professional opportunities that seem like a stretch can be a powerful way to catapult one's career in a positive direction.

8. **Avoid comparisons**. In many ways, academic medicine (and life in general) thrives on comparisons, making faculty (and friends and family?) members insecure about their place and their accomplishments. It's so hard not to get caught up in comparisons. On the other hand, I have never found this to be useful, just maddening. There will always be someone who seems more productive, more efficient, or better funded. Rather than compete with these people, I've found it more useful to set my own benchmarks. This allows me to focus on my own work while celebrating the achievements of my brilliant colleagues.

9. **Test limits and push boundaries**. As a woman of color in academic anesthesia and a scholar using qualitative and mixed methods, I have heard a lot of "we've never done that before," "we've never considered that," or "we don't know how to do that." I've had to remind myself that these statements

do not mean "no." I've had to fight gender and racial socialization to be agreeable in order to advance my research program or to accomplish clinical or administrative goals. This is okay. In fact, men often do this without a second thought. I've been able to get my work done and to advocate for change by respectfully challenging the status quo, asking questions about why things are the way they are (see point #2), and anchoring these conversations on principles rather than merely precedent.

These are my hard-won lessons. As with any pearls, they will not be universally useful; decide which of the pearls should be part of your individual arsenal.

Lessons Learned

- You'll need a lot of help to succeed in academic medicine. Develop a robust network of friends, mentors, sponsors, and cheerleaders who will provide wise counsel and buoy you when the going gets tough.
- Be strategic about what to do and what not to do. There are many pathways to success at work and in your private life, but being indiscriminate or inconsistent is not one of them.
- Know that there is a place for you. Even if there are not a lot of people who do what you do, or look like you do, the academic medicine tent is a big one, and we need everyone we can get to keep our specialty as dynamic, adaptive, and innovative as possible.

Author

Meghan Lane-Fall is chair of anesthesiology at the Columbia University Vagelos College of Physicians and Surgeons. She is a critical care anesthesiologist who conducts research using implementation science and systems engineering to improve patient safety and communication. She is also a dedicated mentor with more than 90 lifetime mentees. She lives in the NYC metro area with her spouse and two children, affectionately nicknamed Tsunami and Bear.

Animals Need Bridges, Too

206

A. M. Coleman Bank, Melissa Butynski, Daniel J. Marcucci, and Catherine Marcucci

Contributor:

Catherine Marcucci, MD

Introduction

Across the world, wildlife crossings are helping animals navigate human-dominated landscapes. In Banff National Park, grizzly bears use overpasses to safely cross the Trans-Canada Highway (Fig. 206.1). In Kenya's Tsavo National Park, elevated railway bridges allow African elephants to pass beneath undisturbed. On the Indonesian island of Java, slow lorises safely traverse roadways thanks to canopy bridges made from ropes and water pipes suspended in the treetops. In Los Angeles, California, the world's largest wildlife crossing structure provides safe passage for mountain lions over the 10-lane Ventura Freeway in the Santa Monica Mountains. What scientific, economic, and policy drivers have made these animal bridges possible?

A. M. Coleman Bank
Virginia Polytechnic Institute and State University, Blacksburg, VA, USA

M. Butynski
University of British Columbia, Kelowna, BC, Canada

D. J. Marcucci
Center for Leadership in Global Sustainability, Virginia Polytechnic Institute and State University, Blacksburg, VA, USA

C. Marcucci (✉)
Department of Transfusion Medicine, Clinical Center, National Institutes of Health, Bethesda, MD, USA

S. Mohamed et al. (eds.), *Anesthesia Bridges*, https://doi.org/10.1007/978-3-032-08294-7_206

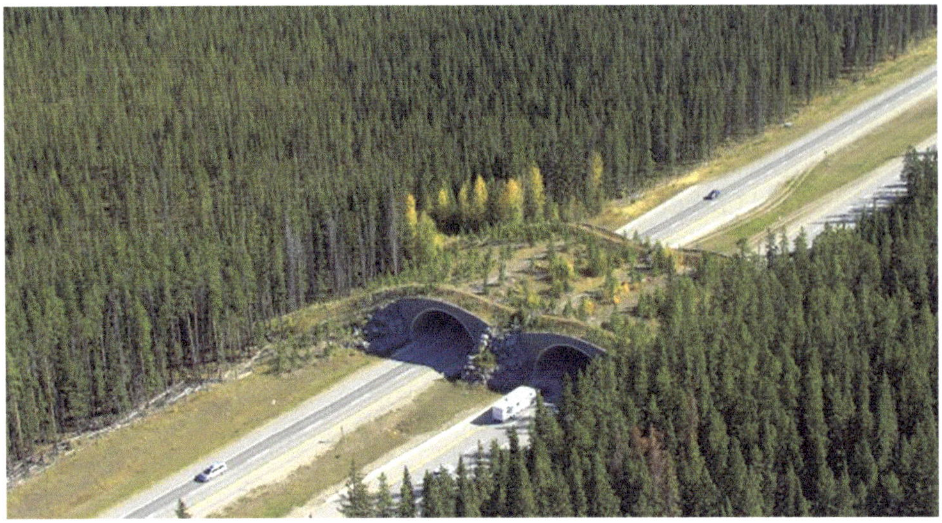

Fig. 206.1 A wildlife overpass in Banff National Park, Canada. Photo: Adam Ford, PhD

Background

Across the globe, the human population grows, and with this, we build more and more infrastructure to connect our cities and towns. While increased transportation connects our lives, the landscapes that other animals rely on become more fragmented as roadways and railways chop animal ranges into smaller and smaller pieces. Tragically, this often leads to fatal results for both wildlife and humans. To mitigate these fragmented landscapes, animals need bridges too.

Each day, approximately one million vertebrate animals are struck and killed by vehicles in the United States [1]. Not only is this a pointless loss of life, but these traffic accidents are extremely dangerous for drivers and also pose an extreme safety risk to passengers. In the United States alone, there are approximately 1.5 million deer-vehicle collisions per year and 200 human fatalities. These collisions make deer the deadliest animals in the US [2].

Fences, concrete barriers, and other precautions have been added to major roadways in an attempt to reduce the number of these animal-based collisions, and research has found an impact in significantly helping to reduce collisions and loss of animal life [3]. With a growing population and an increase in the amount of vehicular traffic, however, there is still considerable pressure on wild animal populations. Life is fraught with danger for the wildlife living next to major roadways, and driving is unsafe for travelers on roads that transect wildlife habitats.

Like humans, wild animals need to move to survive. They need to move across the landscape to find resources such as food or water, shift with changing climate conditions, or disperse to find new mates. The constant creation of new roadways significantly interferes with allowing animals to practice their natural behavior. Wild animals did not evolve to understand what a vehicle is or how it poses a threat to them. Large prey animals such as deer or elk will stand frozen in front of vehicles, as they may not associate the bright headlights with an oncoming vehicle and do not recognize the imminent danger. Instead of attempting to overlook the effects public roads have on our ecosystem, conservationists have developed new and exciting approaches and systems to "bridge" the gap between industry and nature.

Origins

Wildlife bridges, also called "green bridges" or "wildlife crossing infrastructure," stretch over or under roadways and are specifically designed for the safe passage of animals. Originally developed in France during the 1950s, wildlife bridges spread rapidly throughout Europe due to their immediate effectiveness. The Netherlands is currently the world leader in green bridges, with over 600 active overpasses and eco ducts. Reconnecting the Dutch landscape has led to the successful recovery of the European badger. The construction of the first wildlife bridge in the U.S. was completed in 1975 by the Utah Department of Transportation. Since its development, over 1000 wildlife crossing structures have been constructed across the continental United States and Canada. Since 1996, Banff National Park has constructed 38 underpasses and six overpasses across the Trans-Canada Highway, which runs through the park.

Efficacy

Do highway fencing and wildlife bridges make humans safer? The answer is a resounding yes, and there are many studies that demonstrate a positive result in increased traffic safety. For instance, in Banff National Park, there has been a 96% decrease in deer and elk collisions, as well as an 80% decrease in overall animal collisions, making these innovative structures a massive success for transportation ecology [4]. A Montana-based study on the movement patterns of large mammals conducted in 2017 found that animals are 146% more likely to use wildlife bridges as opposed to crossing roads or railroads at random locations [5].

Wildlife bridges or underpasses enhance landscape function by increasing ecological connectivity (Fig. 206.2). One interesting phenomenon occurring throughout the world is that utilization increases gradually in the years after a structure is opened as wildlife becomes adapted to utilizing the structure, especially if fencing had prevented movement prior to construction.

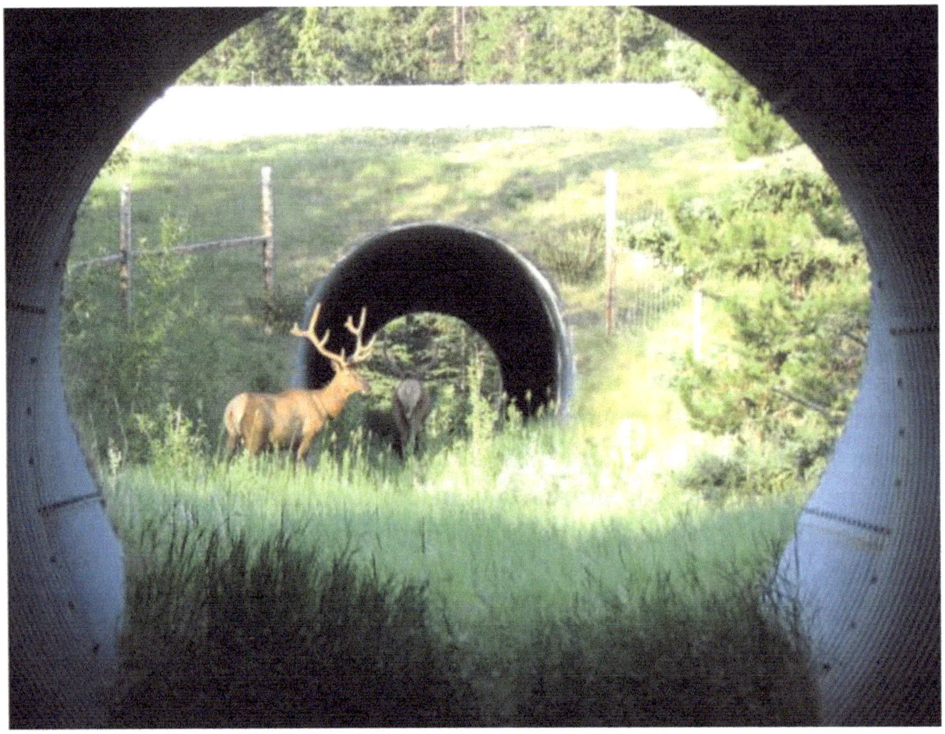

Fig. 206.2 An elk uses a tunnel in the Banff area, one of the wildlife crossings designed to decrease vehicle-wildlife collisions and restore critical migration routes. Photo and caption: Adam Ford, PhD

There is some evidence of predator and prey interaction at wildlife bridges and their associated fencing, and research is ongoing to better understand this. Overall, it is abundantly clear that animals are making the most out of these new ecosystem transit methods and will sometimes even start to use them before they are completed. Wildlife experts in Florida were thrilled to see panthers, bears, and alligators using the same wildlife underpass in the Everglades. So, how will new green bridges and underpasses be funded, and when can we expect to see more of them?

Future Infrastructure Investment

U.S. citizens are likely to see a significant amount of new wildlife crossing structures within the next decade. The Bipartisan Infrastructure Law, signed by President Biden in November of 2021, pledged roughly $350 million towards animal-based infrastructure such as the development of new wildlife bridges, eco ducts, and roadside fencing.

In its first round of grant awards, the Federal Highway Administration awarded $110 million for 19 wildlife crossing projects in 17 states. The Wallis Annenberg Wildlife Crossing, which spans Highway 101 in Los Angeles County, California, is a first-of-its-kind example of a public-private partnership, with a significant portion coming from private donations and philanthropic organizations. Soon to be the world's largest overpass, spanning 210 feet long and 165 feet wide, thousands of animal species will have the ability to safely cross the busiest 10-lane highway in America. The overpass will greatly improve driver safety while seamlessly integrating into the surrounding environment, giving new hope to Southern California's wildlife.

Lessons Learned

- By valuing and accommodating non-human species, we can create landscapes that are functional for multi-species conservation and that reduce human-wildlife conflicts. It is truly a case where good bridges make good neighbors.

The editors and authors of *Anesthesia Bridges* thank Dr. Adam T. Ford and Melissa Butynski, MEM, for their review and assistance with this chapter and permission to use Adam's photographs. Dr. Ford is an associate professor of biology at the BRAES Institute at the University of British Columbia. Melissa Butynski is a PhD student at the University of British Columbia.

References

1. Forman RTT, Alexander LE. Roads and their major ecological effects. Annu Rev Ecol Syst. 1998;29(1):207–31. https://doi.org/10.1146/annurev.ecolsys.29.1.207.
2. Huijser MP, Ament RJ, Bell M, et al. Animal vehicle collision reduction and habitat connectivity pooled fund study—literature review. Nevada Department of Transportation; 2021. Accessed 24 June 2025. http://scholarworks.montana.edu/handle/1/17312.
3. Ford AT, Dorsey B, Lee TS, Clevenger AP. A before-after-control-impact study of wildlife fencing along a highway in the Canadian Rocky Mountains. Front Conserv Sci. 2022:3. https://doi.org/10.3389/fcosc.2022.935420.
4. Stewart L, Russell B, Zelig E, Patel G, Whitney KS. Wildlife crossing design influences effectiveness for small and large mammals in Banff National Park. Case Stud Environ. 2020;4(1):1231752. https://doi.org/10.1525/cse.2020.1231752.
5. Andis AZ, Huijser MP, Broberg L. Performance of arch-style road crossing structures from relative movement rates of large mammals. Front Ecol Evol. 2017:5. https://doi.org/10.3389/fevo.2017.00122.

Authors

Cole Bank graduated *magna cum laude* from Virginia Polytechnic Institute and State University in 2024 with a major in animal science. He has started a short-term career as a medical assistant while applying to medical schools. In his rare free time, he enjoys SCUBA diving, hiking, cars, and martial arts.

Melissa Butynski is a wildlife biologist with a decade of experience and is currently pursuing her PhD with Dr. Adam Ford at the University of British Columbia. For the past seven years, she has focused on large landscape connectivity, with a particular interest in road ecology. Melissa has worked extensively in East Africa and across Asia. She is a co-author of the "Handbook to Mitigate the Impacts of Roads and Railways on Asian Elephants" and "Guiding the Future of Linear Infrastructure Development in Snow Leopard Landscapes".

Dan Marcucci is a landscape architect and regional and urban planner on the faculty at Virginia Tech. He has wide-ranging academic and research interests, but is especially interested in managing and optimizing landscapes that are changing due to increased development. He and his wife, Grace, are the proud parents of three adult children and the super-proud grandparents of three young grandsons. In his spare time, Dan enjoys spending time with friends and family, national and international travel, cooking, and gardening.

Cathy Marcucci is a senior academic anesthesiologist and inveterate anesthesiology educator. She is also fellowship-trained in transfusion medicine. When she is not taking care of patients and/or putting the latest book together, she dedicates her time to writing copy for animal rescues and travelling. The beautiful country around Banff is on her bucket list.

More General Life Wisdom

207

Catherine Marcucci, M. Concetta Lupa, F. Jacob Seagull, Conni Walkup Hull, Bradford D. Winters, and Neil B. Sandson

Contributors:

Ronald S. Bank, MD (RSB)

Rodger E. Barnette, MD (REB)

Carol F. Bodenheimer, MD (CFB)

Austin Brown (AB)

Hon. Christopher C. Conner (CCC)

Kathleen (Cathy) Conroy-Cantilena, MD (KCC)

Conni Walkup Hull, JD* (CWH)

Michael P. Hutchens, MD (MPH)

Deb Waterman Johns, BS (DWJ)

C. Marcucci (✉)
Department of Transfusion Medicine, Clinical Center, National Institutes of Health, Bethesda, MD, USA

M. C. Lupa
Department of Anesthesiology, University of North Carolina – Chapel Hill, Chapel Hill, NC, USA

F. J. Seagull
Center for Bioethics and Social Sciences in Medicine, Michigan Medicine, Ann Arbor, MI, USA

C. W. Hull
Law Office of Conni L. Walkup, Columbia City, IN, USA

B. D. Winters
Department of Anesthesiology and Critical Care Medicine, Johns Hopkins University, Baltimore, MD, USA

N. B. Sandson
Department of Psychiatry, VA Maryland Health Care System, Baltimore, MD, USA

University of Maryland, Baltimore, MD, USA

S. Mohamed et al. (eds.), *Anesthesia Bridges*, https://doi.org/10.1007/978-3-032-08294-7_207

Evan D. Kharasch, MD PhD (EDK)

Kirk Lalwani, MD (KL)

Mark J. Lema, MD PhD (MJL)

Daniel J. McCoy, MD'26 (DJM)

K A Kelly McQueen, MD, MPH, FASA (KAKMcQ)

Rajen V. Nathwani, MBBS BSc (RVN)

Mark Nelson, MD MEd (MN)

Amy J. Robbins, MD MBA* (AJR)

Charles H. Sandson, BS IME (CHS)

Richard G. Sheffield, BS MA (RGS)

Louise Y. Sun, MD (LYS)

Charles J. Yeo, MD* (CJY)

Introduction

This was a really fun topic to put together. We emailed and interviewed the entire roster of authors and editors for their best life advice and got a lot of wisdom—about happiness, families, and how to get to a place of happiness and contentment, which are not the same thing at all, it turns out. The contributors sent us the best things they have read and the thoughts they came up with on their own. We also have the great good fortune to know and have worked with several pros over the years. Both Jake Seagull and Neil Sandson consider themselves good and true friends of the national anesthesia community and shared their favorite wisdom with us as well. Please enjoy this content, and if helpful, feel free to borrow anything that seems helpful or true.

Life Management

- Here is a 'Covey-esque' concept. Be mindful to sharpen the saw. In other words, if you don't spend the down time to sharpen the teeth of the saw, you will work twice as hard and twice as long to accomplish your task. Take time to decompress—even though your work may demand more of your time. A refreshed physician functions more effectively and efficiently. I recall a busy plastic surgeon being able to physically work out routinely. When I asked him how he managed to find the time, he said that he found a fitness center near his practice and had his secretary book himself as a patient clinic visit so he could get to that gym.—**MJL**

- Don't let the doubters discourage you from pursuing your dreams.—**KAKMcQ**

- Like it says in the song, "If it fires you up, you got to let it shine." So be ready when somebody asks you what your superpower is. Yes, it's become a bit of an annoying, predictable interview question. But if you can't answer it—if you can't tell somebody in ten words what your anesthesia superpower is and what your outside superpower is—you need to ask yourself why you are spread so thin.—**CM and Editors**

- The best answer to the superpower question that I ever heard was "needlecrafts." When I asked if this pertained to the practice of anesthesia or life outside anesthesia, the reply was "both." I was so envious!—**CM**

- Nothing good happens after 9 PM.—**CHS and CM**

- If you achieve happiness, success follows. Success is just not always a reliable path to happiness.—**NBS**

- Having money may not make you happy, but accept that it will likely make you less afraid.—**Editors**

- How you spend your days is how you've spent your life.—**Editors**

- It's okay to cry on the way home from work, but you shouldn't be crying on the way to work. That indicates a real problem.—**NBS**

- Contemplating a big change of any type? The two questions you should ask yourself are: am I still young enough to do this? And am I also old enough to do it?—**Editors**

- Harbors are great places, but ships are meant for the ocean.—**MN**

- Forward is almost always the best direction to go—the only question is which way is it?—**MN**

- Excellence and compassion are in the details.—**BMT**

- Success is a platform where all kinds of people gather in all kinds of ways.—**Editors**

- Always remember that a lot of people would love to have our problems.—**MJB**

- Skiers know this—where your head is pointed is where you will go. In other words, you become what you think about.—**MN and NBS**

- Life is about competition. If you find yourself competing for something, resolve that you will either win or get beaten honorably. But don't allow yourself to passively lose.—**NBS**

- Accept that challenges and competitive situations will be present in your life on an ongoing basis. A good matter-of-fact approach to the realities of life: Play the game, win the game, move to the next game.—**NBS**

- Strength is not evidenced through force or conflict; it is demonstrated by our ability to quietly demonstrate our skills, show respect and kindness to others, and lead by example.—**LYS**

- The key to a successful life is the ability to avoid lugging around extra emotions to spend on worthless people.—**Editors**

- Sometimes you have to be comfortable with the gray.—**NBS and Editors**

- How do you get through the unthinkable? You climb up the mountain, and then you climb down the mountain.—**KCC**

- Never do somebody else's emotional work or make yourself responsible for making somebody's world go around. Your minor children are the exception to this, of course.—**Editors**

- Not everyone who rattles a sword is a warrior.—**CWH**

- Leave work at work whenever you can. This may mean staying a little bit longer to look up your patients, finish those emails, or complete your charting. When you are home, be home. Just like watching TV in bed, it is important to have some boundaries.—**MCL**

- Accept that life, and certainly work, is not perfect.—**MCL**

- Seeming impervious to a crisis may become a habitual response; it certainly will be for experienced anesthesiologists. Keep in mind that while it's effective in a professional situation, sometimes in personal situations, it wins no medals. People with stoic personalities are often misunderstood and accused of being cold or indifferent. Many of us have been called 'intimidating' more than once.—**CWH and Editors**

- Remember why you chose what your career is. I keep my med school application essay nearby to look at when I am feeling disenchanted with work. It reminds me of how lucky I am to be where I am and also that not everyone has had the privilege of getting accepted into medical school and living out their dream. This helps on those tougher days when you question the imperfections of a career that will have its ups and downs, and helps recreate a focus.—**MCL**

- In adult life, there are very rarely any complete or true solutions; there are only tradeoffs.—**Editors**

- Once I was standing at the scrub sinks in the old General Operating Rooms at Hopkins, talking to Charlie Yeo—now the Samuel Gross Professor and Chair at Jefferson, but at the time a busy young surgeon on the GI Gold service. I was new to Hopkins, and he wasn't. I was telling him about the issue of the day, and finally, he said to me, "Okay, Cathy, here are my thoughts – first of all, meaningful change can occur without everybody having to see Jesus. Second, places like Hopkins can swamp you a bit. Just find some reasonable way to wade through the water and the weeds while keeping your patients as safe as possible, which you already know. Beyond that, just get yourself to the other side of any issue or controversy without getting too wet." Such simple but great advice.—**CM and CJY**

***Note from the Editors:** Philadelphia is known for its beautiful suburbs, known as the Main Line, with winding roads, shady lawns, and stately houses. We were delighted when we asked Dr. Yeo to scout the Philadelphia suburbs for beautiful little bridges, and he sent us the photos below as a perfect illustration to that long-ago conversation. This creek runs through Gladwyne, PA (Fig. 207.1a and b).

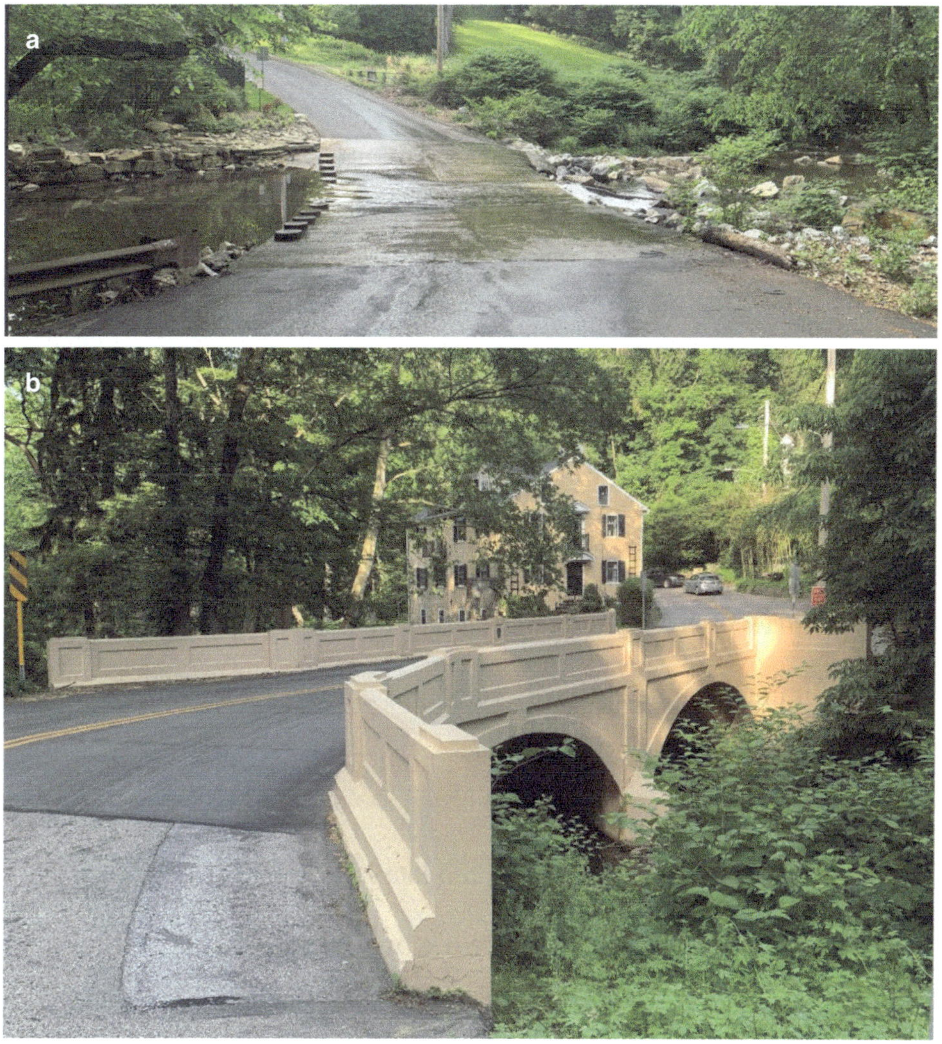

Fig. 207.1 (**a**) Charming creek, but a bit of a problem with the roadbed! (**b**) There's always a way to get through or over. Photo: Charlie Yeo

- Question whether you should remain in situations that have been associated with you, either losing or gaining weight that you didn't need or intend to. Because unwelcome changes in your weight mean unwelcome changes in your health. Is it worth it? Of course, the same is also absolutely true if you find yourself drinking more.—**Editors**

- It's been said that a huge source of stress derives from driving towards goals that you don't really want.—**Editors**

- You don't always need to win to be victorious.—**Editors**

- We are kept from our goal not by obstacles but by a clear path to a lesser goal.—**Robert Brault**

- There is no better goal than to spend more time with your loved ones.—**Editors**

- The *big three questions* from the great **Rabbi Hillel** are below.—**FJS**

   1. If I am not for myself, who will be for me? **Stand up for yourself.**
   2. If I am only for myself, what am I? **Don't be selfish or a bully.**
   3. If not now, when? **Seize the day.**

- It's the little things some days.—**NBS**
- How to get institutional power—make yourself indispensable and inoffensive. And look for tasks that nobody wants to do or can do.—**NBS**
- To paraphrase the Broadway show *Alexander Hamilton:* If you don't stand for something, you'll fall for anything.—**RVN**
- Be really careful around people who do a lot of virtue-signaling of any type. As Ralph Waldo Emerson said, *"The louder he talked of his honor, the faster we counted our spoons."*—**Editors**
- Stop worrying about it until you need to worry about it but work hard to learn when that is.—**MJB and NBS**
- Work ethic beats talent every time.—**MJB**
- Avoid at all costs: too much, too little, too loud, too late.—**Editors**
- We make a living by what we get, but we make a life by what we give.—**MJB**
- Begin with the end in mind.—**Editors**
- Straight roads do not make skillful drivers.—**Paul Coelho**
- Great things are done by a series of small things brought together.—**Vincent Van Gogh**
- A great leader/physician/parent/life partner cares about the result, not the glory.—**NBS**
- Even the boldest plan needs a steering wheel.—**RGS**
- If something precious gets broken, I don't stand over it and wail—I get a broom. Staring at broken pieces only extends the pain. And remember that the river waits for no one.—**CWH**
- When something truly tragic happens to somebody, never say to them that God doesn't give us more than we can handle, that the purpose of heartache is to make us stronger—that's cruel and unkind. Sometimes that person is already stronger than any person should ever have to be.—**CWH**
- I finished college when I was 49 and law school when I was 52. Better late than never, as the saying goes. It's never too late to be what you could have been. If the start of your life wasn't so great, trust me, you still have time. Just live it backward.—**CWH**

***Note from the Editors:** Conni Walkup Hull is a writer and poet that we read as often as we can, and we were delighted to get her permission to use some quotes. We also just happened to ask her if she had any cool bridge photos, and did she ever! It turns out that her husband is a chief engineer in the Merchant Marine (equal in rank to the captain) as well as a trained artist, and he had some great pictures in his files (Figs. 207.2 and 207.3).

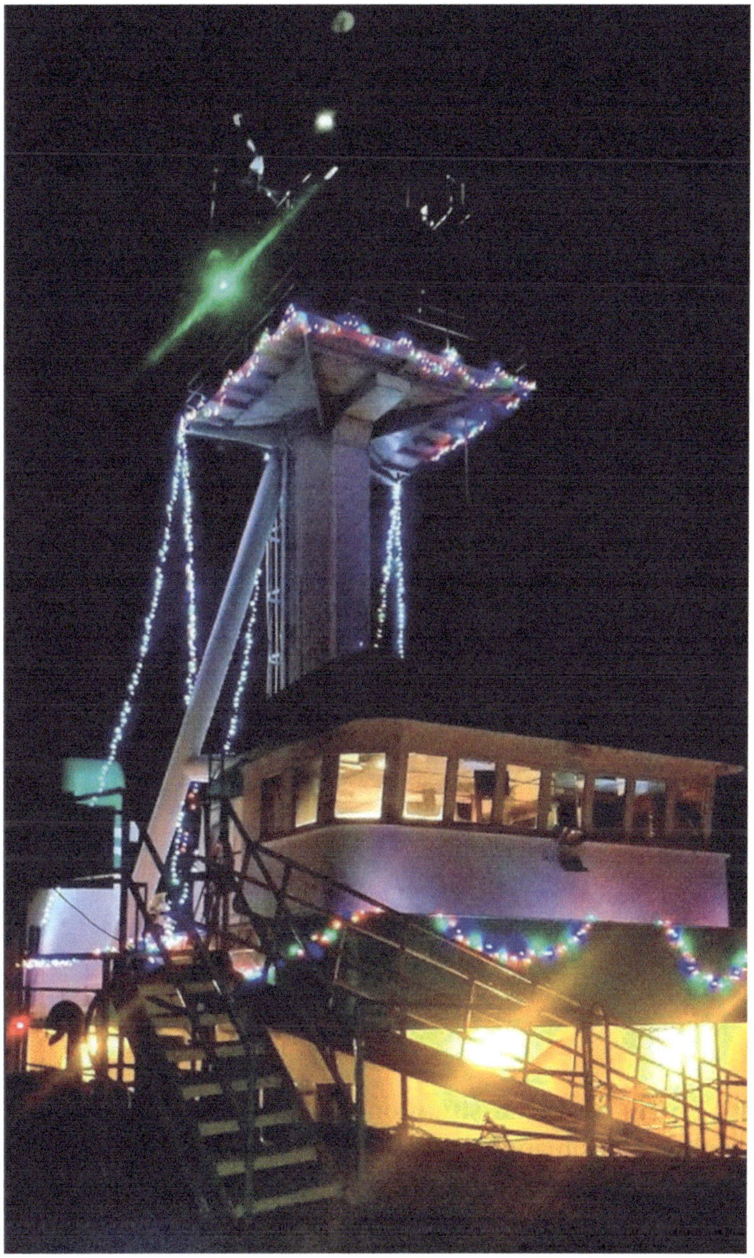

Fig. 207.2 What we might call the "bridge" of a commercial boat is known to the pros as the wheelhouse. This is a photo of the command center of the articulated tugboat *George L. Ostrander*, which carries cement and other industrial commodities between ports on the Great Lakes. Although the Merchant Mariners are away from home during the holiday season, they go all out on the boat with decorations, special food, and even some holiday baking. Photo: Scott Hull

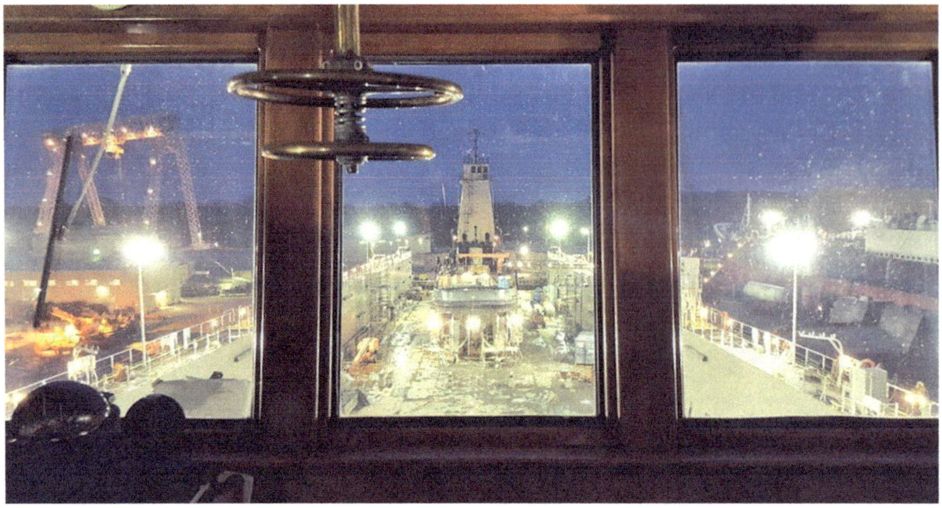

Fig. 207.3 Here is the view *from* the bridge (wheelhouse!) of the *George L. Ostrander*, taken in dry dock in Milwaukee, looking at the wheelhouse of another tug in dry dock. Photo: Scott Hull

Personal and People Management

- To understand where you are trying to get to, you need to understand where you are now.—**RVN**
- We are all in this world to be happy and joyful—but we get there faster if we help each other.—**RVN**
- Remember, nothing is unattainable if you are able to conquer yourself.—**LYS**
- Be careful who you trust. Behavior can change, but not basic character.—**NBS**
- Find your voice. Use it.—**MCL**
- Be your authentic self. Nobody is better at being you than you. It's ok to try to seek self-improvement, but don't ever be sorry for who you are.—**MCL**
- Sometimes you prove your value most when you are not there.—**CHS**
- If not you, then who?—**Editors**
- **Happy people don't create zero-sum situations.** Only unhappy people do that. This is basically because unhappy people set up situations where they can extract value from situations that should be value-neutral. Everybody has to make their own decisions about what is or isn't worth it when deciding who to associate with. But be clear with yourself about what's going on if you see somebody create a zero-sum situation after a zero-sum situation. Do you want to be the unhappy person who finds themself tied to such individuals?—**NBS**

- Never take an action or even ask a question that is solely intended to convey how smart or important you are. It's not a nice thing to do, and usually backfires anyway.—**NBS**
- Loyalty should never come at the expense of your own personal well-being. And do not **EVER** do something for somebody that they would not do for you (if they could).—**Editors**
- Share the problem! Avoid falling into the trap of believing that you must unilaterally craft solutions to systems or group problems. Sharing the problem works for everyone on multiple levels.—**NBS**
- People are always going to be afraid to some extent of the devil they don't know. If you want to motivate and lead people, you must keep this in mind.—**NBS**
- Real people have real problems—be kind and don't be superior.—**NBS**
- Unless they are debilitated, if you are working harder than somebody else to solve one of their problems, then something is wrong.—**NBS**
- If you can't understand someone's maladaptive choices, then ask the question. "How are the behaviors and choices less anxiety-provoking than obvious alternatives?" That should produce some answers, if not for them, at least for you.—**NBS**
- To be early is to be on time, to be on time is to be late, to be late is to be forgotten.—**MJB**
- Sometimes the problem isn't that you are asking the wrong question, it's that you are asking the wrong person.—**Editors**
- The most valuable questions are the ones you ask yourself.—**Editors**
- You hold your life's trajectory in your mouth every time you open it.—**NBS**
- The fastest way (in seconds!) you can derail your life is to say something really destructive, hateful, or offensive.—**NBS**
- **WALK AWAY** from people who don't value you. There is no need to try to prove your worth or give them a second chance, and that rarely works anyway. If you can't distance yourself completely, try to distance yourself an inch. If you can't do even an inch of physical distance, start to remove yourself in your mind.—**CM**
- No one can do more damage to you than you.—**Editors**
- If you don't develop the ability to follow through, it's not so much that you have derailed yourself; it's that you never were on the rails in the first place. Work hard to develop this character trait.—**NBS**
- I was raised military—my dad graduated from West Point, Class of 1953 (Fig. 207.4). I was taught from early childhood that before you even think about following through with actions, you have to clearly think through your decisions in terms of tactics and strategies.—**AJR**

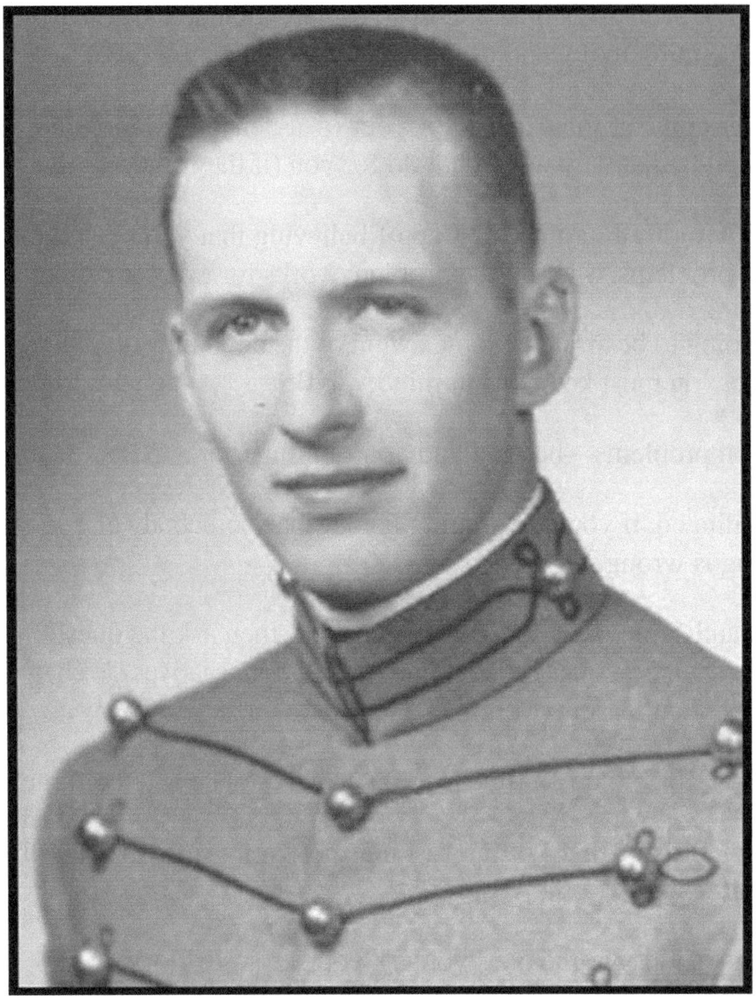

Fig. 207.4 Gary Wayne Robbins, Amy Robbins' father, attended the United States Military Academy at West Point, Class of 1953. He went on to earn his Master of Science in Aerospace Engineering from the Air Force Institute of Technology in 1964 and an MBA from Southern Illinois University. He retired from active duty in the USAF as a Major in 1974. Photo: Collection of the Robbins family

- And then once you have made your decisions, that's what you do. So many people make the mistake of not doing what they have previously decided to do. They promise something, then do something else. This is a gigantic mistake that never stops paying you back. It's just the simple concept of accountability, and the military could not run without it. So, call when you say you will call. And do what you have said you will do.—**AJR, CHS, and NBS**
- I'm not too big on the concept of willpower. But I do believe in discipline. Discipline is nothing more than the ability to prioritize future needs over present needs. That's all it is. But it's incredibly important for a successful life.—**NBS**
- If you are trying to develop discipline, just visualize what it would be like if you had a butler to help you prepare for the next hour, day, and week. Think, "What would Jeeves be doing right now to help me?"—**Editors**

- Don't make it somebody else's job to convince you of what you already know.—**NBS**

- Everybody's career is a little different what they originally envisioned. Success means adapting to those differences. In other words, gracefully bridging the gap between expectation and reality.—**NBS**

- When the floodgates open, make sure you're on high ground.—**Editors**

- "Coping" is predicated in some way, shape, or form on change and the ability to move forward and past a situation. You don't cope with a difficult situation by staying in the exact same circumstances. That's endurance, not coping. And remember that is difficult to heal in the environment where you were wounded.—**NBS**

- As a rehab medicine physician, I believe that resilience is what helps patients overcome physical disability and go on to thrive. But anybody, even those who are not dealing with a disability, would benefit from resilience. What is resilience exactly? **It's the ability to tolerate and even accommodate change over time.** This can mean resolving and coming to terms with an ongoing stream of multiple smaller changes on a longitudinal basis or patiently managing the aspects pertaining to a catastrophic change while advancing on one issue at a time.—**CFB**

- Some people are born with resiliency as an innate character attribute or capacity, but resilience is also a skill that can be learned and practiced.—**Editors**

- "Once" is a pattern.—**Editors**

- Never let yourself be made into the police. Shame doesn't work.—**NBS**

- Old friends are best! I have been friends with *Anesthesia Bridges* authors and/or photographers LouAnn Kopenhaver since 1972; Kit Conner since 1974; Jane Jacobs, Deb Waterman Johns, Christie Gilmartin Waters, Elaine Matte Mut, and Michael Liu since 1975 and 1976; Ruth and Randy Jensen since 1982; Carol Bodenheimer since 1985; Neil Sandson since 1987; Amy Robbins since 1992; and Carolyn Metzler since 2009. Everybody should be so lucky. Besides my family, my friends are the gold in my life.—**CM**

- I met Jane Jacobs on the first day of college at Cornell University in 1975. Forty-six years later, my son helped her daughter move a mini fridge out of a dorm at Goucher College, and Jane and I had a quiet chuckle at the course of life. Make no mistake about it—the wheel turns, and the circle comes around, as my college and I became who we already were.—**CM**

- Know what you feel. Choose what you do.—**FJS**

- It is important to have clarity about your emotions and desires. Don't invalidate your own feelings to be a people pleaser; you can still do nice things if you choose to. Understand your emotions and don't let them control you.—**FJS**

- You can't get good at something unless you are willing to be bad at it for a while first. So, understand the value of determination in accomplishing things.—**FJS**

- There is often a reason people are not remembered much at all. Strive to leave every situation with a positive memory in the minds of your colleagues.—**CCC**

- Aaron Lloyd, who trained at Hopkins with me, told me that when he went to college, his dad told him something that had been passed on to him by his own father: **Do the right thing, don't do the wrong thing, and don't screw up**.—**CM**

- The best marker of success isn't money, or power, or prestige. It's safety. It's not possible to be completely successful, specifically or generally, if you are rendered less safe.—**Editors and NBS**

- Just as important as your bucket list is your **anti-bucket list**. Be very clear in your mind and as firm as you can be in any given moment, what you are working towards *not* doing.—**RGS and Editors**

- And just like any other personal or professional list of action items, you can have whatever you want on your anti-bucket list as long as you provide adequate love and support for the people who depend on you and take competent care of your patients.—**NBS and Editors**

- Don't waste an ounce of energy trying to rebuild trust with someone who has lied to you or about you, especially if it was to escape discomfort or consequences for themselves. Lies, whether by commission or omission, are always for the benefit of the liar. They also indicate profound disrespect. You may find yourself smiling at and being polite to this person, but they've already shown you who they are. If they lie once, they will lie again. Don't invest!—**Editors**

- Don't ever call somebody a fool. It's a terrible insult and one that people really never forget.—**Editors**

- Memories are fickle and so very short. People forget battles they didn't bleed in.—**CWH**

- One of my least favorite types of people is those people who are looking for something for nothing. Avoid them like the plague.—**CM**

- Everything you were taught that counts, does actually count. Manners, tidiness, punctuality—it's hard to be really successful without them.—**CM**

- There is no day that is too busy for 10 minutes of music, especially classical music. The health benefits are well-recognized at this point.—**Editors**

- As a fashion and apparel design professional, I read Dr. Harter's thoughts on "dressing the part" with interest. I agree with his opinions and advice! What people don't understand is that "dressing well" is also done for the benefit of the people you are interacting with. It denotes respect for your companions. Clothes should engender not only comfort in the person who is wearing them but also confidence in the person observing them.—**DWJ**

- Everybody could use a bit more color therapy in their life. It is one of the simplest ways to add a pleasurable feature to a busy and stressful life. Figure out what your favorite color is and make sure that you see it first thing in the morning and last thing at night. Employ your favorite colors in your sock choice, your watch band, and your headband. Physicians, who are often tired, should stay away from colors with a lot of gray tones. I recommend lots of exposure to green since it is the color of trees and grass and apples. The other colors that are great for physicians are the shades of yellow and orange, since these mimic the sun.—**DWJ**

- Deb Waterman Johns and I were talking about doing a study on how patient anxiety before surgery and while donating blood is affected by color exposure. We know that looking at pictures of nature on the ceilings of ICU rooms promotes healing. Deb is pretty convinced that color therapy would work in the preoperative period and procedure rooms as well.—**CM and DWJ**

- It is never too late to become who you might have been.—**MJB**

- You only have one shot at life, and you have to find a way to make it work. We really are not huge believers in living only for today. We agree with the *Anesthesia Bridges* editor and human factors expert Jake Seagull that you have to look far ahead **a lot** and also look back **just enough** so that you don't needlessly repeat mistakes. Always be mindful of what, when you are at the end of the game, you are going to wish you had done and not done.—**DWJ and CM**

- Be more concerned with your character than your reputation.—**John Wooden**

- The "forgiveness" paradigm that is so popular today in pop psychology is misplaced and places too much pressure on those who have been truly wronged. What is more appropriate is to work towards coming to terms with the untoward circumstance. And the most important person to forgive is yourself.—**NBS**

- Sundown and sunrise are the greatest gifts given to humankind—a new day. Remember that tomorrow's mistakes haven't happened yet and so are completely under your control to avoid.—**Editors**

- Never quit on a bad day.—**Editors**

- Sometimes you have to do whatever you need to so that you can settle matters between you and you.—**Editors**

- You will feel some hate about something at some point—you may feel hate about people's suffering, terrible diseases, or being so tired. Do not stuff it down. Try to find ways to get the hate out. If not constructive ways, at least safe ways.—**Editors**

- People treat you according to how you matter to them, where you live in the pecking order. Yes, they do. Take note.—**CWH**

***Note from the Editors:** We think there is only one bridge in the world that deserves as many pictures as we can get, and it is the Mackinac Bridge, which spans the Straits of Mackinac, the body of water that separates Lake Huron from Lake Michigan and the Upper and Lower Peninsulas of Michigan. The bridge is considered an iconic emblem of the state. It is not as long as the Golden Gate, but just as dramatic and beautiful (Fig. 207.5). It is the favorite bridge of a number of *Anesthesia Bridges* editors and authors.

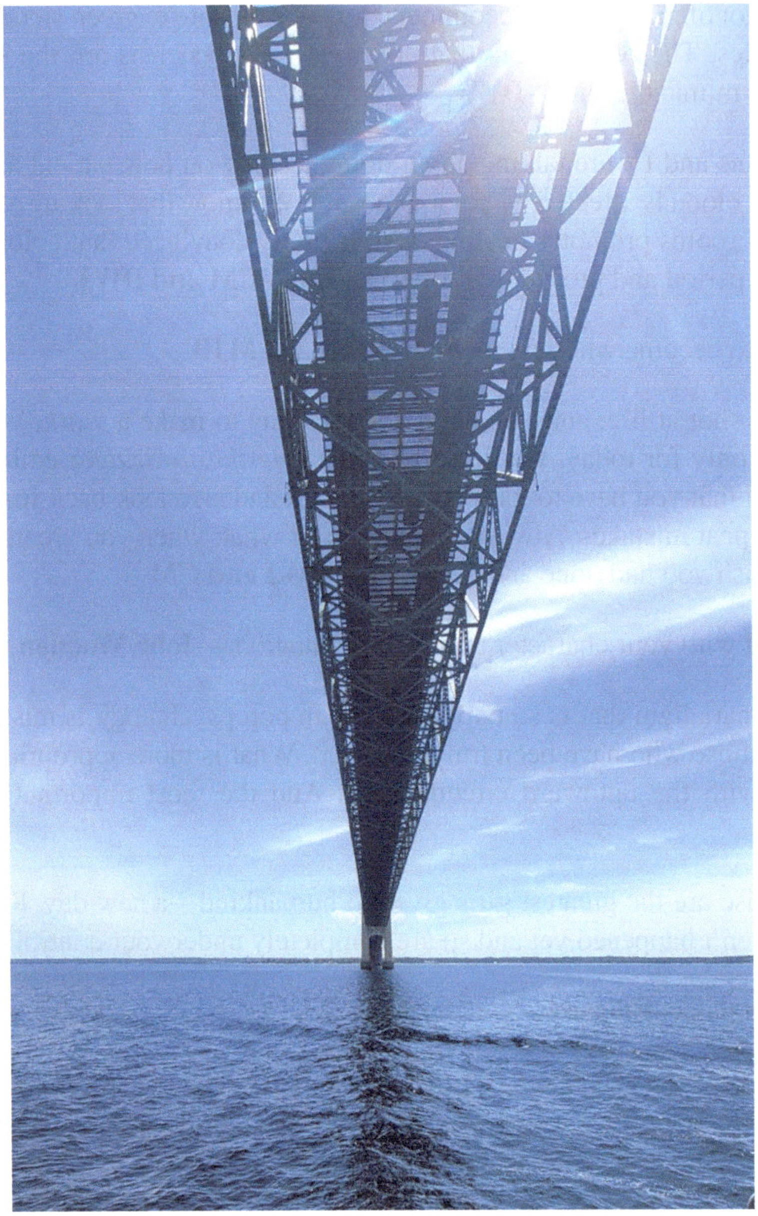

Fig. 207.5 A stunning and unique view of the Mackinac Bridge, captured by the photographer on a day when the sky and sea were a match for each other. Photo: Scott Hull

Family Life

- The advice that most changed my career, and which I repeat to trainees most often (always with attribution, because the attribution is important), is from **Jeff Kirsch**. At a pivotal moment in my family life, Jeff told me, "Nothing works at work when something isn't right with my family. Focus on your family."—**MPH**

- Our previous chairperson, **Harry Kingston**, told us at his retirement faculty meeting that he had been watching his grandkids grow and develop with amazement…until it hit him that he had missed all those milestones in his own kids because he had been too busy working all the time. That was the biggest regret of his life and professional career. So, his advice to us was not to neglect our families, as work will come and go, and someone will always be there to fill in. None of us is that important that the machine will stop if we stop…we are the proverbial cogs in one of the wheels of the mighty machine.—**KL**

- Evolve instead of revolve.—**MJB**

- Every temper tantrum needs an audience. A neutral response will diffuse almost every type of tense situation.—**CFB and NBS**

- You can't make yourself popular by trying.—**Editors**

- Always be honest and never be embarrassed about devoting the time necessary to deal with personal situations and difficulties. You don't have to dish up every last detail to everybody at the hospital, but there is no need to pretend that you do not have things you are dealing with. Everybody has children who need attention—maybe meetings at school or with a medical provider—or a parent who has fallen three times in the last two days. Take exactly the time you need to deal with it, but no more.—**Editors**

- I once heard **Steve Frank** say something that I use to this day. He was coordinating, and somebody couldn't come in for the late shift. He went into a room and said, "The relief person is now on leave for the evening, here's what we are going to do." The anesthesiologist in the room started fussing and fuming—no, it wasn't me. ☺ Steve looked at the person and said, "Severe domestic pressures. I'm not saying anything more about it. So, here's what we're going to do." Severe domestic pressures. Such a short but valuable phrase. Who doesn't know precisely what that means even without knowing a single detail? And who hasn't had such a type of pressure at home?—**CM**

- Similarly, once I was the call attending at Hopkins, and I got a call on a Saturday night in the early evening from one of our favorite junior surgeons—now a chairperson at a major academic department. He had a family pressure of some sort and was hoping to do an elective case 5 AM the next morning, a Sunday, when we typically didn't do elective cases. He didn't try to bully us into doing the case. He didn't post it as an urgent case and demand that it be done. He just called us and was completely honest about the scheduling pressures and asked if we would consider doing the case. And we did.—**CM**

- Neil and I were classmates at Temple Med, so we have always been medical comrades as well as life partners. We purposely kept a low bar between our specialties and careers. I mean, for a shrink, the man knows an astonishing amount about the practice of anesthesiology. The link is our shared love of pharmacology. Our joint publications have also been fun to do. We did socialize with our fellow trainees in both specialties and also always attended all faculty events with each other as well. A faculty member once hosted a restaurant get together for our oral boards study group, and I was sick. Neil went without me.—**CM**

- Neil and I also negotiated and renegotiated home and child duties—and each made decisions to limit our careers—I decided not to travel at all, not even three days at the ASA. Neil turned down several promotions. I do have minor regrets—too much pizza, not enough dusting and vacuuming—but I can honestly say that I do not have regrets about the kids or our family. I really feel that I was fundamentally there for my group in the ways that were most important for us. We had wonderful holidays, my children never once went to school sick, and their clothes and gear were always neat and up to date. And I still managed to put together a satisfying career. It might not have been everybody's idea of a stellar career—the years working in relative obscurity at the VA and the thousands of hours spent doing the books—but, honestly, I don't think I was ever anybody's idea of chairperson material. Which was fine with me; it would not have been my thing, anyway, all the politics and so forth. I wouldn't have minded hiring people, but I would have hated firing them. I was definitely better spending my time in the OR. In the end, I found a way that worked for me. Final assessment: No regrets.—**CM**

- It's great to be endlessly curious and a seeker of knowledge and experiences. But just remember that seekers often find takers.—**Editors**

- You can't expect to be good at everything all the time.—**MCL**

- If you are in a profession that requires you to give of yourself and devote time and true engagement, make sure that you give at least as much thought, care, effort, engagement, and, when possible, time to the people at home and the people you love. You don't want to have the most important people in your life ever have to question whether they matter to you as much, or are getting as much from you, as your patients/audience. Make sure that the people who are first in your heart *always* have strong evidence of that.—**AB and NBS**

- Advice to young families—just go ahead at the beginning of your family life when your kids are little and buy yourself a pop-up sun tent and enough comfortable folding chairs for the whole family. Otherwise, those hot, hot, hot Saturday morning swim meets are just unbearable.—**Editors**

- When the kids were little, we had all kinds of pets—dogs, cats, strays, guinea pigs, birds with broken wings, and fish tanks. We even had African frogs and little mice that were born from school projects—not joking! We were the hang-out house because we fostered puppies for the local dog rescues. All the kids always wanted to come over and play with the puppies. That, plus we were always willing to make lots of pizza happen. Puppies and pizza work really well if you are trying to keep younger kids under supervision and out of trouble.—**AJR**

- Your evening schedule starts before you leave the hospital Call your parents quickly to confirm upcoming plans, use the restroom, or pop an ibuprofen, if you need to, before you leave from work. That way, you can get home and give your whole focus to whomever is there waiting for you.—**MCL**

- I am truly indebted to my wonderful wife, Laura, who takes the brunt of childcare duties—her dedication, love, and patience leave me in awe every day.—**RVN**

- You would think that the shrinks, as they go through their careers, would increasingly see and urge people to see the deep complexities of life and all the shades of gray. But they don't, not really. I've noticed that they tend to see things more and more in black and white. A child psychiatrist told me that he looks for the basics, and he stressed that he meant basics. Was your home free of contempt and violence? Were the adults decently nice to each other and any animals? Can everybody you raised swim and ride a bike? Do they have an occupation that will support them in adult life? Was there something (anything) concrete in their childhood that will allow them to look back and know and feel on a deep level that they were seen and cared about, not for what they did but for who they were? Were the adults present as much as possible, and were they trying? This is what counts.—**CM**

- A different psychiatrist told me something similar about relationships between adults. If there has been no abuse, no infidelity, no addictions, and no other major issues such as criminal involvement, bankruptcy, hoarding, and the like, then most marriages and domestic partnerships stand a fair chance of being saved. As he said, "Usually, if the parties are willing and there is **any** degree of affection and respect remaining, things can be shoehorned back together. Absent the deal-breakers, the first thing I try to get suffering couples to do is not suffer so much."—**CM**

- Accept that risk management in family life might require some negotiation. Because to us, of course, a situation with a 1% risk of a bad outcome seems like a gigantically possible bad outcome. I was never a helicopter parent, but Neil and I finally had to agree to disagree about what was "safe" for the kids to do. Sometimes we did it my way, sometimes we did it his way.—**CM and NBS**

Hobbies and Recreation

- Work hard—play hard!—**RSB**

- **SCUBA** diving is an awesome hobby for anesthesiologists. You'll love the science and physiology behind it. You'll also get to see the big world in a magnificent way that very few do.—**RSB**

- Golf is the best of all sports and the most gentlemanly—that could be a quote from one of Jane Austen's books. In every other sport, there is only one ball—and everyone wants it or wants to control it. But in golf, everyone has their own ball, and it just lies there on the ground waiting for you to come to it.—**REB**

- **Travel!** Travel not to see the objects and things, travel to see the people. Travel to places untraveled, see people unseen. Listen closely to what they say and let them write on your tablet. It is only by seeking to understand others we can understand ourselves.—**MN**

- A great travel rule—always be on vacation, just back from vacation, or planning the next vacation.—**Editors**

- The Robbins-Cooley-Koloski family group is quite a large one. My husband Ray, and I haven't really been able to institute a "Ro-Co-Ko" family travel policy because we are just trying to round everybody up! When you are the parents of young adult children, the question isn't where you are going; the real question is how many of those busy kids can you get together. Once you book the people you want, the place doesn't really matter that much.—**AJR**

- Not only am I a minor league baseball fan, but I recently saw the exhibition Savannah Bananas play in Durham. Baseball meets PT Barnum, and "banana ball" rules apply! For example, games are won by points, not runs. The team that scores the most runs in an inning gets one point; all runs count in the ninth inning. The batter cannot step out of the box or bunt. Foul balls caught by fans count as an out. Each team gets to challenge one play per game, and it can be any play. Walks are now called sprints—after the fourth ball, the player sprints around the bases trying to get to home plate and score a run. The ball remains dead, and the player cannot be tagged out *until* every infielder has touched the ball. And so on. And this is special—all cheerleaders are Medicare-eligible. They are called the "Banana Nanas" of course. Finally, you have to really respect a team that goes out on a world tour to…. Mobile, Alabama. ☺ Banana ball is a blast—I highly recommend it for adults and children alike.—**EDK**

- It's sometimes hard to find a hobby, especially when you are in the early family years, but it will be worth it to do so. Sometimes my hobbies are just things I can do with my kids—like learning to bake new things, learning how to garden, simple stuff. Some hobbies are just for me—exercise. Whatever it is you do, make sure you find something worth doing when the work is done.—**MCL**

- I am now a MAMIL—middle-aged man in Lycra. I have always cycled to work, and now it keeps me sane. Physical activity is a great way to focus in the morning and wind down at the end of the day. Cycling over the lakes in Seattle with views of the mountains makes me appreciate life. It also enables me to keep eating sweet things! No electric bike yet....—**RVN**

- The outdoors always brings a smile to my face. A bad day on the hill is still always better than a good day in the office!—**RVN**

- Being in the outdoors brings us back to our basics—there is something for everybody. Turn your phone off and enjoy being there. A photo never does nature justice.—**RVN**

- The older my three boys get, the more exercise I need to do to be able to keep up.—**RVN**

- We asked *Anesthesia Bridges* author **Brad Winters** to tell us about his model train hobby, thinking he would send back some information on the best sources and prices for model train components. Instead, he sent us the following thoughts, which we organized into an outline. Who knew that underneath that let's-ride-motorcyles-and-never-heard-of-an-action-movie-I-don't-want-to-see exterior, Dr. Winters sort of has the soul of a poet? ☺ And what are railroad tracks, anyway, but bridges on the ground?—**Editors**

  Trains inspire a fascination in kids and adults alike. Perhaps it is the heralding of a simpler time when things moved more slowly and people to time to observe the world around them. Train travel is more civilized than air travel. It is unfortunate that America forsook trains for the automobile, dismantling our once burgeoning passenger rail service. I still prefer a train trip to a car ride or a plane.

  Trains also evoke a sense of human ingenuity, industrial prowess, and progress. Hearing a mournful train whistle through the valley on an early autumn morning. I live in an old railroad town, the first stop on the original Baltimore and Ohio railroad that still has frequent freight trains passing through, and hence that familiar sound always evokes a sense of the small town I grew up in.

As such, model trains remain a popular hobby, though seemingly more so for older people now. I suspect the attraction is the nostalgia, but it also brings together a variety of skills, including understanding electrical systems, exploring history (especially if the model railroad you build is based on a real one), but especially art and design as one designs and creates the landscape environment for the model railroad.

The community of train geeks, like other geek communities, provides friendly advice, knowledge, learning, and a place to turn to for a tacit understanding when others like your spouse wonder why you are spending $500 on a "toy" diesel locomotive with direct digital computer control and built in sound recorded from real trains—it is not a cheap hobby! Not to mention the opportunity to just sit back and enjoy a beer while your trains clickety clack along the track."

Attached is a photo of a diesel locomotive I took, coming through Reed Point, South Dakota, heading to Washington state (Fig. 207.6). The freight train is owned by the Burlington Northern and Sante Fe Railroad (BNSF) which is a merger of the Burlington Northern and Atchison Topeka and Santa Fe railroads.

Burlington Northern is the successor of the Great Northern Railroad, which ran from Chicago to Seattle and other Pacific ports. It was the only 100% privately funded and created railroad in the country at the time, taking no government money. This railroad was instrumental in developing Glacier National Park in Montana, and built the famous national park lodge in that park (to increase passenger rail business on their railroad)

To this day, there is an Amtrak station at that lodge, and one can travel to the park on the Amtrak Empire Builder line—BNSF is a freight-only railroad, but the Empire Builder line was originally Great Northern's service. BNSF currently uses the original color scheme of the Great Northern—orange and black."

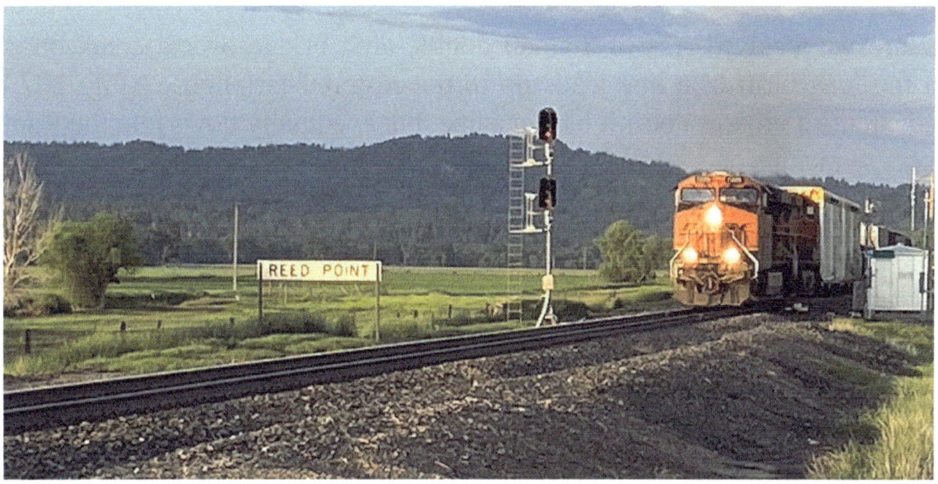

Fig. 207.6 A beautiful shot of a BNSF freight train travelling through the lovely American countryside. Photo: Brad Winters

- We all love pharmacology and physiology. But that's what makes us competent, not what makes us interesting. So get out there and live your life!—**Editors**

- We don't understand why more anesthesiologists don't play bridge**.** It is the best analytical, tactical, and strategic game there is! Like chess, it can be played on an infinite number of skill levels. But it is also a team game and so way more social. It's even been said to possibly stave off dementia. And it's a lot of fun to channel our parents and grandparents and eat nuts and avocado dip and that chocolate candy called bridge mix. Some of our favorite memories from residency are playing social bridge with *Anesthesia Bridges* contributors Herb Chen and Rob Minahan. **Does anybody out there want to learn**? Feel free to get in touch!—**CM and NBS**

Our Personal Bridges

- If we may wax philosophical for a moment, the most important bridges are those that lead to home—be it your physical home, emotional home, or spiritual home.

- One of the editors has a bucket list wish to have her own creek—because creeks are about nothing, if not all about transition and renewal. And her fantasy creek will be traversed by a tiny bridge, if she has her way. Until this happens, she is content to admire other people's bridges. So, she put out a call to the *Anesthesia Bridges* authors for pictures of their personal bridges and the details thereof. She was delighted to receive pictures of three bridges and their stories.

- The first picture we received was of a small double-arch bridge over a creek on a farm in rural Virginia, on the long farm lane that leads up to the restored farmhouse. (Fig. 207.7a and b) The mountain-fed stream it crosses doesn't have a name, but eventually flows into the Rapidan River. It's such a gorgeous, picturesque setting, especially with the green rolling hills in the background. Honestly? If you lived on this beautiful property, how would you ever tear yourself away to go to the hospital to do your cases?

- The next picture she received was this miniature suspension bridge that spans the Black Moshannon Creek in Centre County, Pennsylvania. It is on the grounds of a privately-owned hunting camp (Fig. 207.8). The camp doesn't own the creek per se, but does own the bridge and the creek shoreline for several hundred yards in either direction. Wouldn't it be fun to spend summers and vacations and holidays tiptoeing across this bridge and fishing in this creek?

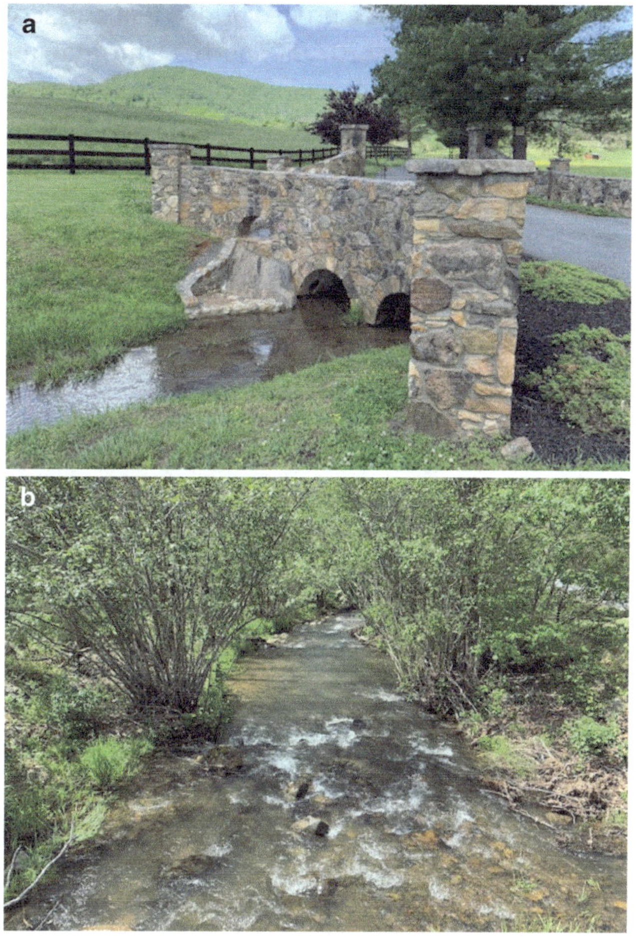

Fig. 207.7 (**a**) A beautiful small stone arch bridge on a historic farm in rural Virginia. (**b**). The creek and tiny rapid downstream from the bridge. Who would not love such a efeature on their property! Photo: Vince Hoellerich

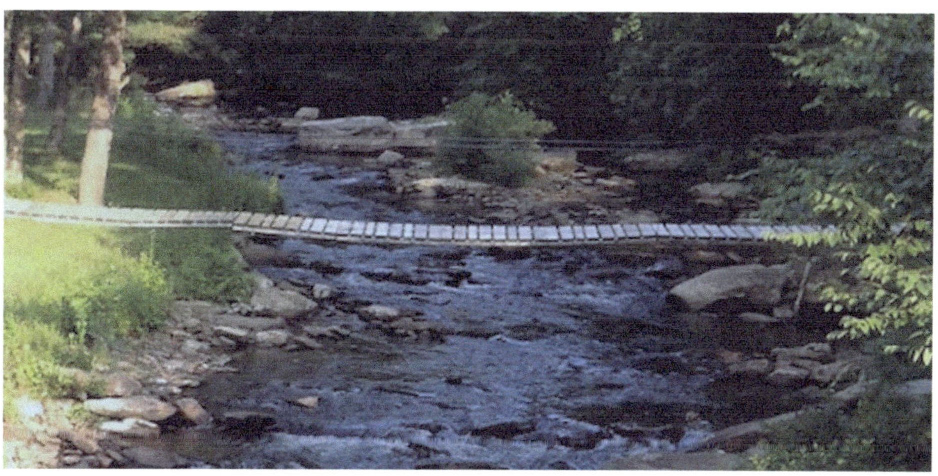

Fig. 207.8 A small suspension bridge serves as a walkway over the Black Moshannon Creek in Centre County, Pennsylvania. Photo: Kit Conner

- Finally, the third set of pictures she got was of a private bridge that crosses the spillway of a small lake on a wonderful property in the South. (Fig. 207.9a and b). Unfortunately, the earthen (and wood) foundation collapsed in a major storm several years ago. So, this bridge illustrates a great point—bridges fall down sometimes, literally and figuratively. And if they do, you must buckle down and put them up again, even stronger than before.

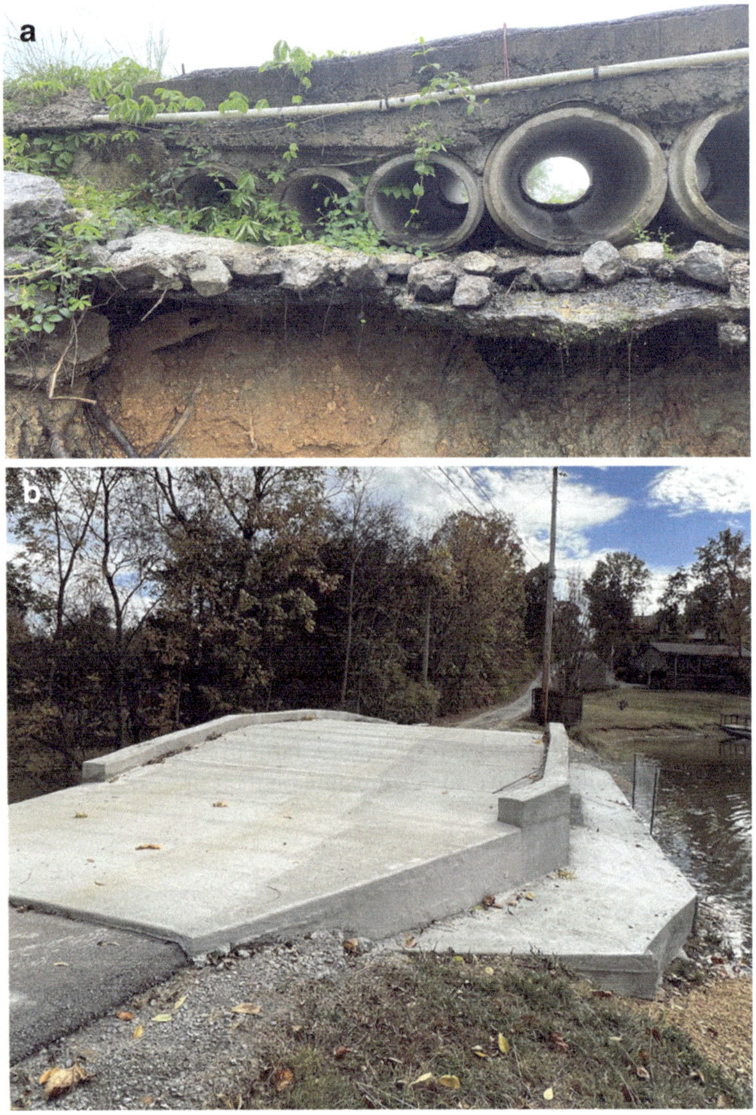

Fig. 207.9 (**a**). Eroded spillway foundation, and we think we see an exposed wooden beam in there! (**b**) Beautifully rebuilt spillway bridge on the lane to the house. There's just nothing like new concrete! Photo: Austin Brown

- The owners of this property parked up at the top of the lane and walked a quarter of a mile back and forth to the house for a year and a half while they took the time for the proper surveys, engineering assessments, permits, and then finding the right contractor to do the restoration. But look at their result—absolutely beautiful!

A Few More Thoughts to Consider

- If fate whispers to you that you can't withstand the storm, whisper back, "I am the storm."—**Folk Saying**
- When things go wrong, don't go with them.—**Elvis Presley**
- Forever is composed of now.—**Emily Dickinson**
- One day, in retrospect, the years of struggle will strike you as the most beautiful.—**Sigmund Freud**
- So, your goal is not to control every possible outcome. Your goal is to live in line with your values.—**Unknown**
- Children are the living messages we send to a time we will not see.—**John F. Kennedy**
- We can choose courage or we can choose comfort, but we can't have both.—**Brene Brown**
- A competent and self-confident person is generally incapable of jealousy. Jealousy is almost always a symptom of neurotic insecurity.—**Anonymous**
- You can't argue people into feeling better with statistics. Numbers and facts and figures can change people's minds, but usually not their hearts.—**David Graham and Editors**
- Some things break your heart but fix your vision.—**Unknown**
- Whatever you are not changing, you are choosing.—**NBS**
- If you are distressed by anything external, the pain is not due to the thing itself, but to your estimate of it; and this you have the power to revoke at any moment.—**Marcus Aurelius Antoninus**
- The key to persuasion isn't debate, it's listening.—**Editors**
- Sometimes you are in the enjoyable process of living your life and creating your story, and sometimes you are just enduring the schedule. And that's okay as long as you can see it clearly and acknowledge it honestly.—**Editors**
- More important than being able to know the truth or tell the truth is the ability to hear the truth.—**Editors**
- It is wise to direct your anger toward problems, not people; to focus your energies on answers—not excuses.—**William Arthur Ward**
- Do what you can, with what you have, where you are.—**Theodore Roosevelt**
- Trust is gained in drops and lost in buckets.—**Proverb**

- You can't succeed if you don't enjoy the journey. The journey is all there is. We all know what the end is.—**JR Roessl**
- There is nothing in the world so irresistibly contagious as laughter and good humor.—**Charles Dickens, A Christmas Carol**
- The human race has only one really good weapon, and that is laughter.—**Mark Twain**
- The home should be the treasure chest of living.—**Le Corbusier**
- To improve is to change; to be perfect is to change often.—**Winston Churchill**
- Sometimes you don't need better aim, you just need a different target.—**Proverb**
- Life is pretty much one continuous audition, and it's a mistake to assume otherwise. For example, if you think about it and are honest with yourself—a first date is really nothing more than a job interview, and a job interview is really nothing more than a first date.—**NBS and Editors**
- You don't get to decide what somebody else's feelings should be or what they feel upset about. Likewise, if somebody else feels insulted, aggrieved or injured, that's not your situation to judge. Everybody gets to own and process their own feelings, as long as this remains within reason. Meaning that you can tell people what to do or not do—in certain circumstances—but not how to feel.—**NBS and Editors**
- The best personal brand is to be known for being nice to everybody.—**Editors**
- **Sometimes the odds can be beaten.** I have beaten long odds several times in both my professional and personal lives. Don't believe me? Well, for example, I applied to med school with a GPA earned years earlier by way of great diligence and hard work, of (wait for it)….**2.37**. I am not joking. Basically, a *C+ average,* and I had the audacity to think I could slip through the doors of a mid-tier American medical school. How in the world did I manage to get accepted?—**CM**
- I think it had something to do with the personal phone call that the chemical engineering professors made to the admissions offices, saying, "No, we think you are not understanding how our course load worked in those years." They then proceeded to explain about the 5-year curriculum crammed into four years and grade deflation, grading curves, and so forth. Somehow this was enough, plus, okay, I did have rock-solid MCAT scores and very, very good grades in my post-baccalaureate pre-med courses, I will admit that, including at least one A+. In the end, I was accepted into two fine medical schools on my first try, and nobody ever said that was a travesty.—**CM**
- People ask me if I am embarrassed by those undergraduate grades. Not one bit! I think it's hilarious, and my kids (both good students) have laughed and laughed about it over the years. Plus I can instantly relate to students who get a bad grade on anything. In the end, I am as impressed by top grades as anybody else, but they are not always strictly necessary.—**CM**
- No less a person than Winston Churchill was also in the habit of emphasizing his schoolboy stupidity. Below is his description of his Latin entrance exam to the famous British school, Harrow.—**Editors**

> I wrote my name at the top of the page. I wrote down the number of question 1. After much reflection, I put a bracket around it, thus (1). But thereafter, I could not think of anything connected with it that was either relevant or true. It was from these slender indications of scholarship that Mr. Weldon drew the conclusion that I was worthy to pass into Harrow. It is very much to his credit.

- And here is what the brilliant Colin Powell said about his college career after reminding people that he graduated honorably in 6 years and "you must remember that it was a four-year degree."—**Editors**

> I've got to tell you, I wasn't considered one of the great successes of the CCNY educational system. The only reason I got out of CCNY was that they included all of my ROTC grades into my grade point average, and when they rolled it in there, it brought me up to 2.0. They said good enough for government work, get him out of here.
>
> Now I'm considered one of the greatest sons the City College of New York has ever had. So those of you who are not graduating with a 3.76 … have faith, my young friends, have faith. It's not where you started in life. It's where you end up and what you did along the way. Did you work hard, never stop learning? Would you believe in yourself? Were you your own role model? Did you believe in this country? Did you dream big?

- If you lived the story, you get to tell it. You're the one who paid the dues.—**CWH**
- Past isn't always prologue. Sometimes your past is just a lesson, perhaps hard-earned. It doesn't always have to be a life sentence.—**Editors**
- As parents, grandparents, and mentors, it is our responsibility, duty, and privilege to ensure that those coming up behind us fully take their place in the sun. Live your life and do your career so that you have something left to give.—**Editors**
- We do not necessarily believe that hardship, deprivation, and struggle make a child, or really anyone, strong. All it does is put you behind.—**Editors**
- Children become strong when they have and can draw on resources and reserves in times of adversity. At the beginning, they do not have the power to create those resources; somebody must do it for them. Later, they will learn the process of creating resources for themselves.—**Editors**
- This does not mean there is no place for boundaries, guidelines, and instruction for children, students, and learners at any stage of life. But these work best in a background of abundance.—**Editors**
- If life, there is often a lot of demoralization and discouragement disguised as stoicism. Be kind to those who appear to be strong but silent. You don't know what they might be hiding.—**Editors**
- Knowing they have loving support behind them gives children the confidence to succeed. It's easier to fly high when you aren't afraid of falling.—**CWH**
- Jealousy over the affections of a child only creates anxiety. Children benefit from having many people who love them.—**CWH**
- Life isn't short if you do it right.—**CWH**
- My view is that the idea that life is short is a fatalistic view. I'm always faintly irritated when people casually toss out that phrase. I've never thought life is short, but infinitely interesting if we choose it to be.—**CWH**

- Because if you live as if you believe life is truly short, you mess it all up because you're always worried about time running out. You waste the time you do have fretting about how little is left.—**CWH**

- Mentorship is more than just career advice. It is the reassurance that you belong.—**DJM and Editors**

- The current and future generations of medical students will come up in an era of rapid technological advancement. They have been raised with instant access to knowledge, social media shaping our perceptions of success, and a culture of constant comparison. It is important to realize, however, that medicine is still an ancient craft—built on mentorship, patience, and experience.—**Editors and DJM**

- Two of the most powerful things said to me so far in my training were six-word sentences. Once, a senior resident pulled me aside after a long shift and said, "You're doing fine. Just keep going." It was a simple statement, but at that moment, I needed to hear it. The other thing I will never forget happened when I was agonizing and devastated when a patient in the ICU that I had spent weeks helping to care for deteriorated. The attending quietly said to me, "Do your best, then let go."—**DJM**

Note from the Editors: *Anesthesia Bridges* editor Dan McCoy is from Fairbanks, Alaska, and he suggested we include a picture of an ice bridge (Fig. 207.10). He tells us that year after year, people drive across what they hope are frozen rivers too late into the spring and end up getting stuck. This is fascinating, as you would think that Alaskans and Canadians would never make this type of mistake, but they do.

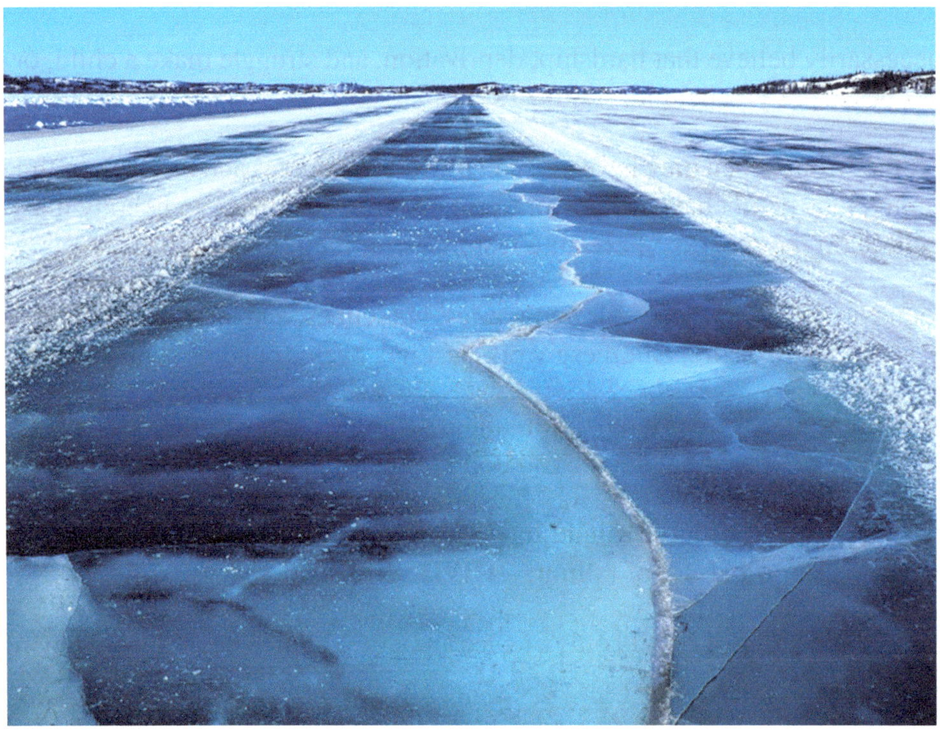

Fig. 207.10 The ice bridge across Great Slave Lake in the Northwest Territories of Canada. Photo: Jessica Harrison, image used under standard license from iStock.com

Some Universal Advice from Our Friends in the Legal Profession and Other Wise Laws

- Never mess with people's money or family unless you want to die on the courthouse steps.—**Conni Walkup Hull**

- Before you can even begin to think about winning a lawsuit, you must first find a way to endure it.—**Proverb**

- Biding one's time is a skill set many people fail to master—so many problems resolve themselves given a little breathing space. But once ego gets involved, you're on the road to disaster.—**Conni Walkup Hull**

- Nothing in this world can take the place of persistence. Talent will not; nothing is more common than unsuccessful people with talent. Genius will not; unrewarded genius is almost a proverb. Education will not; the world is full of educated derelicts. Persistence and determination alone are omnipotent. The slogan "press on" has solved and always will solve the problems of the human race.—**Calvin Coolidge**

- A lion will never have to tell you it's a lion.—**Conni Walkup Hull**

- What are the three laws of medicine?—**Proverb**

  Law No. 1: A strong intuition is more powerful than a weak test

  Law No. 2: "Normals" teach us rules; "outliers" teach us laws

  Law No. 3: For every perfect medical experiment, there is a perfect human bias

- When negotiating, think carefully and deploy the simplest of the Stoic principles. It isn't the situation itself that does people engaged in conflict the most disservice, it's the interpretation—the meaning—they assign to it. Their response will tell you everything you need to know—but understand it works both ways. You won't always be the only shark in the water.—**Conni Walkup Hull**

- There is a litigator in my professional community who has never lost a case, and this includes some very big cases, indeed. How does he do it? I've watched him for years with great interest. What I've observed is that he is never aggressive, he never bluffs, and he never allows ego to gain even the slightest amount of traction on his side of the matter. He is always supremely prepared, and he never overplays his hand. These simple principles have resulted in stunning successes.—**Conni Walkup Hull**

- One of the simplest and most powerful statements you can make in a conflict or negotiation, said without any aggression, threat, or rancor, is "Okay, is that your final offer/answer/decision?" And then say nothing more and see what happens. Sometimes you don't really have to work beyond that to move people's position; they move it themselves.—**Conni Walkup Hull and Editors**

- Don't give someone a pass by making excuses for their bad behavior. In general, people do what they want to do. No matter how much someone may backpedal later, they **understand they meant it.** Just because it's something you would never do doesn't mean it wasn't intentional.—**Conni Walkup Hull**

- Be sure to put your feet in the right place, then stand firm.—**Abraham Lincoln**

- Whatever you choose to do, leave tracks. That means don't do it just for yourself. You will want to leave the world a little better for having lived.—**Ruth Bader Ginsburg**

- You can disagree without being disagreeable.—**Ruth Bader Ginsburg**

- None of us got where we are solely by pulling ourselves up by our bootstraps. We got here because somebody—a parent, teacher, an Ivy League crony, or a few nuns—bent down and helped us pick up our boots.—**Thurgood Marshall**

- If you can't muster courage before the court, at least practice dignity.—**Proverb**

Six Final Quotes

- The price of anything is the amount of life you give away for it.—**Henry David Thoreau**

- Soon or late, everyone sits down to a banquet of consequences.—**Robert Louis Stevenson**

- The meaning of life is to find your gift. The purpose of life is to give it away.—**William Shakespeare**

- He who has a "why" to live can bear almost any "how."—**Friedrich Nietzsche**

- Just keep going. No feeling is final.—**Rainer Maria Rilke**

- We build too many walls and not enough bridges.—**Isaac Newton**

Authors

Cathy Marcucci is a senior anesthesiologist who lives in suburban Baltimore. She is most proud of her children and the family unit she has built with her husband, Neil Sandson. She has abiding interests in cooking, gardening and garden design, travel, antiques, dog rescue, movies (but only happy ones), and duplicate bridge.

Chetta Lupa is a senior anesthesiologist at UNC-Chapel Hill. Besides her family first and foremost, she loves pediatric anesthesiology, teaching and mentoring, North Carolina, and coffee.

Jake Seagull is a senior human factors expert in the University of Michigan system. Also a devoted family man, he enjoys fishing, biking, movies, and games of strategy.

Conni Walkup Hull is a lawyer, writer, and poet living on a small, beautiful lake in northeast Indiana. When not practicing law or writing, she enjoys playing her piano, creating textile art, riding motorcycles, and dancing in the kitchen with her Sailor husband, *Anesthesia Bridges* photographer Scott Hull.

Brad Winters is a senior anesthesiologist and intensivist at Johns Hopkins. He is a devoted family person whose outside interests have included hiking and mountain climbing, motorcycles, movies, travel, and, of course, trains.

Neil Sandson is a senior psychiatrist in the VA Maryland Health Care and the University of Maryland systems. He agrees with Cathy Marcucci that the best thing they ever did was to have their beautiful children! His outside interests include gaming, movies, anime, all things Japan, and playing bridge both online and in person.

208 Lessons from a World War II Soldier

Patricia M. Togioka, Robert D. Togioka,
Brandon M. Togioka, and Catherine Marcucci

Introduction

This chapter and the next one—the last two chapters in the book—are perhaps the most important we have written. They perfectly capture the two messages we are trying to impart to our readers and junior colleagues. First, none of us would be where we are now without the bravery, fortitude, intelligence, integrity, and loyalty of those who went before us. And second, as we will discuss in the next and final chapter, we are here in this specialty to do only one thing—take care of our patients in their hour of need.

In this penultimate chapter, the family of the late Noboru Togioka (1920–2013) tells us about the events that befell him in Italy in 1944, and there is surely no truer test of a person than those that occur on the battlefield. Noboru was, by all accounts, a quiet and modest man, but the lessons his life provides us are indeed valuable for all who practice anesthesia. The operating room has situations that mirror the intensity, life and death circumstances, and consequences of the battlefield. Quick decisions determine outcomes. Experts train for years in order to prepare for conditions that evolve in seconds. Split-second judgments determine the course of lives. What can we learn from a military hero?

***Note from the Editors:** Noboru Togioka was born in Dinuba, California, in 1920, the son of Kango and Fumi Togioka. Here he is as a young man and young soldier (Figs. 208.1 and 208.2).

P. M. Togioka (Retired)
Oregon School for the Deaf, Certified Interpreter for the Deaf and Hard of Hearing, Salem, OR, USA

R. D. Togioka (Retired)
Oregon School for the Deaf, Certified Interpreter for the Deaf and Hard of Hearing, Salem, OR, USA

American Sign Language, Salem-Keizer School District, Keizer, OR, USA

B. M. Togioka
Department of Anesthesiology and Perioperative Medicine, School of Medicine, Oregon Health & Science University, Portland, OR, USA

C. Marcucci (✉)
Departments of Transfusion Medicine, Clinical Center, National Institutes of Health, Bethesda, MD, USA

S. Mohamed et al. (eds.), *Anesthesia Bridges*, https://doi.org/10.1007/978-3-032-08294-7_208

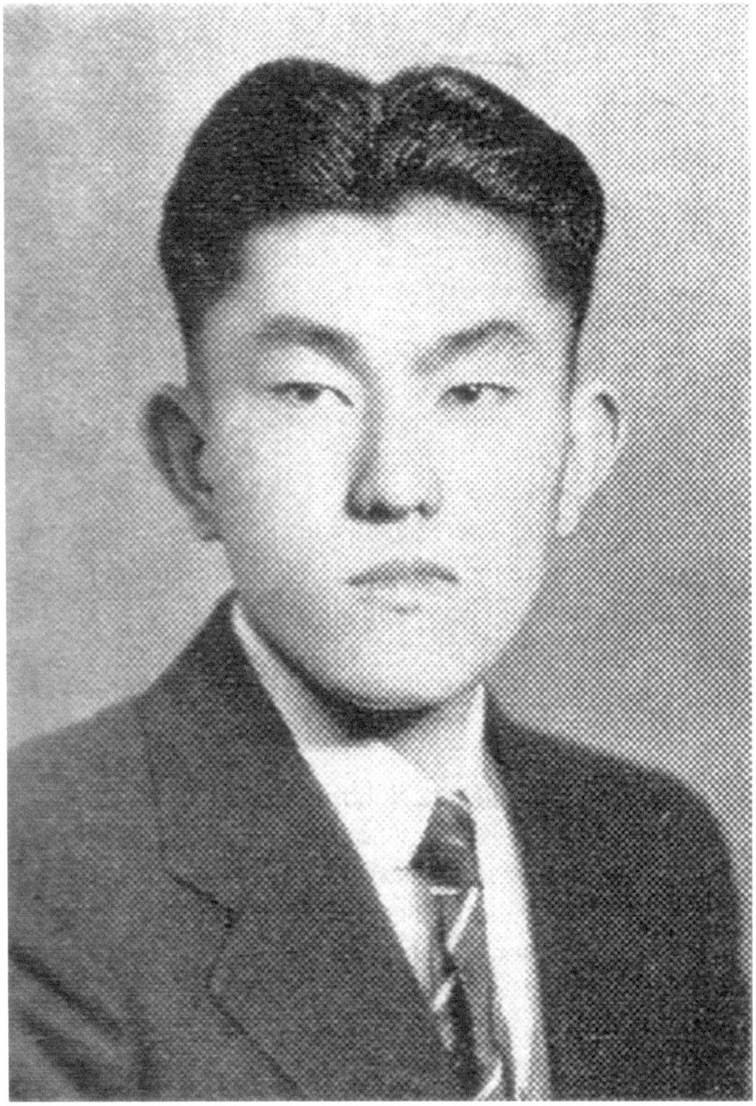

Fig. 208.1 An early formal photo of Noboru, perhaps a graduation photo. Photo: Collection of the Togioka family

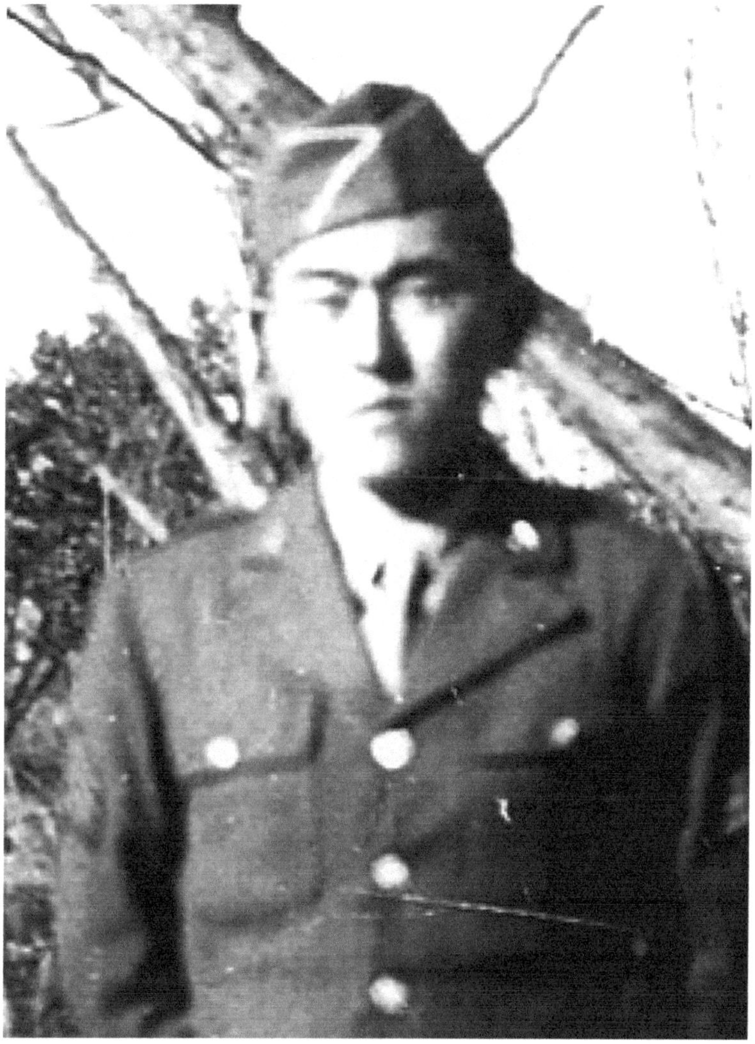

Fig. 208.2 The young soldier and officer. Photo: Collection of the Togioka family

The Battlefield and the Operating Room

In both the operating room and the battlefield, the choices made require long-term training and study, understanding of logistics and situations, skills using required tools, and a complete understanding of the presenting conditions. Before entering the battlefield, whether a military or medical operation, the professional must have already scoped out the possible issues that may arise. Because swift decisions must be enacted, it is vital to have developed a set of remedies: "If this happens…these are possible solutions." Life and death hang in the balance. In both cases, experts must train for years to perform as a smooth functioning team. Hesitation or indecision on the part of a single member can have dire consequences. Mistakes must be minimized as they can lead to serious injury or possible death. Since life or death is determined by assessment, judgment, and action, it takes years to hone the skills necessary to ensure safety, minimize error, and optimize results.

So, what exactly can we learn from a World War II hero who received many awards for valor including a Silver Star, Purple Heart and, as part of his unit, a Congressional Gold Medal?*

***Note from the Editors:** The Togioka family is grateful for the recognition that Noboru received, but as Sgt. Togioka himself might have told us, it's not the medals that made the WWII combat heroes, it's what was inside the men (Fig. 208.3). And it's also likely that he would quietly and simply insist that he was just doing the job he was given to do.

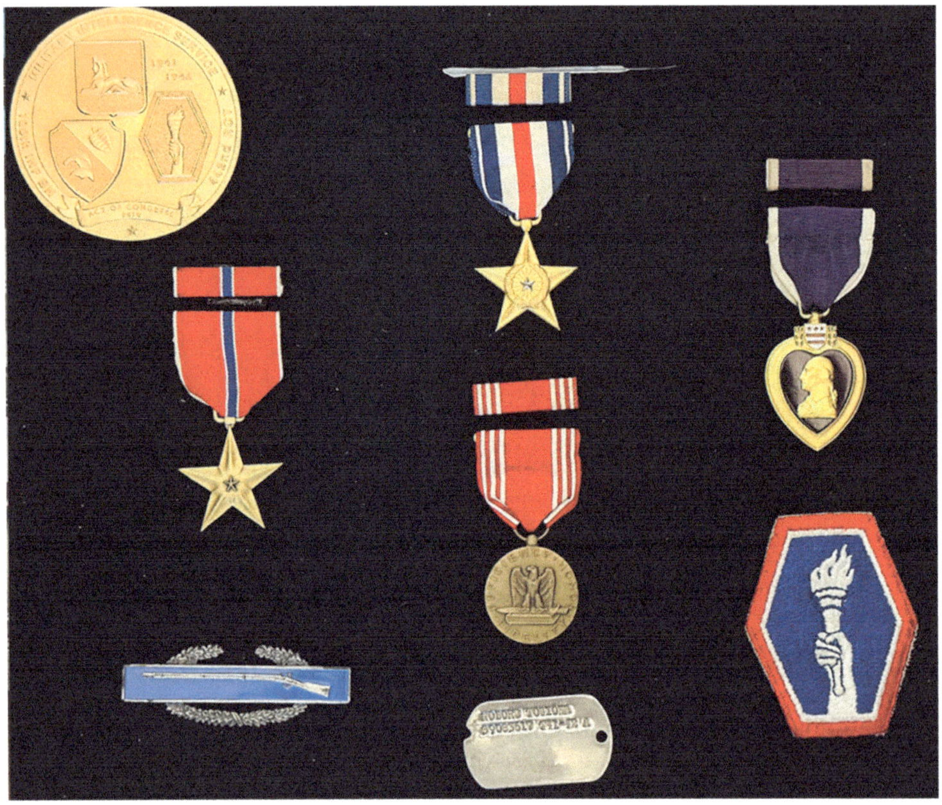

Fig. 208.3 The WW2 citations of Sgt. Noboru Togioka, second Battalion, 442 RCT. The Silver Star medal is top center. The 442nd RCT patch is lower right. Photo: Collection of the Togioka family

Let us share the account of Sergeant Noboru Togioka, our father and grandfather.

The Story of Sergeant Togioka [1, 2]

Sgt. Togioka fought in the Italian Campaign of World War II, by every account a grueling and brutal series of coastal landings and land battles that took place from 1943 to 1945. The campaign was designed to establish Allied air bases on the Southern European continent and divert German forces from Western Europe. On June 26th, 1944, the 2d Battalion of the 442nd Regimental Combat Team was stationed near Suvereto, Italy, as they began their push north towards the entrenched German Gothic Line. Suddenly, heavy German artillery fire rained down. Communications officer Sergeant Noboru Togioka (ASN:

39083617) and his team were responsible for maintaining telecommunications between the command posts and front lines. When the barrage started, Sergeant Togioka got his men to safety in the cover of a dry creek bed.

At this juncture, it was vital to notify the battalion command of the attack; however, the telephone wire had been damaged. The damaged wire was in full view of the enemy and was centered in the area of the heaviest shelling. Several of his men volunteered to help him repair the lines, but he refused. He felt that, on his own, he could be less conspicuous. Prior to leaving to make the critical repairs, Sergeant Togioka was informed that the captain and his clerk had been killed.

The young soldier grabbed a repair kit and started down the path towards the broken telephone wire, fully aware of the danger that it entailed. The closer he got to the broken wire, the more visible he became to the enemy. After walking for about a half mile, Noboru started to hear shells landing behind him. As he approached the broken wire, the sound of the explosions became louder. He saw a culvert and ran toward it, ducking under it. After a while, the shells stopped landing, and he dashed out to find the telephone wire break. He spliced the wires together, then quickly ran back under the culvert. The broken wire was so close to the enemy that he could hear the enemy soldiers speaking German while he fixed it.

Sergeant Togioka repeated this maneuver for over an hour, patrolling the wire and repeatedly making repairs as the telephone line was damaged by artillery fire. During one of the periods of heaviest shelling, the culvert was hit. At first, he felt that he had been hit by a rock. The culvert consisted of many large rocks, and he thought one had fallen on his legs. He looked down and saw blood squirting out, so of course it was an arterial bleed. There were significant shrapnel wounds in one leg and a knee injury on the other side. He used a bandage to stop the bleeding and used his rifle to straighten his leg. Later, the medics were amazed at what he was able to do.

After temporarily slowing the bleeding, Sergeant Togioka was faced with the problem of saving his own life. He was lying under a roadway bridge, severely wounded, isolated from other American troops, in the middle of an intense artillery battle. And he had no weapon since his rifle was splinting his shattered leg. He heard a Jeep traveling down the road, but because he was in enemy territory, he thought it must certainly be German soldiers. He also didn't know how to stop it, so he let it go by. A few minutes later, he heard the same Jeep coming back. With ***no*** good options and knowing he was close to bleeding to death, Sergeant Togioka, from under the culvert, threw his mess kit up on the bridge. The Jeep stopped. Miraculously, the soldiers were American. Sergeant Togioka was retrieved from the culvert, loaded onto the Jeep, and taken to the first aid station.

He then received his first airplane ride and landed in a general hospital in Naples, Italy. In the hospital, **Sergeant Togioka was awarded the Silver Star for "conspicuous gallantry and intrepidity in action against the enemy"** [1]. Later, he was awarded a Purple Heart, and on November 2, 2011, the 442nd Regimental Combat Team, the most decorated military unit in United States history, was awarded a Congressional Gold Medal.* The Congressional Gold Medal is the highest civilian honor in the United States. The first recipient was George Washington.

***Note from the Editors:** Sgt. Noboru Togioka's Silver Star Citation is shown below (Fig. 208.4). How many of us could or would have been able to do what he did on that day? He had just turned 24.

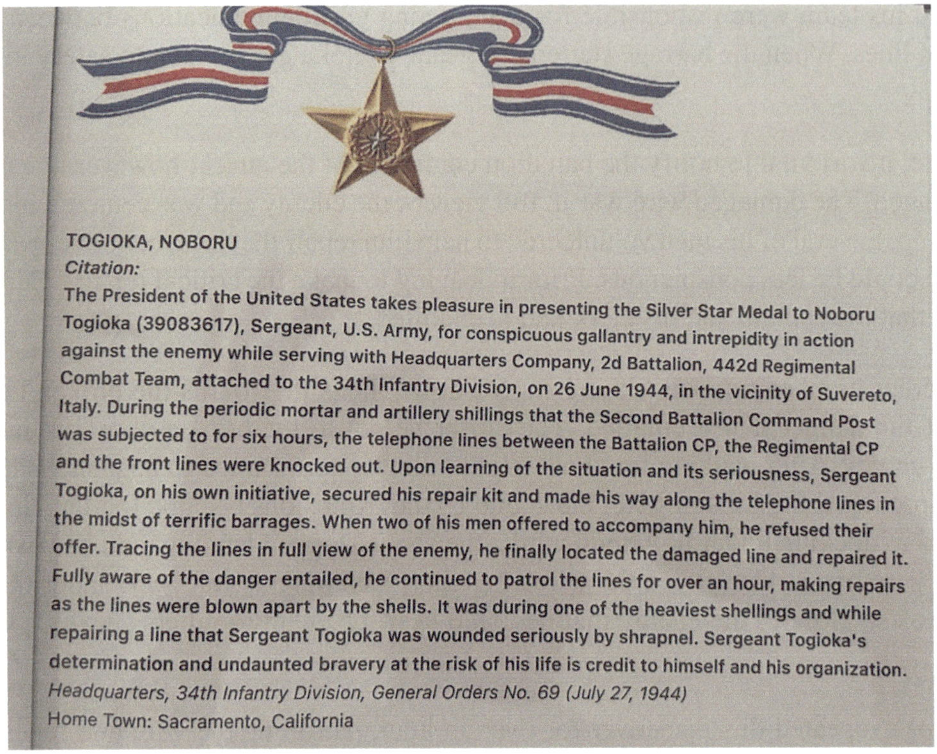

TOGIOKA, NOBORU

Citation:

The President of the United States takes pleasure in presenting the Silver Star Medal to Noboru Togioka (39083617), Sergeant, U.S. Army, for conspicuous gallantry and intrepidity in action against the enemy while serving with Headquarters Company, 2d Battalion, 442d Regimental Combat Team, attached to the 34th Infantry Division, on 26 June 1944, in the vicinity of Suvereto, Italy. During the periodic mortar and artillery shillings that the Second Battalion Command Post was subjected to for six hours, the telephone lines between the Battalion CP, the Regimental CP and the front lines were knocked out. Upon learning of the situation and its seriousness, Sergeant Togioka, on his own initiative, secured his repair kit and made his way along the telephone lines in the midst of terrific barrages. When two of his men offered to accompany him, he refused their offer. Tracing the lines in full view of the enemy, he finally located the damaged line and repaired it. Fully aware of the danger entailed, he continued to patrol the lines for over an hour, making repairs as the lines were blown apart by the shells. It was during one of the heaviest shellings and while repairing a line that Sergeant Togioka was wounded seriously by shrapnel. Sergeant Togioka's determination and undaunted bravery at the risk of his life is credit to himself and his organization.

Headquarters, 34th Infantry Division, General Orders No. 69 (July 27, 1944)

Home Town: Sacramento, California

Fig. 208.4 The Silver Star Citation for Sgt. Noboru Togioka. Photo: Courtesy of the Togioka family

To us, Sergeant Togioka was known as Grandfather.* He was a man with quiet confidence who always carried himself with civility. He modeled a very strong work ethic, growing raisins in the San Joaquin Valley of California for 53 years. He passed away peacefully at the age of 93 and is buried at the San Joaquin National Cemetery.

***Note from the Editors:** Scenes from a life (Figs. 208.5, 208.6, and 208.7).

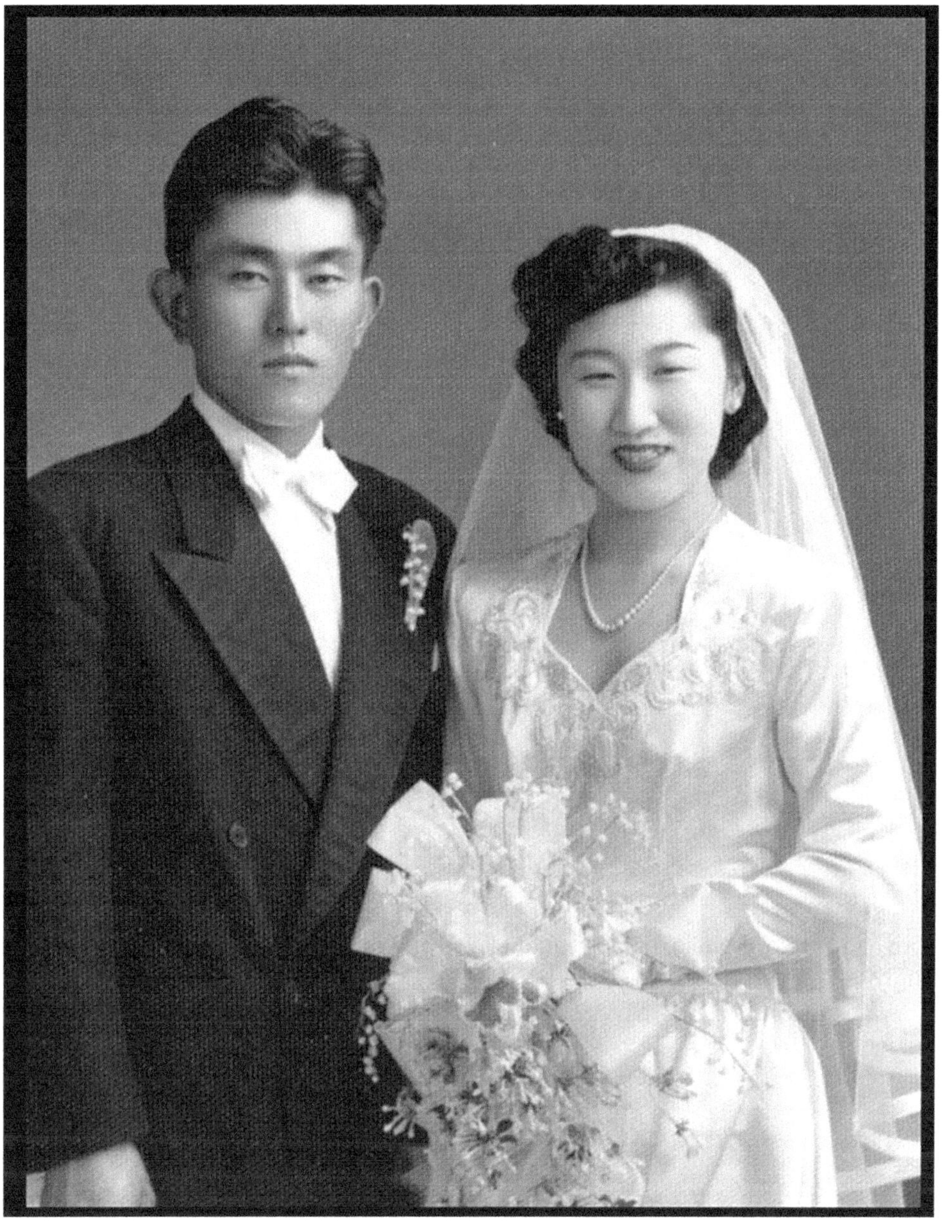

Fig. 208.5 Noboru and Yuriko Togioka on their wedding day, a wonderful picture of the young couple. There probably never was a more beautiful bride than Yuriko in her beautiful 1940s satin wedding gown and pearls. Photo: Collection of the Togioka family

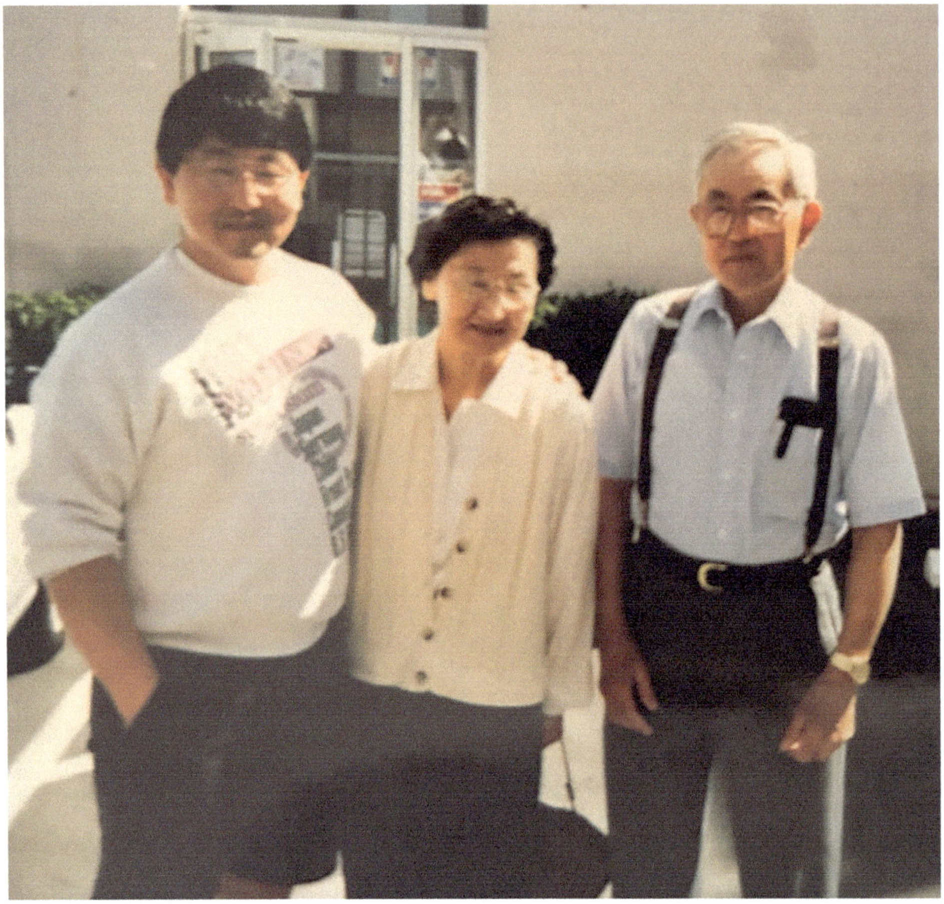

Fig. 208.6 Noboru and Yuriko Togioka, in their middle age, with their son Robert, Brandon's dad. Photo: Collection of the Togioka family

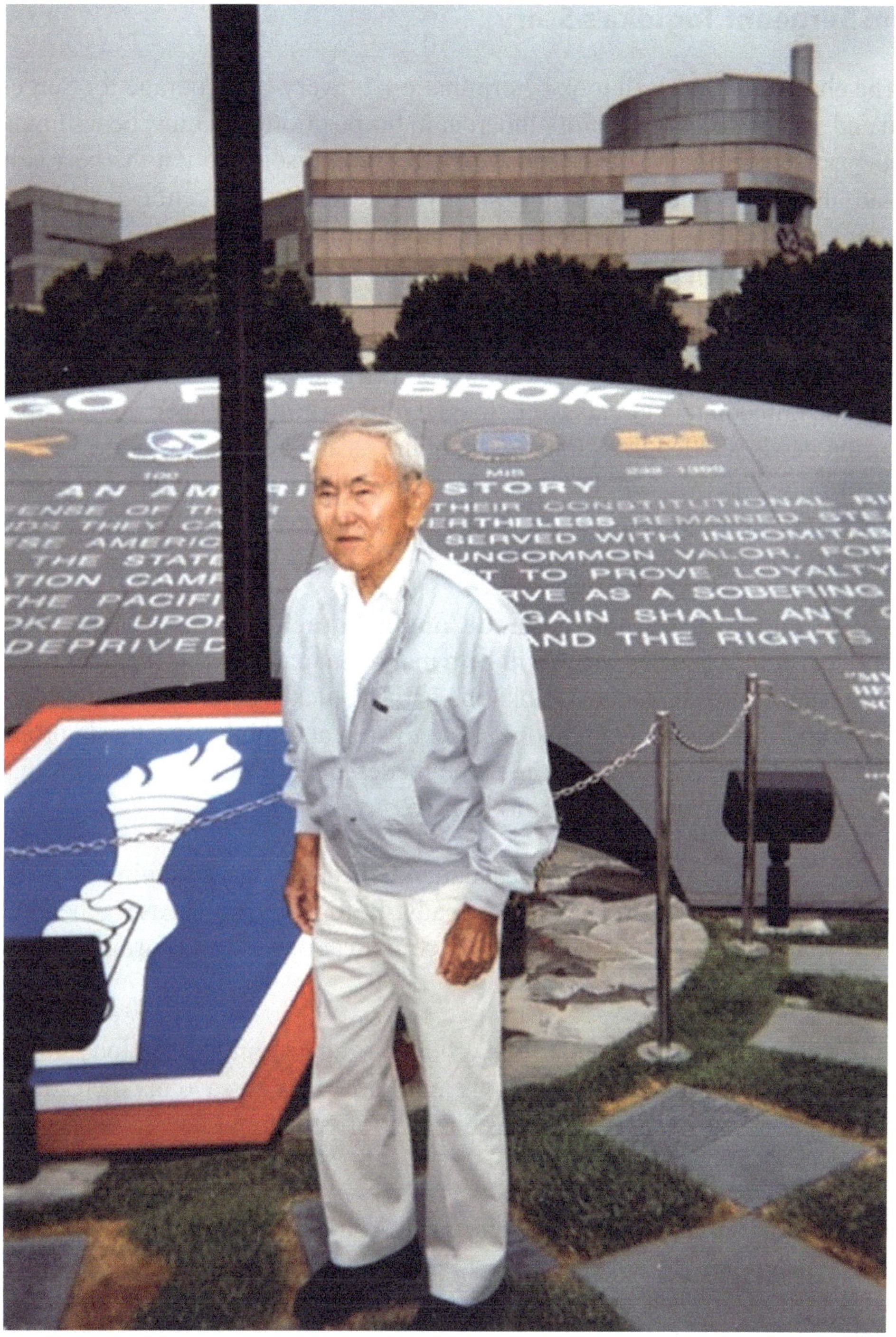

Fig. 208.7 Noboru Togioka in later life. Genuine war hero notwithstanding, could he not also be America's grandpa, with his crisply pressed khaki golf slacks and his zip-front poplin jacket? On this day, he was visiting the 442nd RCT memorial in Los Angeles. The motto of the regiment was "Go for Broke." Photo: Collection of the Togioka family

Lessons from Sergeant Togioka's Story

- **Step up to the challenge.** Just as it took determination, bravery, and courage for Sergeant Togioka to take the lead and accept the responsibility inherent in his position, you must be willing to call the hard shots and put yourself on the line. The most experienced person is often the best suited to manage dangerous and high-risk scenarios. Be clear with your team. Project confidence, even when you are uncertain. Your team needs to believe in you and in your plan to follow your course of action. When the situation in the operating room becomes perilous, the surgical and nursing teams will look to the anesthesiologist for guidance.

- **Know your equipment and have it ready.** When Sergeant Togioka learned the communication wires were cut, he immediately got his well-stocked repair kit. It contained all the supplies he needed to keep repairing newly shelled lines for over an hour. As an anesthesiologist, you never know when an emergency need for specific supplies will occur. Have all the tools you need at your ready disposal prior to starting a difficult surgery or procedure. This is your responsibility. There is often no time to obtain supplies after things start going badly.

- **Be decisive, determine which steps to pursue, and act quickly.** Split-second decisions will define you. One poor decision or one heroic act will help mark your career, your reputation, and your legacy. When difficulties arose for Sergeant Togioka, he had to quickly determine the best course of action for his situation and implement it. He had no time to stop and think. Anesthesia providers are faced with similar life and death decisions that must be made quickly. Hesitancy at a crucial juncture will often make the situation worse and harder to resolve.

- **Be prepared.** Sergeant Togioka was able to act quickly because of his training. Practice and preparation drive out fear and indecision. Have plans ready. Before starting a case, rehearse in your mind. Consider what challenges may lie ahead—what complications may occur, and how am I going to remedy them?

- **Trust your training.** Sergeant Togioka knew how to repair communication cables. He had also learned how to stop bleeding and had the tools and know-how to save his own life. You have been taught and have practiced how to perform each aspect of your job. Practice your skills so that when they are most needed, you are ready.

- **Have faith in your team.** You can't do everything. You aren't the gunner or the infantry person. Know each team member's job duties and trust them to do their part. Be a supportive member of the team. See where help is needed and lend a hand. Lead by example. Bring your tool kit, knowledge, and skills to the medical battle front, ready to do your part.

- **Do your best work—always.** You never know when a little extra effort will mean the difference between a near miss and a bad outcome. Each of us can be a hero by doing our best work with integrity and skill. You won't receive a Silver Star or Purple Heart, but you will receive the best possible outcomes for your patients—and this is the best award there is.

- **Accept setbacks and drive toward better outcomes.** Setbacks are inevitable. Everyone experiences them. Successful people have many setbacks, but they learn from each one and use them to craft their next success.

***Note from the Editors:** Brandon Togioka's maternal grandfather, the late Andrew M. Prischak, also proudly served his country (Fig. 208.8).

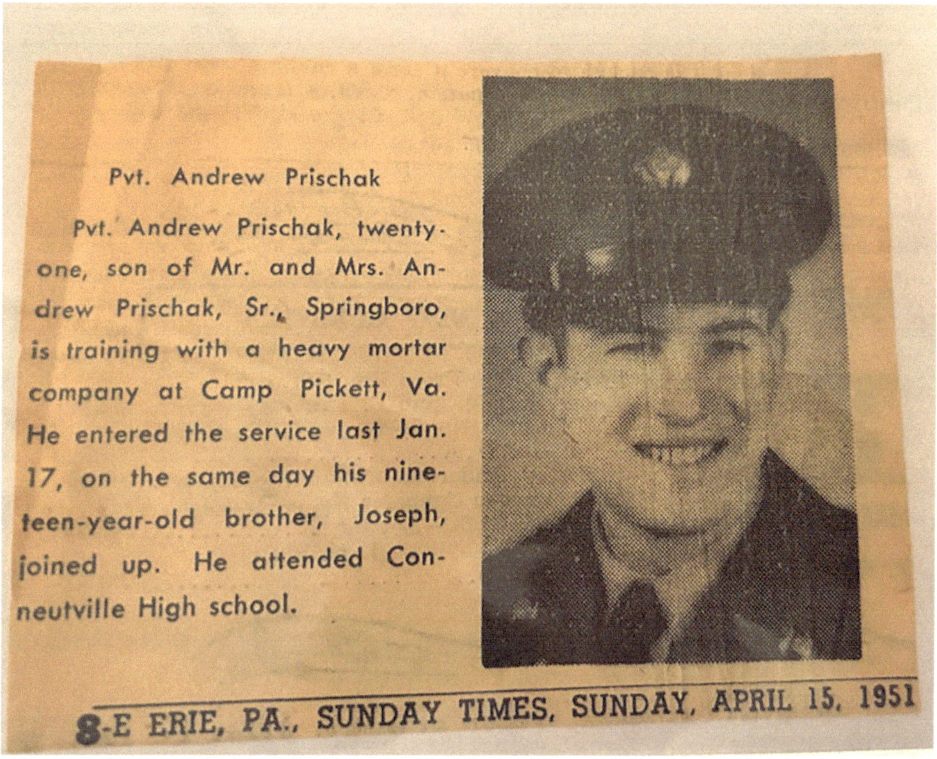
Pvt. Andrew Prischak

Pvt. Andrew Prischak, twenty-one, son of Mr. and Mrs. Andrew Prischak, Sr., Springboro, is training with a heavy mortar company at Camp Pickett, Va. He entered the service last Jan. 17, on the same day his nineteen-year-old brother, Joseph, joined up. He attended Conneutville High school.

8-E ERIE, PA., SUNDAY TIMES, SUNDAY, APRIL 15, 1951

Fig. 208.8 Newspaper item featuring Pvt. Andrew Prischak, Patti Togioka's dad, and Brandon's grandfather. Photo: Collection of the Prischak family

Bonus Content

The 442nd Regimental Combat Team was a segregated fighting unit manned with Nisei—second generation Japanese Americans. If you ever get a moment's extra moment, we urge you to read about this remarkable unit [3]. It is a fascinating chapter of American and military history—both sad due to the blatant racism the soldiers encountered and triumphant at the same time due to the astounding integrity and bravery of the troops.

Their story is even more distressing and complex than the segregation and racism suffered by the soldiers, as many of them had families and loved ones who were imprisoned in the Japanese detention camps during the war, as Yuriko Togioka was.* Many of the soldiers' families lost their farms, properties, and livelihoods as a result of the internments, as the Togioka family did. In spite of these tragic events and circumstances, the men of the 442nd showed incredible loyalty and fought for their country with astonishing dedication and stoicism. They are rightfully recognized as some of the most tenacious and brave of all the men and women who served during WWII.

***Note from the Editors:** Government records pertaining to the detention of Yuriko Katsuki Togioka before her marriage (Fig. 208.9).

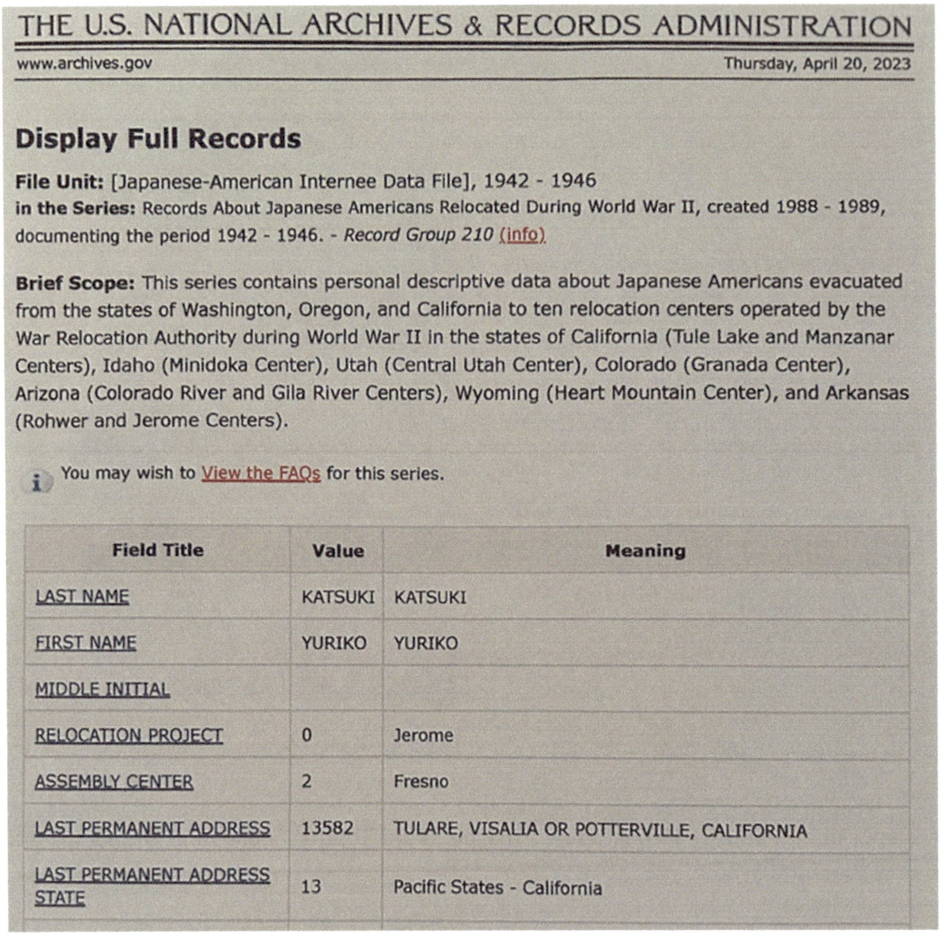

THE U.S. NATIONAL ARCHIVES & RECORDS ADMINISTRATION

www.archives.gov Thursday, April 20, 2023

Display Full Records

File Unit: [Japanese-American Internee Data File], 1942 - 1946
in the Series: Records About Japanese Americans Relocated During World War II, created 1988 - 1989, documenting the period 1942 - 1946. - *Record Group 210* (info)

Brief Scope: This series contains personal descriptive data about Japanese Americans evacuated from the states of Washington, Oregon, and California to ten relocation centers operated by the War Relocation Authority during World War II in the states of California (Tule Lake and Manzanar Centers), Idaho (Minidoka Center), Utah (Central Utah Center), Colorado (Granada Center), Arizona (Colorado River and Gila River Centers), Wyoming (Heart Mountain Center), and Arkansas (Rohwer and Jerome Centers).

You may wish to View the FAQs for this series.

Field Title	Value	Meaning
LAST NAME	KATSUKI	KATSUKI
FIRST NAME	YURIKO	YURIKO
MIDDLE INITIAL		
RELOCATION PROJECT	0	Jerome
ASSEMBLY CENTER	2	Fresno
LAST PERMANENT ADDRESS	13582	TULARE, VISALIA OR POTTERVILLE, CALIFORNIA
LAST PERMANENT ADDRESS STATE	13	Pacific States - California

Fig. 208.9 Detention records of Yuriko Katsuki Togioka during WWII. She, as much as Noboru, passed down her strength and courage to her children and grandchildren. Photo: Courtesy of the Katsuki-Togioka family

Ultimately, though, Noboru and Yuriko persevered and even triumphed over their painful and difficult early life experiences as they built stable and successful lives in the years and decades after the war.* They farmed their own land, travelled, raised a family, and in time were delighted by their expanding family of nieces and nephews and grandchildren and great children.

***Note from the Editors:** More scenes from the lives of Noboru and Yuriko Togioka (Figs. 208.10, 208.11, and 208.12).

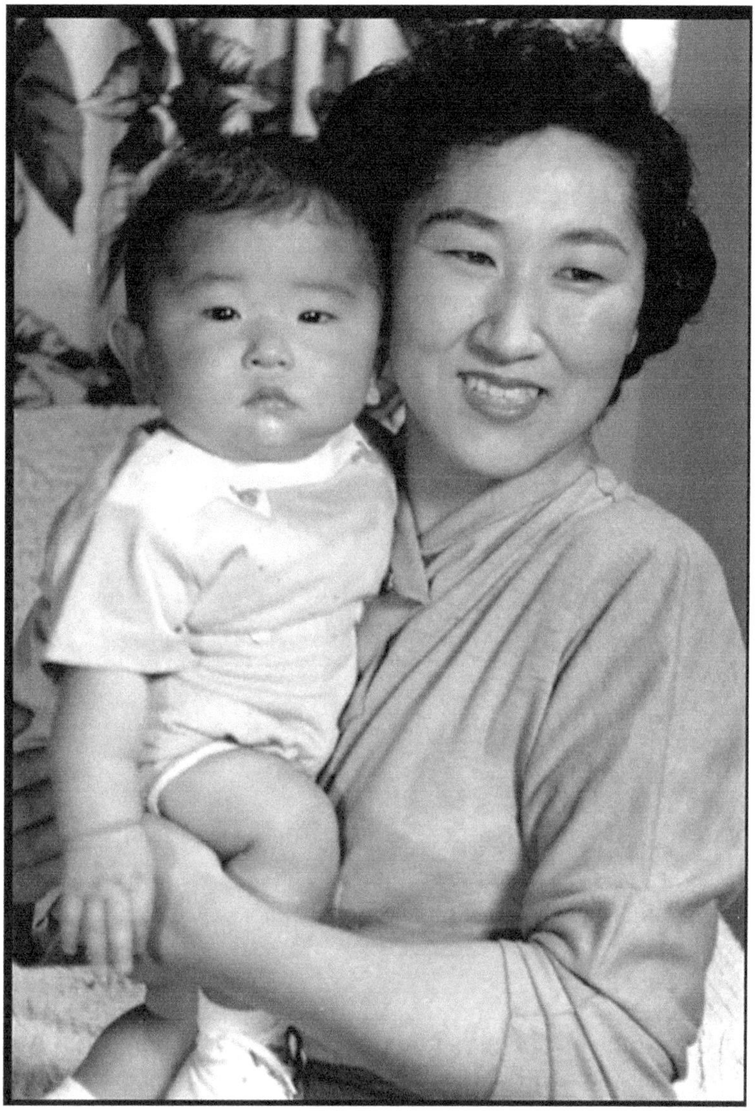

Fig. 208.10 Yuriko as a young mother in an undated photo. Photo: Collection of the Togioka family

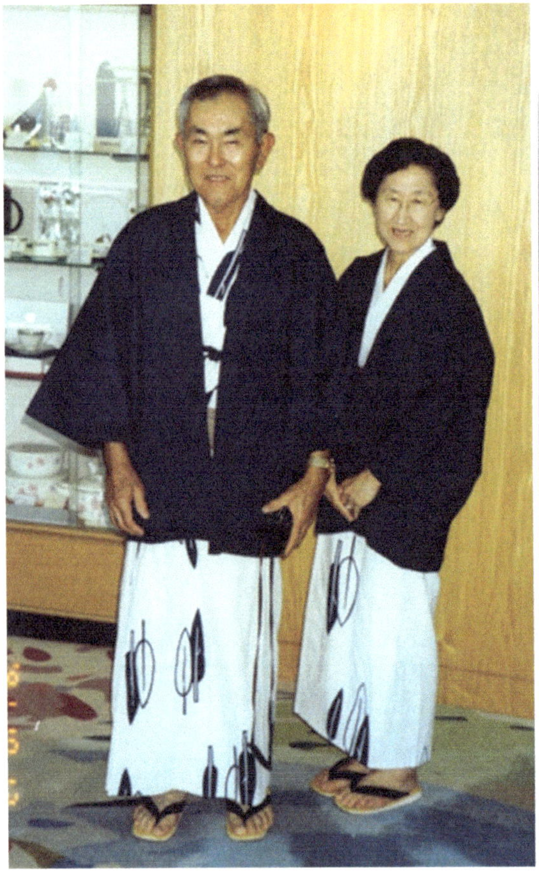
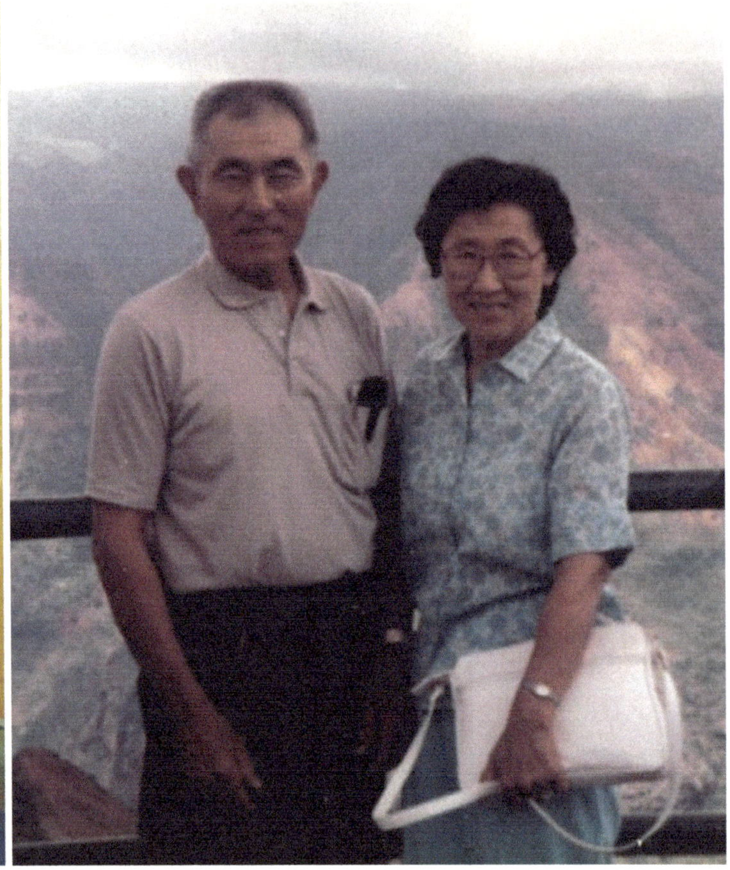

Figs. 208.11 and 208.12 Mr. and Mrs. Togioka on their travels. Photos: Collection of the Togioka family

Finally, remember that a bridge isn't always just to get a traveler from point A to point B. Sometimes it is a life-saving shelter for the soul underneath it, as it was for Noboru on that long-ago and awful day.

References

1. Sterner D. Noboru Togioka. Hall of Valor Project. Sightline Media Group; 2023. [cited 2025 Jul 27]. Available from: https://valor.militarytimes.com/hero/26902
2. Togioka N: narrator, Govan Y: interviewer, Go For Broke National Education Center: publisher. Noboru Togioka oral history interview, part 1 of 4, March 7, 2004. Japanese American Military History Collective. [cited 2025 Jul 27]. Available from: https://ndajams.omeka.net/items/show/105020
3. 442nd Infantry Regiment (United States) [Internet]. Wikipedia; 2021. Available from: https://en.wikipedia.org/wiki/442nd_Infantry_Regiment_(United_States).

Authors

Patricia Togioka is retired and lives in the metropolitan Portland, Oregon area. She is the former superintendent of the Oregon School for the Deaf. In her free time, she takes courses at Portland Seminary and leads women's groups in her community, including a Parkinson's Disease support group. Patricia also interprets American Sign Language when her skills are needed for unique and difficult situations.

Robert Togioka lives in the Portland area with his wife, Patricia. After years of teaching math, he was asked to start an American Sign Language program, which he taught until he was in his early seventies, succeeding as a lauded teacher while battling Parkinson's Disease. Many of his students have gone on to become interpreters or other professionals working with persons who are Deaf. Robert is looking forward to the next chapter in his career as a lifelong educator.

Brandon Togioka is the vice chair of clinical research for Anesthesiology and Perioperative Medicine at Oregon Health & Science University and the former medical director of obstetric anesthesia. He is Noboru Togioka's grandson. He is married to Jennifer Togioka, with whom he has two daughters, Ella and Brynn.

Cathy Marcucci is a senior academic anesthesiologist and inveterate anesthesiology educator. She was an attending anesthesiologist in the VA health care system for 19 years where it was her honor to care for many WWII veterans.

One Final Case

209

Ronald S. Bank and Catherine Marcucci

Introduction

In this final chapter, **Ron Bank** relates a case that perfectly captures what we do and why.

We get up in the morning to come to work to save lives, in whatever way that is required. It is as simple as that.

Emergency!

About 17 years ago, I was taking care of a young, otherwise healthy woman for an electrophysiology (EP) procedure. At the conclusion of the case, we were getting ready to move her over to the stretcher, folks were talking, and all were assuming that all had gone perfectly. Suddenly, the patient went unresponsive. I could not feel a carotid pulse. I loudly voiced that she had likely been arrested to get the staff's attention. We hit the code button and did CPR. We emergently intubated. We did CRP on the stretcher as we went to the cath lab. We had no idea what had happened.

We continued CPR while they established access in the cath lab and shot an angiogram. It turned out that she had a 100% occlusion of, I believe from memory, her RCA. They were able to remove the occlusion via a PTCA and restore her RCA flow. She went up to the CVICU intubated. Hours later, to my absolute delight, she woke up and was extubated. When I asked her how she was doing, she said that her chest hurt, and she wasn't expecting that from her EP procedure. Indeed. I was elated.

Sometime later, I received a beautiful letter from her, which is shown below; the names have been omitted for privacy (Fig. 209.1).

R. S. Bank
Department of Anesthesiology, INOVA Fairfax Hospital, UVA School of Medicine, INOVA Campus, Falls Church, VA, USA

C. Marcucci (✉)
Department of Transfusion Medicine, Clinical Center, National Institutes of Health, Bethesda, MD, USA

S. Mohamed et al. (eds.), *Anesthesia Bridges*, https://doi.org/10.1007/978-3-032-08294-7_209

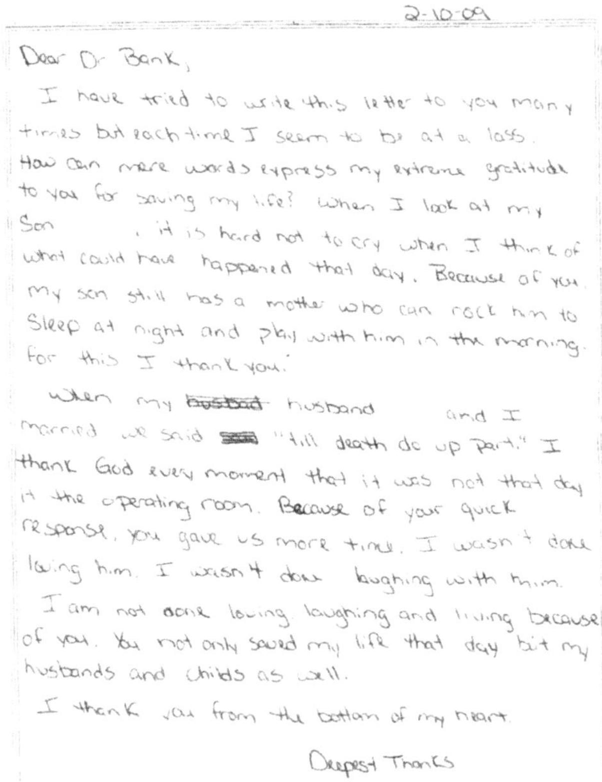

2-10-09

Dear Dr Bank,

I have tried to write this letter to you many times but each time I seem to be at a loss. How can mere words express my extreme gratitude to you for saving my life? When I look at my Son , it is hard not to cry when I think of what could have happened that day. Because of you my son still has a mother who can rock him to sleep at night and play with him in the morning. For this I thank you.

When my ~~husbad~~ husband and I married we said [redacted] "till death do up part." I thank God every moment that it was not that day in the operating room. Because of your quick response, you gave us more time. I wasn't done loving him. I wasn't done laughing with him.

I am not done loving laughing and living because of you. You not only saved my life that day but my husbands and childs as well.

I thank you from the bottom of my heart.

Deepest Thanks

Fig. 209.1 The letter Ron Bank received from a grateful patient. The text of the letter is below. Photo: Ron Bank

Dear Dr. Bank,

I have tried to write this letter to you many times, but each time I seem to be at a loss.

How can mere words express my extreme gratitude to you for saving my life? When I look at my son, it is hard not to cry when I think about what could have happened that day. Because of you, my son still has a mother who can rock him to sleep at night and play with him in the morning. For this, I thank you.

When my husband and I married, we said, "till death do us part." I thank God every moment that it was not that day in the operating room. Because of your quick response, you gave us more time. I wasn't done loving him. I wasn't done laughing with him.

I am not done loving, laughing, and living because of you. You not only saved my life that day but my husband's and my child's as well.

I thank you from the bottom of my heart. Deepest thanks.

Motivation

Sometimes, when I'm down on medicine, I look at this and other letters that I've received—just for motivation. It is an effective strategy.

A couple of years later, I got a call from one of the high-risk obstetricians. He asked if I was around. I said that I was there, but on the way out. He said that one of his patients had asked if I was available and would take care of her for her C-section. Then he told me her name. I remembered that she was the patient from the EP lab per the above. Of course, I stayed and took care of her! After the case, her husband hugged me. He said, "Thank you for my wife's life. Without you there back on that day, there would have been no delivery on this day." It is a moment that I'll never forget.

One of my relatives, who is an extremely wealthy businessman, heard of the entire story when one of my siblings sent him a copy of the patient's letter. He wrote back that, while he makes a lot more than I do, he'll never get a letter like that or do something so meaningful. He said that medicine must be so rewarding.

These events made me reflect on the fact that, despite that many people with far less education make far more than we do (not that we don't do well), our jobs literally save lives and are in many ways far more meaningful and impactful. Ours is truly a noble profession. We are very blessed to be a part of it.

Lessons Learned

- It's wonderful that Ron has this letter to draw strength from on difficult days. You will have your own that are similar or just like this. Whatever you do, keep them in a safe place. Pull them out when the time is right.

- Always keep what this patient wrote to Ron at the top of mind when you go to work. It's one reason why we get up in the morning. This is really what it is all about.

- And **always** keep your eye on your patient. A patient who suddenly stops talking or responding is a life-threatening emergency situation until conclusively established to be otherwise. Everyone expects the acute events to happen in emergency or acute situations and understands that we have to be vigilant. But bad things happen in low-acuity situations as well. **Vigilance always!**

Authors

Ron Bank is a cardiac anesthesiologist at a large hospital in northern Virginia. Nobody who knows him was the least bit surprised to hear about his expert care of this patient.

Cathy Marcucci is a senior academic anesthesiologist and inveterate anesthesiology educator. She is also fellowship-trained in transfusion medicine. When not taking care of patients and/or putting the latest book together, she dedicates her time to mentoring junior colleagues, writing copy for animal rescues, and travel.

Afterword

In conclusion, we urge our readers to ponder a bit the two bridges below, as they are perfect metaphors for the safe passage that we all need for our personal and professional journeys (Figs. 1 and 2).

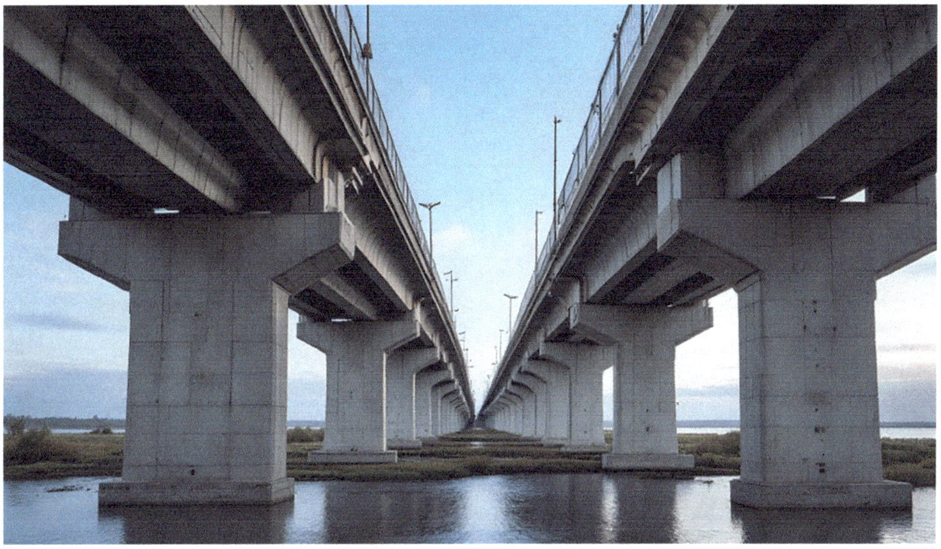

Fig. 1 A massive and sturdy bridge. You could practically trust those foundations hold up the Empire State Building. Use this as a metaphor for your life and career. Photo: Image under standard license from stock.adobe.com

S. Mohamed et al. (eds.), *Anesthesia Bridges*, https://doi.org/10.1007/978-3-032-08294-7

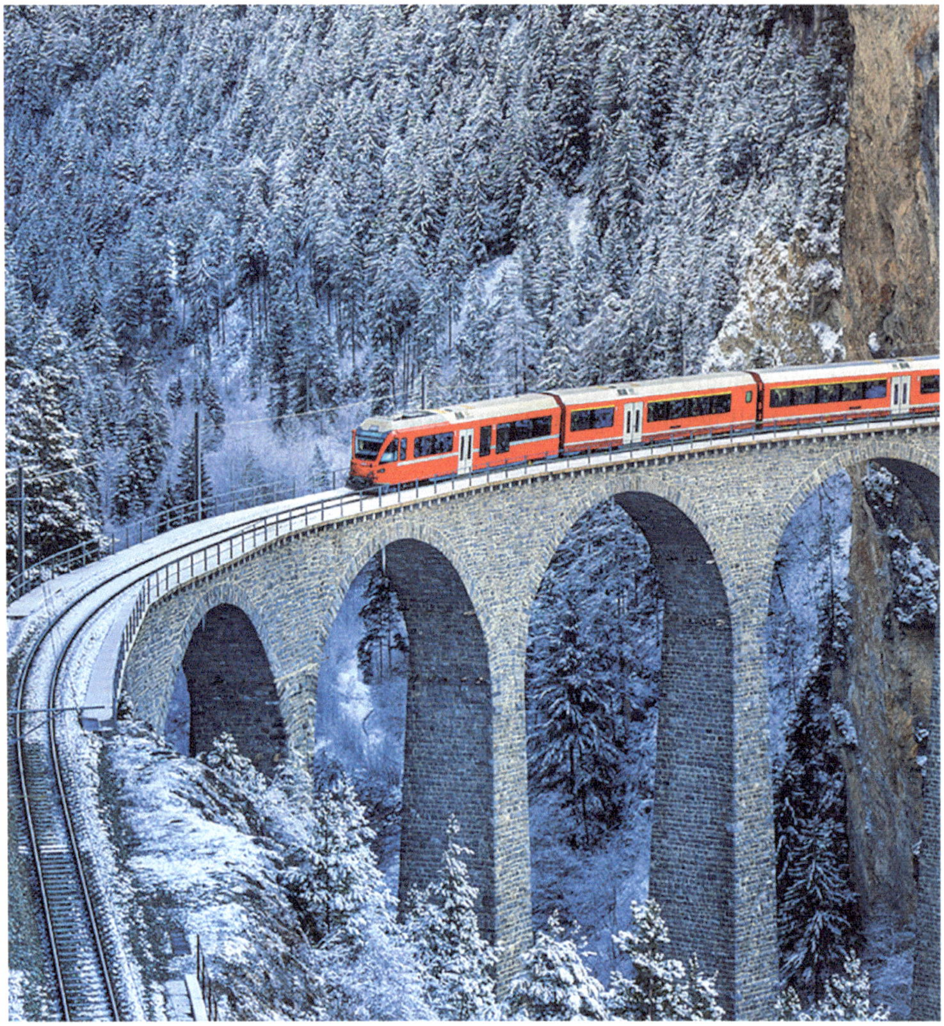

Fig. 2 Aerial view of train passing through the Alps in Filisur, Switzerland. That train doesn't look a bit afraid. Photo: tawatchaiprakobkit, image used under license from iStock.com

We wrote about this earlier in the book, but it bears repeating one last time. You build the solid foundations of your life and career by always working hard, always trying to do the right thing, and always seeking to build bridges and connections with the people you care for and care about.

And when circumstances dictate, just get in your little red train and go where you have to go.

Be well and good luck on all your journeys!

Index

S. Mohamed et al. (eds.), *Anesthesia Bridges*, https://doi.org/10.1007/978-3-032-08294-7

C

D

E

GPSR Compliance

The European Union's (EU) General Product Safety Regulation (GPSR) is a set of rules that requires consumer products to be safe and our obligations to ensure this.

If you have any concerns about our products, you can contact us on ProductSafety@springernature.com

In case Publisher is established outside the EU, the EU authorized representative is:

Springer Nature Customer Service Center GmbH
Europaplatz 3
69115 Heidelberg, Germany

Batch number: 10622478

Printed by Printforce, the Netherlands